For Lisa

The autumn wind touches the mountain
The spring leaf falls to earth

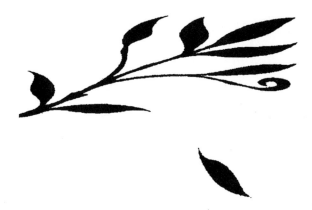

Foreword to the Sixth Edition

The remarkable capacity of humans to communicate emerged in a gradual, evolutionary way. Today it explodes on the scene during the early years of life. As normal communicators, we benefit from the reliability and adaptability conferred by evolution. We could be reminded daily—if we stopped to think about it—of the crucial roles that speech, language, and communication ability play in our social, emotional, intellectual, and working lives.

Of course, we usually don't stop to think about it. Communication is so much a part of our "selves" that the wonder of it becomes apparent only when we choose to study it. Readers of this book probably already have a better sense than most others of the complexity of the processes that make us normal speakers, listeners, readers, writers, and communicators.

Most of you have chosen to embark on an effort to learn about what happens when—because of neurologic disease—the ability to communicate becomes impaired. Such impairments seem to insult and diminish the accomplishments of evolution. Fortunately, neurologic disease does not happen to an entire species. Unfortunately, it does happen to people, often in ways that disable, handicap, and devastate. It is one of life's paradoxes that our speech and language ability permits us to study the effects of its destruction and then share that knowledge with others. Such study should be conducted with a keen awareness that our "subjects" deserve our commitment to use what we learn from them responsibly and productively.

Don't misinterpret the word *introduction* in the title of this book. The contents herein represent more than a handshake. The text provides a solid foundation in the neurology of communication, as well as the causes, symptoms, diagnosis, and management of the most frequently encountered neurologic communication disorders. Serious students will leave this book prepared to study the disorders in greater depth. Aspiring clinicians will leave it prepared to develop the skills necessary to work with people whose lives are affected by the disorders.

Many texts about neurogenic communication disorders have come and gone over the years. Some texts became extinct because of limited substance, some because they failed to communicate their content effectively, and some because their content no longer reflected current knowledge, thinking, or practice. This seventh edition of *Introduction to Neurogenic Communication Disorders* has come to life because it reflects the evolution of several things. First, the assessment, diagnosis, understanding, and management of neurogenic communication disorders and their causes have changed in subtle to dramatic ways. Those changes are reflected in these pages. Second, the range of communication disorders to which we must attend has broadened. When the first edition of this text was published, clinicians were "up to speed" if they knew something about aphasia, dysarthria, and apraxia of speech. We now appreciate, by virtue of their increasing prevalence and careful clinical observation and research, that right hemisphere lesions, traumatic brain injury, and dementia can affect communication in ways that often are not captured by our concepts of aphasia and motor speech disorders. Those changes are also reflected in these pages. Finally, Dr. Brookshire's very special talents as a clinician, researcher, and teacher have evolved. No book reaches a second, let alone a seventh edition, without its author having gotten something right the first time and then building on it in a way that keeps the ever-evolving needs of its readers in mind. The content of this book reflects what a recognized expert believes are the core of "facts" and concepts necessary to a foundation for understanding neurogenic communication disorders. You should also know that you will be learning from someone whose clarity of thought and expression have been, for many years, greatly respected and admired by his colleagues and appreciated by his students.

Be assured that the organization, style, and clarity of this book will meet your needs if you are coming to this complex subject for the first time. I suspect this book also will become a friend and valuable resource to those of you who already have or will develop a lasting interest in neurogenic communication disorders. It almost certainly will contribute to your own evolution as students, teachers, researchers, or clinicians.

Joseph R. Duffy, PhD, BC-NCD
Head, Section of Speech Pathology
Department of Neurology
Mayo Clinic
Professor
Speech Pathology
Mayo Clinic College of Medicine
Rochester, Minnesota

Preface

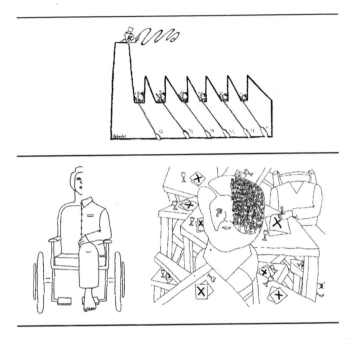

In the early 1980s I attended a conference in Rotterdam, The Netherlands. At that conference, Phillipe Van Eeckhout, a French speech-language pathologist, described his work with Sabadel, a French political cartoonist who at the age of 39 experienced a left-hemisphere stroke that left him aphasic, unable to speak, and paralyzed on his right side. Phillipe described his work with Sabadel and showed us drawings done by Sabadel in the months following Sabadel's stroke. I never forgot those drawings. Van Eeckhout later sent me a book—L'Homme Qui ne Savait plus Parler (The Man Who No Longer Could Speak). The book contains many of Sabadel's drawings from that time. I share with you three drawings. The upper drawing is one of Sabadel's political cartoons, drawn before his stroke, which spoke to the issue of industrialization in France. The lower two drawings were done by Sabadel after his stroke, during the time in which he was essentially without speech. Sabadel's drawings depict the physical and mental aftermath of stroke in ways that words cannot. I trust that they will be as memorable for you as they continue to be for me.

I have written this book to provide readers with a general understanding of neurogenic communication disorders—their causes, symptoms, typical course, treatment, and outcome. I have tried to be practical about what I have included in this book. I have included material that I believe is both important and useful to readers who are beginning their study of neurogenic communication disorders. My decisions regarding what to include and what to leave out no doubt reflect my personal biases about who, how, and why we treat. It also reflects my experiences in 30 plus years of teaching university students about neurogenic communication disorders and my sense of what has seemed important to them.

I have not addressed all controversial issues, and sometimes may have presented my opinions as facts. But facts often prove evanescent. Even such seeming facts as *the pyramidal system* and *apraxia of speech* are in one sense matters of opinion or convenient fictions. What passes for fact in much of the scientific and clinical literature about neurogenic communication disorders (and in literature relating to many other areas of knowledge as well) is in truth opinion, intuition, or someone's best guess about what seems true. The content of this book represents my best guess about what is likely to prove true over time. I trust that I have guessed right more often than not.

I believe that clinical competence comes as much (or more) from one's development of intuitions based on regularities observed across patients as it does from reading the literature. I also believe that treatment of neurogenic communication disorders combines art and science and that many empirically verified facts may prove trivial or irrelevant to helping the neurologically compromised adult become a better communicator.

This book is neither a training manual nor a catalog of techniques. Reading it will not make the reader competent to evaluate, diagnose, or treat patients with neurogenic communication disorders. No book or collection of books can do that. Clinical competence comes from blending knowledge acquired from clinical and scientific literature, supervised clinical training, and independent clinical experience. This book will, I hope, help the student get started on the road to clinical competence by providing a basic understanding of what neurogenic communication disorders are, what the individuals who have them are like, and how neurogenic communication disorders may be measured and treated.

Now an editorial note: The word *aphasic* is an adjective, not a noun. I believe that using the word *aphasic* as a noun, as in *conduction aphasics* depersonalizes those for whom we provide services, in addition to being stylistically deplorable. Therefore readers will not find me referring to *aphasics* in this book, and I trust that readers will, in their own writing, speech, and professional activities, focus on the person and not the condition.

THOUGHT QUESTIONS

I have included a few Thought Questions at the end of each chapter. In the thought questions I have tried to depict realistic situations—situations such as those clinicians may encounter in the course of their professional practice. Your responses to the thought questions will encourage you to combine factual knowledge with logic and intuition to arrive at reasonable responses. There are no correct answers to most of the thought questions, and my responses represent my best guesses and are not necessarily the only reasonable responses. I believe that the process by which readers arrive at responses to the thought questions is more important than the responses themselves, provided that the responses are logically consistent and are based on reasonable interpretations of relevant information. I trust that readers will be challenged and perhaps entertained as they respond to the thought questions and that doing so helps them to practice and sharpen their clinical thinking.

Robert H. Brookshire

Acknowledgments

Few of the ideas in this book are truly my own. The influence of colleagues, students, and the patients I have known and worked with permeates the contents. Without them, my life would have been much less interesting and this book would not exist.

My special thanks:

- To Linda Nicholas for her continuing love, support, tolerance, and understanding while this edition was a work in progress.
- To Kathy Falk, Christie Hart, and Kristin Hebberd, my editors at Elsevier, for their professionalism, patience, impeccable advice, and unwavering good humor during the often arduous process of editing, formatting, scheduling, and getting this edition into print.
- To John Casey, my project manager at Elsevier, for his keenness of eye, his efficiency, and his patience with my stylistic idiosyncracies during final editing and page composition.
- To Katy Gano for her efficiency, thoughtfulness, attention to detail, and word-processing skills in manuscript preparation.
- To Jeanne Robertson, whose drawings illustrate concepts with elegance and clarity.
- To the friends, colleagues, and patients who have made my professional life rewarding, challenging, and a never-ending source of education and enlightenment.

Robert H. Brookshire

Contents

Neuroanatomy and Neuropathology

Most of us have spent time wondering how our brain works. Brain scientists spend their entire lives pondering it, looking for a way to begin asking the question, How does the brain generate mind? The brain, after all, is so complex an organ and can be approached from so many different directions using so many different techniques and experimental animals that studying it is a little like entering a blizzard, the Casbah, a dense forest. It's easy enough to find a way in—an interesting phenomenon to study—but also very easy to get lost. (Allport S. [1986]. Explorers of the black box: The search for the cellular basis of memory.)

This book is about neurogenic cognitive-communicative disorders in adults. *Neuro-* in *neurogenic* means *related to nerves or the nervous system* and *-genic* means *resulting from* or *caused by.* In everyday language, this book is about cognitive-communicative disorders caused by injury, abnormality, or disease in the adult nervous system. Neurogenic cognitive-communicative disorders include several specific abnormalities:

- *Aphasia.* Impaired comprehension and production of language, usually caused by damage in the language-competent brain hemisphere.
- *Right-hemisphere syndrome.* Impaired comprehension and production of abstract language and impaired appreciation of visuo-spatial relationships, usually caused by damage in the non–language-competent brain hemisphere.
- *Traumatic brain injury syndrome.* Impaired attention and memory, impaired appreciation of abstract information, and altered interpersonal behavior, usually caused by diffuse brain damage.
- *Dementia.* Memory impairments, personality changes, and altered behavior, usually caused by damage in brain regions related to memory, attention, and affect.
- *Dysarthria.* Impaired speech production, usually caused by damage in nerves controlling muscles involved in speech or damage in the speech muscles.

Neurogenic cognitive-communicative disorders are an important consequence of nervous system damage. Their features, severity, and outcome reflect the location, magnitude, and nature of the damage. For these reasons clinicians who assess, diagnose, and treat neurogenic cognitive-communicative disorders must have at least rudimentary knowledge of the human nervous system and what can go wrong with it. The intent of this chapter is to provide that knowledge. The chapter begins by describing the anatomy of the parts of the nervous system likely to be affected when neurogenic cognitive-communicative disorders appear. It then describes some of the major nervous system incidents that give rise to the most common neurogenic cognitive-communicative disorders.

Unfortunately for those learning neuroanatomy, the human nervous system is a complex and confusing array of interacting systems. Almost every part of the nervous system has several names, most of them convenient fictions invented by humans to make it easier to describe, analyze, draw, and speculate about the nervous system. The proliferation of names began in the 19th century when the nervous system was under intense study, when communication among investigators was slow and inefficient, and when there was a tendency for explorers of the nervous system, like explorers of the planet, to name their discoveries after themselves.

Eventually practitioners began to call for more descriptive names because the old names were difficult to remember and because most parts of the nervous system had been named, so it was inappropriate for new people to name things after themselves. Nevertheless, there remains some gratification in attaching a name to something, even if that something already has a name. The proliferation of names, although slowing, has not stopped.

Many names for parts of the nervous system seem obscure today, and some have lost currency and perhaps should be abandoned. However, many names, and the concepts that underlie them, are traditional in spite of their scientific faults and need to be understood for purposes of communicating with other professionals.

CENTRAL NERVOUS SYSTEM
Cellular Structures

Glial cells and *neurons* (nerve cells) make up most of the cellular structure of the central nervous system. Glial cells are the bricks and mortar of the brain. Glial cells support neurons and nerve fiber tracts. Glial cells also may serve other functions such as regulating fluid levels, removing foreign substances, and participating in brain metabolism.

Nervous system activity begins with nerve cells, or *neurons*. The activity of pools of neurons distributed throughout the nervous system creates sensations, perceptions, emotions, behaviors, and the actions of muscles, organs, and glands.

All neurons have the same basic structure, but they differ in size and shape. A typical neuron has a cell body and small hairlike projections called *dendrites* and a longer, thicker tubular projection called an *axon* (Figure 1-1). Dendrites receive information (in the form of chemical and electrical changes) from other neurons and transmit the information to the cell body. Axons carry information away from the cell body and connect with the dendrites of other neurons. Most neurons are *multipolar*, meaning that there are many dendrites projecting from the cell body, but some are *unipolar* (have only one dendrite) or *bipolar* (have two dendrites). Neuronal cell bodies

come in various sizes. The largest are about 20 times the size of the smallest. Axons differ in length and diameter. Most are only a few millimeters long, but some, such as those that connect neurons in the cerebral cortex to neurons in the lower spinal cord, are several feet long. Long axons are larger in diameter than short axons—the longest axons in the human nervous system are about 20 times the diameter of the shortest. Longer axons have larger diameters because the speed of neural transmission depends on the thickness of the axon. Axons with the smallest diameters transmit information at about 1 meter per second, whereas axons with the largest diameters transmit information at up to 120 meters per second. Some axons (mostly the longer, thicker ones) are covered with a thin layer of a white fatty substance called *myelin*. Myelin provides electrical insulation for nerve axons, much like the coatings on electrical wires. Myelin allows axons to transmit information at higher rates.

Some neurologic diseases (e.g., multiple sclerosis) are characterized by degeneration and loss of the myelin from neuron axons. Loss of myelin causes weakness and impaired control of muscles served by the affected neurons.

The point at which the axon of one neuron encounters a dendrite of another neuron is called a *synapse*. The tiny space between an axon and a dendrite is called the *synaptic cleft*. Transmission of nerve impulses across the synaptic cleft is a chemical process. A chemical transmitter is released by the axon of one neuron and drifts across the synaptic cleft, where it stimulates the dendrite of a second neuron. The stimulation causes a change in the second dendrite's electric charge. This change (if it is especially strong, or if it is combined with the response of other stimulated dendrites) causes the second neuron to fire, sending a signal down its axon to stimulate the dendrites of one or more additional neurons.

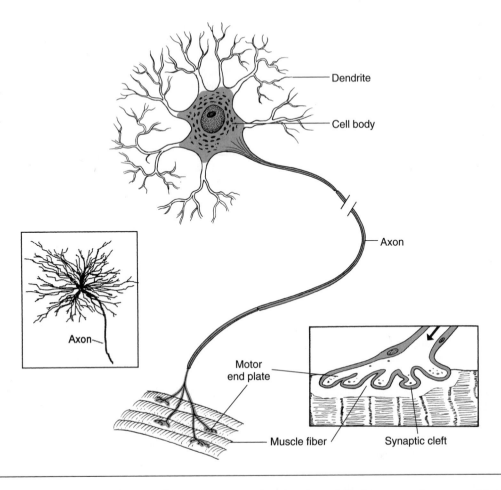

Figure 1-1 ■ A simplified drawing of a motor neuron, showing the cell body, axon, and myoneural (muscle-nerve) junction. A motor end plate (the junction between a neuron and a muscle fiber) is shown on the lower right. The insert on the left shows a tracing of a real spinal motor neuron to show the complexity of dendritic structures relative to the simplified drawings provided in most textbooks.

Neurons traditionally have been categorized according to function. *Sensory neurons* respond to stimulation (such as touch or temperature) or receive input from sensory receptor cells (such as those in the retina or inner ear). *Motor neurons* connect to muscles and glands. *Interneurons* connect other neurons. More than 99% of human neurons are interneurons, and sensory neurons outnumber motor neurons by about 5 to 1.

Anatomists customarily divide central nervous system tissue into *gray matter* or *white matter.* Gray matter consists of neurons and glial cells. White matter is composed primarily of myelinated axons. White matter is white because the myelin around the axons is white. Bundles of axons within the white matter are called by various names, the most common of which is *tract.* The names of many tracts provide information about their origin and destination—

for example, the *corticospinal tract,* which begins in the cerebral cortex and ends in the spinal cord, and my personal favorite, the *habenulointerpeduncular tract.*

Living gray matter is actually pink, because of its rich blood supply. When it loses its blood supply it turns gray. Anatomists call it gray matter because it is gray when it arrives at their dissecting tables.

Functionally related nerve cells cluster into collections of interacting neurons called *nuclei.* Nuclei differ from surrounding tissue by cell type, cell density, and function (e.g., the *nucleus ambiguus,* which sends motor fibers from the brain stem to the pharynx and larynx and plays an important part in swallowing).

Neuroanatomists from the 1800s to the present traditionally have divided the human nervous system into the *central nervous system* and the *peripheral nervous system.* The *central nervous system* is the part of the nervous system inside the skull and vertebrae. It includes the *brain,* the *brain stem,* the *cerebellum,* and the *spinal cord.* The central nervous system supports perception and discrimination of sensory stimuli and expression of emotion, keeps processes such as respiration and heartbeat going, organizes and regulates behavior, and enables us to engage in mental pursuits such as thinking, remembering, and understanding this sentence.

The *peripheral nervous system* is the part of the nervous system outside the skull and vertebrae. Neuroanatomists divide the peripheral nervous system into two functional systems— the *somatic nervous system* and the *autonomic nervous system.* The somatic nervous system enables us to perceive sensory stimuli and carry on volitional motor activity. The autonomic nervous system is a self-regulating system that controls the glands and vital functions such as breathing, heartbeat, and blood pressure.

Protective Envelope

The central nervous system is fragile but well protected from injury by a surrounding bath of fluid and a covering of bone and membranes. Fluid cushions the central nervous system and minimizes stresses on the central nervous system tissues caused by abrupt movements of the head and body. The skull and vertebrae provide a durable envelope. Strong membranes anchor the brain and spinal cord to the skull and vertebrae.

Skull. The skull encloses the brain, brain stem, and cerebellum. Human skulls are roughly symmetrical, although one half usually is slightly larger than the other. The human skull is made up of eight plates, joined together to form a continuous surface (Figure 1-2). The plates of an infant's skull are less firmly joined than those of an adult's, making the infant's skull pliable and elastic (a characteristic for which mothers in childbirth have cause to be thankful). Skull elasticity diminishes across the life span. An 80-year-old person who experiences a blow to the head is much more likely to receive a skull fracture than a 20-year-old. The adult human skull is thin in the front and on the sides (3 to 5 mm) and thick in the back (15 to 20 mm). Blows to the (thinner) front of the skull are much more dangerous than blows to the (thicker) back of the skull.

That human skulls are thicker in back than in front may be at least partially a result of natural selection. A person who falls backward is more likely to strike his or her head than a person who falls forward, because the person who falls forward can break the fall with hands and arms. Those whose skulls were thin in back may have been less likely to survive the perils of prehistoric times than those whose skulls were thick in back.

The space inside the skull is called the *cranial vault.* The ceiling and walls of the cranial vault are smooth, but the floor is irregular, with cavities, openings, partitions, and ridges giving it a craggy appearance (Figure 1-3). The large opening in the base of the cranial vault is called the *foramen magnum* (great opening). It is the opening through which the brain stem passes on its way to the spinal cord.

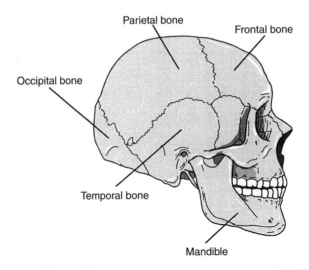

Figure 1-2 ■ A lateral view of the human skull. The four bony plates on each side of the skull are called, reading counterclockwise, the *frontal bone,* the *parietal bone,* the *occipital bone,* and the *temporal bone.*

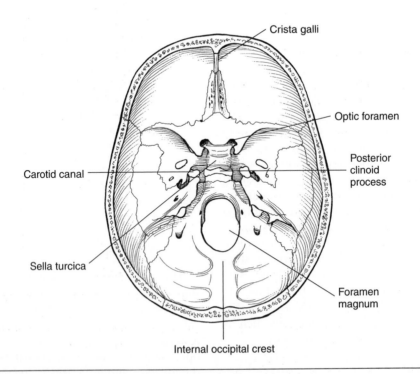

Figure 1-3 ■ The floor of the cranial vault. The crista galli, the clinoid process, and the sella turcica are three of several ridges and projections that arise from the floor of the cranial vault.

Foramen comes from a Latin word meaning *aperture*. In anatomy a *foramen* is an aperture or opening in tissue or bones.

Vertebrae. *Vertebrae* are bony structures supporting and protecting the spinal cord. Humans have 33 vertebrae, divided by neuroanatomists into 5 sets. The uppermost 7 vertebrae are called *cervical vertebrae;* the next 12 are called *thoracic vertebrae;* the next 5 are called *lumbar vertebrae;* the next 5 are called *sacral vertebrae;* and the lowest 4 are called *coccygeal vertebrae* (Figure 1-4). The 5 sacral and the 4 coccygeal vertebrae are fused into 2 larger structures, the *sacrum* and the *coccyx,* respectively.

Sacrum comes from Latin and means, roughly, *sacred bone. Coccyx* comes from Greek, and means *cuckoo,* or more likely *cuckoo's beak.*

The vertebrae are separated by disks of cartilage and are held together and in alignment by muscles, tendons, and ligaments. The lower vertebrae are larger than the upper vertebrae, enabling the lower vertebrae to bear greater weight and resist twisting forces, which tend to converge in the lower back. Through the center of the chain of vertebrae is a roughly circular opening through which the spinal cord passes. Notches between the vertebrae provide spaces through which nerves and blood vessels exit or enter. These notches are called the *intervertebral foramina.*

Pathologic changes in the vertebrae or the intervertebral discs sometimes put pressure on nerves and blood vessels, causing neurologic symptoms such as pain, loss of sensation, weakness, or paralysis. Patients with spinal nerve or blood vessel compression make up a significant part of most neurosurgeons' caseloads, and decompression of spinal nerves and blood vessels is a common neurosurgical procedure.

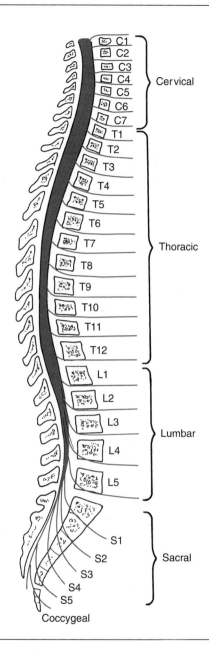

Figure 1-4 ■ The human spine, showing the division of vertebrae into cervical, thoracic, lumbar, sacral, and coccygeal groups.

Meninges. Three membranes, called *meninges,* enclose the central nervous system (the brain, brain stem, cerebellum, and spinal cord). The outer membrane is called the *dura mater.* The middle membrane is called the *arachnoid,* and the inner membrane is called the *pia mater* (Figure 1-5). Because the meninges help to *cushion* the central nervous system, the mnemonic *PAD* (for *p*ia, *a*rachnoid, and *d*ura) may help the reader keep them in order.

The *dura mater* is a tough (DURable), slightly elastic membrane that encloses the brain and spinal cord and lines the inner surface of the skull. The outer surface of the dura mater adheres to the inner surface of the cranial vault, and the inner surface of the dura is attached to the arachnoid. The dura mater has two layers. In most of the dura mater the two layers are fused, but in the *dural venous sinuses* the layers separate to form a complex system of cavities and channels. The dural venous sinuses collect venous blood flowing down from the brain and funnel it into the internal jugular vein for return to the heart and lungs. Some of the venous sinuses are shown in Figure 1-6.

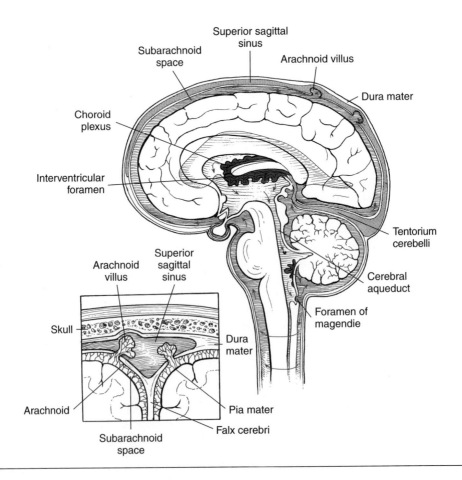

Figure 1-5 ■ The meninges and related structures. Cerebrospinal fluid (CSF) circulates throughout the ventricles and subarachnoid space. Its direction of flow is indicated by arrows. CSF is passed into the blood via the arachnoid villi, which protrude into the venous sinuses.

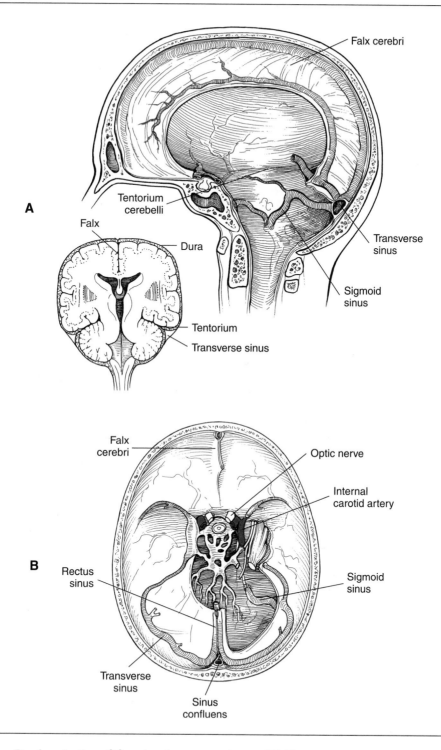

Figure 1-6 ■ Dural projections **(A)** and major venous sinuses **(B)**. The venous sinuses are cavities between sheets of dura into which arterial blood passes on its way back to the heart.

Sinus is from a Latin word meaning cavity or channel. In anatomy, *sinus* means a groove, hollow, or cavity, often for the storage or transport of fluids.

Rigid sheets of dura mater extend into the cranial vault in several places, dividing it into compartments (see Figure 1-6) and providing support for the brain, brain stem, and cerebellum. The two largest dural sheets are the *falx cerebri* and the *tentorium cerebelli*. The *falx cerebri* is a long, crescent-shaped band of dura mater that protrudes downward along the midline of the skull, dividing the cranial vault into two side-by-side compartments occupied by the brain hemispheres. The *tentorium cerebelli* is a dome-shaped sheet of dura mater protruding forward horizontally from the back of the cranial vault, creating two compartments, one above the other. The upper compartment holds the brain hemispheres; the lower compartment holds the cerebellum.

Ordinarily there is no space on either side of the dura, but in some pathologic conditions fluid accumulates between the dura and the skull or between the dura and the arachnoid. The most frequent source of such fluid is bleeding from blood vessels on the surface of the dura mater.

The *arachnoid* is a cobweblike sheet of tissue sandwiched between the dura mater and the pia mater. The arachnoid has no blood vessels and does not conform closely to the contours of the underlying pia mater, thereby creating a space—the *subarachnoid space*. The subarachnoid space is filled with *cerebrospinal fluid* (CSF), a clear, colorless fluid that cushions and protects the central nervous system against trauma, provides a pathway for metabolic and nutritional compounds to reach the central nervous system, and (perhaps) provides a medium for transport of waste products away from the central nervous system. At the base of the brain

are several large spaces between the arachnoid and the pia mater, also filled with CSF. Those large spaces are called *subarachnoid cisterns*.

Arachnoid comes from the Greek *arachne,* which means spider or cobweb. *Cistern* is a generic name for cavities or spaces for the storage of fluids.

The arachnoid protrudes into the venous sinuses at many places. The protrusions are called *arachnoid villi* (see Figure 1-5). The arachnoid villi provide places at which excess CSF is absorbed and removed from the subarachnoid space.

The *pia mater* is fragile, adheres tightly to the brain's surface, and follows the contours of the brain. The outer surface of the pia mater has many blood vessels, and many blood vessels cross the space between the pia mater and the arachnoid.

Pia is from a Latin word meaning *tender* (appropriate here because the pia mater is a fragile membrane, easily torn or cut).

The central nervous system is shaped something like a tree, with a trunk (the spinal cord), branches (nerve fiber tracts), and a canopy (the brain hemispheres). The central nervous system is arranged so that phylogenetically more primitive structures (the spinal cord and the brain stem) are at its base and phylogenetically more advanced structures (the brain hemispheres) are at the apex. For descriptive purposes the central nervous system traditionally is divided into five segments—the *spinal cord,* in the torso; the *brain stem,* atop the spinal cord; the *cerebellum,* behind the brain stem and below the brain hemispheres; the *diencephalon,* deep in the brain hemispheres; and the *cerebrum,* represented by the brain hemispheres, at the top. Neuroanatomists often lump the cerebrum and diencephalon together and call the lump the *brain.*

GENERAL CONCEPTS 1-1

- *Neurons* (nerve cells) are the basic units of the nervous system.
- Neurons receive input from other neurons by way of *dendrites* and transmit output to other neurons by way of *axons*.
- *Nerve fiber tracts* form the white matter in the nervous system. They are made up of bundled axons. Nerve fiber tracts are white because the myelin covering of the axons is white.
- The human central nervous system consists of the *brain, brain stem, cerebellum,* and *spinal cord*. It is enclosed in the *skull* and *vertebrae*.
- The peripheral nervous system lies outside the skull and vertebrae. It consists of *cranial nerves* and *spinal nerves*.
- Three membranes form a covering for the central nervous system. They are called *meninges*. The *dura mater* is the outer membrane; the *arachnoid* is the middle membrane; and the *pia mater* is the inner membrane.
- Rigid sheets of dura mater divide the skull into compartments. Two important dural partitions are the *falx cerebri,* which crosses front to back on the midline of the roof of the cranial vault, and the *tentorium cerebelli,* which crosses the cranial vault horizontally above the cerebellum and below the posterior base of the brain.
- *Cerebrospinal fluid* (CSF) is a clear, colorless fluid that surrounds the central nervous system in the subarachnoid space.

Brain

The *brain* is the largest member of the central nervous system family. It is a gelatinous mass of nerve cells and supportive tissue floating in CSF. An average human brain weighs about 3 pounds and is about three-fourths water. The brain is soft and mushy because of its great water content. A human brain removed from the skull and its supporting membranes and flotation system slowly collapses into a shapeless lump.

> *One of the difficulties in understanding the brain is that it is like nothing so much as a lump of porridge. (Gregory, R.L. [1966]. The eye and the brain: The psychology of seeing.)*

The one fourth of the brain that is not water is made up of glial cells, neurons, and connective tissue. Glial cells support and separate nerve fiber tracts. Glial cells are 5 to 10 times more numerous than neurons and account for about half of the brain's solid mass. Even so, a human brain contains more than 10 billion neurons (50 billion to 100 billion glial cells). The brain is a big spender. It makes up only about 2% of total body mass, but receives 20% of cardiac output and consumes 25% of the oxygen used by the body. The brain is not thrifty. It has no metabolic or oxygen reserves and is completely dependent on a constant supply of oxygen and nutrients. If the brain's blood supply is cut off for more than about 10 seconds the brain's owner loses consciousness; and after about 20 seconds, the brain's electrical activity stops. If blood supply to the brain is interrupted for more than 2 minutes, permanent brain damage is almost certain.

Cerebrum. The cerebrum contains about three fourths of the nervous system's mass. The cerebrum is divided into two halves, or *hemispheres,* by a deep fissure (the *longitudinal cerebral fissure*). The longitudinal cerebral fissure sometimes is called the *interhemispheric fissure* or the *superior longitudinal fissure*. (It seems to be a rule that the more prominent a fissure is, the more names it gets.) The *falx cerebri* extends downward into the longitudinal cerebral fissure. The surface of the hemispheres is covered by a layer of *cortex,* rich in nerve cells and blood vessels. The cortex is crisscrossed by a network of convolutions, making the brain look something like the surface of a pecan. The convolutions (ridges) are called *gyri,* and the depressions (valleys) are called *sulci.* Very deep sulci are called *fissures.*

Gyrus (singular for *gyri*) is from a Greek word meaning *circle. Sulcus* (singular for *sulci*) is from a Latin word meaning *furrow* or *ditch.*

Two prominent fissures mark the lateral surface of each brain hemisphere. One, the *central cerebral fissure,* travels vertically down each hemisphere, dividing it into roughly equal anterior and posterior regions. The central cerebral fissure sometimes is called the *fissure of Rolando,* and sometimes it is known as the *central sulcus.* The second prominent fissure

travels horizontally across the lateral surface of each hemisphere. This fissure is called the *lateral cerebral fissure,* the *fissure of Sylvius,* or the *frontotemporoparietal fissure,* after adjacent brain regions (Figure 1-7). The *calcarine fissure* is a short, less prominent fissure inside the longitudinal cerebral fissure at the back of the brain. It is mentioned here because cortical areas important for vision are adjacent to it. (Note that this short, shallow fissure gets only one name.)

The left and right hemispheres of the human brain are structurally similar but not identical. The left hemisphere in right-handed adults usually is slightly larger than the right hemisphere, and the lateral fissure in the left hemisphere of a right-handed adult usually is slightly longer than the lateral fissure in the right hemisphere

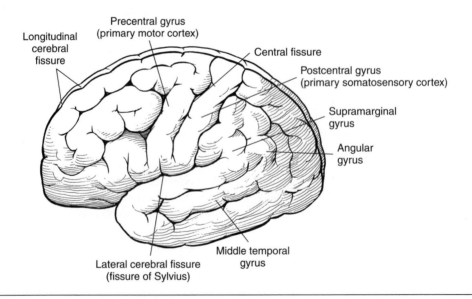

Figure 1-7 ■ Prominent gyri and sulci on the surface of the human brain. The left brain hemisphere is shown. The gyri and sulci on the surface of the right hemisphere are essentially mirror images of those on the surface of the left hemisphere. There is considerable variability across brains in the location, shape, and prominence of the landmarks, sometimes making them difficult to identify.

(von Bonin, 1962). However, right-handers' parietal lobes go in the opposite direction. Right-handers' right-hemisphere parietal lobes are larger than their left-hemisphere parietal lobes (Rubens, 1977). In spite of their structural similarity, however, the two hemispheres are in many respects functionally specialized.

By tradition each hemisphere has been divided into four *lobes*—the *frontal lobe,* the *parietal lobe,* the *occipital lobe,* and the *temporal lobe*—named after the parts of the skull above them (Figure 1-8). The lobes are topographic conventions and do not reflect differences in the structure or functions of the brain. Although different brain regions differ in structure and function, the structural and functional differences do not correspond to the boundaries of the lobes.

The *frontal lobes,* as their name implies, are at the front of the brain. The cortex in the frontal lobes accounts for about one third of all the cortex in the brain. The lateral cerebral (Sylvian) fissure marks the lower boundary for each

frontal lobe, and the central (Rolandic) fissure marks the posterior boundary.

The *parietal lobes* lie behind the central fissure and above the lateral fissure in each hemisphere. The posterior boundary of each parietal lobe is an imaginary line an inch or two forward from the *occipital pole* (farthest back point in the hemisphere).

The *occipital lobes* form the posterior part of each hemisphere. They extend from the imaginary line forming the posterior boundary of the parietal lobe to the longitudinal cerebral fissure at the occipital pole.

The *temporal lobe* makes up approximately the bottom one third of each hemisphere. The lateral cerebral fissure marks its upper boundary, and its lower boundary is on the underside of the hemisphere, near the midline. Its posterior boundary is the imaginary line marking the anterior boundary of the occipital lobe.

The *insula* is a patch of cortex folded into the lateral cerebral fissure. It is hidden from view by folds of the frontal, parietal, and temporal

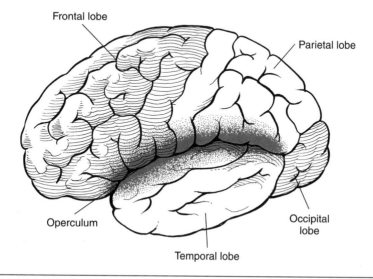

Frontal lobe

Parietal lobe

Operculum

Occipital lobe

Temporal lobe

Figure 1-8 ■ The lobes of the brain. Much of the occipital lobe is hidden from view within the longitudinal cerebral fissure. The lobes are arbitrary divisions and do not represent either architectural or functional differences.

lobes. The insula is sometimes called the *island of Reil*. The folds of cortex that conceal the insula are called the *operculum*.

Operculum is from a Latin word meaning cover or lid; in this case the cortex that folds over and covers the insula.

Cerebral Ventricles. Four *cerebral ventricles* (cavities filled with CSF and connected by narrow channels) lie deep inside the brain. The two largest are the crescent-shaped *lateral ventricles* deep in each hemisphere (Figure 1-9). The *third ventricle* is an irregularly shaped disk-like cavity standing on the edge on the midline below the lateral ventricles. The *fourth ventricle* is a narrow tubular cavity extending down through the brain stem, ending at an opening into the subarachnoid space (see Figures 1-5 and 1-9).

Each lateral ventricle is connected to the third ventricle by an *interventricular foramen (foramen of Munro)*. The third ventricle is connected to the fourth ventricle by the *cerebral aqueduct (aqueduct of Sylvius)*. The ventricles hold about 15% of the CSF in the central nervous system, and the subarachnoid space holds the remaining 85%.

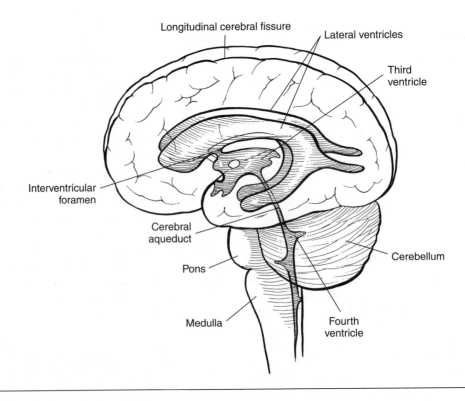

Longitudinal cerebral fissure — Lateral ventricles — Third ventricle — Interventricular foramen — Cerebral aqueduct — Pons — Medulla — Fourth ventricle — Cerebellum

Figure 1-9 ■ The cerebral ventricles. The ventricles form a fluid-filled space in the center of the brain and brain stem. One lateral ventricle is located deep within each brain hemisphere. The third and fourth ventricles are located on the midline. Most of the fourth ventricle is in the brain stem.

As noted earlier, a foramen is an aperture or opening. In physiology, an *aqueduct* is a tube or channel. Aqueducts are tubular; foramina are not.

The ventricles contain the *choroid plexus,* a spongy mass of vascular tissue that is the body's primary producer of CSF. (A small amount of CSF is produced by cells on the surface of the brain.) CSF circulates through the central nervous system from the lateral ventricles to the third ventricle via the interventricular foramina and from the third ventricle to the fourth ventricle via the cerebral aqueduct (see Figure 1-9). CSF drains from the fourth ventricle into the subarachnoid space through the *median aperture (foramen of Magendie)* and the two *lateral apertures (foramina of Luschka).* From there the CSF circulates upward around the brain hemispheres and downward around the spinal cord. Eventually it is resorbed into the blood through the arachnoid villi. In healthy adults the CSF regenerates approximately every 8 hours.

Changes in the chemical composition of CSF may indicate neurologic disease. For example, the presence of blood cells in the CSF suggests bleeding into the subarachnoid space, and reduced glucose levels suggest bacterial infection (the bacteria consume the glucose).

Diencephalon. The diencephalon is located deep in the substance of the brain, at the top of the brain stem. The *thalamus* and the *basal ganglia*—structures that play important roles in movement and sensation—are located in the diencephalon.

The *thalamus* consists of a pair of egg-shaped nuclei, one on each side of the third ventricle (Figure 1-10). The thalamus is a major relay center for motor information coming down from the motor cortex and for sensory information going up to the sensory cortex. The thalamus receives input from many sources— the cerebellum, the basal ganglia, other subcortical regions, and the brain stem—and its fibers project to much of the cortex.

Because of its role as a relay center for information going to the cortex, the thalamus is thought to play a part in regulating the overall electrical activity of the cortex. Many sensory pathways synapse at the thalamus, and perhaps because of this, the thalamus plays an important part in maintaining consciousness, alertness, and attention.

Diencephalon is from Greek, and means, literally, *through-brain. Thalamus* comes from a Latin word, meaning *little nut.*

Several nuclei adjacent to the thalamus form the *basal ganglia* (see Figure 1-10). The number of basal ganglia varies somewhat, depending on who is writing about them. Most writers include the *caudate nucleus,* the *putamen,* and the *globus pallidus* in the basal ganglia. Some add the *subthalamic nucleus* and the *substantia nigra.* To make things even more complicated, the putamen and the globus pallidus often are lumped together and named the *lenticular nucleus.* The lenticular nucleus is separated from the caudate nucleus by a band of nerve fibers called the *internal capsule* (described later). The lenticular nucleus is also separated from the thalamus.

The *subthalamic nucleus,* as its name implies, is located just beneath the thalamus, and the *substantia nigra* is just beneath the subthalamic nucleus. The precise functions of the subthalamic nucleus and the substantia nigra are unknown, although their numerous connections to the other basal ganglia suggest that they collaborate with them in important ways. The substantia nigra, as the name implies, is darkly colored.

Degeneration and fading of the substantia nigra is frequently seen in *Parkinson's disease.*

The basal ganglia receive input from multiple sites in the cortex (almost all in the frontal lobe) and send, or relay, information via the thalamus

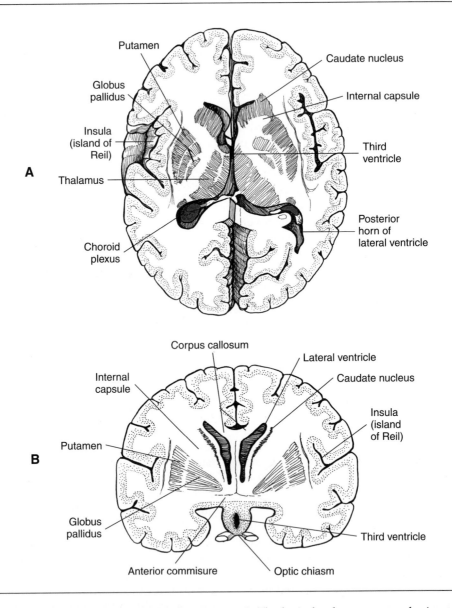

Figure 1-10 ■ The basal ganglia and related structures. **A,** The brain has been cut on a horizontal plane at about the middle of the third ventricle. **B,** The brain has been cut on a vertical plane just anterior to the thalamus. The corpus callosum (B) is the major interhemispheric nerve fiber tract. It forms the roof of the lateral ventricles. The anterior commissure is a minor interhemispheric fiber tract. (See also Figure 1-13.)

to the cortex. The basal ganglia control major muscle groups in the trunk and limbs to produce the postural adjustments necessary for dealing with shifts in body weight and to compensate for inertial forces accompanying movement. Damage in the basal ganglia causes a variety of problems with movement and sensation depending on the location of the damage, but most are characterized by loss of voluntary movements and the appearance of involuntary movements.

Brain Stem

The brain stem provides the communicative and structural link between the brain and the spinal cord, although structurally it is simply a continuation of the spinal cord. The *cranial nerves,* which serve the muscles and sensory receptors of the head, originate here. The brain stem also serves as the only pathway by which motor nerve fibers from the brain reach the spinal cord, and it is the only pathway by which sensory nerve fibers from the periphery reach the brain. For this reason, damage in the brain stem often has important effects on motor and sensory functions.

Brain stem structures regulate some aspects of breathing and heart rate and play a role in integrating complex motor activity. Some brain stem structures help to regulate a person's overall level of consciousness, primarily by means of the *reticular formation* in the brain stem's central core. Because structures in and just above the brain stem control many of the body's vital functions (e.g., breathing, heart rate, and temperature regulation), brain stem injuries may have disastrous—even fatal—results.

For descriptive purposes, anatomists divide the brain stem into three parts—the *midbrain* (upper), the *pons* (middle), and the *medulla* (lower). The *midbrain* (mesencephalon) connects the brain stem with the cerebral hemispheres via the *cerebral peduncles.* Cranial nerves 3 and 4, which connect to muscles that move the eyes, originate in the midbrain.

The word *peduncle* comes from a Latin word meaning *foot. Pedestrian* and *pedal* are more common descendants of that Latin word. In neuroanatomy, *peduncle* refers to various stemlike or stalklike connecting structures in the brain.

The midbrain merges into the pons at the level of the cerebellum. The pons is easily identified by a prominent forward bulge in the brain stem. The pons contains several nuclei involved in hearing and balance, plus the nuclei of three cranial nerves (CN 5, CN 6, and CN 7). Pontine damage typically produces paralysis of muscles responsible for moving the eyes horizontally, but large lesions in the anterior pons may cause *locked-in syndrome,* in which the person is conscious but cannot talk and is quadriplegic (all limbs are paralyzed). Patients with locked-in syndrome may communicate only with eye blinks or by moving the eyes vertically.

The *medulla* is a tapered section of the brain stem connecting the pons and the spinal cord. The medulla contains the nuclei for five cranial nerves (CN 8 through CN 12) and several nuclei concerned with balance and hearing. Nerve fiber tracts for volitional movement cross from one side of the central nervous system to the other in the medulla. The point at which they cross is called the *point of decussation.* Medullary damage typically causes combinations of vertigo (dizziness), paralysis of muscles in the throat and larynx, and various combinations of sensory loss in the limbs and sometimes the face.

Decussation comes from a Latin word meaning *in the form of an X.*

Cerebellum

The cerebellum is just behind the pons and medulla (see Figure 1-9) and looks like a miniature brain. The cerebellum has two hemispheres, each with an outer layer of gray matter called the *cerebellar cortex.* The cerebellum does not initiate movements but coordinates and modulates movements initiated elsewhere (primarily by the motor cortex). The cerebellum plays a major role in regulating the rate, range, direction, and force of movements. Cerebellar damage causes clumsy movements—a condition called *ataxia*.

Spinal Cord

The spinal cord in a normal adult is about 18 inches long. The body of the spinal cord extends from the first cervical vertebra to the first lumbar vertebra, and from there it continues downward as a fine bundle of nerve fibers. This bundle reminded Andreas Laurentius, a 17th-century German physiologist, of a horse's tail. He named the bundle the *cauda equina* (Latin for *horse's tail*), an appellation that has continued to this day.

The spinal cord has an outer layer of *white matter* and a central core of *gray matter* (Figure 1-11). The white matter contains ascending and descending nerve fiber tracts. In cross-section the gray matter resembles a butterfly. It contains motor and sensory neurons. The motor neurons are located primarily in the *anterior horns* of the central gray matter, and most sensory neurons are located in the *posterior horns* (see Figure 1-11). The spinal cord is connected to muscles and sensory receptors by *spinal nerves.* Motor neurons in the anterior horns connect with muscles via *efferent spinal nerves,* and sensory receptors in the body's periphery connect to sensory neurons in the posterior horns via *afferent spinal nerves.*

GENERAL CONCEPTS 1-2

- The human brain is divided into two *hemispheres,* which are structurally similar but functionally different.
- The brain is covered by a thin layer of gray matter called the cerebral cortex. The cerebral cortex is rich in nerve cells and is crisscrossed by ridges *(gyri)* and grooves *(sulci).*

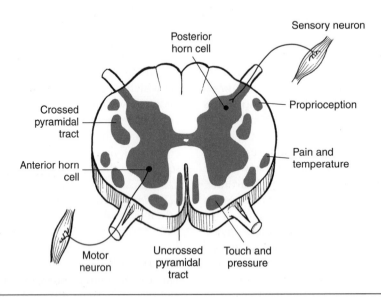

Figure 1-11 ■ Cross-section of the human spinal cord showing motor and sensory fiber tracts. The posterior columns (which contain the posterior horn cells) primarily serve sensory functions, and the anterior columns (which contain the anterior horn cells) primarily serve motor functions.

- Deep sulci are called *fissures*. Two prominent fissures on the human brain are the *central fissure (fissure of Rolando)* and the *lateral cerebral fissure (fissure of Sylvius)*.
- The surface of each hemisphere traditionally is divided into four lobes—the *frontal lobe*, the *parietal lobe*, the *occipital lobe*, and the *temporal lobe*, named after the parts of the skull above them.
- The *cerebral ventricles* are cavities in the brain that are filled with CSF. There are two *lateral ventricles*, one *third ventricle*, and one *fourth ventricle*. They are connected by *foramina* (openings) and an *aqueduct* (tubular channel).
- The diencephalon contains the *thalamus* and *basal ganglia*. The thalamus and basal ganglia modulate, integrate, and regulate motor output and sensory input.
- The brain stem (*midbrain, pons,* and *medulla*) serves as a conduit for all motor output from the central nervous system to the peripheral nervous system and for all sensory input from the peripheral nervous system to the central nervous system.
- The *nuclei* of most cranial nerves are located in the brain stem, as are centers that control vital functions such as respiration and heart rate.
- The *cerebellum* is located behind the brain stem. It resembles a miniature brain and is responsible for controlling the rate, force, direction, and amplitude of volitional movements.
- Most spinal cord motor neurons (*anterior horn cells*) are located in the anterior horns of the spinal cord central gray matter. Most spinal cord sensory neurons (*posterior horn cells*) are located in the posterior horns of the spinal cord central gray matter.

Fiber Tracts

Communication among parts of the central nervous system depends on bundles of nerve axons arranged into nerve fiber tracts. (As noted earlier, these tracts form the *white matter* of the nervous system.) Neuoranatomists have divided central nervous system nerve fiber tracts into three major categories—*projection fibers, commissural fibers,* and *association fibers.*

Projection fibers are the long-distance carriers of the central nervous system. They carry information from the brain to the brain stem and spinal cord, or from peripheral sensory nerves to the brain via the spinal cord.

Projection fibers that carry command and control signals from the brain to muscles and glands are called *efferent (motor) projection fibers.* They originate at neurons in the motor cortex and the premotor cortex and progress down through the brain, the basal ganglia, the brain stem, and the spinal cord to synapse with cranial nerves and spinal nerves.

Projection fibers carrying sensory information from receptors in the periphery to the central nervous system are called *afferent (sensory) projection fibers.* Information from receptor cells is conveyed to the central nervous system by sensory nerves. The sensory nerves synapse with neurons in the spinal cord and brain stem, which send the information up to the brain.

I know of no great mnemonic for remembering efferent vs. afferent. It may help to remember that in the alphabet a precedes e, and that sensations (*a*fferent) often precede responses (*e*fferent).

As the nerve axons making up projection fiber tracts pass through the brain stem and spinal cord, they form a compact and roughly circular band. As they pass between the thalamus and the basal ganglia, the fiber tracts widen and flatten to form the *internal capsule*. From the internal capsule they fan out to destinations in the cortex, primarily in the postcentral gyrus and other parts of the parietal lobe.

The term *capsule,* as in *internal capsule,* is misleading. In ordinary use, the word denotes *enclosure* or *case.* As used here, it denotes a horizontal slice of the motor and sensory fibers passing between the thalamus and basal ganglia. The label *capsule* apparently comes from early dissections, wherein the dense white matter and membranelike appearance of the nerve fibers compared with the gray matter of the basal ganglia and thalamus suggested a capsular structure.

Motor Pathways

Several fiber tracts descend from the brain, midbrain, and brain stem, eventually synapsing with motor neurons at lower levels. The *corticospinal tract* begins in the cerebral cortex and connects with motor neurons in the spinal cord. The spinal cord motor neurons control muscles responsible for volitional movement of the trunk and limbs. The *corticobulbar tract* begins in the cerebral cortex and connects with motor neurons in the brain stem. The brain stem motor neurons are responsible for volitional movement of muscles of the head and neck. The *vestibulospinal tract* begins in the brain stem and connects with spinal cord motor neurons that control muscles responsible for quick movements in response to sudden changes in body position, such as occur in loss of balance or falling. The *descending autonomic tract* begins at structures deep within the brain and connects with motor neurons in the brain stem and spinal cord. These neurons are responsible for modulating autonomic functions such as heart rate and blood pressure.

Sensory Pathways

The sensory pathways in the spinal cord are complex and are the scourge of medical students who must learn them (and of other students who must remember them at least until after the examination). *Pain* and *temperature* sensation share a common pathway to the thalamus and the parietal lobe up the side of the spinal cord opposite to the side of the nerves serving pain and temperature (see Figure 1-11). *Proprioception* (the ability to tell the position of the head and limbs without seeing them) and *stereognosis* (the ability to identify objects by touch) share a pathway up the side of the spinal cord to the brain stem, where the pathway decussates and proceeds up to the cerebellum and the parietal lobe. The pathway for *light touch* ascends in the ventral (anterior) spinal cord to the brain stem and parietal lobe. This pathway contains both uncrossed fibers and fibers that cross at the brain stem.

The complexity of spinal cord sensory pathways, although the bane of students who must learn them, is a blessing for physicians who must deduce what is wrong with patients with sensory abnormalities. A physician often can identify the location—and sometimes can identify the nature—of spinal cord pathology by noting how pain and temperature sense, proprioception, and stereognosis are affected in various parts of the body.

Reflex Arc

Some reflexive motor responses are created by the *reflex arc,* which permits rapid movements without the participation of higher neural systems. The reflex arc has five parts, all in the spinal cord—a *sensory receptor;* an *afferent (sensory) neuron;* an *interneuron;* a *motor neuron;* and an *effector,* usually a muscle (Figure 1-12). Stimulation of the sensory receptor generates an electrical signal, which it sends to the afferent neuron, which sends it to the interneuron (in the posterior column of the spinal cord). The interneuron sends the signal to the motor neuron (in the anterior column of the spinal cord). The motor neuron activates a muscle or gland. Reflexes permit very quick but indiscriminate responses to stimulation. Many of these reflexes serve protective functions—for example, the sneeze, cough, and eye-blink reflexes.

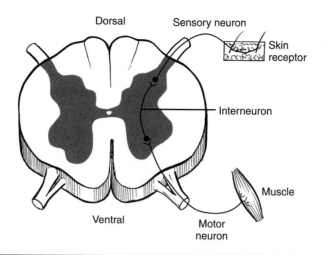

Figure 1-12 ■ The reflex arc. Stimulation of a sensory nerve is transmitted to a motor nerve via an interneuron, making possible rapid responses to stimuli (usually painful ones) without participation of higher centers in the nervous system.

Commissures

Commissural fiber tracts (commissures) are the regional carriers of the central nervous system, providing communicative links between the brain hemispheres. Human brains depend on three commissures for interhemispheric communication—the *corpus callosum,* the *anterior commissure,* and the *posterior commissure* (Figure 1-13).

The *corpus callosum* is the largest and most important commissure, and it is the major player in interhemispheric communication. Anatomically, the corpus callosum is the major structural bridge between the hemispheres. The corpus callosum is crescent shaped, with the open side of the crescent facing down. The anterior third of the corpus callosum is called the *genu;* the central third is called the *rostrum,* or *body;* and the posterior third is called the *splenium.* Nerve fibers crossing through the corpus callosum are spatially arranged to minimize their length. Fibers in the genu connect the anterior frontal lobes. Fibers in the rostrum connect the posterior frontal lobes and anterior

parietal lobes. Fibers in the splenium connect the posterior parietal lobes and the occipital lobes. Damage to the corpus callosum prevents communication between the hemispheres, giving rise to a variety of signs and symptoms, depending on the location of the damage.

The *anterior commissure* and the *posterior commissure* are small bands of fibers crossing between the hemispheres deep in the brain. The anterior and posterior commissures are much smaller than the corpus callosum, and their importance for interhemispheric communication is debated. Given that the anterior commissure and the posterior commissure together are about 1/100th the size of the corpus callosum, it is clear that the corpus callosum is the major player in interhemispheric communication.

Association Fibers

Association fibers are the local carriers in the central nervous system. They connect cortical areas within a hemisphere. If the cortical areas are in the same lobe, the association fibers connecting them are called simply *association*

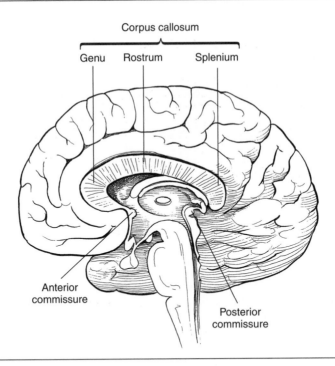

Figure 1-13 ■ The interhemispheric fiber tracts (commissures) of the human brain. The brain hemispheres have been cut apart at the superior longitudinal fissure, and the cut ends of nerve fibers making up the corpus callosum, anterior commissure, and posterior commissure are visible.

fibers. If the cortical areas are in different lobes, the association fibers connecting them get a shorter but harder-to-remember name— *fasciculus,* the plural of which is *fasciculi. Fasciculi* are bundles of nerve fibers connecting nonadjacent regions in a hemisphere. However, they never cross the midline. If they did, they would be commissures.

Fasciculus comes from a Latin word for *bundle. Fascist* comes from that same word.

Neuroanatomists have described three major fasciculi in the human brain—the *uncinate fasciculus,* the *cingulum,* and the *arcuate fasciculus* (Figure 1-14). The uncinate fasciculus is a direct pathway connecting the inferior frontal lobe with the anterior temporal lobe in each hemisphere. The cingulum runs along the top of the corpus callosum and connects deep regions of the frontal and parietal lobes with deep regions of the temporal lobe and midbrain in each hemisphere. The uncinate fasciculus and the cingulum apparently play no major part in speech and language. This is not true for the arcuate fasciculus, sometimes called the *superior longitudinal fasciculus.* The arcuate fasciculus is a crescent-shaped fiber tract in each hemisphere connecting posterior and central regions of the temporal lobe with posterior and inferior regions of the frontal lobe (see Figure 1-14). From its origin in the temporal lobe, the arcuate fasciculus sweeps back and up around the lateral fissure, about an inch below the cortex. Then it curves forward and downward to the frontal lobe. As we shall see, the arcuate fasciculus plays a central role in some models of how the brain deals with language.

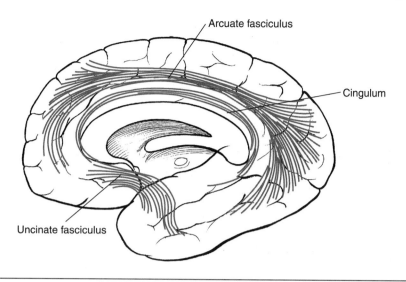

Arcuate fasciculus

Cingulum

Uncinate fasciculus

Figure 1-14 ■ Major fasciculi in the human brain. The arcuate fasciculus is believed to play an important part in many speech and language processes.

GENERAL CONCEPTS 1-3

- *Projection fibers* carry information from motor neurons in the brain to motor neurons in the brain stem or spinal cord *(efferent projection fibers)* or from sensory neurons in the peripheral nervous system to the brain *(afferent projection fibers).*
- The *corticospinal tract* connects motor neurons in the brain cortex with motor neurons in the spinal cord.
- The *corticobulbar tract* connects motor neurons in the brain cortex with motor neurons in the brain stem.
- Sensory pathways in the spinal cord are complex. They ascend in various regions of the spinal cord. Some cross; some do not cross. Those that cross do so at various levels in the spinal cord.
- Some protective reflexes (e.g., sneeze, eye blink) are accomplished within the spinal cord by *reflex arcs.*

- The *internal capsule* is a segment of efferent and afferent projection fibers at the level of the thalamus and basal ganglia.
- *Commissural fiber tracts* cross between the brain hemispheres. The corpus callosum is the primary commissural fiber tract. The anterior commissure and the posterior commissure are minor ones.
- *Association fiber* tracts connect regions within a brain hemisphere. Shorter tracts (those within a lobe) are called *association fibers.* Longer tracts (those connecting regions in different lobes) are called *fasciculi.*
- The *arcuate fasciculus* connects regions in the temporal lobes with regions in the frontal lobes. It is important for some neurophysiologic explanations of language.

Blood Supply to the Brain

As previously mentioned, the brain is a major consumer of oxygen and glucose, both of which get to the brain by way of the blood. At any given time, about 25% of the blood in the body is in the brain. Because the brain is such a massive consumer of oxygen and glucose, and because it has no significant reserves, cutting off the brain's blood supply usually has catastrophic results. Consequently, it is not surprising that interrupted blood supply is a common cause of brain injury.

The mechanical process of getting blood to the brain begins at the heart, where pumping pressure pushes the blood through the arteries.

The heart pumps oxygenated blood into the *aorta,* the major artery from the heart. From the aorta the blood is distributed to two *subclavian arteries,* one on each side of the body. A *common carotid artery* branches off from the right subclavian artery and another *common carotid artery* branches off from the left aorta. The common carotid arteries travel up into the neck where they each divide into an *internal carotid artery* and an *external carotid artery.* (This is going to be complicated. Figure 1-15 may help.) The external carotid arteries provide blood supply to the face. The internal carotid arteries travel to the brain on each side of the neck, near the surface, just behind the angle of

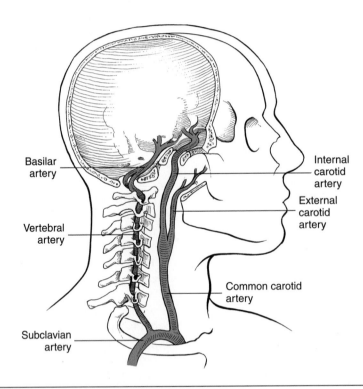

Basilar artery

Vertebral artery

Subclavian artery

Internal carotid artery

External carotid artery

Common carotid artery

Figure 1-15 ■ How the blood gets to the brain. The subclavian arteries branch off from the aorta, which is the major artery from the heart. The right common carotid artery branches off from the subclavian artery; the left common carotid artery branches off from the aorta. Each common carotid artery divides into an external and an internal carotid artery. The external carotid arteries supply blood to the face, and the internal carotid arteries supply the central regions of the brain. The vertebral arteries also branch off the subclavian artery. They supply posterior regions of the brain via the basilar artery.

the jaw. The carotid arteries eventually connect to opposite sides of the *circle of Willis.*

> If you place your open hand on your neck under the angle of your jaw, you should feel a relatively strong pulse near your middle or ring finger. That pulse comes from your internal carotid artery.

Now let's return to the subclavian arteries and follow them to where each branches into a *vertebral artery* (one on each side). The vertebral arteries follow the front side of the medulla upward until they join together (*anastomose*) at the base of the pons to form *the basilar artery.* The basilar artery continues up along the front of the pons and eventually connects into the posterior part of the *circle of Willis.*

The *circle of Willis* is a heptagonal set of arteries centered at the base of the brain (Figure 1-16). The circle of Willis provides blood flow to three paired cerebral arteries—two *anterior cerebral arteries,* two *middle cerebral arteries,* and two *posterior cerebral arteries* (Figure 1-17). The anterior cerebral arteries supply the upper and anterior regions of the frontal lobes and the anterior corpus callosum. The middle cerebral arteries have fan-shaped distributions and supply most of the lateral surfaces of the brain hemispheres, plus the thalamus and basal ganglia. The posterior cerebral arteries supply blood to the occipital lobes and the lower parts of the temporal lobes.

Because the internal carotid arteries and the basilar artery connect to the underside of the circle of Willis, anatomists consider the circle of Willis a common pathway among the two carotid arteries, the basilar artery, and the three pairs of cerebral arteries. If blood flow in a carotid artery or the basilar artery is reduced, the remaining arteries may maintain blood flow to the circle of Willis and from there to the

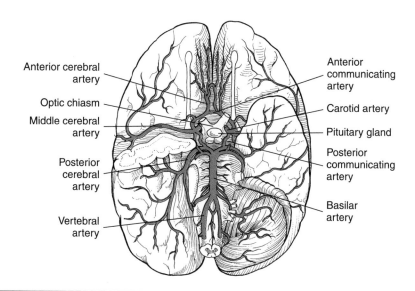

Figure 1-16 ■ How blood is distributed to the brain by the circle of Willis. Occlusions below the circle of Willis may not cause as much damage as occlusions above the circle of Willis, because the circle of Willis provides a common pathway for blood coming from the three major feeder arteries (two internal carotid arteries and the basilar artery) to the cerebral arteries that branch off the top of the circle of Willis.

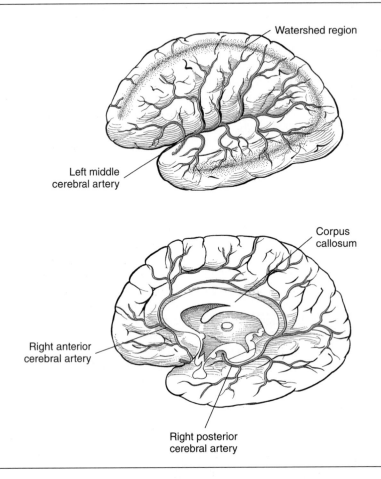

Figure 1-17 ■ The distributions of the cerebral arteries. The watershed region is where the distributions of the cerebral arteries overlap. Occlusions in the watershed region may have relatively small effects on cerebral functions because of collateral circulation from the neighboring artery.

cerebral arteries. This safety valve function works only if the obstruction is below the circle of Willis. Occlusion of a cerebral artery above the circle of Willis almost inevitably causes brain damage because the cerebral arteries share no common source once they leave the circle of Willis.

The compensation provided by the circle of Willis may be less than one might expect because occlusion of a feeder artery is most common in patients with vascular diseases that compromise

blood flow through the entire arterial system. For these patients, collateral flow from the other arteries coming from the heart is likely to be compromised by the vascular disease. Furthermore, the cerebral arteries and the arteries in the circle of Willis may themselves be narrowed or occluded by the disease.

The amount of brain tissue affected by occlusion of a cerebral artery depends on the location of the occlusion in the artery. Occlusions in the trunk or a main branch of a cerebral artery affect large regions of the brain, whereas occlusions in peripheral branches affect smaller regions. Furthermore, the distributions of the cerebral arteries overlap slightly at their boundaries, so that occlusions at the periphery of an artery's distribution may not cause as much brain damage as might be expected because of collateral blood supply from an adjacent artery. These areas of overlapping blood supply are called *watershed areas* (see Figure 1-17).

Now we leave the central nervous system and move to the *peripheral nervous system,* which connects the central nervous system to the world outside.

GENERAL CONCEPTS 1-4

- Two *vertebral arteries* and two *internal carotid arteries* supply blood to the brain. The *basilar artery* connects the vertebral arteries to the *circle of Willis.*
- The *circle of Willis* is a ring-shaped set of arteries at the base of the brain. It connects the basilar artery and the carotid arteries to the *cerebral arteries,* which supply blood to the brain hemispheres.
- The circle of Willis may help to mitigate the effects of occlusion of a feeder artery below the circle of Willis by making it possible for blood supplied by other feeder arteries to reach the cerebral arteries.
- Three pairs of cerebral arteries supply blood to the brain hemispheres. The *anterior cerebral artery* supplies the upper and anterior frontal lobes and the anterior corpus callosum. The middle cerebral artery supplies the posterior frontal lobe, most of the parietal and temporal lobes, plus the thalamus and basal ganglia. The *posterior cerebral artery* supplies the occipital lobe and the inferior temporal lobe.
- Occlusions of the main branch of a cerebral artery are more serious than occlusions in *watershed regions,* where the distributions of the cerebral arteries overlap.

PERIPHERAL NERVOUS SYSTEM

The peripheral nervous system serves as a conduit for sensory information from the body's sensory receptors to the central nervous system, and for motor commands from the central nervous system to the muscles. The major components of the peripheral nervous system are the *cranial nerves* and the *spinal nerves.*

Cranial Nerves

Motor fibers in the *cranial nerves* control muscles in the head and neck. Sensory fibers in the cranial nerves transmit information from sensory receptors in the head and neck to the central nervous system. Most cranial nerves connect with the central nervous system in the midbrain, pons, and medulla.

Cranial nerves 1 (olfactory) and 2 (optic) are sensory tracts that project directly into the brain above the brain stem. Therefore, they probably ought to be considered parts of the central nervous system. However, they were called cranial nerves in the 19th century and the custom persists.

Twelve cranial nerves originate on each side of the central nervous system midline. Each cranial nerve controls muscle groups on its side of the midline or receives sensory input from receptors on its side of the midline. Traditionally the 12 paired cranial nerves are labeled from top to bottom with the Roman numerals I through XII, a labeling system that began with Galen, a Roman physician who died about 200 AD. Contemporary writers (including this one) often substitute Arabic numerals for Roman numerals. The names of the cranial nerves often are abbreviated (e.g., CN 1, CN 3).

Each cranial nerve has been given a name. Some are descriptive: *optic* (CN 1), *olfactory* (CN 2), and *facial* (CN 7). Some are cryptic: *trigeminal* (CN 5) and *vagus* (CN 10). Some serve only motor functions: CN 3, CN 4, CN 6,

CN 11, and CN 12. Some serve only sensory functions: CN 1, CN 2, and CN 8. The remainder serve both motor and sensory functions. The cranial nerves, their names, their motor or sensory functions, and their connection into the central nervous system are summarized in Table 1-1. Several mnemonic devices (most scatological) have been devised by students who must memorize the cranial nerves and their names. I pass along the following socially acceptable (but not very literary) mnemonic:

On old Olympus's towering tops,

A Finn and German vend at hops.

Calling the accessory nerve the *spinal* accessory nerve makes the mnemonic slightly more literary.

On old Olympus's towering tops,

A Finn and German vend some hops.

Table 1-1 shows how these mnemonic devices work.

Spinal Nerves

The spinal nerves provide motor input to or gather sensory information from the viscera, the blood vessels, the glands, and the muscles below the head and neck. The human nervous system contains 31 pairs of spinal nerves, divided into 5 divisions. From top to bottom they are: *cervical* (8 pairs), *thoracic* (12 pairs), *lumbar* (5 pairs), *sacral* (5 pairs), and *coccygeal* (1 pair) (Figure 1-18). Each spinal nerve has a sensory *dorsal root* and a motor *ventral root* connected to the posterior and anterior columns of the spinal cord, respectively. Because of the location of their cell bodies, spinal sensory neurons are called *posterior horn cells,* and spinal motor neurons are called *anterior horn cells.* The anterior and posterior spinal columns sometimes are called the *anterior* and *posterior horns.*

The names of spinal nerves, like the names of the cranial nerves, often are abbreviated. *C3* stands for the third cervical nerve, *T4* for the fourth thoracic nerve, and so on (see Figure 1-18).

TABLE 1-1	The Cranial Nerves				
Nerve	Name	Type*	Function		Mnemonic
1	Olfactory	S	Smell, taste		On
2	Optic	S	Vision		old
3	Oculomotor	M	Eye, eyelid movement		Olympus's
4	Trochlear	M	Eye movement		towering
5	Trigeminal	S,M	Sensation from face; motor to masseters, palate, pharynx		tops
6	Abducens	M	Eye movement		a
7	Facial	S,M	Sensation from anterior tongue; motor to facial muscles		Finn
8	Vestibular	S	Balance, hearing		and
9	Glossopharyngeal	S,M	Sensation from posterior tongue, soft palate, pharynx; motor to pharynx		German
10	Vagus	S,M	Motor to larynx, pharynx, viscera; sensation from viscera		vend
11	Accessory (spinal accessory)	M	Motor to larynx, chest, shoulder		at (some)
12	Hypoglossal	M	Motor to tongue		hops

*S, Sensory; M, motor.

GENERAL CONCEPTS 1-5

- Cranial nerves and spinal nerves are parts of the *peripheral nervous system.*
- Cranial nerves serve structures in the head and neck. Spinal nerves serve structures in the torso and limbs.
- Most cranial nerves arise from nuclei in the brain stem. Spinal nerves arise from nerve cell bodies in the central gray matter of the spinal cord. Each spinal nerve has an *anterior motor (efferent) branch* and a *posterior sensory (afferent)* branch.

CENTRAL NERVOUS SYSTEM FUNCTIONAL ANATOMY

Cerebral Cortex

Neuroanatomists typically divide the cortex of the human brain into two major functional categories—*primary cortex* and *association cortex.* The primary cortex is responsible for specific motor or sensory functions. The association cortex is responsible for combining, refining, interpreting, and elaborating crude sensory information coming from primary cortical sensory areas and for organizing and planning action sequences for the primary motor cortex. In simple terms, the association cortex interprets sensory information and plans motor activity.

Primary Cortex. The first functional region of the primary cortex to be identified by neuroanatomists was the *primary motor cortex*— a narrow strip of cortex located immediately in front of the central fissure in each hemisphere, corresponding roughly to the area of the precentral gyrus. The nerve cells in the primary motor cortex are responsible for initiating and controlling voluntary and precise skilled movements of skeletal muscles *contralateral* to (on the opposite side of the body from) the primary motor cortex.

The *primary somatosensory cortex* is a narrow strip of cortex behind the central fissure

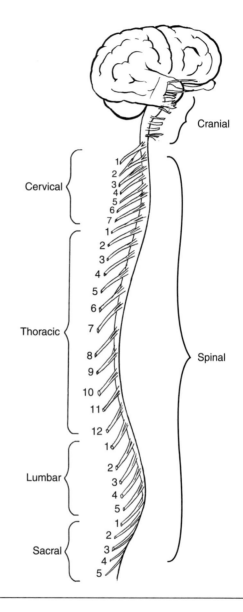

Figure 1-18 ■ The human central nervous system, showing the vertical location of cranial and spinal nerves and the division of spinal nerves into cervical, thoracic, lumbar, and sacral nerves.

in each hemisphere, corresponding roughly to the area of the postcentral gyrus. The primary somatosensory cortex is responsible for *somesthetic* (skin, muscle, joint, and tendon) sensation from the contralateral side of the body. (However, lower structures in the brain also mediate gross perception of pain, temperature, and light touch.)

Some contemporary neurophysiologists (such as Nolte, 1993) combine the motor and *somatosensory cortices* into a single sensorimotor cortex, apparently to illustrate the important role somatosensory information plays in regulation and control of movement. For simplicity's sake I have elected to remain with the traditional division of precentral and postcentral cortex. However, the reader should keep in mind that the somatosensory cortex plays an important role in regulating and controlling almost all volitional movement.

The *primary auditory cortex* is located on the upper surface of the temporal lobes, on the lower lip of the lateral fissures, corresponding roughly to the transverse temporal gyrus (better known as the *gyrus of Heschl*). The auditory cortex in each hemisphere receives input from both ears, and, together, they are responsible for hearing.

The *primary visual cortex* is located in the occipital lobes, surrounding the calcarine fissures, and is responsible for vision. Each visual cortex receives half the visual input from each eye.

The *primary olfactory cortex* is located in the posterior inferior frontal lobe and is responsible for our sense of smell. Figure 1-19 shows the location of these functional areas.

The regions of the primary cortex are organized so that tactile sensations from the skin, visual sensations from the eyes, or auditory sensations from the ears are projected onto their primary cortical regions in topographic arrays, with point-to-point connections between the cortex and tactile receptors in the skin,

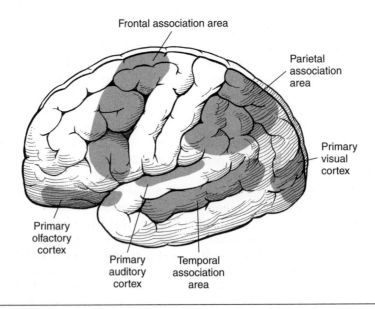

Figure 1-19 ■ The association areas and primary auditory, visual, and olfactory cortices of the human brain. The association areas, like the lobes, represent arbitrary divisions. No differences in brain architecture mark these divisions, and their size and location vary, depending on who is drawing the picture. The right hemisphere contains mirror-image representations of these cortical areas.

visual receptors in the eyes, and auditory receptors in the cochlea. (The olfactory cortex seems not to be arranged topographically.)

Stimulating the primary motor cortex produces gross unrefined movements of major muscle groups, sometimes associated with primitive movements such as licking, chewing, or swallowing. Stimulating the primary somatosensory cortex produces gross unrefined sensations such as numbness, tingling, or electric shock. Stimulating the olfactory cortex produces sensations of peculiar odors and tastes. Stimulating the visual cortex produces subjective flashes of light. Stimulating the auditory cortex produces buzzing or roaring sensations. Damage to the primary motor or sensory cortex impairs the motor or sensory functions previously served by the destroyed cortex.

Association Cortex. Several association areas in the human brain have been described in the literature, of which four are most relevant to language and communication (see Figure 1-19).

- The *frontal association cortex* is a strip of cortex just in front of the primary motor cortex. Sometimes the frontal association cortex is called the *premotor cortex.* It plays an important part in planning and initiating complex volitional movements.
- The *parietal association cortex* participates in processing tactile information and seems to be responsible for position sense, visuospatial processing, and awareness of extrapersonal space.
- The *temporal association cortex* is important for discriminating and processing auditory information and for many language-related processes.
- The *parieto-occipital association cortex* is important for discriminating and processing visual information. The left-hemisphere parieto-occipital association cortex participates in many of the visual processes involved in reading.

Stimulation of association cortex usually causes combinations of sensory phenomena (typically unpleasant) and primitive movements

of muscle groups (e.g., eye closure, twisting of the torso, or limb contraction). Destruction of association cortex does not cause specific motor or sensory deficits, but it impairs discrimination, recognition, or comprehension of categories of stimuli, depending on which region of association cortex has been destroyed. For example, destruction of the temporal association cortex may prevent a person from recognizing the significance of sounds, even though the person's perception of sounds is intact.

Lobes of the Brain

Frontal Lobes. The frontal lobes are intimately involved in planning and executing volitional behavior. The primary motor cortex in the posterior frontal lobes is responsible for initiating complex volitional movements. The premotor cortex, just in front of the primary motor cortex and sometimes called the *frontal association area,* is responsible for planning sequential volitional movements (see Figure 1-19). The anterior frontal lobes regulate general activity levels and play a role in formulating intentions, plans, and patterns for volitional behavior. Some anatomists identify a small patch of cortex inside the superior longitudinal fissure directly in front of the primary motor cortex for the leg as the *supplemental motor cortex.* Stimulation of the supplemental motor cortex causes bilateral limb movements, vocalization, or muteness.

Damage to the primary motor cortex causes weakness or paralysis of muscle groups on the contralateral side of the body. Damage to the premotor cortex causes disruption of complex volitional movement sequences. Damage to the anterior frontal lobes may cause a variety of impairments, including disturbed affect, attentional impairments, and difficulties initiating and maintaining behavior. Whether the left and right anterior frontal lobes serve different cognitive or behavioral functions is not well understood, in part because unilateral damage to otherwise normal frontal lobes is relatively rare (Gainotti, 1991). Consequently, the two frontal lobes usually are lumped together when anterior frontal lobe syndromes are described.

Parietal Lobes. The parietal lobes are important for perception, integration, and mediation of touch, body awareness, and visuospatial information. The primary sensory cortex, responsible for somesthetic sensation, forms the anterior margin of the parietal lobe, and the strip of cortex just behind it appears to be important for interpretation of somesthetic sensory information. Damage in the latter strip of cortex sometimes causes a contralateral phenomenon called *tactile agnosia* (or *astereognosis*), in which a person is unable to recognize objects by touch, despite intact tactile perception. Damage in the association cortex in either parietal lobe typically disturbs position sense and causes various visuospatial impairments in which the patient has difficulty drawing or copying geometric designs, discriminating complex visual stimuli, and appreciating spatial relationships, including attention to locations in extrapersonal space.

Temporal Lobes. The temporal lobes are important for perception and processing of auditory stimuli. The primary auditory cortices are located in the upper temporal lobes, and auditory and auditory-visual association areas are found in the midtemporal and posterior temporal regions, respectively. The anterior temporal lobes appear to be important in pitch discrimination and for separating an auditory signal from a noise background, such as when one engages in conversation at a cocktail party. The association cortex in the left temporal lobe is important for comprehension of verbal material, both spoken and written, and for language processes involving semantics and syntax. The right temporal lobe appears to be important for interpretation of complex nonverbal visual stimuli and for recognition and comprehension of nonverbal sounds, including receptive components of music. Damage in the temporal association cortex sometimes causes *auditory agnosia,* the inability to recognize familiar sounds, although hearing is intact.

Occipital Lobes. The occipital lobes contain the primary visual cortex and the visual association areas. Destruction of the visual cortex in either hemisphere causes blindness in regions of the contralateral visual fields. Damage in the association cortex adjacent to the visual cortex in either hemisphere typically causes *visual agnosia* (the inability to recognize familiar visually presented stimuli, even though visual perception is adequate), and distorted visual perceptions. Damage in the visual association cortex in the left hemisphere usually causes severe reading impairment. Bilateral destruction of the visual cortex results in a phenomenon called *cortical blindness.* Patients who are cortically blind have extreme difficulty discriminating visual shapes and patterns, but remain sensitive to light and dark. A few cortically blind patients may perceive gross characteristics of simple visual stimuli, although they are unable to describe them or incorporate them into other mental activity.

GENERAL CONCEPTS 1-6

- The *primary olfactory cortex* is in the inferior frontal lobes.
- The *primary motor cortex* in each hemisphere is responsible for skilled volitional movement of contralateral muscle groups. Neurons in the left motor cortex connect with muscles on the right side of the body and vice versa.
- The *premotor cortex,* just in front of the primary motor cortex in each hemisphere, is a strip of association cortex responsible for organizing and planning complex volitional movements.
- The *primary sensory cortex* in the anterior parietal lobe of each brain hemisphere is responsible for contralateral skin, muscle, joint, and tendon sensation.
- The *parietal association cortex* is responsible for position sense and for interpreting tactile and visuospatial information.
- The *primary auditory cortices* are in the upper temporal lobes. The temporal association cortices are responsible for interpreting auditory information.

GENERAL CONCEPTS 1-6—cont'd

- The association cortex in the left temporal lobe is responsible for many language-related processes.
- The association cortex in the right temporal lobe is responsible for interpreting nonverbal auditory information, including receptive aspects of music.
- The *primary visual cortex* is in the posterior occipital lobe. The *parieto-occipital region* is responsible for interpreting complex visual stimuli. The left hemisphere parieto-occipital region is important for visual processes involved in reading.

THE MOTOR SYSTEM

Normal motor performance depends on the integrated activity of three systems—the *pyramidal system,* the *vestibular-reticular system,* and the *extrapyramidal system.* Damage in any one system produces characteristic impairment of motor performance that often points to the location—and sometimes to the nature—of the damage.

Pyramidal System

The pyramidal system is responsible for initiating most, if not all, skilled volitional movement. The pyramidal system begins at pyramidal neurons in the cerebral cortex. (They are called pyramidal neurons because they have pyramidal shapes.) The axons of the pyramidal neurons converge into a dense band of nerve fibers that descends through the internal capsule to synapse with neurons in the brain stem and spinal cord.

The pyramidal system is a *direct system. Direct* means that the only synapses in the pyramidal system are where neurons in the brain cortex connect with neurons in the brain stem or spinal cord. (Some of the axons in the pyramidal system are 2 or 3 feet long. The longest axons are those that synapse with the lowermost spinal nerves.) The smaller the

number of synapses in a neural circuit, the faster is the circuit's response time. Pyramidal circuits, being single-synapse circuits, have especially quick response times.

The motor neurons in the pyramidal system are called *upper motor neurons.* The cell bodies of upper motor neurons are located in the primary motor cortex. Their axons pass through the midbrain, brain stem, and spinal cord to synapse with motor neurons in the brain stem and spinal cord (called *lower motor neurons*). The lower motor neurons synapse with muscles at specialized junctions called *motor endplates.*

> The pyramidal system fibers that connect with neurons in the brain stem are called the *corticobulbar tract,* and the fibers that connect with neurons in the spinal cord are called the *corticospinal tract.* In total, the fiber tracts of the pyramidal system are called *projection fiber tracts.*

The neurons in the primary motor cortex are arranged topographically so that a functional map of the motor cortex can be created, showing which cortical areas are responsible for volitional movements of given muscle groups. Such a map, sometimes called a *homunculus* (little man), is shown in Figure 1-20.

> The word *homunculus* dates from the 16th and 17th centuries, when it referred to an exceedingly minute human body that was thought to inhabit each sperm cell. Development of the embryo and subsequent growth from infant to adult were believed to represent the growth of the homunculus.

It can be seen in Figure 1-20 that cortical responsibility for muscle groups is arranged in upside-down fashion on the motor cortex. The motor cortex for the foot and toes is located at the top of the primary motor cortex, and representation for the knee, hip, shoulder, elbow, wrist, hand, and face progresses laterally and downward. The representation of the body in Figure 1-20 looks odd because the size of a

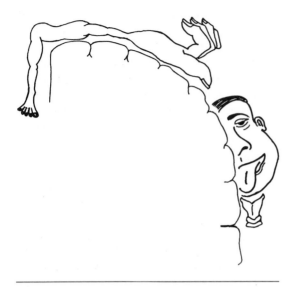

Figure 1-20 ■ A *homunculus* representing the allocation of motor function in the motor cortex. The size of the body part portrayed in the figure represents the amount of cortex devoted to innervation of the muscles in that body part.

body part in the figure represents the amount of motor cortex assigned to various muscle groups and relates in a general way to the precision of movement required from muscle groups. The hand, mouth, tongue, larynx, and lips are allocated large amounts of motor cortex relative to the trunk, legs, and upper arms because the muscles of the hand, mouth, tongue, larynx, and lips are called on to perform more diverse, intricate, and precise movements than are the muscles of the trunk, legs, and upper arms.

The *primary somatosensory cortex* is not part of the pyramidal system, but I describe it here because of its location near the primary motor cortex, its topographic similarity to the motor cortex, and its importance to skilled movement. The primary somatosensory cortex, located just behind the central fissure, is topographically arranged as a mirror image of the motor cortex. Sensation from the face is represented at the lower (lateral) end of the sensory cortex, and

sensation from the foot is represented at the top, inside the superior longitudinal fissure.

Vestibular-Reticular System

The vestibular-reticular system (also not part of the pyramidal system, but related to it) is responsible for balance and orientation of the body in space and for maintaining general states of attention and alertness. The vestibular-reticular system is made up of neurons scattered throughout the brain stem and cerebellum. Like pyramidal system neurons, the neurons in the vestibular-reticular system synapse with lower motor neurons. Unlike the pyramidal system, the vestibular-reticular system is not under volitional control—its functions are largely automatic and preprogrammed. Some writers combine the vestibular-reticular system with the extrapyramidal system. Although they have structural similarities, they serve different functions, so they are described separately here.

Extrapyramidal System

The extrapyramidal system is a diffuse system of subcortical structures and pathways arising from diverse locations in the central nervous system (primarily the basal ganglia) and projecting to cranial and spinal nerves. (According to some neuroanatomists, *extrapyramidal* is synonymous with *basal ganglia*.) The extrapyramidal system is phylogenetically older than the pyramidal system, and it is an *indirect system,* which means that it is made up of networks of neurons, with chains of neurons and multiple synapses between the origin and destination of any extrapyramidal system pathway. The extrapyramidal system does not initiate movements but adjusts muscle tone and posture concurrent with volitional movements. Damage in the extrapyramidal system distorts or abolishes volitional movements and causes involuntary movements to appear.

Because of its diffuseness, some writers dismiss the concept of the extrapyramidal system as a convenient fiction without neuroarchitectural validity.

(The same could be said about many other conventional physiologic divisions.) These writers argue that the concept of the extrapyramidal system should be abandoned, and some contemporary descriptions of the nervous system do not mention it. However, the demise of the extrapyramidal system seems likely to be a slow one, because it has a long history and it provides *a convenient shorthand for two broad classes of motor disorders* (Nolte, 1993).

Because the paths of the pyramidal, vestibular-reticular, and extrapyramidal systems are common throughout much of their course, an injury that affects one usually affects all three. Therefore, we commonly see combinations of pyramidal, extrapyramidal, and sometimes vestibular signs when any of the divisions is damaged.

How the Nervous System Produces Volitional Movement

The process by which the nervous system produces volitional movement is complex and not completely understood. It is clear that several subsystems participate in all but the simplest movements. The following simplified scenario provides a general sense of the process by which the nervous system moves from intention to action.

Activation of cortical regions in the anterior frontal lobes prepares the motor system for movement. The premotor cortex creates a set of neurally coded instructions for the intended movement sequence and transmits the instructions to the primary motor cortex. The primary motor cortex sends the command and control information necessary to execute the plan to the cranial nerves via the corticobulbar tract and the spinal nerves via the corticospinal tract. The vestibular nuclei, midbrain, and reticular formation adjust balance and posture before and during the movement. The cerebellum modulates the rate, force, and direction of the movement. The extrapyramidal system adjusts muscle tone and posture to make the movement smooth and continuous.

GENERAL CONCEPTS 1-7

- The *pyramidal system* is responsible for skilled volitional movement. The pyramidal system begins with neurons in the primary motor cortex *(upper motor neurons)* whose axons synapse with neurons in the brain stem *(corticobulbar tracts)* and spinal cord *(corticospinal tracts).*
- Neurons in cranial nerves and spinal nerves are called *lower motor neurons.* Neurons in the motor cortex are called *upper motor neurons.*
- Muscle groups are represented in the primary motor cortex in topographic arrays. Motor neurons for the face, larynx, and head are represented in the upper part of the primary motor cortex, and motor neurons for the leg and foot are represented at the lower end.
- The amount of cortical representation for a muscle group reflects the precision and complexity of movements performed by the muscle group.
- The *vestibular-reticular system* is a self-regulating system that maintains balance, orientation of the body in space, and general levels of alertness and arousal.
- The *extrapyramidal system* is a diffuse system of subcortical structures and nerve fiber tracts. Its primary function is that of adjusting skeletal muscles concurrent with volitional movement.
- Damage in the extrapyramidal system disrupts or abolishes volitional movements and causes nonvolitional movements to appear.

This section describes some major neurologic causes of adult language disorders, primarily *aphasia,* in which comprehension and production of spoken and written verbal materials is compromised, and the cognitive-communicative impairments exhibited by some adults with right-hemisphere damage. It will not deal with the neurologic causes of *dysarthria* (speech impairments caused by nervous system damage) or *traumatic brain injury* (linguistic and cognitive impairments following traumatic injury to the nervous system). The neuropathology of dysarthria and traumatic brain injury are addressed in later chapters.

STROKE

Stroke is a generic term for brain damage caused by vascular disruptions (loss of blood supply or bleeding). A more technical term for stroke is *cerebrovascular accident (CVA)*. During the past decade public-information campaigns have proposed the label *brain attack* for stroke and CVA. The appellation *brain attack* was adopted because of its resemblance to *heart attack,* presumably to reinforce the public's awareness of the need for immediate medical attention when symptoms of a stroke are experienced. The following are the most common symptoms of a stroke:

- Abrupt weakness or numbness on one side of the body
- Abrupt impairment of vision, especially in one eye
- Abrupt difficulty speaking or understanding speech
- Abrupt episodes of dizziness or falls
- Abrupt severe headache, especially with any of the other symptoms

---

Brain attack has yet to replace *stroke* in health science and the popular press. I will use the traditional label in the remainder of this book.

Stroke is the third leading cause of death in the United States, ranking behind heart disease and cancer, but is the leading cause of long-term disability. Approximately 5 million survivors of stroke are alive in the United States in any given year. Each year about 500,000 U.S. residents experience a first stroke; about 200,000 experience a second or third stroke; and about 150,000 die as a consequence of a stroke. About three quarters of those who experience a stroke are 65 years old or older. About 75% survive for at least 1 month after their first stroke, but only about one third are alive 10 years later (U.S. Centers for Disease Control, 2005). Of those who survive a stroke, from 50% to 75% are able to return to their prestroke living environment, usually with some level of persisting impairment, while 15% are sufficiently impaired to require institutional care (Greenberg, Aminoff, & Simon, 1996). The incidence of stroke differs across regions of the United States. The Southeastern region and lower Mississippi River Valley have considerably greater rates of stroke than other U.S. regions (Figure 1-21).

The brain is remarkably intolerant of sudden changes in its oxygen and glucose supplies. The onset of communicative disorders following strokes almost always is dramatic, with symptoms developing rapidly and becoming maximally expressed within a few minutes to a few hours. During the first few days after a stroke, parts of the brain that are not actually damaged or destroyed may be functionally impaired, unless the stroke is a very small one.

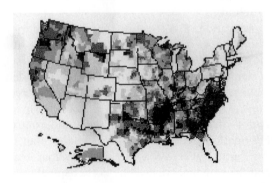

Figure 1-21 ■ Stroke death rates, 1991-1998. Darker shading represents greater incidence of death from stroke. (From National Center for Chronic Disease Prevention and Health Promotion. [2005]. Atlas of stroke mortality. Atlanta: Centers for Disease Control and Prevention.)

Major strokes often yield a pattern in which there is immediate general disruption of cerebral functions, gradually resolving to more limited (focal) disruption of specific processes, depending on what parts of the brain have been permanently damaged.

Strokes can be *ischemic* (a term that means *deprived of blood*) or *hemorrhagic* (a term that means *caused by bleeding*), although the percentage of ischemic strokes (80%) is far higher than the percentage of hemorrhagic strokes (20%).

Ischemic Stroke

Ischemic stroke (sometimes called *occlusive stroke*) occurs when an artery is blocked and part of the brain loses its blood supply. If the occlusion lasts more than 3 to 5 minutes, death *(necrosis)* of brain tissue is likely. (The medical term for death of brain tissue caused by loss of blood supply is *infarct*.) Ischemic strokes may be caused by *thrombosis* or *embolus*. In *thrombotic strokes (cerebral thrombosis),* an artery slowly is occluded by a plug of material accumulating at a fixed location. In *embolic strokes,* an artery abruptly is occluded by material that moves through the blood and blocks the artery.

Most cerebral thromboses occur in the large arteries carrying blood to the brain—the internal carotid arteries, the vertebral arteries, and the basilar artery. A thrombosis typically begins in an area of increased turbulence—locations at which arteries change direction or divide *(bends* and *bifurcations).* Debris in the blood stream tends to accumulate at bends and bifurcations, just as it does in river bends and bifurcations. In rivers the debris may include driftwood, cola bottles, and overturned canoes. In arteries the debris consists mainly of fatty substances *(lipids)* and fibrous material *(atherosclerotic plaque)* that accumulate on the lining of the artery and narrow its diameter. Turbulence and increased blood velocity at the narrowing abrade and roughen the lining of the artery. Plaque forms on these roughened areas

and thickens over the course of years, until it may fill the *lumen* (space within the artery), causing a stroke.

Atherosclerotic comes from a combination of Greek words meaning *paste* (athero-) and hard (sclero-). *Plaque* comes from a French word meaning *plate* or *slab.*

As the size of the lumen diminishes (a condition called *stenosis*), the volume of blood flowing through the narrowed artery decreases (although its velocity increases—the *Bernoulli effect*). Sometimes the plaque in the arterial wall cracks or ulcerates. Blood platelets and fibrin (a protein found in blood) then adhere to the ulceration, accelerating clot development. The clot may eventually occlude the artery, or parts of the clot may break off and become *emboli* traveling through the vascular system, eventually occluding smaller vessels downstream from the original clot, causing a stroke.

Embolic strokes (cerebral embolisms) are caused by a fragment of material that travels through the circulatory system until it reaches an artery smaller than its own diameter, where it lodges, occluding the artery. The material in the embolus may be a blood clot that has broken loose from its original location, a fragment of arterial lining, a piece of atherosclerotic plaque, tissue from a tumor, a clump of bacteria, or other solids that may move through the arteries. The most frequent sources of emboli are fragments from thromboses in the heart, followed by fragments of atherosclerotic plaque from an artery. Patients with atrial fibrillation (heart palpitations) are particularly susceptible to cerebral embolism, because the absence of strong atrial contraction promotes pooling and clotting of blood in the left atrium, which then embolizes. Atrial fibrillations may break off parts of the clot, creating an embolus.

Determining whether the cause of a stroke is thrombosis or embolus is difficult, so a diagnostician may hedge by referring to ischemic strokes as *thromboembolic strokes*. However, thrombotic and embolic strokes differ in their progression. Because embolic strokes are a consequence of sudden blockage of an artery, symptoms are maximally expressed within a few minutes. Because thrombotic strokes are caused by slowly developing occlusion of an artery, they tend to develop in an irregular, stepwise manner, sometimes preceded by transient periods of ischemia (small strokes).

Transient Interruptions of Cerebral Blood Supply. Many stroke patients have a history of *transient ischemic attacks (TIAs)*—temporary disruptions of cerebral circulation accompanied by rapidly developing sensory disturbance, limb weakness, slurred speech, visual anomalies, dizziness, confusion, mild aphasia, or other symptoms, which resolve completely within a few minutes to 24 hours. Most TIAs are thought to be caused by small emboli that temporarily occlude an artery, then break up or dissolve. TIAs sometimes occur when a stationary thrombus has nearly, but not completely, occluded an artery, so that otherwise insignificant decrements in blood pressure may be sufficient to interrupt blood flow through the artery. TIAs occasionally (but rarely) are caused by *cerebral vasospasm* of a nearly occluded artery, in which the muscles of the arterial wall contract, narrowing the lumen and compromising blood flow.

Transient interruptions of blood supply to the brain that last more than 24 hours but completely resolve within a few days sometimes are called *reversible ischemic neurologic deficits (RINDs)*. Interruptions of blood supply to the brain that last more than 24 hours but leave minor deficits after a few days sometimes are called *partially reversible ischemic neurologic deficits (PRINDs)*. The general public, many physicians, and some neurologists forgo these categorizations and call any transient episode of sensory disruption, weakness, slurred speech, visual anomalies, dizziness, confusion, or aphasia caused by temporary interruption of blood supply to the brain a *small stroke*.

Because TIAs, RINDs, and PRINDs are manifestations of cerebrovascular disease, their occurrence often presages a full-blown stroke. About one third of patients who have TIAs or RINDs will have a stroke that leaves them with permanent neurologic deficits within 5 years of the transient ischemic event (Greenberg, Aminoff, and Simon, 1993). However, this percentage may be reduced by treatments and lifestyle changes that control hypertension, lower blood cholesterol, and eliminate smoking.

Hypoperfusion. Insufficient blood supply to the brain sometimes is caused by *hypoperfusion,* in which the brain's blood supply is compromised not by occlusion of arteries but by insufficient blood volume. Insufficient blood volume is most commonly caused by massive bleeding elsewhere in the body or by insufficient cardiac pumping capacity (usually from heart disease). The pattern of cerebral damage caused by hypoperfusion is different from that caused by occlusion. Occlusions usually cause localized regions of dense neuron loss in brain tissue supplied by the affected artery or branch. Hypoperfusion usually causes patchy damage in the watershed regions (border zones) of the cortex supplied by the artery or branch, because the blood does not penetrate into the border zones where vessel diameters are small and flow resistance is high. Although hypoperfusion causes cerebral ischemia, it is not a stroke, and, unlike ischemic strokes, its effects have a gradual onset. I discuss it here because it is a cause of cerebral ischemia (albeit a minor one).

General Effects of Ischemic Stroke. Dobkin and associates (1989), Keefe (1995), Kwakkel, Kollen, and Lindeman (2004), Ruudinger and associates (2000), and Rubens (1977), have described some of the physiologic changes that take place following major ischemic strokes. Within the first few hours after the stroke, neurons deprived of blood supply die. Damaged brain tissue swells. If the damaged area is large, swelling may raise intracranial pressure and cause displacement of brain tissue in regions remote from the site of the stroke. Blood flow to both hemispheres diminishes. Neurotransmitters and other neurotoxins are released, not only into the brain tissues at the site of the stroke, but throughout the brain and into the CSF. Their presence upsets neuronal metabolism and perhaps contributes to reduced cerebral blood flow. Neurons in undamaged parts of the brain that connect with destroyed neurons degenerate because of the lost connections *(transneural degeneration)*. Surviving neurons that have lost some (but not all) of their input from neurons in the damaged region become hypersensitive to residual input from the damaged region *(denervation hypersensitivity)*.

Diaschisis is a phenomenon in which brain function is disrupted in regions away from the site of injury but connected to it by neuronal pathways. It too plays a role in the impairments seen immediately after a stroke. For many years diaschisis was an unproven phenomenon, but imaging studies of cerebral metabolism (e.g., positron emission tomography, functional magnetic-resonance imaging) have confirmed that destruction of brain tissue in one area is followed by reductions in cerebral metabolism in other areas, primarily those that have substantial neuronal connections to the damaged area (Kwakkel, Kollen, and Lindeman, 2004; Metter and associates, 1983, 1984; Ruudinger and associates, 2000).

Brain swelling, reduction in cerebral blood flow, neurotransmitter release, transneural degeneration, denervation hypersensitivity, and diaschisis, individually or in combination, create diffuse impairment of brain functions, behavior, and mental status, which gradually resolves over time. In the first hours and days after the patient's stroke, the symptoms generated by this diffuse impairment are superimposed on the more focal symptoms caused by death of tissue at the site of the stroke. As time passes, cerebral swelling diminishes, cerebral blood flow to undamaged tissue is restored, and neurotransmitters and neurotoxins are excreted

or resorbed. Axons in brain tissue near the infarct establish new connections with neurons that have lost direct connections with the infarcted area *(collateral sprouting)*. As these physiologic repairs take place, the patient gradually improves, with diffuse impairment of behavior, bodily function, and mentation resolving to a more specific *(focal)* collection of symptoms reflecting the permanent loss of neurons in the infarcted area.

Predictions about a patient's eventual neurologic recovery (or predictions of their residual level of impairment) during the first few days after a stroke often prove unreliable because the permanent effects of the tissue destruction caused by the stroke are masked by the stroke's temporary effects on brain chemistry and function. For this reason, experienced clinicians often refrain from making predictions about a patient's eventual level of recovery until these temporary effects have diminished—usually within 2 weeks to a month.

Hemorrhagic Stroke (Cerebral Hemorrhage)

Cerebral hemorrhages are caused by rupture or leakage of cerebral blood vessels. Cerebral hemorrhages may be the result of weakness of a vessel wall, traumatic injury to a vessel, or (rarely) extreme fluctuations in blood pressure. Hemorrhages from the blood vessels in the meninges or on the surface of the brain are called *extracerebral hemorrhages* because the bleeding is outside the brain. Hemorrhages into the brain or brain stem are called *intracerebral hemorrhages* because the bleeding is in the brain tissues.

To complicate matters further, extracerebral hemorrhages can be described as *subarachnoid, subdural,* or *epidural,* depending on where the blood accumulates. If the bleeding is under the arachnoid, between the arachnoid and the pia mater, it is called a *subarachnoid hemorrhage*— the most common extracerebral hemorrhage. If the bleeding is under the dura mater, it is called a *subdural hemorrhage;* and if it is above the dura, between the dura mater and the skull, it is called an *epidural hemorrhage.* After the bleeding stops, patients are left with a *subarachnoid, subdural,* or *epidural hematoma*—accumulation of clotted or partially clotted blood in the space created by the hemorrhage.

Hemorrhages involving the dura mater (subdural or epidural) usually are caused by traumatic head injuries in which dural blood vessels are torn or lacerated. Subarachnoid hemorrhages usually come from leaking or ruptured blood vessels on the surface of the brain, brain stem, or cerebellum—often the result of *aneurysm.*

Aneurysms are pouches formed in weakened arterial walls. Blood pressure in the artery causes the weakened section of the arterial wall to stretch, much like an inflating balloon. The resulting malformations are sometimes called *berry*

aneurysms or *saccular aneurysms* because of their berrylike or saclike appearance (Figure 1-22). The stretched arterial walls in aneurysms are thin, weak, and susceptible to rupture.

About half of all berry aneurysms develop in the arteries at the base of the brain (the vertebral arteries, basilar artery, internal carotid arteries, and the circle of Willis). Most of the remainder develop in the anterior and middle cerebral arteries. Very few (2% to 3%) develop in the posterior cerebral artery. An aneurysm detected before it ruptures may be surgically repaired by clamping or tying off the neck of the aneurysm, by wrapping it, or by tying off the artery that supplies it with blood. A leaking aneurysm may be repaired, but a ruptured aneurysm often is impossible to repair. Ruptured aneurysms are dangerous and carry substantial risk of death or irreversible brain damage.

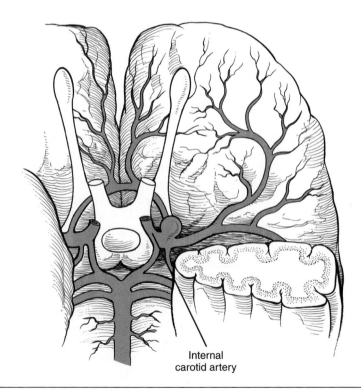

Internal
carotid artery

Figure 1-22 ■ A *berry aneurysm* on the left anterior communicating artery in the circle of Willis. Aneurysms are most common in the arteries at the base of the brain.

Some subarachnoid hemorrhages arise from *arteriovenous malformations (AVMs)*. AVMs are collections of dilated, thin-walled veins connected to a tangled mass of fragile arteries (Figure 1-23). AVMs can develop in many locations in the brain, brain stem, and spinal cord, but most large AVMs appear deep in the cerebral hemispheres. The vessel walls in AVMs, like those in aneurysms, are weak and likely to rupture. Almost all AVMs are present at birth and become larger over time. As an AVM grows it presses on and displaces brain tissue, causing headache, blurred vision, or other signs of cerebral dysfunction. If an AVM is identified before it ruptures, it may be surgically excised, or the blood vessels that connect to it may be tied off or plugged. According to Adams & Victor (1981), the risk of bleeding from AVMs is about 1% to 2% per year, which suggests that a patient with an AVM is unlikely to reach the age of 60 or 70 without a hemorrhage.

Almost all *intracerebral hemorrhages* (about 90%) occur in patients who have high blood pressure *(hypertension)*. The most obvious reason for this relationship is the pressure on arterial walls caused by hypertension. A less obvious reason is that chronic hypertension leads to degenerative changes in the small penetrating arteries deep in the brain, weakening them and creating *microaneurysms.* These microaneurysms may rupture and leak blood into the brain. The resulting microhematomas cause brain swelling and put pressure on adjacent vessels, which then rupture, leading to a cascade of events in which the hemorrhage slowly grows as adjacent blood vessels are affected. The most common sites for intracerebral hemorrhages are the thalamus and basal ganglia, but the brain stem (especially the pons) and the cerebellum also are potential sites for these hemorrhages.

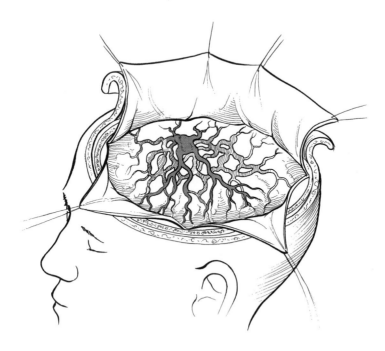

Figure 1-23 ■ An arteriovenous malformation (AVM). AVMs are tangled masses of arteries and veins that gradually increase in size with the passage of time. The greatest risk to patients with AVMs is rupture and subsequent hemorrhage.

Intracerebral hemorrhages destroy brain tissue next to white matter tracts, but they usually do not destroy the tracts themselves. Some intracerebral hemorrhages may decompress by bleeding into the ventricles or subarachnoid space. Because of their location, most intracerebral hemorrhages are not surgically repairable, and surgery usually is considered only if the bleeding is life threatening. Medical management usually includes reducing blood pressure, maintaining adequate respiration, and regulating fluid intake.

Recovery from Ischemic and Hemorrhagic Strokes

Patients with ischemic or hemorrhagic strokes recover at different rates. The pattern of recovery depends largely on whether the stroke is ischemic or hemorrhagic, and the eventual level of recovery depends largely on the amount of brain tissue destroyed and the location of the destruction.

Neurologic recovery from ischemic strokes usually is greatest in the first 2 weeks and diminishes over time until the patient's condition stabilizes (Figure 1-24).

Recovery from ischemic strokes is greatest for patients in the middle severity ranges. If a patient remains severely impaired when the acute effects of the stroke have dissipated (2 to 4 weeks poststroke), the patient's limited recovery usually means that he or she has substantial destruction of brain tissue. Such patients usually remain severely impaired for years or for life. Patients with very mild impairments during the first few days after an ischemic stroke do not benefit much from neurologic recovery because they have little to recover— small amounts of improvement bring them back to or near their premorbid levels.

No one knows exactly how long neurologic recovery from ischemic stroke goes on. We do know that most neurologic recovery takes place in the first 2 to 4 weeks after stroke, and that most recovery of language takes place during the first 3 months after stroke (Culton, 1969; Sarno and Levita, 1971).

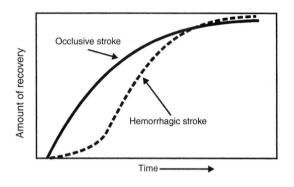

Figure 1-24 ■ The general course of neurologic recovery from stroke. The graph represents the average pattern of recovery for groups of patients. The recovery of individual patients often differs from the group average. These patterns are based primarily on clinical experience and anecdotal evidence because there is little empirical evidence documenting patterns of neurologic recovery for groups of patients with occlusive or hemorrhagic strokes.

Neurologic recovery from hemorrhagic strokes usually follows a different course from that for occlusive strokes. Patients with hemorrhagic strokes often show little improvement for the first few weeks after the stroke, followed by a period of relatively rapid recovery (see Figure 1-24). Recovery then slows and stabilizes, usually at a level above that for ischemic stroke patients with equivalent deficits at onset. For most patients, neurologic recovery is essentially complete by 6 months after onset (Basso, Capitani, and Vignolo, 1979), although some slow neurologic recovery may continue for additional months or years (Caplan, 1993).

That hemorrhagic strokes do not destroy white matter (nerve fiber tracts), whereas ischemic strokes do destroy it, may explain the reason that patients with hemorrhages tend to experience better recovery than patients with ischemic strokes. Greater amounts of cerebral swelling caused by hemorrhages may explain why patients with brain hemorrhages take longer to begin their recovery than do patients with ischemic strokes.

GENERAL CONCEPTS 1-8

- *Stroke* is a label for loss of blood supply to the brain. Strokes may be caused by occlusion of a cerebral artery *(thrombosis, embolus)* or by bleeding *(hemorrhage).*
- *Thromboses* are slow accumulations of material within an artery that cause its gradual occlusion.
- *Emboli* are fragments of material that travel through cerebral arteries and lodge in branches that are smaller than the emboli.
- Symptoms of *thrombotic strokes* tend to develop gradually over hours to days, often in stepwise fashion. Symptoms of *embolic strokes* tend to appear suddenly with maximal symptoms within a few minutes.
- Many strokes are preceded by transient episodes of sensory disturbance, weakness, slurred speech, or other symptoms, most of which resolve within minutes to hours. *Transient ischemic attacks (TIAs)* are the most common of these transient episodes.
- Low blood volume or low blood pressure may lead to *hypoperfusion,* in which blood does not penetrate into small-diameter arteries in border zones of arterial supply.
- Major strokes usually are followed by temporary (days to weeks) disruption of cerebral function, caused by *brain swelling, neurotransmitter release, diminished cerebral blood flow, transneural degeneration, denervation hypersensitivity,* and *diaschisis.*

The diffuse effects of these processes eventually resolve, leaving the patient with residual focal impairments.
- *Extracerebral hemorrhages* may be *epidural* (between the dura mater and the skull), *subdural* (between the dura mater and the arachnoid), or *subarachnoid* (between the arachnoid and the pia mater).
- *Subarachnoid hemorrhages* usually come from ruptured *aneurysms* (weakened balloonlike pouches in cerebral artery walls). Some come from *arteriovenous malformations (AVMs),* which are tangled masses of thin-walled cerebral arteries and veins.
- Most *intracerebral hemorrhages* occur in people with high blood pressure. Most are caused by a combination of increased arterial pressure and the formation of *microaneurysms* on penetrating cerebral arteries deep within the brain hemispheres.
- Recovery from ischemic strokes tends to be most rapid in the first days and weeks poststroke, with gradual slowing of recovery thereafter. Recovery from hemorrhagic strokes often is slow during the first 4 to 8 weeks poststroke, followed by a period of rapid recovery, which then slows and stabilizes.
- Recovery from either ischemic or hemorrhagic strokes is essentially complete by 6 months poststroke.

OTHER NEUROLOGIC CAUSES OF COGNITIVE-COMMUNICATIVE DISORDERS

Most other neurologic conditions that may cause cognitive-communicative impairments are insidious, rather than abrupt, in onset (excluding traumatic brain injury, discussed later in this book). Insidious conditions make their presence known slowly over a period of time, sometimes with intermittent periods of stabilization or remission, until the patient receives treatment, becomes incapacitated, or dies. The major insidious conditions that affect the central nervous system are:
- Intracranial tumors
- Hydrocephalus
- Infections and toxins
- Nutritional and metabolic disorders

Any of these conditions can cause impaired communication. However, when these conditions are the cause, dementia or personality disruptions usually precede or accompany the communication impairment. Insidious conditions often do not have a clearly definable time of onset. A patient often does not see his or her physician when the first symptoms of an insidious condition appear because the symptoms are mild and appear innocuous, so the condition has progressed by the time the patient first seeks medical attention.

Intracranial Tumors

Tumors affecting brain tissues may be either *primary* (originating there) or *secondary* (originating elsewhere and migrating to intracranial locations). The process by which a tumor appears at a secondary site in the body is called *metastasis,* and such tumors are called *metastatic tumors.*

Primary intracranial tumors most often affect the cerebrum and the cerebellum. They occur at all ages, but are most common in adults from 25 to 50 years old. The causes of most primary intracranial tumors remain a mystery. Some appear to be related to previous injuries, and there is a tendency for some kinds of intracranial tumors to occur in families.

Intracranial tumors, whether primary or secondary, have similar effects on the central nervous system. The tissue around the tumor swells. This swelling is one of the major causes of observable symptoms in patients with cerebral tumors. If the tumor exerts pressure on circumscribed areas of the brain or brain stem, localized symptoms (e.g., motor impairments, sensory loss) may follow. If the tumor causes swelling of the brain and brain stem, widespread symptoms of cerebral dysfunction related to pressure and displacement of brain tissue appear. Localized symptoms commonly appear in the early stages of tumor growth, with increasing and more generalized dysfunction as tumor growth and swelling of brain tissue cause intracranial pressure to rise.

When cerebral swelling is severe, *herniation* may occur. Large masses in the brain hemispheres (or smaller ones in the brain stem) may force the brain stem downward through the foramen magnum, or may squeeze parts of the brain against dural projections such as the falx cerebri or the tentorium, causing compression, shearing, and bleeding of brain tissues. Pang (1989) described four major types of herniation.

Subfalcine herniation is most common and least ominous. It occurs when one brain hemisphere is pushed against the falx cerebri, the rigid sheet of dura that projects downward into the superior longitudinal fissure (Figure 1-25, *B*). Subfalcine herniation does not generate focal neurologic symptoms unless the anterior cerebral artery is compressed, in which case the patient may complain of numbness and weakness in the contralateral leg.

Lateral transtentorial herniation usually occurs as a consequence of masses in the temporal lobe. The mesial surface of the temporal lobe is squeezed against the tentorium, the rigid sheet of dura that separates the space occupied by the brain from the space occupied by the cerebellum (Figure 1-25, *C*). The herniation creates pressure on CN 3, causing ipsilateral pupillary dilation. The pressure also forces brain tissues downward into the foramen magnum, compressing tissues and stretching blood vessels at the base of the brain and in the brain stem. The resulting brain stem ischemia may lead to coma, and if the brain stem hemorrhages, to irreversible coma or death.

Central transtentorial herniation is caused by swelling near the apex of the brain or in the frontal lobes. The brain is pushed against the tentorium and downward into the foramen magnum. As in lateral transtentorial herniation, tissues and blood vessels at the base of the brain and in the midbrain are compressed, stretched, and distorted, leading to impairment of vital functions. Irreversible coma or death are common outcomes.

Tonsillar herniation is caused by swelling in the cerebellum, pons, or medulla. The cerebellar

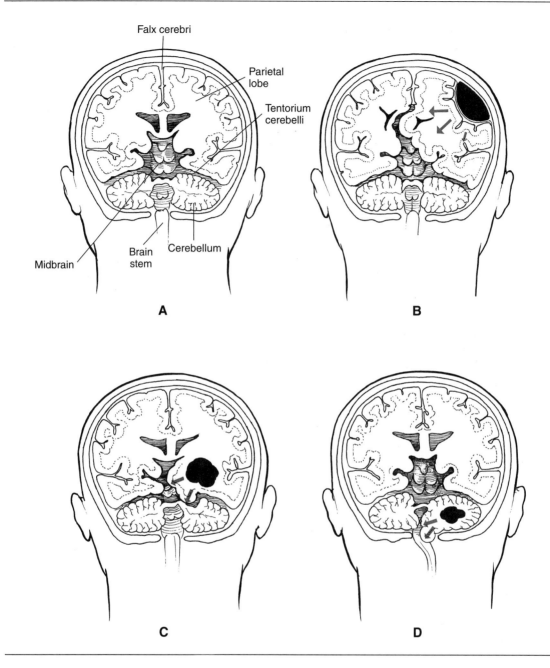

Figure 1-25 ■ Examples of herniation syndromes. **A,** A cross-section of a normal brain and skull. **B,** Displacement of brain tissue caused by a mass above the right parietal lobe that pushes adjacent regions of the right hemisphere under the falx cerebri (subfalcine herniation). **C,** Displacement of the mesial temporal lobe around the tentorium cerebelli by a mass in the temporal lobe (transtentorial herniation). **D,** Displacement of the right cerebellar tonsil downward into the foramen magnum by a mass in the right cerebellar hemisphere (tonsillar herniation).

tonsils (hence the name *tonsillar*) are extruded through the foramen magnum, where they exert pressure on the medulla (Figure 1-25, *D*). The brain stem is displaced downward, with shearing and distortion of tissues. Respiration is compromised; heart rate decreases; blood pressure rapidly increases; and coma soon follows.

Patients with intracranial tumors typically experience gradual intensification of symptoms. In the early stages of tumor growth, when intracranial pressure is low, the patient may complain of nonspecific alterations in mental function such as forgetfulness, lack of initiative, drowsiness, blurred or double vision, lightheadedness, or vertigo. About one third of patients report headaches early in the course of tumor development. Such headaches can take several forms, but most are not affected by analgesics. Vomiting sometimes occurs in the early stages of tumor growth, and seizures are common when a tumor is within the brain itself.

Tumor patients with elevated intracranial pressure almost always have cognitive impairments, are lethargic, and may be stuporous. Most experience unremitting bifrontal and bioccipital headaches unaffected by analgesics and present day and night. Vomiting is common, as are motor unsteadiness and clumsiness.

The number of symptoms and the rate at which symptoms progress is determined by the size, rate of growth, and location of the tumor. Large tumors generate more extreme symptoms. Faster-growing tumors produce symptoms more quickly than slower-growing ones, because the brain adapts to slowly developing masses better than to quickly developing ones. If a slowly growing tumor is located in or near areas that serve important functions (e.g., the sensory or motor cortex, the brain stem), a relatively small tumor may quickly generate major symptoms. If the tumor is located in a "silent" area of the brain, it may grow to surprising size before generating symptoms.

Different kinds of intracranial tumors have different rates of growth and differ in malignancy. *Gliomas* are the most common. Gliomas can be divided into several subtypes, but the two most important ones are *astrocytoma* and *glioblastoma multiforme*. Astrocytomas are the most common and the most benign (nonmalignant) of the gliomas. They usually grow slowly, and symptom development may span 5 or 6 years. Postoperative survival of 10 or more years is common. In some cases, astrocytomas may be completely removed, and the patient is considered cured. However, even benign astrocytomas may cause substantial neurologic impairments or kill the patient if the tumor is strategically located (for example, in the brainstem).

Glioblastoma multiforme is the second most common glioma. It is also one of the most malignant and rapidly growing of all intracranial tumors. Symptoms typically develop during a period of 3 months to 1 year, and the average postsurgical survival is only about 6 to 9 months.

Meningiomas are relatively common tumors, and, as the name implies, arise from the meninges. They are among the most benign of all intracranial tumors because they are slow growing, well defined, and do not usually invade the brain substance. For this reason they often can be completely removed. The symptoms of meningiomas are slow to develop because meningiomas are slow growing. Because they produce pressure at specific places on the brain and rarely cause general increases in intracranial pressure, when symptoms do appear, meningiomas are among the most localizable of intracranial tumors.

Secondary intracranial tumors (metastatic carcinomas) are tumors that form from cancerous cells that have migrated (usually through the bloodstream) from the primary tumor site to the brain, where they settle and grow. The primary sources for metastatic carcinoma of the brain are, in decreasing order of frequency, the breast, the lungs, and the pharynx and larynx. Metastatic carcinomas of the brain usually are grossly well defined, but multiple sites of metastasis within the brain are common.

Metastatic tumors usually cause substantial local swelling around the tumor site. The prognosis for most metastatic brain tumor patients is poor. The average survival after diagnosis of metastatic brain tumor is 2 to 6 months.

Hydrocephalus

Hydrocephalus is a condition in which the cerebral ventricles are enlarged, either as a result of increased pressure in the ventricles or as a result of brain atrophy (shrinkage). *Obstructive hydrocephalus* is caused by obstruction of the interventricular passageways through which CSF circulates. The obstruction blocks the flow of CSF from the ventricles into the subarachnoid space. Sometimes obstructions are caused by material circulating in the CSF (plugs of bacteria, bits of floating tissue), but more often they are caused by swelling of nearby brain tissue. Because CSF is formed in the cerebral ventricles, anything that blocks the exit of CSF from the ventricles causes the pressure in the ventricles to rise. As the pressure rises the ventricles enlarge, the brain is compressed against the skull, and the patient becomes mentally dulled, lethargic, and hyporesponsive.

The most frequent site of obstruction is the *cerebral aqueduct,* which connects the third and fourth ventricles. The cerebral aqueduct is the longest and narrowest of the passageways between the ventricles and, consequently, is the most susceptible to obstruction (usually because of swelling of adjacent brain tissues or displacement of brain tissue by tumors).

The primary medical treatment for obstructive hydrocephalus is *intraventricular shunt.* A cannula (hollow needle connected to a small flexible tube) is passed through the brain into a ventricle. Excess CSF is then forced by intraventricular pressure through the shunt, lowering the pressure in the ventricles. The tube may be passed into the neck or the abdominal cavity, where the excess fluid is allowed to drip away. The patient's response to shunt placement usually is dramatic with few long-term residual deficits, unless intracranial pressure has reached exceptionally high levels or has continued for weeks or months.

Nonobstructive hydrocephalus is a generic label for several conditions that cause ventricular enlargement but do not involve obstruction of interventricular passageways. One of the most common causes of nonobstructive hydrocephalus is cerebral atrophy. Nonobstructive hydrocephalus is not accompanied by elevated intracranial pressure.

Infection

The central nervous system ordinarily is resistant to bacterial or viral infection, but such infections sometimes occur. The major bacterial infections are *bacterial meningitis* and *brain abscess*. In *bacterial meningitis* the pia, arachnoid, and CSF become infected with bacteria, causing inflammation, swelling, and fluid exudate from the meninges. The patient becomes feverish, chilled, lethargic, and complains of headache, drowsiness, and stiff neck. If the infection is severe, the patient may progress into coma. Bacterial meningitis progresses quickly and can be fatal if not promptly treated. The standard treatment is antibiotic medication, which usually cures the infection, although neurologic sequelae may persist.

Brain abscess is caused by introduction of bacteria, fungus, or parasites into brain tissues from a primary infection site elsewhere in the body. Transmission may be through the blood or by migration through tissues. The primary sources of infection are the nasal sinuses, middle ear, or mastoid cells in about 40% of cases. The sources are the lungs or cardiovascular tissue in about 30% of cases. Symptom development in brain abscess is slower than in bacterial meningitis, and brain abscesses tend to generate localized symptoms (such as visual anomalies or sensory loss) rather than the generalized symptoms of meningitis. However, patients with brain abscess, like those with meningitis, complain of fever, chills, headache, lethargy, and drowsiness. The usual treatment is surgical drainage of the abscess in combination with antibiotic medication. Recovery usually is dramatic, although the patient may be left with chronic deficits related to destruction of brain tissue by the abscess.

Numerous viruses may infect the central nervous system. The two major sources of central nervous system viral infections are general infections such as mumps or measles, and viruses transmitted by insect or animal bites, such as equine encephalitis or rabies. The progression of a viral infection depends on the virus. Sometimes, as in viral meningitis, symptoms develop quickly, followed by gradual improvement. Sometimes symptoms develop slowly, followed by gradual improvement (for example, when the body's immune system successfully eliminates the infection). Sometimes, as in acquired immunodeficiency syndrome (AIDS), symptoms develop slowly and continue to worsen, often ending in death. In some cases, as in rabies, symptoms develop quickly and dramatically, invariably ending in death. A few antiviral medications that are not toxic to the body may be of benefit. Otherwise, treatment of viral infections is palliative—directed toward maintaining the patient's vital functions, providing adequate nutrition, and regulating fluid balance to help the patient's natural defenses rid the body of the virus.

Toxemia

Toxemia is caused by the introduction into the nervous system of substances that inflame or poison nerve tissue. Toxemia may be caused by drug overdoses, drug interactions, bacterial toxins (tetanus, botulism, diphtheria), or heavy metal poisoning (lead, mercury). The course of heavy metal or chemical poisoning, such as may occur in occupational exposure, usually is one of decreasing mentation and increasing lethargy, with motor or sensory disruptions generally occurring only in advanced stages of poisoning. Poisoning with bacterial toxins usually follows a more rapid course, with symptoms developing quickly, followed by slow recovery, unless the poisoning ends in death. Treatment usually is directed toward removal of the source of the toxin, and, sometimes, purging the toxin from the system.

Metabolic Disorders

Metabolic disorders are common causes of central nervous system dysfunction, but, as in other insidious processes, rarely cause isolated communication disorders. Severe hypoglycemia may cause deterioration of cerebral function, leading to confusion, stupor, or coma. Thyroid disorders may create central nervous system symptoms (apathy, confusion, and intellectual deterioration). Treatment of metabolic disorders usually involves correcting or compensating for the metabolic imbalance, and symptoms usually regress or resolve when the metabolic disturbance is corrected.

Nutritional Disorders

Though rare in the United States, nutritional disorders sometimes cause central nervous system dysfunction and may occasionally generate cognitive-communicative impairments. One classic nutritional deficiency syndrome is *Wernicke's encephalopathy,* caused by thiamine deficiency, and usually associated with alcoholism. The primary symptoms of Wernicke's encephalopathy are paralysis of some of the eye muscles; clumsy, staggering gait; and mental confusion. Other vitamin deficiencies, including deficiencies in vitamin B_{12} and nicotinic acid, may cause variable neurologic symptoms. Neurologic syndromes associated with vitamin or mineral excess may also be seen (for example, overdose of vitamin A). In the case of nutritional deficiencies, treatment usually involves replenishment of the deficient compound by medication, together with dietary adjustment. In the case of vitamin or mineral excess, treatment is directed toward reducing the patient's intake of those compounds.

GENERAL CONCEPTS 1-9

- *Intracranial tumors* cause displacement of cerebral tissue. Some also destroy cerebral tissue.
- When displacement of cerebral tissues is severe, *herniation* may occur. In herniation, brain tissue is pressed against or pushed across rigid partitions, such as the falx cerebri, or through apertures, such as the foramen magnum.
- *Subfalcine herniation* (a brain hemisphere is pressed against the falx cerebri) is the least dangerous form of herniation. *Transtentorial herniation* (the brain is pushed downward against the tentorium cerebelli) and *tonsillar herniation* (the cerebellum and brain stem are pushed downward through the foramen magnum) are much more dangerous because of risk to brain stem structures that control vital functions such as respiration and heartbeat.
- *Meningiomas* and *astrocytomas* are relatively benign (nonmalignant) cerebral tumors. *Glioblastoma multiforme* is among the most dangerous (malignant).
- *Obstructive hydrocephalus* (enlarged cerebral ventricles) usually is caused by blockage in the cerebral aqueduct, which connects the third ventricle to the fourth ventricle. Obstructive hydrocephalus raises intracranial pressure and may displace brain tissue.
- *Nonobstructive hydrocephalus* is not caused by blockage of CSF transit in the ventricular system. It does not increase intracranial pressure.
- *Bacterial or viral infections, toxemia, metabolic disorders,* or *nutritional disorders* sometimes cause neurogenic cognitive-communicative disorders as part of a larger complex of behavioral and cognitive decline. Medical treatment usually resolves these conditions, together with any associated speech, language, or cognitive impairments.

THOUGHT QUESTIONS

Question 1-1 Mr. Johnson is a 72-year-old right-handed man who has just suffered a thrombotic stroke in the posterior branch of his middle cerebral artery. Mrs. Redmond is a 53-year-old right-handed woman who has just suffered a thrombotic stroke in the posterior watershed region of her left middle cerebral artery. Describe the probable nature and magnitude of their impairments and describe any differences that you might expect in their neurologic recovery.

Question 1-2 Mr. Carillo arrives in the emergency room complaining of double vision, slurred speech, weakness in his left arm, back pain, and a severe headache. He states that he has been in good health for the last several years except for mild hypertension, for which he takes medications, and denies previous episodes suggestive of neurologic problems. He states that he works as a mechanic in a local garage and that his symptoms began shortly before lunch time. He denies falling or any workplace accidents. He states that the back pain began as he was helping a co-worker move a heavy transmission, but that he noticed no other symptoms at that time. At lunch about an hour later his head began to ache. He finished his lunch, but he noticed left arm weakness as he began work. His headache became progressively worse, and he notified his supervisor, who brought him to the emergency room. What happened to create Mr. Carillo's symptoms?

Question 1-3 Patients who are experiencing subfalcine herniation often complain of weakness and sensory loss in one leg. Why does this symptom appear? Which leg will be affected?

Question 1-4 Harry Lang, age 46, appeared at his dentist's office (Dr. Payne) complaining of increased sensitivity to heat and cold in his left upper molars. He reported that he had had some sensitivity to heat and cold in the affected teeth for many months, but that within the past day the sensitivity had suddenly increased to the point that either hot or cold substances touching the teeth caused sudden, stabbing pain that radiated from his jaw up into his left cheek. "It feels like someone ran a red-hot poker up inside my head." Harry's dentist checked over Harry's teeth and found moderate abrasion at and above the gum line in the affected teeth. He explained to Harry that the abraded areas probably permitted heat and cold to reach the nerves within the teeth and recommended that Harry switch to a toothpaste for sensitive teeth. Harry switched to the recommended toothpaste, but his symptoms persisted. He called his dentist, who told Harry, "Well I guess you'll just have to live with it." Harry decided to see Dr. Luck, another dentist. Harry described his symptoms to Dr. Luck, and after examining Harry, Dr. Luck recommended that Harry see a neurologist. Why do you think Dr. Luck made that recommendation?

Question 1-5 There is an interesting difference between the United States and England in the laterality of Bell's palsy (paralysis of muscles on one side of the face, caused by inflammation or damage in the facial nerve—CN 7). In the United States, Bell's palsy affects the left side of the face significantly more often than it affects the right side of the face. In England, Bell's palsy affects the right side of the face significantly more often than it affects the left side of the face. What might explain this puzzling phenomenon?

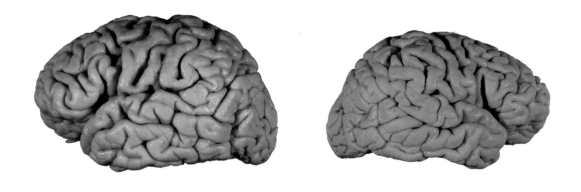

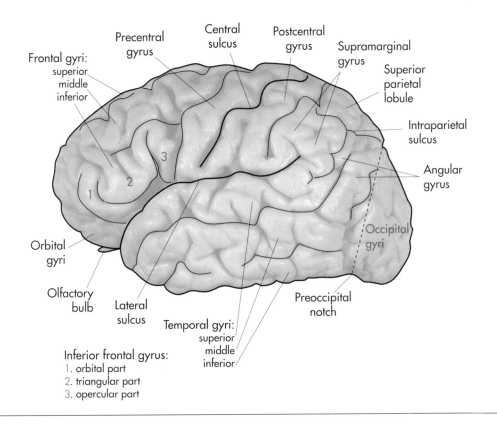

Precentral gyrus

Central sulcus

Postcentral gyrus

Supramarginal gyrus

Frontal gyri:
superior
middle
inferior

Superior parietal lobule

Intraparietal sulcus

Angular gyrus

3

2

1

Orbital gyri

Occipital gyri

Olfactory bulb

Lateral sulcus

Temporal gyri:
superior
middle
inferior

Preoccipital notch

Inferior frontal gyrus:
1. orbital part
2. triangular part
3. opercular part

From Nolte, J., & Angevine, J. B. (2000). *The human brain in photographs and diagrams* (2nd ed.). St. Louis, MO: Mosby. (Dissections courtesy of Grant Dahmer, Department of Cell Biology and Anatomy, University of Arizona College of Medicine.)

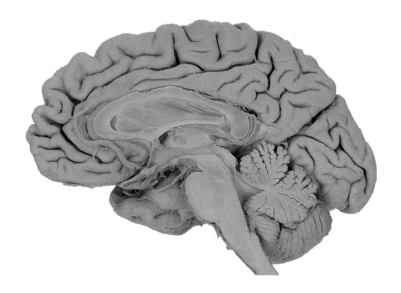

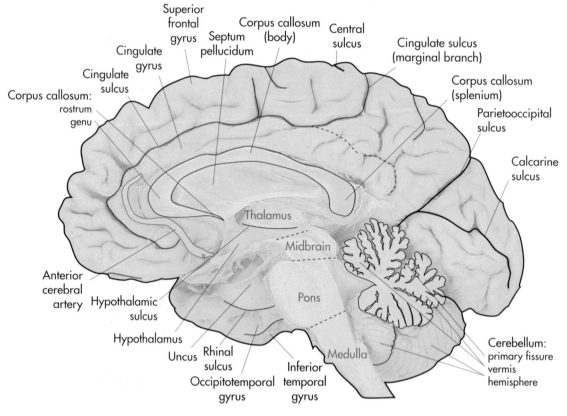

Superior frontal gyrus
Cingulate gyrus
Septum pellucidum
Corpus callosum (body)
Central sulcus
Cingulate sulcus (marginal branch)
Cingulate sulcus
Corpus callosum (splenium)
Corpus callosum: rostrum genu
Parietooccipital sulcus
Calcarine sulcus
Thalamus
Midbrain
Anterior cerebral artery
Hypothalamic sulcus
Pons
Hypothalamus
Medulla
Uncus
Rhinal sulcus
Inferior temporal gyrus
Cerebellum: primary fissure vermis hemisphere
Occipitotemporal gyrus

From Nolte, J., & Angevine, J. B. (2000). *The human brain in photographs and diagrams* (2nd ed.). St. Louis, MO: Mosby. (Dissections courtesy of Grant Dahmer, Department of Cell Biology and Anatomy, University of Arizona College of Medicine.)

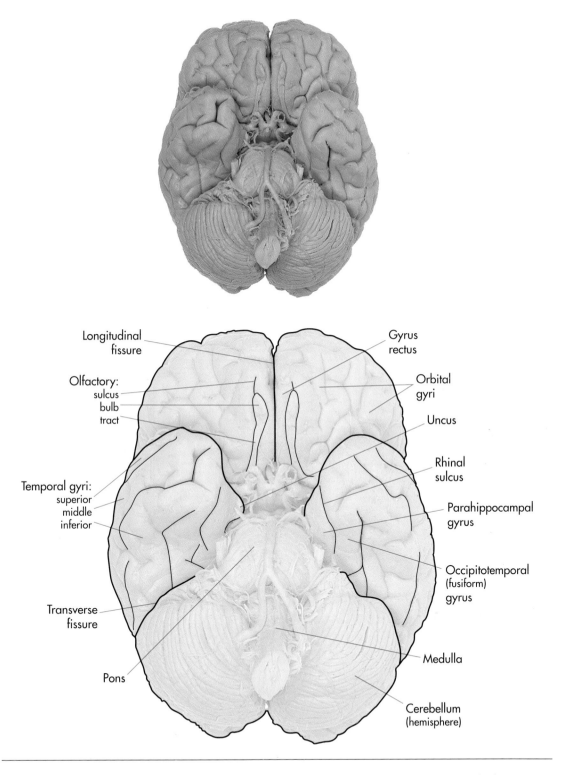

Longitudinal
fissure

Gyrus
rectus

Olfactory:
 sulcus
 bulb
 tract

Orbital
gyri

Uncus

Rhinal
sulcus

Temporal gyri:
 superior
 middle
 inferior

Parahippocampal
gyrus

Occipitotemporal
(fusiform)
gyrus

Transverse
fissure

Medulla

Pons

Cerebellum
(hemisphere)

From Nolte, J., & Angevine, J. B. (2000). *The human brain in photographs and diagrams* (2nd ed.). St. Louis, MO: Mosby. (Dissections courtesy of Grant Dahmer, Department of Cell Biology and Anatomy, University of Arizona College of Medicine.)

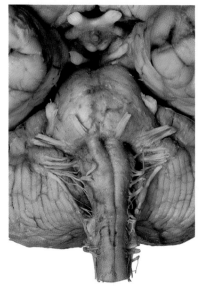

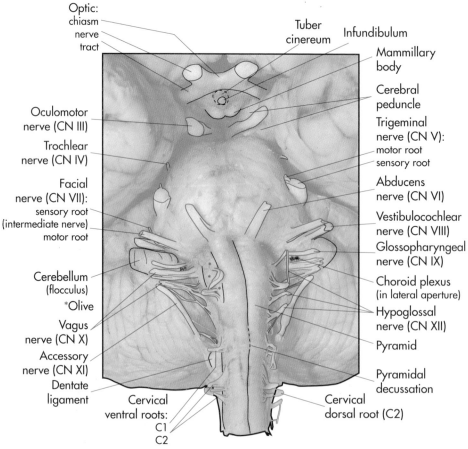

Optic:
chiasm
nerve
tract

Tuber
cinereum

Infundibulum

Mammillary
body

Cerebral
peduncle

Oculomotor
nerve (CN III)

Trigeminal
nerve (CN V):
motor root
sensory root

Trochlear
nerve (CN IV)

Facial
nerve (CN VII):
sensory root
(intermediate nerve)
motor root

Abducens
nerve (CN VI)

Vestibulocochlear
nerve (CN VIII)

Glossopharyngeal
nerve (CN IX)

Cerebellum
(flocculus)

Choroid plexus
(in lateral aperture)

*Olive

Hypoglossal
nerve (CN XII)

Vagus
nerve (CN X)

Pyramid

Accessory
nerve (CN XI)

Pyramidal
decussation

Dentate
ligament

Cervical
ventral roots:
C1
C2

Cervical
dorsal root (C2)

From Nolte, J., & Angevine, J. B. (2000). *The human brain in photographs and diagrams* (2nd ed.). St. Louis, MO: Mosby. (Dissections courtesy of Norman Koelling, Department of Cell Biology and Anatomy, University of Arizona College of Medicine.)

CHAPTER

2

Neurologic Assessment

The greatest mistake in the treatment of diseases is that there are physicians for the body and physicians for the soul, although the two cannot be separated. (Plato)

Most patients with neurogenic communication disorders are examined by a physician (usually a neurologist) before they arrive at the speech-language pathologist's door. The physician's report of the examination provides important information about the origin, nature, and potential course of the neurologic problems underlying a patient's communication disorders. Understanding the content of the neurologic examination and related reports is vital for speech-language pathologists who participate in a patient's care. Speech-language pathologists who serve patients with neurogenic communication disorders must understand the causes and characteristics of a patient's neurologic impairments and take them into account when designing or performing testing or treatment. Speech-language pathologists who wish to get and keep the respect of physicians and other healthcare professionals must be conversant with medical terminology, the physical and neurologic examination, and the laboratory tests commonly ordered for patients with neurogenic communication disorders.

This chapter provides an overview of how a physician goes about examining a patient with suspected neurologic involvement, summarizes the information gathered in the examination, and tells how the results of the examination and related laboratory tests are reported in a patient's medical record.

The physician typically begins the neurologic examination by interviewing the patient and family members to find out what brought the patient to the medical facility, how the patient's symptoms first expressed themselves, and how the symptoms changed over time. Then the physician evaluates the patient's motor, sensory, and mental status. After examining the patient, the physician may order laboratory tests or imaging studies to answer unresolved questions about the nature and severity of the patient's nervous system abnormalities.

THE INTERVIEW AND PHYSICAL EXAMINATION
Symptom Development

Many diseases and pathologic processes exhibit characteristic progressions of symptom development that point toward a diagnosis. Gradual and uninterrupted development of symptoms over months to years suggests a slowly progressive degenerative disease, such as Huntington's disease, or a slowly growing tumor. Rapid and uninterrupted development of symptoms over days to weeks suggests infection, a rapidly growing tumor, or a progressive degenerative disease, such as amyotrophic lateral sclerosis. Rapid development of symptoms over minutes to hours suggests occlusive vascular disease of large arteries. Gradual development of symptoms over months or years, punctuated with periods of remission ranging from weeks to months, suggests occlusive vascular disease of small arteries or a slowly developing degenerative disease, such as multiple sclerosis (Figure 2-1).

Family History

Some neurologic diseases are hereditary or familial. *Hereditary diseases* have a definite genetic inheritance pattern; *familial diseases* have a greater-than-expected occurrence in families but do not exhibit a definite inheritance pattern. Several progressive neurologic diseases are hereditary (e.g., Huntington's disease, myotonic dystrophy, Friedreich's ataxia). Some dementing illnesses and some forms of epilepsy may be familial. When a disease is hereditary and the inheritance pattern is known, the family history and the patient's complaints may lead directly to a diagnosis. When a disease is known

to exhibit familial patterns, the history may point to a probable diagnosis, in which case the patient's symptoms and the results of the neurologic examination and laboratory tests serve primarily to confirm or refute the diagnosis.

THE NEUROLOGIC EXAMINATION

In the neurologic examination the physician systematically evaluates the functional state of each part of the nervous system. The physician assimilates, integrates, and analyzes information from the patient's medical history, the patient's current symptoms and complaints, and the neurologic examination to arrive at a diagnosis of the nature and location of nervous system pathology. There is no standard neurologic examination, and different physicians go about the examination in different ways. However, all cover the major components of the nervous system—the motor system, the sensory system, equilibrium, consciousness, and mentation. Most begin with assessment of the motor and sensory functions served by the cranial nerves.

The Cranial Nerves

History and Current Complaints. Patients with pathology affecting sensory cranial nerves or the sensory branches of mixed cranial nerves typically complain of diminished or distorted sensation. Some patients report sensory hallucinations in the modality of the affected nerve (ringing or buzzing sounds, flashes of light, tingling or shocklike sensations). Patients with pathology affecting motor cranial nerves or the motor branches of mixed cranial nerves complain of diminished strength or paralysis (sometimes called *palsy*) of the muscles served by the nerve. Cranial nerve or cranial nerve nucleus pathology creates motor and sensory deficits on the same side of the body as the damaged nerve or nucleus. When the pathology is in fibers connecting the cranial nerve to the brain (the corticobulbar tract), motor and sensory impairments are on the side of the body opposite the damaged nerve fibers.

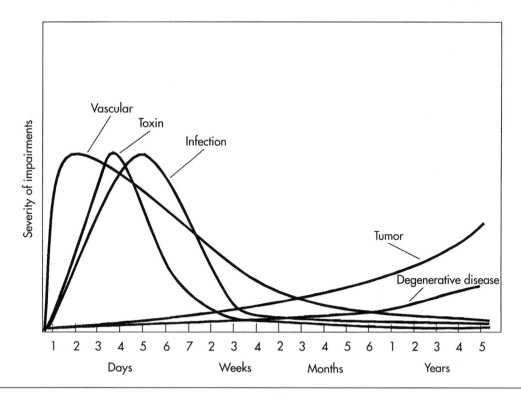

Figure 2-1 ■ The progression of symptoms in major categories of neurologic disease. These curves represent overall trends. Specific diseases within a category may differ from the trend for the category in which the disease is located. For example, multiple sclerosis is a degenerative disease with an overall pattern of gradual increasing severity, but there may be periods of exacerbation and remission.

A general rule of thumb: Central nervous system damage to motor or sensory nerves above the medulla (where pyramidal fibers decussate) causes impairment on the side of the body opposite the damage. Central nervous system damage to motor or sensory nerves below the medulla causes impairment on the same side as the damage.

Cranial Nerve Function. The physician typically begins examination of the cranial nerves (CNs) at the top, with CN 1, and works down to CN 12. The physician may forgo evaluation of the olfactory nerve (CN 1) in routine neurologic examination unless there is reason to believe that CN 1 has been injured. Injury to the olfactory nerve causes loss of the sense of smell *(anosmia).* If the physician suspects olfactory nerve injury, he or she tests its function by asking the patient to identify odors such as cloves, peppermint, coffee, or tobacco.

Most injuries to the olfactory nerve are caused by traumatic injuries, especially falls in which the back of the person's head strikes a hard surface. The impact stretches and shears the olfactory nerve. The person loses the sense of smell and also loses appreciation of complex taste sensations that depend on olfaction but retains perception of elementary taste sensations (sweet, sour, salty, and bitter) that depend on sensory receptors on the tongue. Occasionally a frontal lobe tumor may press on the olfactory bulb and cause loss of the sense of smell.

The *optic nerve* (CN 2) carries visual information from the eyes to the visual cortex. Pathology affecting the optic nerve may cause loss of visual acuity, blindness in portions of the visual field, or impairment of color vision, especially red and green. Sensory information transmitted by the optic nerve is necessary for the *pupillary light reflex*—constriction of the pupil when a bright light is shined on the eye. The muscles that accomplish the pupillary light reflex are innervated by CN 3.

The physician assesses the function of the optic nerve by testing the patient's visual acuity, color vision, and visual fields. The physician also estimates the size and symmetry of the pupils and tests their responsiveness to light— the pupillary light reflex. The physician uses an ophthalmoscope to evaluate the condition of the optic disc (a yellowish, oval region of the retina located at the back of the eye). Examining the optic disc provides information about a variety of conditions, most of which do not involve the optic nerve. Optic disc swelling *(papilledema)* may suggest increased intracranial pressure, inflammation, or an ischemic condition. Fading *(pallor)* of the optic disc and impaired visual acuity or visual field blindness suggests optic nerve malfunction, often caused by inflammation, nutritional deficiency, or degenerative disease.

Next the physician tests the cranial nerves that innervate the external muscles of the eyes. The muscles are called, collectively, the *extraocular muscles.* The extraocular muscles are served by three cranial nerves—the *oculomotor nerve* (CN 3), the *trochlear nerve* (CN 4), and the *abducens nerve* (CN 6). The extraocular muscles act together to move the eyes laterally and vertically and to keep the eyes

fixed on the same spatial location. At rest, equal and opposing actions of the extraocular muscles (six for each eye) keep the eyes looking straight ahead. When the eyes move, the extraocular muscles act together to keep the eyes moving in synchrony.

When the function of an extraocular muscle is disrupted (a condition called *ophthalmoplegia*), the eye served by the affected muscle cannot be moved in the direction of the affected muscle and may deviate in the opposite direction because of the unopposed action of the other extraocular muscles. Patients with extraocular muscle weakness or paralysis often complain of double vision *(diplopia)* because the affected eye is not looking in the same direction as the unaffected eye. The diplopia often disappears when the patient looks in the direction in which the affected eye deviates because that brings the two eyes into alignment.

Injury to the oculomotor nerve (CN 3) causes the patient's eyelid on the affected side to droop *(ptosis)* because the muscles that raise the eyelid are paralyzed. Oculomotor nerve injury also causes chronic downward and outward deviation of the affected eye because the muscles that rotate the eye upward and inward (the medial rectus, superior rectus, and inferior oblique muscles) are paralyzed and do not counteract the action of the lateral rectus muscle, which is innervated by the abducens nerve (CN 6). Patients with oculomotor nerve injury often experience diplopia, except when looking downward and outward (when both the affected and unaffected eyes are looking in the same direction). The oculomotor nerve innervates the muscle that changes the pupillary opening. Injury to the oculomotor nerve disrupts the pupillary light reflex and the *pupillary accommodation reflex* (constriction of the pupils when the eyes converge to focus on a near object).

Injury to the trochlear nerve (CN 4) paralyzes the muscle that moves the eyes downward (the *superior oblique muscle*), causing chronic upward and outward deviation of the affected eye because of the unopposed action of the other extraocular muscles. The patient experiences diplopia when looking down because the affected eye cannot follow the unaffected eye downward. Patients with trochlear nerve injury often have trouble descending stairs because of this diplopia. Some learn to tilt their head down and away from the side of the affected eye, thereby bringing the eyes into alignment and eliminating diplopia.

Injury to the abducens nerve (CN 6) paralyzes the lateral rectus muscle, causing inability to rotate the eye outward. The affected eye deviates inward at rest because of the unopposed action of the other extraocular muscles. The patient experiences diplopia when looking toward the side of the affected eye. Figure 2-2 and Table 2-1 summarize the effects of extraocular muscle paralysis on eye movements.

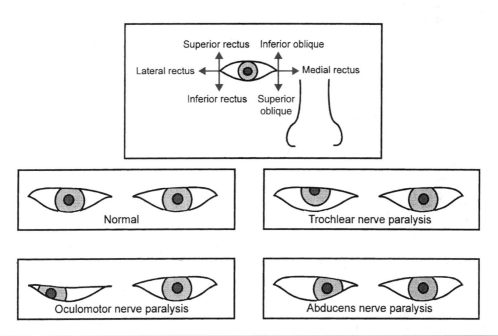

Figure 2-2 ■ Summary of symptoms generated by paralysis of extraocular muscles.

TABLE 2-1   How Paralysis of Extraocular Muscles Affects Eye Movements

Muscle	Cranial Nerve	Movement*	Deviation at Rest	Diplopia[†]
Medial rectus	3	Inward	Outward	Inward
Superior rectus	3	Upward	Downward and inward	Upward and outward
Inferior rectus	3	Downward	Upward and inward	Downward and outward
Inferior oblique	3	Upward	Downward and outward	Upward and inward
Superior oblique	4	Downward	Upward and outward	Downward and inward
Lateral rectus	6	Outward	Inward	Outward

*Movement: primary direction in which a muscle moves the eye.
[†]Diplopia occurs when the patient looks in this direction.

The physician's evaluation of the extraocular muscles considers the smoothness of eye movements as the patient looks ahead, up, down, laterally, and medially. *Nystagmus* (abnormal, involuntary oscillation of the eyes) during movement sometimes appears when extraocular muscles are weak. Nystagmus appearing when the patient looks in specific directions *(gaze-evoked nystagmus)* suggests weakness in the muscles that move the eyeball in the direction of the nystagmus. Nystagmus appearing when the patient looks in any direction *(multidirectional gaze-evoked nystagmus)* usually is caused by anticonvulsant or sedative drugs, but it can be a sign of cerebellar or vestibular disease.

The *trigeminal nerve* (CN 5) is the next nerve to receive the physician's attention. The trigeminal nerve innervates muscles and sensory receptors in the face and oral cavity. The sensory branch of the trigeminal nerve carries information from sensory receptors in the skin of the face, the oral and nasal mucosa, the eyeball, and the teeth and gums. The motor branch innervates the muscles of mastication.

The physician begins evaluation of the trigeminal nerve by testing two reflexes that depend on the trigeminal nerve—the *corneal reflex* (blinking when the eyeball is touched with a wisp of cotton) and the *jaw-jerk reflex* (elicited when the examiner taps the mandible of the patient's partially opened mouth). Exaggeration of the corneal and jaw-jerk reflexes implicates corticobulbar tracts above the CN 5 nucleus. Abolition of the corneal reflex and the jaw-jerk reflex implicates CN 5 on the affected side. The physician tests the function of the motor branch of the trigeminal nerve by asking the patient to open and close the jaw against resistance. Weak jaw muscles and deviation to one side upon opening and closing suggest involvement of the motor branch of the trigeminal nerve.

The physician tests the sensory branch of the trigeminal nerve by assessing the patient's sensitivity to touch (light touch or stroking), pain (pinprick), and temperature in the face

and anterior scalp. The sensory branch of the trigeminal nerve has three divisions— *ophthalmic, maxillary,* and *mandibular* (Figure 2-3). The ophthalmic division provides sensation to the eye, cornea, upper eyelid, bridge of the nose, and anterior scalp. The maxillary division provides sensation to the cheeks, nose, upper teeth and lip, hard palate, and nasopharynx. The mandibular division provides sensation to the skin of the lower jaw, outer ear, lower teeth and gums, lower lip, floor of the mouth, and inside surfaces of the cheek. Injury in any of the three divisions causes loss of sensation in the regions served by that division. Injury to the main trunk of the trigeminal nerve or to its nucleus causes loss of sensation in all three branches. Irritation of the trigeminal nerve causes severe paroxysmal facial pain (called

Trigeminal neuralgia usually develops spontaneously in the middle to late years of life. The most common cause is pressure on the trigeminal nerve by an enlarged artery or vein. Less common causes include tumor, inflammation of the trigeminal nerve, and multiple sclerosis. Treatment begins with medication. If medication is ineffective, surgery may be performed to decompress the nerve. In extreme cases, partial destruction of the nerve may be necessary to relieve the patient's symptoms.

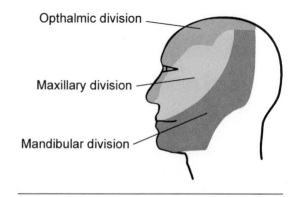

Figure 2-3 ■ The three sensory divisions of the trigeminal nerve (CN 5).

trigeminal neuralgia, or *tic douloureux)* and may cause abnormal contraction of the muscles of mastication *(trismus).*

Now the physician evaluates the muscles responsible for facial expression, which are served by the *facial nerve* (CN 7). Injury to the facial nerve causes weakness or paralysis of the muscles of facial expression on the side of injury. Patients with facial nerve damage cannot close the eye on the affected side, cannot wrinkle the forehead or pucker the lips, and may lose taste in the anterior two thirds of the tongue. When the patient's facial muscles are at rest, paralysis of muscles causes the eyelid on the affected side to droop, the nasolabial fold on the affected side to flatten, and the lips on the affected side to droop. The unopposed action of muscles on the unaffected side may cause the patient's lips to draw upward on that side when the facial muscles are at rest (Figure 2-4).

Damage in the facial nerve or its nucleus causes paralysis of all the facial muscles (upper face and lower face) on the same side as the damage (a condition called *peripheral 7th nerve palsy).* Damage in the corticobulbar tracts above the facial nerve nucleus causes paralysis of the lower facial muscles on the side opposite the damage (a condition called *central 7th nerve palsy).* The physician tests facial nerve function by asking the patient to wrinkle the forehead, close and open the eyes, pucker, smile, and perform other movements of facial muscles, both passively and against resistance. If the results of the motor examination suggest cranial nerve pathology, the physician may test taste sensation in the anterior part of the patient's tongue.

> Because assessing taste sensation requires an array of substances with various tastes, physicians tend not to test taste sensation unless the examination suggests facial nerve or olfactory nerve pathology.

The *acoustic-vestibular nerve* (CN 8) serves aspects of audition, balance, and position sense. The acoustic (cochlear) branch of CN 8 provides the pathway by which auditory information reaches the brain, and the vestibular branch serves balance and position sense. The

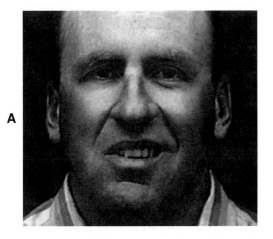
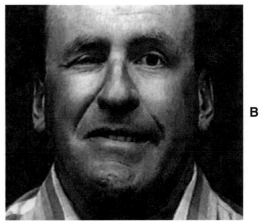

Figure 2-4 ■ A patient with right-side facial weakness caused by pathology affecting his right facial nerve (CN 7). In **A,** the man is spontaneously smiling. He has slight droop on the right side of his mouth. In **B,** he is volitionally retracting his lips. The muscular effort required to retract his lips on the right causes his right eye to close. (From Duffy, J.R. [2005]. *Motor speech disorders: Substrates, differential diagnosis, and management* [2nd ed]. St. Louis: Mosby.)

physician evaluates the function of the acoustic branch of CN 8 by testing the patient's hearing acuity for whispered speech, ticking clocks or watches, and the sounds made by tuning forks. If the patient complains of vertigo, the physician may assess the function of the vestibular branch of CN 8 by *caloric testing*, in which water is injected into the ear canal and the appearance of nystagmus is monitored. Normally, nystagmus appears within 20 seconds after the water enters the ear canal. If the vestibular branch of CN 8 is compromised, nystagmus may fail to appear, appear later than usual, or disappear earlier than usual.

The neurologic examination becomes more relevant to communication as the physician moves on to examine the *glossopharyngeal nerve* (CN 9) and the *vagus nerve* (CN 10). The physician tests the sensory functions of the glossopharyngeal and vagus nerves by evaluating the patient's sensitivity to touch on the posterior wall of the pharynx and the presence of gag and swallowing reflexes when the posterior tongue and pharynx are stimulated. Diminished or abolished sensation in the posterior pharyngeal wall, loss of taste sensation in the posterior third of the tongue, and loss of the gag or swallow reflexes implicates the sensory branches of CN 9 and CN 10.

If the glossopharyngeal nerve is affected, the vagus and the accessory nerves usually are affected also, because they travel through the same small opening in the skull. They are tested together because they share control of some muscle groups.

The physician tests the motor function of CN 9 and CN 10 by asking the patient to swallow and by observing the position of the velum (soft palate). Injury to the glossopharyngeal nerve causes the midline of the velum to be displaced away from the side of the injured nerve, both at rest and when the patient phonates (because of the unopposed action of contralateral muscles). Vagus nerve injury causes widespread dysfunction of muscles of the soft

palate, pharynx, and larynx. Injury to the recurrent laryngeal nerve, which arises from the vagus nerve, causes weakness or paralysis of the ipsilateral vocal fold.

Perception of sweet, sour, salty, and bitter tastes depends on sensory receptors (taste buds) in the tongue. The facial nerve (CN 7) innervates taste buds in the anterior two thirds of the tongue and permits perception of sweet, salty, and sour tastes. The glossopharyngeal nerve (CN 9) innervates taste buds in the posterior one third of the tongue and permits perception of bitter tastes. Patients with facial nerve (CN 7) or glossopharyngeal nerve (CN 9) pathology often lose these aspects of taste sensation on one side of the tongue.

The *spinal accessory nerve* (CN 11) moves muscles of the neck and shoulders. The physician tests the spinal accessory nerve by assessing the patient's ability to turn the head, to resist the physician's attempts to rotate the patient's head, to shrug the shoulders, and to elevate the shoulders against resistance. Injury to CN 11 causes the shoulder on the affected side to droop, interferes with arm movements above the shoulder on the affected side, and interferes with head turning away from the side of the injured nerve (the left sternomastoid muscle rotates the head to the right).

The *hypoglossal nerve* (CN 12) provides motor input to tongue muscles that protrude, retract, and curl the tongue. The physician evaluates the hypoglossal nerve by testing the patient's ability to protrude the tongue and move it from side to side, both freely and against resistance. Injury to CN 12 causes the patient's tongue to deviate toward the side of the injured cranial nerve on protrusion. This happens because the muscles that pull the tongue forward on the side of the injured cranial nerve are weak or paralyzed. Injury to CN 12 also prevents the patient from volitionally moving the tongue to the corner of the mouth on the side of the injured nerve and prevents the patient from pushing the tongue into the cheek on the affected side (because the muscles that pull the tongue toward that side are weak or paralyzed).

> Speech-language pathologists often carry out similar evaluations of cranial nerve function with patients who have speech impairments caused by weakness, paralysis, or incoordination of muscle groups involved in speech.

The physician's active testing of muscle strength and movement during evaluation of cranial nerve functions is accompanied by observation of muscles at rest to look for signs of involuntary movements *(fasciculations, fibrillations)* and wasting away *(atrophy)*, all of which are signs of compromised innervation. These phenomena are discussed later in this chapter.

Visual Fields. As noted previously, the physician's examination of CN 2, the optic nerve, usually includes assessment of the patient's visual fields. The presence of visual field blindness suggests damage in an optic nerve, the optic tract, or the visual cortex.

> The nerve fibers serving vision are called the *optic nerve* between the eye and the optic chiasm, and the *optic tract* between the optic chiasm and the visual cortex.

The nature of a patient's visual field blindness provides the physician with important clues about the location of damage in the visual system. This is true because of how the human visual system is arranged. In the human visual system, fibers from the right side of each retina project to the visual cortex in the right hemisphere, and fibers from the left side of each retina cross the midline (at the *optic chiasm*) and project to the visual cortex in the left hemisphere (Figure 2-5).

Because light rays travel in straight lines, light rays that pass into the eyes from right-side visual space strike the left side of each retina. From there the visual information is sent to the left-hemisphere visual cortex. Light rays from

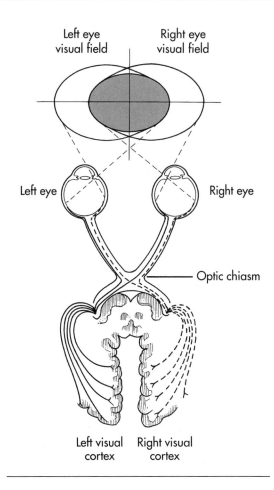

Figure 2-5 ■ The human visual system. Each hemisphere receives visual input from contralateral visual space. Visual fibers from the nasal (inner) half of the retina in each eye cross at the optic chiasm and project to the visual cortex in the contralateral hemisphere. Visual fibers from the temporal (outer) half of each retina do not cross and project to the visual cortex in the ipsilateral hemisphere.

left-side visual space strike the right side of each retina, and from there the visual information is sent to the right-hemisphere visual cortex (see Figure 2-5).

A *confrontation visual field test* may be performed to determine if the patient has damage in the eyes or visual pathways. In a confrontation visual field test the examiner covers one of the patient's eyes and asks the patient to look straight ahead while the examiner introduces visual stimuli (usually the examiner's wiggling index finger) into various locations in the patient's field of vision. Patients with blindness in parts of the visual field do not report stimuli when they are presented in the affected regions of the visual field. Blindness in certain regions of a patient's visual field may suggest or confirm the location of the lesion or lesions responsible for the patient's deficits.

If a lesion destroys one optic nerve (as in Figure 2-6, A), the patient is blind in that eye. If a lesion destroys the crossing fibers at the optic chiasm (as in Figure 2-6, B), the patient exhibits *bitemporal hemianopia* (blindness in the lateral visual fields for both eyes) because the fibers that transmit visual information from lateral visual space in both eye fields are destroyed. Bitemporal hemianopia is a rare phenomenon, most frequently caused by tumors that press on the optic chiasm.

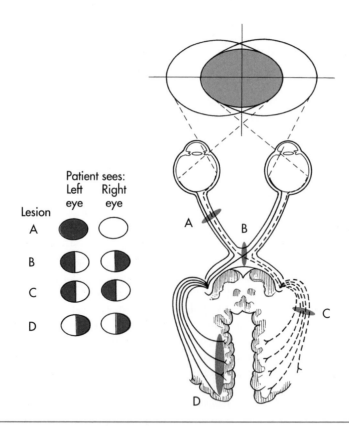

Figure 2-6 ■ How damage in the human visual system affects vision. **A,** Lesions in the optic nerve cause blindness in the eye served by the nerve. **B,** Lesions that destroy the optic chiasm cause loss of vision in both lateral eye fields because they destroy the crossing fibers from the nasal half of the retina in each eye. **C** and **D,** Lesions posterior to the optic chiasm cause contralateral visual field blindness because they interrupt the fibers from the nasal half of the retina in the contralateral eye and the fibers from the temporal half of the retina in the ipsilateral eye or destroy the visual cortex in one hemisphere.

If a lesion destroys the optic tract posterior to the optic chiasm (as in Figure 2-6, *C*), the patient is blind in the contralateral visual half-field. Such blindness is called *homonymous hemianopia* (or *hemianopsia*) and occurs following deep lesions in the temporoparietal region. Destruction of the visual cortex in one hemisphere (as in Figure 2-6, *D*), also causes contralateral homonymous hemianopia.

> *Homonymous* means that the same part of the visual field is affected in each eye. *Hemianopia* means literally *half blindness.* The first known description of a hemianopia is by Hippocrates in the fifth century BC.

Sometimes visual field blindness affects less than half of a visual field. Such partial blindness is called *quadrantanopia (quadrantic hemianopia).* Technically, quadrantanopia means that vision in one fourth of the visual field is lost, but in practice this label is applied to blindness affecting anywhere from about one third of the visual field to patches comprising less than one eighth of the visual field. Quadrantanopia typically is caused by damage in the upper or lower optic radiations on their way to the visual cortex. Lesions in the inferior parietal lobe may damage the upper optic radiations and cause blindness in the lower quadrant of the contralateral visual field. Lesions in the temporal lobe may damage the lower optic radiations and cause blindness in the upper quadrant of the contralateral visual field. (Inferiorly placed lesions posterior to the optic chiasm produce contralateral superior quadrant blindness, and vice versa.)

> As a general principle, lesions posterior to the optic chiasm cause contralateral visual field blindness, and lesions anterior to the optic chiasm cause ipsilateral visual field blindness. Lesions high in the optic radiations produce blindness in the inferior regions of the visual fields, and lesions low in the optic radiations produce blindness in the superior regions of the visual fields.

A physician who is uncertain about the presence or extent of a patient's visual field blindness may request a *tangent screen examination* or a *perimetry examination.* In a tangent screen examination the patient sits in front of a screen that has a visual fixation point in the center. The patient looks at the fixation point while the examiner moves pinheads of various sizes and colors into and out of the patient's peripheral visual fields. The patient reports each time he or she sees a pinhead and each time a pinhead disappears from sight. The patient's reports are used to create a graphic representation of the patient's visual fields.

In perimetry examinations the patient looks into a concave dome at a central fixation point. A computer-driven program flashes small points of light at various locations on the dome's surface. The patient presses a button whenever he or she sees a light. The locations at which the patient sees or does not see the stimuli are recorded and tallied by a computer. Perimetry examinations yield a graphic depiction of the patient's visual fields. Some examples of perimetry plots are shown in Figure 2-7.

A phenomenon called *macular sparing* is common in visual field blindness. The *macula* is a small circular area near the center of the retina. It is the area of greatest visual acuity. In *macular sparing,* vision in the center of the visual field for a hemianopic eye (the part of the visual field served by the macula) is spared. Macular sparing is common in hemianopia caused by posterior cerebral artery occlusions wherein the visual cortex is damaged. Macular sparing occurs because a large area of the visual cortex is devoted to the macula relative to the peripheral retina, and the distributions of the posterior cerebral artery and the middle cerebral artery overlap near the cortical area serving the macula, making collateral blood supply available to this region of the cortex. Macular sparing does not occur if the optic tract is destroyed.

Patients with visual field blindness often mistakenly conclude that they have lost vision in

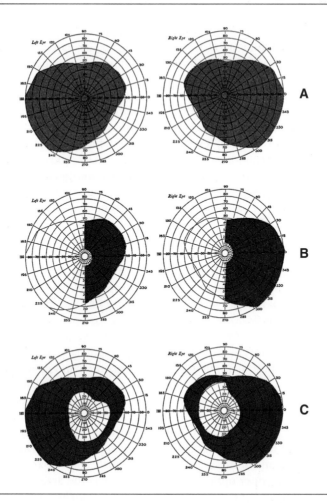

Figure 2-7 ■ Examples of three perimetry plots. **A,** Normal visual fields. The lightly shaded areas show the area of vision for each eye. **B,** Right homonymous hemianopsia (blindness in the right visual field of both eyes). The dark areas show the area of blindness for each eye. **C,** Bitemporal hemianopsia (blindness in the lateral visual fields of both eyes).

the eye on the side of the vision loss, assuming, logically but erroneously, that the right eye sees everything to the right of the midline and that the left eye sees everything to the left of the midline.

Sixty-two-year-old Rosalina Vasquez arrived at her ophthalmologist's office complaining that she couldn't see out of her left eye and saying that it started 3 days ago. As part of his examination of Ms. Vasquez, the ophthalmologist assessed her visual fields and found evidence of left homonymous hemianopia. He referred Ms. Vasquez to a neurologist who confirmed the presence of left hemianopia but also found signs of weakness in her left arm and leg. Subsequent brain imaging tests revealed evidence of a small stroke in Ms. Vasquez's right temporal lobe.

Bilateral destruction of the visual cortex causes cortical blindness. Patients who are cortically blind cannot discriminate shapes and patterns but may be sensitive to light and dark. Sometimes a cortically blind patient's perception of simple visual stimuli may be preserved, although the patient usually has difficulty reporting them or incorporating them into mental activity. Occasionally patients with cortical blindness may claim that they can see, and produce elaborate confabulations when asked to describe their surroundings. This condition is called *Anton's syndrome,* or *visual anosognosia* (*anosognosia* means denial of illness).

When confronted with evidence that he could not see, one 45-year-old cortically blind patient responded, "Well, it's no wonder that I can't tell you what color your shirt is. It's almost dark in here. Let's go out where the light's better, and I'll tell you what color it is."

GENERAL CONCEPTS 2-1

- The pattern of symptom development and the patient's family history often provide information that leads to a diagnosis of a patient's neurologic impairments.
- Assessment of cranial nerve functions is an important part of the neurologic examination. Assessment of cranial nerve function typically begins with CN 1 and progresses to CN 12.
- The function of cranial sensory nerves is estimated by testing the patient's perception of visual and auditory stimuli and sensitivity to touch, pain, and temperature in the face, scalp, and oral structures.
- The function of cranial motor nerves is estimated by testing the integrity of the pupillary, corneal, and jaw-jerk reflexes; by assessing the range of movement of the extraocular muscles; and by assessing the strength and range of movement of the muscles of facial expression, velum, tongue, jaw, neck, and shoulders.
- Active testing of cranial nerve function is supplemented with observation of muscles at rest to detect signs of atrophy or involuntary movements.
- Injury to the optic nerve or optic tract produces characteristic patterns of blindness affecting portions of the patient's visual fields.
- Injury to the optic nerve (anterior to the optic chiasm) causes blindness in the eye on the side of the injury.
- Destruction of one optic tract (posterior to the optic chiasm) causes blindness in the visual field contralateral to the side of injury (*homonymous hemianopia*).
- Destruction of lower optic radiations causes blindness in the upper part of the contralateral visual field. Destruction of upper optic radiations causes blindness in the lower part of the contralateral visual field (*quadrantanopia*).
- Bilateral destruction of the visual cortex causes *cortical blindness.*

The Motor System

History and Current Complaints. The patient's description of problems with movement and motor control help the physician determine the potential involvement of the motor cortex, neural pathways, the cerebellum, the extrapyramidal system, or nerve-muscle junctions—information that subsequently can be embellished by the neurologic examination. Patients with damage in upper motor neurons or the motor cortex complain of general weakness on one side of the body or of arm, hand, finger, or leg weakness. Patients with leg weakness often report episodes of falling. Patients with cerebellar damage complain more of clumsiness than of weakness—complaints such as slurred speech and clumsy arms, hands, fingers, legs, and feet. Patients with damage in the basal ganglia typically complain of stiffness, difficulty initiating movement, and tremor of the hands and fingers. Patients with lower motor neuron damage typically complain of weakness in muscles innervated by damaged cranial or spinal nerves. Patients with disturbances of nerve-muscle transmission usually complain of excessive fatigue, double vision, slurred speech, or a combination of such symptoms.

Movement. At the beginning of the examination the physician watches as the patient enters the room and sits down. The physician observes the patient's general appearance, posture, gait, and behavior and notes characteristics that may suggest abnormalities in the patient's motor system—stooped or slumping posture; slow, effortful, clumsy, or unintentional movements; diminished or hyperactive spontaneous movement; or muscle atrophy (wasting away). After these observations (which usually take only a few minutes and may be completed during the interview) the physician systematically evaluates the patient's motor system. During this part of the examination the physician systematically evaluates the patient's *reflexes, muscle tone, muscle strength,* and *range of movement* (the range over which the patient's muscles can be stretched or flexed).

Reflexes. Nervous system pathology often abolishes, diminishes, or exaggerates reflexes that normally are present and it may cause the appearance of abnormal reflexes that should not be present in adults. The physician evaluates both *superficial* and *deep* (tendon) reflexes by comparing the presence and magnitude of reflexes on one side of the body with the presence and magnitude of reflexes on the other side. Many physicians use the following rating scale to quantify the presence and magnitude of reflexes:

    0 Absent
    1+ Diminished
    2+ Normal

    3+ Brisk (faster, greater amplitude)
    4+ Clonus (rhythmic contraction, relaxation)

Superficial reflexes are elicited by stroking, touching, or brushing the surface of body parts. Normal superficial reflexes include the *gag reflex* (gagging or retching when the back of the tongue or the oropharynx is stimulated), the *swallow reflex* (swallowing movements when the back of the tongue and pharyngeal walls are stimulated), the *corneal reflex* (blinking when something touches the cornea), and the *plantar flexor reflex* (bending downward of the toes when the sole of the foot is stroked).

Pathologic superficial reflexes include the *plantar extensor (Babinski) reflex,* the *palmar (grasp) reflex,* and the *sucking reflex.* The plantar extensor reflex is elicited by forcefully stroking the sole of the foot, at which time the toes bend upward and fan out, in contrast with the normal plantar flexor reflex, in which the toes bend downward and do not fan. The palmar reflex is elicited by stroking the palm, which causes the hand to close involuntarily. If the grasp reflex is strong, the patient may be unable to voluntarily release objects held in the affected hand (such as the physician's hand). The sucking reflex, as its name implies, consists of reflexive sucking movements. It is elicited by touching or stroking the patient's lips. Pathologic superficial reflexes sometimes are called *primitive reflexes,* in part because many of them are present in infants and disappear as the infant matures.

Deep reflexes (sometimes called *tendon reflexes* or *deep tendon reflexes*) are elicited by tapping or suddenly stretching muscles or tendons, which causes contraction of the muscle whose tendon is tapped or stretched. Perhaps the best known tendon reflex is the *patellar reflex (knee-jerk reflex),* elicited by tapping the patellar tendon below the kneecap.

Tendon reflexes may be exaggerated, diminished, or absent. Exaggerated reflexes, either alone or in combination with pathologic superficial reflexes, suggest damage in contralateral upper motor neurons (corticobulbar and corticospinal tracts). The damage releases the reflexes from the inhibitory control ordinarily maintained by the cortex and midbrain structures. Diminished or absent reflexes—a condition called areflexia—suggest damage in the peripheral nervous system (lower motor neurons, sensory fibers, the reflex arc) or the muscles themselves.

Muscle Tone and Range of Movement. The physician evaluates *muscle tone* (the tension remaining in a relaxed muscle or muscle group) by squeezing individual muscles, moving the patient's limbs while the patient neither assists nor resists the movement *(passive movement)*, and sometimes by shaking one or more limbs. The physician evaluates *range of movement* by moving each limb through its full range while the patient keeps the muscles relaxed, noting any resistance or the patient's reports of pain during movement.

Increased resistance to passive movement is called *hypertonia.* There are two major categories of hypertonia—*spasticity* and *rigidity.* Spastic muscles feel hard to the touch and resist stretching, especially fast stretching. If the examiner moves a patient's spastic limb slowly there is little resistance, but if the examiner abruptly increases the rate at which she or he moves the limb, the limb's resistance to movement increases—a phenomenon called the *spastic catch.* If the examiner moves a patient's spastic limb fast enough to create resistance and continues to move the limb at the same rate, the limb's resistance to movement diminishes—the *clasp-knife phenomenon.*

A *clasp knife* is a pocket knife with one or more folding blades. When the knife is open a spring holds the blade firmly in place. As the blade is folded into the handle, the spring's resistance to blade movement decreases as the blade nears the handle.

In *rigidity* the relaxed limb evenly resists movement in any direction because of increased resting tone of the muscles. Rigid muscles are hard to the touch and resist active and passive movement. Rigidity affects flexor muscles more than extensor muscles. Consequently, patients with rigidity stand in a stooped posture with curled fingers. Tendon reflexes are not increased by rigidity. The amplitude of tendon reflexes actually may be diminished by the patient's increased muscle tone. If rigidity affects the facial muscles, the patient exhibits an expressionless, masklike countenance called *masked facies,* which is a prominent feature of advanced Parkinson's disease. Rigidity is a prominent characteristic of many extrapyramidal diseases, including Parkinson's disease.

Decreased resistance to passive movement is called *hypotonia* or *flaccidity.* When shaken, flaccid limbs flop to and fro (the *rag doll phenomenon*). Tendon reflexes usually are diminished by hypotonia. Flaccid muscles provide little or no resistance to passive movement; therefore, limbs with flaccid muscles often can be hyperextended by the examiner. Diminished muscle tone arises from many diseases affecting the nervous system or the muscles, so the presence of hypotonia does not in itself point to a specific disease. However, hypotonia of the muscles in the distribution of a specific cranial nerve or spinal nerve almost always signifies damage to the nerve or its nucleus.

Muscle Strength. The physician evaluates the strength of a patient's muscles by asking the patient to contract them and to maintain their contraction against pressure exerted by the examiner. The strength of muscle groups usually is quantified on a 6-point scale recommended by the Medical Research Council (below).

5 Normal strength
4 Active movement against resistance and gravity
3 Active movement against gravity but not resistance
2 Active movement only when gravity is eliminated
1 Flicker or trace of contraction
0 No contraction

Muscle weakness may indicate damage at many locations—the brain, the brain stem, the spinal cord, the extrapyramidal system, the neuromuscular junction, or the muscles themselves. Damage in the brain, brain stem, or spinal cord above the level at which corticobulbar or corticospinal fibers decussate (i.e., in upper motor neurons) causes contralateral motor impairment. Several muscle groups or all of the muscles on one side of the body usually are affected, and the affected muscles are spastic.

Damage in cranial nerves or spinal nerves (i.e., in lower motor neurons) typically produces ipsilateral hypotonia and weakness or flaccid paralysis of individual muscle groups. For example, damage to CN 7 (the facial nerve) causes flaccid paralysis in the muscles of the lower face on the side of the nerve damage. Table 2-2 summarizes the signs of damage to upper motor neurons and lower motor neurons.

Diseases of muscles *(myopathy)* and diseases of neuromuscular junctions create no right-left division between affected and unaffected muscles. Instead, the patient experiences general weakness or weakness of large muscle groups in which the weakness is not related to the midline of the body. The muscles in the upper limbs may be weaker than those in the lower limbs, or distal muscles in the hands and feet may be affected more than proximal muscles.

In general, motor impairments that respect the midline of the body (affecting only muscles on one side of the midline) suggest nervous system damage, rather than damage to the muscles themselves. Central nervous system damage typically causes motor impairments contralateral to the damage, and peripheral nervous system damage typically causes motor impairments ipsilateral to the damage.

Paralysis or severe weakness of one limb is called *monoplegia*. Paralysis of both limbs on the same side is called *hemiplegia*. Paralysis of both legs is called *paraplegia*, and paralysis of all four limbs is called *quadriplegia*. The suffix denoting weakness is *-paresis*. Substituting *-paresis* for *-plegia* yields labels for limb weakness—*monoparesis, hemiparesis, paraparesis,* and *quadriparesis.*

Paraplegia and quadriplegia almost always are caused by spinal cord injuries (trauma, infection, or vascular accidents). Paraplegia is caused by pathology affecting the lumbar and sacral spine. Quadriplegia is caused by pathology affecting the cervical spine. Monoplegia usually is caused by upper motor neuron damage, but occasionally follows focal spinal cord pathology. Hemiplegia almost always is caused by upper motor neuron damage.

TABLE 2-2	Differences in Neurologic Signs between Upper Motor Neuron Pathology and Lower Motor Neuron Pathology	
Sign	Lower Motor Neuron	Upper Motor Neuron
Weakness, paralysis	Flaccid	Spastic
Atrophy	Present*	Absent†
Tendon reflexes	Diminished or absent	Increased
Pathologic reflexes‡	Absent	Present
Fasciculations, fibrillations	Often present	Absent

*Muscle atrophy develops over time and may not be obvious in early stages.
†Muscle atrophy sometimes develops because of prolonged disuse, but muscles remain spastic.
‡Plantar extensor (Babinski) reflex, grasp reflex, sucking reflex, etc.

Volitional Movements. The physician evaluates the speed, accuracy, and coordination of the patient's volitional movements next. Slowness of volitional movements can come from many sources. Common nervous system sources include lower motor neuron disease (flaccidity), upper motor neuron disease (spasticity), extrapyramidal disease (rigidity), and peripheral myopathy (weakness). Diminished accuracy of volitional movements in the absence of deficits in strength or sensation usually suggests damage in the cerebellum or the extrapyramidal system. Besides producing overall slowing of volitional movements, extrapyramidal damage frequently produces involuntary movements called *dyskinesia.* These involuntary movements are superimposed on and sometimes replace volitional movements. The form of the involuntary movements often provides the physician with helpful clues to which parts of the nervous system are damaged.

Tremor denotes cyclic, small-amplitude involuntary movements primarily affecting the arms, legs, and head. *Distal muscles* (farthest from the trunk) are more likely to be affected by tremor than are *proximal muscles* (nearest the trunk). Some tremor is present in normal muscles (called *benign* or *physiologic tremor*) but is so slight that usually it is not visible. Pathologic tremor may appear in relaxed muscles *(resting tremor),* during certain postures *(postural tremor),* or only during movement *(intention tremor). Resting tremor* is a characteristic sign of Parkinson's disease. It often begins in the patient's hand or foot, and over the years it gradually spreads to other muscle groups, causing rhythmic flexion and extension of the fingers, hands, feet, or both. When it affects the fingers, the thumb and fingers are flexed and the thumb tips rub against the finger tips, giving the tremor its characteristic *pill-rolling* quality.

Chorea (from the Greek word for *dance*) refers to quick, forceful, and abrupt involuntary movements *(choreiform movements).* At rest, the muscles of patients with chorea are hypotonic but with normal muscle strength. When a patient's hand muscles are affected, sustained muscle contraction may be interrupted by involuntary movements. (Neurology textbooks refer to the result of these involuntary movements in the hands as *milkmaid's grasp.*) Patients with mild chorea appear persistently restless and their choreiform movements often resemble clumsy volitional movements. *Ballism* (or *hemiballism* if it affects only one side of the body) is an extreme form of chorea. In ballism, the involuntary limb movements are violent and the limbs are flung wildly about, risking injury to the patient's limbs and to anyone who may be nearby.

Some patients with chorea attempt to disguise the involuntary movements by incorporating them into voluntary movements. However, the strategy usually fails because the combination of voluntary and involuntary movements appears grotesque and exaggerated.

Like other varieties of pathologic movements, choreiform movements disappear during sleep. Chorea often is a manifestation of hereditary neurologic disease, but sometimes it appears as a consequence of anoxia, brain hemorrhage, toxemia, cerebrovascular disease, or damage in the basal ganglia or other parts of the extrapyramidal system.

Athetosis refers to a condition in which resting muscle groups are disturbed by slow, writhing, sinuous movements that increase with emotional tension and disappear during sleep. Athetosis is especially prominent in neck muscles and proximal limb muscles. Athetoid movements are involuntary and purposeless and appear to flow from one muscle group to another. Patients with chorea sometimes experience a combination of choreiform movements and athetoid movements, a condition called *choreoathetosis.* Athetosis usually is caused by birth trauma or anoxia that causes damage in the basal ganglia or extrapyramidal system.

Athetosis is from a Greek word meaning *without position or place.*

Dystonia is a condition in which muscle groups (especially muscles in the limbs and neck) undergo sustained involuntary muscle contractions. Because the contractions persist and cause gross postural deformation, dystonia sometimes is called *torsion spasm.* In its less severe forms, dystonia may resemble athetosis, and the terms are sometimes used interchangeably. Dystonia is caused by damage in the basal ganglia or extrapyramidal system. Dystonia often is inherited but may sometimes be a result of prolonged medication or overmedication with various psychoactive drugs such as tranquilizers or drugs for the control of Parkinson's disease such as levodopa.

Myoclonus denotes a condition in which individual muscle groups contract in short, irregular bursts causing abrupt, brief, twitching movements of the muscle group. The contractions may range from nearly imperceptible movements of a single muscle group to contractions of multiple muscle groups that cause overt movements of the limb, neck, or facial muscles. Myoclonic movements typically are irregular in duration and rate and are most easily observed when the affected muscles are at rest. Persisting myoclonus occurs in epilepsy, dementia, and some cerebellar disorders. Occasional episodes of myoclonus sometimes occur in persons with no detectable nervous system disease (a jumping leg, the whole-body jerk of light sleep).

Fasciculations are fine, rapid, irregular, twitching movements caused by contractions of groups of muscle fibers. The contractions are not large enough to cause overt limb, head, or facial movements but are observable as dimpling or rippling of the skin over the fasciculating muscle fibers. The presence of fasciculations in combination with weakness, muscle atrophy, or both suggests damage in lower motor neurons (spinal nerves or anterior horn cells in the spinal cord, cranial nerves or cranial nerve nuclei in the brain stem). Transient fasciculations often are experienced by normal persons, and, when not accompanied by muscle weakness or atrophy, they are not considered a sign of nervous system pathology.

Fibrillations are contractions of a single muscle fiber or a small group of fibers. They are too small to be seen but are measurable with sensitive instruments. Like fasciculations, they may signify damage in lower motor neurons, but they often are experienced by persons without nervous system pathology. However, persisting fasciculations or fibrillations often are the first signs of lower motor neuron (cranial nerve or spinal nerve) disease.

Tics (sometimes called *habit spasms*) are stereotypic, repetitive movements such as blinking, coughing, throat clearing, or sniffing. Tics usually appear when the affected person is nervous or under stress. Tics can be volitionally inhibited, but when the person's attention is no longer focused on them, they reappear. Tics have no known relationship to nervous system pathology.

The characteristics of abnormal movements and their common sources are summarized in Table 2-3.

Central nervous system pathology sometimes causes clumsiness or incoordination of volitional movements in the presence of normal muscle strength—a condition called *ataxia.* Several forms of ataxia have been described in neurology literature, but by far the most frequently occurring is *cerebellar ataxia* (caused, not surprisingly, by cerebellar damage). In cerebellar ataxia the average speed and velocity of ataxic movements is essentially normal, but acceleration at the beginning of movements is slowed, and braking at the end of movements lags, causing overshoot of the target. If an ataxic patient is asked to hold a limb in position against resistance and the resistance is abruptly removed, the patient characteristically is unable to relax the muscles quickly, and the limb swings uncontrollably in

TABLE 2-3	Characteristics and Common Causes of Abnormal Movements*	
Disorder	**Characteristics**	**Frequent Causes**
Intention tremor	Slow (3-5 cycles per second)	Cerebellar pathology
	Appears during volitional movement or is accentuated by it	Sometimes toxicity, medications
Resting tremor	Moderate rate (4-6 cycles per second)	Extrapyramidal disease, especially Parkinson's disease
	Present when muscles are at rest	
	Diminishes or disappears during volitional movements	Sometimes heavy metal poisoning
Chorea	Quick, irregular muscle contractions occurring involuntarily and unpredictably in different muscle groups	Basal ganglia or extrapyramidal pathology caused by hereditary diseases, drug toxicity, anoxia, cerebrovascular disorders
Athetosis	Slow, sinuous, writhing movements	Pathology affecting basal ganglia and extrapyramidal system
	May move from muscle group to muscle group	
	Increases with emotional tension	Drug toxicity, anoxia
	Disappears during sleep	
Dystonia	Sustained involuntary contractions of muscle groups, often causing postural distortion *(torsion spasm)*	Pathology affecting basal ganglia and extrapyramidal system
		Drug toxicity, anoxia
Myoclonus	Abrupt, rapid, nonrhythmic twitching movements of individual muscle groups	Occasionally occurs in normal persons
	Often large enough to cause movement of limbs or other body parts	Extrapyramidal disease, metabolic disorders, infectious disease
Fasciculations	Rapid, irregular, small twitching movements of small groups of muscle fibers	Occasional fasciculations are common in normal persons
	Does not cause overt movement but can be seen by dimpling or rippling of skin over affected muscles	May be caused by degenerative diseases of anterior horn cells, spinal nerve compression, peripheral nerve disease
Fibrillations	Microscopic contractions of small groups of muscle fibers	Occasional fibrillations are common in normal persons
		May be caused by primary muscle disease, anterior horn cell disease, spinal nerve disease
Tics (habit spasms)	Stereotypic behaviors (blinking, coughing, throat clearing, etc.) appearing when the individual is under stress	Not known to be related to nervous system pathology

*Tremor, chorea, athetosis, dystonia, and myoclonus usually are associated with extrapyramidal system pathology. Fasciculations and fibrillations usually are associated with lower motor neuron (cranial nerve, spinal nerve) pathology.

the direction of the previous resistance (the *rebound phenomenon*).

Ataxia comes from Greek, and means, literally, *out of order.*

Complex volitional movements or movements requiring rapid changes in direction are the most dramatically affected by ataxia. Complex movements often are broken down into a succession of individual movements with a jerky, segmented quality (called *decomposition of movement*). Rapid alternating movements—such as alternately turning the hands palm up, then palm down—are slow and awkward, and their range and force are distorted *(dysmetria)*. Ataxic limb movements often are compromised by a slow, coarse tremor that appears as a rhythmic oscillation at right angles to the direction of the movement.

Gait. If a patient can stand and walk, observation of the patient's standing and walking often provides screening information that may help the physician determine the nature and location of a patient's nervous system pathology.

Patients with *unilateral corticospinal damage* (hemiplegia or severe hemiparesis) walk with what is called *circumducted gait*—the patient tilts toward the unaffected side and swings the paralyzed leg out and forward from the hip without flexing the knee (this movement is called *circumduction* of the leg). The patient's spastic arm is flexed and held close to the body. Patients with mild hemiparesis may swing the affected leg normally, but drag the foot because of weakness in the muscles that lift the leg. (These patients often become regular customers at a shoe repair shop because the shoe on the affected side wears excessively.)

Patients with *lower motor neuron disease* or *peripheral myopathy* may have difficulty standing and may be unable to maintain erect posture if their leg and hip muscles are affected. If the muscles in the front of the lower leg are affected, the patient may exhibit *foot drop,* in which the toes hang down as the foot is lifted, leading the patient to lift the leg abnormally high to allow the toes to clear the ground *(steppage gait)*. If the patient's trunk and hip muscles are involved, the patient may walk with *waddling gait* by tipping the pelvis toward the non-weightbearing side.

Patients with impaired position sense in the legs also may exhibit steppage gait. They lift their feet higher than necessary because they cannot tell how far their feet are lifted. However, their toes do not dangle as they step.

Patients with *extrapyramidal damage* often have abnormal sitting and standing posture and unusual walking patterns because of dyskinesia. Patients with chorea, if they can walk at all, do so in irregular fashion, their progress interrupted by sudden dipping and lurching produced by irregular involuntary contractions in the leg and trunk muscles. Patients with athetosis or dystonia may have difficulty maintaining erect posture because of involuntary movements or contractions of arm and leg muscles. (Patients with severe athetosis or dystonia cannot stand or walk unaided.) Patients with Parkinson's disease often assume a stooped, forward-leaning posture on standing, and when asked to walk they have difficulty starting and stopping. Patients with Parkinson's disease typically shuffle for a few steps before making normal but still shortened strides. When a patient with severe Parkinson's disease walks, his or her steps become progressively shorter and more rapid until the patient is nearly running with tiny shuffling steps (called *festinating gait*).

Patients with *cerebellar disease* who can walk typically do so with their feet wide apart. They lurch from side to side, and their steps are clumsy and irregular in length and rhythm. They turn with difficulty and have a tendency to fall to one side. Walking heel-to-toe is very difficult and usually impossible for these patients.

GENERAL CONCEPTS 2-2

- The integrity of the patient's motor system is evaluated by testing *reflexes, muscle tone, muscle strength*, and *range of movement*.
- Exaggerated reflexes or the appearance of primitive reflexes suggest damage in *upper motor neurons* (corticobulbar or corticospinal tracts). Diminished reflexes suggest damage in *lower motor neurons* (cranial nerves or spinal nerves).
- *Muscle spasticity* suggests injury to upper motor neurons. *Muscle flaccidity* suggests injury to lower motor neurons, neuromuscular junctions, or the muscles themselves. *Muscle rigidity* suggests injury to the extrapyramidal system.
- Injury to upper motor neurons above the medulla and after decussation causes contralateral muscle weakness and exaggerated reflexes. Injury to upper motor neurons in the brain stem or spinal cord prior to decussation causes ipsilateral muscle weakness and exaggerated reflexes.
- Injury to lower motor neurons (cranial nerves, spinal nerves, and their nuclei) causes ipsilateral muscle weakness and diminished reflexes.
- Extrapyramidal damage often produces involuntary movements (*dyskinesia*).
- *Tremor* is characterized by rhythmic, small-amplitude movements. Resting tremor is a sign of Parkinson's disease.
- *Chorea* is characterized by quick, forceful, and abrupt involuntary movements.
- *Athetosis* is characterized by slow, writhing, sinuous involuntary movements.
- *Dystonia* is characterized by prolonged involuntary contractions of muscle groups.
- *Myoclonus* is characterized by quick, irregular contractions of individual muscles.
- *Fasciculations* are visible fine, rapid, irregular contractions of small groups of muscle fibers.
- *Fibrillations* are irregular contractions of individual muscle fibers or small groups of fibers. The contractions are too small to be seen.
- Cerebellar injury disrupts the force, velocity, and targeting of movements (a condition called *ataxia*) causing jerky, segmented movements (*decomposition of movement*).
- Patients with hemiplegia or severe hemiparesis often walk with *circumducted gait*. Patients with lower motor neuron disease or peripheral myopathy often walk with *steppage gait* or *waddling gait*. When patients with dyskinesia walk, their progress is interrupted by involuntary movements. Patients with Parkinson's disease often walk with *festinating gait*.

The irregular dipping and lurching of choreic patients' walking sometimes resembles the movements in some forms of dance, leading some practitioners to label it *dancing gait*. Because the clumsy, staggering gait of patients with cerebellar disease resembles that of intoxicated people, they are sometimes mistakenly thought to be intoxicated by those they meet in public.

Somesthetic Sensation

History and Current Complaints. Patients with abnormality in the regions serving somesthetic (bodily) sensation usually complain of pain, numbness, or abnormal sensations. Pain usually poses the most difficult diagnostic problem because it is one of the body's generic responses to tissue damage. Pain is an important symptom in many diseases, not only those involving the nervous system. Not all pain is a sign of disease, and not all pain is a consequence of tissue damage (e.g., the pain associated with muscle cramps, intestinal gas pains, and most headaches).

The patient's history usually provides the physician with clues to the cause of the pain. The neurologic examination defines the extent to which pain is caused by nervous system involvement. Knowing what relieves or exacerbates pain may help the physician determine its source. When pain is exacerbated with movement or effort, or if it changes with changes in posture, its source may be mechanical (compression of nerves, inflammation of joints). If pain is unaffected by movement, effort, or posture, its source may be inflammation of peripheral nerves or lesions affecting sensory pathways in the central nervous system.

Other kinds of unusual sensations also give the physician clues to the location and nature of nervous system abnormality. Numbness or loss of sensitivity usually point to damage in cranial nerves, spinal nerves, or sensory nerve fiber tracts. Abnormal sensitivity to stimulation (*hyperesthesia*) or abnormal sensations such as tingling or burning in the absence of stimulation (*paresthesia*) suggest a disturbance in the peripheral nerves or central sensory pathways. Sensory loss in an entire limb or on one side of the body suggests damage in ascending spinal cord tracts or the sensory cortex. (Complete loss of sensation is called *anesthesia*; partial loss is called *hypesthesia*.) Patterns of sensory loss that are inconsistent with what the physician knows about the sensory system may suggest a functional rather than an organic cause.

Assessment. The physician assesses the patient's somatic sensation by systematic stimulation of sensory receptors. Sensory abnormalities may affect *deep sensation* (from the muscles, tendons, and joints), *superficial sensation* (from the skin), or both. *Deep sensation* includes *joint sense* (the ability to tell the position of the limbs without seeing them) and *sensitivity to vibration. Superficial sensation*

includes the perception of light touch, superficial pain (pinprick), and temperature. Evaluation of these categories of sensation helps the physician identify pathology affecting the spinal cord. The categories of sensations affected by spinal cord pathology and the parts of the body exhibiting sensory disruption permit the physician to predict the level in the spinal cord at which the pathology exists (spinal cord lesions typically produce sensory deficits below the level of the lesion) and to tell if the lesion affects the front, back, middle, or sides of the spinal cord.

Patients who suffer spinal cord transection lose all sensation below the level of the transection, are paralyzed in all muscles served by spinal nerves below the level of the transection, and lose bowel and bladder reflexes (these reflexes usually return). Fortunately, transection of the spinal cord (Figure 2-8) is rare; it is usually the result of traumatic injury.

The posterior columns of the spinal cord, which travel up the back of the spinal cord at the midline, carry well-localized sensations of fine touch, vibration, two-point discrimination, and proprioception (position sense) from skin and joints (Waxman, 2000). However, some tactile information travels by other pathways. Pathology affecting the posterior half of the spinal cord (including the posterior columns; see Figure 2-8) causes impairment of precise tactile sensation (crude tactile sensation remains) plus impairment of vibration and joint sense on both sides of the body. Pain and temperature sensation are unaffected.

The *spinothalamic tracts,* which travel up the sides of the spinal cord, carry pain and temperature sensations and some light touch sensation. Pathology affecting one side of the spinal cord (*hemitransection syndrome,* or *Brown-Sequard syndrome*) causes loss of sensation relative to the midline (see Figure 2-8). Precise tactile sensation, vibration, and joint sense on the side of the spinal cord pathology are lost at and below the level of the injury. (This happens because the posterior columns,

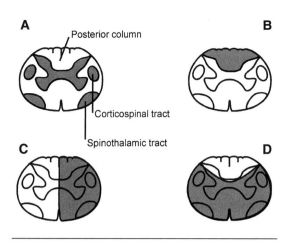

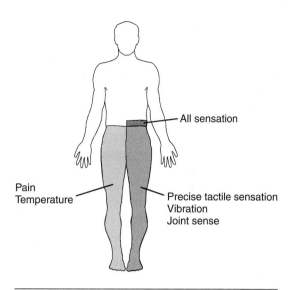

Figure 2-8 ■ Three spinal cord pathology syndromes. Posterior column syndrome **(B)** causes loss of precise tactile sensation and loss of vibration and joint sense. Pain and temperature sensation are spared. Hemitransection syndrome (Brown-Séquard syndrome) **(C)** causes ipsilateral loss of precise tactile sensation, vibration, and joint sense, and contralateral loss of pain and temperature sensation. Anterior myelopathy **(D)** causes loss of pain and temperature sensation and subtle impairment of light touch on both sides of the body. Precise tactile sensation, vibration, and joint sense are preserved. Muscles on both sides of the body below the level of spinal cord injury are paralyzed.

Figure 2-9 ■ Brown-Séquard (hemitransection) syndrome. Pain and temperature sensations are lost contralateral to the side of spinal cord injury, and precise tactile sensation, vibration, and joint sense are lost ipsilateral to the side of spinal cord injury. All ipsilateral sensation is lost at the level of the injury, caused by destruction of all sensory fibers entering the spinal cord at that level. Ipsilateral muscles below the level of spinal cord injury are paralyzed.

which carry tactile sensation, position sense, and vibration information, travel up the spinal cord on the same side as the spinal nerves that connect into them.) Pain and temperature sense on the side opposite the spinal cord pathology are lost at and below the level of the injury. (This happens because sensory nerves carrying pain and temperature information cross the spinal cord and connect into the spinothalamic tract at approximately the level at which the nerves enter the spinal cord.) The sensory impairments are accompanied by spastic hemiplegia at and below the level of the hemitransection because of destruction of one corticospinal tract (Figure 2-9).

Sometimes a neurosurgeon will cut nerve fibers in a patient's spinothalamic tract to relieve intractable pain—an operation called *cordotomy*. The patient also loses temperature sensation below the level of the cordotomy.

Pathology affecting the anterior spinal cord *(anterior myelopathy)* causes loss of pain and temperature sensation and subtle impairment of light touch on both sides of the body, attributable to transection of both spinothalamic tracts. Precise tactile sensation, vibration, and joint sense (conveyed by posterior columns) are preserved. The sensory impairments are accompanied by paralysis of muscles on both sides of the body, at and below the level of the spinal cord pathology because of damage to both corticospinal tracts (see Figure 2-8). Anterior myelopathy most often is associated with occlusion of the anterior spinal artery, which supplies the anterior two thirds of the spinal cord.

Regional loss of superficial sensation, rather than loss on one side of the body or loss below a given level of the spinal cord, suggests damage in cranial nerves or spinal nerves. Knowing the usual distribution of sensory regions for the cranial and spinal nerves (the regions are called *dermatomes*) helps the physician decide which nerves are affected (Figure 2-10). When the sensory impairment matches the dermatome for a cranial nerve or a spinal nerve, the physician can conclude that the patient's neuropathology involves the cranial nerve or spinal nerve.

When the sensory fibers of a cranial nerve or a spinal nerve are destroyed, all skin sensation is lost in the central part of the sensory field for the damaged nerve. However, some sensation usually remains at the periphery because of overlap with adjacent sensory nerves.

The physician may detect slight impairments in sensory function by stimulating two symmetric points on the body (e.g., simultaneously touching the right forearm and the left forearm), a procedure called *double simultaneous stimulation*. If sensory function on one side is impaired, the patient reports only the stimulus on the less-impaired side. Inability to detect stimulation on the impaired side during double

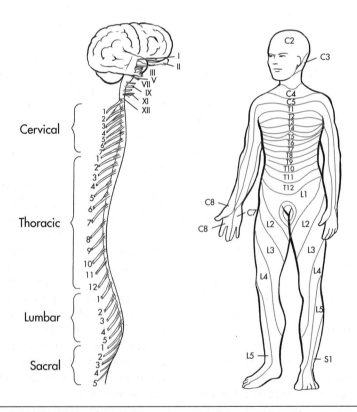

Figure 2-10 ■ The pattern of skin sensation as it relates to cranial nerves and spinal nerves. Each cranial nerve and spinal nerve serves a specific region. (These regions are called *dermatomes.*)

simultaneous stimulation is called *extinction* and typically is associated with cortical damage, usually in the contralateral parietal lobe.

Some patients lose the ability to identify objects by touch even though superficial tactile sensation is unimpaired. They report light touch and pinprick without error yet cannot identify common objects (e.g., a comb or a key) when the objects are placed, out of sight, in either hand. Such problems in recognition of objects by touch are called *astereognosis.* Astereognosis usually is caused by damage in or around the sensory cortex of the contralateral parietal lobe.

Stereo is from Greek. One of its meanings is *three dimensional. Gnosis* also is from Greek. It translates as *knowledge.*

Equilibrium

History and Current Complaints. Patients with impairments of equilibrium usually complain of feeling dizzy or light-headed or report subjective illusions of movement. When a patient complains of dizziness, the physician is likely to ask questions to find out what the patient means by dizziness. Some patients may be referring to *vertigo*—the sensation that the body or the environment is moving (usually rotating) when it is not. Vertigo usually is caused by problems in the inner ear, the vestibular branch of the acoustic nerve (CN 8), or the brain stem. The presence of persisting or recurring vertigo may suggest involvement of the vestibular system or, less frequently, the brain stem or cerebellum. Severe vertigo with sudden onset often is a result of vascular problems in the brain stem or cerebellum. Episodic vertigo may be caused by transient insufficiency of cerebral blood flow or may reflect Meniere's disease (increased pressure in inner ear structures that play a role in equilibrium). Progressive vertigo may be caused by toxicity, some vitamin deficiencies, or degenerative neurologic disease. Except for mild cases, attacks of true vertigo are most often accompanied by nausea, vomiting,

pallor, and sweating, and head movements increase the severity of the attack. Most patients with true vertigo quickly learn that they must remain immobile during an attack.

Some patients may complain of light-headedness, faintness, or giddiness. Such sensations sometimes are experienced by normal healthy individuals, in which case they may be related to anxiety, hyperventilation, sudden changes in head position, or other transitory conditions.

Stance, Gait, and Nystagmus. The patient's stance, gait, and nystagmus often provide clues that point toward the source of a patient's problems with equilibrium. Patients with disequilibrium typically stand with feet wide apart, are reluctant to stand with their feet close together, and may be unable to bring their feet completely together without falling. Patients whose disequilibrium is caused by loss of proprioceptive feedback from the legs and feet compensate by relying on visual input to maintain balance. When these patients close their eyes, they become increasingly unsteady and may fall *(Romberg's sign).* Patients whose disequilibrium is caused by cerebellar pathology are unsteady with eyes open or closed, although unsteadiness is worse when they close their eyes.

Patients with disequilibrium typically walk with a wide-based gait. When a patient's disequilibrium is caused by loss of proprioceptive feedback, the patient is likely to walk with *steppage gait* (see *Gait,* page 70). Patients with vestibular disease and patients with loss of proprioceptive feedback usually walk better when provided support (a cane or the examiner's arm), and both do much worse when walking in the dark or with eyes closed. Having patients with disequilibrium walk with their feet close together or having them walk heel-to-toe along a straight line always exaggerates their symptoms.

Nystagmus (abnormal and involuntary oscillation of the eyes, either at rest or when tracking a visual target) commonly is seen in patients with vestibular disorders. *Caloric testing*, in which cold water is introduced into the ear canal, often produces characteristic patterns of nystagmus in patients with vestibular pathology. The relationships between the nature of a patient's nystagmus and the nervous system pathology that causes it are too complex to be dealt with here, but these relationships often point directly to the site of the patient's nervous system pathology.

Consciousness and Mentation

History and Current Complaints. Changes in consciousness or mentation may be caused by a variety of diseases and pathologic states. In general, changes in consciousness or mentation implicate the brain hemispheres, and to a lesser extent, the brain stem. Changes in consciousness and mentation may be experienced by patients with cerebrovascular disease, head injury, alcohol or drug abuse, central nervous system infections, brain tumors, brain abscesses, metabolic disturbances, nutritional deficiencies, dementing illness, and several other diseases and conditions. Consequently, changes in consciousness or mentation rarely point unequivocally to a diagnosis, but when combined with information from the history and neurologic examination, such changes may point toward a diagnosis with relative certainty.

Altered Mental State. The physician may summarize the assessment of a patient's consciousness and mentation by assigning one of several labels that signify in a general sense the nature of the patient's condition:

- *Confusion.* Patients with confusion (*delirium* or *acute confusional state*) have normal or slightly lowered levels of consciousness but are impaired in their orientation to the environment (e.g., where they are and what day it is). Confused patients' attention spans are short, their memory for recent events is poor, and they cannot think clearly. Acute confusional states are transitory, but a period of confusion may evolve to a more circumscribed but longer-lasting syndrome. For example, a

stroke patient may exhibit confusion immediately following the stroke, with the confusion gradually clearing, leaving the patient not confused but aphasic. Confusional states arise from a variety of causes, including drug or alcohol intoxication or withdrawal, endocrine disturbances, nutritional disorders, infections, cerebrovascular disorders, head trauma, and psychiatric illness.

- *Lethargy* or *somnolence.* Lethargic or somnolent patients are drowsy, fall asleep at inappropriate times, sleep longer than usual, and are difficult to wake. Lethargy and somnolence may be transitory and separated by periods of normal alertness and attention, or they may be progressive, ending in coma and death. Lethargy and somnolence, like confusional states, arise from many causes, such as those listed for confusional states. (Falling asleep during a tedious lecture or in a particularly boring movie is not considered a sign of nervous system abnormality and rarely ends in coma or death.)

- *Syncope.* Syncope (fainting spells) denotes transitory loss of consciousness caused by reduced blood supply to the brain. Syncopal episodes usually appear together with autonomic irregularities—rapid respiration; rapid and feeble pulse; pallor; perspiration; and cold, clammy skin. Syncope may be caused by diminished cardiac output, abnormally low blood pressure, dehydration, drugs, or stress and anxiety.

- *Fugue state.* Fugue state is a temporary disturbance of consciousness lasting from a few minutes to several days. During a fugue state the patient engages in normal activities of daily life. However, the patient later does not remember the events or activities that took place during the fugue state. Fugue states are seen in combination with psychiatric illness and (rarely) as a consequence of epilepsy.

- *Amnesia.* Amnesia denotes complete loss of memory for a limited time period. Amnesic patients usually are aware of the missing memories and distressed by them. Amnesic states often are present in psychiatric illness and are a common consequence of traumatic brain injury.

Seizures. Although seizures involve loss of consciousness, they are more dramatic, and their relationship to nervous system pathology is more straightforward than the changes in consciousness and mentation described above. Seizures are caused by abnormal patterns of neuronal discharge in the brain. The discharges interfere with normal brain activity and cause periods of depressed mental function, confusion, uncontrollable muscle contraction and relaxation, and usually loss of consciousness. Seizures usually signify pathology in the brain hemispheres but may be caused by alcohol or drug withdrawal, central nervous system infections, hypoglycemia (abnormally low blood sugar), or other diseases. Seizurelike phenomena (called *pseudo-seizures*) sometimes occur as a component of psychiatric conditions.

Seizures have been divided into two major categories, reflecting differences in what happens to the patient during the seizure:

- *Generalized seizures* are seizures in which the patient loses consciousness. In *tonic-clonic seizures* (sometimes called *grand mal seizures* or *convulsions)* there is massive discharge of neurons in the brain, causing contraction of almost all the muscles in the body, followed by a series of intermittent *clonic jerks.* Tonic-clonic seizures last from 1 to 3 minutes on average and are never remembered by the patient (perhaps because the patient loses consciousness). In *absence seizures* (formerly called *petit mal seizures*), the loss of consciousness lasts only a few seconds and the patient usually does not fall. The patient may stare, stop moving and talking, drop things, or move his or her head and limbs aimlessly and involuntarily during the seizure.
- *Partial seizures* (sometimes called *focal seizures*) are seizures in which there is localized discharge of neurons in the brain,

with the pattern of discharge differing widely across patients. The patient who experiences a partial seizure usually experiences clonic movements of individual muscle groups, but does not lose consciousness (although typically there is some clouding of consciousness and disruption of mental activity). Partial seizures may last for a few seconds to several minutes or even (rarely) hours. The magnitude of the seizure activity is related to how much of the brain is involved in abnormal neuronal discharge. Partial seizures suggest localized areas of abnormal discharge, and generalized seizures suggest that major regions of both brain hemispheres are involved.

Occasionally an individual goes into a state of unremitting seizure activity or experiences a chain of seizures in which seizures occur so frequently that the patient does not regain consciousness between seizures. This condition is called *status epilepticus* and is a medical emergency, demanding preservation of the patient's airway and administration of intravenous antiseizure medications.

Mental Status. Standard neurologic examinations usually provide for rudimentary assessment of a patient's level of consciousness, attention and concentration, orientation and memory, mood and behavior, thought content, and language and speech. In the physician's report of the examination, the physician typically comments on the patient's level of arousal (e.g., awake and alert, lethargic, somnolent, stuporous, or comatose) and the patient's responsiveness to stimulation (e.g., responsive, unresponsive, appropriate, inappropriate). The physician describes the patient's attention and concentration in terms of the patient's performance in tasks requiring low levels of mental effort, such as counting backward or reciting the alphabet backward. The physician describes the patient's orientation in terms of the answers to questions about himself or herself (person); where he or she is (place); and day, date, and time of day (time). If the patient is considered oriented to person, place, and time, the physician may describe the patient as *oriented X3.*

The physician's report also addresses the patient's mood and behavior (e.g., apathetic, elated, depressed, stable, variable) and describes the patient's thought content (e.g., its appropriateness and rationality; whether hallucinations or delusions are present). The physician tests the patient's memory by asking the patient to recall short lists of numbers or words. The physician evaluates the patient's language and speech by asking the patient to carry out simple spoken commands, repeat words and phrases, name pictures or objects, read words and sentences, and write words and short sentences.

Several more or less standardized screening tests of mental status have been published. One of the most widely used by physicians is the *Mini Mental State Examination* (MMSE) (Folstein, Folstein, & McHugh, 1975) or the *Modified Mini Mental State Examination* (3MS)

(Teng & Chui, 1987). The MMSE contains 11 items to screen orientation to time and present location, immediate memory for a 3-word list, attention (counting backward by 7, spelling a word backward), object naming, phrase repetition, comprehension of spoken instructions, writing a sentence, and copying a geometric figure. The MMSE usually takes from 5 to 10 minutes to administer and normal adults typically score from 25 to 30 points (of a possible 30). Scores below 25 usually are considered an indication of compromised mental status.

The 3MS samples a broader range of performance across a wider range of difficulty than the MMSE and provides for more sensitive scoring. The 3MS adds four items to the MMSE (date and place of birth, naming four-legged animals, similarities, and delayed recall) and broadens the range of scores (0 to 100) by providing scaled scores for original MMSE items and adding scores for the new items. Table 2-4 gives examples of items found in screening tests of mental status.

TABLE 2-4	Examples of Items That Typically Are Included in Screening Tests of Mental Status
Orientation to self	Answer questions: *Where were you born? What is the date of your birth?*
Orientation to time	Answer questions: *What year is it now? What is today's date? What day of the week is it? What time is it right now?*
Orientation to place	Answer questions: *What state are we in? What city are we in? What is the name of this place? Are we in a _____ (hospital, school, home)?*
Memory	Recall a list of words, typically a 3-word list Test immediately and after one or more intervening tasks
Attention, concentration	Count backward from 20 Say the alphabet backward Spell a word backward
Mental flexibility	Describe similarities: *How are a table and a chair alike?*
Naming	Name common objects to confrontation Categorical naming (e.g., *four-legged animals, articles of clothing*)
Repetition	Repeat words and phrases
Auditory comprehension	Follow sequential commands: *Take this paper in your left hand, fold it in half, and give it to me.*
Reading comprehension	Follow printed instructions: *Close your eyes. Make a fist.*
Writing	Write to dictation: *Write on this paper, "I would like to go out."*
Visuospatial ability	Copy simple geometric forms

GENERAL CONCEPTS 2-3

- A standard neurologic examination includes evaluation of *deep sensation* (joint sense, deep pain sensation, sensitivity to vibration) and *superficial sensation* (light touch, superficial pain, and temperature).
- The distributions of sensory regions for cranial and spinal nerves are called *dermatomes*.
- *Double simultaneous stimulation* may reveal slight impairments in sensory function.
- *Confusion* (delirium, acute confusional state), *lethargy* (somnolence), *syncope*, and *fugue state* represent disturbances of consciousness and mentation. *Amnesia* represents the inability to remember past experiences, often for a circumscribed time interval.
- *Seizures* are caused by abnormal patterns of neuronal discharge in the brain. In *generalized seizures* and *absence seizures* the patient loses consciousness. In *partial seizures* the patient does not lose consciousness.
- Assessment of mental status usually includes assessment of the patient's level of consciousness, attention and concentration, orientation and memory, mood and behavior, thought content, and language and speech. The assessment often is conducted using a standard screening test such as the *Mini Mental State Examination (MMSE)*.

LABORATORY TESTS

Laboratory tests provide information about the patient that cannot be obtained from the interview and the physical examination. In addition to standard laboratory tests such as analysis of blood and urine, the physician may order special tests to aid diagnosis of a patient's neurologic disorder. Imaging procedures, which permit visualization of internal body structures, are among the most frequently ordered special tests.

Imaging Procedures

Before the end of the nineteenth century, physicians could visualize internal body structures only by cutting into the body and looking at them. The situation changed in 1895, when Wilhelm Roentgen first demonstrated the use of radiation from a primitive cathode ray generator to visualize bones inside the body. Roentgen called the radiation from his cathode ray generator *x-rays* to indicate that they were a new and mysterious kind of radiation. (X-rays are called *Roentgen rays* in many parts of the world). By 1896, crude x-ray machines *(radiographs)* were being used by surgeons to guide surgery and by battlefield physicians to locate bullets in wounded soldiers.

In *x-ray imaging,* x-rays are passed through body tissues onto a sheet of photographic film to create a negative image of internal body structures. The x-rays pass readily through low-density tissues but are blocked by dense tissues such as bone. Low-density tissues appear as dark areas on the x-ray plate, and higher-density tissues appear as brighter images. Sometimes fluid containing a substance that blocks x-rays (called *contrast medium*) is injected into internal structures (such as veins or arteries) that ordinarily would not appear on an x-ray image. The images obtained from such tests are said to be *contrast enhanced.*

Standard x-ray images of the skull, spine, or both may provide useful information regarding the probable causes of a patient's symptoms. X-ray images of the skull *(skull films)* may show fractures, abnormal deposits, or calcification of structures inside the skull (Figure 2-11). X-ray images of the spine *(spine films)* may show congenital deformities, fractures, displacement of intervertebral disks, degenerative changes, or tumors involving the vertebrae and spinal cord (Figure 2-12).

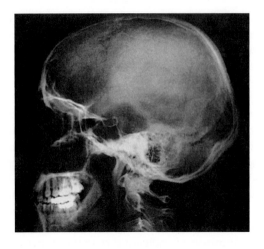

Figure 2-11 ■ X-ray image of a normal adult skull. (From Ballinger, P.W. [1991]. *Merrill's atlas of radiographic positions and radiologic procedures* [8th ed.]. St. Louis: Mosby.)

Myelograms are x-ray procedures in which contrast medium is injected into the subarachnoid space around the spinal cord, after which one or more x-ray images of the spine are obtained (Figure 2-13). Myelograms permit direct visualization of the subarachnoid space surrounding the spinal cord and indirect visualization of the spinal cord and spinal nerves, which are silhouetted against the contrast medium. Myelograms are useful in diagnosing spinal cord or spinal nerve compression, structural abnormalities of the spine, and tumors or deformities of the spinal cord or spinal nerve roots. However, CT or MRI scanning of the spine (see below) often provide a simpler and less invasive procedure for obtaining the information provided by myelography.

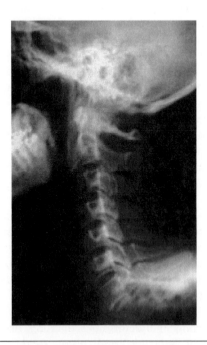

Figure 2-12 ■ X-ray image of a normal human cervical spine.

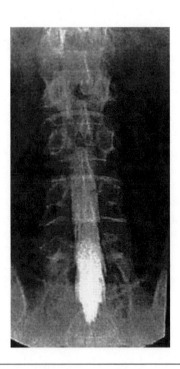

Figure 2-13 ■ A myelogram of a normal human spine (lumbar and sacral regions). The bright region represents contrast material injected into the space surrounding the spinal cord.

Computerized tomography (CT scanning, also called CAT scanning, or computerized axial tomography), a computer-based radiographic procedure, was developed in the early 1970s. In CT scanning the patient is placed in the center of a circular arrangement of x-ray generators and detectors, which rotate axially around the patient. X-rays pass through the parts of the patient's body being scanned and are picked up by detectors on the other side of the circle. The signals from the detectors are sent to a computer that analyzes them and generates photograph-like images that represent cross-sections of the body (Figure 2-14). The scanner moves up or down the parts of the body being scanned in regular steps so that a series of images representing consecutive "slices" of that part of the body are obtained.

The combination of a narrow beam of x-rays, sensitive detectors, and computer enhancement of signals in CT scanning permits visualization of soft tissues not visible on standard x-ray images. In many instances CT scanning has replaced other tests because it provides better visualization of internal structures with less risk to the patient. The primary drawback of CT scanning is that it exposes the patient to radiation. Consequently, CT scans are not a routine part of the neurologic examination. Within the past decade several imaging procedures that do not require exposure to radiation have been developed. Some have replaced CT scanning for some purposes.

Magnetic resonance imaging (MRI) was introduced into medicine in the late 1970s. MRI creates photograph-like images that look somewhat like the images generated by CT scans. However, MRI has two important advantages over CT: MRI does not expose the patient to radiation, and MRI provides images with greater detail.

MRI depends on the fact that the nuclei of hydrogen atoms behave like small bar magnets, so that if they are placed in a strong magnetic field, they orient themselves in line with the magnetic field. The body part to be imaged is placed inside a strong magnetic field. Then, when the hydrogen nuclei in the body tissues have aligned themselves with the magnetic field, a short pulse of electromagnetic energy is introduced into the field, causing the hydrogen nuclei to deflect from alignment. As the nuclei swing back into alignment with the magnetic field, they emit miniscule electromagnetic signals. A set of detectors measures these signals and sends them to a computer that constructs a photograph-like image from the signals (Figure 2-15).

In MRI, as in CT, the detectors are moved in steps along the axis of the body to yield images representing consecutive layers or "slices" of

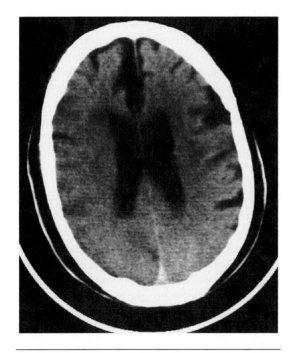

Figure 2-14 ■ A CT scan of a patient with a long history of neurologic problems. The lateral ventricles (butterfly-shaped dark areas in center) are enlarged, and the sulci are widened, suggesting atrophy of brain tissues. Dark areas in the anterior left hemisphere near the midline and in the lateral aspect of the right frontal lobe suggest regions of tissue destruction, probably by strokes.

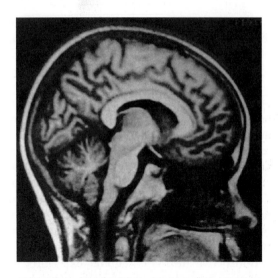

Figure 2-15 ■ A magnetic resonance image of the head. This image shows a vertical "slice" at the midline of the brain. The brain hemisphere, cerebellum, corpus callosum, and brain stem are visible. (From Oldendorf, W., & Oldendorf, W., Jr. [1991]. *MRI primer.* Philadelphia: Lippincott-Raven.)

the body parts scanned. MRI is sensitive to differences in the chemical composition of tissues, whereas CT is sensitive to differences in the density of tissues. For this reason, MRI can show differences between tissues that have similar density but different chemical composition, such as gray matter and white matter in the brain—differences that cannot be seen in CT images.

MRI is superior to CT for imaging the temporal lobes, brain stem, cerebellum, and spinal cord and for detecting multi-infarct disease, multiple sclerosis, degenerative brain disease, arteriovenous malformations, aneurysms, and recent stroke. As mentioned above, MRI requires no radiation, and so far there is no evidence that the magnetic fields used in MRI are a risk to patients. However, MRI cannot be used when patients have metal (e.g., pins, plates, pacemakers) in their body because of the magnetic field. MRI scans take a long time, and the patient

must remain motionless in a noisy, confining space, sometimes leading to claustrophobia and blurring of the MRI image because of patient movement *(movement artifacts)*.

Strokes are visible on MRI images obtained a few hours after a stroke but do not appear on CT images until several days later.

Cerebral angiography (sometimes called *cerebral arteriography*) is an x-ray procedure that provides an image of the veins and arteries of the brain and brain stem (Figure 2-16). A contrast medium is injected into one of the arteries supplying blood to the brain, and a series of x-rays of the head is taken. The contrast medium fills the artery and its branches and eventually makes its way into the cerebral veins, so that when the sequential x-ray plates are developed the physician can visualize the rate of circulation through the cerebral vessels.

Angiograms are useful in detecting occlusions of arteries or their branches because occluded vessels do not fill with contrast medium, and, consequently, they do not appear on the angiogram image. Blood vessels that are narrowed but not occluded (a condition called *stenosis*) fill slowly. Slow filling of vessels is detected by evaluating the progress of the contrast medium through the blood vessels from the beginning to the end of the series of X-ray plates. Angiography may show the presence of space-occupying lesions such as tumors or abscesses if a lesion displaces cerebral blood vessels from their usual locations.

A recently developed procedure, called *digital-subtraction angiography,* provides improved image quality and lessens the amount of contrast medium that must be injected into the vascular system. Digital-subtraction angiography uses a computer-averaging technique, in which the signals from nonvascular structures are deleted from the image, yielding an enhanced image of vascular structures (Figure 2-17).

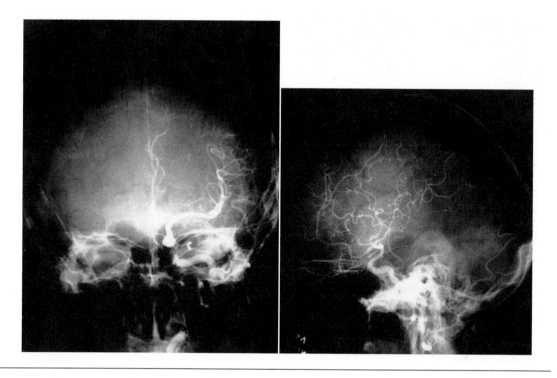

Figure 2-16 ■ A normal cerebral angiogram. The image on the left is taken from the front of the head. The anterior cerebral artery travels upward on the midline, and the middle cerebral travels laterally and upward on the right side of the image. The image on the right is taken from the side of the head. The middle cerebral artery and portions of the posterior cerebral artery can be seen. The carotid artery is visible in both views.

The physician may detect signs of carotid artery stenosis during the physical examination of the patient by putting a stethoscope over the carotid artery and listening to the sound of the blood moving through the artery. Blood moving through a narrowed artery creates an abnormal rushing sound (called *bruit*) that can be heard through a stethoscope.

B-mode carotid imaging (sometimes called *echo arteriography*) is a procedure for visualizing carotid arteries that requires neither radiation nor the injection of a contrast agent. A transducer that emits high-frequency sound waves is placed against the neck over the carotid artery. The sound waves are transmitted into the neck, where some are reflected back, depending on the acoustic absorption characteristics of the tissues under the transmitter. A detector picks up the reflected sound waves, and a computer analyzes the variations in the waves to create an image of the carotid arteries. Echo arteriograms are useful for detecting stenosis or ulceration in the carotid arteries, but they cannot reliably differentiate between severe stenosis and complete occlusion and do not always show blood clots.

Doppler ultrasound provides an indirect measure of carotid artery abnormality by measuring the rate of blood flow through the artery. High-frequency sound waves are transmitted into the head from a probe attached to a computer. The computer manipulates the

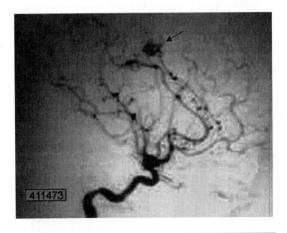

Figure 2-17 ■ A digital-subtraction angiogram. The middle cerebral artery in the right hemisphere is shown. The angiogram indicates the presence of a vascular malformation in the upper posterior frontal lobe *(arrow)*.

characteristics of the sound waves to target a particular artery. If the blood within the artery is moving, the frequency of the reflected sound waves is altered in a predictable way (the *Doppler effect*). A detector picks up the reflected sound waves and passes them to the computer. The computer analyzes changes in the frequency of the reflected waves and calculates the rate at which blood flows through the artery. Lower-than-normal rate of blood flow suggests partial occlusion. Absent blood flow suggests complete occlusion.

The Doppler effect is experienced in everyday life when a rapidly moving vehicle with horn or siren blaring passes a bystander. As the vehicle passes, the pitch of the sound made by the horn or siren drops. This happens because the movement of the vehicle away from the listener adds to the distance between the cycles of the sound wave at the listener's ear, lowering its perceived frequency.

The foregoing laboratory tests provide static images of internal structures or estimate the static characteristics of internal structures from mathematic manipulation of physical measurements such as the Doppler effect. The next group of laboratory tests estimate dynamic processes such the electrical activity of the brain cortex, nerve conduction velocity, and blood flow in the brain.

Electrophysiologic Procedures

Several diagnostic procedures yield recordings of electrical activity in parts of the nervous system. Electrodes are placed at strategic locations to monitor electrical activity in tissue near the electrodes. This low-voltage activity is amplified and sent to a recording device (usually a pen on a moving strip of graph paper), which generates a visual representation of the electrical activity.

The *electroencephalogram* (EEG) yields a graphic record of the electrical activity of the cerebral cortex. An array of recording electrodes is attached to the scalp. The electrodes detect the tiny electrical signals generated by the brain cortex. The signals are amplified until they can operate pens that write the signals out on a moving strip of paper. The activity from a number of electrodes is traced on the paper, so that tracings of electrical activity at several cortical locations (usually 16) are obtained. The amplitude and pattern of the waveforms in the tracings, together with the location of anomalous patterns of activity, permit the physician to make inferences about what is happening physiologically in the patient's brain.

Localized brain lesions often cause focal disturbances in the EEG record in the vicinity of the lesion. The disturbance usually takes the form of aberrations in rhythm and amplitude (Figure 2-18). EEG recording is particularly useful for detecting and locating the source of seizure activity. Sometimes an EEG may permit a physician to tell if a stroke is in or near the cortex or deeper in the brain. If the EEG record from a stroke patient is normal, the stroke is likely to be subcortical; if the EEG is abnormal, the stroke is likely to be cortical. When a patient is in deep coma, EEG recordings may be used to

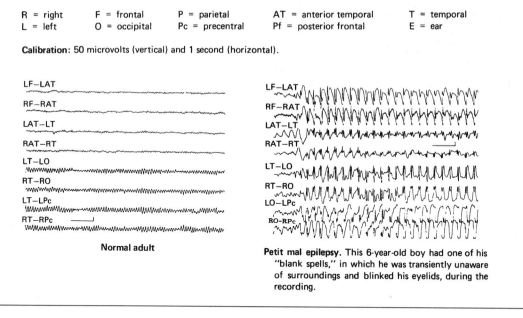

R = right	F = frontal	P = parietal	AT = anterior temporal	T = temporal
L = left	O = occipital	Pc = precentral	Pf = posterior frontal	E = ear

Calibration: 50 microvolts (vertical) and 1 second (horizontal).

LF–LAT

RF–RAT

LAT–LT

RAT–RT

LT–LO

RT–RO

LT–LPc

RT–RPc

Normal adult

LF–LAT

RF–RAT

LAT–LT

RAT–RT

LT–LO

RT–RO

LO–LPc

RO–RPc

Petit mal epilepsy. This 6-year-old boy had one of his "blank spells," in which he was transiently unaware of surroundings and blinked his eyelids, during the recording.

Figure 2-18 ■ Examples of normal and abnormal EEGs. On the left is a recording from an adult with no EEG abnormalities. On the right is a recording from a patient with petit mal epilepsy, showing general disruption of cortical activity. (From Waxman, S. [2000]. *Correlative neuroanatomy* [24th ed.]. New York: McGraw-Hill.)

estimate the severity of the patient's brain injury and to predict whether the patient will return to consciousness.

An adaptation of EEG recording, called *evoked response testing,* is a computerized version of EEG testing. The patient is placed in a quiet, dark room with recording electrodes on her or his scalp. When the patient's EEG has stabilized, tactile, auditory, or visual stimuli are presented and the electrical activity of the cortex is measured. The computer calculates the cortical activity occurring within each of many time intervals following each stimulus. Changes in activity that regularly follow each stimulus are added together, and irregular (random) changes are ignored. A graphic printout of cortical activity attributable to stimulation is then generated. Alterations of computed waveforms for the visual evoked response (elicited by visual stimulation), the brain stem evoked response (elicited by auditory stimula-

tion), and the somatosensory evoked response (elicited by weak electrical stimulation of peripheral sensory nerves) suggest damage to the central nervous system conduction pathways serving those sensory modalities—damage that may not be detectable by clinical neurologic examination.

In *electromyography* fine-needle electrodes are inserted into muscles to record their electrical activity. Relaxed muscles normally produce no spontaneous electrical activity, but when muscles contract they produce bursts of electrical activity that are fairly predictable in terms of amplitude, frequency, duration, and pattern. Spontaneous discharges in resting muscles (fibrillations, fasciculations) may indicate peripheral nerve disease. Other variations in amplitude, frequency, duration, or pattern may indicate disease in anterior horn cells, disease affecting neuromuscular junctions, or disease affecting the muscles themselves.

Nerve conduction studies are performed when peripheral neuropathy is suspected. In nerve conduction studies a nerve fiber (either motor or sensory) is stimulated at one point, and the response is measured at another point along the fiber. The time between the stimulation and the response is called the *nerve conduction velocity*. Variations in nerve conduction velocities sometimes are helpful in diagnosing the nature and extent of peripheral nerve damage.

Brain Mapping Procedures

The next group of laboratory tests indirectly identifies regions of elevated neuronal activity by measuring cerebral blood flow. The generic name for these tests is *regional cerebral blood flow (rCBF)* measurement. As its name implies, rCBF is a procedure for estimating blood flow in regions of the brain. It takes advantage of the relationship between cerebral blood flow and brain metabolism, wherein regions of increased neuronal activity also are regions of increased metabolism, marked by increased glucose uptake and elevated blood oxygenation. The changes in glucose uptake and blood oxygen provide indirect indications of cerebral metabolism rather than static images of brain tissue. rCBF can be measured in several ways, most of which require introduction into the blood of compounds called *tracers* that emit small amounts of radioactivity. The tracers are introduced into the bloodstream either directly by injection of a liquid or indirectly by having the patient breathe air containing small amounts of a slightly radioactive gas, which is absorbed into the blood. When the tracer reaches the brain, specialized scanners detect the subatomic particles (photons, positrons) emitted by the tracer, convert these events into electrical signals, and send the signals to a computer that analyzes them and constructs a series of images representing the blood flow in various brain regions.

Positron-emission tomography (PET) was one of the first imaging procedures to be adapted to visualize metabolic activity in the brain. In the PET procedure a solution of metabolically active material (usually glucose) tagged with a positron-emitting isotope (oxygen, fluorine, carbon, or nitrogen) is introduced into the patient's body either by injection or by a fluid drunk by the patient. The glucose and the isotope make their way to the brain, where the glucose is metabolized, carrying the tracer with it. The glucose and the isotope concentrate at areas of high metabolism and high levels of neuronal activity. As the isotope decays it emits positrons, which strike nearby electrons, producing photons (similar to gamma rays). The photons are sensed by a set of detectors, the signals are amplified and sent to a computer, and the computer processes them to generate an image representing the regional metabolic activity of the brain (Figure 2-19).

PET scanning was introduced in 1975, and until the late 1980s was primarily a research tool, limited to institutions with large medical research operations and budgets that could bear the enormous expense of operating a PET scanning facility. During the 1990s, PET scanning made its way into regular clinical use, but only at large regional clinical facilities. (Most clinical uses of PET are underwritten by companies that supply the tracers used in PET scanning.) PET scans are expensive because the scanning facility requires a cyclotron and physicists and chemists to prepare the isotope. PET scans permit visualization of hypofunction in damaged brain regions in which blood flow is not compromised but in which brain metabolism is altered, even though no structural damage may be visible on standard CT scans.

Single-photon emission computed tomography (SPECT) scanning is another procedure for estimating blood flow in the brain. SPECT scanning of the body was first described in 1963 but did not come into widespread research and clinical use until the 1970s. The SPECT scanning procedure is similar to PET scanning in that a radioactive tracer is introduced into the body by injection, a scanner detects the photons

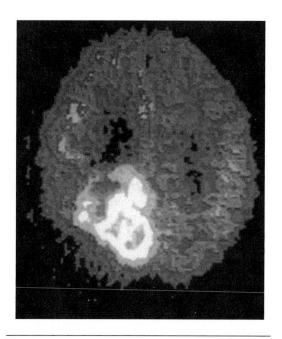

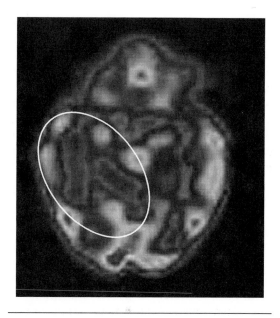

Figure 2-19 ■ A grayscale reproduction of a color positron-emission tomography (PET) scan showing the presence of a tumor in the left parieto-occipital region of the brain. The different shades of gray represent different levels of metabolic activity. Because tumors are metabolically more active than surrounding tissue they appear as enhanced regions in images that depict metabolic activity in tissues. (From NCI Visuals Online, National Cancer Institute, Bethesda, Md. Source: Cedars-Sinai Medical Center.)

Figure 2-20 ■ A grayscale reproduction of a color single-photon emission computed tomography (SPECT) scan of a patient who had experienced a stroke in the distribution of the left middle cerebral artery. The SPECT scan shows a region of hypometabolism in the central region of the left hemisphere (ellipse). (From NASA Remote Sensing Tutorial, National Aeronautics and Space Administration [*http://rst.gsfc.nasa.gov*].)

emitted by the tracer, and a computer uses information from the scanner to construct images of the tissues scanned (Figure 2-20). SPECT scanning, like PET scanning, is sensitive to blood flow, permitting visualization of regions with increased or diminished blood flow, and by inference, regions of increased or diminished neuronal activity. SPECT scans require less costly and complex equipment and personnel than PET scans, making them available at more medical facilities.

Functional magnetic resonance imaging (fMRI), introduced in the mid 1970s, is a modification of the standard MRI procedure. Standard MRI permits visualization of brain structures but does not give information about metabolically active brain regions. Like PET and SPECT, fMRI produces images depicting neural activity in brain regions. Unlike PET and SPECT, fMRI produces the images without the use of tracers. fMRI exploits the response of blood hemoglobin to the magnetic field used in MRI studies. The increased blood flow typical of neurally active brain tissue increases the concentration of oxygen-rich hemoglobin in the tissue. The increase in oxygen-rich hemoglobin causes a change in the MRI signal much like that produced by the tracers used in PET and SPECT procedures. Computerized image processing procedures are used to produce images in which regions with increased oxygen-rich hemoglobin (regions with increased blood flow) appear as enhanced regions in the fMRI image. Sophisticated image-processing procedures convert these very subtle changes in oxygenation into photograph-like images of brain tissues (Figure 2-21). fMRI now largely dominates functional brain imaging because of its low invasiveness, absence of radiation exposure, and relatively low cost.

Analysis of Body Tissue or Fluids

Sometimes diagnosis of nervous system pathology requires laboratory analysis of a sample of nervous system tissue or fluids. A *lumbar puncture* (sometimes called *spinal tap*) may be performed if the physician suspects infection or hemorrhage in the patient's central nervous system. A hypodermic needle

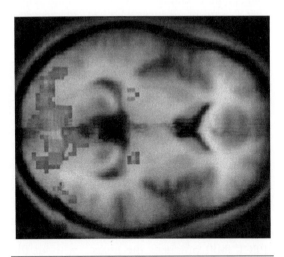

Figure 2-21 ■ A grayscale reproduction of computer-averaged functional magnetic resonance imaging (fMRI) composite color scan representing regions of increased metabolic brain activity in a group of non–brain-injured adults during a visual tracking task. Enhanced areas represent activation of occipital-lobe regions serving vision. (From Wikipedia, the Free Internet Encyclopedia *[http://en.wikipedia.org/wiki/ Functional_magnetic_resonance_imaging].*)

is inserted into the subarachnoid space in the lumbar spine below the level of the spinal cord, and a sample of cerebrospinal fluid (CSF) is taken for analysis. When the needle is inserted, the pressure with which the fluid flows into the syringe is measured. Increased pressure may suggest blockage in the circulation of CSF, the presence of space-occupying pathology such as a tumor or abscess, or swelling of brain tissue.

The CSF obtained from the lumbar puncture is analyzed for the presence of blood cells, bacteria, parasites, or viruses, and its chemical composition is determined, including the amount of glucose and protein in the fluid. The presence of red blood cells or a yellowish color *(xanthochromia)* are signs of bleeding into the ventricles, into the meningeal spaces, or into the spinal canal. The presence of bacteria, parasites, or viruses proves infection. Increased protein content suggests meningeal inflammation, a tumor, or obstructions in the spinal canal. CSF glucose levels often are lowered by bacterial infections. (The bacteria consume the glucose.)

Biopsies (removing a sample of tissue for laboratory analysis) may be performed when less invasive procedures do not yield a diagnosis. Most biopsies of nervous system tissue are *needle biopsies* (sometimes called *aspiration biopsies*) in which a hollow needle is inserted into the tissue of interest and a small amount of tissue is removed by applying suction to the needle. Sometimes *open biopsies* (surgical removal of tissue samples) may be performed if the tissue is accessible to the surgeon's scalpel.

Biopsy of brain tissue may be ordered to determine the nature of brain tumors, to identify the nature of an infection (as in brain abscess), or to diagnose degenerative disease. Muscle biopsy may be ordered to determine if muscle weakness is caused by neuropathy or by disease of the muscle itself. Biopsy of nerve tissue occasionally may be ordered to determine the underlying nature of peripheral neurologic disease. Arterial biopsy may be ordered to identify inflammatory or degenerative diseases affecting the arteries.

RECORDING THE RESULTS OF THE NEUROLOGIC EXAMINATION

The report of the neurologic examination is placed in the patient's medical record, where it usually is the first entry in the record of the patient's care. The report usually ends with a *problem list*, in which the patient's significant medical problems are recorded, and a *plan* for the first phase of the patient's care. The report, the problem list, and the plan provide important information for everyone contributing to the patient's care. An example of a neurologic examination report for a patient with right hemiplegia and aphasia follows.

Report of Neurologic Examination

The patient was seen in the emergency room following reported sudden onset of right-side muscle weakness and slurred speech approximately 2 hours prior to my examination. The patient was alert and cooperative, but his speech was grossly distorted and limited to single words. Observation indicated apparent right hemiparesis and paralysis of lower facial muscles on the right. Neurologic examination of the patient yielded the following results:

Cranial Nerves

- *Olfactory:* Not tested.
- *Optic:* The optic discs were flat, with no evidence of exudates or hemorrhages. Venous pulsations were visible, and retinal vessels were grossly normal. The macular area appeared normal, with perhaps some age-related minimal degenerative changes.
- *Oculomotor, trochlear, abducens:* The pupils were round, equal, and responsive to light and accommodation. The extraocular muscle movements were intact. No nystagmus was observed. Visual fields were normal.
- *Trigeminal:* The patient's jaw opened on the midline but deviated to the right when opened against resistance. Masseter muscle strength was moderately decreased on the right. Corneal reflexes were brisk and equal. Upper facial sensation was intact to pinprick and light touch. Lower facial sensation was intact on the left, moderately diminished on the right.
- *Facial:* No ptosis was observed. Forehead wrinkling appeared normal on both sides. There was mild to moderate facial droop on the right, and the right side of the patient's mouth did not retract on smile or showing teeth.

- *Acoustic:* Hearing appeared intact to sound of ticking watch at 3 feet. Bone conduction not tested.
- *Glossopharyngeal, vagus:* The patient's gag reflex was strong and prompt. The patient's soft palate was lower on the right on passive observation. On phonation the palate elevated on the left but not the right side.
- *Spinal accessory:* Strength of the sternocleidomastoid and trapezius muscles was slightly diminished on the right.
- *Hypoglossal:* The tongue deviated to the right on protrusion. Right-to-left movement was normal to left, restricted to right. No tremor, fasciculations, or atrophy noted.

Motor and Coordination

The patient was unable to stand or walk. Finger-to-finger, finger-to-nose, and rapid alternating movements on the left were within normal limits. Not tested on right because of paralysis. Strength was normal on left, diminished on right (contraction but no movement, upper and lower R extremities). Spasticity and exaggerated reflexes were present on the right but not on the left. Plantar extensor reflex elicited on the right but not on the left. No tremor, involuntary movements, fasciculations, or atrophy were observed. Biceps, triceps, brachioradialis, and ankle jerks were normal on the left, exaggerated on the right (3+), but without sustained clonus.

Sensation

Light touch, pinprick, vibration, and position sense were intact on the left. Light touch and pinprick diminished on the right. Vibration and position sense were intact on right.

Continued

Report of Neurologic Examination—cont'd

Vascular
Carotid pulses present bilaterally. Bruit present on left but not on right.

Impression
Stroke in anterior zone of left middle cerebral artery, probably thromboembolic.

Problem List
1. Right hemiplegia.
2. Aphasia: nonfluent, severe.

Plan
1. Rule out hemorrhage (CT scan, MRI).
2. Medications: anticoagulate if thrombotic or embolic. Dilantin 100 mg. t.i.d.
3. Baseline measures of speech, language, mentation. Speech therapy consult.
4. Begin rehabilitation program. PT, OT consults.

GENERAL CONCEPTS 2-4

- *X-ray imaging* produces visual images of internal bones and tissues that block or attenuate the passage of x-rays.
- *Myelography* is an x-ray procedure that provides visualization of the spinal cord and surrounding space. Myelography is useful for detecting structural changes in the spinal cord or spinal nerve roots.
- *Computerized tomography (CT scanning)* is an x-ray procedure that produces computer-generated photograph-like images of cross-sectional "slices" of internal structures based on their resistance to the passage of x-rays.
- *Magnetic resonance imaging (MRI)* produces computer-generated photograph-like images of cross-sectional "slices" of internal structures by placing them in a strong magnetic field and introducing a burst of electromagnetic energy. MRI images reflect the chemical composition of tissues (particularly their water content).
- *Cerebral angiography (arteriography)* is an x-ray procedure that permits visualization of cerebral veins and arteries. Angiography is useful for detecting narrowed or occluded arteries.
- *B-mode carotid imaging (echo arteriography)* and *transcranial Doppler ultrasound* yield computer-generated images of cerebral blood vessels derived from analysis

of sound waves transmitted into the head and neck.
- *Electroencephalography (EEG)* produces a graphic record of the electrical activity of the cerebral cortex. EEG recording is useful for detecting and localizing seizure activity.
- *Evoked-response testing* is an encephalographic procedure in which a computer is used to analyze the electrical activity of the brain cortex in response to stimulation.
- *Electromyography* produces a record of the electrical activity in muscles. Electromyography is useful in diagnosing diseases of peripheral nerves, neuromuscular junctions, or muscles.
- *Nerve conduction studies* measure the speed of neural transmission. They are useful in diagnosing pathology affecting peripheral nerves.
- *Positron emission tomography (PET)* produces computer-generated images of cross-sectional "slices" of internal tissues that reflect the metabolism taking place in various brain regions. PET requires ingestion of mildly radioactive tracers by the patient.
- *Single-photon emission computed tomography (SPECT)* produces computer-generated maps of the metabolic activity in brain tissues. Increases in metabolic

GENERAL CONCEPTS 2-4—cont'd

activity signify increased neuronal activity. SPECT requires ingestion of mildly radioactive tracers by the patient.

- *Functional magnetic resonance imaging (fMRI)* produces computer-generated maps of the metabolic activity in brain tissues by measuring blood hemoglobin levels. fMRI does not require ingestion of radioactive tracers.

- In *lumbar puncture (spinal tap)* a sample of CSF is removed to analyze it for the presence of blood cells and infectious organisms and to detect abnormal levels of glucose and proteins, all of which are signs of central nervous system pathology.

- *Biopsy* (removal of tissue for laboratory analysis) may be performed when less invasive procedures do not yield a diagnosis.

THOUGHT QUESTIONS

Question 2-1 A 74-year-old man with a 20-year history of heart disease and two previous myocardial infarcts (heart attacks) is brought to a hospital emergency room with a sudden onset of slurred speech and right-sided limb weakness. The neurologist who evaluates the patient in the emergency room makes the following observations:

- Moderate right hemiparesis, arm greater than leg
- Fluent aphasia, consistent with Wernicke's aphasia
- Left homonymous hemianopia

What do you think caused the patient's current problems? Do you see a potential connection between the patient's medical history and his current problems? Where do you think the damage in the patient's central nervous system is? Are the neurologist's observations what you would expect? If not, why?

Question 2-2 A neurologist is administering a mental status examination to a patient with a suspected left-hemisphere stroke. The mental status examination has a memory test in which the examiner tells the patient three words that the patient is to repeat immediately and again later in the examination.

> **Examiner**: Here are three words. I want you to say them back to me. Remember the words, because I will ask you for them later in this examination. The words are

watch, pen, and *key.* Now say them back to me.

> **Patient**: Flimmer, kidder, kadder.
> **Examiner**: No, listen. Here they are again—*watch, pen, key.*
> **Patient**: Kalder, kammer, mander.

What do you think may account for this patient's performance on this test? Suggest a way in which the neurologist might test this patient's memory for the three words.

Question 2-3 A neurologist examines a patient who complains of sensory loss on the left side of her body. She states that the sensory loss was present when she awoke several days ago and has remained essentially unchanged since that time. During the examination the patient consistently fails to report touch, pinprick, heat, or cold in all regions to the left of her body's midline. The neurologist tests the patient's sense of vibration by placing a vibrating tuning fork on bony structures on both sides of the midline of the patient's body. The patient consistently reports the vibration on the right of the midline, but does not report it at any point to the left of midline. The patient's muscle strength and coordination are normal on both sides of her body, and the remainder of the neurologic examination is within normal limits. The neurologist concludes her report of this patient's neurologic examination with, "The symptoms reported by this patient are not consistent with an organic etiology. Additional testing should seek to rule out a psychogenic origin." What led the neurologist to her conclusion?

Question 2-4 Patients with cerebellar pathology (ataxia), patients with loss of sensation and position sense in the legs, and patients with vestibular abnormalities all typically stand with feet wide apart and become unsteady and may fall if forced to stand with feet close together. A neurologist who examines a patient with such a pattern of behavior may ask the patient to stand with feet close together with eyes open and then with eyes closed. What information might the neurologist gain by asking such a patient to close his or her eyes?

Question 2-5 A 56-year-old man is brought to the neurologist's office by his wife. The man complains of a constant dull headache above his eyes that began several weeks ago and is not helped by analgesics. He comments that his vision has slowly become worse and that perhaps he needs a new prescription for eyeglasses. His wife reports that during the past 2 months her husband has become increasingly impulsive and distractible and has made numerous inappropriate comments to family and friends. The neurologic examination yields the following findings:

- The patient has normal visual acuity in the right eye but has impaired acuity in his left eye.
- The patient's left optic disc is abnormally pale.
- The patient has normal olfaction in the right nostril but complete loss of olfaction in his left nostril.
- The muscles of the patient's lower face have normal strength on the left but are weak on the right.
- The patient's tendon reflexes are slightly exaggerated on his right side compared with his left side.

What do you think caused the patient's neurologic signs and the symptoms reported by the patient and his wife?

Assessing Adults Who Have Neurogenic Cognitive-Communicative Impairments

The solution of any clinical problem is reached by a series of inferences and deductions—each an attempt to explain an item in the history of an illness or a physical finding. Diagnosis is the mental act of integrating all the interpretations and selecting the one explanation most compatible with all the facts of clinical observation. (Adams & Victor, 1981).

Adults who have neurogenic cognitive-communicative impairments are fascinating and challenging. Fascination comes from the seemingly endless array of signs, symptoms, and syndromes associated with neurogenic cognitive-communicative impairments. The challenge comes as the clinician organizes, refines, interprets, and draws conclusions from complex, confusing, and sometimes contradictory information to arrive at a diagnosis and to formulate a plan of care. Challenge also comes from the behavioral, cognitive, and emotional consequences of brain injury, which affect how brain-injured patients respond to unusual, unexpected, or demanding situations such as interviews with strangers in white coats or tests with unfamiliar or difficult materials.

According to Stedman's Medical Dictionary, a *symptom* is "any morbid phenomenon or departure from normal in function, appearance, or sensation, experienced by the patient and indicative of disease." A *sign* is "any abnormality discoverable by the physician at his examination of the patient." A *syndrome* is "a concurrence of symptoms." Symptoms are subjective data reported by the patient; signs are objective data observed by the physician. Syndromes represent inferences made by an examiner, based on patterns of signs and symptoms.

THE PROCESS OF ASSESSMENT AND DIAGNOSIS

Novice clinicians can be intimidated by the complexity of cognitive-communicative disorders and the seeming impossibility of making sense of a bewildering array of signs and symptoms. Watching a skilled clinician evaluate a brain-injured patient may be a mystifying experience for the novice. The novice watches the skilled clinician take the patient through an array of tests that share no discernible common purpose, terminate some tests before completion, modify others without apparent reason, improvise new tests on the spot, arrive at a diagnosis of the patient's cognitive-communicative disorder, offer a prognosis, and decide on the advisability and nature of treatment.

A skilled clinician's idiosyncratic approach to assessment comes from training and clinical experience. The skilled clinician is familiar with the signs, symptoms, and usual course of many cognitive-communicative disorders. The skilled clinician is adept at synthesizing test results and patient behaviors into a pattern that points to a syndrome or a diagnostic category. When a skilled clinician recognizes an emerging pattern of test results, she or he deviates from the standard test routine and focuses on tests that add depth and detail to the pattern. Each test result that fits the expected pattern increases the clinician's confidence that the patient's signs and symptoms represent the suspected syndrome, whereas conflicting information moves the clinician toward an alternative diagnosis.

Skilled clinicians use their clinical knowledge without consciously thinking about it, and they cannot verbalize much of what they know. Add to that the likelihood that much of what they do is based as much on intuition as on rules or principles, and it is not surprising that clinical methods are learned as much or more by observation, practice, and imitation as by direct instruction.

Although there is no substitute for experience, some general principles guide the collection and analysis of clinical data. The principles relate in a general way to the well-known *scientific method,* formalized by John Dewey in the 1930s and repackaged by numerous authors for clinical purposes. The new package is called the *clinical method.*

Practitioners using the clinical method usually use a seven-step procedure to guide clinical decision-making:

1. Gather information about the patient's impairments from the referral, history, and examination of the patient.
2. Evaluate the patient's subjective reports (symptoms) and the objective test results (signs) to identify those that are relevant to the patient's current problems and to the practitioner's plan of care.
3. Determine if a distinctive cluster of symptoms and signs, representing a syndrome, exists.
4. Look for correlations among symptoms and signs to identify the parts of the body or the underlying physical or mental processes responsible.
5. If the patient's symptoms and signs represent a syndrome for which information about the course and eventual outcome of the patient's condition is available, decide on a prognosis.
6. Use information from the patient's history, examination of the patient, and knowledge of the patient's life situation to formulate a conclusion about the effects of the patient's condition on the patient's daily life competence and independence.
7. Use the entire corpus of information about the patient, plus other relevant sources of information (e.g., clinical experience and the clinical and scientific literature) to estimate the potential effects of treatment and, if treatment is indicated, the nature of an appropriate treatment program.

The clinical method requires careful assimilation of information and informed decision-making. Clinical experience helps a skilled clinician sort through an abundance of facts about a patient and select those that are relevant to the clinician's purpose. A clinician who learns that a patient is male, is 55 years old, is hypertensive, has a rash on his chest, complains of numbness on the right side of his face, is missing his left index finger, and misarticulates consonant sounds might select hypertension, facial numbness, and misarticulation as suggesting a stroke and disregard the other signs as not relevant to the clinician's purpose.

As each fact about the patient becomes evident, the clinician evaluates its meaning and relates it to other facts. The process of selection and elimination continues until the clinician understands the nature of the patient's problems, at which time she or he may apply a diagnostic label, consider a prognosis, and make decisions about management.

Clinicians gather facts from the history, the medical record, the interview with the patient and family members, and test results. With each new fact the clinician looks for relationships that might suggest a diagnosis. As additional facts become known, the clinician evaluates the consistency of the new facts with the working diagnosis. When new facts suggest that the working diagnosis is no longer valid, the clinician considers alternative diagnoses and may change tests or examination procedures to gather facts relevant to the new diagnosis. When alternative explanations for the pattern of facts have been eliminated, the clinician settles on the diagnosis most compatible with the facts of the history, interview, and examination.

Harvey Johns, McKusick, and associates (1988; p. 2) summarize the principles of the clinical method:

- The collection and analysis of clinical information are essentially the application of the scientific method to the solution of a clinical problem.
- These methods can be taught and learned; it is not an art in which one is either gifted or not. Proficiency can be improved by consciously considering the meaning of each piece of information as it is received.
- The process is rapidly iterative. The cycle is repeated within the time interval of asking

a few questions or making physical observations. This explains the mystery of why the novice fails to ask the key question or seek the key physical finding.
- The process is an ongoing one. There are no irrefutable hypotheses, only unrefuted hypotheses. In clinical terms, the physician should not arrive at a diagnosis and abandon any further consideration of alternative explanations. The physician must remain alert for information that does not fit with his current hypothesis and for sources of new information that might suggest a new hypothesis. When uncertain, the physician should continue to seek ways of testing the tentative diagnosis.
- Consideration of a diagnosis that can be neither confirmed nor excluded fails to advance the decision-making process. Such a diagnosis is directly parallel to a scientific hypothesis that cannot be tested.
- Finally, clinical problem solving is as sensitive to flawed or missing information as are scientific experiments. A major difference lies in the fact that clinical decisions must often be made on what is acknowledged to be incomplete evidence.

SOURCES OF INFORMATION ABOUT THE PATIENT

The Referral

Physicians recruit specialists into a patient's program of care by means of *consultation requests* (sometimes called *referrals*). Patients with cognitive-communicative disorders usually arrive at the speech-language pathologist's office by means of a physician's referral. Consultation requests typically include the following information about the patient:

- Who the patient is (e.g., the patient's name, birth date, medical file number)
- Where the patient is housed (e.g., hospital ward, service, unit)
- The purpose of the request (what the physician wants from the consultant)

Consultation requests also include the referring physician's name and phone or pager numbers and provide space for the consultant's response.

Consultation requests span a range of completeness, accuracy, and legibility. The good ones are legibly written, describe the patient's major current problems, provide a diagnosis (sometimes provisional), and include a brief statement of the services requested. Most contain numerous abbreviations, both standard and nonstandard, and many are telegraphic.

The advent of computerized consultation and referral procedures has had a positive side effect in that consultation requests are typed into a central computer and printed out on a form. Consequently, those receiving the request no longer are burdened with deciphering the scrawl of handwritten requests. Unfortunately, computerized referrals have had little effect on the arcane and nonstandard abbreviations and terminology used by some physicians, nor have they had any measurable salutary effects on spelling, clarity of style, or literary merit.

Figure 3-1 gives an example of a consultation request for assessment of an aphasic patient's language and communication. The shaded areas contain information provided by the physician.

The consultation request was sent from Dr. Ericcson, a neurologist on a neurology ward. The provisional diagnosis suggests that a patient named Mr. Shaw has had a stroke involving the left middle cerebral artery and that he exhibits severe aphasia. The *Reason for Request* section, when decoded, yields the following information:

Mr. Shaw is a 55-year-old right-handed male who yesterday had a stroke in his left middle cerebral artery. He has right arm and right leg weakness and appears globally aphasic. He has a history of diabetes mellitus and hypertension.

Consultation requests such as this provide an important first look at the patient, the patient's history, the nature and severity of the patient's neurologic impairments, and (sometimes) the probable future course of the patient's condition. By making inferences from the information in the consultation request, the recipient may develop an impression of the patient that goes well beyond the sketchy information provided. Consider the consultation request for Mr. Shaw. The information given there suggests several hypotheses about Mr. Shaw and his cognitive-communicative impairments.

- Mr. Shaw is right-handed and has damage in the distribution of the left middle cerebral artery. He is likely to be aphasic—a hypothesis supported by the neurologist's description.
- Mr. Shaw is weak but not paralyzed on his right side, suggesting that the stroke did not affect major regions of the left hemisphere. He is unlikely to be globally aphasic, as the neurologist's description suggests.
- Mr. Shaw's stroke is recent. The next few weeks should be a period of rapid spontaneous recovery.
- Mr. Shaw is 55 years old. He probably was employed at the time of his stroke. Therefore, his stroke may have important financial consequences.
- Mr. Shaw is diabetic and hypertensive—medical problems that could complicate his physical recovery.
- Mr. Shaw is on a neurology ward. His stay on the neurology ward may be only a few days. Mr. Shaw's short stay may restrict how much testing, family education, and counseling can be accomplished before he is discharged.
- Mr. Shaw and his family are likely to be coming to grips with the personal and familial effects of the stroke. They will need education, support, and reassurance to deal with what has happened and to plan for the future.

Sometimes patients with severe Broca's or Wernicke's aphasia are reported by physicians to be globally aphasic because their severe comprehension impairments and vague, empty, circumlocutory speech give an impression of globally impaired language. Physicians sometimes call patients with severe Broca's aphasia globally aphasic because their inability to talk makes testing

Medical Record	Consultation Request/Referral	
To: Speech Pathology	**From**: Ward 2N Neurology	**Date**: 8/12/07 14:36
Provisional Diagnosis: LMCA CVA, global aphasia		
Requested by: Ericsson, G. 4498	**Place:** Consultant's choice	**Urgency:** Routine
Reason for Request: 55 y/o R-H M 1 day s/p recent L MCA CVA. RUE, RLE weakn. Globally aphasic. Pls eval pt's sp & lang & make recs.		

Consultation Report

Signature and Title:			Date:
ID#:	Organization/Service:	Reg #:	Ward:
Patient Identification: Shaw, Arthur 5/17/52 XXX-XX-9680 2K435-32-NEU			**SF 522 5/07 Consultation Request**

Figure 3-1 ■ The consultation request for Mr. Shaw. The shaded areas contain information provided by the referring physician.

of comprehension (which usually is relatively good) difficult. Globally aphasic patients usually are paralyzed on one side. That Mr. Shaw is weak but not paralyzed on his right side suggests that he is not globally aphasic.

This referral shows how information contained in a consultation request permits inferences that go well beyond the explicit information in the consultation request. Inference making is in many ways an idiosyncratic process that depends on experience, knowledge, and talent for making inferences. What a clinician infers from a consultation request may be idiosyncratic, but the information supporting the inferences is fairly consistent.

Source of the Consultation Request. The source of the request often has implications for a patient's probable length of stay, physical and medical condition, and the speech-language pathologist's role in a patient's care.

Patients in *intensive care units (ICUs)* typically are weak, seriously ill, or comatose. Some have tracheotomies in place (openings into the trachea to provide an alternative airway or to facilitate treatment of respiratory impairments). Patients in ICUs are confined to bed, usually with feeding, medication, or drainage tubes or monitoring equipment attached. Patients in ICUs usually remain there only until their medical condition stabilizes and they no longer need intensive around-the-clock monitoring and care, although a few seriously ill patients may remain there for several weeks. When patients leave the ICU, most are transferred to a medical-surgical ward.

Patients in ICUs usually are referred to a speech-language pathologist because they cannot communicate basic needs or because they have known or suspected swallowing impairments. The speech-language pathologist's typical role is to establish a means by which the patient can communicate basic needs to unit personnel, to evaluate the patient's swallowing, or both.

Most patients on *medical-surgical wards* (including neurology wards, which are a sub-

category of medical wards) are discharged in 3 to 5 days, although some with serious illnesses or those recovering from major surgery may stay longer. Patients on medical-surgical wards usually have acute or evolving medical problems (e.g., recent stroke, pneumonia, or recent surgery). Most can get out of bed, and many are ambulatory, although some may require a cane, crutches, a walker, or a wheelchair to get around.

The primary meaning of *ambulatory* is "capable of walking about." Its secondary meaning is "not confined to bed." I use the word in the latter sense.

Patients on medical-surgical wards are referred to speech-language pathologists for many reasons—for an opinion regarding the presence and severity of a cognitive-communicative or swallowing impairment; for assessment of a patient's speech, language, and cognitive status; for an opinion about the potential benefits of treatment; or for help in resolving a diagnostic question. The speech-language pathologist's focus for patients on medical-surgical wards tends to be on assessment and diagnosis because patients often are discharged before treatment of cognitive-communicative impairments becomes an important part of the plan of care.

Patients on *rehabilitation wards* usually stay for several weeks. Few are acutely ill and almost all are ambulatory, although most get around with the help of canes, crutches, a walker, or a wheelchair. Most receive occupational therapy, physical therapy, recreational therapy, or other therapies while they are on the ward. Speech-language pathologists serving patients on a rehabilitation ward are likely to be on a treatment team with the patient's physician and rehabilitation therapists. Because of their relatively long stays, patients on rehabilitation wards often can get started on treatment of cognitive-communicative impairments before leaving the primary care facility.

Patients in *extended care centers* usually stay for weeks or months. Almost all are ambulatory.

Few are acutely ill, but most have chronic medical problems (e.g., stroke-related impairments or pulmonary disease), and some may be receiving continuing treatment for chronic disease (e.g., kidney dialysis, radiation therapy, or chemotherapy). The focus for these patients is likely to be treatment, although some may require only an assessment and diagnostic work-up.

Most *outpatients* seen in speech-language pathology clinics are persons who have been discharged from a primary care facility but need continuing treatment for cognitive-communicative impairments. Most are ambulatory. Not many are acutely ill, but many have chronic low-level medical problems such as diabetes, cardiovascular disease, or pulmonary disease. Some may have degenerative disease such as multiple sclerosis or cerebellar degeneration. Some may be recovering from strokes, neurologic incidents, or surgery. Physicians refer outpatients to speech-language pathology for many reasons, but most often they wish to know the cause and nature of a patient's cognitive-communicative impairments, to know if treatment of a patient's cognitive-communicative impairments is appropriate, or both.

Patient Demographics. Demographic information from the referral is another source of information about the patient's communication history and potential communicative needs. The patient's age may indicate whether the patient is working or retired and whether dependent children live at home. Younger patients are more likely than older patients to be working, and the families of younger patients are likely to suffer more dramatic financial stresses. Older patients often have multiple medical conditions and physical infirmities that add to the burden of caregivers, and many do not have a living spouse, forcing the burden of care onto children or other family members. If no caregiver is available, the patient may have to go into an extended care center on discharge from the primary care facility.

Medical Diagnosis. The medical diagnosis often suggests the nature and severity of the patient's impairments and potential for recovery by specifying the cause, location, and severity of a patient's nervous system abnormality. Stroke, traumatic brain injury, and degenerative disease yield different predictions about the pattern and degree of a patient's recovery. Damage in the brain hemispheres, for example, may compromise language and cognition, whereas brain stem damage may compromise motor and sensory functions but spare language and cognition. The severity of a patient's nervous system damage usually is indicated by the number and severity of the patient's symptoms, and, in a less direct way, to the outcome of treatment. For example, massive damage in the central zone of the language-dominant hemisphere causes more profound, pervasive, and permanent language impairment than does damage in peripheral regions of the hemisphere.

Services Requested. The services requested in the referral specify the speech-language pathologist's potential role in the patient's care. A physician may refer a patient with progressive neurologic disease and ask for baseline measures of speech, language, and cognition against which the progression of the patient's disease may be measured. A physician may refer a patient with a questionable neurologic diagnosis and ask for testing to clarify the diagnosis. A physician may refer a brain-injured patient whose competence to make financial and legal decisions has been questioned to ascertain whether and how much the patient's communicative and cognitive impairments affect his or her financial and legal competence.

Occasionally a consultation request will focus on one aspect of a patient's care but neglect other aspects of care to which the speech-language pathologist may contribute. For example, a patient with a brain stem stroke may be referred for evaluation of swallowing with no mention of coexisting dysarthria. The speech-language pathologist who knows that dysarthria is a common consequence of brain stem injuries may suggest extending the evaluation to include speech as well as swallowing.

The patient's physician retains primary responsibility for the patient's overall plan of care. Changes or additions to the plan of care prescribed by the physician can be made only with the physician's knowledge and consent.

The Medical Record

The medical record is a legal document that contains a complete record of the patient's medical care. How the information in a medical record is organized depends on the medical facility in which the record is created, but most conform in general to the arrangement described in the following sections. The clinician's review of the medical record almost always provides important indications about the nature and severity of the patient's potential cognitive-communicative impairments.

Patient Identification. Patient identification (name, date of birth, ward, and diagnostic or other codes) usually is printed at the bottom of each page in the record.

Personal History. The patient's personal history contains demographic information about the patient (occupation, marital status, children, where the patient lives and with whom, vocation, and work history). Information about the patient's emotional and social history also may appear here—for example, the presence of previous or current emotional or personal problems; the nature of the patient's relationships with others; and whether the patient has a history of depression, mental illness, alcoholism, or substance abuse.

Medical History. The medical history is written by a physician who interviews the patient or other informant and summarizes the interview in the patient's medical record, sometimes adding information from previous medical records. The medical history describes the patient's previous illnesses, injuries, and medical conditions and the patient's current disabilities and complaints. The medical history documents past medical signs, symptoms, and diagnoses

such as stroke, disorientation, confusion, slurred speech, loss of consciousness, or seizures and lists chronic medical conditions such as diabetes, vascular disease, heart disease, or pulmonary disease.

Figure 3-2 shows the neurologist's summary of Mr. Shaw's medical history, a characteristic one for stroke patients. Diabetes and hypertension increase the risk of stroke, and when they appear in combination, the risk is greater than when either appears separately. Mrs. Shaw's description of the March, 2006 incident, plus Mr. Shaw's history of diabetes and hypertension, suggests a transient ischemic attack at that time.

The events that brought Mr. Shaw to the hospital (see Figure 3-2, *Background*) also are characteristic of a stroke, and their nature and progression suggest an occlusive stroke rather than a brain hemorrhage. Occlusive strokes tend to occur early in the day and are not related to physical exertion. The symptoms usually increase gradually, often in a stepwise manner. Hemorrhagic strokes tend to occur during physical exertion, and symptom development typically is rapid and often is accompanied by headache, nausea, and sometimes vomiting. Mr. Shaw's history of smoking and moderate alcohol consumption are unlikely to have much to do with his current symptoms.

Physical and Neurologic Examination. The neurologist's report of Mr. Shaw's physical and neurologic examination (see Figure 3-2) follows a standard format. It begins with observation of Mr. Shaw's appearance, mood, and orientation (*oriented X3* means oriented to *person, place,* and *time*) and continues with a summary of Mr. Shaw's physical examination. Mr. Shaw's *vital signs* are within normal limits, except for slightly elevated blood pressure. The remainder of the physical examination is unremarkable. (*Lymphadenopathy* means "*enlarged lymph glands;*" *thyromegaly* means "*enlarged thyroid gland.*" *Bruit* is the rushing sound blood makes in a constricted or roughened artery—in this case the carotid artery in Mr. Shaw's neck. *S1, S2, gallop,* and *murmur* are heart sounds.

MEDICAL RECORD	NEUROLOGIC EXAMINATION

Personal History: Mr. Shaw is a 55-y/o accountant (college grad). Married, with two children; son 28, daughter 24, neither living at home. Wife (Florence) is a secondary-school teacher. Nonsmoker x 10 yrs. Occasional social ETOH -- non-abuser. Both parents deceased (mid-80s), apparently of natural causes. Employed at time of apparent neurologic incident.

Medical History: Past medical history includes adult-onset diabetes mellitus diagnosed in 1991, hypertension diagnosed 1993, and a possible TIA in March of last year. The patient's wife reports that at the time of the apparent TIA they were watching television when the patient became confused, did not answer questions, and seemed not to understand. The patient's symptoms apparently cleared in an hour or two, and they did not seek medical advice or assistance. Medications on admission include tolbutamide 500 mg twice a day, chlorothiazide 500 mg twice a day, which apparently control the patient's hypertension and diabetes, and occasionally aspirin.

Background: The patient was accompanied to this medical center by his wife, who provided this information. The patient apparently was in good health until this apparent neurologic event, which occurred at approximately 0815 hrs this day. The patient was getting dressed for work when he experienced a sudden onset of speech difficulties and leg weakness. The patient did not vomit, lose consciousness, or report double vision, nausea or vertigo. He arrived at the emergency room at this medical center at 0905 hrs. The neurologic examination began at approximately 0920 hrs.

Habits: The patient is an ex-smoker (0.5 ppd x 10 years) and has not smoked for approximately the past 10 years. The patient apparently drinks three or four glasses of wine per week and other alcoholic drinks occasionally but his wife reports that he has never been a heavy drinker.

Physical Examination: The patient looks his stated age and is in no apparent distress. He appears alert and is oriented x 3. **Vital signs:** Blood pressure 162/89, pulse 72, temperature 98.6, respiration 18. **HEENT exam:** No signs of trauma or deformation. Moist mucous membranes. Neck negative for lymphadenopathy or thyromegaly. No carotid bruit. **Cardiovascular exam:** Normal S1, S2, without gallop or murmurs. **Lungs:** clear to auscultation. **Abdomen:** soft and nontender. No organomegaly or palpable masses. **Lower extremities:** no pedal edema.

Neurologic Examination: The patient is globally aphasic. Listening comprehension evaluation showed that he is able to follow very simple commands like "close your eyes" or "open your mouth." He is unable to give yes-no answers to questions. He is a little bit confused as to right/left commands. He is unable to do complex commands. Reading evaluation showed the patient unable to identify a letter. He had paraphasic errors in single-word identification (example: "wrisp" for "wrist"). The patient was unable to follow commands on reading because of inability to comprehend. Expression evaluation showed that the patient was unable to read a narrative. He was unable to repeat "no ifs, ands, or buts." He was also unable to name objects like watch or pin. **Cranial nerve examination:** It was difficult to examine the patient's visual acuity because of his aphasia. Acuity appears within normal limits, but the patient exhibits a questionable right-sided field cut. Funduscopic examination showed no evidence of papilledema. His pupils are 3 to 4 mm bilaterally, round, equal, and reactive to light and accomodation.. He had intact extraocular movements. His corneal reflexes are present bilaterally. His jaw jerk was +1. He had symmetrical nasolabial folds and wrinkles. His tongue is midline and so is his uvula. He has symmetrical gag reflex bilaterally. He has symmetrical strength in his shoulders bilaterally. **Motor examination:** The patient has no pronator drift and no involuntary movements. His muscle tone is normal bilaterally. His strength appears 5/5 on the left and 4/5 in the right upper extremity and 3/5 in the right lower extremity. Grasp reflex on right. He had external rotation in his right lower extremity. His coordination exam was unremarkable for dysmetria. Deep tendon reflexes are +2 on the left and +3 on the right, except +1 in both ankles. Plantar reflex on right. **Sensory examination:** Impossible to establish accurately because of patient's aphasia. However, the patient withdraws both lower and upper extremities to pinprick stimuli. **Gait:** The patient walks slowly, but with symmetrical arm swings bilaterally. Mild dragging of right foot.

Problem List:
1. Probable LH stroke.
2. Aphasia
3. Hypertension
4. Adult-onset diabetes mellitus.

(Signed)

G. Ericsson

Date: 8/11/07

G. Ericsson, M.D.

Patient ID
Shaw, Arthur 5/17/52
XXX-XX-9680
2K435-32 NEU

MEDICAL RECORD

NEUROLOGIC EXAMINATION

Figure 3-2 ■ The report of the neurologist's examination of Mr. Shaw.

Auscultation refers to "listening to the sounds of various body structures," usually by means of a stethoscope. *Organomegaly* means *"enlarged organs." Palpable* means *"detectable by touch." Pedal edema* means *"swelling of feet or ankles."*)

The neurologist's description of Mr. Shaw's speech and comprehension suggests that Mr. Shaw is aphasic and that he has severely impaired comprehension. Because little information about Mr. Shaw's speech is provided, it is not clear from the neurologist's report whether Mr. Shaw truly is globally aphasic or has severe Wernicke's aphasia.

The neurologist's examination of Mr. Shaw's cranial nerve functions follows the standard top-down format, beginning with visual acuity (CN 2) and moving on to eye movements and pupillary responses (CN 3, CN 4, CN 6); face (CN 5, CN 7); tongue, larynx, and pharynx (CN 9, CN 10, CN 12); and neck and shoulders (CN 11). The results of testing Mr. Shaw's cranial nerves do not suggest cranial nerve damage. Symmetric nasolabial folds and symmetric facial wrinkles suggest that there is no significant damage in corticobulbar tracts serving the lower face, which in turn suggests no major frontal lobe involvement and slightly diminishes the probability that Mr. Shaw is globally aphasic. The neurologist reports a slightly diminished jaw-jerk reflex—of minor significance, given the negative results of other cranial nerve function tests.

The neurologist's omission of CN 1 testing is typical. CN 1 is rarely tested in routine neurologic examinations unless the physician has reason to suspect pathology in the olfactory nerve or the olfactory cortex.

The neurologist's examination of Mr. Shaw's motor functions reveals slight weakness on Mr. Shaw's right side. Mr. Shaw's leg is somewhat weaker than his arm. Reflexes are brisk on his right side but diminished in both ankles. Mr. Shaw has a grasp reflex in his right hand, and a probable plantar extensor (Babinski) reflex

in his right foot. These findings are consistent with damage affecting Mr. Shaw's left-side corticospinal tract. That Mr. Shaw's weakness is not severe is consistent with damage that spares most corticospinal fibers.

A *grasp reflex* is an involuntary closing of the hand when the patient's palm is stroked. It is a sign of upper motor neuron damage in the contralateral corticospinal tract. *Pronator drift* is a sign of muscle weakness. It appears when the patient is asked to hold out his or her arms with palms up and eyes closed. Weakness in arm muscles causes the weak arm to rotate toward a more natural palms-down position, and sometimes the weak arm sags in response to the pull of gravity. Mild weakness in leg muscles sometimes causes the leg to rotate outward, especially when the patient is lying down.

The neurologist's examination of Mr. Shaw's somesthetic sensory functions and gait are generally unremarkable, except for a slight right foot drag, which is consistent with the motor examination. Overall, the neurologic examination suggests that Mr. Shaw has had a stroke involving the posterior left hemisphere, with possible scattered damage extending into the frontal lobe. The most probable communication diagnosis appears to be one of Wernicke's aphasia.

The results of the physician's examination of the patient (including the neurologic examination) are reported here. The physician's report of the examination usually ends with a *problem list,* in which relevant preexisting and current symptoms and the patient's complaints are summarized.

Doctor's Orders. Doctor's orders are written by the patient's primary physician and other professionals to establish the conditions for the patient's care, including medications, special precautions, tests and consultations, diet, monitoring of fluid or caloric intake, and rehabilitation services. Information from the doctor's orders gives an overall sense of the plan of care for the patient, including laboratory tests ordered, medications prescribed, diet modifications or restrictions ordered, therapies requested, and specialists consulted. Each order is signed and dated by the person who writes the order. The person who performs the order initials it and writes the time at which it was performed.

Figure 3-3 shows the neurologist's orders for the period immediately following Mr. Shaw's admission. The first order is for a computerized tomography (CT) scan of Mr. Shaw's head to rule out cerebral hemorrhage. Head CT scans are one of the first laboratory tests ordered for patients with probable strokes because the medical treatment of hemorrhagic strokes is markedly different from that of occlusive strokes. Treatment of occlusive strokes often entails administration of blood thinners (anticoagulants), and blood thinners worsen hemorrhagic strokes. Consequently, ruling out cerebral hemorrhage is a critical concern in the early phase of treatment. The neurologist's next order is for an electrocardiogram, perhaps to rule out coronary artery disease or atrial fibrillations as a source of emboli.

Atrial fibrillations are irregularities in the heartbeat in which the normal rhythmic contractions of heart muscles are replaced by rapid and irregular contractions. The rapid and irregular contractions may cause blood clots or fragments of tissue to break loose and travel through the blood stream.

The next order gives permission for Mr. Shaw to be out of bed and sitting in a chair, but not to walk unassisted—a routine precaution for patients in the first day or two poststroke. The next order prescribes continuation of the medications Mr. Shaw has been taking for his hypertension and diabetes. The neurologist prescribes a standard low-fat, low-salt diet. (In most medical facilities a dietician sees all newly admitted patients and recommends diets to meet their nutritional and hydration needs.) The last order on Day 1 is for laboratory tests of coagulation time and sedimentation rate,

which reflect the time it takes Mr. Shaw's blood to clot. Shorter-than-normal coagulation time and faster-than-normal sedimentation rate suggest a risk of blood clots in the vascular system and may be an indication that anticoagulant therapy is needed.

On Day 2 the neurologist orders a carotid ultrasound to determine if Mr. Shaw has stenosis (narrowing) of his carotid arteries. The order suggests that the neurologist is moving toward a diagnosis of occlusive stroke. Neurologists often order carotid ultrasound tests early in the care of patients with suspected occlusive strokes. If the results show stenosis, the probability that the patient's stroke is occlusive increases. If the stenosis is severe, the neurologist may order a follow-up cerebral angiogram to get a more precise indication of the location, severity, and nature of the stenosis than can be ascertained from the somewhat fuzzy image provided by the carotid ultrasound.

The neurologist also orders referrals to speech-language pathology, social work, and rehabilitation medicine and amends his previous day's order to permit Mr. Shaw to move around the ward without assistance, probably in response to observations that walking poses him no risk. Finally, the neurologist orders laboratory analysis of a sample of Mr. Shaw's blood to determine if the level of fatty compounds that play a part in atherosclerosis is elevated.

Progress Notes. Progress notes are written by patient care personnel to provide a chronologic record of the patient's physical, behavioral, and mental status. The admitting physician writes the first progress note, which includes a brief description of the patient, a summary of the patient's history, and a summary of significant aspects of the physical and neurologic examination. The physician's opening progress note usually ends with conclusions about diagnostic issues and a plan for the patient's care.

Entries in the progress notes by physicians, nurses, ward personnel, and other specialists provide information about the patient's alert-

MEDICAL RECORD	DOCTOR'S ORDERS

DATE AND TIME	PROB. NO.	ORDERS	NURSE'S INITIALS
8/11/07 1035	1	**Lab:** Head CT with contrast. R/O hemorrhage vs occlusion *Ericsson*	KEG 1045
8/11/07 1035	1	**Lab:** EKG. 55-y/o male with probable CVA, aphasia. *Ericsson*	MRB 1045
8/11/07 1035	1	Activity: Up in chair as tolerated. *Ericsson*	KEG 1045
8/11/07 1035	3, 4	Meds: chlorothiazide 0.5g. b.i.d. tolbutamide 0.5g. b.i.d. *Ericsson*	KEG 1055
8/11/07 1035	1,3	Diet: Low fat, no added salt. *Ericsson*	MRB 1055
8/11/07 1035	1	**Lab:** coag time, sed rate. *Ericsson*	MRB 1100
8/12/07 0905		**Lab:** Carotid u/s. R/O stenosis *Ericsson*	MRB 0930
8/12/07 1420	2	Speech Pathology consult: 55 y/o R-H M 1 day s/p L MCA CVA. RUE, RLE weakn. Globally aphas. Hx DM, HTN. Pls eval pt's spch & lang & make recs. *Ericsson*	MRB 1435
8/12/07 1420	1, 2	Social work consult: 55 y/o M 1 day s/p L MCA CVA. Globally aphasic. Pls assist with d/c planning. *Ericsson*	MRB 1440
8/12/07 1420	1	Rehab consult: 55 y/o M 1 day s/p L MCA CVA. Globally aphasic. RUE, RLE weakness. Pls assess and make rec's. *Ericsson*	MRB 1440
8/12/07 1600	1	Activity: No restrictions on ward. Pt. not to leave ward w/o supervision. *Ericsson*	KEG 1620
8/12/07 1600	1	**Lab:** serum triglycerides, cholesterol. *Ericsson*	KEG 1620

Patient Identification:
    Shaw, Arthur 5/17/52
    XXX-XX-9680
    2K435-32 NEU   **DOCTOR'S ORDERS**

Figure 3-3 ■ Excerpts from the physician's orders for Mr. Shaw's care.

ness, orientation, and mood and the patient's responses to caregivers and behavior toward other patients on the ward; they also may indicate whether the patient can walk, dress, bathe, and accomplish other activities of daily living. Reports and recommendations from specialists such as psychologists, social workers, and physical therapists provide insights into aspects of the patient's condition not covered by the physical and neurologic examination.

Figure 3-4 gives a page of progress notes from Mr. Shaw's medical record. The first entry is the neurologist's admitting note. A summary of the neurologic examination follows. The A/P (assessment/plan) section describes the neurologist's diagnostic hunches and plans for the patient's care. From the neurologist's plans for carotid ultrasound and a magnetic resonance imaging (MRI) angiogram, it appears that he suspects an occlusive stroke but has decided not to anticoagulate Mr. Shaw (because he first wants to see the results of the CT scan). If the CT shows no hemorrhage, the neurologist plans to administer anticoagulant medications. The neurologist also plans to include rehabilitation medicine, speech-language pathology, social work, and ophthalmology in Mr. Shaw's care, no doubt to deal with his weakness, aphasia, post-hospital placement, and potential visual field blindness, respectively.

The progress notes continue with several entries by nursing personnel, which give a picture of Mr. Shaw as ambulatory, alert, and oriented but with significant communication impairments. Several comments suggest that Mr. Shaw is aphasic, with significant problems in understanding what others say *(understanding seems to be a major problem, tends to ramble, doesn't appear frustrated or even acknowledge the communication block, doesn't always get what you say)*. However, he appears to be pleasant, cooperative, and helpful, suggesting that behavioral abnormalities are unlikely to be a major management issue. The last entry is by the speech-language pathologist, who acknowledges receipt of the consultation request,

gives her initial impressions, and directs those reading the progress note to a language-screening assessment reported elsewhere in the progress notes.

Laboratory Reports. Most medical records have a separate section for laboratory reports. Results of procedures such as blood tests, CT scans, and electroencephalographic (EEG) reports are found in this section of the medical record. The laboratory tests ordered by the physician often provide insights into the physician's diagnostic hunches and the nature of the physician's concerns about the patient's medical needs.

Figures 3-5 and 3-6 contain examples of two reports from the *laboratory reports* section of Mr. Shaw's medical record. Figure 3-5 shows the neuroradiologist's report of a head CT scan. It suggests that Mr. Shaw has had an occlusive stroke in the white matter beneath the left temporo-parietal cortex and that the stroke extends into the cortex. The stroke apparently was caused by occlusion in a posterior branch of the middle cerebral artery. Importantly, there is no evidence of hemorrhagic stroke.

Figure 3-6 shows the radiologist's report of Mr. Shaw's carotid ultrasound test. It indicates that Mr. Shaw has thickening of the arterial walls and atherosclerotic plaque distributed throughout both carotid arteries. Neither Mr. Shaw's left nor right common carotid arteries are significantly narrowed, but both internal carotid arteries show significant stenosis, the right carotid artery having greater stenosis than the left. Mr. Shaw's left external carotid artery also may be narrowed, as indicated by increased blood velocities during the systolic phase of Mr. Shaw's heartbeat.

Figure 3-7 shows how information from Mr. Shaw's medical record is transferred to a form used in a speech and language clinic. The form includes personal information about Mr. Shaw, labels his communication disorder, and summarizes the information from Mr. Shaw's medical record. The information in such forms provides a quick reference for speech pathology

MEDICAL RECORD	PROGRESS NOTES

Date, Time	Note
8/11/07 1015	Neurology Admit Note: 55-y/o man s/p L MCA stroke 8/11/07 approx. 8:15 a.m. Pt apparently in good health previously. Sudden onset RUE, RLE weakness, slurred speech. Brought to MC by wife. No apparent preceding symptoms or headache. **PMH:** AODM, x 5 yrs. HTN x 3 yrs. Poss. TIA 3/95. **PE:** BP 162/89. P 72. T 98.6 R 18. Lungs clear. Neck supple, Mental Status: Pt awake & responsive, though inappropriate. Responds "I'm fine." Cannot give name or repeat. Follows midline commands -- close eyes, open mouth. Cannot follow complex commands. CN: EOM full, no nystagmus. Pupils equal, reactive. Face symmetric. Tongue midline. Palate midline, elevates symmetrically. Motor. Unable fo follow specific commands. Appears to give normal resistance in arms and legs. Can walk with support. R leg externally rotated when lying. Inc. grasp, plantar on R. Coordination: able to follow and locate moving target. **A/P:** Pt presents with acute alteration in language and comprehension. Also subtle signs of motor deficit on R. Obtain CT or MRI to r/o bleed. Stroke vs TIA most likely diagnosis. Obtain carotid ultrasound for risk factors. Consider MRI angiogram for vascular abnormalities. No clear indication for anticoagulation. Consider ASA or ticlopidine if CT shows no bleed. Will consult rehab, spch, sw, opth. G. Ericsson, M.D.
8/11/07 1105	**Nursing Admission Note**. Pt. alert, oriented in no apparent distress. Wife present, participated in orientation to ward. Pt. is responsive to stimulation, but unable to respond with appropriate answers. Can transfer from bed to chair w/o assistance. Sits upright w/o tipping. Walks with assistance, but seems to have no problems with strength, balance, judgment. No signs of confusion. Continent x2. May need assistance with ADLs for a few days. Not an apparent fall risk. Patient can talk, but doesn't always make sense. Can say name, "I'm fine," "o.k." etc. Understanding seems to be a major problem. L Smith, RN
8/11/07 1245	**Nursing note.** Pt. alert, oriented. Pleasant & cooperative. Tends to ramble. Needs to be kept on one subject as much as possible. Wife came in with pt. Very concerned. Needs reassurance, support. L Smith, RN
8/11/07 1500	**Nursing note.** Pt. ambulating w/o assistance. Had late lunch. Appetite good. Pleasant and helpful. Offers no complaints. M Benson, RN
8/11/07 1805	**Nursing note.** Patient seems to have severe receptive and expressive communication probs. Doesn't appear frustrated or even acknowledge the communication block. Needs seem to be met. No problems with ADLs. M Benson, RN
8/11/07 2200	**Nursing note.** Pt sleeping calmly. No apparent prob's. G Taylor, RNA
8/12/07 0610	**Nursing note.** Slept all night. No complaints. Awake and alert. Carried out ADLs w/o assistance. Doesn't always get what you say. Sometimes helps to repeat, remind pt. of topic. L Smith, RN
8/12/07 1000	**Speech-Language Pathology Note:** Consultation request received. Pt. seen briefly @ bedside. Impression: moderate-severe Wernicke's aphasia. Full report to follow. G Becker, M.A., CCC-SLP

Patient ID
   Shaw, Arthur 5/17/52   **MEDICAL RECORD**
   XXX-XX-9680
   2K435-32 NEU   **PROGRESS NOTES**

Figure 3-4 ■ A series of progress notes from Mr. Shaw's medical record. The notes are not necessarily continuous. Ordinarily several notes would be entered on a patient's first day on the ward. (See *Appendix* for definitions of medical abbreviations.)

MEDICAL RECORD
RADIOGRAPHIC REPORT

NAME: Shaw, Arthur   **WARD:** 2N, Neur

ID#: XXX-XX-9680   **REQ. M.D.:** Ericsson

AGE: 55   **CASE #** 3937

DATE OF EXAMINATION : August 12, 2007: 1433

EXAMINATION: CT HEAD WITH CONTRAST

Clinical History:
55-year old mate with suspected EH stroke 8/11/07. Rule out hemorrhage.

Comparisons: There are no previous studies available for comparison.

Findings: Enhanced CT scan of the head. A new area of decreased attenuation in the left temporo-parietal white matter and extending into the overlying cortex, consistent with a new occlusive infarct. No evidence of hemorrhage. The ventricles are at midline position without evidence of mass effect.

Impressions: New area of infarction in the left temporo-parietal region consistent with occlusion of posterior branch of left middle cerebral artery. See above findings.

Films were read by: *Mary C. Richman*

                    Mary C. Richman, M. D., Neuroradiologist

Figure 3-5 ■ A computerized tomography (CT) scan report from Mr. Shaw's medical record.

MEDICAL RECORD
RADIOGRAPHIC REPORT

NAME: Shaw, Arthur   **WARD:** 2N, Neuro
ID#: XXX-XX-9680   **REQ. M.D.:** Ericsson
AGE: 55   **CASE #:** 2302

DATE OF EXAMINATION: August 13, 2007: 0803
EXAMINATION: NON-INVASIVE CAROTID W IMAGING

Clinical History:
55-year old male with suspected LH stroke 8/11/07. Rule out carotid stenosis.

Comparisons: There are no previous studies available for comparison.

Findings: Intimal thickening and focal areas of soft plaque are identified throughout both carotid systems.

The right common carotid artery has no associated hemodynamically significant stenosis. The right internal carotid artery has increased peak systolic velocities of 160cm per second. This is consistent with a severe stenosis (60% to 79%) of the right internal carotid artery. The right external carotid artery demonstrates no hemodynamically significant stenosis.

The left common carotid demonstrates no associated hemodynamically significant stenosis. The left internal carotid artery has slightly increased peak systolic velocities of 130 to 140 cm per second with a diastolic velocity of 40 cm per second. This is consistent with a mild to moderate stenosis (20 to 59%) of the left internal carotid artery. There are increased peak systolic velocities in the left external carotid artery consistent with an underlying stenosis.

Impressions:
1. Severe stenosis (60 to 79%) of the right internal carotid artery.
2. Mild to moderate stenosis (20 to 59%) of the left internal carotid artery.
3. Increased peak systolic velocities of left external carotid artery consistent with underlying stenosis.
4. Right vertebral artery not visualized on this examination.

Films were read by: W. E. Davies

                    Warren E. Davies, M.D., Radiologist

Figure 3-6 ■ A report of a carotid ultrasound test from Mr. Shaw's medical record.

SPEECH PATHOLOGY SERVICE

Patient Information

Patient Name: Shaw, Arthur	**Soc Sec Number:** XXX-XX-9680	**Referral Date:** 8/12/07
Home Address:	**Occupation:** Accountant	**Physician:** Ericsson 4498
6877 Lakeview Court	**Marital Status:** M (Florence)	**Med Diagnoses:**
Riverview, MN 55444-1212	**Education:** College (B.A.)	L MCA CVA, aphasia
Birthdate: *5/17/52*	**Home Phone:** 612/ 555-9888	
Referring Ward: 2N (Neuro)	**Referring Service:** Neurology	**SPS File #:** 6888

Communication, Swallowing Disorders

Problem #1: Aphasia	**Date of Onset:** 8/11/07
Problem #2:	**Date of Onset:**
Problem #3:	**Date of Onset:**

Medical Information

Previous Medical History: Adult onset diabetes mellitus diagnosed 1991. Controlled by oral medications.
Hypertension diagnosed November 1993. Pt's wife mentioned brief episode of numbness in pt's RUE in March, 2006 – MD: "possible TIA."

History of Present Illness: The patient apparently was in good health until the morning of August 11. He was dressing for work when he experienced sudden onset of right-sided weakness and slurred speech. He alerted his wife who called an ambulance which brought him to the emergency room at this medical center. On arrival he exhibited extreme weakness and exaggerated reflexes on his right side. His speech apparently was fluent with verbal paraphasias and some jargon, and his comprehension was grossly impaired. Since that time he apparently has been improving slowly, although he seems still to have a substantial aphasia. Nursing notes suggest that he is oriented and alert.

Laboratory Results: CT Scan: "New area of decreased attenuation in the left temporo-parietal white matter, extending into cortex, c/w new occlusive infarct. No evidence of hemorrhage. Carotid u/s: Severe stenosis R ICA (60-79%), mild-moderate stenosis LICA (20-50%).

BP: 162/89.

Medications: tolbutamide, chlorothiazide

Other: Low fat low salt diet. Consult to SW: "Pls assist with d/c planning." Consult to Rehab: "RUE, RLE weakness, pls assess and make rec's."

Clinician: G. Becker, Ph.D, CCC-SLP   **Signature:** *G. Becker*
SPEECH-LANGUAGE PATHOLOGIST   **Date:**   8/12/07

Figure 3-7 ■ A form used by the speech-language pathologist to record information from Mr. Shaw's medical record.

clinic personnel who may be involved in Mr. Shaw's care and serves as a record of Mr. Shaw's medical history and current problems should that information be needed in the future if his medical records are not available.

The speech-language pathologist's review of a patient's medical record provides information about the patient's medical and neurologic problems, potential cognitive-communicative impairments, and behavioral and emotional state—information that may help to organize assessment of language and communication. The impressions gleaned from the patient's medical record are firmed up by an interview with the patient and assessment of the patient's cognition, language, and communication. Then the speech-language pathologist writes a response to the consultation request (Figure 3-8).

The response to the consultation request follows a common format. It begins with subjective observations, describes the results of objective tests, interprets the test results, and offers an opinion regarding the nature of the patient's problems and their probable time course. It concludes with recommendations for dealing with the problems noted in the referral. The response to the consultation request is brief and to the point (most physicians and other healthcare personnel are reluctant to read long and complex reports). Tests are described in everyday language, and examples of test items are provided. (The names of most tests of cognitive-communicative ability and scores on such tests have little meaning to most persons who are not speech-language pathologists.) The format of the report makes it easy for the person reading the consultation request to get information from the report.

GENERAL CONCEPTS 3-1

- Skilled clinicians use a structured approach when they evaluate adults who have neurogenic cognitive-communicative impairments. Most use some form of what is called the *clinical method*. The clinical method is a structured procedure for making clinical decisions about diagnosis, testing, prognosis, and treatment.

- The *referral* (consultation request) gives the speech-language pathologist an important first look at the patient. The referral usually provides personal information about the patient together with indications of the patient's medical, physical, and behavioral condition, medical diagnoses, probable length of stay, and the physician's plans for the patient's care.

- *Medical records* typically are divided into sections, with each section containing a different kind of information about a patient:

- *Patient identification:* Personal information about the patient, plus diagnostic or other codes
- *Medical history:* Information about previous medical conditions and a summary of the patient's current symptoms
- *Physical and neurologic examination:* The physician's findings from examination of the patient
- *Doctor's orders:* Orders, instructions, special precautions, consultation referrals, requests for medications, and requests for special tests
- *Progress notes:* Descriptions of the patient's physical, behavioral, and mental status; descriptions of significant events or incidents (e.g., falls, emotional outbursts)

Continued on page 112

Medical Record	Consultation Request/Referral	
To: Speech Pathology	**From**: Ward 2N Neurology	**Date**: 8/12/07 14:36

Provisional Diagnosis: LMCA CVA, global aphasia

Requested by: Ericsson, G. 4498	**Place:** Consultant's choice	**Urgency:** Routine

Reason for Request: 55 y/o R-H M 1 day s/p recent L MCA CVA. RUE, RLE weakn. Globally aphasic. Pls eval pt's sp & lang & make recs.

Consultation Report

Mr. Shaw's speech and language was evaluated in the Speech Pathology Clinic on 8/14/07.

Subjective Observations: Mr. Shaw is a 55-year-old man who experienced a left middle cerebral artery CVA on August 11, 2007. Mr. Shaw was brought to the speech pathology clinic in a wheelchair, although he later claimed that he can walk, although "I guess I'm a little unsteady on my feet." During the evaluation he was cooperative, attentive, alert, and task-oriented, although the presence of a severe auditory comprehension impairment markedly compromised his conversational and test-taking abilities.

Objective Measures: Several speech and language tests were administered. Mr. Shaw's performance suggested:
- Severe impairment of listening comprehension. Mr. Shaw can correctly identify drawings of common objects named by the examiner on about 50% of trials. He can follow one-step commands ("Pick up the spoon") with about 50% accuracy, but cannot follow 2-step commands ("Point to the pencil and give me the key.")
- Severe impairment of speech production. Mr. Shaw's speech, both in conversation and during testing, is vague, devoid of meaning, and littered with verbal paraphasias ("chair" for "table") and literal paraphasias("spomb" for "comb"). Occasional neologisms (nonwords) are also observed. However, the mechanics of Mr. Shaw's speech production are relatively unaffected -- he speaks smoothly and effortlessly, with essentially normal rate, intonation, and stress patterns.
- Severely compromised reading ability. Mr. Shaw can read a few simple concrete words ("man," "dog") but cannot read multisyllabic words or longer units. Failed attempts are characterized by paraphasias and neologisms.
- Severely compromised writing ability. Mr. Shaw could copy his name, with effort, but could write nothing intelligible either spontaneously or to dictation.

Impressions and Conclusions: Mr. Shaw currently exhibits symptoms consistent with severe Wernicke's (receptive) aphasia. Because of the recent onset of Mr. Shaw's aphasia, the severity of his language impairments should diminish during the next several weeks, although he is likely to remain moderately aphasic even when full neurologic recovery has taken place. His return to employability appears, at this time, unlikely.

Recommendations:
1. Additional assessment of Mr. Shaw's listening comprehension to determine the extent and nature of his comprehension impairments.
2. A period of trial treatment to improve auditory comprehension and self-monitoring to determine Mr. Shaw's potential to benefit from treatment.
3. Speech-language pathologist to meet with Mr. Shaw's wife and other concerned family members to answer questions and discuss Mr. Shaw's potential return home.

The patient was examined: [x] yes   [ ] no
The patient's medical record was reviewed: [x] yes   [ ] no

Signature and Title: *G Becker* G. Becker, Ph.D., CCC Speech-Language Pathologist	**Date:** 8/14/07	
ID#: 133591	**Organization/Service:** Speech Pathology	**Reg #:** -	**Ward:** -
Patient Identification: Shaw, Arthur 5/17/52 XXX-XX-9680 2K435-32-NEU	**SF 522 5/98** **Consultation Request**	

Figure 3-8 ■ The speech-language pathologist's response to the consultation request by Mr. Shaw's physician.

GENERAL CONCEPTS 3-1—cont'd

- *Laboratory reports:* Results of tests such as x-ray imaging, CT scans, and analysis of blood or tissues
- Responses to consultation requests follow a common format. Results of objective tests are described first, followed by the consultant's interpretation of the test results, and it concludes with the consultant's recommendations. Responses to consultation requests are succinct, well-structured, and written in everyday language.

INTERVIEWING THE PATIENT

The interview provides the first direct look at the patient's cognitive-communicative abilities, physical condition, orientation and attention, visual and hearing acuity, behavioral inclinations, and other characteristics that might affect how (or if) assessment of cognition, language, and communication is carried out. Getting the interview off to a good start is as important as its information-gathering function. There is no single best way to do this, and different clinicians may approach a given patient in different ways with equivalent results. The most successful, however, share two common attributes—they are dedicated to helping the patient, and they treat the patient with respect. In addition to dedication and respect, good interviewers follow several basic principles that govern the form and content of the interview. The principles are described as follows:

- *Do your homework before the interview.* Review the patient's medical record to get a sense of the patient's personal history, medical history, and medical problems. Talk with the patient's physician and with nursing staff to gain insights that may not be in the medical record. The homework helps you ask the right questions during the interview, and it will help you focus on the most relevant information for testing diagnostic hunches.

It also may help you avoid topics that may make the patient feel upset, apprehensive, or threatened.

- *Conduct the interview in a quiet place, free from distractions.* Many first interviews are held at the patient's bedside. A bedside interview is fine if the room has no distractions. If the patient's room is not free of distractions, find another place nearby— a day room, a conference room, an empty patient room, or, if nothing is available on the patient's ward, move the interview to a quiet room off the ward.
- *Tell the patient who you are.* In teaching hospitals, patients are seen by a confusing mix of physicians, residents, medical students, interns, and others, many of whom pop in and out of the patient's room without introduction or explanation. Helping the patient sort this mix usually makes for a more relaxed and less stressed patient. Regrettably, physicians sometimes neglect to tell patients that they are referring them to other specialists, so patients are surprised and concerned when the specialist arrives unannounced. Therefore, it is important that you make certain that the patient knows who you are and why the physician asked you to see them. Introduce yourself and tell the patient why you are there:

> *I'm Ms. Smith. I'm from the speech clinic. Dr. Jones said that you might be having some problems speaking. I'll be working with you to find out if you do, and we'll talk about what we might be able to do about them.*

Tell the patient your role in the patient's care:

> *Your doctor will take care of your medical problems. The physical therapist will work on your walking and help you regain strength in your arm. I'll be working with you on talking, writing, and understanding.*

Boll (1994) recommends that the interviewer begin by asking the patient why the patient's physician has referred him or her to the specialist. According to Boll, the patient's response gives the interviewer a sense of the patient's comprehension of the circumstances, his or her level of interest and motivation, his or her comfort with the arrangements, and the adequacy with which the referral has been handled by the person making the referral. According to Boll, it also gives the interviewer a sense of whether the patient has been informed about the nature of the interview, and whether the information has been understood, ignored, or forgotten.

- *Make the patient comfortable.* Spend a few minutes in conversation to allow the patient to relax and talk about familiar topics. Ask the patient some general questions: *Where are you from? What kind of work do you do? Are you married? Do you have children/grandchildren?* This usually helps put the patient at ease, especially if the interviewer can discover common ground, such as knowledge of the patient's home town, culture, or mutual interests.

Some patients (in my experience, not many) react emotionally to questions about family and occupation because of concern about compromised family and work relationships and responsibilities. The interviewer must be sensitive to the potential effect of such topics and should be prepared to move away from them if the patient shows signs of emotional upset.

- *Sit down during the interview.* A standing interviewer conversing with a seated or recumbent patient can be intimidating. Regardless of the length of the interview, standing during the interview may give the patient a feeling that you are on the way to somewhere more important and that the patient is an unwelcome intrusion into your busy schedule. Try to give the patient the sense that you are getting to know him or her, that his or her concerns are important to you, and that there

is nothing that you would rather be doing than talking with him or her.

- *Get the patient's story.* Begin with a general question: *How are you feeling today?* Follow with additional questions or commentary that seems appropriate: *I'm glad you're feeling better. It's nice to see you up and out of bed.* Then move on to the patient's cognitive-communicative problems: *Are you having difficulty talking? Tell me about it.* Find out how the patient feels about the problems. Some patients may be traumatized about impairments that most would consider minor annoyances, whereas others are unconcerned about dramatic impairments. Make mental notes of what the patient says and pursue any interesting leads. Note significant aspects of the patient's condition and behavior—whether the patient is ambulatory and able to sit up and attend for the length of time needed for testing; the patient's mood, orientation, and mental status; the patient's visual and auditory acuity; and whether the patient wears dentures, eyeglasses, or a hearing aid.

- *Be a patient, concerned, and understanding listener.* Give the patient time to tell his or her story. Don't interrupt and don't lead, unless the patient gets bogged down in trivial details or goes off on tangents unrelated to the purpose of the interview. Ask questions to follow up on potentially meaningful information, but do not steer the patient to provide the answers you expect based on your preconceptions. Don't be overly solicitous and overly sympathetic. Adult patients don't need (and often resent) overdone expressions of concern and sympathy. Receive what the patient says objectively and treat the interview as a problem-solving collaboration between the patient and the interviewer.

Talk to the patient at the patient's level. Use everyday language. Avoid jargon and technical terminology that may confuse or intimidate the patient. Monitor the patient's alertness and understanding. Repeat and paraphrase if necessary. Pay careful attention to the patient's eye contact, facial expression, and body language as indicators of frustration, anxiety, or failure to comprehend. Talk *with* the patient, not *at* the patient. Treat the patient as a partner. Accommodate the patient's interaction style, but avoid excessive familiarity. Be friendly but objective. Use humor sparingly and judiciously, but do not avoid it. Judiciously used and properly timed humor can humanize the interview, dissipate tension, and reassure the patient, without minimizing the seriousness of the patient's condition.

• *Treat the patient as an adult who merits respect.* Never ask questions or convey an attitude that makes the patient feel inadequate, juvenile, or incompetent. Sometimes it helps to point out to the patient that his or her medical condition may make it difficult or impossible to do some of the things that used to be easy, but that many other abilities remain unaffected. If a topic or line of questioning appears to embarrass the patient or make the patient anxious, it may be time to move on to a different topic. If the abandoned line of questioning is important, come back to it later and lead into it more carefully.

An important but subtle indicator of respect is the way in which the clinician addresses the patient. It is not appropriate to address a patient by first name in the first visits, but use of the patient's first name may be appropriate later, when the clinician and the patient have gotten better acquainted. The clinician always should ask the patient how she or he would prefer to be addressed. Some older patients resent the use of their first names by those involved in their care, especially when the person providing care is appreciably younger than the patient.

• *Prepare the patient for what comes next.* If you plan more testing, prepare the patient. Give the patient a general idea of the kinds of tests you plan to administer and why you are going to administer them. Tell the patient the day and time of testing if you know them. Answer the patient's questions and deal with the patient's expressed concerns.

• *Reassure the patient.* Be objective and straightforward about the patient's impairments, but emphasize the patient's retained abilities. If you believe that the patient will improve as time passes, say so, but do not give false hope by offering an unduly optimistic prognosis. Discuss options for treatment and point out that all members of the patient care team are there to help the patient regain physical, cognitive, and communicative abilities.

By the end of the interview the patient and the clinician should be comfortable with each other, and the patient should be comfortable with the idea of being tested. The clinician should have a good idea of where to begin testing and the approximate level of difficulty of the first few tests. Information from the referral, the patient's medical record, and the interview helps to determine which tests are selected. The clinician's experiences with the patient during the interview largely determine the level of difficulty at which testing begins.

• *Include family members or significant others in the interview.* Family members and significant others should be invited to participate in the interview, especially if the patient's cognitive-communicative impairments are severe. If the patient's impairments are mild or moderate, family members and significant others can corroborate what the patient says and can help the patient remember, produce, or clarify information. If the patient's impairments are severe, family members and significant others may be the primary (or only) source of information. If a patient is able to communicate only rudimentary information, and that with great difficulty, the speech-language pathologist may schedule some additional time with family members and significant others to get the information the patient cannot provide.

TESTING THE PATIENT

Most testing is done in a private testing room, although screening tests may be administered in the patient's room. Before testing begins, the clinician takes a few minutes to explain the purpose of the tests, answer the patient's questions, and obtain the patient's consent to testing. Lezak, Howieson, and Loring (2004) provide guidelines regarding what the patient should be told before any test is administered:

- Explain the purpose of testing (e.g., to determine if the patient has a communicative impairment, to understand the patient's communicative problems, to decide on the need for treatment, to decide how to treat the patient's communicative problems, or to measure the patient's progress).
- Tell the patient why testing is necessary and how the information from the tests will be used.
- Tell the patient what will be done to protect his or her privacy and the confidentiality of test results. Usually this means that only persons who are involved in the patient's care will have access to the results of testing, and that access will be given to others only with the written permission of the patient or the patient's legal representative.
- Tell the patient who will report test results to the patient and family and when they will report them. This usually is the speech-language pathologist, but it may be the physician or another professional.
- Give the patient a brief explanation of test procedures and explain the purpose of testing: *I will be asking you to do some things to help us find out what we can do to help you with your speaking, listening, reading, and writing.* Reassure the patient: *Some of the things I ask you to do will be easy, and some may be hard, but don't worry if you have trouble with some of them. That will tell us what we may need to work on.* Tell the patient how long the testing will take: *We'll probably need about half an hour*

to finish. Tell the patient his or her right to terminate testing: *If you get tired or want to stop, just let me know, and we'll stop.* Answer the patient's questions and deal with his or her concerns: *Do you have any questions?* Get the patient ready: *Are you ready to begin?*

- Find out how the patient feels about taking the tests. Some patients may be uneasy or apprehensive about testing because they fear that poor performance will be seen as weakness, lack of intelligence, or childishness. Reiterating the purposes of testing may dispel the uneasy patient's concerns. However, the patient (or the patient's legal representative) always has the right to refuse any or all testing.

If audiotape or videotape recordings of the patient's test performance are made, the examiner must explain the purposes of the recording (e.g., to monitor the patient's progress); who will have access to the recordings (e.g., the speech-language pathologist, the patient's physician, and student trainees); and what will be done with the recordings when the patient no longer is receiving speech-language pathology services (e.g., given to the patient or erased). Most facilities require that the patient, the patient's legal representative, or both, read and sign a printed consent form giving permission for the recordings.

GENERAL CONCEPTS 3-2

- The speech-language pathologist's initial interview with the patient provides a general sense of the patient's abilities and disabilities, personality, behavior, emotional state, attention, and alertness. It also provides information about the nature and severity of the patient's communicative impairments.
- During the interview the clinician may support, inform, counsel, and educate the patient and family members about the nature of the patient's communicative

Continued

impairments; tell them how, when, and by whom decisions about treatment will be made; and provide them with a preliminary estimate of outcome.

- The speech-language pathologist's interview with the patient provides information that helps him or her decide what tests to give, the level of difficulty at which to begin testing, and what modifications of test procedures might be necessary. The interview may also permit the speech-language pathologist to make preliminary decisions regarding treatment.
- Testing brain-injured adults should be a collaborative effort between the speech-language pathologist and the patient. The speech-language pathologist ascertains the patient's primary concerns and discusses

options for testing and treatment with the patient.

- The speech-language pathologist explains the purpose of each test and how each test relates to the patient's problems and concerns.
- Before testing begins, the speech-language pathologist tells the patient why she or he will be tested, what kinds of tests will be given, who will have access to test results, and who will communicate the results to the patient and family members.
- The speech-language pathologist ascertains how the patient feels about being tested and asks the patient to consent to the testing.
- If audiotape or videotape recordings are made, the patient or the patient's legal representative must give consent to the recording.

Some General Principles for Testing Adults with Brain Injuries

Testing adults who have brain injuries poses special challenges. Because brain-injured adults often exhibit an array of behavioral, cognitive, linguistic, and psychologic abnormalities, those who test them are called on to exhibit unusual levels of patience, empathy, and understanding, in addition to being expert in test administration and skilled at interpreting patients' responses to test items. There is no substitute for experience in testing brain-injured adults, just as there is no substitute for experience in other complex activities, such as making a soufflé, composing a symphony, or driving a taxicab in New York City, but a few general principles, outlined in Box 3-1 and explained below, may help beginning clinicians compensate for lack of experience.

- *Do your homework.* The conscientious clinician comes to the first test session with a plan for assessing the patient's cognition and communication, largely based on information from the patient's medical record and the interview. From the medical record

Box 3-1	*Testing Adults with Brain Injuries*

- Do your homework.
- Choose an appropriate place for testing.
- Schedule testing to maximize the patient's performance.
- Make testing a collaborative effort.
- Select tests that are appropriate for the patient.
- Let the patient's performance guide what and how you test.
- Use standardized tests and test procedures judiciously and purposefully.
- Consider the validity of standardized tests.
- Consider the adequacy of norms for standardized tests.
- Evaluate the representativeness of the normative sample.
- Obtain a large enough sample of the patient's behavior to ensure test-retest stability.

the clinician has learned something about the patient's background, life situation, and current problems; from the interview the clinician has gotten a sense of the patient's cognitive abilities, personality, social behavior, and communicative impairments. The clinician may have formulated a tentative diagnosis and usually will have in mind a plan for where to begin and how to proceed with testing. A plan ensures that testing is systematic and efficient, that each test builds on the one before, and ensures that all necessary tests, but no unnecessary tests, are administered.

- *Choose an appropriate place for testing.* The test environment should be quiet, well-lit, and free from distractions. Furnishings should be comfortable but functional. Test materials should be accessible to the examiner but out of sight until they are needed. If audiotape or videotape recordings are made, microphones and cameras should be in unobtrusive locations.
- *Schedule testing to maximize the patient's performance.* Most hospitalized patients have surprisingly busy schedules. Laboratory tests, appointments with counselors and social workers, physical and occupational therapy sessions, and other such activities fill the patient's day. To compound the problem, most brain-injured patients no longer have the stamina they had before their injury, and by late morning or early afternoon they are exhausted and need nothing so much as a nap. Consequently, the shrewd speech-language pathologist schedules testing sessions early in the day while the patient is still fresh, and if testing sessions must be scheduled later in the day, ensures that the patient has had a chance to rest before the test session.
- *Make testing a collaborative effort.* The clinician must never forget that the patient is an adult who may be anxious, apprehensive, bewildered, and perhaps frightened by his or her changed physical and mental condition. The clinician should point out that the purpose of testing is to get a sense of the nature and severity of the patient's impairments and a sense of what the patient can still do, so that both difficult and easy tests are necessary. The clinician should prepare the patient

for potential failure on difficult tests by pointing out that failure is the result of what has happened to the patient and does not represent the patient's competence or value as a person.

The clinician should approach testing objectively but compassionately. Suggesting that the clinician and patient will be working together to understand the patient's problems and to help the patient deal with his or her problems may help the patient feel more like an active participant than an object of study. Schuell, Jenkins, and Jimenez-Pabon (1964) claim therapeutic benefits for testing approached as a joint effort by the clinician and the patient:

> "... searching exploration of aphasic disabilities can be a therapeutic rather than a traumatic procedure. This is true because the process of testing establishes communication on a level that is highly meaningful to the patient. As a result, he feels less isolated and less anxious. By means of the tests, the examiner leads the patient toward objectivity by helping him understand the nature of his problems and their limits. The patient discovers things he is able to do, which tends to restore confidence and alleviate depression. Patients become less and less defensive as confidence in the clinician increases." (p. 168)

- *Select tests that are appropriate for the patient.* Skilled clinicians usually have a general sense of the nature of the patient's probable impairments and the likely level of the patient's impairments before testing begins. This knowledge helps the clinician focus testing and ensures that testing begins at an appropriate level of difficulty.

The assessment often begins with administration of a generic test battery (e.g., a standardized aphasia test battery). Generic test batteries provide a general description of a patient's' performance in a variety of tasks and at various levels of difficulty within tasks. They are useful for identifying communicative or cognitive disabilities, estimating their severity, and describing their nature. Some can be used to assign patients to diagnostic categories. Some can be used to predict the eventual level of a patient's recovery. Generic test batteries provide broad coverage of a domain of linguistic, cognitive, or behavioral attributes in a reasonable amount of time. Generic test batteries provide clinicians with a look at many aspects of a patient's cognition and communication performance, but the look often is one-dimensional. Generic test batteries in some respects function as screening devices because they are good at detecting impairments but are not good at specifying the exact nature or severity of the impairments.

Weisenberg and McBride (1935), Schuell (1965), and Porch (1967) have discussed requirements for test batteries for brain-injured adults. The following list is a blend of their recommendations:

- The test battery should sample performance at different levels of difficulty in several related tasks so that all potentially disturbed performances are evaluated.
- The test battery should allow the clinician to determine the level at which performance is error-free, the level at which performance completely breaks down, and several intervening levels within each test or subtest.
- The test battery should sample in a consistent way the input modalities through which test instructions are delivered, the mental processes needed to perform the tasks, and the output modalities necessary for carrying out the tasks.
- The test battery should be standardized so that results are reliable from test to test and examiner to examiner. It should control relevant variables such as method of stimulus presentation, nature of test stimuli, instructions to the patient, and response scoring.
- The scoring system should record patient performance in such a way that the

quality of responses as well as their correctness is recorded.
- Subtests in the test battery should include enough items to permit the user to determine a patient's average performance on each subtest and to control for the effects of sporadic fluctuations in the patient's performance.
- The test battery should suggest the reasons for a patient's deficient performance.
- The test battery should permit predictions regarding a patient's recovery.

Because no two brain-injured patients exhibit exactly the same pattern of deficits, clinicians do not rely on a single generic test battery to evaluate every patient in a diagnostic category. Most clinicians begin with all or parts of a generic test battery to get a general impression of a patient's performance under well-controlled test conditions and to establish the general pattern and severity of the patient's impairments. Then they branch off with standardized or nonstandardized tests appropriate for exploration of the patient's unique pattern of impairments. The generic test battery samples the patient's performance under standardized test conditions, permits comparison of the patient's performance with that of norm groups, and establishes reliable baseline levels of performance. The follow-up testing identifies and quantifies the patient's unique pattern of impairments.

- *Let the patient's performance guide what and how you test.* Skilled clinicians are alert to signals suggesting that they should branch off from the usual test routine. The signals come from many sources—the patient's history, the diagnosis, the clinician's previous experience with similar patients, the patient's current test performance, and sometimes from a clinical hunch. When skilled clinicians receive such signals, they depart from the test routine to follow up on leads suggested by the patient's performance. They modify standard tests or improvise new tests to identify the variables that affect the patient's performance. This sometimes requires that the focus of testing change as testing progresses until the nature and magnitude of the patient's impairments become clear.

An important aspect of testing brain-injured adults is what Lezak, Howieson, and Loring (2004) call *testing the limits*. Clinicians test the limits by going beyond standard procedures for administering a test to explore the reasons for a patient's deficient performance. For example, a clinician might allow a patient who fails a test of written spelling to spell the same words orally. Normal oral-spelling performance would show that the patient's deficient performance on the standard test was not because the patient could not spell, but perhaps because the patient could not write. If the patient were to fail the oral spelling test, the clinician might allow the patient to choose correctly spelled words from sets of printed words in which the correctly spelled word is shown with incorrectly spelled foils. According to Lezak, Howieson, and Loring (2004):

"The limits should be tested whenever there is suspicion that an impairment of some function other than the one under consideration is interfering with an adequate demonstration of that function." (p. 116).

Increased efficiency is an important benefit of personalizing tests to the patient. Clinicians do not spend time on tests in which the patient's performance is normal, nor do they spend time on too difficult tests in which the patient experiences only failure. Tests in which a patient either makes no errors or makes only errors are of little diagnostic or therapeutic use, and administering them may be a waste of precious clinic time. Administering tests that are outside the patient's range also may have negative consequences for the patient. Too easy tests may be boring or insulting, and too difficult tests may be frustrating or anxiety-provoking.

- *Use standardized tests and test procedures judiciously and purposefully.* Skilled clinicians do not avoid standardized tests and test batteries, although standardized tests rarely provide the detail needed to understand a particular patient's pattern of performance. There is no substitute for standardized tests when the clinician wishes to compare a patient's test performance with that of other patients or with that of non–brain-injured adults, to compare a patient's performance across several test occasions, or to communicate about the patient with other professionals. For any of these purposes, uniform test procedures are necessary, and standardized tests are more likely than nonstandardized tests to have them.

  Standardized tests can contribute to efficiency in testing—most are structured to minimize redundancy, maximize precision, and ensure consistency in test administration, scoring, and interpretation. However, standardized test batteries may contribute to inefficiency by forcing the patient to undergo more testing than necessary. Skilled clinicians often enhance efficiency by administering selected subtests to focus on aspects of performance that are most important for a particular patient. This method of testing is most practical when norms are available for individual subtests in a test battery. Subtest norms permit a clinician to compare a patient's performance with that of groups of individuals—usually a group of normal adults and one or more groups of adults representing various diagnostic categories (e.g., adults with aphasia)—subtest by subtest.

- *Consider the validity of standardized tests.* Most standardized tests come with information about their validity—the degree to which they actually measure what they purport to measure. Various kinds of validity have been described in the literature, but the most important for our purposes are *content validity* and *construct validity*. There is some overlap, but in general *content validity* relates to how well the content of a test (items, tasks, or questions) represents the domain of concern (e.g., intelligence), and *construct validity* relates to how well the content of a test represents an underlying theory, model, or concept of a process or structure. Clinicians tend to be concerned more with content validity than with construct validity. They want to know that a test of auditory comprehension actually tests comprehension, that a test of memory actually tests memory, and that a test of sustained attention actually tests a patient's ability to maintain attentiveness over time.

- *Consider the adequacy of norms for standardized tests.* Scores on a test are of limited value unless there is a way of relating a patient's performance to the performance of normal adults or to the performance of other adults in the same diagnostic category. Such comparisons are made possible by *norms.* Unfortunately, not all published tests provide norms, and the norms provided in some published tests are insufficient or inappropriate. It is not always easy to tell if the norms in a test manual are adequate and appropriate. However, the following general principles should help identify the very deficient ones:

  Evaluate the size of the norm group. The size of the norm group must be large enough to ensure that the sample is representative of the population to which the norms apply and to ensure that statistics calculated on performance of the norm group are reliable. There is no simple answer to the question of how large a normative sample must be. It depends partly on how much variability in performance there is in the norm group and partly on how much error users are willing to tolerate in comparing individuals with the norm group. When there is little variability in performance among individuals in the norm group, a relatively small sample may suffice. This sometimes happens when a group of non–brain-injured adults takes a test designed for assessing adults with brain injuries—few of the non–brain-injured adults make any errors on the test, and those who make errors make very few. Because the performance of the non–brain-injured adults is very homogeneous, increasing the size of the norm group beyond that necessary to establish that non–brain-injured adults rarely make errors adds little, if anything, to the accuracy of the norms.

  The situation changes when the performance of a norm group spans a wide range, as is true with brain-injured adults. Brain-injured adults are a heterogeneous group. Their performance on standardized tests spans a wide range, from individuals who perform near the bottom of the test's range to individuals who perform at or near the top. For this reason, tests designed for brain-injured adults need large norm groups—often 50 to 100 individuals.

  Evaluate the representativeness of the normative sample. The individuals in the normative sample must be representative of the population from which the sample is drawn. Which characteristics of a normative sample are important depends to some extent on the nature of the test and on the population represented by the sample, but characteristics that may affect test performance are the most important. When the norm group represents an impaired population, the severity and nature of the impairments of those in the norm group should match the severity and nature of the impairments in the population with the impairments. When the norm group represents a normal population, the norm group should resemble the population on any variables that are likely to affect test performance. For tests of language, communication, and cognition, these variables almost always include age, education, and intellect.

Obtain a large enough sample of the patient's behavior to ensure test-retest stability. When brain-injured adults are tested with materials that challenge but do not overwhelm them, their performance often fluctuates from item to item within tests. For example, a patient asked to name a set of 10 line drawings on three successive presentations of the set may miss three items on the first presentation, five on the second, and two on the third. In general, increasing the number of items reduces test-to-test variability, at least up to a point, after which increasing the number of items minimally affects the stability of performance.

There is no answer to the question: *How many items are enough?* Most test designers and clinicians would agree that 10 items in a subtest are adequate for testing most brain-damaged adults. Most also likely would agree that tests containing five or fewer items are too short to ensure adequate test-retest stability.

GENERAL CONCEPTS 3-3

- Experienced clinicians observe several principles when testing adults who have brain injuries:
  - They come to the first test session with a plan, based on previously acquired information about the patient.
  - They choose a quiet place for testing and schedule testing to minimize the effects of patient fatigue.
  - They make testing a cooperative effort between the clinician and the patient.
  - They select tests that are at an appropriate level of difficulty and focus on the patient's likely areas of impairment.
  - They permit the patient's performance to guide them in selecting tests and follow leads revealed by the patient's performance.
  - They are prudent in their use of standardized tests so that the patient is not subjected to more testing than necessary and so that important aspects of the patient's performance are measured.
  - They obtain a large enough sample of patient performance to ensure test-retest stability.
- Generic test batteries function best as general screening instruments that permit the speech-language pathologist to sample patient performance in several domains and at several levels of difficulty. The results of a generic test battery provide a basis for in-depth testing in which the speech-language pathologist may test the patient's limits in key areas.
- Standardized tests are necessary if the clinician wishes to relate a patient's performance to that of other patients or to groups representing a population, including the population of normal adults.
- Generic test batteries should:
  - Sample performance at different levels of difficulty with a range of tests that covers all potentially important aspects of a patient's performance
  - Allow the clinician to determine a basal level (where performance is normal), a ceiling level (where performance breaks down), and several intervening levels within each subtest
  - Systematically sample performance across the input modalities for instructions and test stimuli, the mental processes required to perform test tasks, and the output modalities involved in the patient's responses
  - Possess interexaminer reliability and test-retest reliability. Control variables such as test stimuli, instructions, and scoring of responses
  - Permit recording the quality of responses as well as their accuracy

Continued

GENERAL CONCEPTS 3-3—cont'd

- Include enough items to control for response variability
- Suggest reasons for a patient's deficient performance
- Contribute to decisions concerning treatment and predictions of outcome

Purposes of Testing

The speech-language pathologist may test patients with neurogenic cognitive-communicative disorders for several reasons. The most common are to:

- Diagnose a patient's cognitive-communicative impairments
- Arrive at a prognosis for a patient's recovery
- Determine the nature and severity of a patient's impairments
- Make decisions about the appropriateness and potential focus of treatment
- Measure a patient's recovery
- Measure the efficacy of treatment

The initial evaluation of a patient's cognitive-communicative abilities typically is directed toward some combination of the first four reasons, and it may be impossible to separate them. Determining the severity and nature of a patient's impairments usually has implications for the diagnosis, the prognosis, and the decisions about treatment. A diagnosis may have prognostic implications and may affect decisions regarding treatment, such as when a patient's pattern of impairments suggests degenerative neurologic disease. Nevertheless, the speech-language pathologist now and then may have a more limited objective in testing a patient—for example, when a patient with mild cognitive-communicative impairments is referred by a physician who needs help in determining if the patient has an underlying neurologic disease. In such a case the emphasis is on diagnosis. Prognosis and treatment are secondary, or perhaps not considered at all.

Deciding on a Diagnosis. Diagnosing a patient's cognitive-communicative disorder means attaching a label to it. Diagnostic labels are devices for summarizing a collection of related symptoms. Diagnostic labels are an efficient way of communicating large amounts of information about a patient in a few words, provided, of course, that those reading the diagnostic labels understand their implications.

Diagnosis by speech-language pathologists takes several forms. Sometimes the intent is to differentiate a patient's cognitive-communicative disorder from disorders that might resemble it (a process called *differential diagnosis*). For example, diagnostic testing might be designed to determine if a patient's pattern of impairments represents aphasia, dysarthria, apraxia of speech, or some form of dementing illness.

Sometimes the speech-language pathologist knows, based on a patient's history and medical record, that the patient's pattern of impairments represents a general class of disorders, but he or she wishes to arrive at a more specific diagnosis. For example, a speech-language pathologist may conclude that a patient is dysarthric based on the location of the patient's brain injury and the neurologist's description of the patient's speech, but he or she may wish to determine which of several dysarthria syndromes best fits the patient's speech characteristics.

Labeling a patient's cognitive-communicative disorder often suggests the location of the nervous system abnormality responsible for the patient's symptoms. For example, the label *Wernicke's aphasia* suggests injury to the temporal lobe of the language-dominant hemisphere, and the label *hypokinetic dysarthria* suggests abnormality in the extrapyramidal system. It is true, however, that the diagnosis of the nature and location of a patient's brain injury rarely depends on the word of the speech-language pathologist because often the neurologic examination and the results of imaging studies have localized the patient's brain injury well before the patient gets to the speech-language pathologist.

Speech-language pathologists sometimes make a provisional diagnosis of a patient's cognitive-communicative disorder based on information in the patient's medical record before they actually see the patient. If, for example, a patient's medical record shows that he or she has had a brain stem stroke, it is likely that the patient will be dysarthric and may have swallowing problems, but the patient will not be aphasic and will not be demented (unless there is a history of previous stroke or other neurologic disease affecting the brain). Davis (1993) was discussing aphasia when he wrote:

> "In clinical practice, a test is seldom used to diagnose aphasia, in the sense that a clinician has no idea what the disorder is until the test is analyzed. ... Having read a patient's chart, an experienced clinical aphasiologist need only talk to a patient before reaching an initial conclusion about not only the presence of aphasia but also the type of aphasia." (p. 211)

Davis's assertion is true not only for patients with aphasia, but also for patients with other cognitive-communicative disorders. By the time an experienced speech-language pathologist has reviewed a patient's medical record and interviewed the patient, the speech-language pathologist usually has a diagnosis in mind. Subsequent testing may only confirm or elaborate on the preliminary diagnosis.

For most speech-language pathologists the act of attaching a diagnostic label to a neurologically impaired patient's cognitive-communicative impairment is less important than determining the nature and severity of the patient's impairments and making decisions about the appropriateness and content of treatment. This does not mean, however, that diagnostic labeling has no place in the speech-language pathologist's professional repertoire. The physician who refers a patient may expect a diagnostic label. A diagnostic label in a report may take the place of a lengthy description. For example, reporting that a patient exhibits behaviors consistent with *conduction aphasia* communicates, in

two words, extensive information about the nature of the patient's speech, the patient's comprehension of language, and the probable location of the brain injury responsible for the patient's aphasia. Likewise, reporting that a patient exhibits *flaccid dysarthria* communicates information about the patient's articulatory impairments and the probable location of nervous system abnormality. Some diagnostic labels have implications for treatment planning. For example, reporting that a patient exhibits *multi-infarct dementia,* which usually increases in severity in stepwise fashion, suggests not only the general nature of treatment, but also that treatment may have to be adjusted as the severity of the patient's impairments increases.

Making a Prognosis. A prognosis is a prediction about the course (sometimes) and the eventual outcome (usually) of a disease or condition. A prognosis may represent no more than a clinician's best guess, based on clinical experience and intuition, or it may represent a more objective probability statement, based on actuarial information from studies of groups of individuals who have had the disease or condition. Such actuarial information usually comes from prospective or retrospective prognostic studies.

In *prospective prognostic studies* patients in the early stages of a disease or condition are identified, and selected characteristics of the patients (the prognostic variables) are assessed at the beginning of the study. The patients then are followed to determine outcome. At some predetermined time the outcomes are tallied, and the relationships between prognostic variables and outcomes are evaluated to identify the prognostic variables most strongly related to outcome.

In *retrospective prognostic studies* the records of a group of patients who have reached the outcome stage are reviewed to evaluate the relationships between various prognostic variables (determined from the records) and outcome (also determined from the records). Retrospective studies are scientifically less robust than prospective studies because in retrospective studies the prognostic variables are not defined in advance, the data are not collected using standardized procedures, and the definitions of outcome measures tend to be less precise than the definitions of outcome measures in prospective studies.

Most studies of prognostic variables related to recovery of communication and cognition by patients with nervous system abnormalities are retrospective. The records of groups of brain-injured patients who have recovered various levels of communicative or cognitive abilities are reviewed and the relationships between patients' recoveries (usually defined as scores on standardized tests) and various prognostic variables (e.g., age, education, or severity of brain injury) are evaluated.

Numerous studies and opinion pieces have been published in the search for prognostic variables that might predict brain-injured adults' recovery of communication or cognition. These variables fall into three categories—*neurologic findings, associated conditions,* and *patient variables.*

Neurologic Findings. In addition to their function as shorthand for communicating information about the patient, many neurologic diagnoses have prognostic significance. Longstreth, Koepsell, Nelson, and Van Belle (1992) link diagnosis, prognosis, and treatment when they assert:

> "A diagnosis that has no prognostic implications does little more than describe a constellation of patient characteristics. Prognosis links diagnosis to outcomes and identifies the diseases that warrant treatment. Treatment becomes an intervention intended to modify prognosis. Thus...the concepts of diagnosis, prognosis, and treatment are inseparable, with prognosis as the keystone." (p. 29)

This opinion might be regarded by some as extreme because the prognostic implications of many diagnostic labels for communicative or cognitive disorders are fuzzy at best. For example, diagnosing a patient's communication

disorder as *Wernicke's aphasia* implies little in the way of prognosis, except that as a group, patients with Wernicke's aphasia recover slightly less well than those with Broca's aphasia (Benson, 1979a; Goodglass, 1993; Kertesz, 1979). Many neurologic diagnoses carry considerably more prognostic weight because the time-course and outcome of many neurologic conditions are well documented.

The speech-language pathologist who wishes to predict a patient's recovery of communication and cognition pays close attention to the neurologic diagnosis, because changes in a patient's communicative and cognitive abilities often parallel changes in the patient's physical and medical condition. When the usual course of a patient's neurologic disease is well-known and highly predictable, the prognosis for recovery of communication and cognition also is likely to be quite accurate (although perhaps redundant, once the neurologic diagnosis has been made).

Notes or comments in a patient's medical record relating to the location and extent of damage in a patient's nervous system often affect prognosis. The location of the damage is important because damage affecting parts of the nervous system that are directly involved in language and cognitive processes carry greater negative implications than damage affecting peripheral regions. For example, damage in the central zone of the language-dominant hemisphere typically creates more severe and persistent aphasia than damage in peripheral regions. Likewise, unilateral brain stem damage often causes severe and persistent dysarthria, whereas unilateral damage in fiber tracts above the brain stem usually produces less dramatic effects.

The extent of nervous system abnormalities also affects prognosis. Large lesions, multiple lesions, and damage disseminated throughout the nervous system or throughout parts of the nervous system are ominous. For example, a speech-language pathologist might revise downward the estimated communicative recovery for a patient with a confirmed recent left-hemisphere stroke on learning that the patient's CT scan showed a previous stroke in the right hemisphere. Sometimes indicators of the extent of nervous system damage are indirect. For example, the presence and duration of coma are considered important prognostic indicators for patients with traumatic brain injuries (Jennett, Teasdale, Braakman, & associates, 1979), and, to a lesser extent, for patients with aphasia caused by stroke (Caronna & Levy, 1983). Longer intervals of coma suggest greater destruction of brain tissue, greater impairment, and a poorer prognosis.

The neurologic diagnosis and the location and extent of the nervous system abnormalities responsible for a patient's impairments provide two reasonably dependable prognostic indicators. Other prognostic indicators, although less dependable, often play a part in determining a patient's prognosis. These indicators may represent *associated conditions* or *patient characteristics.*

Associated Conditions. Associated conditions are medical conditions or physical findings that do not directly affect cognition or communication but have indirect effects on the magnitude of a patient's impairments and may compromise a patient's recovery and response to treatment. Several associated conditions have been shown to affect recovery of communication and cognition following nervous system injury.

A patient's *general health* may have important effects on his or her recovery of communicative and cognitive abilities. Illnesses such as diabetes, heart disease, pulmonary disease, or other such chronic diseases impede physiologic and behavioral recovery from brain injury and limit potential benefits from treatment (Candelise, Landi, Orazio, & Boccardi, 1985; Eisenson, 1964; Marshall & Phillips, 1983).

Associated sensory and motor impairments also have some prognostic significance. The presence of hemiplegia, perceptual disturbances, seizures, or motor impairments have

been identified as negative prognostic indicators (Keenan & Brassell, 1975; Van Buskirk, 1955), although some investigators have reported no relationship between the presence of hemiplegia or seizures and recovery of cognitive-communicative abilities (Glonig, Trappl, Heiss, & Quatember, 1976; Smith, 1972). The presence of sensory or motor impairments may be an indirect indicator of the severity of nervous system abnormalities, especially where combinations of such impairments are present.

Patient Characteristics. Several patient characteristics (age, gender, education, occupation, premorbid intelligence, handedness, personality, and emotional state) reputedly affect brain-injured adults' recovery of communication and cognition. However, the relationships between specific patient characteristics and recovery of communication and cognition are weak, and most have been subject to contradictory findings. (See Darley, 1982; Davis, 1993; and Rosenbek, LaPointe, & Wertz, 1989) for reviews of these findings.) The most that can be said in their favor is that they appear to have some weak effects on recovery, but the effects of any single patient characteristic easily are overshadowed by the more potent effects of variables such as the location and severity of nervous system injury.

The nature of a patient's communicative or cognitive impairment often has prognostic significance. For example, there is evidence that patients with Broca's aphasia recover somewhat better than those with Wernicke's aphasia when aphasia severity is equivalent, and that patients with traumatic brain injuries recover better than those with brain injuries caused by stroke. (That patients with traumatic brain injuries usually are younger than stroke patients no doubt makes an important contribution to this relationship.) The overall severity of a patient's communicative or cognitive impairment at the time of testing is a reasonably dependable indicator of future recovery. In general, patients with severe impairments recover less well than those with milder impairments, although there may be striking exceptions. However, making a prognosis based on the overall severity of a patient's cognitive-communicative impairment is in many respects a subjective process because the predictive validity of the standardized tests for measuring the severity of a patient's communicative or cognitive impairments has not been established (Tompkins, 1995).

The relationship between severity of impairments and outcome is weak in the first days (and sometimes weeks) following nervous system injury but becomes stronger as the diffuse and transitory effects of nervous system injury resolve, allowing the permanent effects of destroyed nervous system tissue to become visible. Most clinicians hedge their prognostic bets in the early postinjury period and defer their ultimate prognosis until the patient's neurologic condition has stabilized.

A few tests provide systematic procedures for making prognostic statements based on patients' test performance. Some make use of a *patient profile approach,* in which a test battery is administered and a profile of the patient's performance is developed. The clinician then matches the patient's profile with the profiles of previously studied groups of patients whose recovery is known, expecting that the patient's recovery should match that of previously studied patients with the same profile.

The *Minnesota Test for Differential Diagnosis of Aphasia* (MTDDA; Schuell, 1972) is an example of the patient profile approach to prediction. The MTDDA permits clinicians to assign aphasic patients to one of five major and two minor groups based on their test performances. The MTDDA test manual gives a prognosis for each group, based on the recovery of previously studied patients. For example, MTDDA Group 1 usually has "*excellent recovery of all language skills*" (Schuell, 1972, p. 9), whereas for MTDDA Group 5 "*language does not become functional or voluntary in any modality*" (Schuell, 1972, p. 14).

Other tests permit the use of a more sophisticated *statistical prediction approach* (Porch, Collins, Wertz, & Friden, 1980). The statistical prediction approach, like the other approaches, makes predictions based on the characteristics of previously studied patients. Unlike the other approaches, the statistical prediction approach uses statistical analyses to determine the relative contribution of multiple variables, alone and in combination, to observed recovery. The statistical procedures provide quantitative information about which variables are most strongly related to recovery and which combinations of variables provide the most accurate predictions. They also permit predictions regarding the actual level of recovery to be expected. However, the predictions are not perfect—there is always some error in prediction associated with even the strongest prognostic variables.

A good example of the *statistical prediction approach* is Porch's (1981a) *HOAP* (for *high-overall prediction*) procedure for predicting recovery from aphasia. In the HOAP procedure, the patient is tested at 1 month postonset with the *Porch Index of Communicative Ability* (PICA; Porch, 1981a), which has 18 subtests. The clinician then calculates an average score for the nine subtests with the highest scores. This average then is used to enter a table in the PICA manual, from which the patient's 6-month overall PICA performance can be predicted.

Predicting brain-injured adults' recovery of communication and cognition can be an uncertain business. No prognostic variables have been linked unequivocally to recovery of communication and cognition, and many have been subject to conflicting claims in the literature. Even sophisticated *patient profile* and *statistical prediction* approaches, which are fairly accurate when predicting the average recovery of groups of patients, often yield inaccurate predictions for individual patients (Aten & Lyon, 1978; Porch & Callaghan, 1981; Wertz, Dronkers, & Hume, 1993). For this reason, many clinicians offer some patients a few sessions of *prognostic treatment* (Rosenbek, LaPointe, & Wertz, 1989) to increase predictive precision. In prognostic treatment the clinician and patient spend several sessions working together to find out if the patient can benefit from treatment.

Present-day restrictions on reimbursement may make it impractical for a clinician to spend many sessions in prognostic treatment because third-party payers may refuse to pay for it. However, it is true that the first few treatment sessions with a patient often serve diagnostic and prognostic purposes, although diagnosis and prognosis are not listed as formal objectives.

Regardless of how it is done, predicting newly referred patients' recovery (or loss) of communicative or cognitive abilities is an important skill. Patients and their families, concerned about the potential effects of a patient's disabilities on familial, social, and financial conditions, may press for a prognostic opinion. Physicians and other healthcare workers may need the prognosis to help them plan a patient's discharge and arrange for follow-up care. Social workers may need a prognostic opinion to make appropriate social and vocational arrangements for a patient and the patient's family. Attorneys may request a prognostic opinion to establish a patient's legal competence or lack thereof. Funding agencies may require evidence for a favorable prognosis before consenting to pay for a patient's treatment. Finally, the speech-language pathologist must have a sense of the potential benefits of treatment before deciding whether to offer treatment.

Measuring Recovery and Response to Treatment

Measuring patient performance across time is an important part of the clinical management of patients with neurogenic communicative or cognitive impairments. Measuring performance across time permits clinicians to establish baselines against which the effects of treatment can be measured and permits clinicians to describe changes in a patient's performance during treatment. Well-defined baselines are the principal element in studies of the evolution of neurologic diseases, and they are key elements in documenting the progression of a particular patient's impairments and in predicting outcome for that patient.

Defining a baseline for a patient with a neurogenic cognitive-communicative disorder typically entails administering a test or set of tests at regular intervals to measure the patient's performance in the domain of interest. A patient with progressive dementia might be evaluated with a story-retelling test at 1 month intervals to evaluate the degree to which organization, recall, and production of story elements are affected by the patient's dementia. A semicomatose patient might be evaluated with daily tests of alertness and attention to determine when she or he might be a candidate for a more comprehensive evaluation. A patient with progressive muscle weakness might be evaluated with monthly tests of articulatory proficiency to monitor the course of the disease and to determine the effects of treatment on the patient's dysarthria.

Figure 3-9 shows how a speech-language pathologist used baseline measurements to help a neurologist decide on a diagnosis for a 63-year-old woman who was brought to the neurology clinic with vague complaints about difficulty concentrating and memory lapses. The patient's neurologic examination was unremarkable, and she scored within normal limits on a screening test of memory and cognition. The neurologist referred the patient to speech-language pathology with a request for help in determining if the patient had a progressive condition, and if so, whether the patient was in the early stages of dementia.

The speech-language pathologist chose three tests as baseline measures—a test of *proverb interpretation,* a *story-retelling test,* and a *picture-naming test.* He reasoned that performance on the proverb-interpretation and story-retelling tests should be sensitive to dementing

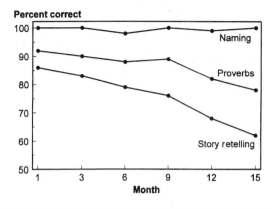

Figure 3-9 ■ Baseline measurements for a patient who was eventually diagnosed as having dementia. Naming performance remained stable throughhout the period of baseline measurement, while performance on tests of proverb interpretation and story-retelling gradually worsened.

illness because they require analytic skills, abstract reasoning, and memory—all of which typically are affected early in the course of dementia. The speech-language pathologist included a picture-naming test because he knew that picture naming rarely is affected in the early stages of dementia. If the patient's performance on the proverb-interpretation and story-retelling tests declined while her performance on the picture-naming test remained stable, a diagnosis of early dementia would become plausible.

The speech-language pathologist tested the patient at 3-month intervals, concurrent with her appointments in the neurology clinic. The graph in Figure 3-9 shows the patient's performance across five test sessions. The patient's naming performance remained stable and within the normal range across all five tests, but her proverb-interpretation and story-retelling performance gradually declined. The patient's neurologic examination remained unremarkable across the five test sessions, except for a questionable decline in performance on screening tests of cognition in the sixth session. The

patient's baseline pattern of performance led the neurologist to conclude that the patient was in the early stages of progressive dementia, a diagnosis which was confirmed by subsequent evaluations during the following year.

Measuring the Effects of Treatment

Careful testing is crucial for establishing baseline performance, for measuring patients' responses to treatment, and for alerting the clinician to the need for changes in treatment procedures. Well-planned and well-executed testing helps clinicians determine the outcome of treatment and tell if changes in performance in treatment generalize in a meaningful way to a patient's daily life. These aspects of assessment become more important as providers consider the social, psychological, and environmental effects of intervention and as healthcare agencies become increasingly preoccupied with balancing the costs of rehabilitation against its positive effects on patients' daily life independence. The concepts of *efficacy* and *effectiveness* are central to these considerations.

EFFICACY AND EFFECTIVENESS

The terms *efficacy* and *effectiveness* appeared in the medical literature in the 1970s. In the medical parlance of the time, *efficacy* denoted the effects of treatment under carefully controlled (and often artificial) conditions in which selected participants were treated, tested, and monitored more rigorously than is usual in standard clinical practice. *Effectiveness* denoted the effects of treatment given in routine clinical practice, wherein patients did not receive specialized testing, treatment, or education because of their participation in a study. Studies of treatment efficacy were designed to answer the question: *Does this treatment have a measurable effect under ideal conditions?* whereas studies of treatment effectiveness were designed to answer the question: *Does this treatment work in the real world?*

In the rehabilitation literature *efficacy* and *effectiveness* have been used in a different sense. *Efficacy* relates to the existence of a measurable change in a patient characteristic as a result of treatment, whether the treatment was administered as part of a research investigation or as part of standard clinical practice. *Effectiveness* relates to the effects of treatment on a patient's daily life well being. In speech-language pathology, efficacy usually is defined as a positive change on a standardized test of cognition, language, or communication. Effectiveness is usually defined by subjective reports of patients or family members or by observation of patients in daily life activities.

That a treatment is efficacious does not necessarily mean that it is effective. Consider, for example, a treatment that produces a significant increase in an aphasic patient's performance on the *Boston Naming Test* (Kaplan, Goodglass, & Weintraub, 2001), which requires the tested person to name drawings representing common and uncommon objects. If one's measure of efficacy were improvement on the *Boston Naming Test,* the treatment would be considered efficacious. Whether the treatment was effective is unknown because we do not know if improved picture naming provides any meaningful benefit in daily life. To decide if a treatment is efficacious, one asks, "*What happened to the patient's test performance?*" To decide if a treatment is effective, one asks, "*What happened to the patient's daily life well being?*"

A treatment could conceivably be effective although not efficacious. This unusual situation could occur if, for example, one chose performance on the *Boston Naming Test* as the measure of efficacy for a treatment program that provided broad-based language stimulation and no naming training. One might then see no significant change in patients' *Boston Naming Test* scores (the measure of efficacy) but find a meaningful positive change in ratings of the patient's communicative success in daily life activities (a measure of effectiveness).

The issues of efficacy and effectiveness are exemplified by a study of aphasia therapy by Wertz, Weiss, Aten, and associates (1986). In that study a *clinic group* of aphasic adults received 12 weeks of treatment followed by 12 weeks of no treatment. A *deferred group* received 12 weeks of no treatment followed by 12 weeks of treatment. At the end of the first 12 weeks, the *clinic group's* overall percentile score on the *Porch Index of Communicative Ability* (PICA; Porch, 1981a) was about six points higher than that of the *deferred group*— a statistically significant difference. The change in PICA scores permitted Wertz, Weiss, Aten, and associates to conclude that the treatment was efficacious—it yielded a statistically significant change in the chosen measure of treatment effect (PICA overall percentile). Whether the treatment was effective is not clear because we do not know if an improvement of six percentile points on the PICA overall score signifies a meaningful change in aphasic persons' daily life communicative functioning.

Most treatment studies in which participants are adults who have neurogenic cognitive-communicative disorders are *efficacy* studies. The indicators of treatment effects are changes in performance on standardized tests of cognition and communication, perhaps because these tests are sensitive and reliable indicators of the cognitive-communicative performance of adults under carefully controlled test conditions. Few treatment studies of adults with neurogenic cognitive-communicative disorders have incorporated measures of daily life benefit, perhaps because few standardized effectiveness measures with proven sensitivity, reliability, and validity were available when the studies were done.

In contrast, many medical studies of treatment effects have incorporated measures that speak both to efficacy and to effectiveness. For example, a study of the effects of treatment for hypertension (Veterans Administration, 1972) compared the effects of antihypertensive medication with the effects of a placebo administered to large groups of adults with hypertension. The measures of treatment effects were the frequencies of five adverse events—

sudden death, heart attack, congestive heart failure, increased hypertension, and *ruptured aneurysm,* all known to be consequences of hypertension. At the end of the study 9% of the group given the antihypertensive medications had experienced one or more adverse events, whereas 22% of the group given the placebo had experienced such events. Because the occurrence of these adverse events is likely to have profound negative effects on patients and their families, it is reasonable to conclude that the treatment regimen was both *efficacious* (the difference in the rate of adverse events between the groups was statistically significant) and *effective* (the treatment improved patients' daily life well being).

> Although no direct measures of effectiveness were included in the hypertension study, few would argue that decreasing the occurrence of death, heart attack, heart failure, hypertension, and ruptured aneurysm would not have positive effects on the daily lives of patients and their families. The design of the study also supports the efficacy of the treatment. The study was a multi-center clinical trial in which the treatment regimen resembled the customary medical treatment for hypertension at the time.

The word *functional* has come to replace *effective* in the rehabilitation literature and in some medical literature. In this context *functional* means *affecting the patient's daily life competence or well being.* Thousands of articles and dozens of measuring instruments with *functional* in their titles have appeared in the literature in the past 30 years, and it is now true that in speech-language pathology an emphasis on functionality in writing clinical goals and outcomes is almost mandatory.

Despite the frequency of the word *functional* in contemporary clinical writings and practice, no standard definition of the term exists, and its meaning depends on who is using the word and what their purposes are. The label *functional communication* has

been used by speech-language pathologists to describe an approach to assessment and treatment that focuses on patients' daily life communicative success or lack thereof. It emphasizes the means by which patients get messages across, and it represents a movement away from a traditional emphasis on *language* to an emphasis on *communication*—the successful transfer of information from speaker or writer to listener or reader. This movement has been especially evident with regard to aphasia, but the emphasis on functional communication has spilled over to other neurogenic cognitive-communicative disorders as well. The general idea is that successful communication does not depend on the linguistic or phonologic accuracy of messages, but that speakers (and writers) can communicate successfully in spite of errors in word choice, syntax, or the phonologic-graphemic form of messages. It is this sense of the term that underlies several *"functional"* approaches to treatment, such as *Promoting Aphasics' Communicative Effectiveness* (Davis & Wilcox, 1985). Functional treatment approaches typically rely on activities that are structured to resemble the patient's daily life communication environment and focus on socially relevant aspects of communication, such as social conventions (greetings, farewells, and the like) and adherence to conversational rules.

When used by organizations that manage and pay for healthcare, *functional* often means *able to communicate basic needs and wants.* Because these organizations may be unwilling to pay for treatment to move patients beyond this level, defining the term in this way may save them money by eliminating their obligation to pay for treatment of patients with mild or moderate cognitive-communicative impairments (because the patients already can communicate basic needs and wants), and by ending payment for patients with more severe impairments as soon as they reach the minimal level of communicative competence represented by the provider's definition of functional.

In 1990 an advisory group to the American Speech-Language-Hearing Association (ASHA) proposed an operational definition of functional communication:

> "...the ability to receive or convey a message regardless of the mode; to communicate effectively and independently in natural environments." (p. 2)

The advisory group described assessment of functional communication as follows:

> "The extent of the ability to communicate with others in a variety of contexts, considering environmental modifications, adaptive equipment, time required to communicate, and listener familiarity with the client. Special accommodation of the communication partner to either receive or enhance the reception must be considered." (p. 2)

Simmons-Mackie and Damico (1996) commented, however, that functional communication entails more than simply conveying or receiving messages—it also serves to establish and maintain social relationships. Parr (1996) questioned inclusion of the word *independently* in ASHA's definition of functional communication, suggesting that *autonomous* would be a better choice.

Not all disabled people seek functional independence. Disabled persons often define independence in terms of autonomy and personal control in decision-making, thought, and action. A disabled person may be physically dependent on others in many aspects of everyday life but retain responsibility for other aspects of life such as managing finances, managing personal affairs, and maintaining social relationships.

IMPAIRMENT, DISABILITY, AND HANDICAP

Until the 1970s the medical model of disability dominated thinking about disability and its effects. The medical model considered disability a health problem caused by the physiologic effects of disease, injury, or physical abnormality on a person's body or mind. The purpose of intervention was to cure the disease, repair the injury, or correct the abnormality. The medical model ignored the potential contributions of a patient's physical and social environment to the disabling process. Regardless of how functional communication is defined, it has become clear that assessment of functional communication now must go beyond identifying and quantifying specific communicative or cognitive impairments to measuring the effects of such impairments on social and interpersonal relationships in natural settings.

In the 1970s many began to criticize the medical model for ignoring the effects of a disabling condition on the person's daily life competence and well being. Recognition of the medical model's limitations led some to argue for a *functional limitations* model of disability, which expanded the concept of disability to include nonmedical aspects—especially the affected person's ability to perform activities of daily life and to participate in social and community affairs.

In 1980 the World Health Organization (WHO) published the *International Classification of Impairment, Disability, and Handicap* (ICIDH), a system for coding aspects of disability based on a conceptual model of disablement. The ICIDH broadened the concept of disability to include not only the physiologic effects of a health condition but also the social effects of a disabling condition on a person's daily life competence and well being.

The World Health Organization is an international health agency established by the United Nations in 1948. WHO's stated mission is to support attainment of the highest levels of health by all peoples. The WHO Constitution defines *health* as complete physical, mental, and social well being, and not merely the absence of disease or infirmity. WHO publishes several international classification systems, the best known of which is the *International*

Statistical Classification of Diseases and Related Health Problems (ICD-10) which is used around the world for classification by diagnosis of diseases and other adverse health conditions.

The ICIDH summarized the effects of a disabling condition with the concepts of *impairment, disability,* and *handicap. Impairment* represented a structural abnormality (e.g., brain injury) or functional abnormality (e.g., hemiplegia) within a person. *Disability* represented the effects of an impairment or collection of impairments on a skill or ability. *Aphasia* and *poor ambulation* are examples of disabilities caused by brain injury and hemiplegia (their respective underlying impairments). *Handicap* represented the effects of one or more disabilities on a person's ability to carry out daily life roles. *Diminished ability to function as a spouse or parent* is one handicap that may be caused by brain injury. A single impairment may cause multiple disabilities and multiple handicaps; a single disability may cause multiple handicaps. For example, brain injury (an *impairment*) may cause hemiplegia, somatosensory loss, and visual-field blindness *(disabilities).* Hemiplegia (a *disability*) may prevent a person from resuming previous employment, preclude participation in recreational sports, and compromise activities such as playing a musical instrument or word processing *(handicaps).* The ICIDH classification system conceptualized disability as a linear process beginning with an underlying cause, leading to disability, leading in turn to handicap.

Before 1980, assessment of brain-injured adults focused on what the WHO called *impairments*—abnormalities in specific functions such as auditory comprehension, speech production, memory, and attention. The focus on assessing at the impairment level was consistent with prevailing attitudes toward treatment, which focused on remediation of specific functions. Publication of the ICIDH began a movement toward assessment that reflects the effects of brain injury on the affected person's successful participation in activities of daily living. The objectives of assessment moved from *efficacy* (changes in performance on impairment-level tests) to *effectiveness* (changes in performance on measures reflecting daily life communicative performance). The effects of these conceptual changes on assessment practices in speech-language pathology will be considered in Chapter 4.

GENERAL CONCEPTS 3-4

- Speech-language pathologists may test a patient with a neurogenic communication disorder to:
  - Diagnose a patient's communication impairments
  - Arrive at a prognosis for a patient's recovery of communication
  - Determine the nature and severity of a patient's communication impairments
  - Make decisions about treatment
  - Measure a patient's recovery of communication abilities or assess the efficacy of treatment

- Diagnostic labels are a convenient shorthand for summarizing several patient characteristics in a few words. Diagnostic labels, in themselves, do not lead directly to decisions about treatment, but they may convey information that suggests generic characteristics of treatment.
- Clinicians consider several categories of information when deciding on a prognosis:
  - *Neurologic findings.* The location and extent of nervous system abnormalities often have dramatic effects on a patient's recovery.

GENERAL CONCEPTS 3-4—cont'd	
• *Patient health.* A patient's general health and the presence of sensory and motor impairments also strongly influence recovery. • *Patient characteristics.* A patient's age, education, and premorbid intelligence have relatively weak effects on recovery. • The *patient profile approach* and the *statistical prediction approach* are two formalized procedures for generating prognoses. Both have greater accuracy for predicting the recovery of groups of patients than for predicting the recovery of individual patients. • Establishing stable performance baselines followed by periodic testing of performance is an objective way to measure a patient's recovery of communicative abilities or response to treatment. • In rehabilitation, the word *efficacy* refers to whether a treatment has a meaningful positive effect on a disease or condition. Efficacy	often is defined as change in performance on a standardized test. The word *outcome* refers to whether a treatment has a meaningful positive effect on a patient's daily life competence. • The word *functional* has no single established meaning in the rehabilitation literature, but usually means *affecting the patient's daily life competence or well being.* • The *International Classification of Impairment, Disability, and Handicap* (ICIDH) is a system for coding aspects of disability. It defines disability as the physiologic and social effects of a health condition on an individual's daily life competence and well being. • The ICIDH summarizes the effects of a disabling condition with the concepts of *impairment* (structural abnormality), *disability* (effects of impairments on skills or abilities), and *handicap* (diminished ability to carry out daily life roles).

THOUGHT QUESTIONS

Question 3-1 You receive the following referral from a neurologist on a patient named Mrs. Olson: *63-year old female 1 day postonset of suspected right-hemisphere stroke. Evaluation and recommendations please.*

You go to the patient's ward and find that Mrs. Olson's medical record is temporarily off the ward at a care-planning meeting. The nurse tells you that the patient is in her room, so you decide to do a preliminary screening at bedside. When you enter the patient's room she is lying in bed with her eyes closed. You touch her on the shoulder and she opens her eyes and looks at you. You introduce yourself and ask her how she is feeling. She gestures weakly with her left hand and closes her eyes. You say, "*Are you Mrs. Olson?*" She shakes her head without

opening her eyes. You touch her on the shoulder. She opens her eyes and looks at you. You say, "*Are you Mrs. Olson?*" She mumbles something incomprehensible and closes her eyes. You touch her on the shoulder. She does not respond.

What would you do next? What are some potential reasons for Mrs. Olson's unresponsiveness?

Question 3-2 Describe some ways in which not having a sufficient number of items in a test might lead to inaccuracy in describing a patient's true performance. What are some ways in which a patient's performance might fluctuate over time? How might those fluctuations interact with the number of test items to affect the accuracy with which a patient's true performance is specified?

Question 3-3 The following items make up a screening test of oral reading for use with brain-injured adults. The test instructions are, "*Now I'll show you some words on these cards. I want you to read each word aloud when I show it to you.*" What potential problems do you see in interpreting the results of the test?

1. cat
2. umbrella
3. dog
4. she
5. perambulator
6. the
7. yellow
8. seventy-two
9. its
10. slowly

Question 3-4 Consider the following inter-change between a clinician and a brain-injured patient:

Clinician: O.K. Mr. Chambers, now I'm going to say some words and sentences, and I want you to...

Mr. Chambers: O.K., fine, fine...

Clinician: ...and I want you to say them after me.

Mr. Chambers: Say them after you. O.K. O.K.

Clinician: Are you ready?

Mr. Chambers: Yes, yes, O.K. O.K.

Clinician: Here's the first one...

Mr. Chambers: Fine, fine, O.K. O.K.

Clinician: The boy has...

Mr. Chambers: The boy...

Clinician: The boy has a dog.

Mr. Chambers: The boy has...something or other.

What do you think is happening here? What potential explanations do you see for Mr. Chambers's pattern of responses? What would you do next if you were the clinician?

Assessing Cognition

I stood among them, but not of them, in a shroud of thoughts which were not their thoughts.
(Byron, L. Childe Harold)

Brain-injured adults may exhibit a confusing mix of cognitive and communicative impairments, ranging from disturbances in elementary cognitive processes such as attention and memory to disruption of complex cognitive and linguistic processes such as thinking, reasoning, language, and interpersonal communication. Perhaps no two brain-injured adults exhibit the same combination of impairments and severity of impairment. Consistent patterns do exist, however, making assessment less an unguided foray and more a systematic exploration of a brain-injured adult's unique pattern of impairments.

The nature and severity of a brain-injured adult's cognitive and communicative impairments are determined largely by the location and severity of the person's brain injury. Persons who have lost large amounts of brain tissue often experience impairments of basic processes such as attention and perception plus impairments of higher-level processes such as language, reasoning, and abstract thinking.

Persons who have localized or patchy brain injuries are likely to experience impairments of higher-level processes but not impairments of basic processes. However, severity is not the only determinant of what a brain-injured person can or cannot do. Location also matters. Cortical brain injuries are more likely to affect higher-level processes than are subcortical injuries. Frontal lobe injuries characteristically cause problems with initiation and regulation of purposeful behavior. Posterior language-dominant-hemisphere injuries characteristically cause problems with comprehension and production of language. Posterior non-language-dominant-hemisphere injuries characteristically cause problems with affect, interpersonal behavior, and attention to certain regions of extrapersonal space.

Sorting through a brain-injured person's collection of impairments and retained abilities requires patience, persistence, logic, intuition, and carefully chosen, reliable tests. In this chapter I will summarize some of the general relationships among brain injuries and cognitive impairments, and I will describe some of the many tests that may be used to identify and quantify the cognitive impairments experienced by brain-injured adults. In later chapters I will discuss assessment of specific brain injury syndromes—aphasia, nondominant-hemisphere syndrome, traumatic brain injury, dementia, and motor speech disorders. I begin with a basic process that underlies all purposeful behavior—the process of attention.

Although perception may be more basic than attention, I begin with attention because attentional impairments are common in brain-injured adults regardless of the location of brain injury. Perceptual impairments, on the other hand, tend to be related to specific regions of brain injury. For these reasons I will discuss perceptual impairments as they appear in the various brain injury syndromes.

ATTENTION

Tell me to what you pay attention and I will tell you who you are. (Jose Ortega y Gasset)

Investigators, theorists, and practitioners have discussed attention for decades but have not agreed on a definition. They have defined attention in a multitude of ways, and dozens of models purporting to explain attention have been proposed since the time of Wilhelm Wundt and William James, who first drew psychologists' attention to attention in the late 1800s. Most contemporary models portray attention as a chain of cognitive processes organized more or less hierarchically, with lower-level processes more time-limited and modality-bound than later processes.

Wilhelm Wundt (1832-1920) and William James (1842-1910) are considered the fathers of modern psychology. Each established schools of psychology with psychology laboratories—Wundt in Germany and James in the United States. Both schools were housed in departments of philosophy. At that time psychology was considered a branch of philosophy.

Although contemporary models of attention differ in specifics, most partition attention into components reflecting progressively increasing levels of cognitive workload, from elementary responsiveness to management of attentional resources during complex cognitive processing. Most models of attention consider *alertness*—the organism's physiologic and behavioral readiness to respond to stimulation—the foundation of all higher-level attentional processes.

Van Zomeren, Brouwer, and Deelman (1984) divided alertness into two forms, which they called *tonic alertness* and *phasic alertness*. They defined *tonic alertness* as an individual's readiness to respond over long time intervals (minutes to hours). Diurnal rhythms, drowsiness in monotonous tasks, and the midafternoon slump are examples of changes in tonic alertness. Lowered tonic alertness is a common consequence of brain injury. Brain-injured patients who drift off or fall asleep during testing or treatment do so because of lowered tonic alertness. Tonic alertness has much in common with *sustained attention (vigilance)*. Van Zomeren, Brouwer, and Deelman defined *phasic alertness* as an individual's momentary, rapidly occurring (within milliseconds) changes in receptivity to stimulation. Increased alertness in response to warning signals or to novel, interesting, or threatening stimuli are examples of changes in phasic alertness.

Diminished tonic alertness is an inconvenience and may slow brain-injured persons' progress in rehabilitation, but diminished phasic alertness usually is a greater hindrance to rehabilitation and usually causes greater impairment in daily life. Patients with diminished phasic alertness often miss initial items in testing or treatment tasks, fail to perceive brief stimuli, and fail to accommodate to changes in stimuli or response requirements. In daily life these patients often miss key elements in conversations and respond slowly or inappropriately to rapidly changing stimuli such as traffic signals.

Subsequent investigators have elaborated on Van Zomeren, Brouwer, and Deelman's model by partitioning attention into several types. Sohlberg and Mateer (2001), for example, recommended a clinically relevant model of attention that divides attentional processes into five categories, any or all of which may be affected by brain injury:

- *Focused attention* (sometimes called *orienting*) denotes basic responsiveness to simulation (e.g., looking toward the source of auditory, visual, or tactile stimuli). Focused attention has much in common with *phasic alertness,* discussed earlier.
- *Sustained attention* (sometimes called *vigilance*) denotes attention maintained over time. Although sustained attention and vigilance denote similar concepts, vigilance implies sustained attention over comparatively long time intervals in tasks in which targets to be detected occur randomly and infrequently relative to nontarget stimuli.
- *Selective attention* denotes attention maintained in the presence of competing or distracting stimuli or attending to individual stimuli in an array.
- *Alternating attention* denotes attention shifted from one stimulus to another in response to changing task requirements or the person's changing intent.
- *Divided attention* denotes attending to more than one activity concurrently (e.g., driving an automobile while talking on a cell phone).

Assessing Attention

Alertness. Clinicians usually do not directly test *tonic alertness* but estimate a patient's tonic alertness during interviews; from reports of family members, caregivers, and associates; or during tests of other cognitive and communicative abilities, especially tests requiring responsiveness maintained over long time intervals.

Reaction-time testing gives the most direct indication of phasic alertness. In reaction-time tests the patient responds (usually by pressing a key or a pushbutton) each time he or she perceives a specified stimulus (e.g., a flash of light or a brief sound). The time between the onset of each stimulus and the patient's response is measured. Incorporating warning signals (e.g., a tone preceding each target stimulus) into reaction-time tests may identify patients with impaired phasic alertness. Patients with impaired phasic alertness do much better when warning signals are provided than when no signals are given. (Persons with normal phasic alertness also do better when warning signals are provided, but the differences between no-warning-signal and warning-signal conditions are much greater for persons with impaired phasic alertness.)

Sustained Attention (Vigilance). Sustained attention typically is assessed with strings of computer-presented auditory or visual stimuli (e.g., tones, numbers, letters, or words) presented over relatively long and purposely monotonous intervals. The patient is instructed to indicate when she or he perceives a specified target by tapping, pressing a key on a keyboard, raising a hand, or saying *yes.*

Selective Attention. Selective attention typically is assessed with paper-and-pencil *cancellation tasks* in which the test taker must scan printed arrays of numerals, letters, or symbols and cross out or circle each occurrence of a designated target (Figure 4-1). The difficulty of cancellation tasks may be increased by adding conditions to the specification of targets (e.g., *Cross out the number 6 when it follows a letter*) or by adding competing or distracting visual material to stimulus arrays, as in Figure 4-1.

The *Stroop Test* (Golden, 1978) is a popular test of visual selective attention. In the Stroop test the test taker first reads aloud color names printed in black ink, then names the colors of groups of *X*s printed in different colored inks, and finally reads aloud color names printed in colors that conflict with the color names (e.g.,

ᖜᖷᖷ☆ᖷᖜᖷ☆ᖳᖷᖜᖜᖜ☆ᖳ

"Cross out each star."

JL19N6MO765PZ64AFK858PGAX6736RMC92

"Cross out each number that immediately follows a letter."

JL19N6MO765PZ64AFK858PGAX6736RMC92

"Cross out each number that immediately follows a letter."

Figure 4-1 ■ Cancellation tasks. A simple cancellation task *(top)*. A more difficult cancellation task *(middle)*. A cancellation task with superimposed distracting visual material *(bottom)*.

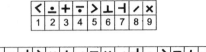

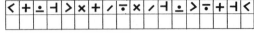

Figure 4-2 ■ Test items similar to those in the *Symbol Digit Modalities Test* (Smith, 1982). The test taker writes numbers in the blank cells according to the key above.

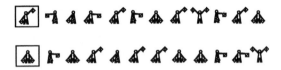

Figure 4-3 ■ A cancellation task with changing targets (in boxes) for each line.

the word *red* printed in blue ink). Large differences in speed and accuracy between the first two tasks and the third task are considered indications of impaired selective attention.

Selective attention sometimes is assessed with tasks like those used to test sustained attention, but with competing or distracting stimuli added. *Choice reaction-time tests* are tests in which the tested person is instructed to respond each time he or she perceives a stimulus matching a specified criterion (e.g., a 500 *Hz* tone embedded in a string of higher-pitched or lower-pitched tones). Performance is quantified as the number of correct and incorrect responses and as the person's reaction times to target stimuli.

> The distinction between sustained attention and selective attention is in some respects artificial because even in simple sustained-attention tasks the test taker must selectively attend to the test stimuli and not to some other aspect of the task such as the label on the computer monitor, the background noise on the auditory stimulus tape, or the pattern on the clinician's neckwear.

The *Symbol Digit Modalities Test* (*SDMT;* Smith, 1982) is a paper-and-pencil test that requires visual scanning plus sustained attention and selective attention. The SDMT has 110 blank squares in which the test taker writes the numerals 1 through 9 according to a key

(Figure 4-2). Impaired performance on the SDMT is not necessarily a sign of brain injury. SDMT performance also declines as a consequence of normal aging. Mean SDMT scores of persons who are 15 to 24 years old are almost 20 points higher than SDMT scores of persons who are 65 to 74 years old.

Alternating Attention. Tests of alternating attention require the test taker to change attentional focus in response to changing task requirements. Most tests of alternating attention are sustained-attention tests in which response requirements periodically change. For example, the test taker may have to perform a cancellation task in which targets in lines of letters, numerals, or other symbols must be crossed out, with a new target designated for each line (Figure 4-3).

Another alternating-attention test format requires the test taker to begin the test by crossing out the odd numbers in a long list of randomly arranged numbers. When the test taker's performance stabilizes, the examiner says *even,* and the test taker switches to crossing out even numbers. The test continues for several cycles in which the examiner changes the target response each time the test taker's performance stabilizes.

Serial calculation tests are challenging tests of alternating attention. The test taker begins by subtracting a specified number (e.g., 5) from a number specified by the examiner, then subtracts that number from the remainder, and so on. When the test taker's performance stabilizes the examiner says *add,* and the test taker reverses direction and begins adding by 5. The test continues with the examiner changing the test from addition to subtraction or vice versa each time the test taker's performance stabilizes.

Divided Attention. Divided-attention tests come in two forms. In one form the test taker must retain information in memory while performing mental operations on the information. *Digits backward* is a relatively easy divided-attention test with this format. The examiner says a group of single-digit numbers and the test taker repeats them in reverse order. Other tests with this format include counting backward; saying the alphabet, days of the week, or months of the year in reverse order; spelling words backward; counting backward by 2s, 3s, 4s, or 5s; or saying letters and words alternatively in sequence (*A-1-B-2-*).

The second form of divided-attention tests (called *dual-task format*) requires the test taker to perform two concurrent tasks. In a typical dual-task test the test taker listens to a tape recording in which a speaker reads aloud a list of randomly arranged letters and the test taker says *yes* whenever she or he hears a designated letter, while simultaneously performing a paper-and-pencil cancellation task by crossing out occurrences of a target letter in strings of random letters.

The *Paced Auditory Serial Addition Test* (*PASAT;* Gronwall, 1977) is a challenging divided-attention test in which the test taker hears strings of single-digit numbers, adds each number to the preceding number, and says the result. (For example, the string *3-6-5-1-9* requires the response *9-11-6-10*). Lezak, Howieson, and Loring (2004) have commented that the PASAT is stressful even for non-brain-injured adults, who experience great pressure and a sense of failure even when they are doing well. Consequently, Lezak, Howieson, and Loring reserve the PASAT for detection of subtle attentional impairments. They recommend that persons being tested be forewarned that the PASAT may be stressful and that they may believe they are failing when they are not.

Attention in Daily Life. Most tests of attention call on cognitive processes in addition to attention (e.g., visual search, scanning, tracking, short-term memory, and appreciation of verbal or mathematical concepts). The ecologic validity of such tests—whether they represent what individuals need in daily life—is unknown. Some (e.g., Ponsford & Kinsella, 1992; Sbordone, 1998; Kerns & Mateer, 1998) have argued that because standard tests of attention are highly structured they are not sensitive to impairments that may be present in less structured daily life environments. In response to these concerns, Robertson, Ward, Ridgeway, and Nimmo-Smith (1994, 1996) designed the *Test of Everyday Attention (TEA)* as an ecologically valid test of attention, using everyday materials such as maps and telephone directories.

There are eight subtests in the TEA, assessing *sustained attention, selective attention,* and *alternating attention,* with and without distraction. Subtests are administered in the order shown in Table 4-1.

Although the TEA is based on a neuropsychological model of attention and includes subtests to assess selective attention, sustained attention, alternating attention, and divided attention, it remains to be seen whether the TEA provides ecologically more valid estimates of attention than standard tests. Bate, Mathias, and Crawford (2001) have suggested that the TEA has much in common with traditional tests of attention. They compared the TEA performance of adults who had severe traumatic brain injuries with the performance of age-matched and education-matched adults without brain injury. Brain-injured participants' performance on most

TABLE 4-1	Subtests in the *Test of Everyday Attention*	
Subtest	**Attentional Component**	**Description**
Map search	Selective attention	The test taker searches for designated symbols on a map.
Elevator floor counting	Sustained attention	The test taker pretends to be in an elevator whose floor indicator is out of order. The test taker must keep track of floors by counting tape-recorded tones simulating tones used in elevators to announce arrival at a floor.
Elevator floor counting with distraction	Selective attention	The situation is the same as the elevator counting task, but the test taker must ignore higher-pitched distractor tones interspersed with the tones heard in the previous elevator counting task.
Visual elevator floor counting	Alternating attention	Rows of drawings of elevator doors are divided into sets by up or down pointing arrows. The test taker must count floors up or down according to the directions of the arrows.
Auditory elevator floor counting with reversal	Alternating attention	The test taker hears tape-recorded medium- or high-pitched tones and must count up for each high-pitched tone and down for each low-pitched tone.
Telephone directory search	Selective attention	The test taker searches for designated symbols in a simulated telephone directory.
Telephone directory search —dual task	Divided attention	The test taker searches a simulated telephone directory for designated symbols while concurrently counting tape-recorded sequences of tones.
Lottery	Sustained attention	The test taker listens to tape-recorded sets of two letters plus three numbers and writes down the two letters preceding any number ending in 55.

Data from Robertson, J.H., Ward, T., Ridgeway, V, and Nimmo-Smith, I. (1996). The structure of normal human attention: The test of everyday attention. *Journal of the International Neuropsychological Society, 2,* 525-534.

subtests of the TEA correlated significantly with their performance on standard tests of attention, except for *elevator floor counting* and *elevator floor counting with distraction.* The TEA *map search* best discriminated between participants with traumatic brain injuries and participants with no brain injuries.

Bate, Mathias, and Crawford did not directly test the ecologic validity of the TEA. However, the TEA, like traditional tests of attention, is structured and administered in a distraction-free environment. Although the TEA tries to mimic daily life by using materials resembling daily life, the structured TEA test environment differs markedly from unstructured daily life environments. At this time the ecologic validity of the TEA has yet to be established.

GENERAL CONCEPTS 4-1

- Major cognitive processes supporting communication include *attention, memory,* and *executive function.*
- Attention may be partitioned into components reflecting progressively increasing levels of cognitive workload.
  - *Alertness* denotes an individual's physiologic and behavioral readiness to respond.
  - *Tonic alertness* denotes an individual's readiness to respond maintained over long intervals (minutes to hours). Clinicians usually assess a brain-injured patient's tonic alertness during interviews and tests or from reports of family members or caregivers.

GENERAL CONCEPTS 4-1—cont'd

- *Phasic alertness* denotes an individual's momentary, rapidly occurring (within milliseconds) readiness to respond. Reaction-time testing is the primary way to test phasic alertness. Diminished phasic alertness usually causes more daily life problems for brain-injured individuals than does diminished tonic alertness.
- *Focused attention* denotes basic responsiveness to stimulation (e.g., looking toward the source of auditory or visual stimuli).
- *Sustained attention* denotes attention maitained over time (minutes to hours). Sustained attention may be assessed by presenting strings of auditory or visual stimuli over long and monotonous intervals and requiring the patient to report each occurrence of a stimulus.
- *Selective attention* denotes attention maintained in the presence of competing or distracting stimuli or attention to individual stimuli in an array. Selective attention may be assessed with paper-and-pencil cancellation tasks or with choice reaction-time tests. The *Stroop Test* and the *Symbol Digit Modalities Test (SDMT)* are popular tests of visual sustained and selective attention.
- *Alternating attention* denotes attention shifted from one stimulus to another in response to changing task requirements or the person's changing intent. Alternating attention may be assessed with paper-and-pencil cancellation tasks with changing targets or with serial calculation tasks that alternate between addition and subtraction.
- *Divided attention* denotes attending to more than one activity concurrently (e.g., carrying on a conversation while cooking dinner). Divided attention may be assessed with dual-task tests in which the test taker must respond to two concurrent tasks or with tests in which the test taker must perform mental operations on material held in memory. The *Paced Auditory Serial Addition Test (PASAT)* is a challenging divided-attention test in which the test taker hears strings of single-digit numbers and must add each number to the preceding number and say the result.
- The *Test of Everyday Attention (TEA)* is said by its authors to be an ecologically valid test of attention with content resembling daily life. However, the *TEA* is structured and is administered in a distraction-free environment that does not mirror daily life. Consequently, the ecologic validity of the *TEA* is unknown.

MEMORY

If any one faculty of our nature may be called more wonderful than the rest, I do think it is memory. There seems something more speakingly incomprehensible in the powers, the failures, the inequalities of memory, than in any other of our intelligences. Memory is sometimes so retentive, so serviceable, so obedient; at others again, so tyrannic, so beyond control! We are, to be sure, a miracle in every way; but our powers of recollecting and forgetting do seem peculiarly past finding out. (Jane Austen, Mansfield Park)

Philosophers, scientists, novelists, and poets have been entranced and perplexed by the mystery of human memory for more than 200 years. Memory has been romanticized by novelists and dissected by philosophers, usually with more sound than substance. During the past 50 years, however, scientists studying how normal persons store and recall information have developed and tested theoretically based models of memory that possess considerable explanatory merit. Some of these models have been used to explore how brain injury affects memory and how models of normal memory may or may not explain the memory impairments of persons with brain injuries.

Impaired memory is an important consequence of brain injury. Memory disturbances afflict most brain-injured persons throughout recovery, and for many, memory never fully returns. Severe memory impairments consign brain-injured persons to a life of dependence on others. Mild memory impairments compromise independence in daily life, success in school, and competence at work.

Models of Memory

A voluminous literature concerned with how we process, retain, and recall information and experiences has emerged during the past three or four decades. During the 1960s, *stages models* of memory were popular. Stages models conceptualized memory as a series of phases through which information passed on its way to permanent storage. The phases were given different names in different models, and different models assigned slightly different characteristics to the phases, but the differences among models were mainly in details and not in general form. Most contemporary models of memory are elaborations on a basic three-stage model. *Three-stage models* divide memory into two stages of short-term storage and one stage of long-term storage.

The first stage in three-stage models is called the *sensory register* (or *sensory memory*). The sensory register is a mental space where incoming information is retained in modality-specific form (auditory, visual, or tactile after-images), a process called *registration*. The sensory register has limited capacity, and its contents decay within 1 or 2 seconds, after which the information is lost unless it has been transferred to the next stage. Registration is the means by which perceptions are introduced into the memory system by a combination of perceptual, attentional, and encoding processes, which occur more or less automatically and are not under volitional control.

The second stage in three-stage models is called *immediate memory* (sometimes called *short-term memory* or *primary memory*). Immediate memory has limited capacity, and information in immediate memory decays within a few seconds unless it is rehearsed. Rehearsal enables an individual to maintain information in memory for intervals ranging from minutes to hours. (Information in the sensory register cannot be rehearsed.) In early models of memory, immediate memory was considered a passive storage space through which information passed on its way to permanent storage in long-term memory.

The idea that immediate memory is the only path by which information can get to long-term memory has been challenged by studies of some brain-injured persons who perform poorly in immediate-memory tasks but have no obvious long-term memory impairments (Baddeley, 1996).

Immediate-memory capacity may be quantified as *retention span,* or the number of items of discrete information (e.g., numbers, letters, or words) that can be held in immediate memory at one time—for average normal adults, 7 ± 2 units. Immediate memory provides temporary mental space where a person making a telephone call can retain a telephone number between looking it up in the directory and dialing it, where a stenographer can retain what is said between hearing it and typing it, and where a carpenter can retain the dimension of a board between reading the plan and cutting the board. When the caller has dialed the restaurant, the stenographer has typed the phrase, or the carpenter has cut the board, the information in immediate memory decays unless rehearsed, freeing space for new information.

The third memory stage is called *long-term memory* (or *secondary memory*). Long-term memory has very large (perhaps infinite) capacity. Long-term memory is considered a static repository for knowledge acquired from schooling, books, movies, television, radio, and everyday experiences. Information in long-term memory decays slowly, if at all. Long-term memory permits us to remember that Vilnius is the capital of Lithuania, that winds blow counterclockwise around low-pressure systems, that a red signal light means *stop*, and that Heathcliff is a character in *Wuthering Heights.*

Some models of memory (such as that of Craik & Lockhart, 1972) dismiss the *stages* concept of memory in favor of a continuous *depth-of-processing* explanation. The general theme of depth-of-processing models is that the durability of information stored in memory is a function of the amount of active mental processing the information receives prior to storage. However, the general sense of how comprehension proceeds in depth-of-processing models is similar to that for stages models.

Contemporary cognitive science has largely replaced the concept of immediate memory with the concept of *working memory* (Baddeley, 1986; Baddeley & Hitch, 1974; Shallice & Warrington, 1970; and others). Working memory resembles immediate memory in that it is a limited-capacity system in which information decays within a few seconds unless rehearsed. Unlike immediate memory, which was considered a static repository for information on its way to long-term memory, working memory is considered a mental space in which the temporary outcomes of cognitive operations are stored during complex cognitive processing. For example, a person mentally performing an arithmetic calculation such as: *(12 + 14) − (8 + 7)* calculates the intermediate sums *26* and *15* and stores them in working memory before subtracting *15* from *26,* after which the results of the intermediate calculations are discarded and the final result is retained in working memory. Working memory is thought to play a central role in cognition by providing a means for storing and manipulating information needed for complex cognitive activities including reasoning, comprehension, abstract thinking, and problem solving.

The best known model of working memory is that of Baddeley & Hitch (1974). Baddeley and Hitch's model replaced unitary immediate memory with a three-part system—a *central executive* or *attentional controller* and two slave systems (a *phonologic loop,* which retains speech-related information, and a *visuospatial sketch pad,* which retains mental images of visual stimuli).

The *phonologic loop* is considered a temporary storage system for memory traces of phonologic input. Unless refreshed by rehearsal, the memory traces decay in 2 or 3 seconds. The phonologic loop is assumed to depend on subvocal articulation, which can maintain phonologic memory traces indefinitely provided the information does not exceed the capacity of the phonologic loop. If the information exceeds the capacity of the phonologic loop, the first items decay before the last items are processed, creating the well-known limit to immediate memory span (7 ± 2 units of information).

> Long words apparently take up more space in the phonologic loop than short words. More short words, such as *dog, boy, big,* and *day,* than long words, such as *convention, establishment, maintenance,* and *caravan,* can be retained in the phonologic loop without rehearsal. Most adults can remember about as many words as they can say in 2 seconds.

The *visuospatial sketch pad* is conceptualized as a temporary storage system for visual and spatial information. The visuospatial sketch pad is thought to be the means by which we visualize and mentally manipulate images. Some models of working memory divide the visuospatial sketch pad into visual and spatial subsystems, wherein the visual system processes aspects of color, shape, and texture and the spatial system processes aspects of location and distance. Empiric confirmation of the existence and character of the visuospatial sketch pad has proved difficult (Baddeley, 1996). The mechanism by which visual images are maintained in the visuospatial sketch pad has yet to be explained, and its functional significance has yet to be determined.

The *central executive* is the least well-defined and least well-understood of the three working-memory subsystems. The central executive is said to be responsible for selecting, initiating, and terminating cognitive processing operations and for coordinating the activities of the visuospatial sketch pad and the phonologic loop. The central executive is thought to control exchange of information between the phonologic loop and the visuospatial sketch pad and between working memory and other components of memory. The central executive is said to play a crucial role in logical reasoning, mental calculation, and comprehension of spoken and printed language. The concept of the central executive appears to have much in common with the concept of *executive function,* to be discussed later.

Recent Memory and Remote Memory

Discovery of patients in whom memory for the recent past (the last few hours to several months) is affected differently from memory for the distant past (years ago) led investigators to divide long-term memory into *recent memory* and *remote memory.* Recent memory and remote memory cannot be separated in normal adults but may be differently affected by brain injury. Persons with dementia, for example, often have no memory of events from the past few hours, days, or weeks but accurately remember events from childhood and growing-up years.

Retrospective Memory

Retrospective memory denotes retention and recall of information about past experiences and events. Most standardized memory tests assess retrospective memory. Retrospective memory was for many years considered a unitary phenomenon, but discovery of brain-injured persons who had severely impaired memory for past events and experiences but retained well-learned behavior patterns led investigators to divide retrospective memory into *declarative memory* and *procedural memory.* **Declarative Memory.** Declarative memory denotes *what we know about things.* Knowl-

edge of who we are, our parent's names and birthdates, the capital city of Poland, how many eggs make a dozen, the composition of a protein molecule, the names of the cranial nerves, and other such material is stored in declarative memory. Information in declarative memory can be brought to conscious awareness and verbally reported.

Tulving (1972) suggested that declarative memory in turn can be divided into *episodic memory* and *semantic memory.* Tulving characterized *episodic memory* as memory for personally experienced events that are specific to time and place. Our knowledge of who we were with and what we were doing at certain times comes from episodic memory, as does our sense of relationships between events that took place at different points in time. In many respects our sense of who we are comes largely from information in episodic memory.

Semantic memory contains our organized knowledge of the world, including most of what we learned in educational settings (facts, dates, names, and places). Semantic memory contains information that permits us to report that Thomas Jefferson was the third President of the United States, that there are 12 eggs in a dozen, that gasoline stations usually are found on busy highways, or that some barking dogs do bite. Semantic memories are not localizable in time and place.

However, one's knowledge that some barking dogs bite may be based on one or more incidents stored in episodic memory, which illustrates the interactions and overlap between episodic memory and semantic memory. It also shows that much of what we remember actually is constructed rather than remembered, but that is another (too long) story.

Procedural Memory. *Procedural memory has been described as* a collection of habits which can be applied automatically without having to think about new response strategies *(Garner & Valadka, 1994, p. 92). Procedural* memory can be loosely characterized as *knowing how to do things.* Remembering how to perform previously learned behavioral routines (e.g., driving an automobile, making a tuna salad sandwich, repairing a television set, or doing a neurologic examination) calls on information in procedural memory. Information in procedural memory cannot be brought to conscious awareness, but must be accessed via performance of the activity to which the information relates.

One's memory of having performed a procedure can be brought into consciousness and the steps in the procedure verbally reported. However, one's knowledge of the exact sequence, timing, amplitude, and other characteristics of the behaviors in the procedure can be accessed only by performing the procedure. Every good mechanic can tighten a nut on a bolt tightly enough so that it will not loosen but not so tightly that it breaks the bolt, but none can tell a novice how to do it, and a novice can learn how only by doing it many times.

Brain injury sometimes affects procedural memory less than declarative memory. There are reports of brain-injured patients who learn and use newly trained procedural routines although they are not aware of learning them and cannot verbally describe them (Ewert, Levin, Watson, & associates, 1989; Parkin, 1982; Verfaelli, Bauer, & Bowers, 1991). Even brain-injured persons who have severely impaired declarative memory usually remember how to perform well-learned procedures such as dressing, eating, and playing familiar card games.

Prospective Memory

As noted earlier, retrospective memory (which includes declarative and procedural memory) relates to past experience. *Prospective memory* permits intentions formed in the past to govern present behavior (remembering to remember). Prospective memory denotes remembering to do things at specific times—keep an appointment, show up for class, prepare dinner, or feed the cat. Some writers, including Lezak, Howieson,

and Loring, 2004, suggest that impaired prospective memory is not actually an impairment of the memory system, but arises because a person fails to recognize contextual cues that ordinarily would trigger recall of specific memories. For example, a person with impaired prospective memory might see an empty feeding dish on arising in the morning and not recall that the cat customarily is fed first thing in the morning. (Presumably the hungry cat would provide stronger and more salient cues on finding the dish empty.) Many brain-injured persons who have functional declarative memory are handicapped in daily life by faulty prospective memory. They miss appointments, forget to take medications, fail to pay bills, and do not acknowledge significant life events such as birthdays or anniversaries.

Table 4-2 summarizes the types of memory discussed in this section.

Assessing Memory

Retrospective Memory. For a patient who can tolerate the testing, clinicians are likely to administer a comprehensive retrospective memory test battery to assess the patient's retention span, retention and recall of new information, retrieval of information from remote memory, and visual memory.

Retention Span. *Retention span* denotes the amount of information an individual can store in memory after a single exposure to the information. Retention-span testing usually assesses *immediate retention,* in which the test taker's retention of information is tested immediately after the information is presented, and *short-term retention,* in which the test taker's retention of the information is tested following a delay interval of a few seconds to a minute or more.

The most common way of testing immediate retention span is *digit span testing,* in which the test taker repeats lists of randomly arranged single-digit numbers read aloud by the examiner. Digit-span testing typically begins with two-digit or three-digit lists, the number of digits

TABLE 4-2	**Divisions of Memory**
Divisions of Memory	Description
Sensory register	Very brief storage of stimulus traces in modality-specific form. Information cannot be manipulated or maintained by rehearsal.
Immediate memory	Limited capacity. Information decays in a few seconds unless consciously maintained by rehearsal.
Working memory	Contemporary replacement for the concept of short-term memory. An active working space in which intermediate products of cognitive processes are temporarily stored. May contain three components—the phonologic loop, the visuo-spatial sketch pad, and the central executive.
Long-term memory	Long-lasting storage of information. Information in long-term memory decays slowly, if at all.
Retrospective memory	Memory for past experiences, events, and information.
Declarative memory	Memory for what we know about things.
Episodic memory	Memory for past events that are specific to a time and a place.
Semantic memory	Organized knowledge of the world, including knowledge gained in educational settings.
Procedural memory	Knowledge of how to perform behavioral routines learned in the past.
Prospective memory	*Remembering to remember*—remembering to carry out previously scheduled actions.

in successive lists increasing until the patient cannot repeat a list without error. Digit-span tests are found in several memory test batteries and in most general-intelligence tests. Lists of random letters or lists of unrelated words also may be used to measure immediate retention span. Normal spans for digits, letters, and words are similar, and range from five to seven items. (Average retention span is seven digits, six letters, or five words.)

The number of elements that can be remembered in retention-span tests increases if the elements in the list to be remembered are related. Semantic relationships among words (e.g., knife, fork, spoon, plate, cup, saucer, breakfast, lunch, dinner) or familiar number patterns (e.g., 1492, 911, 365) permit test takers to "chunk" elements, thereby increasing the number of elements that can be retained.

Digit-span, letter-span, and word-span tests are *auditory-verbal tests,* in that the patient must comprehend, retain, and repeat digits, letters, or words spoken by the examiner. Patients with impaired auditory comprehension or impaired speech production may do poorly on such tests because of their comprehension or speech-production impairments and not because of impaired retention. For these patients, retention-span tests with nonverbal stimuli may provide a better estimate of their true retention span. The most common nonverbal retention-span tests are *block-tapping tests.* A set of blocks is placed before the test taker, and the examiner taps some of them in prearranged order. The test taker then is asked to tap the blocks in the order tapped by the examiner. The number of blocks in the sequence increases until the test taker no longer can duplicate the examiner's tapping patterns without error. The *Knox Cube Test* (Arthur, 1947) is the best known block-tapping test. However, the cubes in the Knox Cube Test are arranged in a row, permitting resourceful test takers to number them mentally. The *Corsi*

Block-Tapping Test (Milner, 1971) prevents that strategy by placing the blocks in a random array.

Short-term retention typically is assessed with retention-span tests in which a delay of a few seconds to a few minutes is inserted between the examiner's presentation of each test item and the test taker's opportunity to respond. Language-competent test takers typically retain the items in short-term retention tests by mentally rehearsing the information (most often by subvocally repeating the items). Some retention-span tests prevent rehearsal by requiring the test taker to count backward or say the alphabet backward during the delay interval. The intervening activity is called *interference*. Normal adults whose retention performance is errorless with unfilled delays of up to 30 seconds recall only about 60% to 75% of items after a 10-second delay with interference (Lezak, Howieson, and Loring, 2004). The performance of adults with brain injuries is even more strongly affected by interference. For some, imposing a 3-second filled delay completely disrupts short-term retention.

Short-term retention tests come in two forms. In *subspan* retention tests the examiner repeats a list of words until the patient can produce them without error. The examination continues with other activities, and after several minutes the examiner asks the patient to say the words in the list. The examiner may prompt the patient for unremembered words by saying a related word or a category name, or by saying words the patient has failed to remember mixed in with new words and asking the patient to identify the words previously heard.

In *supraspan* retention tests the examiner reads aloud a list of words that exceeds the patient's immediate retention span (usually 15 or more words). After the first reading the examiner asks the patient to repeat as many of the words as he or she can remember. Then the examiner reads the list again and asks the patient to say as many as he or she can remember. This procedure continues until the patient has learned the list or for a predetermined number of trials (usually four or five). Sometimes a recognition trial is provided after the final recall trial for patients who have not learned the list in the prescribed number of trials. The *Auditory-Verbal Learning Test* (Rey, 1964) and the *California Verbal Learning Test* (2nd ed.; Delis, Kramer, Kaplan, & Ober, 2000) are frequently administered supraspan retention tests.

Remote Memory. In *remote-memory* tests the examiner asks the patient for personal information such as birthplace, school attendance, and employment history. It is not always necessary to administer a separate test of remote memory because some items in screening tests of mental status test remote memory. Biographic information that depends on remote memory also may be obtained during the patient interview or as part of routines for gathering patient information when filling out test forms.

Visual Memory. In typical tests of *visual memory* the examiner shows the patient cards on which geometric designs such as the one shown in Figure 4-4 are printed and asks the patient to draw them from memory. Many such tests are available, but the *Memory for Designs*

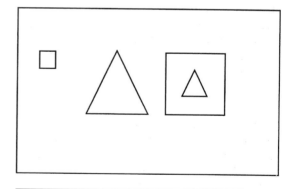

Figure 4-4 ■ A plate from the *Revised Visual Retention Test*. The inclusion of smaller figures in the periphery makes these designs sensitive to visual inattention. (From Benton, A.L. [1992]. *The Revised Visual Retention Test* [5th ed.]. San Antonio, TX: The Psychological Corporation.)

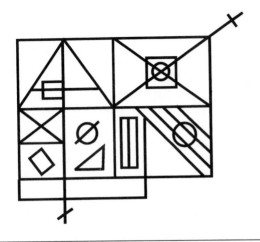

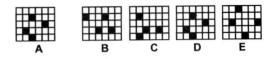

Figure 4-6 ■ A test item similar to those in the *Visual Retention Test* (Warrington & James, 1967). The test taker is shown a stimulus figure **(A)** for several seconds. Then the test taker is shown several figures **(B, C, D, E)**, one of which is the one previously seen. The test taker must identify the previously seen figure.

Figure 4-5 ■ A complex figures test item. The test taker first copies the figure, then must draw it from memory after an intervening activity.

Test (Graham & Kendall, 1960) and the *Benton Visual Retention Test* (5th ed.; Benton, 2003) are popular with clinicians for testing brain-injured adults. The Benton test differs from the others in that test items are sensitive to the presence of attentional impairments affecting one side of visual space (see Figure 4-4).

Complex-figure tests are challenging tests of visual perception, organization, and memory. The test taker is shown a complex geometric drawing such as the one in Figure 4-5 and is asked to copy the design on a blank sheet of paper. After a short delay (1 to 3 minutes) the test taker is asked to draw the design from memory. After a longer delay (20 to 30 minutes) the test taker again is asked to draw the figure from memory. Several complex-figure tests have been published, the best known of which is the *Rey-Osterrieth Complex Figure Test* (Rey, 1941; Osterrieth, 1944).

If a patient fails a drawing-from-memory test, the clinician may administer a visual memory test in which the patient is asked to recognize rather than draw previously presented visual stimuli. In most visual recognition memory tests the patient is shown a series of cards, each con-taining a different drawing or picture. Then a second set of cards containing the previously seen items mixed with new items is shown to the patient, and the patient indicates the items she or he has seen before. Some visual recognition memory tests resemble visual reproduction tests in which the stimuli are geometric designs (i.e., the *Recurring Figures Test,* Kimura, 1963; and the *Visual Retention Test,* Warrington & James, 1967). In other visual recognition memory tests the stimuli are drawings of real objects, as in the *Continuous Recognition Memory Test* (Hannay, Levin, & Grossman, 1979), in which the stimuli are plants, sea creatures, and animals. Figure 4-6 shows designs similar to those included in the *Visual Retention* test.

Prospective Memory. Tests of retrospective memory are not sensitive to impaired prospective memory (Sunderland, Harris, & Baddeley, 1983), but few tests of prospective memory are available. The primary exception is the *Rivermead Behavioural Memory Test (RBMT;* Wilson, Cockburn, and Baddeley, 1985). The RBMT provides for limited testing of prospective memory, with six items to test retrospective memory and two items to test prospective memory (Box 4-1).

A second version of the RBMT, called the *Rivermead Behavioural Memory Test—Extended (RBMT-E),* was published in 1999 (Wilson, Cockburn, & Baddeley, 1999). The RBMT-E doubles the amount that must be remembered, but test items and administration are similar to the original RBMT.

Box 4-1	**The Rivermead Behavioral Memory Test**

- *(Retrospective memory)* The examiner shows the patient a photograph and tells the patient the pictured person's name (e.g., *Catherine Taylor*). After several intervening test items the examiner again shows the patient the photograph and asks the patient to give the person's name.
- *(Prospective memory)* The examiner borrows a possession from the patient, hides it in a drawer or cupboard in view of the patient, and tells the patient to ask for the belonging at the end of the session and to tell the examiner where it is hidden. At the end of the session the examiner announces that the test is over. If the patient does not spontaneously ask for the hidden possession, the examiner prompts the patient (e.g., *You were going to ask me…*).
- *(Prospective memory)* The examiner sets a timer to sound an alarm in 20 minutes and tells the patient to ask about his or her next appointment when the alarm sounds. If the patient does not spontaneously ask about the next appointment when the alarm sounds, the examiner asks the patient what he or she was to do when the alarm sounded.
- *(Retrospective memory)* The examiner shows the patient 10 line drawings of common objects and asks the patient to name each one. After an intervening test item, the examiner shows the patient the 10 line drawings mixed with 10 new drawings and asks the patient to identify those seen before.
- *(Retrospective memory)* The examiner reads aloud a short narrative and asks the patient to retell it. After several intervening test items, the examiner again asks the patient to retell the story.
- *(Retrospective memory)* The examiner shows the patient five pictures of faces, one at a time, and asks the patient to tell the examiner whether the person is male or female and under or over 40 years old. The examiner tells the patient that he or she is to remember the faces. After an intervening test item the examiner shows the patient the five pictures mixed with five new ones and asks the patient to identify those seen before.
- *(Retrospective memory)* The examiner walks a short route in the room (e.g., to the door, bookshelf, sink, desk, chair) and leaves an envelope at one place on the route while the patient watches. The examiner then retrieves the envelope and gives it to the patient and asks the patient to walk the same route and leave the envelope in the same place as the examiner did. After three intervening test items the examiner again asks the patient to retrace the route and put the envelope in the same place as before.
- *(Retrospective memory)* The examiner asks the patient 10 questions that assess orientation to person, place, and time.

Data from Wilson, B.A., Cockburn, J., & Baddeley, A. (1985). *The Rivermead behavioural memory test.* Suffolk, England: Thames Valley Test Company.

Lezak, Howieson, and Loring (2004) comment that the RBMT lacks sensitivity at both high and low ends. It is too difficult for patients with severely impaired memory and too easy for patients with mild memory impairments. Lezak, Howieson, and Loring consider the RBMT most appropriate for patients with midrange memory impairments—impairments that are too severe to permit the patient to be fully independent but not so severe that the patient requires custodial care.

GENERAL CONCEPTS 4-2

- *Stages models* of memory conceptualize memory as a series of phases through which information passes on its way to permanent storage. *Three-stage models,* which divide memory into two stages of short-term storage and one stage of long-term storage, are the most common stage models of memory.

Continued

- The *sensory register* (also called *sensory memory*) is the first stage in most three-stage models. The sensory register is a place where incoming information is retained in modality-specific form. The sensory register has limited capacity, and its contents decay within 1 or 2 seconds.
- *Immediate memory* (also called *short-term memory* or *primary memory*) is the second stage in most three-stage models of memory. Immediate memory has limited capacity, and information in immediate memory decays within a few seconds unless rehearsed. Immediate memory capacity may be quantified as retention span—the number of discrete items of information that can be retained without rehearsal. Retention span for normal adults is 7 ± 2 items.
  - *Long-term memory* (also called *secondary memory*) is the third stage in most three-stage models of memory. Long-term memory has very large (perhaps infinite) capacity, and information in long-term memory decays slowly, if at all. Long-term memory is where we retain knowledge acquired in school or from everyday experiences.
- Cognitive science has largely replaced the concept of immediate memory with the concept of *working memory*—a limited-capacity space in which information decays within a few seconds unless rehearsed. Working memory is considered a mental space for storing temporary outcomes of cognitive operations during complex cognitive processing.
  - The most popular model of working memory includes three components—a *central executive,* a *phonologic loop,* and a *visuospatial sketchpad.*
- Most tests of memory are designed to test *retrospective memory*—retention and recall of information about past experiences.

- Retrospective memory can be divided into *declarative memory* and *procedural memory.* Declarative memory is memory for past events and experiences. Procedural memory is memory of how to perform procedures such as preparing a meal or driving an automobile. Brain injury often affects procedural memory less than it affects declarative memory.
- Declarative memory can be divided into *episodic memory* and *semantic memory.* Episodic memory is memory for personally experienced events specific to time and place. Semantic memory contains our knowledge of the world, including what we learn in educational settings.
- *Prospective memory* denotes remembering to do things such as keeping appointments and preparing meals. Impaired prospective memory may represent failure to recognize contextual cues that ordinarily stimulate recall of intended actions. In daily life many brain-injured persons are severely handicapped by faulty prospective memory.
- Assessment of retrospective memory typically includes tests of retention span, retention and recall of new information, retrieval of information from remote memory, and visual memory.
  - The most common test for retention span is a *digit-span test. Letter-span* and *word-span tests* also may be used to test immediate retention span. *Block-tapping tests* offer a nonverbal alternative to verbal digit-span testing.
  - Short-term retention may be assessed with retention-span tests administered with a delay between each test item and the patient's opportunity to respond. Retention-span tests may prevent rehearsal by requiring the test taker to count or say the alphabet backward during the delay interval (called *interference*).

- Most screening tests of mental status include items that test remote memory. Remote memory also may be assessed during interviews or when the examiner asks a patient for information needed to complete forms and reports.
- In tests of visual memory the patient is shown a series of geometric designs and must draw each design from memory. Tests of visual memory range from tests with relatively simple figures to tests with complex figures that challenge visual perception, organization, and memory.
- Tests of retrospective memory are not sensitive to impaired prospective memory. The *Rivermead Behavioural Memory Test (RBMT)* contains some items that test retrospective memory and some items that test prospective memory. Lezak has commented that the RBMT is too difficult for patients with severely impaired memory and too easy for patients with mild memory impairments.

EXECUTIVE FUNCTION

Everyone complains of poor memory. No one complains of poor judgment. (François de la Rochefoucauld)

The concept of *executive function* grew out of work by Norman and Shallice (1986), who incorporated a *supervisory attentional system* into a model of attentional processes. Shallice (1988) summarized the role of the supervisory attentional system as follows:

> ...the supervisory system has access to a representation of the environment and of the organism's intentions and cognitive capacities. It is held not to operate by directly controlling behavior but by activating or inhibiting particular schemata. It would be involved in the genesis of willed action and [is] required in situations where the routine selection of actions is unsatisfactory. (p. 335)

Since the time of Norman and Shallice the concept of executive function has proliferated. My February, 2006 search of the Medline database using the search term *executive function* yielded more than 4000 citations.

Executive function is doing what must be done to solve a problem or achieve one's goals. Executive function incorporates aspects of attention, memory, planning, reasoning, and problem solving to organize and regulate purposeful behavior. Executive function includes:

- Initiating intentional behavior
- Planning behavioral routines to accomplish intentions
- Maintaining and regulating goal-directed behavior
- Monitoring and modifying behavior in response to situational variables

Impaired executive function is a common consequence of brain injury, especially injury to the frontal lobes. Persons with impaired executive function perform poorly in situations in which they must plan behavioral routines to achieve a goal, monitor progress toward a goal, modify behavior in response to changing circumstances, or sustain behavior until the goal is reached.

Patients with impaired executive function do not spontaneously initiate purposeful activity. Those with severe impairments may not independently act to satisfy wants and needs unless instructed by others or impelled by discomfort such as thirst, bladder pressure, or cold temperature. Patients with severe impairments of executive function may sit alone in a room and stare at a wall, indiscriminately watch television from morning to night, or wander aimlessly from room to room. They may eat when food is put before them but may not independently eat or prepare meals even if hungry.

Patients with less severe impairments may carry out familiar and highly practiced activities such as meal preparation and housecleaning but do not spontaneously perform activities requiring planning and long-term goals. Activities of daily life (shopping, home maintenance, driving, or managing medications) may be impossible for these patients even though their attention, memory, and physical abilities are adequate. Even patients with mild executive function impairments have difficulty following directions, judging the adequacy and appropriateness of their behavior, staying on task, and carrying activities through to completion. Patients with mild executive function impairments are compliant but passive. They respond appropriately to requests, especially in highly structured situations. Some may talk at length about intentions, plans, and projects but never actually carry them out.

Patients with mild to moderate impairment of executive function often forget the purpose of what they are doing, are distracted by irrelevant events, wander off on mental tangents, or become caught up in one aspect of an activity and never finish. Because patients with impaired executive function are capable of doing more than they actually do, family members, caregivers, and others may consider them lazy, obstinate, or noncompliant, adding interpersonal conflict to the mix of psychosocial, cognitive, and communicative problems.

The concepts of executive function and the central executive are important elements of *resource-allocation models* of cognitive processing, in which mental resources are allocated to cognitive processes based on the demands of a task and the intentions of the person engaged in the task. Several resource-allocation models of mental processes have been described in the literature (Friedman & Polson, 1981; Kahneman, 1973; Norman & Bobrow, 1975). Clark and Robin (1995); McNeil and Kimelman (1986); McNeil, Odell, and Tseng (1990); Murray,

Holland, and Beeson (1997); Nicholas and Brookshire (1995b); Tompkins (1990); and Tompkins, Bloise, and Timko (1994) have related resource allocation to adults who have brain damage. The basic concept of resource allocation is that human brains have a limited pool of resources available for carrying out mental operations such as perceiving incoming stimuli, comprehending messages, storing information in memory, and formulating responses.

Any mental operation is believed to draw resources from the pool. More complex mental operations draw more resources than do less complex mental operations. If several mental operations are active at the same time, each draws resources from the pool. Consequently, the amount of resources drawn from the pool depends both on the number of mental operations and their complexity. If the demand for resources exceeds the resources available, some mental operations may be shut down or shortchanged, and performance suffers.

If the demands of ongoing mental operations reach the limit of available resources, calls for more resources cannot be honored by the central executive. If processing demands exceed the capacity of the pool, calls for more resources from individual mental operations may be ignored, or resources may be diverted from other active mental operations to the one making the call. In either case, performance deteriorates.

Those who have applied the concept of resource allocation to the performance of brain-injured adults assume that brain injury reduces the amount of processing resources in the pool, disrupts allocation of resources from the pool, or interferes with the use of resources gotten from the pool. They speculate that brain-injured adults' impaired performance may emanate from lack of resources, inefficient allocation of resources, or compromised access to resources. Whether brain injury reduces the amount of resources in the pool or compromises access to resources without diminishing the volume of the pool is not known. In

Box 4-2	**Effects on Performance of Brain-injured Adults**

A clinician was testing an aphasic woman's comprehension and recall of information from printed stories. She began by asking the patient to read a story aloud. Then she asked the patient questions about information in the story. The patient, who was troubled by phonologic selection and sequencing problems in her speech, read the stories slowly and with frequent phonologic errors that she tried to correct—usually without success. When she was questioned about information in the stories, the patient recalled almost nothing except the general theme of each story.

The clinician sensed that the patient's speech production problems interfered with her comprehension of the stories. In resource-allocation lingo, the mental resources required by the patient's effortful oral reading depleted the pool, leaving insufficient resources to be allocated to comprehension. The clinician then eliminated oral reading from the task by permitting the patient to read the stories silently. Under these conditions the patient's recall of information from the stories was equivalent to that of normal adults.

either case the effects on performance would be similar, although not identical in all situations (Box 4-2).

The resource allocation concept formalizes relationships that clinicians, psychologists, and teachers have recognized for many years—that when individuals are working at or near their limit, adding workload either by increasing the difficulty of what the person is doing or by adding another task, causes performance to deteriorate. The concept of resource allocation is nevertheless useful for clinicians because it provides a structured way to manage manipulation of variables when testing or treating brain-injured adults.

Assessing Executive Function

Most standard tests of cognition and communication are not sensitive to impaired executive function because the structure, predictability, and control of distractions associated with standard testing minimize the need for cognitive flexibility and executive control on the part of the test taker. Patients with impaired executive function who perform well on standard tests often break down when called on to perform similar tasks in less structured, more complex, and less protected real-life environments.

Because executive function encompasses underlying cognitive processes such as attention, memory, response flexibility, planning, reasoning, problem solving, and abstract thinking, conclusions about a patient's executive function typically come from the patient's performance on tests reflecting those processes. Assessment of attention and memory were discussed earlier. Assessment of response flexibility, planning, reasoning, problem solving, and abstract thinking are discussed next.

Response Flexibility. Some brain-injured patients have no trouble initiating behavior, but they have difficulty inhibiting, modifying, or stopping behavior once it has begun. They seem to be trapped by their first impressions and fail to appreciate subtle or abstract aspects of events or situations. They have difficulty adapting their behavior to changing tasks or response requirements. These patients often show a pattern of test performance in which the first few responses in a new task are less accurate than later responses in the same task. The problem may represent slowness in reallocating attention when situational requirements change or slowness at developing a strategy for dealing with changing task requirements. Response flexibility may be assessed with paper-and-pencil tasks in which the patient is asked to draw continuations of repetitive patterns such as those shown in Figure 4-7. Impaired response flexibility often appears as *perseveration*—excessive repetition of pattern elements caused by inability to shift from element to element within a pattern. Perseveration in such paper-and-pencil tasks is common in patients with severe brain injuries, in patients with right-hemisphere damage, in

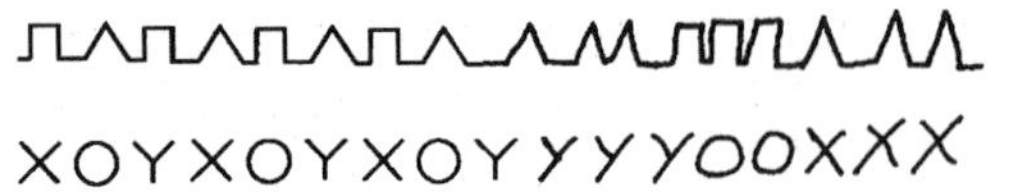

ЛЛЛЛЛЛЛ∿ЛЛ∿∿∿ЛЛ∿∿ЛЛ

XOYXOYXOYYYYOOXXX

Figure 4-7 ■ An example of perseveration in a test in which the test taker must draw continuations of repetitive patterns. Excessive repetitions of the same pattern of elements are considered perseveration.

patients with diffuse damage caused by traumatic brain injuries, and in patients with dementia. Verbal perseveration (inappropriate repetition of words or phrases) is common in many aphasia syndromes, as when a patient who has correctly named a pencil calls the next several objects pencils, or when a patient who has correctly given her name in response to the examiner's request continues to give her name in response to the examiner's questions about her address and vocation. Perseveration often appears in the first days and weeks following brain injury, but often diminishes and sometimes disappears as the patient recovers.

Planning. Planning may be assessed with *cancellation tests* (described previously) or with *trail-making tests* and *maze tests*. In *trail-making tests* the patient is given a sheet of paper on which sequences of letters, numbers, or a combination of letters and numbers are printed in a quasi-random array (Figure 4-8). The patient is asked to draw lines connecting the letters or numbers in sequence, according to a rule (such as 1-A-2-B, and so on). In *maze tests* the patient is asked to draw a continuous line to trace a path from the beginning to the end of the maze (Figure 4-9). Both tasks require the patient to maintain a mental representation of the appropriate path and to monitor progress as he or she draws. Making the paths longer and more complex increases the difficulty of the tasks.

The *Five-point Test* (Regard, Strauss, & Knapp, 1982) is a test of planning that also requires sustained attention, response flexibility, self monitoring, and rule following. The test consists of a

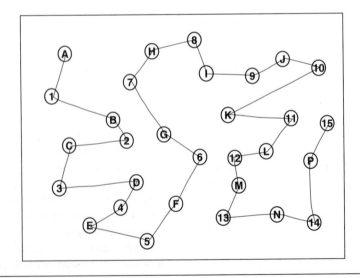

Figure 4-8 ■ A trail-making test. The test taker draws a path by alternately connecting letters and numerals in alphabetic and numeric order.

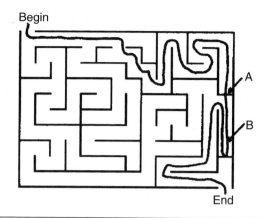

Begin

A

B

End

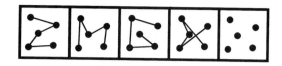

Figure 4-10 ■ Stimuli similar to those in the *Five-point Test* (Regard, Strauss, & Knapp, 1982). The test taker is instructed to create as many different designs as she or he can in 5 minutes by connecting the five dots *(right)*. The *Five-point Test* contains eight rows of identical five-element dot patterns such as these.

Figure 4-9 ■ A maze test item. The test taker must draw a continuous line from the beginning to the end of the maze without crossing maze lines *(A)* or retracing *(B)*.

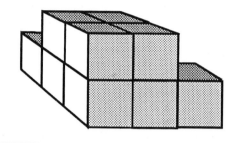

Figure 4-11 ■ An example of a block-counting test stimulus. The difficulty of a block counting test item depends on the number of blocks and the number of blocks hidden from view.

page on which an array of 40 squares is printed. Each square contains five identically arranged dots (Figure 4-10). The test taker is given 5 minutes to make as many different designs as possible by connecting the dots in each square with straight lines.

Reasoning. According to Lezak, Howieson, and Loring (2004), tests of reasoning assess an individual's capacity for logical thinking, appreciation of relationships, and practical judgment. Reasoning tests may focus on *verbal reasoning, arithmetic and numerical reasoning,* or *visuospatial reasoning.*

Verbal reasoning tests include:
- Reasoning and judgment tests in which the patient responds to questions such as, *What would you do if you found an unmailed letter on the street?*
- Verbal absurdities tests in which the patient identifies the logical inconsistencies in statements such as, *Bill Jones's feet are so big that he has to pull his trousers on over his head.*
- Logical relationship tests in which the patient must arrive at a conclusion based on analysis of logical relationships presented in a short narrative such as, *Fred is taller than Bill but shorter than Oliver. George is taller than Fred. Is George taller than Bill?*

Arithmetic and numerical reasoning tests include:
- Arithmetic problems in which the patient solves story problems such as, *Jill has 8 pencils. Katy has 4 times as many pencils as Jill. How many pencils do they have together?*
- Block-counting tests in which the patient counts the number of blocks depicted in drawings of three-dimensional stacks (Figure 4-11)

Visuospatial reasoning tests include:
- Picture-completion tests in which the patient tells what is missing from drawings of common objects, human figures, or animal figures with missing parts (Figure 4-12)

- Picture-arrangement tests in which the patient arranges scrambled pictures to portray a storylike sequence of events (Figure 4-13)
- Picture-absurdities tests in which the patient tells what is wrong with pictures depicting bizarre or impossible relationships or situations (Figure 4-14)

Raven's *Standard Progressive Matrices* (Raven, 1960), and *Coloured Progressive Matrices* (Raven, 1965) are tests of visuospatial analysis, integration, and reasoning with low verbal loadings, making them useful for estimating reasoning skills of brain-injured patients who have language impairments. The progressive matrices are multiple-choice tests in which the patient is shown visual patterns in which a part of each pattern is missing. The patient is asked to choose from a set of six or eight choices the one that completes the stimulus (Figure 4-15). The *Standard Progressive Matrices* includes many difficult items that may require verbal reasoning for their solution. The

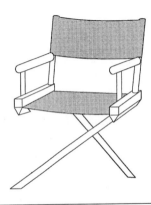

Figure 4-12 ■ An example of a picture-completion test stimulus. The person taking the test tells what is missing from the test stimulus.

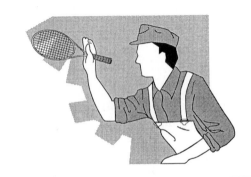

Figure 4-14 ■ A picture-absurdities test item. The person taking the test tells what is wrong with the picture.

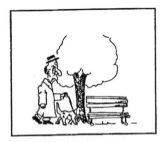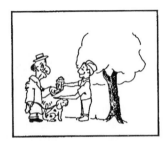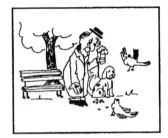

Figure 4-13 ■ An example of a picture-arrangement test stimulus. The person taking the test rearranges the pictures to tell a story. The pictures are shown in story order. The examiner gives them to the person taking the test in scrambled order.

Coloured Progressive Matrices are easier and are a better choice for brain-injured patients, except patients with very mild impairments.

Problem Solving. Problem solving calls on several abilities, including thinking ahead, understanding the consequences of actions, considering alternatives, and making choices—all components of executive function. Impairment of any of these abilities can disrupt problem solving. Few standardized tests of cognitive abilities are exclusive to problem-solving skills, although success in most requires some degree of problem solving. The *tower tests* (Shallice, 1982; Glosser & Goodglass, 1990; Saint-Cyr & Taylor, 1992) and the *Tinkertoy test* (Lezak, Howieson, & Loring, 2004) test problem solving as well as planning, organization, and maintenance of goal-directed behavior.

In the *tower tests* the test taker must rearrange colored rings, beads, or blocks on upright dowels to end with a specified arrangement (Figure 4-16). Performance is scored as the number of moves required to get from the starting position to the specified final arrangement.

In the *Tinkertoy test,* the patient is given 50 pieces of a standard Tinkertoy set and is told to make whatever he or she wants with them. The patient is given 5 minutes to plan and execute

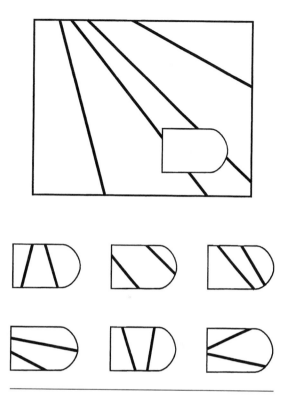

Figure 4-15 ■ An example of a *Progressive Matrices* task. The person taking the test chooses the pattern segment at the bottom that best completes the overall pattern at the top.

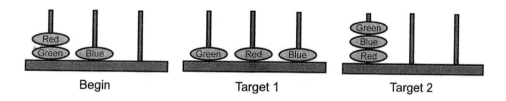

Begin   Target 1   Target 2

Figure 4-16 ■ A tower test. The test taker starts with the blocks arranged in a pattern by the examiner (*Begin*). Then he or she is given a drawing that shows the blocks rearranged in a new pattern and is asked to move the blocks to create the new pattern with the smallest number of moves possible. The number of moves the test taker makes to create the new pattern is recorded. *Target 1* can be created with two moves. *Target 2* cannot be created with fewer than five moves. (Data from Shallice, T. (1982). Specific impairment of planning. *Philosophical Transactions of the Royal Society of London, 298,* 199-209.)

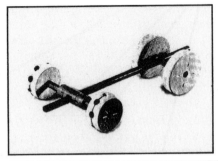

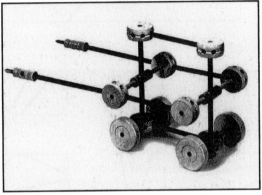

Figure 4-17 ■ A Tinkertoy construction by a brain-injured adult *(top)* and by a neuropsychologist presumably with no brain injury *(bottom)*. (From Lezak, M. D. [1995] *Neuropsychological assessment.* New York: Oxford.)

Tinkertoys are collections of small dowels of various lengths and colors, plus connectors, wheels, and other parts that can be assembled into constructions of considerable complexity.

Abstract Thinking. Impaired abstract thinking is almost a universal consequence of brain injury. Lezak (1995) describes impaired abstract thinking as, "...inability to think in useful generalizations, at the level of ideas, or about persons, situations, events not immediately present (past, future, or out of sight)." (p. 602). Lezak comments that tests of other cognitive processes such as planning, organizing, problem solving, and reasoning also supply information about abstract thinking. Adults with moderate to severe brain injuries do poorly on tests of abstract thinking regardless of the modality in which test items are presented or the nature of the responses required. Those with less severe injuries may perform well on some tests and poorly on others, depending on the complexity of the test and whether the test addresses an impaired stimulus or response modality.

Commonly administered verbal tests to assess abstract thinking include *proverb interpretation,* in which the patient tells the meaning of common proverbs such as *Don't put the cart before the horse,* and *similarities and differences,* in which the patient tells how two words are similar (orange/banana) or different (bird/dog).

Categorization and sorting tests provide another way to assess abstract thinking. In categorization and sorting tests the patient must determine the rules for assigning stimuli to categories by means of a trial-and-error process in which the examiner tells the patient only *right* or *wrong* following correct or incorrect assignments, respectively. The *Wisconsin Card Sorting Test* (*WCST*; Grant & Berg, 1948) is a widely used categorization and sorting test. In the WCST the test taker is given a deck of cards, each of which contains one to four symbols (triangle, cross, star, circle). The symbols on each card are printed in one of four colors (red, green, yellow, blue). The test taker is instructed

the construction, after which the examiner asks, *What is it?* and writes down the patient's response. The construction is scored with a seven-category system that takes into account the number of elements in the construction; whether it has moving parts; whether it is free-standing and three-dimensional; the appropriateness of the name given by the patient; and the number of misfits, incomplete fits, and failed fits. According to Lezak, Howieson, and Loring, the Tinkertoy test allows patients to initiate, plan, and structure a potentially complex activity and independently carry it out. Figure 4-17 shows a Tinkertoy construction by a brain-injured adult and a construction by an adult with no brain injury.

to sort the cards into four stacks according to the examiner's feedback.

When the test begins, color is the principle governing the sort, and the examiner says *right* whenever the patient sorts a card by its color. When the test taker has deduced the color-sorting principle (10 consecutive correct placements), the principle for sorting changes to form. (The only signal of the change to the test taker is a change in the feedback provided for sorting responses.) When the test taker has deduced the form-sorting principle, the principle changes to number, and so on, for two cycles of color-form-number.

Tests Specifically Designed for Assessment of Executive Function. Several procedures for directly estimating executive function have been published during the past 2 decades. The procedures attempt to assess behavior in tasks that require initiation, planning, problem solving, organization, control, and monitoring of performance, often in tasks that simulate real-life situations. One of the first of these procedures was the *Six Elements Test* (*SET*; Burgess & Shallice, 1991). The SET is made up of six open-ended tasks, divided into three sets of two tasks each:

- Make up and tell two stories—one's best holiday or birthday, and one's most memorable experience.
- Solve two sets of 30 easy arithmetic problems.
- Write the names of two 30-item sets of line drawings depicting common objects.

The test taker is told that she or he has 10 minutes to complete the test, but that it is impossible to complete all six tasks within the time limit. The test taker also is told that she or he must follow two rules during the test: (1) complete at least part of all six tasks, and (2) work on at least one different task before working on the second set of any task. Scoring penalties are imposed for not working on every task, unequally apportioning time among the tasks, or otherwise breaking the rules.

Burgess and Shallice (1997) developed the *Hayling Sentence Completion Test (HSCT)* as a stand-alone test of executive function. The HSCT has two parts. In Part A, the examiner reads a set of 15 sentences in which the final word of each sentence is missing and asks the test taker to say a word that completes the sentence so that the sentence makes sense, as in, *He mailed a letter without a...(stamp)*. In Part B, the examiner reads a different set of 15 sentences and asks the test taker to say a word that makes no sense as the final word: *He opened the door and turned on the...(carrot)*. The HSCT yields two scores: error responses (words unrelated to sentence contexts in Part A or related to sentence contexts in Part B) and response latencies in Part B minus response latencies in Part A (which, according to Burgess and Shallice, represents the additional time needed to inhibit high-probability responses and to think of and say a nonsensical alternative).

Wilson, Alderman, Burgess, and associates (1996) published a test of planning, organization, reasoning, problem solving, and self-monitoring called *The Behavioural Assessment of the Dysexecutive Syndrome (BADS)*. The BADS includes six subtests that, according to the authors, simulate everyday activities.

- *Rule Shift* (cognitive flexibility). The test taker names the colors or the values of red or black playing cards according to the examiner's instructions, which periodically change during the test.
- *Action Programme* (planning). The test taker removes a cork from a narrow plastic tube while following a set of rules.
- *Key Search* (planning, organization). The test taker plans a strategy to find a key lost in a field.
- *Temporal Judgment* (reasoning). The test taker estimates the length of everyday time intervals, such as the average life of a dog.
- *Zoo Map* (planning). The test taker plots a route on a map according to a set of rules.
- *Modified Six Elements Test* (planning, organization, self-monitoring). This test is a modified version of the Shallice and Burgess (1991) *Six Elements Test*. The test taker must apportion the available time among three

tasks (picture naming, arithmetic, and dictation) while following a set of rules.

The BADS also includes two *Dysexecutive Questionnaires,* each containing 20 items describing behaviors related to executive function. One version is completed by the patient, and the other is completed by a family member or someone who knows the patient well. The 20 items address changes in emotion, personality, motivation, behavior, and cognition. Discrepancies between the responses of the patient and the family member or associate are considered evidence of the patient's lack of insight or awareness.

Norris and Tate (2000) evaluated the ecologic validity of the BADS compared with six other commonly used tests of executive function. Their findings supported the ecologic validity of the BADS but not the ecologic validity of the other six tests. Norris and Tate also evaluated the reliability of the Dysexecutive Questionnaires and reported disappointing results because of variability in the ratings of patients and family members or associates. Norris and Tate concluded that, "The results of this study support the inclusion of the BADS in the tests available for the assessment of executive abilities." (p. 42), but they did not consider the BADS an adequate replacement for other commonly used tests. Sohlberg and Mateer (2001) commented that the BADS may be appropriate for a broad range of brain-injured patients but usually is not sensitive to impaired executive function in high-functioning patients.

Chamberlain (2003) cautioned that two issues must be kept in mind by those using the BADS. First, the BADS shares the weakness of other standardized tests in that it is administered in a structured environment with no distractions, thereby limiting the characteristics that lead to failures of executive function in everyday situations. Second, the BADS does not identify the abilities required for success in the BADS tasks, making it difficult to interpret test scores and to identify the kinds of daily life tasks that might prove difficult for a test taker.

A few observational procedures for assessing executive function in less structured environments have been proposed. The *Multiple Errands Task* (Shallice & Burgess, 1991) is one such procedure. The task takes place in an everyday environment such as a shopping mall. The tested person must complete a specified set of errands in a specified time while following a set of rules. The errands require the tested person to carry out a sequence of activities (e.g., get a copy of a daily weather forecast, buy an envelope and a stamp, obtain a pen, address the envelope to a specified recipient, and mail the weather forecast to the recipient). An observer follows the tested person and records information about how she or he performs the tasks.

The *Executive Route-Finding Task* (Boyd & Sauter, 1994) is another such observational procedure. The task requires the tested person to find a specified place (e.g., an office in the medical center or rehabilitation facility). An observer follows the tested person and rates the tested person's understanding of the task, use of information sources, retention of directions, error detection and self-correction, and on-task performance.

Emotional and Psychological Effects of Brain Injury on Cognition

Brain injury often has emotional and psychological effects that may influence the efficiency and accuracy of test performance. These emotional and psychological effects can affect perception, cognition, and motor performance. Clinicians who test brain-injured persons should be alert to the potential for these effects, recognize them, and compensate for them in testing.

Self-Doubt. Some brain-injured persons behave as if they do not trust their perceptions and doubt their ability to handle challenges. Self-doubt makes them hesitant, indecisive, and slow to respond when they feel challenged or threatened. Excessive caution affects these persons' test-taking performance, wherein they often perform below their true abilities. Excessive caution may lead them to withdraw from all but the most comfortable and predictable daily life relationships and activities. Persons with mild brain injury are most likely to be excessively cautious, perhaps because they are aware of minor lapses that would not be noticed by patients with more severe brain injury.

Emotional Lability. Brain injury sometimes contributes to exaggerated swings in emotional expression, a condition called *emotional lability.* Emotionally labile patients' expression of emotion is appropriate (they express sadness and happiness in appropriate contexts), but excessive. The magnitude of their emotional response is out of proportion to the event or situation that elicits the emotional response. Emotional lability usually appears as uncontrollable crying in response to neutral or mildly emotional stimuli—for example, the patient who breaks into tears when asked if he has children. Emotional lability sometimes appears as inappropriate laughter in situations that are not humorous, or excessive laughter in response to mildly amusing stimuli, especially when the patient feels stressed, challenged, or threatened. Neurologists and others sometimes call this phenomenon *pseudobulbar affect,* because it is common following bilateral damage to corticospinal and corticobulbar tracts above the pons. (As mentioned earlier, the pons is sometimes called the *bulb;* hence the term *pseudobulbar.*) For these patients, lability may represent loss of cortical inhibition of emotional responses originating in lower, phylogenetically more primitive structures.

Emotional lability can occur in association with, or as a consequence of, conditions that have nothing to do with brain injury—for example some psychiatric states, intoxication, or as a reaction to stress, confusion, or embarrassment.

Some brain-injured patients are prone to emotional outbursts as a consequence of lowered frustration tolerance. They explode emotionally when stressed or pushed to their limits

or beyond—a response that Schuell, Jenkins, and Jimenez-Pabon (1964) called *catastrophic reaction.* There are several differences between emotionally labile patients and patients with low frustration tolerance. Emotionally labile patients can be pushed into emotional breakdown by innocuous or mildly stressful events, but patients with low frustration tolerance typically lose control only when pushed too far. The emotional outbreaks of emotionally labile patients appear suddenly and without warning, but patients with low frustration tolerance often give visible signs of an impending explosion, becoming progressively more agitated and showing other signs of autonomic arousal as they approach the threshold for an outburst. Those who live and work around patients with low frustration tolerance learn to recognize the precursors to emotional outbursts and may prevent the outbursts by changing the situation or by otherwise lowering the patient's level of arousal.

Concreteness. Concreteness, or what Goldstein (1948) referred to as *loss of the abstract attitude* is a common consequence of brain injury, especially when damage is diffusely distributed throughout the brain. Goldstein was referring to brain-injured patients' failure to appreciate the abstract or implied meaning of events, situations, language, or visual images. These patients fail to appreciate the true meaning of figurative language such as idiom and metaphor (e.g., *having a heavy heart* or *seeing the handwriting on the wall*) and fail to grasp the implications of humor, sarcasm, and proverbs, wherein literal interpretations do not portray intended meanings.

Concreteness may contribute to some brain-injured patients' tendencies toward *egocentrism* (inability to appreciate another's point of view). Concreteness often has major effects on brain-injured patients' problem solving because they see only the simplest and most obvious solutions. Sometimes what seems to be concreteness may actually represent impulsiveness, but more often concreteness reflects an underlying cognitive impairment that prevents the patient from appreciating the implied meaning of abstract material.

CONCLUSIONS

Cognitive processes supporting communication span a range of interacting and overlapping processes—from basic processes such as attention and memory to higher-order processes represented by the label *executive function* (initiating, planning, organizing, monitoring, problem solving, reasoning). Assessment of these cognitive processes requires judicious selection and application of tests sufficient to identify and quantify each patient's unique pattern of impairment, supplemented by observation of a patient's performance in unstructured naturalis-

tic situations in which subtle impairments of executive function may become apparent.

There is no standard test battery for these aspects of a brain-injured adult's' cognitive function. Assessment typically involves basic tests of attention, memory, and executive function, supplemented by in-depth assessment of impairments considered important for diagnosis, prognosis, or rehabilitation. Findings from these tests are supplemented by observation of the patient in natural settings and by ratings and subjective impressions from the patient's family members, associates, and caregivers. Objective test results, structured observations, and subjective impressions are combined to provide an accurate and comprehensive representation of a brain-injured patient's current strengths and weaknesses in attention, memory, and executive function.

GENERAL CONCEPTS 4-3

- *Executive function* denotes the ability to plan, organize, and regulate behavior to solve a problem or achieve one's goals.
- Executive function includes initiating intentional behavior, planning behavioral routines to accomplish intentions, maintaining and regulating goal-directed behavior, and monitoring and modifying behavior in response to situational variables.
  - Impaired executive function is a common consequence of brain injury, especially injury to the frontal lobes.
  - Patients with severe impairments of executive function do not initiate purposeful activity and do not act independently to satisfy wants and needs.
  - Patients with less severely impaired executive function may perform familiar and highly practiced behavioral routines but do not spontaneously perform activities requiring planning and appreciation of long-term goals.

- Executive function depends on cognitive processes such as attention, memory, response flexibility, planning, reasoning, problem solving, and abstract thinking.
  - Response flexibility may be assessed with paper-and-pencil tasks in which the patient is asked to draw continuations of repetitive patterns.
  - Planning may be assessed with *cancellation tests, trail-making tests,* or *maze tests.*
  - *Reasoning tests* may focus on verbal reasoning, arithmetic and numerical reasoning, or visuospatial reasoning. Verbal reasoning tests include *reasoning and judgment tests, verbal absurdities tests,* and *logical relationship tests.* Arithmetic and numerical reasoning tests include *arithmetic story problems* and *block-counting tests.* Visuospatial reasoning tests include *picture-completion tests, picture-arrangement tests,* and *picture absurdities tests.*

GENERAL CONCEPTS 4-3—cont'd

- Raven's *Progressive Matrices* are tests of visuospatial analysis, integration, and reasoning with low verbal loadings. They are useful for estimating reasoning skills of brain-injured patients with language impairments.
- Problem solving requires the capacity to think ahead, to understand the consequences of actions, to consider alternatives, and to make choices. The *tower tests* and the *Tinkertoy test* are tests of problem solving that also require planning, organization, and maintenance of goal-directed behavior.
- Impaired abstract thinking is almost a universal consequence of brain injury. Tests of abstract thinking include *proverb interpretation tests, similarities and differences tests,* and *categorization and sorting tests.* The *Wisconsin Card Sorting Test (WCST)* is a widely used categorization and sorting test.
- Standard tests of cognition and communication are not sensitive to impaired executive function. Patients with impaired executive function often perform well on structured tests given in a supportive environment but break down when asked to perform similar tasks in less structured and more complex real-life environments.
- Tests to directly estimate executive function assess behavior in tasks requiring initiation, planning, problem solving, organization, control, and monitoring of performance in situations that are designed to mimic daily life. The *Six Elements Test (SET),* the *Hayling Sentence Completion Test (HSCT),* and the *Behavioural Assessment of the Dysexecutive Syndrome (BADS)* are three such tests.
- Observational procedures to provide information about executive function in realistic daily life environments include the *Multiple Errands Task* and the *Executive Route-Finding Task.*
- The concepts of executive function and the central executive are important elements of *resource allocation models* of cognitive processing.
  - The basic concept of *resource allocation* is that human brains have a limited pool of resources available for carrying out mental operations. The amount of resources drawn from the pool depends on the number of mental operations and their complexity. If the demand for resources exceeds the amount available, performance deteriorates.
  - We do not know if brain injury reduces the amount of resources in the pool or compromises access to resources without diminishing the volume of the pool.
- A combination of objective test results, structured observations, and subjective impressions of the clinician, caregivers, and family members is necessary for accurate and comprehensive assessment of a brain-injured patient's strengths and weaknesses in attention, memory, and executive function.

THOUGHT QUESTIONS

Question 4-1 You administer a retention-span test to a patient who experienced a mild concussion 5 days previously after striking his head in a fall from a scaffold at a building site. You read aloud a list of numbers at a one-per-second rate and ask the patient to repeat the numbers in the order you say them. Then you read aloud a list of words and ask the patient to tell you the words in the order you say them. Here are the two lists and the patient's responses to each list:

List 1: 7, 5, 1, 9, 6, 3, 8, 2
Patient's response: 6, 3, 8, 2
List 2: dog, me, red, car, tree, cup, boy, night
Patient's response: car, cup, boy, night

Something about this pattern of responses is unusual. What is it? What do you think is the reason for this pattern of responses?

Question 4-2 A patient with a left-hemisphere brain injury produces the following responses in a test of written spelling:

Test Word	Patient's Response
before	befor
bring	being
seven	sebing
here	bere
away	away
green	green
never	greever
there	greer
live	live
fast	last

What does the patient's pattern of responses suggest? How might you modify the test to improve the patient's performance?

Question 4-3 A man is suing a medical facility for damages. He claims that he has brain damage because he was deprived of oxygen during gallbladder surgery. He is a college graduate who, prior to the surgery, was an elementary school teacher. As part of a cognitive-communicative assessment he is asked to take a test in which he writes words dictated to him by the clinician. Here are the list of words and his written responses:

Test Word	Written Response
architect	rchitekt
license	licens
everyone	everion
birthday	birtdai
farmer	farmr
thought	thoght
afternoon	aftrnun
eight	aght
example	egsampl
campground	kampground
believe	biliev
cowboy	kowboi
understand	undrstand
today	tudai
heartache	hartach

What do the test results suggest to you?

Assessing Language

The limits of my language mean the limits of my world. (Ludwig Wittgenstein)

Assessing brain-injured adults' language usually entails administering a comprehensive language test, but assessment does not always begin there. Many brain-injured adults are first seen at bedside, where the speech-language pathologist conducts a brief interview and may administer a screening test. The interview gives the speech-language pathologist a general sense of the patient's background, problems, and concerns. The screening test gives the speech-language pathologist a general sense of the nature and severity of the patient's communicative impairments and sets the stage for more comprehensive testing.

SCREENING TESTS OF LANGUAGE

Several screening tests for assessing brain-injured adults' communicative abilities are on the market (Crary & associates, 1989; Fitch-West & Sands, 1987; Helm-Estabrooks, Ramsberger, Morgan, & associates, 1989; Keenan & Brassell, 1975; Sklar, 1973). Davis (1993), however, suggests that published screening tests are not needed for screening brain-injured adults' language at bedside:

> We do not need one of these tests to evaluate a patient's language abilities at bedside. All we need is a concept of what needs to be assessed, a few common objects, a pen, and some paper. We have the patient answer some yes/no questions, point to things, and name and describe some other things. If the patient cannot converse, we want to see if he or she can count or recite the days of the week. (p. 215)

Davis subsequently comments that published screening tests have advantages over informal tests because standardized administration ensures consistency in measurement and interpretation. Although it is no doubt true that a skilled clinician can improvise a satisfactory bedside screening examination with a few common objects, something to write with, and something to write on, such informal approaches may lead the examiner to miss important signs and may prevent comparison of the patient's performance with that of other patients or with the performance of the same patient on subsequent tests.

Many experienced clinicians forgo published screening tests in favor of locally designed tests, but few are content with idiosyncratic screening methods. Most speech and language clinics have formalized procedures for screening patients with impaired communication—usually with separate procedures for patients with aphasia, motor speech disorders,

right-hemisphere syndrome, traumatic brain injury, or dementia. The use of standard screening procedures ensures that everyone in the clinic does the screening in the same way and that the results obtained by one clinician are equivalent to the results obtained by other clinicians.

Figure 5-1 shows a screening protocol for patients with suspected language impairment. The protocol takes 10 to 20 minutes to administer and provides a general sense of the patient's orientation and memory, auditory and reading comprehension, production of automatized sequences, repetition, naming, oral reading, writing, and conversational speech.

Screening tests such as the one in Figure 5-1 serve several purposes. Sometimes they identify patients for whom no additional testing is appropriate—patients who have no significant communicative impairments; patients who have complicating conditions such as advanced dementia, confusion, or illness that would render formal assessment impossible or meaningless; or patients with severe and irreversible impairments. More often screening tests help a clinician decide which tests to administer during full-scale testing and the level of difficulty at which full-scale testing will begin. Screening tests also provide enough information about the nature and severity of the patient's linguistic or communicative impairments to permit the clinician to write initial impressions, diagnoses, and recommendations in a progress note. (Some screening forms such as the one in Figure 5-1 are progress notes that can be placed in a patient's medical record.)

COMPREHENSIVE LANGUAGE TESTS

Comprehensive language tests permit clinicians to measure patients' communication performance in the two primary input modalities (vision and audition) and three output modalities (speech, writing, and gesture) at various levels of difficulty within modalities or combinations of modalities. Comprehensive language tests permit clinicians to identify and describe

Language screening assessment

Date:	**Reason for referral, significant history**

Orientation, memory

What year is it? _____ [__]   What day of the week is it? _____ [__]

What time is it right now? _____ [__]   What city are we in? _____ [__]

Three-word recall: _____ _____ _____ [__]   **Number Correct [__ /5]**

Auditory comprehension

Single-word ("Point to the. . .")

Chair[__]   Ring[__]   Shoe[__]   Key[__]   Pencil[__]   **Number correct[__ /5]**

Yes-no questions

Personal information: (1) Is your first name (correct name)?[__]   (2) Is your last name (incorrect name)?[__]

Immediate environment: (3) Are we in a bus station right now?[__]   (4) Is it nighttime right now?[__]

Factual information: (5) Is a dime worth ten cents?[__]   (6) Do carrots grow on trees?[__]   **Number correct [__ /6]**

Sentence comprehension ("Point to the one that best matches what I say.")

A shoe.[__](shoe)   A standard comb.[__](comb)   Children play with this one.[__](ball) It has rubber on one end and a point on the other.[__](pencil)   The flat surface of this one is ideal for doing a jigsaw puzzle.[__](table)   **Number correct [__ /5]**

Reading comprehension

Word to picture matching (foils are in parentheses)

Fox (box, coat)[__]   Frog (flag, fish)[__]   Cup (spoon, cap)[__]   Letter (city, ladder)[__] Television (thermometer, camera)[__]   **Number Correct[__ /5]**

Patient identification:

Speech Pathology: language screening assessment (Page 1 of 2)

Figure 5-1 ■ A language screening assessment form that may be placed in a patient's medical record.

Continued

Automatized sequences

Counting: 1[__] 2[__] 3[__] 4[__] 5[__] 6[__] 7[__] 8[__] 9[__]
10[__]

Days of week: Sunday[__] Monday[__] Tuesday[__] Wednesday[__]
Thursday[__] Friday[__] Saturday[__]   **Number correct [__ /17]**

Repetition

Words: Boy[__] Dog[__] Cowboy[__] Gingerbread[__] Artillery[__]
Number correct [__ /5]

Sentences: It was raining.[__] Bill went to the store.[__] Please put the groceries in the
refrigerator.[__] Arthur was an oozy, oily sneak.[__]
Number correct [__ /4]

Confrontation Naming: Pictures

dog[__] broom[__] airplane[__] igloo[__] tambourine[__] **Number correct [__ /5]**

Oral Reading

Words   Man[__] Book[__] Forever[__] Understanding[__] Conventional[__]
Number correct [__ /5]

Sentences: It was raining.[__] Mary baked a pie.[__] Under the table in the dining room. [__]
The little girl was happy to see the new puppy. [__]   **Number correct [__ /4]**

Rating of connected speech

Fluency: Fluent[__] Nonfluent[__]

Average phrase length (words): 1-2[__] 3-4[__] 5-6[__] >6[__]

Literal paraphasia: Absent[__] Infrequent[__] Frequent[__]

Verbal paraphasia: Absent[__] Infrequent[__] Frequent[__]

Word-finding in connected speech: Normal[__] Moderate impairment[__]
Severe impairment[__]

Writing

Name[__]
Letters to dictation: F[__] M[__] D[__] X[__] Q[__] **Number correct [__ /5]**
Words to dictation: Man[__] Today[__] Carrot[__] Venture[__]
Number correct [__ /4]

Comments and impressions:

_____   _____
Speech-language pathologist   Date
                          Speech pathology: language screening assessment
                          (Page 2 of 2)

Figure 5-1, cont'd ■ A language screening assessment form that may be placed in a patient's medical record.

communication impairments and to estimate their severity. Some permit prediction of a patient's recovery. Most help clinicians make a diagnosis. All include subtests for assessing component language skills—auditory and reading comprehension, speech production, and written expression.

AUDITORY COMPREHENSION

All comprehensive language tests include auditory comprehension subtests, and several freestanding tests devoted to auditory comprehension have been published. Some assess comprehension of single words in isolation or at the end of short carrier phrases. Some assess comprehension of single-sentences, questions, or instructions. A few assess comprehension of spoken narratives.

Single-Word Comprehension

The simplest word-comprehension tests require the patient to point to body parts (e.g., *show me your elbow; show me your knee*) or objects in the environment (e.g., *point to the door; point to the ceiling*). These simple tests often are used by physicians, speech-language pathologists, and others as part of a bedside screening examination because they do not require special materials and they give a quick indication of a patient's comprehension of single words and simple spoken directions.

Most standard word-comprehension tests use a select-from-an-array procedure. The examiner shows the patient an array of everyday objects (e.g., spoon, comb, pencil, toothbrush, cup, and key) or an array of drawings of everyday objects, then says the name of each object or drawing and asks the patient to point to or touch each as it is named. In most word-comprehension tests the examiner says the test word at the end of a short carrier phrase, such as *Point to the _____*. Such tests are tests of single-word comprehension and not sentence comprehension because the carrier phrase quickly becomes redundant. Figure 5-2 shows an array of pictures for a select-from-an-array word-comprehension test.

Some word-comprehension tests assess verb comprehension with an array of drawings or photographs representing actions (e.g., running, painting, riding, and swimming). Figure 5-3 shows an array of drawings for testing verb comprehension.

Some word-comprehension tests assess comprehension of color, form, and number names, perhaps reflecting the influence of a study by Goodglass and associates (1966), which sug-

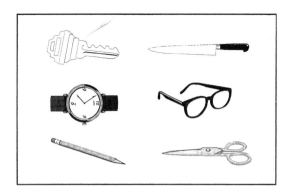

Figure 5-2 ■ A picture plate for testing single-word auditory comprehension. The examiner says the names of the items in random order, and the patient points to a picture as the examiner names it.

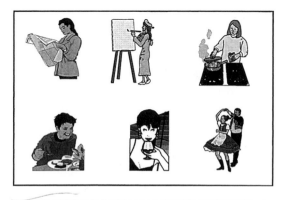

Figure 5-3 ■ A response plate for testing verb comprehension. The examiner names an action represented by a drawing, and the patient points to the appropriate drawing.

gested that aphasic adults comprehend object and action names better than color, form, or number names. Color, form, and number word-comprehension tests also may reflect the influence of several case reports of patients with unusual impairments in comprehending specific categories of words (e.g., color names). Although it may be clinically interesting and theoretically important to find a patient who comprehends color or letter names better (or worse) than the names of objects and actions, the relevance of such a finding to treatment planning or to estimation of the patient's daily life communicative competence is enigmatic. Many clinicians forgo testing of form, color, and number word comprehension unless they have reason to suspect an unusual pattern of word comprehension or see an opportunity for a published case report.

The single-word comprehension performance of most brain-injured adults who are tested using select-from-an-array procedures is not strongly affected by whether the items in the array are real objects, drawings, or pictures, although brain-injured adults with impaired visual perception or impaired visual discrimination tend to do better when real objects are used. Patients with brain injuries affecting the visual cortex or visual association cortex often do better when tested with real objects than when tested with pictorial representations of the objects. Patients with confusion or dementia also may perform better when tested with real objects.

Helm-Estabrooks (1981) contrasted real objects with line drawings in a test of aphasic adults' word comprehension. She tested comprehension in three conditions. In the *array condition,* 12 familiar objects were shown as line drawings printed on 12 separate cards. In the *composite condition,* smaller versions of the same 12 drawings were presented on a single card. In the *environment condition,* the 12 objects were distributed around the testing room. Somewhat surprisingly, the aphasic adults performed significantly better when pointing to pictures than when pointing to real objects. Their performance was not significantly affected by whether the drawings were presented on individual cards or in an array on a single card.

Helm-Estabrooks's findings illustrate the effects of array size and spatial distribution on performance in select-from-an-array tasks. As the number of items in an array increases or as items are distributed across larger areas of visual space, the time needed to locate items in the array increases. For non-brain-injured adults it may not matter if an array contains 6 items or 12 items or if the items are picture cards on a table or objects in a room. Their pointing response usually is unaffected.

Large and visually complex arrays may cause problems for brain-injured adults with compromised short-term retention because increasing the time spent in visual search also increases the time during which the test word must be retained in memory. In most select-from-an-array word comprehension tests the same array of test items is used to test all items in the array, so the effects of array size usually diminish as a patient becomes familiar with the location of items in the array. Some patients with compromised short-term retention compensate for their memory impairment by repeating test words over and over as they search an array for a matching item. Requiring these patients to perform an activity that prevents rehearsal (e.g., counting aloud) causes their performance to deteriorate.

No free-standing tests of single-word auditory comprehension for brain-injured adults have been published, although picture vocabulary tests such as the *Peabody Picture Vocabulary Test-Third Edition* (PPVT-III; Dunn & Dunn, 1997) are, in a way, tests of single-word comprehension. However, picture vocabulary tests differ in content and purpose from single-word auditory comprehension tests for brain-injured adults. Picture vocabulary tests contain unfamiliar low-frequency words such as *lancinate* and *bumptiously,* which are known by few normal adults, whereas single-word comprehension tests for brain-injured adults focus on common words.

The most common words represented by the early items of picture vocabulary tests may be equivalent to the words in single-word comprehension tests for brain-injured adults. Brain-injured adults often make scattered errors on vocabulary test items representing common words, followed by uninterrupted strings of errors when they reach less common words. The early scattered errors probably represent something other than limited vocabulary, such as word retrieval failure, stimulus uncertainty, or momentary inattention. Strings of consecutive errors when less common items are reached probably represent the limit of the individual's true listening vocabulary.

Norms for picture vocabulary tests are based on the entire test, making partially completed picture vocabulary tests of limited value to clinicians who wish to compare an individual patient's performance with that of a norm group. A patient's performance on the common items in a picture vocabulary test could, however, serve as a baseline measure against which to measure his or her response to the same items following treatment. The patient's performance on the complete test may provide an estimate of his or her available listening vocabulary, including a school grade level.

Items in the last one third to one half of most vocabulary tests rarely occur in everyday communicative interactions. Consequently, impaired performance on those items may not suggest significant handicap in daily life interactions.

Although word comprehension tests occupy a prominent place in comprehensive language tests, their results may not imply much about a patient's daily life language comprehension. Single-word utterances in daily life usually are supported by situational or linguistic context. (e.g., *Where in the world did you see that? Television.*) It is well known that brain-injured adults' comprehension of language is enhanced by context. Thus it seems unlikely that their performance on tests in which they are asked to comprehend isolated single words presented with no context implies much about their daily life comprehension. Add to this the strangeness (in a daily life sense) of being asked to point to objects or pictures as they are named, and the relevance of word comprehension tests to daily life becomes even less apparent.

Nevertheless, most clinicians assess single-word comprehension as part of their testing routine for brain-injured adults. Tests of single-word comprehension are quick and easy to administer. The results of single-word comprehension tests may suggest unusual patterns of impaired performance, leading the clinician to revise a diagnosis or a treatment plan. For patients whose single-word comprehension is preserved, single-word comprehension tests may provide a comfortable lead-in to more challenging sentence-level and paragraph-level tests. For patients with severely impaired comprehension, the results of testing at the single-word level may be the only indicator of the patient's spoken language comprehension.

Variables That May Affect Single-Word Comprehension

Frequency of Occurrence. A word's frequency of occurrence in the language usually affects the ease with which brain-injured listeners comprehend it (Figure 5-4). This effect can be seen in aphasic adults' performance on listening vocabulary tests such as the PPVT-III, wherein most have inordinate difficulty with infrequently occurring words.

A patient's failure to comprehend infrequent words may not relate strongly to daily life comprehension of spoken language, because most words used in daily life are words with high frequency of use in English. Data from Hayes (1989) show that everyday spoken language contains many more high-frequency words than low-frequency words (Figure 5-5). More than 80% of the words used in daily life interactions are among the 1,000 most frequent words in English. *Semantic or Acoustic Similarity between Target Words and Foils.* Semantic similarity between target words and foils often confuses

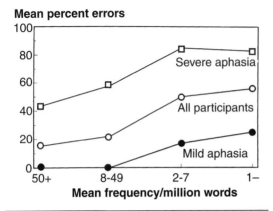

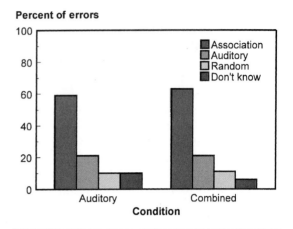

Figure 5-4 ■ The effects of word frequency on aphasic adults' single-word comprehension. As word frequency declines, error rates increase. (Data from Schuell, H.M., Jenkins, J.J., & Landis, L. [1961]. Relationship between auditory comprehension and word frequency in aphasia. *Journal of Speech and Hearing Research, 4,* 30-36.)

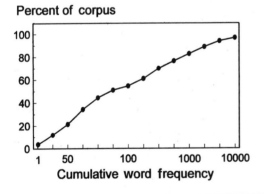

Figure 5-5 ■ Word frequency of occurrence in everyday conversations of normal adults in the United States. (Data from Hayes, D. P. [1989]. *Guide to the lexical analysis of texts.* [Tech. Rep. Series 89-96]. Ithaca, NY: Cornell University Department of Sociology.)

brain-injured adults, especially those who are aphasic. Schuell and Jenkins (1961), for example, reported that semantic confusions (such as *mother* for *father*) are far more frequent than either acoustic confusions (such as *dime* for

Figure 5-6 ■ Performance on a test of single-word comprehension by a group of aphasic adults. *Association errors* are errors in which an individual chose a semantically related foil. *Auditory errors* are errors in which an individual chose a foil that sounded like the target word. *Random errors* are errors in which an individual chose a foil that had no semantic or acoustic similarity to the target. In *auditory condition,* the examiner said the target word, and the aphasic individual chose one of two pictures. In *combined condition,* the examiner showed the aphasic individual a card on which the target word was printed and said the target word. (Data from Schuell, H. M., & Jenkins, J. J. [1961]. Reduction of vocabulary in aphasia. *Brain, 84,* 243-261.)

time) or random errors (such as *motorcycle* for *cigarette*) when aphasic patients match spoken words to pictures (Figure 5-6).

Part of Speech. Part of speech affects some brain-injured adults' single-word comprehension, although the effect is highly variable across individuals. Miceli, Silveri, and Nocentini (1988) studied aphasic adults' comprehension of nouns and verbs and found all possible patterns of noun and verb comprehension. Some comprehended nouns better than verbs, some comprehended verbs better than nouns, and some comprehended nouns and verbs equally well (or poorly). Miceli and associates' findings show that part of speech may affect a brain-injured adult's single-word comprehension, but the

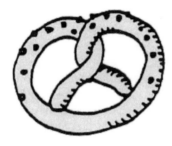

Figure 5-7 ■ An example of a line drawing *(pretzel)* that is ambiguous for some brain-injured persons, who may see it as a snake, worm, rope, or hose.

nature of the effect can be determined only by testing the patient.

Referent Ambiguity. Ambiguity in pictured referents for spoken words often affects brain-injured adults' performance when they are asked to match spoken words to pictures. If pictorial referents are ambiguous or unclear, patients may respond inaccurately, not because they cannot comprehend the words, but because they cannot tell what the pictures represent (Figure 5-7).

Fidelity. The fidelity of spoken messages (from words to discourse) can have important effects on brain-injured listeners' comprehension (and, if the loss of fidelity is serious, on that of non-brain-injured listeners, too). Most brain-injured adults' comprehension of spoken materials deteriorates in noisy listening environments or when speech is acoustically distorted. Answering the telephone can be a challenge for many, because telephones are low-fidelity instruments and many produce background noise.

Sentence Comprehension

Sentence Comprehension Subtests in Comprehensive Language Tests. All major comprehensive language tests include sentence comprehension subtests. Most require patients to perform gestural or manipulative responses to spoken commands. Sometimes the patient must point to one or more items in sets of pictures, objects, or body parts (e.g., *Point to the [pictured] dog, garage, and ladder. Point to the ceiling and then to the floor. Show me the one used for fixing hair. Point to your left ear and your right knee.*). Sometimes patients must manipulate objects or body parts. (e.g., *Ring the bell, close the box, and give me the key. Tap each shoulder twice with two fingers, keeping your eyes closed.*)

Most comprehensive language tests include subtests for assessing comprehension of spoken yes-no questions. The yes-no questions in these tests may assess comprehension of different kinds of information. Some test personal information (e.g., *Is your last name Smith?*). Some test awareness of the surrounding environment (e.g., *Are the lights on in this room?*). Some test knowledge learned in school (e.g., *Was Abraham Lincoln the first President of the United States?*). Some ask for opinions, inferences, or abstractions (e.g., *Should children disobey their parents?*). Some test general knowledge (e.g., *Do apples grow on trees?*). Questions that test general knowledge may test comprehension of temporal relationships (e.g., *Does March come before June?*), numerical relationships (e.g., *Are there seven days in a week?*), or comparative relationships (e.g., *Are towns larger than cities?*).

Free-Standing Tests of Sentence Comprehension. The *Token Test* (DeRenzi & Vignolo, 1962) and its variants are the most widely used free-standing tests of sentence-level auditory comprehension. In the original DeRenzi and Vignolo version, 62 spoken commands direct the patient to touch or manipulate 20 tokens (5 large circles, 5 small circles, 5 large rectangles, and 5 small rectangles in each of 5 colors—red, yellow, green, white, and blue). There are 5 levels in the original *Token Test.* The length and complexity of commands increases from level 1 to level 5 (Box 5-1). Responses are scored correct or incorrect. The maximum score is 62. No norms are provided in DeRenzi and Vignolo (1962), although norms for adults and children can be found elsewhere (Gaddes & Crockett, 1973; Noll & Lass, 1972; Spreen & Benton, 1977; Wertz, Keith, & Custer, 1971).

Box 5-1	Token Test Levels (Original DeRenzi and Vignolo Version)

Level 1: Touch the red circle.
Level 2: Touch the large blue rectangle.
Level 3: Touch the red rectangle and the blue circle.
Level 4: Touch the large white circle and the small green rectangle.
Level 5: When I touch the green circle, you take the white rectangle.

Several modified versions of the *Token Test* have been published. One is a subtest of the *Neurosensory Center Comprehensive Examination for Aphasia* (NCCEA; Spreen & Benton, 1977). It contains 39 test commands similar to those in the original *Token Test* divided among 6 levels of length and complexity. The easiest level in the Spreen and Benton version contains commands such as *Show me a square* and *Show me a red one,* which permits testing patients at a lower level than is possible with the original *Token Test* and also permits identification of patients with specific impairments in comprehension of color or shape names. The Spreen and Benton version of the *Token Test* allows users to score patients' responses according to how accurately they represent the critical elements in test commands. For example, the command *Point to the small white circle* is worth 3 points—1 each for *small, white,* and *circle.* A perfect score on the Spreen and Benton version of the *Token Test* is 163 points. Norms for brain-injured adults, nonaphasic but brain-injured adults, and non-brain-injured adults are provided in the NCCEA manual.

Spreen and Benton replaced rectangles with squares, which brings the Token Test shape names closer together in terms of their frequency of occurrence in English. Rectangle occurs approximately 10 times per million words; circle and square each occurs approximately 140 times per million words. Most users of the original version of the Token Test also replace rectangles with squares.

The Spreen and Benton version of the *Token Test* appears to be as sensitive to the presence of impaired auditory comprehension as the original DeRenzi and Vignolo version, is quicker to administer, score, and interpret, and gives partial credit for responses that include some but not all of the critical elements in test commands. Consequently, the Spreen and Benton version is more widely used in the United States and Canada than is the original DeRenzi and Vignolo version.

The *Revised Token Test* (RTT; McNeil & Prescott, 1978) is a longer and more elaborate version of DeRenzi and Vignolo's test. The RTT has 10 subtests, each with 10 equally difficult test commands. The first 4 subtests in the RTT are similar to the first 4 parts of the original *Token Test.* Tests 5 through 8 each consist of 10 items that test comprehension of positional relationships (e.g., in front of, behind, above, below, to the right of). Tests 9 and 10 test comprehension of complex grammatic relationships (e.g., instead of, unless, if, either). Patients' responses to RTT items are scored with a multidimensional system similar to the scoring system for the *Porch Index of Communicative Ability* (Porch, 1981a). Profiles for five *auditory processing deficits* are provided in the test manual. Several procedures for scoring and analyzing patients' responses are described in the RTT manual.

The RTT takes longer to administer, score, and interpret than the other versions (usually more than an hour). Its comprehensiveness and its psychometric integrity make it a powerful research tool, but its length and complexity may preclude its use in routine clinical evaluation of brain-injured adults.

The *Token Test* and its variants are sensitive measures of sentence comprehension. Even patients with mild comprehension impairments have difficulty on higher-level token test commands. However, this sensitivity makes the token tests difficult or impossible for patients with severe comprehension impairments. A few patients have inordinate difficulty with token tests, compared with their performance on other tests of auditory comprehension. Some have specific difficulty with color, shape, and size descriptors. Others have temporal sequencing impairments that prevent them from maintaining the temporal order of the responses required by test commands. (These patients typically point to the correct tokens but in the wrong order.) A few patients may have motor planning impairments *(limb apraxias)* that prevent them from making the required pointing responses, even though they understand the commands.

In my experience, few patients have such severe limb apraxia that they cannot point sequentially to test tokens. However, it should be kept in mind as a potential cause of poor performance on token tests and on other tests requiring sequential pointing, gestural, or manipulative responses.

To rule out problems with comprehension of color, shape, and size descriptors, patients can be pretested by asking them to point to *a red one, a circle, a small one,* and so on (a procedure included as the first level in the Spreen and Benton version of the *Token Test* and as a pretest for the RTT). To rule out temporal sequencing impairments and limb apraxias as the causes of deficient performance, the examiner can ask the patient to imitate sequences of pointing responses modeled by the examiner. If the patient is successful, temporal sequencing impairments and limb apraxia become unlikely explanations for the deficient performance.

Some patients with poor comprehension improve their performance on tests that require them to point to items in an array by visually fixating on items as they are named by the examiner, thereby using visual strategies to compensate for impaired auditory retention. These patients' performance deteriorates if the target items are covered while the commands are spoken. If the examiner suspects that a patient is relying on a visual strategy in tests of comprehension with an array of visual stimuli, covering the array while test commands are spoken

ensures that a patient's performance reflects only auditory comprehension and retention.

For patients with subtle comprehension and retention impairments, an examiner can increase the difficulty of sentence comprehension tests by imposing a delay between each test sentence and the opportunity for a patient to respond. A 10-second or 20-second delay usually reveals even the most subtle auditory retention impairments. However, testing patients with nonstandard test procedures precludes comparison of their performance with norms based on the standard procedures.

The *Token Test* and its variants test comprehension of a limited range of syntactic structures and provide little information about a patient's listening vocabulary. For examiners who wish a more detailed picture of a patient's sentence comprehension, a sentence comprehension test designed for children—such as the *Northwestern Syntax Screening Test* (NSST; Lee, 1971) or the *Test for Auditory Comprehension of Language-Third Edition* (TACL-3; Carrow-Woodfolk, 1999)—may be used, but most do not provide norms for adults. These tests do, however, show how grammatic and syntactic characteristics of sentences affect comprehension, and for this reason may be used to test brain-injured adults, even though the brain-injured adults cannot be compared with an adult norm group.

Variables That May Affect Sentence Comprehension

Length and Syntactic Complexity. Although several variables affect brain-injured listeners' comprehension of spoken sentences, two of the strongest are *sentence length* and *syntactic complexity.* As spoken sentences become longer or syntactically more complex, they become more difficult to comprehend, provided other sentence characteristics do not change. Syntactic complexity seems to have stronger negative effects on comprehension than either sentence length or vocabulary difficulty (Shewan & Canter, 1971; Goodglass & associates, 1979; Nicholas & Brookshire, 1983).

Goodglass, Blumstein, Gleason, and associates (1979), for example, compared the effects of sentence length and syntactic complexity on aphasic listeners' comprehension of two sets of spoken sentences. The sentences in one set were syntactically complex (e.g., *The man greeted by his wife was smoking a pipe.*). The sentences in the other set were syntactically simpler forms of the complex sentences (e.g., *The man was greeted by his wife, and he was smoking a pipe.*). The aphasic listeners comprehended the syntactically simpler sentences better than the syntactically complex ones, even though the simple sentences were longer than the complex ones.

Increasing sentence length may facilitate brain-injured adults' comprehension if the increased length also adds redundancy—something clinicians should keep in mind when designing treatment procedures.

Brain-injured adults usually exhibit the same pattern of difficulty across syntax types as do non-brain-injured adults, although they take longer to comprehend the sentences and they make more errors. Syntactically simple active sentences (e.g., *The dog bit the boy.*) are easier than passive sentences (e.g., *The boy was bitten by the dog.*). Conditional sentences (e.g., *If the cup is blue, give it to me.*), negative sentences (e.g., *The dog is not chasing the rabbit.*), sentences with locational or directional statements (e.g., *Put the cup behind the box.*), and comparative or relational sentences (e.g., *The boy is taller than the girl.*) are difficult for many brain-injured listeners. Embedded clause sentences (e.g., *The letter the girl wrote is on the table.*) are impossible for most brain-injured listeners (and for many non-brain-injured listeners). Data reported by Caplan, Baker, and DeHaut (1985) suggest that brain injury affects the quantitative characteristics but not the qualitative characteristics of sentence comprehension. (Brain-injured persons make more errors, but the pattern of their errors across sentence types matches that of non-brain-injured persons.) The data also

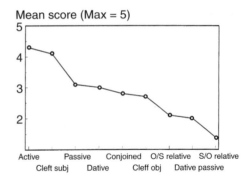

Mean score (Max = 5)

Active: The student hit the beggar.
Cleft subject: It was the student that hit the beggar.
Passive: The beggar was hit by the student.
Dative: The student gave the paper to the beggar.
Conjoined: The student hit the beggar and pushed the mailman.
Cleft Object: It was the beggar that the student hit.
Object/Subject Relative: The student that hit the beggar pushed the mailman.
Dative/ Passive: The paper was given to the beggar by the student.
Subject/Object Relative: The beggar that the student hit pushed the mailman.

Figure 5-8 ■ Performance of a group of aphasic adults on a test of sentence comprehension in which the syntactic complexity of sentences was manipulated. As syntactic complexity increased, the performance of the aphasic adults declined. (Data from Caplan, D., Baker, C., & DeHaut, F. [1985]. Syntactic determinants of sentence comprehension in aphasia. *Cognition, 21,* 117-125.)

show that the syntactic structure of sentences affects aphasic listeners in the same way, regardless of aphasia severity (Figure 5-8).

Fortunately for brain-injured listeners, sentences with complex syntax are not common in daily life. Most sentences in daily life are active sentences (e.g., *I am going to the store.*) or simple interrogatives (e.g., *Have you eaten yet?*). Many are truncated sentences that depend on the listener's ability to fill in missing words based on context (e.g., *Over there.* in response to *Where did you put the paper?*). Interestingly, most brain-injured listeners with mild to moderate comprehension impairments have little difficulty comprehending such truncated sentences, perhaps because of the contextual support associated with daily life interactions.

Plausibility and Predictability. In some sentences (called *reversible sentences*) subject and object may be transposed without making the sentence implausible (e.g., *The man is kissing the woman.* becomes *The woman is kissing the man.*). In other sentences (called *nonreversible sentences*) transposition of subject and object creates an implausible sentence (e.g., *The man is carrying the book.* becomes *The book is carrying the man.*). Subject and object transposition in some sentences creates an improbable, but not implausible, sentence (e.g., *The dog is chasing the cat.* becomes *The cat is chasing the dog.*).

Caramazza and Zurif (1976) investigated the effects of reversibility on aphasic listeners' comprehension of embedded-clause sentences (e.g., *The apple the boy is eating is red.*). They concluded that aphasic listeners' sentence comprehension was poorer when sentences were reversible than when they were not; although their major finding was that aphasic listeners, like nonaphasic listeners, relied heavily on plausibility to comprehend syntactically complex sentences.

Brain-injured listeners, like non-brain-injured listeners, apparently use general knowledge to deduce the meaning of spoken language. A listener who knows that books never carry humans and that cats rarely chase dogs need not rely on laborious syntactic analysis to decide who did what to whom but can use knowledge of what is likely, customary, or possible to deduce the meanings of such sentences. Other kinds of daily life sentences are predictable from general knowledge. For example, the relationships conveyed by comparative sentences (e.g., *The man is stronger than the boy.*) can be deduced based on a listener's knowledge of the relative strengths of men and boys without the need for deeper syntactic analysis. Such use of general knowledge to facilitate comprehension (called *top-down processing*) offers a convenient shortcut to the meaning of sentences— a shortcut often taken by non-brain-injured and brain-injured listeners alike.

Personal Relevance. The personal relevance of questions affects their difficulty for brain-injured listeners, especially those who have moderately to severely impaired comprehen-

sion. Gray, Hoyt, Mogil, and associates (1977) and Busch and Brookshire (1982) evaluated aphasic adults' responses to three categories of spoken yes-no questions. Questions in one category tested nonpersonal factual information (e.g., *Do apples grow on trees?*). Questions in the second category referred to the immediate environment (e.g., *Are we in a hospital?*). Questions in a third category referred to personal information (e.g., *Is your name Smith?*). In both studies aphasic adults' responses to personal information questions most often were accurate. Their responses to questions about the immediate environment were more often accurate than their responses to questions about nonpersonal factual information.

Semantic Variables. Schuell, Jenkins, and Jimenez-Pabon (1964) reported that semantic confusions among words are much more common in aphasic adults' test performance than either phonemic or visual confusions. Butterworth, Howard, and McLoughlin (1984) also reported that semantic errors are common in comprehension tasks performed by brain-injured adults. Goodglass (1993) commented that breakdown of semantic boundaries among words prevents brain-injured persons from recognizing distinctions between semantically related words that are easily recognized by non-brain-injured adults. Because of their semantic impairments, brain-injured adults often make errors in sentence comprehension when factual questions are falsified by substituting a semantically related word for a word that makes the sentence true. *Does the sun rise in the west?* will trip up many patients, whereas *Does the sun rise in the kitchen?* would mislead only those with severely impaired comprehension (or those who have very large kitchens).

Reasoning and Inference. Questions that require reasoning or inferences (e.g., *Is it possible for a good swimmer to be drowned?*) are more difficult for language-impaired persons than questions in which reasoning or inference are not required, if the length, vocabulary, and syntactic structure of the sentences are equivalent. Answering inferential questions adds to the processing load in comprehension by requiring that the listener (1) recognize that implied information is not in memory in verbatim form, (2) construct the implied information, using preexisting knowledge, (3) relate the implied information to the question, and (4) produce the answer. Brain-injured adults may perform poorly on questions requiring inferences because they do not realize that an inference is called for, are unable to identify or retrieve from memory information relevant to the inference, are unable to deduce the inference, or cannot produce the answer. Questions such as *Why should children attend school?* also require longer and more complex responses than yes-no or short-answer questions, making them especially difficult for brain-injured adults with impaired speech formulation or production.

Rate. A study by Salvatore, Strait, and Brookshire (1978) showed that changes in the rate at which clinicians say the sentences in sentence comprehension tests can have clinical consequences. Salvatore and associates asked experienced and inexperienced examiners to administer a token test to two groups of brain-injured adults. One group had mild comprehension impairments, the other group had severe comprehension impairments. Salvatore and associates reported that the experienced examiners spoke test commands at a slower rate than the inexperienced examiners, that both experienced and inexperienced examiners spoke test commands at a slower rate when they tested severely impaired patients than when they tested mildly impaired patients, and that both experienced and inexperienced examiners spoke test commands at a slower rate following patients' errors than following patients' correct responses.

Redundancy. The lexical redundancy of spoken sentences affects comprehension for many brain-injured adults. West and Kaufman (1972) compared brain-injured and aphasic listeners' comprehension of token-test-like commands in which some commands repeated key words (e.g., *Show me the big **blue circle** and the little **blue circle**.*) with their comprehension of

commands that did not repeat key words (e.g., *Show me the big blue circle and the small red square.*). The lexically redundant commands were easier for the aphasic listeners than the lexically nonredundant commands. Gardner, Albert, and Weintraub (1975) reported that aphasic listeners comprehended semantically redundant sentences (e.g., *You see a cat that is furry.*) better than semantically neutral sentences (e.g., *You see a cat that is nice.*), although the statistical analyses did not strongly support their conclusion.

Number, Similarity, and Nature of Response Choices. The number of choices available for pointing or manipulation and similarity among the choices may affect the difficulty of tasks in which brain-injured listeners point to or manipulate tokens, objects, or pictures in response to spoken directions. In general, increasing the number of possible choices increases the difficulty of the task. *Point to the red circle.* is less difficult if there are three choices (e.g., red circle, blue square, yellow circle) than if there are six (e.g., red circle, blue circle, yellow circle, red square, blue square, yellow square). Increasing the semantic similarity among choices also increases the difficulty of the task. *Point to the knife.* is more difficult if the targets are semantically related (e.g., fork, knife, spoon) than when they are not (e.g., train, knife, horse).

The chance probability of correct responses diminishes as the number of choices increases. When a patient has only two response choices, one of which is correct, about half of the patient's responses would be correct if the patient were to respond randomly. Increasing the number of choices to four lowers the chance probability of correct responses to 1 in 4 (25%). The chance probability of a correct response in a 10-item array is 1 in 10 (10%), and so on.

There is some evidence that brain-injured adults' performance on point-to tests of spoken-sentence comprehension is slightly better when the choice stimuli are real objects rather than tokens (Kreindler, Gheorghita, & Voinescu, 1971; Martino, Pizzamiglio, & Razzano, 1976; LaPointe, Holtzapple, & Graham, 1985). However, the differences between performance on token tests and picture or object tests usually are small, and the performance of individual subjects often does not match the performance of the group. For most brain-injured adults it probably makes little difference whether tokens, pictures, or objects are used in point-to tests of sentence comprehension. Their scores on token tests are likely to be slightly worse than their performance on picture tests or object tests. This makes token tests slightly more sensitive to the presence of subtle comprehension impairments but also causes token tests to underestimate most patients' daily life comprehension.

Sentence Comprehension and Comprehension in Daily Life

The items in most sentence comprehension tests are not very representative of what adults experience in daily life. In most sentence comprehension tests, the listener hears a series of minimally redundant sentences with no relationship among sentences in the series. The listener must remember the information from each sentence long enough to answer a question or point to tokens or a picture but can then forget it because each sentence is unrelated to preceding sentences. In this respect sentence comprehension tests are similar to immediate-memory tests in which the examiner reads lists of numbers or words and the listener must recognize or reproduce them after a delay of a few seconds.

Adult listeners in daily life rarely hear strings of nonredundant sentences with no relationship to each other or to the listener's prior knowledge. Listeners in daily life usually need only remember the gist of sentences and not their verbatim form, and they do not have to remember the gist for more than a few seconds. Speakers in daily life relate new information to what they assume the listener already knows and relate what they say to preceding utterances and to a topic, creating a semantic context for individual utterances. Single-sentence compre-

hension tests eliminate that context, no doubt to the detriment of the patient tested, because brain-injured listeners, like non-brain-injured ones, use context to help them comprehend what they hear (Stachowiak & associates, 1977; Waller & Darley, 1978; Pierce 1989; and others).

The results of several studies confirm the tenuous relationship between performance on sentence comprehension tests and comprehension of spoken discourse (Stachowiak, Huber, Poeck, & Kerschensteiner, 1977; Brookshire & Nicholas, 1984; Wegner, Brookshire, & Nicholas, 1984; and others). These studies show that sentence comprehension test scores do reasonably well in predicting scores on other *sentence-level* tests of comprehension, but they are poor at predicting scores on tests of *discourse* comprehension. Clinicians should be cautious in making inferences about brain-injured listeners' daily life comprehension competence based on single-sentence comprehension tests. Most brain-injured listeners are likely to perform better in daily life than their single-sentence comprehension test scores suggest that they should.

Comprehension of Spoken Discourse

Discourse Comprehension Subtests in Comprehensive Language Tests. Some comprehensive language tests include subtests to assess comprehension of spoken discourse in a limited way, with paragraphs read aloud by the examiner followed by spoken questions about the paragraphs. Some are short storylike narratives, such as the following, from the *Boston Diagnostic Aphasia Examination* (BDAE; Goodglass, Kaplan, & Barresi, 2001a).

A customer walked into a hotel carrying a coil of rope in one hand and a suitcase in the other. The hotel clerk asked, "Pardon me, sir, but would you tell me what the rope is for?" "Yes," responded the man. "That's my fire escape!" "I'm sorry, sir," said the clerk, "but all guests carrying their own fire escapes must pay in advance."

Was the customer carrying a suitcase in each hand?

Did the clerk trust this guest?

Other subtests include expository paragraphs such as the following excerpt from the *Minnesota Test for Differential Diagnosis of Aphasia* (MTDDA; Schuell, 1972).

Gold was first discovered in California by a millwright named James Marshall. Marshall was building a sawmill on the banks of the American River. One morning in January, 1848, as he was walking along the millrace, he saw some bright flakes at the bottom of a ditch. Marshall picked up a handful and took them back to the fort to show his partner, John Sutter. They turned out to be pure gold. Marshall and Sutter tried to keep the discovery a secret.

In this story, did Marshall discover gold on the Rio Grande?

Did Marshall and Sutter try to spread the news of the discovery?

Tests with expository paragraphs tend to be more difficult for brain-injured listeners (and for those without brain injuries) than tests with storylike narratives because the questions about expository paragraphs usually ask for details such as names, places, and dates, whereas the questions about storylike narratives usually ask for salient information such as topic, theme, and main ideas. Numerous studies have shown that both brain-injured and normal listeners comprehend and remember main ideas from discourse better than they comprehend details (Meyer, 1975; Meyer & McGonkie, 1973; Kintsch, 1974; Brookshire & Nicholas, 1984; Wegner, Brookshire, & Nicholas, 1984; Nicholas & Brookshire, 1995b; and others).

A Test of Discourse Comprehension. The *Discourse Comprehension Test* (DCT; Brookshire & Nicholas, 1993) is a standardized test for assessment of brain-injured adults' spoken discourse comprehension. The DCT contains 10 tape-recorded narrative stories controlled for number of words and sentences, mean sentence length, speech rate, number of unfamiliar words, listening difficulty, and grammatic complexity.

Eight questions for each story test the patient's comprehension and retention of information. Four questions test main ideas, and four questions test details. Two of the main idea questions and two of the detail questions test information that is directly stated in the story. The remaining two main idea and two detail questions test information that is implied by information in the story, so that patients must make inferences to answer them correctly. Box 5-2 contains a story and questions from the DCT. *Variables That May Affect Comprehension of Spoken Discourse.* Many of the variables mentioned earlier as affecting sentence comprehension also affect discourse comprehension, but not necessarily to the same degree. Because discourse permits listeners greater use of heuristic processes, variables such as word frequency and syntactic complexity, which have strong effects on language-impaired listeners' comprehension of sentences, do not have equally strong effects on their comprehension of discourse. Several discourse-specific variables do have important effects on comprehension of discourse. Two of the most important are *salience* and *directness.*

Heuristic processes in comprehension are processes in which the listener or reader uses world knowledge and previous experience to arrive at the meaning of spoken or printed materials. Heuristic processing is sometimes called *top-down processing* because the listener or reader begins with assumptions about the general meaning of spoken or printed materials and uses those assumptions to guide lexical and syntactic analyses.

Salience. Speakers and writers make information salient by means of devices such as repetition, elaboration, and paraphrase and by creating syntactic and semantic relationships among parts of the discourse. In this way speakers and writers make important information stand out (the main ideas) relative to information that is less important to the sense of the

Box 5-2	*Sample DCT Narrative Story and Questions*

One day last fall, several women on Willow Street decided to have a garage sale. They collected odds and ends from all over the neighborhood. Then they spent an entire day putting prices on the things that they had collected. On the first day of the sale, they put up signs at both ends of the block and another one at a nearby shopping center. Next they made a batch of iced tea and sat down in a shady spot beside the Anderson's garage to wait for their first customer. Soon a man drove up in an old truck. He looked around and finally stopped by a lumpy old mattress that was leaning against the wall. He gestured to it and asked how much they wanted for it. Mrs. Anderson told him that it wasn't for sale. Then she added that they were going to put it out for the trash collectors the next day. The man asked if he could have it. Mrs. Anderson said that he could. Then she asked, "Why do you want such a terrible mattress?"

"Well," he said, "my no-good father-in-law is coming to visit next week, and I don't want him to get too comfortable."

Questions

1. Did several women have a party? (No) [Stated main idea]
2. Were there a large number of things at the garage sale? (Yes) [Implied main idea]
3. Did the women put up a sign at a shopping center? (Yes) [Stated detail]
4. Was it cold the day of the garage sale? (No) [Implied detail]
5. Was the man driving a car? (No) [Stated detail]
6. Was the mattress in terrible condition? (Yes) [Stated main idea]
7. Was the man married? (Yes) [Implied detail]
8. Was the man fond of his father-in-law? (No) [Implied main idea]

---

discourse (the details). As noted earlier, both normal listeners and brain-injured listeners comprehend and remember main ideas in discourse better than they comprehend details.

Directness. Normal speakers do not always specify all the information needed for listeners to understand the speaker's meaning and intent (Clark & Haviland, 1977) but leave informational gaps, expecting the listener to construct inferences and make assumptions to fill in the gaps. For example, a speaker might say:

When I looked out the window, I saw the garage in flames. It took the firemen 20 minutes to get here, but by then it was too late.

and expect the listener to infer that the speaker called the fire department right away and that the garage was destroyed.

Several studies have assessed the effects of directness (whether information is directly stated or implied) on brain-injured adults' comprehension of information in spoken discourse (Nicholas & Brookshire, 1986; Nicholas & Brookshire, 1995b; Katsuki-Nakamura, Brookshire, & Nicholas, 1988). Brain-injured adults in these studies, like those without brain damage, had more difficulty with questions that tested implied information and less difficulty with questions that tested stated information. The differences between questions about stated information and questions about implied information were greatest when the required inferences went beyond simple paraphrase of information in the discourse and required listeners to retrieve relevant information from memory and connect it with information provided by the speaker (Nicholas & Brookshire, 1986).

Redundancy. Repetition, elaboration, and paraphrase increase the redundancy of discourse and highlight important information, making it easier for listeners to establish the overall theme or point of the discourse, organize it in memory, and recall it later. The main ideas in discourse become main ideas thanks to repetition, elaboration, and paraphrase. Repetition, elaboration, and paraphrase also contribute to the relatedness of information in discourse (its cohesion) and to the overall unity of the material (its coherence).

Cohesion and Coherence. *Cohesion* denotes the relationships among semantic units in discourse. Cohesion is created by linguistic devices called *cohesive ties*. Many kinds of cohesive ties have been described in the literature (Halliday & Hasan, 1976), but a few examples will suffice:

- *Pronominal ties* are pronouns that refer back to a previously mentioned referent (e.g., *The boy was lost.* **He** *stood in the center of the plaza, crying.*).
- *Conjunctive ties* are conjunctions (e.g., *The horse ran fast* **but** *lost the race.*).
- *Lexical repetition ties* are repeated words or their synonyms in adjacent propositions (e.g., *The man and the woman got on the train. The* **man** *carried a large black suitcase. The* **woman carried** *flowers.*).

Coherence denotes the overall unity of discourse. Multiple variables, which are not readily quantified, contribute to coherence. Cohesion and coherence contribute to heuristic, top-down comprehension processes, making cohesive and coherent discourse easier for both normal and brain-injured listeners to comprehend and retain in memory than discourse lacking cohesion and coherence.

Speech Rate and Emphatic Stress. Most language-impaired adults complain that they can no longer mentally keep up with what others say.

> I'm not as quick as I used to be. Mentally, I mean. When people talk—especially when they talk fast—and most do—I get lost. I'm okay for the first sentence or two, but then I get behind. By the time I've figured out the first sentence, I'm already three or four sentences behind. I may get bits and pieces from then on, but most of the time I don't have the foggiest idea what they're saying. Everybody talks too fast. Sometimes I feel like I'm in a foreign country.

Slowing speech rate and adding emphatic stress may improve brain-injured listeners' comprehension of discourse. Pashek and Brookshire (1982) assessed aphasic adults' comprehension of spoken paragraphs at slow (120 wpm) or normal speech rate (150 wpm), with either normal stress or exaggerated stress (extra prosodic emphasis on important words). They found (1) that slow rate and exaggerated stress facilitated aphasic listeners' comprehension of the paragraphs, (2) that slow rate was slightly more effective than exaggerated stress in improving comprehension, and (3) that comprehension was best when slow rate and exaggerated stress were combined. Kimelman and McNeil (1987) replicated Pashek and Brookshire's study and reported similar results.

Several studies have reported beneficial effects of slowed speech rate on auditory comprehension of brain-injured adults (Parkhurst, 1970; Liles & Brookshire, 1975; and others), but not all aphasic listeners' comprehension of discourse improves when speech rate is slowed, and sometimes an aphasic listener benefits from slowed speech rate at one time and not at another. Nicholas and Brookshire (1986) played tape-recorded narrative stories to aphasic listeners at slow (120 wpm) and fast (200 wpm) speech rates. The aphasic listeners' comprehension was tested twice, with a week or more between tests. Slow speech rate improved comprehension for the group in the first session. The facilitating effects of slow speech rate had essentially disappeared by the second session. Individual group members often failed to match rate effects exhibited by their group. Nevertheless, Nicholas and Brookshire commented that slowed speech rate helps many brain-injured listeners and rarely worsens comprehension, making it a useful management device for clinicians.

GENERAL CONCEPTS 5-1

- Screening tests help clinicians identify patients for whom treatment is not appropriate, plan subsequent testing, and respond to consultation requests. Although a commercially marketed language screening test may not be necessary, a standard procedure for screening brain-injured patients is necessary to assure uniformity across users within a facility.
- Most comprehensive language tests contain subtests to assess *single-word comprehension*. Single-word comprehension typically is tested by asking the patient to point to common objects or pictures of common objects named by the examiner. Most brain-injured adults' performance is not greatly affected by whether the test stimuli are objects or pictures.
  - *Picture vocabulary tests* are not valid tests of single-word comprehension for brain-injured adults because they contain large proportions of low-frequency words that are not common in daily life. Picture vocabulary tests are designed to estimate an individual's receptive vocabulary and not daily life word comprehension.
  - Single-word comprehension tests may not be dependable indicators of brain-injured adults' daily life comprehension. Single-word utterances are not common in daily life and usually are supported by linguistic and situational context, which enhances comprehension.
  - Single-word comprehension of most brain-injured adults is not strongly affected by whether items in stimulus arrays are real objects, drawings, or pictures. Individuals with impaired visual perception or discrimination may perform better when tested with real objects rather than with drawings or pictures.
  - Large, visually complex arrays may affect single-word comprehension test scores of patients with impaired short-term memory because the time spent in visually searching arrays increases the burden on short-term memory.
- Several variables may affect brain-injured adults' single-word comprehension, including the following:
  - *Frequency of occurrence.* Low-frequency words are more difficult for most brain-injured adults.
  - *Semantic or acoustic similarity* between target words and foils. Semantic similarity has stronger effects for most brain-injured adults.
  - *Part of speech.* Nouns and verbs are perhaps easier than other parts of speech, but there is great variability across brain-injured adults.
  - *Referent ambiguity.* Ambiguous pictured referents compromise most brain-injured adults' performance.
  - *Fidelity.* Low fidelity of spoken test stimuli may compromise brain-injured adults' performance.
- *Sentence comprehension* typically is tested by asking patients to perform gestural or manipulative responses to spoken instructions or to answer spoken yes-no questions.
  - *Yes-no questions* may test personal information, perception of surroundings, knowledge learned in school, or general knowledge. General knowledge questions may test temporal, numeric, or comparative relationships. Some yes-no questions ask for opinions or inferences that require extended speech, thereby compromising the performance of patients with speech production problems.
  - The *Token Test* is a widely used test of sentence comprehension for brain-injured adults. It requires manipulation of large and small colored circles and squares in response to the examiner's instructions. The Spreen and Benton version is shorter and permits scoring of critical elements within commands.

Continued

- Several variables affect the difficulty of sentence comprehension tests for brain injured adults:
  - *Length and syntactic complexity.* Longer and syntactically more complex sentences are more difficult. Syntactic complexity usually has stronger effects than length.
  - *Reversibility and plausibility.* Semantically reversible sentences are more difficult than nonreversible sentences. Plausibility may allow patients to use general knowledge to enhance comprehension.
  - *Predictability.* Syntactic or semantic constraints on sentence content contribute to ease of comprehension.
  - *Personal relevance.* Sentences about personally relevant material are easier for most brain-injured adults to comprehend than sentences about less personal material.
  - *Semantic relationships.* Sentences that are falsified by substituting a semantically related word for a key word in the sentence are difficult for many brain-injured adults to identify as false.
  - *Reasoning and inference.* Requiring reasoning and inference increases the difficulty of sentence comprehension for most brain-injured adults.
  - *Rate.* Slow rate helps many brain-injured patients comprehend spoken sentences, but the effects of slow rate may be variable across patients and within patients across time.
  - *Redundancy. Lexical redundancy* (repeating key words) and *semantic redundancy* (providing semantically related words) enhances sentence comprehension for many brain-injured adults.
  - *Response choices.* Adding foils and increasing the similarity of foils and targets makes sentence comprehension more difficult. The nature of response choices (tokens versus pictures versus objects) has minor effects on most brain-injured adults' sentence comprehension.
  - Performance on sentence-comprehension tests usually does not predict brain-injured adults' comprehension in daily life.
- Some comprehensive language tests include subtests to assess *comprehension of spoken discourse* in a limited way, with short paragraphs that are read aloud by the examiner, who then asks questions about the paragraphs. Some are storylike, and some are expository. Expository paragraphs tend to be more difficult for brain-injured adults.
- The *Discourse Comprehension Test* is a standardized test for assessment of discourse comprehension, including comprehension of main ideas, details, stated information, and implied information.
- Several variables affect brain-injured adults' comprehension of spoken discourse:
  - *Salience.* Brain-injured adults comprehend and remember important information (the *main ideas*) better than incidental information (the *details*).
  - *Directness.* Brain-injured adults comprehend and remember directly stated information better than implied information.
  - *Redundancy.* Repetition, elaboration, and paraphrase increase the redundancy of discourse and make it easier for brain-injured adults to comprehend and remember it.
  - *Cohesion and coherence.* Cohesive ties within discourse make it easier for brain-injured adults to comprehend and remember information in the discourse. Cohesive ties contribute to the overall unity of discourse—its coherence.
  - *Speech rate and emphatic stress.* Slow speech rate and exaggerated emphatic stress usually enhance brain-injured patients' comprehension of discourse, although the effects may differ across patients and across time within patients.

READING
Reading Subtests in Comprehensive Language Tests

All comprehensive language tests contain reading subtests. A few include *visual matching subtests,* in which the patient is shown a series of cards showing geometric forms, letters of the alphabet, or words. The patient chooses a matching form, letter, or word from a card containing a test stimulus plus several foils. The test stimuli and target choices are visually identical, permitting selection of the correct target based on visual form alone. When the test stimuli are letters or words, this means that patients can make correct choices by matching the visual form of stimuli and targets without translating either into alphabet letters or words. Consequently, such letter-matching or word-matching subtests are best characterized as tests of visual perception and discrimination rather than as reading tests. Figure 5-9 shows typical geometric-form-matching, letter-matching, and word-matching stimulus cards and response plates.

Most comprehensive language tests assess *oral reading of printed words and sentences.* The patient is shown cards on which words or sentences are printed and is asked to read aloud the words or sentences. Such oral-reading subtests provide an indication of a patient's ability to convert the graphemic forms of words into their phonologic equivalents and to encode and produce the phonologic equivalents. They do not necessarily test reading comprehension because graphemes can be converted to phonemes without accessing the semantic representations of words.

Single-word comprehension tests are the simplest tests of actual reading comprehension. Single-word comprehension tests come in several forms. In the most common form the examiner places a card containing several drawings or photographs before the patient and shows the patient a card on which the name of one of the drawings or photographs is printed. The patient points to the drawing or photograph that matches the printed word *(word-to-picture matching).* Usually the drawings or photographs depict common objects, but sometimes they depict verbs, colors, numbers, or geometric forms. In another form of single-word reading comprehension tests, the patient is shown the printed name of an object and chooses the

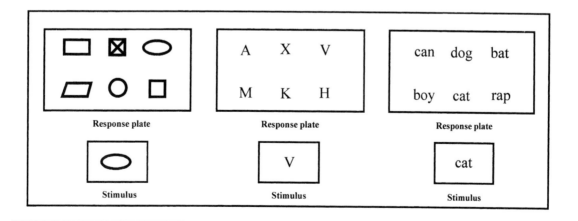

Figure 5-9 ■ Stimulus cards and response plates representing form-matching *(left)*, letter-matching *(center)*, and word-matching tasks *(right)*. These tasks can be completed successfully without comprehending the linguistic value of the letters and words.

named object from a set of real objects *(word-to-object matching)*.

Some tests of single-word reading comprehension employ a reversed version of word-to-picture matching by showing the patient a drawing or photograph and asking them to choose the printed name of the drawing or photograph from a card containing the correct name plus several other names *(picture-to-word matching)*. For most brain-injured adults it makes little difference which format is used to test single-word reading comprehension. Word-to-picture and picture-to-word matching usually give equivalent results, and most patients perform similarly regardless of whether the printed words are matched to pictures or to real objects. (The exception is patients with impaired visual perception and discrimination, who may perform better with real objects.)

Figure 5-10 gives an example of a word-to-picture test item and a picture-to-word test item in which foils represent semantically similar, visually similar, and unrelated choices. Tests that categorize potential responses in this way provide information about the underlying reasons for impaired performance. As noted earlier, most brain-injured adults have difficulty discriminating semantically similar material. Consequently, when they choose the wrong picture they tend to choose one that is semantically related to the test stimulus. Patients with compromised visual processing tend to choose a foil that is visually similar to the test stimulus. Choosing foils with no obvious relationship to the test stimulus is considered by many practitioners a sign of confusion or dementia.

Some comprehensive language tests assess single-word reading comprehension with cards, each of which has a drawing and two words printed on it. One of the words matches the drawing. Nonmatching words often are selected so that errors can be identified as semantic confusions (lion/tiger), auditory confusions (mail/sale), visual confusions (horse/house), or irrelevant responses (grapes/chair). Because there are only two response choices for each item, patients can get half correct by chance. Figure 5-11 gives an example of this test format.

Matching printed words to spoken words is another way of testing single-word comprehension. The most common form is one in which a card with several words printed on it is

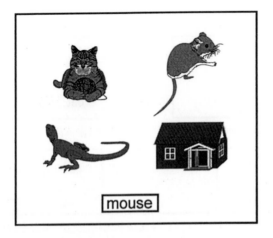 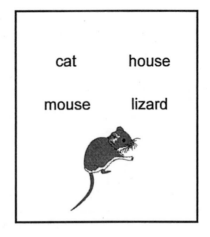

Figure 5-10 ■ An example of a word-to-picture matching task *(left)* and a picture-to-word matching task *(right)*.

shown to the patient, the examiner says the words in the test in random order, and the patient points to each word as the examiner says it (Figure 5-12). These tests are somewhat more difficult than picture-to-word matching subtests for most brain-injured adults because they require auditory comprehension and retention as well as word reading.

Tests for assessing *comprehension of printed sentences* also come in several forms. In one form the sentences are yes-no questions (e.g., *Do eggs come from chickens?*). Like spoken yes-no questions, printed yes-no questions may relate to personal information, common knowledge, knowledge acquired in school, or opinions, inferences, and abstractions. And, like spoken yes-no questions, the general knowledge questions can be separated into questions that test comparative, temporal, or numeric relationships. The relative difficulty of these sentence types matches that for spoken sentences—common knowledge questions typically are

easiest, and comparative-relationship, temporal-relationship, and numeric-relationship questions typically are most difficult.

In another form of printed-sentence comprehension tests, patients complete unfinished sentences by choosing from a list of words, as in:

A cowboy rides a...			
cow	horse	house	candlestick

(Foils often represent semantic, visual, or unrelated errors, as in this example.)

In yet another form of printed-sentence comprehension tests, the patient is given cards on which instructions for manipulating test objects (or, less frequently, pictures) are printed. In the *Porch Index of Communicative Ability* (Porch, 1981a), for example, patients are given cards with instructions such as *Put this card to the left of the cigarette.* or *Put this card under the one used for picking up food.* Sometimes the printed instructions are similar to those in

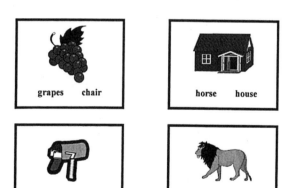
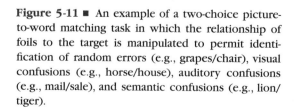

Figure 5-11 ■ An example of a two-choice picture-to-word matching task in which the relationship of foils to the target is manipulated to permit identification of random errors (e.g., grapes/chair), visual confusions (e.g., horse/house), auditory confusions (e.g., mail/sale), and semantic confusions (e.g., lion/tiger).

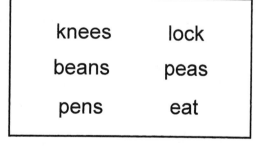

Figure 5-12 ■ A response plate from a single-word comprehension test in which the examiner says a word and the patient points to the word. The target for this card is *peas*. Foils represent auditory confusion (knees), semantic confusion (beans, eat), and visual confusion (pens). (*Beans* represents a *semantic category* error; *eat* represents a *semantic function* error.)

spoken-sentence comprehension tests (e.g., *Pick up the pencil, knock three times, and put it back.*).

Several comprehensive language tests provide subtests for assessing *comprehension of printed texts.* In the most common form, the patient is given one or more short passages to read. The final sentence in each passage is incomplete, and several phrases that might complete the passage are printed below it, as in the following item from the BDAE.

In the early days of this country, the functions of government were few in number. Most of the functions were carried out by local town and county officials, while centralized authority was distrusted. The growth of industry and of big cities has so changed the situation that the farmer of today is concerned with…

  local affairs above all
  the price of lumber
  the actions of the government
  the authority of town officials

A few comprehensive language tests contain expository passages similar to those found in elementary school reading materials. The following item is a portion of the paragraph-reading subtest of the MTDDA. The patient circles, underlines, or points to *yes* or *no* for each question.

Lawrence Griswold, a writer and scientist who lives in Minnesota, states that dragons really exist. In 1934, he and a classmate camped for 8 months on Komodo, an island in Indonesia. Here they found dragons 18 feet long who walked on their hind feet like the ancient dinosaurs…

  Did Griswold go to Komodo in 1943? **Yes No**
  Did he find dragons in Indonesia?   **Yes No**

The Discourse Comprehension Test (Nicholas & Brookshire, 1993) includes a reading comprehension subtest to assess brain-injured adults' reading comprehension of the 10 stories described earlier in this chapter.

A Free-Standing Test of Reading Comprehension for Aphasic Adults

One free-standing test of brain-injured adults' reading comprehension is currently on the market. As the title suggests, the *Reading Comprehension Battery for Aphasia-Second Edition* (RCBA-2, LaPointe & Horner, 1998) is designed for evaluating aphasic adults' reading abilities but may be appropriate for testing brain-injured persons in other diagnostic categories. The core section of RCBA-2 contains 10 subtests with 10 items in each subtest. Subtests 1, 2, and 3 assess single-word reading from preschool to Grade 3 vocabulary levels. Subtest 4 tests functional reading of signs, labels, menus, calendars, recipes, and other such daily life material (Figure 5-13).

Subtest 5 is a reading vocabulary subtest in which the test-taker chooses synonyms for five common verbs and five common nouns, half abstract and half concrete. In Subtest 6 the test-taker reads each of 10 five-word sentences and chooses, from a set of three pictures, the one that best illustrates the meaning of each sentence (Figure 5-14).

Weather forecast
Turning much colder beginning today
Wednesday fair and cold
High today low 60s
Low tonight near 30
Chance of rain: 70%

Point to the part that tells how cold it will get tonight.

Figure 5-13 ■ A functional reading test item from the *Reading Comprehension Battery for Aphasia—Second Edition.* (From LaPointe, L.L., & Horner, J. [1998]. *Reading comprehension battery for aphasia* [2nd ed.]. Austin, TX: Pro-Ed.)

Subtest 7 contains 10 two-sentence, 25-word paragraphs in which the second sentence directs the test-taker to choose, from a set of three pictures, the one identified by the paragraph (Figure 5-15).

Subtests 8 and 9 each present five paragraphs with four sentence-completion test items for each paragraph to assess comprehension of stated information (Subtest 8) and implied information (Subtest 9) (Figure 5-16).

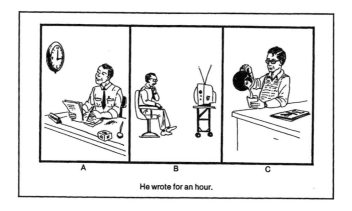

He wrote for an hour.

Figure 5-14 ■ A sentence comprehension test item from the *Reading Comprehension Battery for Aphasia— Second Edition*. (From LaPointe, L.L., & Horner, J. [1998]. *Reading comprehension battery for aphasia* [2nd ed.]. Austin, TX: Pro-Ed.)

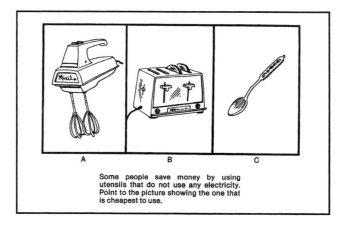

Some people save money by using utensils that do not use any electricity. Point to the picture showing the one that is cheapest to use.

Figure 5-15 ■ A two-sentence-paragraph comprehension item from the *Reading Comprehension Battery for Aphasia—Second Edition*. (From LaPointe, L.L., & Horner, J. [1998]. *Reading comprehension battery for aphasia* [2nd ed.]. Austin, TX: Pro-Ed.)

Goose down

The soft and light feathers from the underside of a goose have so many uses. This material is called *down*, and it is used to fill some pillows. Goose down is used to fill sleeping bags and cold weather clothes, also. That is why you see so many naked geese walking around.

Soft goose feathers are called:

| Down | | Up | | Pillows |

This material is used to fill:

| Weather | | Sleeping bags | | Time |

A down-filled coat would be best in:

| Summer | | Winter | | Cars |

Goose down equipment can be used for:

| Swimming | | Music | | Camping |

Figure 5-16 ■ A longer paragraph comprehension item from the *Reading Comprehension Battery for Aphasia—Second Edition*. (From LaPointe, L.L., & Horner, J. [1998]. *Reading comprehension battery for aphasia* [2nd ed.]. Austin, TX: Pro-Ed.)

According to the RCBA-2 manual, correct answers are not obvious from the command sentence alone. However, in several items (including the ones in Figure 5-15 and 5-16) the correct answer seems obvious from the command sentences alone.

Subtest 10 is a sentence-to-picture matching task in which the subject chooses one of three sentences that best describes a picture (Figure 5-17). The choice sentences differ in syntax, ranging from active declarative (e.g., *The player is hitting the ball.*) to object embedded (e.g., *She threw the boys' dog the leash.*)

The supplemental section of the RCBA-2 contains seven subtests to test skills related to reading: *single-letter visual discrimination, letter naming, letter recognition, lexical deci-*

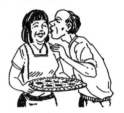

A. The man is kissing the woman who is holding the pizza.

B. The woman is kissing the man who is holding the pizza.

C. The man who is holding the woman is kissing the pizza.

Figure 5-17 ■ A sentence-comprehension item from the *Reading Comprehension Battery for Aphasia—Second Edition*. (From LaPointe, L.L., & Horner, J. [1998]. *Reading comprehension battery for aphasia* [2nd ed.]. Austin, TX: Pro-Ed.)

sion (discriminating valid words from nonsense trigrams), *semantic categorization* (deciding if two words semantically go together), *oral reading of single words*, and *oral reading of sentences.*

Reading Tests for Non-Brain-Injured Adults and Children

The reading tests in comprehensive language tests and the RCBA-2, which were designed for brain-injured adults, are good screening tests to identify patients with moderate to severe reading impairments, but most do not provide enough detail to enable clinicians to detect subtle reading impairments or to describe the nature of a patient's reading impairment. For these purposes clinicians usually turn to standardized reading tests. Standardized reading tests provide a comprehensive look at the severity and nature of a patient's reading impairments and permit a clinician to compare a patient with normal readers. Because brain-injured adults' reading abilities range from single-word reading to college-level reading, clinicians who assess brain-injured adults' reading need tests that span a range from primary grades to college level.

The *Gates-MacGinitie Reading Tests* (Mac-Ginitie, MacGinitie, Maria, & Dreyer, 2000) span a range of reading skills from kindergarten through post–high school. The tests from Level 3 (third grade) through Level AR (adult reading) span a range that permits testing most brain-injured adults. All have vocabulary and comprehension sections. Items in the vocabulary sections consist of short phrases with one word in the phrase underlined. The test-taker chooses one of four definitions that follow each phrase, as in this item from Level 3:

The others *peered* at it
☐ looked closely
☐ smiled
☐ pecked
☐ made loud noises

Items in the comprehension sections consist of reading passages taken from published works representing fiction, nonfiction, science, and social studies and are written in a variety of styles. Passage content is selected to represent the interests and experiences of test-takers at a given grade level. Consequently, passages intended for testing lower grades tend to have juvenile themes which some brain-injured adults may consider demeaning, as in the following excerpt from Level 3.

When I come home from school, my mother and father are still at work, so Gogo takes care of me. Gogo calls me her little tail because I follow her everywhere. She lets me carry her beautiful blue cloth bag in which she keeps her important things…

Why does Gogo take care of the girl who is telling the story?
☐ The girl has no parents.
☐ Gogo gets lonely by herself.
☐ Gogo is the girl's' mother.
☐ The girl's parents have jobs away from home.

Comprehension items at Level 7 and above have more adultlike content and would be suitable for testing most brain-injured adults who can read material at this level. The following excerpt is from Level 7.

My earliest clear memory of my mother is her tall figure standing alone in the center of the lawn behind the house, looking down at the grass, turning in a slow circle, scanning the ground. I knew this to be a mild sign of trouble for my mother, trouble for the family…

What was the author doing?
☐ Watching
☐ Helping his mother
☐ Copying his mother
☐ Trying to stop his mother

The reading comprehension subtest of the *Peabody Individual Achievement Test-Revised* (Markwardt, 1989) can be used to test the sentence-level reading comprehension of brain-injured patients representing a range of reading impairments. The clinician shows a page containing a printed sentence to the patient, then covers it with another page that contains four pictures, one of which represents the meaning of the sentence. The patient responds by pointing to one of the pictures. Sentences increase in length (from 5 to 30 words) and difficulty of vocabulary as the test progresses. Norms (grade equivalents and percentiles) are provided for non-brain-injured children and adults up to 23 years old. Most brain-injured patients can complete this test in less than 30 minutes, making the test useful for moderately impaired to severely impaired brain-injured adults who might not tolerate longer tests.

The *Nelson-Denny Reading Test* (NDRT; Brown, Fisehco, & Hanna, 1993) may be useful for testing brain-injured adults with mild reading impairments. The NDRT uses reading materials selected from high school through college level humanities, social science, and science textbooks. Like the Gates-MacGinitie tests, the NDRT has vocabulary and paragraph comprehension sections. The NDRT permits users to classify paragraph comprehension test items according to whether they test *literal* (stated) *information* or *interpretive* (implied) *information,* as in the following test item, in which the first item tests literal information and the second item tests interpretive information.

One of Jung's best-known contributions is his personality typology of two basic attitudes, or orientations, toward life: extraversion and introversion. Both orientations are viewed as existing simultaneously in each person, with one usually dominant. The extravert's energy is directed toward external objects and events, while the introvert is more concerned with inner experiences…

The concept of extraversion and introversion was one of Jung's:

☐ earliest contributions
☐ most controversial contributions
☐ most widely known contributions

You would infer that extraverts would most likely be:

☐ speakers
☐ listeners
☐ readers

Reading Rate and Capacity

In their standard administration, reading tests are given with a time limit, and norms for the test are based on scores obtained within the time limit. Clinicians who are interested in brain-injured patients' reading usually want to know how much a patient can read and comprehend within the time limit *(reading rate),* so that their performance can be compared with the performance of the norm group. They also wish to know how much a patient can read and comprehend if permitted to work without time constraints *(reading capacity).* Reading rate tells the clinician how much the patient can read and understand under normal time constraints and allows comparison of the patient with norm groups, whereas reading capacity

tells the clinician how much the patient can read under optimal conditions. Most brain-injured adults' reading rate is slower than their premorbid rate, even when their vocabulary, word recognition, and single-word comprehension seem intact. Estimates of reading rate and reading capacity are important in planning treatment programs and in counseling the patient and family about the patient's probable daily life reading competence.

Reading rate and capacity are measured in the following way. The patient begins the test and works for the amount of time prescribed by the test manual. At the end of that time the examiner marks the last item completed by the patient and the patient continues until he or she completes the test or can go no further. The examiner records the time at which the patient finishes the test and marks the last item completed.

Component Skills

One weakness of most reading comprehension tests for adults is that they do not measure component skills that may be necessary for different aspects of reading comprehension (e.g., *sound-to-letter conversion, getting main ideas, using context*). After administering most adult reading tests, the examiner has a test score, perhaps a percentile rank, and a reading grade level, but no real sense of which component skills are compromised and which are preserved.

There is no universal list of component skills for reading, but the *Specific Skill Series* of remedial reading materials (Boning, 1990) provides materials suitable for getting a look at some of the more important ones: *symbol-to-sound correspondences, following directions, using context, locating answers, getting facts, getting main ideas, drawing conclusions, recognizing sequences,* and *identifying inferences.* The *Specific Skill Series* includes materials at 10 levels of graded difficulty within each skill. Box 5-3 gives examples of items from *following directions, getting main ideas, drawing conclusions,* and *identifying inferences.*

Box 5-3	*Examples of Reading Items from the* **Specific Skill Series**

Following Directions
Directions
There are four words in the left-hand column. To the right of each word are two more words. Choose the one that is opposite in meaning to the word at the left. Circle it.

listen	speak, hear
below	beside, above
everyone	lately, nobody
many	few, some

Getting the Main Idea
There is a plant in our country that doesn't have any green leaves. This plant grows about 8 inches tall. At the end of each stem is a white flower. The stem is also white. The plant looks like many clay pipes. It is called the Indian Pipe.

The story tells mainly:
(A) why American Indians smoke pipes
(B) why American Indians named plants
(C) what the plant called the Indian Pipe looks like

Drawing Conclusions
Horses don't live as long as people. A horse that lives to the age of 30 is very old. One year of a horse's life is equal to 3 years of a person's. A 30-year-old horse is as old as a person who is 90.

A horse of 10 is equal in age to a:
(A) 10-year-old child
(B) 30-year-old person
(C) 3-year-old baby

Identifying Inferences
"That's a pretty jewel you have in your ring," said Karen.

"Thank you," said Martha. "It was given to me as a present. I have other rings, but this is my favorite. My mother always gives me things that I really like."

Martha has more than one ring.

          True   False   Inferred*

The ring was given to Martha by her mother.

          True   False   Inferred

Karen didn't like Martha's ring.

          True   False   Inferred

From Boning, R. A. (1990). Specific skill series (4th ed.). New York: Macmillan/McGraw-Hill.

*True items are facts that are directly stated in the story. *False* items are not true, based on information in the story. *Inferred* items are probably true, based on the story and the reader's experience.

The reading materials in the *Specific Skill Series* cover a wide range of reading levels (preschool to Grade 8). Some selections have juvenile themes, but the incidents and situations portrayed are sufficiently interesting that most adult readers should not find them demeaning. With its separation of the reading process into component skills and its wide range of reading levels within skills, the *Specific Skill Series* provides a useful collection of materials for assessing and treating brain-injured adults' reading impairments.

Reading Test Format
Those who design standardized reading tests for normal adults and children assume that potential test-takers have essentially normal (for their age) memory, organizational skills, problem-solving skills, and visual perception and are able to attend to and follow spoken directions. These assumptions permit users of the tests to conclude that impaired test performance signifies reading impairment and not impairment of some underlying or related ability. Because reading tests for normal children and adults were designed with these assumptions in mind, the format of some may be unsatisfactory for testing brain-injured adults who may have memory impairments, impaired organizational or problem-solving skills, visual perceptual impairments, or difficulties in following instructions.

Most standardized reading tests for normal adults and children do not require written answers to test items but allow the test-taker to check off, circle, or underline their choice from an array of possible multiple-choice answers.

Consequently, brain-injured adults with mild to moderate impairments are likely to have little difficulty with the responses required. Tests with answer sheets that are scored by machine, in which the person taking the test must read a stimulus item, choose the correct answer from a group of possible answers, remember the number of the test item and the number or letter of the correct choice, find the corresponding set of response choices on the answer sheet, and blacken the appropriate area on the answer sheet often cause transcription and bookkeeping errors, even for adults with no brain injury. Consequently, they should be not be used to test brain-injured adults unless the response format can be changed to eliminate demands on skills other than reading.

Passage Dependency

Passage dependency is a term coined by Tuiman (1974) to reflect the extent to which readers must rely on information from printed texts to answer test questions correctly. Questions that can be answered without reading the related texts are said to be *passage independent* because they do not depend on the test-taker's comprehension of the text. When reading-test items have low passage dependency, the test is more likely a test of single-sentence reading skills than a test of multiple-sentence reading comprehension. When you look at the following example, try to answer the questions before you read the passage. If you can answer a question correctly without reading the passage, the question is not passage dependent.

Obesity is:
- [ ] not prevalent in the United States
- [ ] a major social and medical problem in the United States
- [ ] a condition that primarily affects older people

Some consequences of obesity are:
- [ ] increased resistance to communicable disease
- [ ] increased risk of strokes, heart attacks, and diabetes
- [ ] increased ability to tolerate cold weather

Obesity is a major social and medical problem in the United States. More than one half of the United States population is considered overweight, and about 30% are considered obese (excessively fat). Obesity increases risk of strokes, heart attacks, diabetes, and several other medical problems. Billions are spent in the United States every year for diet books and over-the-counter diet drugs, but experts assert that eating less and exercising more is the best and surest way to lose weight.

Nicholas, MacLennan, and Brookshire (1986) reported that the validity of most multiple-sentence reading tests for brain-injured adults is compromised by low passage dependency. They evaluated the performance of non-brain-injured adults and aphasic adults on reading test items from the multiple-sentence reading subtests from the BDAE, the MTDDA, *Examining for Aphasia* (EFA; Eisenson, 1974), the *Western Aphasia Battery* (WAB; Kertesz, 1982), and the *Reading Comprehension Battery for Aphasia* (RCBA; LaPointe & Horner, 1979). First they had participants respond to the test questions without having previously read the passages to which the questions referred. On average, aphasic adults correctly answered beyond chance level 58% of the test questions, and non-brain-injured adults correctly answered 64% without having read the test passages. Only the questions from one of the two RCBA subtests had acceptable passage dependency. However, the reading passages in this subtest are only two sentences long and would be unlikely to predict performance on longer passages.

Tuiman (1974) suggested that passages for which test-takers can answer not more than 40% to 50% of test questions without reading the passages have acceptable passage dependency.

It seems inappropriate, however, for clinicians to shun the multiple-sentence reading tests in language test batteries because they have questionable passage dependency. These tests no doubt are sufficiently sensitive and have sufficient validity to make them acceptable screening tests of multiple-sentence reading comprehension. These tests appear well suited for identifying patients with reading impairments who then can be tested with a more comprehensive free-standing reading test, if appropriate. These tests also may be appropriate for estimating changes in a brain-injured patient's multiple-sentence reading ability over time, although their test-retest reliability is unknown. Repeated exposure to the same few test passages seems likely to decrease their passage dependency and inflate test scores. Consequently, standardized reading tests with alternate test forms would be a good choice for repeated testing.

GENERAL CONCEPTS 5-2

- Most comprehensive language tests include subtests to assess *oral reading* and *reading comprehension.*
- *Oral reading tests* typically require the patient to read lists of words and sentences. Success in oral reading does not require comprehension of what is read.
- Most comprehensive language tests assess several aspects of *reading comprehension:*
  - *Comprehension of single words.* Single-word reading comprehension typically is assessed by asking the patient to match printed words to pictures or to match printed words to spoken words.
  - *Comprehension of sentences.* Comprehension of printed sentences typically is assessed by asking the patient to respond to printed yes-no questions, to complete unfinished sentences, or to follow printed instructions requiring gestural or manipulative responses.
- Several comprehensive language tests contain subtests to assess *comprehension of printed texts.* The patient is given one or more short passages to read and answers questions about information in the passages. The passages may consist of storylike narratives or expository prose. As with spoken discourse, printed expository prose usually is more difficult than storylike narratives for brain-injured adults to comprehend.

- The *Reading Comprehension Battery for Aphasia* is a standardized test of reading comprehension. It permits assessment of brain-injured adults' comprehension of single-words, sentences, signs, labels, and short paragraphs and provides supplemental tests for letter and word skills related to reading. It is an appropriate screening test of reading for brain-injured patients but it may be too easy for patients with mild reading impairments.
- Reading tests for non-brain-damaged children and adults provide for more comprehensive assessment of brain-injured adults' reading than is possible with items from comprehensive language tests or the *Reading Comprehension Battery for Aphasia.* Most permit assessment of reading vocabulary and paragraph comprehension and allow calculation of a reading grade level.
- The *Nelson-Denny Reading Test* may be appropriate for patients with mild reading impairment. It permits assessment of a patient's ability to answer questions related to *literal information* or *interpretive information.*
- Measuring brain-injured patients' *reading rate* (how much the patient reads and understands under normal time constraints) and measuring *reading capacity* (how much the patient reads and understands if given unlimited time to finish) are important for

Continued

GENERAL CONCEPTS 5-2—cont'd

understanding the adequacy of brain-injured patients' reading ability.

- Materials that permit measurement of component reading skills (*following directions, using context, getting main ideas, drawing conclusions,* and *identifying inferences*) are a useful adjunct to standardized tests of reading and permit clinicians to tailor remedial programs to a patient's specific pattern of impairment.

- A straightforward and easy-to-understand test format is important when choosing a reading test for use with brain-injured adults, who may not be able to comprehend and follow complex instructions and test format.

- The passage dependency of reading test materials in comprehensive language tests is relatively low, suggesting that these materials may test patients' general knowledge as much as their reading comprehension.

SPEECH PRODUCTION

Speech production subtests are prominent in all comprehensive language tests, and several free-standing tests of speech production for brain-injured adults are available. Speech production tests cover a wide range of content, from repetition of syllables and words to self-generated connected speech. Patients with severely compromised communication usually can do the easiest tests reasonably well, whereas the most difficult tests challenge even patients with mild speech impairments.

Simple Speech Production Tests

The simplest speech production tests are useful for testing patients with moderate to severe speech production impairments. They call on patients to *produce rhymes, recitations, and automatized sequences; complete sentences;* and *repeat words, phrases, and sentences* after the examiner.

Recitations, Rhymes, and Automatized Sequences. These tests are among the easiest speech-production tests for most brain-injured adults. They require the patient to produce highly practiced material such as counting or reciting the days of the week, the months of the year, or the alphabet. Even severely brain-injured patients who produce little or no volitional speech often can produce highly practiced material. Those who cannot produce such

material in response to the examiner's request often can continue if the examiner helps them get started.

> **Clinician:** *Now, Mrs. Ryder, I'd like you to count from one to ten for me.*
> **Patient:** *Ah...umm...lahti...lahti...*
> **Clinician:** *Can you count from one to ten?*
> **Patient:** *Lahti...lahti...lahti...*
> **Clinician:** *Let's count from one to ten. Are you ready? One, two...*
> **Patient:** *...three...four...five...six...seventy...eighty ...ninety...tenty.*

Sentence Completion. Sentence completion tests usually are more difficult than tests calling for recitation, rhymes, and automatized sequences, but most brain-injured adults can perform them with reasonable success. The stimuli in these tests are short, syntactically simple sentences, minus the final word, which is highly predictable from the rest of the sentence (*I'd like a cup of... Roses are red, violets are...*).
Speech Repetition. Speech repetition tests span a range of difficulty, from monosyllabic words (e.g., *boy*) to simple phrases (e.g., *up and down*) to phonologically complex phrases and sentences (e.g., *Please put the groceries in the refrigerator.*). The longer and more phonologically complex the phrase or sentence, the more difficult it is for most patients to produce.

Patients with conduction aphasia or apraxia of speech often become tied in knots when asked to repeat phonologically complex materials. Their responses often contain multiple phonologic errors. Patients with conduction aphasia or apraxia of speech usually recognize their errors and try to correct them, often to no avail. Patients with Wernicke's aphasia sometimes have difficulty with such materials, not because of the phonological complexity of the materials but because of their short retention span. They often fill in with semantically related material when they fail to remember sentence elements.

> A patient with conduction aphasia, when asked to repeat *please put the groceries in the refrigerator,* responded with:
> *Pease put the gripperies in the...pease put the gorsheries in the refligalator...the frerigerator...*
> A patient with Wernicke's aphasia, when asked to repeat the same phrase, responded with:
> *Please put the...please put the...please put the bread, etcetera in the shopping cart.*

Naming

Naming Subtests in Comprehensive Language Tests. Naming subtests are found in all the major comprehensive language tests and provide information about patients across the aphasia severity continuum. Naming subtests take several forms. The most common is *picture or object naming* (sometimes called *confrontation naming*), in which the patient is shown a series of pictures or objects and is asked to say the name of each. The stimuli in most confrontation naming subtests are drawings or objects, but naming subtests in which the stimuli are geometric shapes, colors, numbers, or body parts are included in some comprehensive aphasia tests.

> Letter naming tests are also found in some comprehensive aphasia tests. However, I would categorize these as low-level oral reading tests.

Two variants on confrontation naming subtests are seen in some comprehensive language tests. In *responsive naming tests,* the examiner asks a question that can be answered with one or two words (e.g., *What do you write with? What do you do with soap? What color is snow?*). In *generative naming tests* (sometimes called *category naming tests*), patients are given a specified time interval (usually 1 minute) to say as many words as they can think of that either begin with a certain letter or represent certain semantic categories (e.g., *animals* or *tools*).

Free-Standing Tests of Naming. Several free-standing tests for assessing brain-injured adults' naming have been published or described in the literature. One of the oldest is a generative naming test called the *Word Fluency Measure* (Borkowski, Benton, & Spreen, 1967), which is a subtest of the *Neurosensory Center Comprehensive Examination for Aphasia* (NCCEA; Spreen & Benton, 1977). In the *Word Fluency Measure,* the patient is allowed 1 minute in which to say as many words that begin with a specified letter of the alphabet as the patient can think of. The letter (either *F, A,* or *S*) is specified by the examiner. The patient's score is the total of all appropriate words spoken in the 1-minute interval.

> The letters *F, A,* and *S* yield the largest numbers of correct responses from non-brain-injured adults (Borkowski, Benton, & Spreen, 1967). No equivalent information is available for semantic categories.

The *Word Fluency Measure* is a sensitive indicator of brain injury, but it does not discriminate among aphasia syndromes or between aphasia syndromes and other neurogenic impairments of communication or cognition. A patient's performance on the word fluency measure has marginal value for planning treatment because the task is unusual, with little relationship to daily life communication. Some clinicians make up informal generative naming tests in which the patient is asked to produce words within functional categories (e.g., furniture, foods, or flowers). Although no norms are available for these informal tests, they can provide useful insights into a patient's word retrieval, speech production, and semantic knowledge.

Aphasic adults almost always produce far fewer appropriate words in generative naming tasks than non-brain-injured adults (and fewer than adults with right-hemisphere brain injury). One potential problem for clinicians who wish to use generative naming tasks in treatment is that there is great variability in the number of names that non-brain-injured adults produce. For example, one group of non-brain-injured adults produced, on the average, 23 animal names in a 1-minute interval, but the scores of individuals ranged from 9 to 41 words (Goodglass & Kaplan, 1983).

The *Boston Naming Test* (BNT; Kaplan, Goodglass, & Weintraub, 2001) is a picture naming test in which the examiner shows the person being tested each of 60 line drawings and asks him or her to name each drawing. *Word familiarity* (the frequency of occurrence of target names) decreases as the test progresses. Each response is scored for latency, correctness, and whether a cue was given. The BNT manual provides brief instructions for administering the BNT and for scoring responses, but neither administration nor scoring instructions are explicit enough to ensure interexaminer or test-retest reliability, and the manual does not report either. Nicholas, Brookshire, and associates (1989) subsequently published more explicit procedures for administering and scoring the BNT, together with intrajudge and interjudge reliability for their more explicit procedures.

The *Test of Adolescent/Adult Word Finding* (TAWF; German, 1990) is a comprehensive test of word retrieval with norms for non-brain-damaged persons from age 12 to age 80. The TAWF provides for assessment of word retrieval in five tasks: *noun picture naming, verb picture naming, sentence completion* (e.g., *The farmer milked the...*), *naming to description* (e.g., *Something you write with*), and *category naming* (e.g., *Bananas, oranges, and apples are...*). The TAWF can be administered in 20 to 30 minutes for normal adults and should take no more than 1 hour for most brain-injured adults. A short version of the test takes less than 20 minutes for normal adults and should take no more than 30 minutes for most brain-injured adults.

Variables That May Affect Naming Accuracy

Frequency of Occurrence. A word's frequency in the language usually affects the ease and accuracy with which brain-injured adults name objects or pictures (Weigel-Crump & Koenigsknecht, 1973; Rochford & Williams, 1965; Tweedy & Schulman, 1982; and others). More frequent words are easier than less frequent words. However, confounding variables—length, abstractness, age of acquisition, and phonologic complexity of words—and the ambiguity or uncertainty of pictures have not been controlled in most studies, making conclusions about the effects of word frequency alone ambiguous.

As noted earlier, published word-frequency counts are based on frequency of occurrence in printed materials. Hayes (1989) has shown that published word-frequency counts do not accurately represent frequency of occurrence in everyday speech because printed materials contain greater proportions of low-frequency words than everyday speech does. Investigators also generally agree that word-frequency norms based on printed materials do not accurately represent the familiarity of words to normal adults. Brookshire and Nicholas (1995) had normal adults rate the familiarity of the words in the BNT. Then they tested a group of aphasic adults and a group of non-brain-injured adults with the test. The correlation between word frequency and aphasic adults' naming performance was $r = .37$, whereas the correlation between judged familiarity and aphasic adults' naming performance was much stronger ($r = .71$). Figure 5-18 shows the performance of the two groups according to word familiarity.

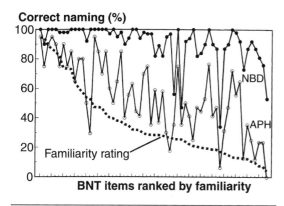

Correct naming (%)

BNT items ranked by familiarity

Figure 5-18 ■ Non-brain-damaged '(NBD) adults' and aphasic '(APH) adults' performance on the *Boston Naming Test* (BNT), with test items arranged in order of diminishing familiarity. (Neither the frequency of occurrence or the familiarity of BNT items diminishes uniformly across the test.)

Correlation coefficients range from 0 to 1.00. Larger correlation coefficients indicate stronger relationships. A correlation coefficient of .37 explains about 10% of the overall variability in scores. A correlation coefficient of .71 explains about 50%.

Length and Phonologic Complexity. Goodglass, Kaplan, Weintraub, & associates (1976) found that aphasic adults' naming success decreased as the number of syllables in words increased. The true culprit, however, may not be number of syllables but articulatory complexity because the number of syllables in a word is related to the ease with which it can be articulated. Word length and articulatory complexity affect the mechanical production of words, unlike variables such as word frequency or stimulus uncertainty, which are more likely to affect accessing words and retrieving them from memory. Patients with motor speech impairments *(apraxia of speech)* and phonologic selection and sequencing impairments *(conduction aphasia)* are most likely to be adversely affected by word length and phonologic complexity.

Semantic Categories. The semantic characteristics of items to be named may slightly affect how readily some brain-injured adults name pictures and objects. Goodglass, Klein, Carey, and associates (1966) evaluated aphasic adults' ability to name and comprehend words representing five semantic categories—*objects, actions, colors, numbers,* and *letters.* They reported that object names were hardest for aphasic adults to produce and that letters were easiest. The spoken names of objects were easiest to comprehend, and spoken letter names were hardest to comprehend. However, the difference between object-naming and letter-naming was only 2 points of a possible 18, and it is almost certain that not every participant's performance pattern matched that of the group. Consequently, clinicians undoubtedly will choose to evaluate the strength of the effects of semantic categories on individual patients' naming before incorporating manipulation of semantic categories into their treatment procedures.

Form of Visual Stimuli. During the 1970s several investigators set out to determine if the form of visual stimuli (objects, pictures, photographs, or line drawings) affected the naming performance of brain-injured adults. Benton, Smith, and Lang (1972) asked aphasic adults to name real objects and line drawings of real objects and found a small but statistically significant difference in favor of real objects. Bisiach (1966) asked aphasic adults to name either realistic colored pictures or line drawings of common objects. He reported a small but significant difference in favor of realistic colored pictures. Corlew and Nation (1975) reported contradictory results. They asked aphasic adults to name either real objects or line drawings representing the objects. They found no meaningful difference between participants' object naming and their ability to name objects and their ability to name drawings.

Most brain-injured adults are unlikely to perform much differently if they are asked to name objects, colored photographs, or line drawings. However, as in the case of comprehension tests, differences in the form of visual stimuli used in naming tests may be important for severely impaired patients or for patients with visual-perceptual impairments. For these patients, real objects may elicit better naming performance than pictures or drawings, and realistic photographs may elicit better performance than line drawings.

The naming performance of some brain-injured patients improves in object-naming tasks if they are permitted to pick up the objects to be named. Apparently the tactile information supplied by handling adds information that enhances retrieval.

Context. Context seems to have stronger effects on naming performance than the nature of the stimuli to be named. For many brain-injured adults, naming of drawings, pictures, or objects improves when they are portrayed in a natural context. For example, a brain-injured adult who cannot name a drawing of a horse portrayed in isolation may name it if the horse is shown harnessed to a cart. A patient who has difficulty naming cups, plates, knives, and forks presented in isolation or in an array of unrelated items may name them more easily if they are arranged in a place setting like those experienced in daily life.

Williams and Canter (1982) reported conflicting findings with regard to the effects of context on aphasic adults' naming. They asked aphasic adults to name line drawings of objects that were shown either in isolation or in a pictorial context. Adults with Broca's aphasia were better at naming the drawings of objects in isolation, and adults with Wernicke's aphasia were better at naming them in contexts. Other groups of aphasic adults exhibited no overall preference for contextual or acontextual pictures, although Williams and Canter reported that individual aphasic adults in all groups showed marked differences in performance between the two conditions.

The presence of context can have negative effects on the naming performance of some

patients who have right-hemisphere brain injury, traumatic brain injury, or dementia. These patients may focus on trivial or tangential details of the context, with negative effects on their naming performance. For these patients highly structured test procedures with minimally contextual stimuli may yield better performance than less structured procedures with contextually rich stimuli.

Sentence Production

Sentence Production Subtests in Comprehensive Language Tests. Sentence production subtests are included in all comprehensive language tests. They take several forms. In *word definition tests,* the examiner provides a word and asks the patient to tell what the word means (e.g., *Tell me what* onion *means.*). In *make-a-sentence-from-a-word tests,* the examiner says a word and asks the patient to say a sentence containing the word (e.g., Today. *Tell me a sentence that includes the word* today.). In *expressing ideas tests,* the examiner asks the patient to produce a sentence or two in response to the examiner's request (e.g., *Tell me three things you did today* [MTDDA]; *As completely as possible, tell me what you do with each of these* [PICA].)

Free-Standing Tests of Sentence Production. The *Reporter's Test* (DeRenzi & Ferrari, 1978) is a sentence-production version of the *Token Test.* In the *Token Test,* the examiner asks the patient to manipulate large and small colored tokens. In the *Reporter's Test,* the examiner manipulates the tokens and the patient describes the examiner's actions.

There are five levels in the *Reporter's Test,* similar to the five levels in the *Token Test.* In Level 1 (four items), only large tokens are present, and the examiner touches a single token (e.g., *You touched the green circle.*). In Level 2 (four items), large and small tokens are present, and the examiner touches one of them (e.g., *You touched the small white circle.*). In Level 3 (four items), only large tokens are present, and the examiner touches two in succession (e.g., *You touched the red circle and the green* square.). In level 4 (four items), all tokens are present, and the examiner touches two in succession (e.g., *You touched the large red circle and the small green square.*). In Level 5 (10 items) only the large tokens are present, and the examiner manipulates them in several ways (e.g., *You put the red circle on the green square. You touched all the circles except the green one.*). DeRenzi and Ferrari assert that the *Reporter's Test* is more sensitive to the presence of language impairment than is confrontation naming, word fluency, picture description, or sentence repetition.

Wener and Duffy (1983) compared the *Reporter's Test* with other measures of speech production and language comprehension for English-speaking aphasic adults. Their results support DeRenzi and Ferrari's assertions about the test's sensitivity to language impairments. However, Wener and Duffy concluded that the *Reporter's Test* in combination with other tests is more sensitive to the presence of sentence-production impairments than the *Reporter's Test* alone.

Discourse Production

Discourse Production Subtests in Comprehensive Language Tests. The most common test format for eliciting discourse in comprehensive language tests is *picture description,* in which the examiner shows the patient a drawing depicting several characters engaged in activities that should be familiar to most adults and asks the patient to describe the picture. The BDAE, the MTDDA, and the WAB include such picture description subtests. Figure 5-19 shows the pictures used to elicit speech in those tests.

The picture from the MTDDA is less storylike and more likely to elicit enumeration (naming of items in the picture) and is less likely to elicit narrative than the WAB and BDAE pictures (Correia, Brookshire, & Nicholas, 1990).

Story retelling sometimes is used to elicit connected speech from brain-injured adults.

The patient reads (or, less frequently, hears) a narrative and retells it to the examiner. Story retelling makes heavy demands on comprehension and verbal memory. Consequently, poor performance on story retelling tasks may not always be attributable to impaired speech formulation or production. Other connected speech tasks that do not tax comprehension and memory usually are a better choice if the clinician's concern is with speech formulation and production and not with comprehension and memory.

The Boston Diagnostic Aphasia Examination (BDAE) and the Western Aphasia Battery (WAB) base judgments of patients' aphasia type primarily on the characteristics of the speech they produce in an interview.

The BDAE provides a useful *Rating Scale Profile of Speech Characteristics* (Figure 5-20) for rating melodic line, phrase length, articulatory agility, grammatic form, paraphasia, repetition, and word finding in connected speech (from the interview, conversation, and picture-description). The rating scale can be used to construct a speech profile that may be compared with profiles for major aphasia syndromes. (Auditory comprehension also is included in the rating scale, although it is not a speech characteristic.)

Examiners using the BDAE also focus on connected speech when they rate the patients' overall aphasia severity with the following rating scale.

0 No usable speech or auditory comprehension.

1 All communication is through fragmentary expression: There is great need for inference, questioning, and guessing by the listener. The range of information that can be exchanged is limited, and the listener carries the burden of communication.

2 Conversation about familiar subjects is possible with help from the listener. There are frequent failures to convey the idea, but the patient shares the burden of communication with the examiner.

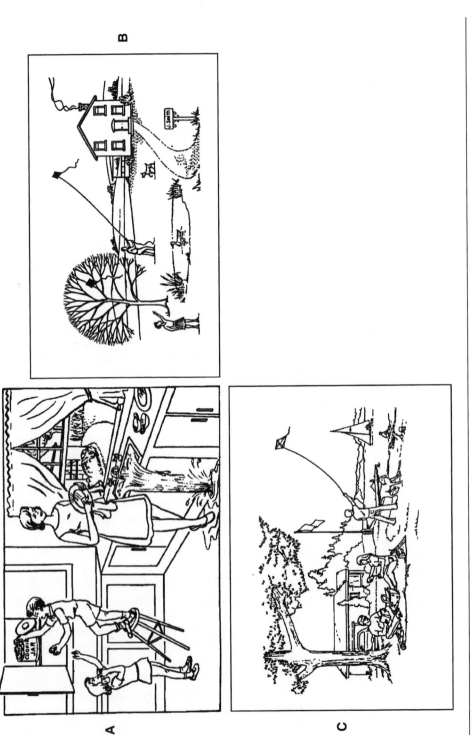

Figure 5-19 ■ The connected-speech elicitation pictures from the *Boston Diagnostic Aphasia Examination* (**A**), the *Minnesota Test for Differential Diagnosis of Aphasia* (Schuell, 1965) (**B**), and the *Western Aphasia Battery* (**C**). (**A** from Goodglass, H., Kaplan, E., & Barresi, B. [2001]. *The assessment of aphasia and related disorders* [3rd ed.]. Philadelphia: Lippincott Williams & Wilkins, now owned by Pro-Ed [Austin, Texas]. **B** from Schuell, H.M. [1965]. *The Minnesota test for differential diagnosis of aphasia.* Minneapolis: University of Minnesota Press. **C** from Kertesz, A. [1982]. *Western aphasia battery,* New York: Grune & Stratton.)

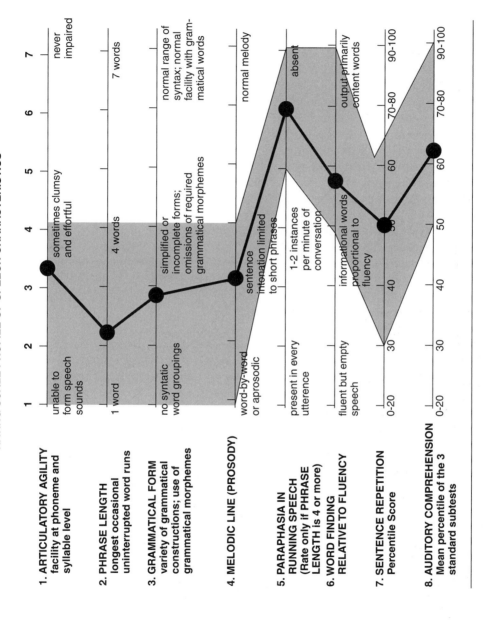

Figure 5-20 ■ *A Rating Scale Profile of Speech Characteristics from the Boston Diagnostic Aphasia Examination for a patient with Broca's aphasia.* (From Goodglass, H., Kaplan, E. & Barresi, B. [2001]. *The assessment of aphasia and related disorders* [3rd ed]. Philadelphia: Lippincott Williams & Wilkins, now owned by Pro-Ed [Austin, Texas].)

3 The patient can discuss almost all everyday problems with little or no assistance. However, reduction of speech and/or comprehension make conversation about certain material difficult or impossible.

4 Some obvious loss of fluency in speech or facility of comprehension, without significant limitation on ideas expressed or form of expression.

5 Minimal discernible speech handicaps; the patient may have subjective difficulties that are not apparent to the listener.

(I often have used excerpts from the BDAE rating scale in consultation reports and progress notes because they are written in nontechnical language and efficiently convey fundamental information about a patient's speech communication.)

The WAB provides two 11-point (0-10) scales for rating the speech elicited in the WAB connected-speech subtest: one for rating information content and the other for rating fluency and grammaticality. Speech fluency is important in Kertesz's taxonomic approach in which patients are assigned to neurodiagnostic categories such as Broca's aphasia or Wernicke's aphasia according to their WAB performance. Trupe (1984) has questioned the reliability of the WAB procedures for scoring spontaneous speech, as well as the validity of assigning patients to diagnostic categories based on spontaneous speech scores.

Interviews and conversations are important parts of some comprehensive language tests. The examiner asks the patient for personal information such as the patient's name and address and asks questions about the patient's complaints, problems, or history (e.g., *How are you today? Tell me why you are here. What kind of work do you do?*).

Free-Standing Procedures for Assessing Discourse Production. Several free-standing procedures for eliciting and scoring discourse produced by language-impaired adults have been described in the literature (Glosser & Deser, 1990; Glosser, Wiener, & Kaplan, 1988; Golper, Thorpe, Tompkins, & associates, 1980; Hier, Hagenlocker, & Shindler, 1985; Nicholas & associates, 1985). These elicitation and scoring procedures are not actually tests of discourse. However, their materials and procedures may be useful for clinicians concerned with measuring and treating brain-injured adults' discourse impairments.

Yorkston and Beukelman (1980) published a system for measuring the amount of information conveyed by brain-injured adults as they described the *cookie theft* picture from the BDAE (see Figure 5-19). The central measure in their system is what Yorkston and Beukelman called *content units,* which they defined as elements of information that were mentioned by at least 1 of 78 non-brain-injured adults who described the BDAE picture.

Yorkston and Beukelman's 1-of-78 criterion seems too permissive to me. It seems to me that including information mentioned by only 1 of 78 judges risks including tangential, irrelevant, or unimportant informational elements. Making the criterion more stringent (e.g., requiring mention by at least 10 of 78 judges) would, I think, provide a list of content units with greater validity when applied to a population of speakers.

Yorkston and Beukelman reported that *content units per minute* differentiated the speech of aphasic adults from that of non-brain-injured adults. (The aphasic adults produced fewer content units per minute.) Results reported by Yorkston and Beukelman for one aphasic adult suggested that both *number of content units* and *content units per minute* are sensitive measures of change in connected speech as a result of treatment.

Others have modified or expanded on Yorkston and Beukelman's content unit measures (Golper & associates, 1980; Shewan, 1988). However, the content units measure and its variants are limited in application because they can be used only to analyze speech elicited with the BDAE *cookie theft* picture.

Nicholas and Brookshire (1993, 1995a) published a standard protocol for eliciting and scoring discourse from brain-injured adults, using several kinds of elicitation stimuli:

- The speech elicitation pictures from the BDAE and the WAB (see Figure 5-19)
- Two *single pictures* depicting storylike situations with a central focus and interactions among picture elements (Figure 5-21)
- Two *picture sequences*, each of which contains six pictures portraying a short story (Figure 5-22)
- Two *requests for personal information* (e.g., *Tell me what you usually do on Sundays.* and *Tell me where you live and describe it to me.*). Two *requests for procedural information* (e.g., *Tell me how you would go about doing dishes by hand.* and *Tell me how you would go about writing and sending a letter.*).

Nicholas and Brookshire provided rules for scoring *words, correct information units,* and *main concepts* in speech samples elicited with the protocol. They defined *correct information units* as words that are accurate, relevant, and informative relative to the eliciting stimulus. They defined *main concepts* as statements that convey the most important information about a stimulus.

Nicholas and Brookshire (1993) reported that *words per minute, correct information units per minute,* and *percentage of words that are correct information units* reliably discriminate aphasic adults from those without aphasia, but suggested that combining a speech rate measure *(words per minute)* with an informativeness measure *(percentage of words that are correct information units)* provides a better description of brain-injured adults' connected speech than any single measure. They also reported that the number of main concepts mentioned did not reliably discriminate aphasic speakers' performance from that of non-brain-injured

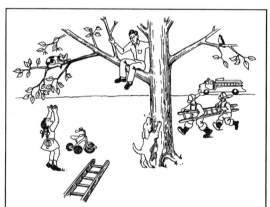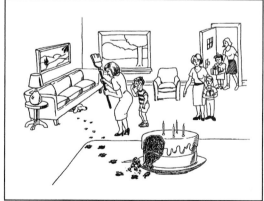

Figure 5-21 ■ Connected speech elicitation pictures. (From Nicholas, L.E., & Brookshire, R.H. [1993]. A system for quantifying the informativeness and efficiency of the connected speech of adults with aphasia. *Journal of Speech and Hearing Research, 36,* 338-350.)

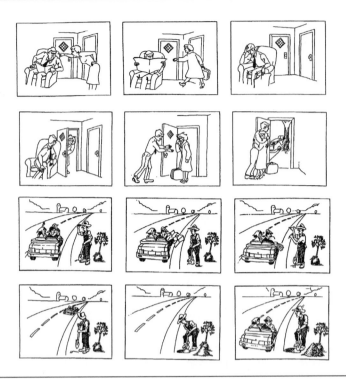

Figure 5-22 ■ Prompted story telling pictures. (From Nicholas, L.E., & Brookshire, R.H. [1993]. A system for quantifying the informativeness and efficiency of the connected speech of adults with aphasia. *Journal of Speech and Hearing Research, 36,* 338-350.)

speakers. The *accuracy* and *completeness* of the main concepts aphasic speakers produced did, however, reliably discriminate them from non-brain-damaged speakers (Nicholas & Brookshire, 1993).

Brookshire and Nicholas (1995a) also described a rule-based system for scoring what they called *performance deviations* in the speech of brain-injured adults. They defined performance deviations as *features that make the connected speech of brain-injured adults distinctive (e.g., inaccurate or vague words, revised utterances)...* (p 118), and described nine categories of those features (Table 5-1).

Several categories of performance deviations distinguished non-brain-injured adults from those with aphasia. Non-brain-injured adults produced fewer inaccurate words, false starts, and part-words or unintelligible productions than did the aphasic adults. The non-brain-injured adults also produced fewer instances of unnecessary exact repetition than did fluent aphasic adults and fewer instances of the word *and* and less nonword filler than did nonfluent aphasic adults. There were no significant differences between a group of non-brain-injured adults and a group of aphasic adults in the frequency with which they produced nonspecific words, filler words, or off-task words.

Brookshire and Nicholas suggested that measuring performance deviations in brain-injured adults' connected speech provides a useful supplement to measures of communicative informa-

TABLE 5-1	**Performance Deviation Categories***	

Performance Deviations	Definition	Examples
Non-CIU Categories		
Inaccurate	Not accurate with regard to the stimulus, and no attempt to correct.	...on a **chair** (for stool)
False start	False start or abandoned utterance.	...on a **chair..no**, a stool
Unnecessary exact repetition	Exact repetition of words, unless used purposefully for emphasis or cohesion.	...on a..**on a** stool
Nonspecific or vague	Nonspecific or vague words or words lacking an unambiguous referent.	...on a **thing** ...on **it** (with no referent for *it*)
Filler	Empty words that do not communicate information about the stimulus.	...on a, **you know**, stool
The word *and*	All occurrences of the word *and*.	...a boy **and** a stool
Off-task or irrelevant	Commentary on the task or the speaker's performance.	**I've seen this one before.** **I can't say it.**
Nonword Categories		
Part-word or unintelligible production	Word fragment or production that does not result in a word that is intelligible in context.	...on a **st..sk**..stool ...on a **frampi**
Nonword filler	Utterances such as *uh* or *um*.	...on a..**um**..stool..**uh**.

*Data from Brookshire, R. H., & Nicholas, L.E. (1995). Performance deviations in the connected speech of adults with no brain damage and adults with aphasia. *American Journal of Speech-Language Pathology, 4*, 118-123.

NOTE: In the examples, only nonwords and words printed in boldface italics are scored as performance deviations.

tiveness and efficiency. Although Brookshire and Nicholas studied only aphasic adults, their categories of performance deviations and their scoring system are appropriate for quantifying the connected speech of brain-injured adults in other diagnostic categories.

Speech Fluency

Several methods for assessing brain-injured adults' speech fluency have been described in the literature. None has been standardized, and their reliability remains to be documented, but they do provide procedures with which speech fluency can be assessed in more or less systematic fashion.

Wagenaar, Snow, and Prins (1975) described 30 measures for quantifying various characteris-

tics of brain-injured adults' connected speech. Among their conclusions were the following:

- The most useful measure for classifying aphasia patients on the basis of their speech production is fluency.
- Patients can be classified as fluent or nonfluent on the basis of *speech tempo* (words per minute) and mean length of utterance.
- Telegraphic speech and empty speech are separate syndromes.
- Grammatic errors and articulatory errors are separate factors and not directly related to fluency.

Wagenaar, Snow, and Prins's procedures are too unwieldy for routine clinical use, but their list of measures and their findings may help clinicians develop procedures for analyzing brain-injured patients' spontaneous speech.

GENERAL CONCEPTS 5-3

- *Speech production tests* in comprehensive language tests range from word and syllable repetition to self-generated connected speech.
  - *Recitations; rhymes; automatized sequences; sentence completion;* and *repeating short, simple phrases* are the easiest speech production subtests in comprehensive language tests. Patients with moderate to severe speech production impairments often perform acceptably (though not without error) in these subtests.
  - *Sentence completion* tests are more difficult than tests requiring brain-injured patients to produce rhymes, recitations, or automatized sequences, but most brain-injured patients can perform them reasonably well.
  - *Speech repetition tests* range from monosyllabic utterances to phonologically complex phrases and sentences. Long and phonologically complex material proves difficult for many brain-injured patients.
- In tests of *confrontation naming,* patients name pictures, drawings, or objects. In tests of *responsive naming,* patients give one-word answers to questions such as *What color is snow?*
- The *Word Fluency Test* is a standardized test of generative naming in which the patient says all the words he or she can think of that begin with a certain letter (usually *F, A,* or *S*).
- The *Boston Naming Test* (BNT) is a standardized test of confrontation naming. The words in the first part of the BNT are more common than the words in the last part.
- The *Test of Adolescent/Adult Word Finding (TAWF)* is a comprehensive test of naming. It permits assessment of naming in five tasks: naming pictured nouns, naming pictured verbs, sentence completion, description naming, and category naming.

- Several variables affect the ease with which brain-injured adults can retrieve and produce words in tests of naming:
  - *Frequency of occurrence.* Frequently occurring words usually are easier to retrieve and produce.
  - *Length and phonologic complexity.* Shorter and less complex words usually are easier to retrieve and produce. Phonologic complexity is most likely to affect patients with speech motor control or phonologic selection and sequencing problems.
  - *Semantic characteristics.* Nouns may be slightly easier than verbs for brain-injured adults.
  - The *form* of stimuli to be named (drawings, photographs, real objects) has little effect on most brain-injured adults' naming performance.
  - Providing *context* for pictorial stimuli to be named has stronger effects than the form of the stimuli, although there is considerable variability in the effects of context among brain-injured adults.
- Comprehensive language tests typically assess *sentence production* by requiring patients to define words, make sentences from words supplied by the examiner, or express simple ideas.
- The *Reporter's Test* is a free-standing test of sentence production in which the patient describes manipulations of tokens carried out by the examiner.
- Picture description is the primary means by which *discourse* is elicited with comprehensive language tests. Some comprehensive language tests also contain *story telling* or *story retelling tests.* However, brain-injured patients' performance in story retelling tests may be compromised by impaired comprehension of and memory for the stories.

- *Interviews* and *conversations* are important speech production tasks in some comprehensive language tests. Patients' performance in the interview and conversation is an important aspect of classifying patients with these tests.
- Several free-standing procedures for assessing brain-injured adults' discourse production have been reported in the literature. Measuring the *informativeness* (percent of words that are informative) and the *content units per minute* (rate at which information is produced) provides a measure of communicative efficiency.
- Measuring *performance deviations* helps to capture qualitative aspects of brain-injured adults' spoken discourse.
- Several methods for assessing *speech fluency* have been described in the literature, but they are not standardized and do not have confirmed reliability.
- *Speech intelligibility* usually is not a major problem for adults with unilateral brain injury.

Intelligibility

The speech of most patients with neurogenic language disorders caused by unilateral brain injury is intelligible, although its content may be anomalous. Consequently, assessment of intelligibility usually is not an important concern in evaluating these patients. When intelligibility is a concern, *Assessing Intelligibility of Dysarthric Speech* (Yorkston & Beukelman, 1981) permits its measurement. Yorkston and Beukelman's procedure is described in Chapter 13 of this book.

WRITTEN EXPRESSION
Writing Subtests in Comprehensive Language Tests

All major comprehensive language tests include subtests for assessing written expression at several levels, but no standardized free-standing tests designed for assessment of brain-injured adults' writing are currently available. The writing subtests in comprehensive language tests permit clinicians to assess written expression at four levels—*generating automatized sequences, copying, writing to dictation,* and *writing self-formulated material.* However, there are minor differences in test content within levels, and some comprehensive language tests include writing subtests not seen in the others.

In *generating automatized sequences subtests,* the patient is asked to write overlearned sequences (usually the alphabet and numbers from 1 to 20 and sometimes the patient's name). Scoring of patients' responses differs across tests, but it usually involves counting misspellings, omissions, transpositions, and illegible productions. Producing automatized sequences usually is the easiest writing subtest for most brain-injured adults. Many can write strings of consecutive numbers and letters when they can produce little else in the way of written material. Signing one's name is a highly automatized activity for most adults, and many brain-injured adults who cannot generate strings of letters or numbers can write their name fluently and with little effort.

Sometimes patients who cannot generate strings of letters or numbers or write their name in response to spoken requests can complete letter and number strings and complete their written name if given the first few letters or numbers in the series. Completing such automatized sequences often proves surprisingly easy for patients who seem completely at a loss when asked to generate them in response to the examiner's requests.

Copying subtests require patients to copy geometric forms, symbols, letters, printed words, or printed sentences. Adults with posterior brain injury often have unusual difficulty with copying subtests, perhaps because of impairments in visual perception and discrimination. Brain-injured adults usually do well at copying simple stimuli such as forms, symbols, and letters, but their performance deteriorates when they copy words and sentences, wherein spelling errors, syntactic errors, and word substitutions may appear. Brain-injured adults who are weak or paralyzed in their preferred hand and arm usually produce distorted representations of stimuli in copying tests because of the mechanical difficulty of producing forms or letters.

Writing to dictation subtests usually follow a letter-to-word-to-sentence progression. Patients are asked to write letters, then words, then sentences to dictation.

In *letter or number transcription subtests,* the patient writes nonconsecutive strings of letters or numbers (e.g., *R...C...Y...M...G...*) dictated by the examiner, who pauses after each letter or number to give the patient time to write it. Sometimes the examiner spells words aloud, pausing after each letter to give the patient time write it (e.g., *T...O...O...T...H...B...R...U...S...H*).

> Sometimes the examiner spells words aloud by saying one letter per second without waiting for the patient to write each letter. Such tests are extremely difficult for patients with restricted auditory retention span unless they recognize the word and can spell it from memory.

Most comprehensive language tests include subtests in which patients write words to dictation. The examiner may say a phrase with emphatic stress on the target word and then repeat the target word (e.g., *I went to the dentist. Write went.*), but most often the examiner simply explains the procedure to the patient, then says the target words one at a time. (*Now I'll say some words, one at a time. I want you to write each word after I say it. Write*

banana.). Tests in which patients write words to dictation are primarily tests of spelling ability, although performance may also be affected by impaired auditory retention, compromised visual perception, or limb weakness or clumsiness.

> The difficulty of write-a-sentence-given-a-word tests depends greatly on the nature of the stimulus words provided. It is easier for brain-injured adults (and non-brain-injured adults) to write sentences when the stimuli are nouns or verbs than to write sentences when the stimuli are adjectives, adverbs, prepositions, or function words. Composing a sentence containing the word *man* requires much less mental effort than composing a sentence containing the word *slowly.*

Most comprehensive language tests include subtests in which patients write material for which the examiner provides no spoken model. The easiest for most brain-injured patients are *written confrontation naming subtests* in which the patient is shown a drawing or an object and asked to write its name. Some comprehensive language tests include subtests requiring *writing self-formulated sentences—* for example, writing sentences containing each of several specified words (e.g., *Write a sentence containing the words* little, boy, *and* dog.) or writing sentences describing the functions of everyday objects (e.g., *Write a sentence that tells what you use a pencil for.*). Several comprehensive language tests contain written versions of oral picture description subtests in which the patient is asked to write a paragraph about the picture they have described orally. (See Figure 5-19 for the pictures used in these subtests.)

Writing words and sentences to dictation is easier for most brain-injured patients than writing self-formulated sentences or paragraphs. However, a few patients may do better when their responses are not constrained to reproduce exactly what the examiner says but are free to choose their own words to construct sentences and to communicate their own thoughts and ideas.

Free-Standing Tests of Written Expression

Few free-standing writing tests are commonly used in evaluation of brain-injured adults' language, perhaps because the subtests in comprehensive language tests are sufficient for most clinical purposes. However, written spelling tests such as the spelling subtest of the *Wide Range Achievement Test* (Wilkinson, 1993) sometimes are used to evaluate brain-injured adults' written spelling. Using these tests permits the examiner to calculate a spelling grade level and sometimes a percentile rank for a patient's spelling performance.

LANGUAGE PRAGMATICS

Comprehensive language tests focus on the content and structure of language but give little insight into how language is used to communicate in daily life—an aspect of language called *pragmatics. Language pragmatics* denotes how language is used to communicate thoughts, ideas, wishes, opinions, and intentions in social interactions. The domain of language pragmatics includes:

(a) *speech acts,* such as greeting, asserting, questioning, denying, requesting, and informing
(b) *social behaviors,* such as facial expression, posture, gesture, eye contact, and turn-taking
(c) *conversational behaviors,* such as initiating interchanges, maintaining topics, and repairing breakdowns
(d) *conversational rules and conventions,* such as informativeness, efficiency, truth, relevance, and clarity

Some writers also include in the domain of language pragmatics *receptive skills,* such as appreciation of implied meanings associated with indirect requests, humor, sarcasm, and metaphor and the ability to resolve ambiguity and construct inferences.

Assessing pragmatic language skills is a challenge. A few standardized tests of pragmatic language are on the market, including the *Test of Pragmatic Language* (TOPL; Phelps-Terasaki & Phipps-Gunn, 1992), a 44-item test designed to assess six aspects of pragmatic language—physical setting, audience, topic, purpose, visual-gestural cues, and abstraction. Adams (2002) comments, however, that the TOPL "goes well beyond the boundaries of pragmatics and is more akin to a test of high-level language competence, incorporating elements of complex vocabulary, semantics, and verbal reasoning" (p. 976). Existing standardized tests of pragmatic language focus on appreciation of nonliteral meanings, making inferences, resolving ambiguity, and producing narratives but largely neglect the social-interactional dimensions of pragmatics.

The social-interactional dimensions of pragmatics are observable only in social interactions, and social interactions are by nature fluid and spontaneous because the behaviors of each participant are influenced by the behaviors of other participants. It may be difficult or impossible to construct valid standardized tests of language pragmatics that capture the full range of potential pragmatic behavior. Standardized tests have the merit of being efficient to administer and permit comparison of individuals with normative groups, but language pragmatics may not be amenable to quantification with procedures that separate the behaviors from the natural contexts in which they typically occur.

Checklists of pragmatic behavior offer an alternative to standardized tests. Checklists permit users to describe, quantify, and categorize the pragmatic behavior of an individual. Checklists often are organized so that a completed checklist provides a profile of the pragmatic behaviors exhibited by an individual across various categories of behavior (e.g., speech acts, social behaviors, and conversational behaviors). Prutting and Kirchner's *Pragmatic Protocol* (1987) is a popular checklist of this kind. Raters who use the *Pragmatic Protocol* score the occurrence of inappropriate pragmatic behaviors while the person being rated participates in 15 minutes of conversation with a familiar partner. Inappropriate pragmatic behaviors are assigned to one of 30 categories, representing verbal aspects such as speech acts, topic maintenance, turn-taking, and communicative

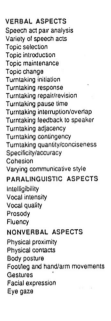
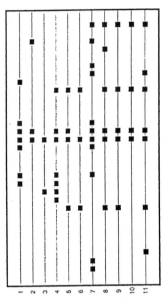
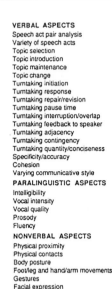
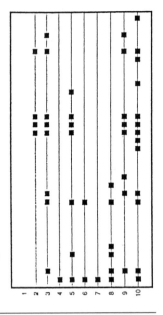

Figure 5-23 ■ Patterns of performance on the *Pragmatic Protocol* for adults with left-hemisphere brain injuries and adults with right-hemisphere brain injuries. Adults with left-hemisphere injuries *(left)* tend to be deficient in pause time, quantity, conciseness, specificity and accuracy of speech, and speech fluency. Adults with right-hemisphere injuries *(right)* tend to be deficient in adjacency, contingency, quantity and conciseness of turns, prosody, and eye gaze.

style; paralinguistic aspects such as vocal intensity and quality, prosody, and fluency; and nonverbal aspects such as physical proximity, posture, and eye contact (Figure 5-23).

The scoring procedures for the *Pragmatic Protocol* overemphasize violations because any occurrence of inappropriate behavior in a category causes that category to be marked deficient, even though the person being evaluated may have had several occurrences of appropriate behavior in the same category. The person being evaluated is penalized for a single occurrence of inappropriate behavior in a category but gets no credit for appropriate behaviors in the same category, even when the appropriate behaviors outnumber the inappropriate ones.

In its published form, the *Pragmatic Protocol* seems best used as a screening instrument to

identify problem areas that can then be evaluated in greater detail by counting both appropriate and inappropriate behaviors. Prutting and Kirchner apparently agree, because they suggested that a patient's performance on the *Pragmatic Protocol* should lead to detailed assessment of the patient's pragmatic performance, focusing on inappropriate pragmatic behaviors identified by the *Pragmatic Protocol*. They also recommend that clinicians use the results of the detailed assessment to determine the probable impact of the inappropriate behaviors on daily life interactions.

Rating scales for assessing pragmatic language are included in some tests designed for assessment of persons with right-hemisphere brain injuries (e.g., the *Right Hemisphere Language Battery* [RHLB; Bryan, 1989] and the *Rehabilitation Institute of Chicago Evaluation* of Problems in Right-Hemisphere Dysfunction —Revised [RICE-R; Halper, Cherney, Burns, & associates, 1996]). The RHLB and the RICE-R are described in Chapter 10. Such rating scales also may be useful for assessing the pragmatic skills of persons with language impairments related to other neurologic conditions.

STANDARDIZED APHASIA TESTS

Assessment of language has for many years relied on comprehensive language tests that contain an assortment of subtests with which to assess language production and comprehension at various levels of difficulty in major input and output modalities. Most comprehensive language tests for adults are designed for aphasic adults but can be used to assess language performance of adults with other linguistic or communicative impairments. Some comprehensive language tests provide norms for other populations such as adults with right-hemisphere damage or adults with dementia.

Detailed assessment of brain-injured adults' language requires comprehensive testing across a range of language skills spanning a range of difficulty levels within each skill. Standardized aphasia tests are designed to provide such detailed assessment, although they differ in the number of skills addressed and the depth to which they evaluate each skill. The major standardized aphasia tests are similar in content but have important differences in intent, scoring, and interpretation. Some of these differences are illustrated in the following summary of standardized aphasia test batteries that are in general use in the United States.

Minnesota Test for Differential Diagnosis of Aphasia

The *Minnesota Test for Differential Diagnosis of Aphasia* (MTDDA; Schuell, 1972) is one of the pioneers in aphasia testing. It was one of the first tests for aphasia to emphasize the importance of qualitative scoring of responses rather than simply counting errors. According to its

authors, the MTDDA was designed to do the following:

- Permit users to explore differences in the behavior of aphasic adults in all language modalities
- Include tests of graduated difficulty within each language modality
- Include a variety of nonlanguage tasks to measure processes underlying language behavior
- Be comprehensive and detailed enough to identify clinical syndromes caused by brain damage

The MTDDA is one of the longest and most detailed standardized aphasia tests, with 47 subtests divided among five sections—auditory disturbances (9 subtests), visual and reading disturbances (9 subtests), speech and language disturbances (15 subtests), visuomotor and writing disturbances (10 subtests), and numerical relations and arithmetic processes disturbances (4 subtests). The MTDDA is heterogeneous with regard to the number of items in subtests and the pattern of difficulty within subtests. The number of items within subtests ranges from 5 to 32. In some subtests, items increase in difficulty across the subtest; in others, the items are of approximately equal difficulty. Because of its length and the time it takes to administer and score the entire MTDDA (3 to 6 hours), clinicians who are pushed for time (most are) tend not to administer the complete test.

Schuell recognized the need for a shortened version of the MTDDA, and in 1957 suggested a *baseline-ceiling* procedure for shortening the test. The examiner first estimates the patient's probable level of performance in each performance category (listening, speaking, reading, writing, and calculating), then selects a performance category (e.g., listening) and begins testing with the most difficult subtests the examiner thinks the patient can complete with no more than one error. If the patient makes more than one error on a subtest, the examiner administers progressively easier subtests until the patient performs a subtest without error. This defines the patient's *baseline*. Then the examiner administers progressively more difficult subtests until the patient makes 90% errors, at which point testing ends (the *ceiling*), and the examiner moves on to another category.

Schuell's baseline-ceiling procedure resembles that used by many clinicians to shorten testing and to avoid administering too easy tests, in which a patient makes no errors, or too difficult tests, in which a patient makes only errors. The results of tests in which a patient makes no errors or makes only errors are uninformative about the nature of the patient's language processing impairments.

Most responses to MTDDA test items are scored plus-minus (correct-incorrect) with some longhand notation, although errors made in two subtests, (matching printed words to pictures, matching printed to spoken words) can be categorized as semantic confusions, auditory confusions, visual confusions, or irrelevant responses.

The MTDDA provides few standardized procedures for interpreting patients' performance. The test manual provides mean scores, standard deviations, and subtest-by-subtest percentages of errors for a group of 50 nonaphasic adults and six groups of aphasic adults representing five major categories of aphasia and one minor syndrome (see following). The norm group of aphasic adults ranges from 31 to 157 patients, depending on the subtest. Most subtests are normed on 75 aphasic adults. The test manual provides a list of signs and most discriminating tests which enable the user to assign patients to one of five major and two minor categories of aphasia, but it does not provide standardized and reliable procedures for making the assignment. The seven MTDDA categories are as follows:
- Simple aphasia
- Aphasia with visual involvement
- Aphasia with sensorimotor involvement
- Aphasia with scattered findings compatible with generalized brain damage

- Irreversible aphasic syndrome
- Minor syndrome A: aphasia with partial auditory imperception
- Minor syndrome B: aphasia with persisting dysarthria

The MTDDA manual provides no standardized prognostic procedures, although general descriptions of expected recovery patterns for the seven categories are included. The subjective nature of procedures for assigning patients to diagnostic categories gives users of the MTDDA considerable latitude in making these decisions, which may contribute to unreliability. The MTDDA manual provides no procedures for profiling patterns of impairment and provides no percentiles, either for individual subtests or the MTDDA as a whole, although some statistical information can be found in Schuell, Jenkins, and Jimenez-Pabon (1964). The test manual also provides no information about interexaminer reliability or the reliability of its patient-categorization procedures.

The MTDDA is somewhat dated. Its length and lack of psychometric sophistication have diminished its popularity in favor of psychometrically better-designed tests. Some individual MTDDA subtests continue in fairly wide use, even though few clinicians administer the entire MTDDA.

Porch Index of Communicative Ability

The *Porch Index of Communicative Ability* (PICA) was designed to satisfy

> …the pressing need for a tool which could sensitively and reliably quantify the patient's ability to communicate, for only if such a tool were available could an experimenter measure the effects of treatment, drugs, surgery, time, and the myriad of other variables of communication. (Porch, 1981a)

The PICA differs from other aphasia test batteries in several ways. With 180 test items in 18 subtests, it is one of the shortest aphasia tests. Most aphasic adults can be tested with the PICA in about 1 hour. The PICA is unique among aphasia tests because the same 10 test stimuli (pen, pencil, matches, cigarette, key, quarter, toothbrush, comb, fork, and knife) are used in all 18 subtests. The order in which PICA subtests is given also differs from that of other aphasia tests. In other aphasia tests, subtests are administered in groups representing different communicative abilities (e.g., listening, reading, speaking, writing), but Porch arranged the subtests in the PICA to minimize the amount of information early test items provide about later test items. (If, for example, Subtest 12, in which the patient repeats the names of test items after the examiner, were given before Subtest 4, in which the patient names each test object, the patient's naming in Subtest 4 may be enhanced by having previously heard the names in Subtest 12.)

Another result of this ordering of PICA subtests is that the subtests are arranged in general order of decreasing difficulty. Because of this arrangement, the patient's initial experience is on tests in which failure is most likely, which may prove discouraging to some patients. Porch (1981a) comments, however, that "administering the tests in order of decreasing complexity, or increasing information, progressively increases the chance of the patient being motivated by a successful performance as he moves from test to test" (p. 16).

The PICA also differs from other standardized aphasia test batteries in the constraints it places on test procedures. Instructions to the patient are specified word-by-word for each subtest, and the circumstances under which the examiner can repeat a test instruction or offer a prompt or cue are stipulated. Every patient response is scored with a 16-category, binary-choice system (Table 5-2). A set of diacritic markings (circles, squares, and triangles around scores; marks through scores; superscript letters) can be used to augment the 16-category system, thereby increasing the descriptiveness of PICA scoring. (For example, drawing a square around a score shows that the response was produced

with motoric distortion or awkwardness.) The complexities of administering and scoring the PICA require that new users be trained to administer and score the PICA. The training, together with tightly controlled administration and scoring procedures, ensures high reliability across clinicians and clinics.

A mean score for the entire PICA (the *Overall Score*) can be calculated, as well as modality mean scores for writing, copying, reading, pantomime, verbal, auditory, and visual subtests. Profiles may be plotted on a *Rating of Communicative Ability* form (Figure 5-24), which groups subtests according to each of the modalities. Profiles may also be plotted on a *Ranked Response Summary* graph (Figure 5-25), which plots subtest scores in order of decreasing subtest difficulty across the page. Changes in a patient's performance over time can be recorded on an *Aphasia Recovery Curve* form (Figure 5-26), on which the overall percentile score and the variability of scores among subtests can be graphed.

The PICA is normed on 357 left-hemisphere-damaged adults, 96 right-hemisphere-damaged adults, and 100 bilaterally damaged adults. Duffy, Keith, Shane, and Podraza (1976) have published norms for a group of 130 non-brain-injured adults.

The PICA manual provides procedures for predicting the recovery of aphasic patients by plotting recovery curves that allow predictions of a patient's eventual recovery of communicative ability based on PICA performance 1 month or more after the onset of aphasia. Porch calls this method *high overall prediction (HOAP)*. The HOAP procedure is described in Chapter 3. A variant of the HOAP method, called the *HOAP slope method*, can be used to predict recovery for patients tested at more than 1 month post-onset. The patient is tested with the PICA, and an average score for the nine subtests with the highest scores is calculated. The average score is used to place the patient on one of several recovery curves to predict the patient's overall score at 6 months postonset.

| TABLE 5-2 | The 16-Category, Binary-Choice Scoring System Used in the *Porch Index of Communicative Ability* |

Score	Level	Description
16	Complex	Spontaneous, accurate, fluent elaboration about the test item.
15	Complete	Complete, accurate, fluent response to test item.
14	Complete-distorted	Complete, accurate, response to test item but with reduced facility of production.
13	Complete-delayed	Complete, accurate response to test item but significantly slowed or delayed.
12	Incomplete	Accurate response to test item but lacking in completeness.
11	Incomplete-delayed	Accurate, incomplete response to test item, which is significantly slowed or delayed.
10	Corrected	Accurate response to test item self-correcting a previous error by request or after a prolonged delay.
9	Repeated	An accurate response after a repetition of instructions, by request, or after a prolonged delay.
8	Cued	Accurate response to test item stimulated by a cue, additional information, or another test item.
7	Related	An inaccurate response to test item which is closely related to a correct response.
6	Error	An inaccurate response to the test item.
5	Intelligible	An intelligible response, which is not associated with the test item, such as perseverative or automatic responses or an expressed indication of inability to respond.
4	Unintelligible	Differential responses to the test item, which are unintelligible.
3	Minimal	Undifferentiated, unintelligible responses.
2	Attention	Patient attends to the test item but gives no response.
1	No response	Patient exhibits no awareness of the test item.

From Porch, B.E. (2001). *Porch index of communicative ability* (4th ed.). Albuquerque, NM: Pica Programs.

Shortened versions of the PICA have been described in the literature (Disimoni, Keith, & Darley, 1980; Disimoni, Keith, Holt, & Darley, 1975; Lincoln & Ellis, 1980). However, Holtzapple, Pohlman, LaPointe, and Graham (1989) reported significant differences between full PICA scores and scores on the Disimoni, Keith, and Darley version for a group of 19 aphasic adults. They commented:

> We believe that as difficult as it is to obtain reliable retest results using the same measure, it is demonstrably more difficult when you eliminate a good portion of the test... Our current recommendations are for caution. (p. 140)

Boston Diagnostic Aphasia Examination

The *Boston Diagnostic Aphasia Examination —Third Edition* (BDAE-3; Goodglass, Kaplan, & Barresi, 2001) permits users to assign patients to classical aphasia syndromes such as Broca's aphasia, Wernicke's aphasia, and conduction aphasia. According to Goodglass, Kaplan, and Barresi, the BDAE permits clinicians to:
- Determine the presence of aphasia and the type of aphasia syndrome
- Make inferences concerning cerebral localization, linguistic processes that may have been damaged, and the strategies a patient uses to compensate for the damage

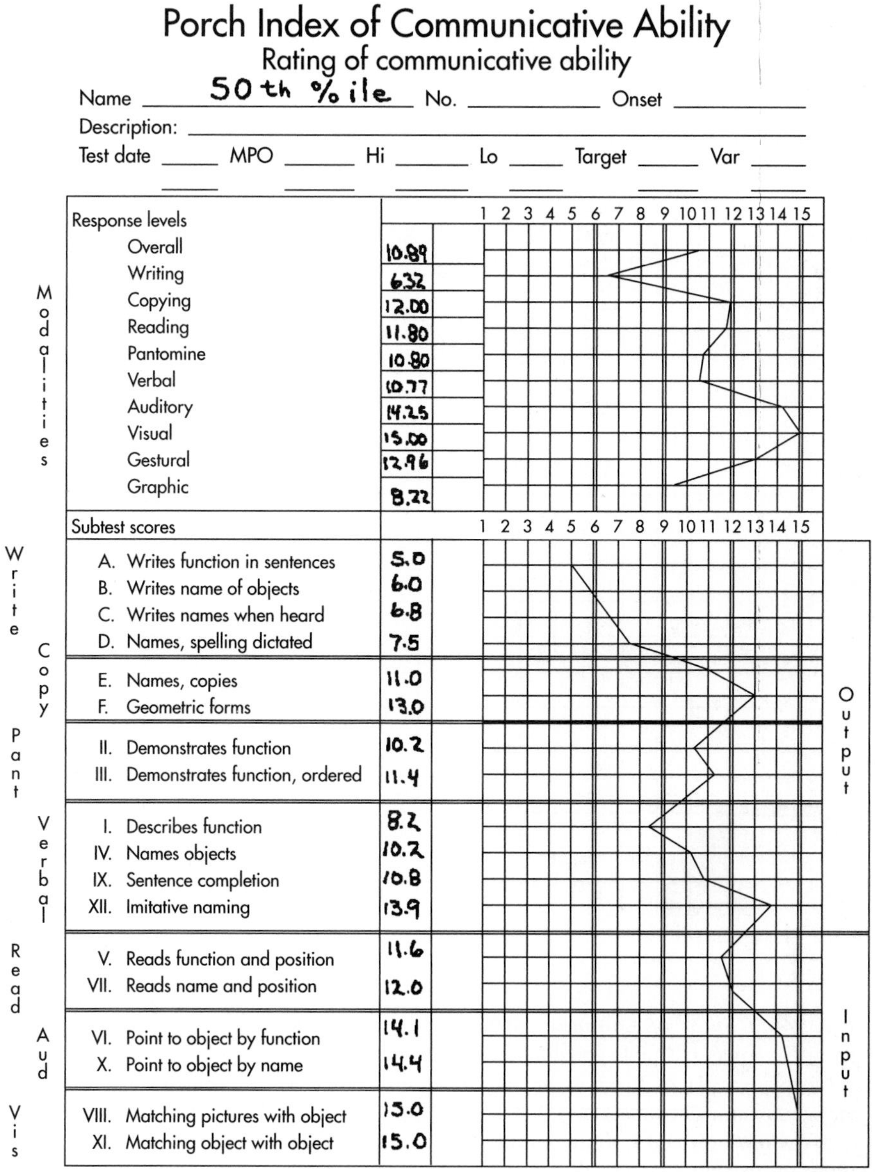

Porch Index of Communicative Ability

Rating of communicative ability

Name 50th %ile No. ______ Onset ______

Description: ______

Test date ____ MPO ____ Hi ____ Lo ____ Target ____ Var ____

Response levels		1 2 3 4 5 6 7 8 9 10 11 12 13 14 15
Overall	10.89	
Writing	6.32	
Copying	12.00	
Reading	11.80	
Pantomine	10.80	
Verbal	10.77	
Auditory	14.25	
Visual	15.00	
Gestural	12.96	
Graphic	8.22	

Subtest scores			1 2 3 4 5 6 7 8 9 10 11 12 13 14 15	
Write	A. Writes function in sentences	5.0		Output
	B. Writes name of objects	6.0		
	C. Writes names when heard	6.8		
	D. Names, spelling dictated	7.5		
Copy	E. Names, copies	11.0		
	F. Geometric forms	13.0		
Pant	II. Demonstrates function	10.2		
	III. Demonstrates function, ordered	11.4		
Verbal	I. Describes function	8.2		
	IV. Names objects	10.2		
	IX. Sentence completion	10.8		
	XII. Imitative naming	13.9		
Read	V. Reads function and position	11.6		Input
	VII. Reads name and position	12.0		
Aud	VI. Point to object by function	14.1		
	X. Point to object by name	14.4		
Vis	VIII. Matching pictures with object	15.0		
	XI. Matching object with object	15.0		

Figure 5-24 ■ A *Porch Index of Communicative Ability (PICA) Rating of Communicative Ability* form for a patient with moderate aphasia. Mean scores (using the 16-category PICA scoring system) are written in the middle column and graphed in the cells on the right. (From Porch, B.E. [2001]. *Porch Index of Communicative Ability* [4th ed.]. Albuquerque, NM: Pica Programs.)

Porch Index of Communicative Ability
Ranked response summary

Name _50th %ile_ _____ Case No. _____

Description: _____ Onset _____

Test dates: Test 1 _____   Test 2 _____   Test 3 _____

MPO	Target	OA	Writ	Copy	Read	Pant	Verb	Aud	Vis	Gest	Graph
1 ___		10.89	6.32	12.00	11.90	10.80	10.17	14.25	15.00	12.96	8.22
2 ___		___	___	___	___	___	___	___	___	___	___
3 ___		___	___	___	___	___	___	___	___	___	___

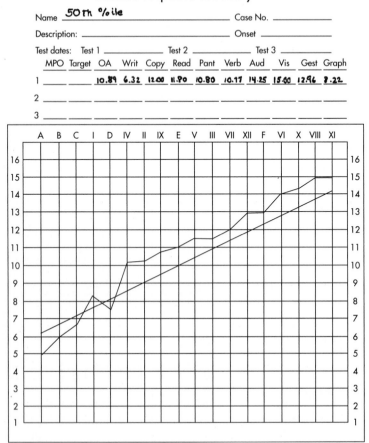

Figure 5-25 ■ A *Porch Index of Communicative Ability (PICA) Ranked Response Summary Form* for a patient with moderate aphasia. The diagonal line represents the hypothetical performance of a group of patients whose PICA performance places them at the 50th percentile of a large group of aphasic adults. The PICA subtests are arranged from right to left in order of decreasing difficulty. (From Porch, B.E. [2001]. *Porch Index of Communicative Ability* [4th ed.]. Albuquerque, NM: Pica Programs.)

- Measure a patient's level of performance across a wide range of tasks and several levels of difficulty within each task, both for initial evaluation and measurement of change over time
- Assess a patient's assets and liabilities in all language skills as a guide to treatment

The BDAE-3 is a long test. The standard form consists of a structured interview, 27 subtests, a free-standing 60-item confrontation naming test (*The Boston Naming Test;* Kaplan, Goodglass, & Weintraub, 2001), and 9 rating scales. Administering the standard form of the

Porch Index of Communicative Ability
Aphasia recovery curve

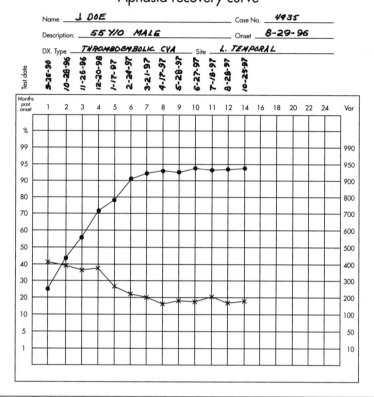

Name ___J DOE___   Case No. ___4935___

Description: ___55 Y/O MALE___   Onset ___8-29-96___

DX. Type ___THROMBOEMBOLIC CVA___ Site ___L. TEMPORAL___

Figure 5-26 ■ A *Porch Index of Communicative Ability (PICA) Aphasia Recovery Curve* for a hypothetical aphasic patient with a left temporal lobe stroke. The circles denote the patient's overall mean percentile on the PICA, and the Xs denote the patient's overall response variability on the PICA. The patient's overall PICA performance increases for the first 6 months, then plateaus. The patient's overall response variability gradually decreases during the first 8 months, after which it stabilizes. (From the Administration, Scoring and Interpretation Manual of the Porch Index of Communicative Ability; Porch, B.E. [1981]. *Porch Index of Communicative Ability.* Palo Alto, CA: Consulting Psychologists Press.)

BDAE-3 takes from 1 to 5 hours. The average for aphasic adults is about 2 hours. A short form consists of selected items from 21 subtests of the standard form and takes from 40 to 60 minutes to administer. Individual subtests from a 28-subtest *Extended Testing* section can be added to the standard form of the BDAE-3 for more detailed assessment of particular functions (e.g., story telling, comprehension of syntacti-cally complex sentences, naming in categories, oral spelling). A patient's BDAE-3 subtest scores and an overall severity rating can be entered in a *Subtest Summary Profile* (Figure 5-27) from which percentile ranks for each subtest score can be read. Norms for the BDAE-3 are based on a sample of 85 aphasic adults and 15 elderly normal volunteers tested at several clinics in the United States.

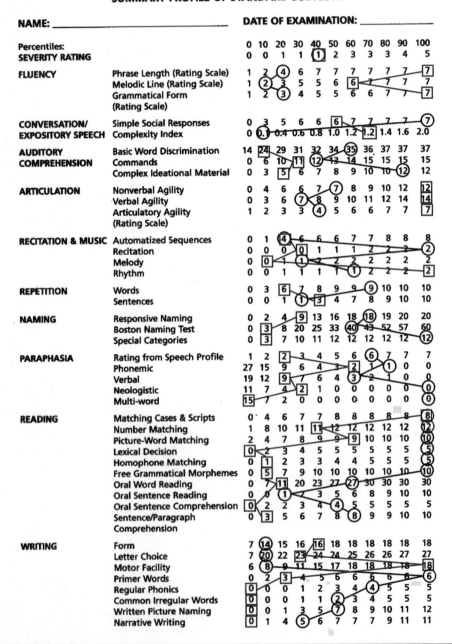

Figure 5-27 ■ A *Boston Diagnostic Aphasia Examination (BDAE) Subtest Summary Profile* for a patient with Broca's aphasia (black circles) and a patient with Wernicke's aphasia (color squares). (From Goodglass, H., Kaplan, E., & Barresi, B. [2001]. *The assessment of aphasia and related disorders* [3rd ed.]. Philadelphia: Lippincott Williams & Wilkins, now owned by Pro-Ed [Austin, Texas].)

The BDAE-3 is a comprehensive test of language and associated processes that permits clinicians to compare the performance of any aphasic patient with the performance of a large group of aphasic adults and to assign aphasic patients to neurodiagnostic aphasia syndromes based on their BDAE-3 performance. However, users should be aware that many patients cannot be unambiguously classified on the basis of their BDAE-3 performance.

Western Aphasia Battery

The *Western Aphasia Battery* (WAB; Kertesz, 1988) is shorter and psychometrically more sophisticated than the BDAE-3, which it resembles in many respects, including an emphasis on classifying patients according to classic neurodiagnostic syndromes. The WAB employs what Kertesz calls a *taxonomic* approach to classification, in which patients are assigned to diagnostic categories (e.g., Broca's aphasia and Wernicke's aphasia) according to their scores on four language subtests—spontaneous speech, auditory comprehension, repetition, and naming (Figure 5-28). The WAB also includes subtests for evaluating reading and writing; one apraxia subtest; and several subtests for assessing constructional, visuospatial, and calculation abilities.

Nonfluent			
Broca			
Global			
Isolation syndrome			
Transcortical motor			
Poor Comprehension		**Fair Comprehension**	
Global		Broca	
Isolation syndrome		Transcortical motor	
Poor Repetition	**Fair Repetition**	**Poor Repetition**	**Fair Repetition**
Global	Isolation syndrome	Broca	Transcortical motor

Fluent			
Wernicke			
Anomic			
Conduction			
Transcortical sensory			
Poor Comprehension		**Fair Comprehension**	
Wernicke		Conduction	
Transcortical sensory		Anomic	
Poor Repetition	**Fair Repetition**	**Poor Repetition**	**Fair Repetition**
Wernicke	Transcortical sensory	Conduction	Anomic

Figure 5-28 ■ How the *Western Aphasia Battery* (WAB) assigns aphasic adults to classic neurodiagnostic categories. (From Kertesz, A. [1982]. Western Aphasia Battery. New York: Grune and Stratton.)

No normative information is given in the WAB test manual. The reader is referred to Kertesz (1979) and Shewan and Kertesz (1980) for information on standardization of the 1977 version of the WAB. Subtest mean scores and their standard deviations are reported in Kertesz (1979) for 365 aphasic and 162 nonaphasic adults from two standardizations of the WAB. The first, in 1974, included 150 aphasic and 59 control subjects. The second, in 1979, added 215 aphasic and 63 control subjects. Information on the reliability and validity of the WAB are provided in Kertesz (1979).

A patient's scores on the auditory comprehension and speech subtests can be used to calculate an *aphasia quotient,* and both language and nonlanguage subtest scores are used to calculate a *cortical quotient.* The aphasia quotient is said by Kertesz to be a reliable measure of the severity of language impairment. The cortical quotient is said to be a measure of cognitive functions. Shewan and Kertesz (1984) described an additional summary score, called the *language quotient.* The language quotient is based on the oral language subtest scores that contribute to the aphasia quotient, plus scores from the reading and writing subtests (Box 5-4).

The accuracy and reliability of WAB procedures for classifying patients has been questioned. Swindell, Holland, and Fromm (1984) compared the WAB classifications of 69 aphasic adults to subjective classifications made by clinicians who had been trained to identify neurodiagnostic aphasia syndromes. They reported that the clinicians' judgments matched the WAB classification only 54% of the time. Wertz, Deal, and Robinson (1984) compared WAB and BDAE classifications for 45 aphasic adults. The two tests agreed on patients' classification only 27% of the time; 28 patients were unclassifiable with the BDAE, but only 5 were unclassifiable with the WAB. The WAB has been criticized for forcing

Box 5-4	Aphasia, Language, and Cortical Quotients

Aphasia Quotient
- Spontaneous speech (rating of information content, fluency)
- Auditory comprehension

Language Quotient
- Spontaneous speech (rating of information content, fluency)
- Auditory comprehension
- Reading, writing

Cortical Quotient (entire test)
- Spontaneous speech (rating of information content, fluency)
- Auditory comprehension
- Reading, writing
- Praxis (limb, buccofacial)
- Construction (drawing, block design, calculation, *Raven's Progressive Matrices*)

Data from Kertesz, A. (1982). *Western aphasia battery.* New York: Grune & Stratton.

patients into diagnostic categories. This may be one reason for the lack of agreement between WAB and BDAE classifications.

Other Aphasia Test Batteries

The BDAE, the MTDDA, the PICA, and the WAB are well-known and widely used in the United States. Several other tests, though less widely used, are marketed in the United States and are the tests of choice for some clinicians. They include the *Neurosensory Center Comprehensive Examination for Aphasia* (NCCEA; Spreen & Benton, 1977), *Examining for Aphasia* (Eisenson, 1974), the *Aphasia Language Performance Scales* (Keenan & Brassell, 1975), the *Psycholinguistic Assessment of Language Processing in Aphasia* (Kay, Lesser, & Coltheart, 1992), and the *Boston Assessment for Severe Aphasia* (Helm-Estabrooks & associates, 1989).

GENERAL CONCEPTS 5-4

- Comprehensive language tests typically assess brain-injured adults' ability to produce written language by asking them to write automatized sequences, copy, write to dictation, and write self-formulated material. Copying usually is easier for brain-injured adults than is writing to dictation. Most brain-injured adults are better at writing to dictation than they are at writing self-generated material.
- *Language pragmatics* denotes how language is used and how ideas and intentions are communicated in social contexts.
  - Language pragmatics includes speech acts, social behaviors, conversational behaviors, and conversational rules and conventions.
  - Standardized tests of pragmatic language focus on appreciation of nonliteral meanings, making inferences, resolving ambiguity, and producing narratives but largely neglect the social-interactional dimensions of pragmatics. Most standardized tests of pragmatic language isolate pragmatic behavior from the natural contexts in which it typically occurs.
  - Checklists and rating scales such as the *Pragmatic Protocol* offer an alternative to standardized tests. Rating scales for assessing pragmatic language are included in some tests designed for persons with right-hemisphere brain injuries and may be appropriate for other categories of brain-injured persons.

- Comprehensive language tests provide a general sense of an individual's speech, auditory comprehension, reading, and writing. Most help clinicians identify communication impairments and plan treatment. Some help clinicians make a diagnosis and predict recovery.
  - The *Minnesota Test for Differential Diagnosis of Aphasia* (MTDDA) contains 47 subtests and takes 3 to 6 hours to administer. It permits users to assign patients to one of five major and two minor categories of aphasia.
  - The *Porch Index of Communicative Ability* (PICA) uses the same 10 test stimuli in each of its 18 subtests. Users score responses with a 16-category, binary-choice scoring system. The PICA provides several procedures for charting patients' performance and predicting recovery.
  - The *Boston Diagnostic Aphasia Examination* (BDAE) contains 27 subtests in its standard form, which takes from 1 to 5 hours to administer. A 21-subtest short form takes about 1 hour to administer. The BDAE permits users to assign patients to classic neurodiagnostic aphasia syndromes and to measure patients' performance across a large number of tasks.
  - The *Western Aphasia Battery* (WAB) resembles the BDAE but is shorter and psychometrically more sophisticated. Those who use the WAB may classify patients into classic aphasia syndromes with a taxonomic procedure.

THOUGHT QUESTIONS

Question 5-1 Andante Portofino, a right-handed patient with Broca's aphasia following a stroke exhibits the following signs:

Right hemiparesis, arm greater than leg

Good auditory comprehension (85th percentile)

Poor oral reading (25th percentile)

Poor reading comprehension (30th percentile)

Is this pattern of performance what one would expect? Justify your answer.

Question 5-2 Corrina Aldeberan is a right-handed woman who has had a left-hemisphere stroke and has been diagnosed as aphasic. She is given a list of words to read aloud. The following is a sample of her performance:

Stimulus Word	Patient Reads
house	horse
cliff	stiff
tomorrow	tomorrow
store	stone
mother	mother
stand	stain
newspaper	newspaper

Speculate as to the reasons for Ms. Aldeberan's performance. What would you expect the nature of her aphasia to be?

Question 5-3 You administer the Token Test shown on the facing page to Jennie Smith, an aphasic patient. She receives the following scores:

Part A	(7 points possible)	7	(100%)
Part B	(8 points possible)	8	(100%)
Part C	(12 points possible)	12	(100%)
Part D	(16 points possible)	13	(81%)
Part E	(24 points possible)	8	(33%)
Part F	(96 points possible)	85	(89%)
Total		133	(82%)

(Words struck out denote parts of the commands that Ms. Smith missed. Underlined words are characteristics that are scored in Ms. Smith's response—1 point per characteristic correctly identified. The number of points possible in each part are in parenthesis in the score boxes.)

There is something unusual about Ms. Smith's performance. Tell what it is and speculate about the reasons for the unusual performance.

Question 5-4 The following speech samples represent transcripts of two adults talking about the birthday party picture. They are typed without punctuation. The number of dots indicate the relative durations of pauses.

Mrs. Bloom produces the following speech sample (she produces 105 words per minute):

> *and..um..what do you call it....but I guess the cat got into it and..uh he's hiding under the sitter and the mother is gonna......trying to get him out of there...and he cleaned up the rug and..uh the rest of the birthday cake ...those ones there....children...boys and girls ...are arriving and it's....um not too good a deal I'd say...*

Mr. Jones produces the following speech sample (he produces 40 words per minute):

> *um...um...uh.....cake..and..um..and..and dog.....dog ate cake..and..and...trouble..... mom is mad....and..and..um..um..kid is crying...and ..and...neighbors.....neighbors is coming*

Is Mrs. Bloom aphasic? Is Mr. Jones aphasic? If so, what aphasia syndrome do they represent?

QUESTION 5-3: TOKEN TEST SCORE SHEET

Patient Name: _____ J. Smith _____

Date of Evaluation: _9/9/07_ **Examiner:** _____ J. Doe ___

Part A

#	Item	Score
1	Show me a circle.	1
2	Show me a square.	1
3	Show me a yellow one.	1
4	Show me a red one.	1
5	Show me a blue one.	1
6	Show me a green one.	1
7	Show me a white one.	1

Total: A (7)	7
Time (sec)	90

Part B

#	Item	Score
8	Show me the yellow square.	2
9	Show me the blue circle.	2
10	Show me the green circle.	2
11	Show me the white square.	2

Total: B (8)	8
Time (sec)	85

Part C

#	Item	Score
12	Show me the small white circle.	3
13	Show me the large yellow square.	3
14	Show me the large green square.	3
15	Show me the small blue square.	3

Total: C (12)	12
Time (sec)	95

Part D

#	Item	Score
16	Show me the red circle and the green square.	4
17	Show me the yellow square and the blue square.	3
18	Show me the white square and the green circle.	2
19	Show me the white circle and the red circle.	4

Total: D (16)	13
Time (sec)	125

Continued

QUESTION 5-3: TOKEN TEST SCORE SHEET

Part E

#	Item	Score
20	Show me the ~~large white~~ circle and the ~~small green~~ square.	2
21	Show me the ~~small blue~~ circle and the ~~large yellow square~~.	1
22	Show me the large green square and the ~~large red~~ square.	3
23	Show me the ~~large white~~ square and the ~~small~~ green ~~circle~~.	2

Total: E (24)	8
Time (sec)	140

Part F

#	Item	Score
24	Put the red circle on the green square.	6
25	Put the white square behind the ~~yellow~~ circle.	5
26	Touch the blue circle with the red square.	6
27	Touch the blue circle and the red square.	6
28	Pick up the blue circle or the red square.	6
29	Move the green square away from the ~~yellow square~~.	4
30	Put the white circle in front of the blue square.	6
31	If there is a black circle, pick up the red square.	6
32	Pick up all the squares except the yellow one.	6
33	Put the green square beside the red circle.	6
34	Touch the squares slowly and the circles quickly.	6
35	~~Put~~ the red circle ~~between~~ the ~~yellow square~~ and the ~~green square~~.	2
36	Touch all the circles except the ~~green~~ one.	5
37	Pick up the red circle --- no --- the white square.	6
38	Instead of the white square, pick up the yellow circle.	6
39	Together with the yellow circle, pick up the blue ~~circle~~.	5

Total: F (96)	85
Time (sec)	190

Total: A - F (163)	133
Time (min/sec)	725 / 12:05

Assessing Functional Communication and Quality of Life

Communication is not only the essence of being human, but also a vital property of life. (John A. Piece)

FUNCTIONAL COMMUNICATION
Influence of the World Health Organization

As noted in Chapter 3, publication of the *International Classification of Impairments, Disabilities, and Handicaps (ICIDH)* by the World Health Organization (WHO) powerfully affected how practitioners regarded issues of health and disability by broadening the concept of disability to include not only the physical effects of a health condition but also the effects of a disabling condition on a person's daily life success and well-being. The ICIDH summarized the effects of disabling conditions with the concepts of *impairment* (structural or functional abnormality), *disability* (the effects of impairments on skills or abilities), and *handicap* (the effects of disabilities on daily life). The ICIDH conceptualized disability as a three-stage linear process:

Impairment → Disability → Handicap

As experience with the ICIDH accrued, it became apparent that the relationship between the domains of impairment, disability, and handicap was not linear and that other important contributions to health and well-being (e.g., psychological, social, and environmental influences) were not identified by the ICIDH classification system.

In 1997 the WHO revised its classification system and changed its terminology to reflect changes in attitudes toward the labels *impairment, disability,* and *handicap,* which were thought to have negative connotations. In the 1997 version of the classification system *(International Classification of Impairments, Disabilities, and Handicaps: ICIDH-2), body functions and structures* replaced *impairment, activity restriction* replaced *disability,* and *participation restriction* replaced *handicap.* The ICIDH-2 defined *body functions* as *the physiological or psychological functions of body systems;* it defined *body structures* as *anatomic parts of the body such as organs, limbs, and their components;* it defined *activity* as *the execution of a task or involvement in a life situation in a uniform environment;* it defined *participation* as *the execution of a task or involvement in a life situation in an individual's current environment.* The WHO intended the new labels to be socially neutral terms that permit recording both positive and negative effects of health conditions.

The terms *uniform environment* and *current environment* are crucial distinctions. A *uniform environment* is one in which the full capabilities of the individual can be expressed. It provides neither hindrances nor enhancements that might affect the individual's performance. The individual's *current environment* is the context in which the individual currently lives, including society's response to the individual's performance in that environment. Performance in the uniform environment represents the individual's performance achieved under environmentally neutral conditions. Performance in the current environment represents the individual's performance in his or her current living environment, which may contain hindrances to performance or facilitators of performance.

Figure 6-1 shows the conceptual model underlying the ICIDH-2.

In 2001 the WHO revised the ICIDH-2 and published it as the *International Classification*

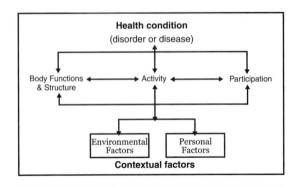

Figure 6-1 ■ The conceptual model for the International Classification of Impairment, Disability, and Handicap (ICIDH).

of Functioning, Disability, and Health (ICF). The intent of the ICF was to shift the conceptual focus from illness and death to how people live with their health conditions and how health conditions can be managed to assure a productive and fulfilling life. The ICF considers disability and functioning the product of interactions between *health conditions* (e.g., diseases, disorders, and injuries), *personal factors* (e.g., age, education, experience, coping styles), and *environmental factors* (e.g., social attitudes, legal and social policies, building design, climate).

The ICF retains much of the terminology of the ICIDH-2 but gives greater emphasis to the social aspects of disabling conditions than did the ICIDH-2 by providing more extensive documentation of the effects of a person's social and physical environment on his or her daily life functioning. These changes reflect the belief that reductions in the severity of disabling conditions in a population can be achieved both by enhancing affected persons' functional capacity and by modifying affected persons' social and physical environment. Table 6-1 summarizes the classification system used in the ICF. The classification system identifies three levels of functioning—*the body or body part, the person,* and *the person in a social context.* Disability results from dysfunction at one or more

TABLE 6-1	Components of the *International Classification of Functioning, Disability, and Health*		
Component	**Subcomponent**	**Definition**	
Body functions		Physiologic functions of body systems (including psychologic functions)	
Body structures		Anatomic parts of the body such as organs, limbs, and their components	
	Impairment	Problems in body function or structure such as a significant deviation or loss	
Activity		Execution of a task or action by an individual	
	Activity limitation	Difficulties an individual may have in performing activities	
Participation		Involvement in a life situation	
	Participation restriction	Problems an individual may experience related to involvement in a life situation	

Data from World Health Organization (WHO). (2001). *International classification of functioning, disability and health.* Geneva, Switzerland: WHO.

of these levels, yielding *impairments, activity limitations,* and *participation restrictions.*

The ICF adds two qualifiers to *activity level* and *level of participation.* The qualifiers reflect the concepts of *uniform environment* and *current environment* as defined in the ICIDH-2. The *performance qualifier* attempts to capture the life situation or lived experience of people in their actual living environments by describing what a person does in his or her current environment, which may include prosthetic or assistive devices or assistance by others. The *capacity qualifier* describes a person's ability to perform a task or an activity in environmentally neutral conditions. *Capacity* indicates a person's highest probable level of functioning without help from prosthetic or assistive devices and without assistance from other persons.

The ICF is now the world standard for collection of information on disability. In addition to its data collection role, the ICF is influencing the nature of assessment and outcome measures in the same way as did its predecessors, the ICIDH and the ICIDH-2. Publication of the ICIDH, the ICIDH-2, and the ICF encouraged professionals concerned with disability to reexamine the philosophical and conceptual foundations

of assessment and treatment for disabling conditions. For speech-language pathologists it became apparent that most of the standardized tests traditionally used to assess brain-injured adults' communication and cognition provided detailed information about impairments but said little about disabilities and handicaps (ICIDH) or activity limitations or participation restrictions (ICIDH-2, ICF). As speech-language pathologists incorporated the concepts of the ICIDH, the ICIDH-2, and the ICF into clinical practice, it became apparent that the codes provided in these instruments do not accurately reflect daily life communication and are not sensitive to changes in daily life communicative competence. In response to these shortcomings of the WHO measures, practitioners began to develop instruments to measure *functional communication* (communication in contexts resembling daily life) in greater detail.

Measures of Functional Communication

The *Functional Communication Profile (FCP;* Sarno, 1969) antedates the ICIDH, the ICIDH-2, and the ICF. The FCP was the first measure of functional communication to be widely used by speech-language pathologists for evaluating functional communication. The FCP is a rating scale that is filled out by someone who knows the person whose communication is rated (often a family member, sometimes the speech-language pathologist). The items in the FCP are intended to quantify the communication behaviors a person actually uses when interacting with others, regardless of the severity of the person's communicative impairment. The person who fills out the FCP estimates the rated person's competence in five categories of communication behavior considered common in everyday life (Table 6-2). The behaviors are rated on a 9-point scale in which the rated person's current ability is rated as a proportion of premorbid ability.

The *Communicative Effectiveness Index* (*CETI;* Lomas, Pickard, Bester, & associates, 1989) is a more recent rating scale for estimating aphasic adults' ability to communicate in several daily life situations. Lomas and associates selected the situations in the CETI based on interviews with stroke survivors and spouses. The stroke survivors and spouses were asked to identify situations in which a stroke survivor has to *get his meaning across and to understand what someone else means* (p. 115). Lomas and associates then partitioned the responses into four categories:

1. Basic needs (e.g., toileting, eating, grooming, positioning)
2. Life skills (e.g., shopping, home maintenance, using the telephone, understanding traffic signals)
3. Social needs (e.g., dinner conversation, playing cards, writing to a friend)
4. Health threats (e.g., calling for help, giving or receiving information about one's medical condition)

The list of situations generated by the stroke survivors and spouses then was refined to yield a list of 16 items (Table 6-3).

Lomas and associates do not identify which items in the CETI represent each category, and it is clear that the 16 items in the CETI are not distributed

equally across the four categories. I counted 4 or 5 *basic need* items, 10 *social need* items, 1 *health threat* item, and 0 or 1 *life skills* item, using my own intuitions about which behaviors represented each category.

Results reported by Lomas and associates suggest that the CETI has acceptable internal reliability (CETI items test the same domain), adequate test-retest reliability (CETI results do not change unpredictably from test to test), and acceptable interexaminer reliability (different examiners rating the same patient agree). The procedures used to select items for the CETI support its face validity (it appears to measure what it was intended to measure), although strong evidence for its validity as a measure of daily life communication performance (e.g., correlations between CETI ratings and actual daily life performance) is not provided in the published report.

Lomas and associates reported strong and significant correlations between spouses' CETI ratings of their aphasic partner and spouses' ratings of their aphasic partner's overall communicative ability and considered those correlations evidence of CETI's construct validity. However, it seems that strong correlations would be expected because the same people did both ratings, apparently in the same rating session.

Limitations of Subjective Rating Scales

The FCP and CETI are subjective rating scales. Subjective rating scales are susceptible to unreliability from test to test and from rater to rater because they rely on raters' subjective judgments. Most subjective rating scales also suffer from lack of sensitivity to small changes in opinions, attitudes, or behavior, making them of limited value in tracking changes over time. Because rating scales consider a limited set of generic functions, they may not represent the true everyday experiences of individuals, and they do not account for individual differences in

TABLE 6-2	Abilities Rated with the Functional Communication Profile
Category	Behavior
Movement	Ability to imitate oral movements
	Attempt to communicate
	Ability to indicate *yes* and *no*
	Indicating floor to elevator operator
	Use of gestures
Speaking	Saying greetings
	Saying own name
	Saying nouns
	Saying verbs
	Saying noun-verb combinations
	Saying phrases (nonautomatic)
	Giving directions
	Speaking on the telephone
	Saying short complete sentences (nonautomatic)
	Saying long sentences (nonautomatic)
Understanding	Awareness of gross environmental sounds
	Awareness of emotional voice tone
	Understanding of own name
	Awareness of speech
	Recognition of family names
	Recognition of names of familiar objects
	Understanding action verbs
	Understanding gestured directions
	Understanding verbal directions
	Understanding simple conversation with one person
	Understanding television
	Understanding conversation with more than two people
	Understanding movies
	Understanding complicated verbal directions
	Understanding rapid, complex conversation
Reading	Reading single words
	Reading rehabilitation program card
	Reading street signs
	Reading newspaper headlines
	Reading letters
	Reading newspaper articles
	Reading magazines
	Reading books
Other	Writing name
	Time orientation
	Copying ability
	Writing from dictation
	Handling money
	Using writing in lieu of speech
	Calculation ability

Data from Sarno, M.T. (1969). *The functional communication profile.* New York: NYU Medical Center Monograph Department.

TABLE 6-3	Situations Rated by the *Communicative Effectiveness Index (CETI)*

Item	Situation
1	Getting someone's attention
2	Getting involved in group conversations about him/her
3	Giving *yes* and *no* answers appropriately
4	Communicating his/her emotions
5	Indicating that he/she understands what is being said to him/her
6	Having coffee time visits and conversations with friends and neighbors
7	Having a one-to-one conversation with you
8	Saying the name of someone whose face is in front of him/her
9	Communicating physical needs such as aches and pains
10	Having a spontaneous conversation
11	Responding to or communicating anything (including *yes* or *no*) without words
12	Starting a conversation with people who are not close family
13	Understanding writing
14	Being a part of a conversation when it is fast and there are a number of people involved
15	Participating in a conversation with strangers
16	Describing or discussing something at length

Data from Lomas, J., Pickard, L., Bester, S., & associates. (1989). The communicative effectiveness index: Development and psychometric evaluation of a functional communication measure for adult aphasia. *Journal of Speech and Hearing Disorders, 54,* 113-124.

the frequency of specific functions or their importance to individual patients.

> The multidimensional nature of everyday communication is not sufficiently captured by traditional functional communication assessments that, by necessity, reduce communication to a number of items that are rated on a checklist. (Worrall & associates, 2002, p. 119)

Ratings made by patients who are receiving treatment or ratings by family members of patients receiving treatment are susceptible to *ratings creep*—an increase in positive ratings in the absence of true changes in the characteristics rated. Ratings creep in such situations may be attributable to a rater's belief that treatment should make a positive difference, or to a rater's desire not to offend the person providing the treatment. Ratings creep is similar to the placebo effect in medicine. The *placebo effect* is common in medical studies in which parti-cipants in one group are given a medication, and participants in another group are given a visually identical inert substance. Up to one third of those who are given a placebo and believe it to be medication experience improvements like those experienced by participants who are given the medication.

In the 1940s and 1950s patients with chest pain caused by insufficient blood supply to the heart were treated by *ligating* (tying off) the internal mammary artery—a surgical procedure believed to increase blood supply to the heart. The surgical procedure was a common remedy for chest pain throughout the 1940s and 1950s. About 90% of patients reported reduced chest pain following the surgery. In 1959 a group of cardiac surgeons published the results of a placebo-controlled study of internal mammary artery ligation. Half the participants received standard mammary artery ligation; the other half received a sham operation. Participants receiving the sham operation were anesthetized and a chest incision was made, but no artery ligation was done. The sham operation worked as well at reducing chest pain as the real operation. Internal mammary artery ligation turned out to be no more than a placebo and was soon abandoned.

An Objective Measure of Functional Communication

Communicative Activities in Daily Living (*CADL;* Holland, 1980) and *Communicative Activities in Daily Living—Second Edition* (*CADL-2;* Holland, Frattali, & Fromm, 1999) differ from the FCP and the CETI in that a patient's performance in an interview and in various simulated daily life communication activities are objectively scored rather than subjectively rated. Holland and associates validated the CADL and CADL-2 by observing the daily life communication of aphasic and nonaphasic adults and by interviewing family members of the aphasic adults.

> The fact that the CADL is scored relative to getting a message across rather than to correctness or incorrectness *per se* is one of its major departures from traditional tests of language and communication. The CADL's other major departure is in its conceptualization of test items. Rather than being a series of acontextual attempts addressed to isolating a number of language modalities (speaking, reading, writing, comprehension, etc.), most CADL items are molecular communicative interactions not easily described by language modality. Additionally, many items are richly supplied with context and often require understanding of the context for appropriate communicating. Finally, a number of nonverbal communicative events are sampled. (Holland, 1980, p. 29).

CADL-2 testing begins with an interview. The examiner says, *Hello, Mr./Mrs. _____* and waits for a response. The examiner then requests personal information from the patient, occasionally making mistakes (e.g., saying, *Your first name is* [wrong name], *isn't it?*) and noting if the patient corrects the examiner. Following the interview the examiner asks the patient to respond to various test items relating to daily life activities by pointing to pictures (e.g., *Here's a bus schedule. What time in the afternoon does bus #3 leave Maintown?*) or by speech or gesture (e.g., *How would you let someone know you are cold?*).

Next the examiner gives the patient an appointment card for a pretend visit to a doctor's office and, by means of questions and pictorial props, tests the patient's understanding of the appointment card and estimates the patient's ability to carry out the appointment. For example, the patient is shown a picture of the control panel of an elevator while the examiner says, *Remember, Dr. Clark's office is on the third floor. Here's the elevator. What do you do after you step into the elevator?* (Pointing to the *3* button in the picture or an appropriate verbal response are both acceptable.)

The next CADL-2 items are supported by pictorial or object props. The items relate to traveling by car, grocery shopping, making change, and using a telephone and a telephone directory (e.g., *Make a list of three things you might need from the grocery store. Here's a map. How do you get from the bank to the post office? Please call time and temperature and let me know what time it is and what the temperature is.*).

The CADL-2 was standardized on a sample of 175 adults with neurogenic communication impairments. The test manual contains information about test-retest reliability, interexaminer reliability, and test validity. Information about the standardization of the original CADL (Holland, 1980) also is included.

Functional Communication and Program Evaluation

Some measures of functional communication are designed for *program evaluation* rather than for *patient evaluation*. The primary objective in *program evaluation* is to identify the most efficient providers of healthcare service— *those who provide the greatest amount of functional improvement over the shortest period of time for the least cost* (Warren, 1992, p. 63). The concept underlying program evaluation is that, in a competitive market, healthcare providers who reduce costs, maintain the quality of services, and produce good outcomes survive and prosper, whereas those who do not are destined to vanish (a concept called *managed care*). The emphasis in program evaluation is on the financial health of the program rather than on treatment outcomes for individual patients.

Program evaluation typically depends on information from rating scales. Patients' functional abilities in the domain(s) of interest are rated when they enter the program and again when they leave. Judgments about the quality of the program are based on the amount of improvement in ratings of functionality between entry and exit and on patients' average level of functionality upon completing the program. Rating scales used in program evaluation are not specific to a given disease or condition such as stroke and are not specific to a given discipline such as speech-language pathology. They usually provide for global ratings of broadly defined categories of abilities likely to be important in daily life (e.g., ambulation, self-care). Most rating scales are insensitive to small changes in a patient's level of performance and typically do not capture changes in component skills (e.g., attention and memory) that may underlie broadly defined categories of performance (e.g., social participation).

The best known and most widely used measure of functional outcome in rehabilitation is a rating scale called the *Functional Independence Measure* (*FIM*; Uniform Data System for Medical Rehabilitation, 1996). The FIM was developed to measure outcome in rehabilitation medicine programs. It provides a 7-point ordinal scale to assess self-care, sphincter control, mobility, locomotion, communication, and social cognition in 18 activities of daily life (Figure 6-2).

The scale is divided into three levels. At the *independent* (no helper) level, patients do not need assistance to carry out an activity. At the *dependent* (helper) level, patients need help to carry out an activity. The dependent level is in turn divided into two levels (*modified dependence* and *complete dependence*), based on the frequency with which assistance is needed by a patient.

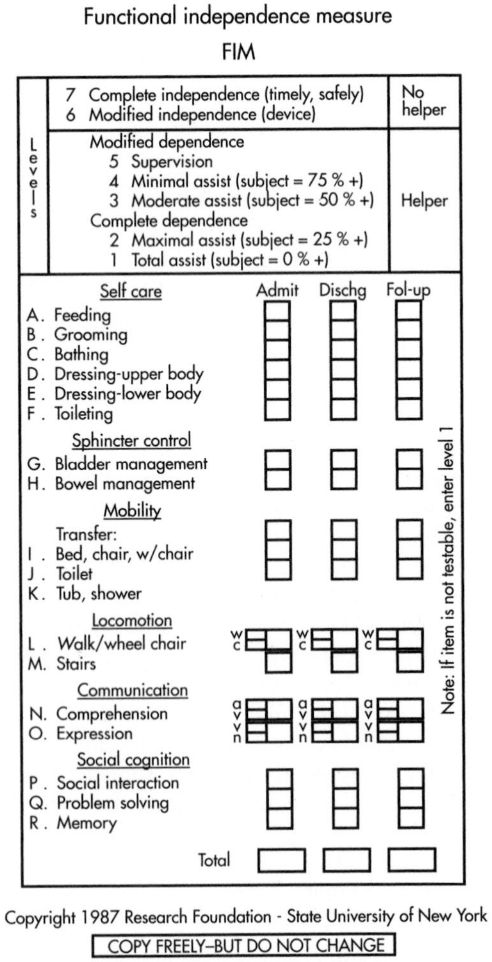

Figure 6-2 ■ The *Functional Independence Measure (FIM)*. (Copyright 1987, Research Foundation, State University of New York, Buffalo, NY.)

The FIM has been criticized for poor reliability in rating levels of independence (Adamovich, 1990), and its use for rating functional independence in communication has been criticized because of its insensitivity to changes in communication abilities (Warren, 1992; Frymark, 2003). Nevertheless, it remains the principal outcome measure for program evaluation in rehabilitation medicine.

The combination of increased emphasis on functional outcome by healthcare providers and dissatisfaction with the FIM as a measure of communicative adequacy led the American Speech-Language-Hearing Association (ASHA) to develop a measure of functional communication called *ASHA Functional Assessment of Commu-nication Skills for Adults (ASHA FACS;* Frattali, Thompson, Holland, & associates, 1995). ASHA FACS permits users to rate a patient's communicative adequacy in four domains: social communication, communication of basic needs, daily planning, and reading/writing/number concepts (Table 6-4). The communicative adequacy of each behavior shown in Table 6-4 is estimated with a 7-point *Scale of Communicative Independence* which, like the FIM, rates behaviors in terms of how much assistance is needed to perform them:

- Does with no assistance (7)
- Does with minimal assistance (6)
- Does with minimal to moderate assistance (5)
- Does with moderate assistance (4)

TABLE 6-4	**Assessment Domains for *ASHA Functional Assessment of Communication Skills for Adults (FACS)***		
Social Communication	Communication of Basic Needs	Daily Planning	Reading/Writing/ Number Concepts
Uses names of familiar people	Recognizes familiar faces/voices	Tells time	Understands environmental signs
Expresses agreement/ disagreement	Makes strong likes/ dislikes known	Dials telephone numbers	Uses reference materials
Explains how to do something	Expresses feelings	Keeps scheduled appointments	Follows written directions
Requests information	Requests help	Uses a calendar	Understands printed material
Participates in telephone conversations	Makes needs/wants known	Follows a map	Prints/writes/types name
Answers yes-no questions	Responds in an emergency		Completes forms
Follows directions			Makes short lists
Understands facial expression/ tone of voice			Writes messages
Understands nonliteral meaning and intent			Understands signs with numbers
Understands conversation in noisy surroundings			Makes money transactions
Understands TV/radio			Understands units of measurement
Participates in conversations			
Recognizes/corrects errors			

Data from Frattali, C.M., Thompson, C.K., Holland, A.L., & associates (1995). *Functional assessment of communication skills for adults: ASHA FACS.* Rockville, MD: American Speech-Language-Hearing Association.

ASHA, American Speech-Language-Hearing Association.

- Does with moderate to maximal assistance (3)
- Does with maximal assistance (2)
- Does not do, even with maximal assistance (1)
- No basis for rating

In addition to ratings of the individual communication behaviors shown in Table 6-4, ASHA FACS permits users to rate the adequacy, appropriateness, promptness, and communicative sharing aspects of a patient's overall performance in each of the four ASHA FACS domains.

The FIM and ASHA FACS, like most instruments designed for program evaluation, yield general estimates of functional ability in a small number of domains chosen because they are likely to be important in determining independence in daily life. These instruments may provide reasonably accurate estimates of daily life independence and self-sufficiency in the domains addressed, but they are not sensitive to small differences in specific abilities and do not provide enough detail about specific abilities to make them valid measures of an individual patient's actual functional competence. However, instruments designed for program evaluation are important because they affect the reimbursement policies of organizations that pay for healthcare, determine who is eligible for care, and provide instruments for measuring the quality of healthcare. Some of the most striking effects of program evaluation scales are likely to be on the scope and complexity of assessment and diagnostic procedures.

> Functional assessment has gained popularity in rehabilitation and long-term care in the United States, not as a direct result of its clinical usefulness, but rather as a reaction to cost pressures and broader quality of care issues. (Frattalli, 1992, p. 64)

Organizations that pay for healthcare services want treatments that endure, create rapid and substantial gains in functional activities of daily living, improve quality of life, contribute to longevity, and promote good health. Payers tend to restrict reimbursement to life-sustaining and life-enriching procedures that yield immediate and lasting returns, dramatically affect quality of life, and keep recipients from returning for care again and again (Lyon, 2000). Most payers now require documentation of functional goals and documentation of patients' initial and current functional status. Most payers will authorize payment for treatment only if there is a reasonable probability of meaningful improvement in a patient's overall functional performance.

> It has become almost impossible to write a treatment plan or submit a claim to a third-party payor without using the word *functional*. A speech-language pathologist must identify *functional* goals, using *functional* tasks, and show *functional* gains, or reimbursement for treatment is likely to be denied. (Elman & Bernstein-Ellis, 1995, p. 1)

The positive side of current reimbursement policies is that they reward efficiency. Efficient providers make a profit, and inefficient ones go out of business. The negative side of current reimbursement policies is that the emphasis on reducing costs can compromise the quality of care. Physicians may be encouraged to forgo expensive tests that might provide potentially important information about the nature of a patient's medical problems; may be instructed to substitute cheaper, but less effective, treatments for more expensive and more effective ones; and may be pressured to postpone elective procedures or to change their traditional way of caring for patients to better fit the financial imperatives of the provider.

Effects of Managed Care on Clinical Practice

The effects of managed care are not confined to physicians. Psychologists, social workers, occupational and physical therapists, speech-language pathologists, and other allied-health practitioners also are affected. Shortened in-hospital lengths of stay can make assessment something of a race, with practitioners competing for the limited number of appointment times available during a patient's stay. Assessments that at one time could be spread across several sessions now may have to be completed in a single session. Comprehensive assessment of a patient's impairments may be replaced by selective testing of a patient's most obvious deficits. Treatment options may be reduced. Some groups of patients who traditionally have received treatment may not receive it. Patients who do receive treatment may get less of it.

For the speech-language pathologist concerned with assessment and diagnosis of brain-injured adults' communicative and cognitive impairments, test administration time is likely to become increasingly important, given contemporary pressures from employers and healthcare funding agencies to increase efficiency and decrease costs. In a healthcare system that emphasizes economy and efficiency, tests requiring 2 to 6 hours to administer, score, and interpret will be at a significant disadvantage relative to shorter and quicker tests.

> One of the more often reported complaints from clinicians in recent months is the virtual elimination of standardized test batteries in patient assessments. Clinicians feel they no longer have the time to conduct the kind of comprehensive evaluations they were accustomed to and have been trained to do. (Golper & Cherney, 1999, p. 3).

There is no acceptable substitute for standardized tests that have documented reliability and validity, permit comparison of a patient with other patients in a diagnostic category, and permit comparison of a brain-injured patient's performance with the performance of persons without brain injury. As third-party payers impose limits on the scope of assessment, sensitive and reliable screening tests to detect communication impairments and give a general sense of the pattern of those impairments will become increasingly important. Comprehensive

test batteries may have to be shortened and made more efficient, perhaps by providing norms for individual subtests or combinations of subtests. Some existing language test batteries provide subtest-by-subtest norms (e.g., the *Porch Index of Communicative Ability*, the *Boston Diagnostic Aphasia Examination*). Because they permit subtest-by-subtest comparisons of a patient with norms, language test batteries with subtest-by-subtest norms may prove appealing to clinicians who wish to shorten a long standardized test.

Some test developers and publishers are creating short versions of standardized tests. The third edition of the *Boston Diagnostic Aphasia Examination* (*BDAE-3;* Goodglass, Kaplan, & Barresi, 2001) includes a short version that reduces testing time from the 3 to 5 hours required for the full BDAE to about 1 hour. CADL-2 is shorter and requires less administration time than the first edition of the CADL. The *Discourse Comprehension Test* (Brookshire & Nicholas, 1993) includes a short version that cuts test administration and interpretation time in half. Short forms of several standardized tests have been described in the literature, including the *Boston Naming Test* (*BNT;* Tombaugh & Hurley, 1997), the *Western Aphasia Battery* (*WAB;* Crary & Rothi, 1989), and the *Porch Index of Communicative Ability* (*PICA;* Disimoni, Keith, & Darley, 1980; Disimoni, Keith, Holt, & Darley, 1975; Lincoln & Ellis, 1980). Most contemporary language test batteries could stand (and perhaps benefit from) some pruning. The danger is that the pruning may lop off too much, leaving clinicians with incomplete or inaccurate descriptions of their patients' impairments.

The days of comprehensive language testing may be numbered. If they are, practitioners must work to ensure that gains in economy and efficiency do not come at the expense of understanding their patients' impairments and do not compromise practitioners' ability to provide the most efficacious treatment for those impairments.

Forming an accurate diagnosis and prognosis, and confidently arriving at a plan for treatment that will benefit the patient requires more information than can be gathered through cursory screening assessments, impressions gained from talking with family, or informal conversations with the patient. Further, the benefit of treatment is best determined through periodic testing. It is not appropriate to rely on cursory screening protocols to make a prognosis or design a treatment plan likely to benefit the patient, nor should cursory assessments be used to gauge treatment effects. (Golper & Cherney, 1999, p. 3).

Measures of functional communication are becoming increasingly important as changes in the way healthcare is provided and paid for underscore the need for reliable, sensitive, and valid indicators of daily life communication performance. Those who are paid for services to patients with cognitive-communicative disorders must now show that the services provide meaningful benefits to patients in daily life. Treatment planning and treatment procedures must explicitly address daily life cognitive-communicative performance. Consequently, continuing development of efficient, sensitive, reliable, and valid indicators of daily life cognitive-communicative performance is an important professional responsibility for speech-language pathologists. Frattalli (1998) reminds us, however, that impairment-level assessment and treatment still has a place in clinical and research practice.

Both clinicians and clinical researchers need to be discerning consumers of functional measures. Their current popularity in clinical practice and outcomes research should not overshadow the importance and distinct roles for standardized impairment measures. Each type of assessment was designed for different but complementary purposes—impairment measures for differential diagnosis and identification of patients' specific strengths and weaknesses, functional measures for determination of performance of daily life activities and participa-

tion in society. Perhaps most importantly, the sometimes skewed emphasis on *functional* does not mean that treatment aimed at improving impairment-level skills should be neglected (p. 219).

GENERAL CONCEPTS 6-1

- The World Health Organization (WHO) concepts of *impairment, disability,* and *handicap* have had strong effects on assessment of brain-injured adults. *Impairment* denotes a structural or functional abnormality in a person. *Disability* denotes the effect of impairments on a skill or ability. *Handicap* denotes the effects of disability on a person's ability to carry out daily life activities. In 1997 the WHO replaced the labels *impairment, disability,* and *handicap* with the labels *body function and structures, activity,* and *participation,* respectively.
- Publication of the *International Classification of Impairment, Disability, and Handicap (ICIDH, ICIDH-2)* by the WHO stimulated movement away from treatment focused on impairments to treatment intended to improve disabled persons' successful participation in activities of daily living.
- The *International Classification of Functioning, Disability, and Health (ICF)* considers disability and function as products of interactions among health conditions, personal factors, and environmental factors.
- The *Functional Communication Profile (FCP)* and the *Communicative Effectiveness Index (CETI)* are rating scales designed for subjectively estimating daily life communicative performance.
- *Communicative Activities of Daily Living—Second Edition (CADL-2)* is a standardized measure that estimates daily life communicative performance based on performance in simulated everyday situations.

GENERAL CONCEPTS 6-1—cont'd

- The *Functional Independence Measure (FIM)*, a rating scale for measuring outcome, is widely used for program evaluation in rehabilitation medicine programs. It focuses on self-care activities such as bathing and personal care, and for that reason is not sensitive to changes in cognitive-communicative abilities.
- The *ASHA Functional Assessment of Communication Skills for Adults (ASHA FACS)* is a rating scale designed to capture changes in cognitive-communicative abilities in four domains: social communication, communication of basic needs, daily planning, and reading/writing/number concepts.
- Increasing regulation and restrictions on reimbursement by funding sources make measurement of outcome increasingly important to practitioners who provide diagnostic and therapeutic services to brain-injured adults.
- The current emphasis on functional outcome and funding sources' restrictions on payment should not lead clinicians to abandon standardized tests with documented validity, reliability, and sensitivity.

QUALITY OF LIFE

The quality, not the longevity, of one's life is what is important. (Martin Luther King, Jr.)

Conceptual Background

The term *quality of life* became common in the late 1940s following World War II. It was first used in the United States to denote accumulation of material possessions (e.g., houses in suburbia, patio furniture, barbeque grills, fondue sets, Italian wines). During the 1960s the focus shifted to personal values (e.g., family relationships, emotional health, personal freedom). In the 1970s attention to quality of life made its way into medicine, as concern for *the whole patient* began to affect medical practice. The term *health-related quality of life* now is common in the medical literature.

Concern with health-related quality of life reflects recognition that the effects of intervention are not limited to reductions in the severity and frequency of disease, illness, or physical ailments but also include the effects of intervention on daily life well-being. Concern with quality of life also represents a movement away from the traditional belief that the purpose of healthcare is to treat or cure specific impairments (e.g., hypertension, anxiety, aphasia) to a belief that the purposes of healthcare include helping the person adapt to or compensate for the physical, psychologic, and social effects of disease or physical ailments, as well as helping the person resume a productive and rewarding role in daily life.

The WHO's broadening of the concept of disability to include social and environmental effects, as set forth in the ICF, plus the appearance of social approaches to management of brain-injured adults' communicative-cognitive disabilities, have broadened the focus of assessment to include personal well-being or *quality of life*, which the WHO defines as follows:

> …an individual's perception of their position in life in the context of the culture and value systems in which they live and in relation to their goals, expectations, standards, and concerns. It is a broad-ranging concept affected in a complex way by the person's physical health, psychological state, personal beliefs, social relationships, and their relationship to salient features of their environment. This definition highlights the view that quality of life is subjective, includes both positive and negative facets of life and is multi-dimensional. (WHOQOL group, 1995, p. 1405)

Despite the popularity of the quality-of-life concept in healthcare, publications using the term often neglect to define it or define it narrowly (e.g., as physical mobility, freedom from pain, or living independently). Consequently, measurement of health-related quality of life lacks a unifying theme. The term *quality of life* sometimes refers to objective conditions such as physical or mental functioning, living conditions, and access to services; sometimes it refers to subjective indicators such as satisfaction with life conditions and overall satisfaction with life.

Quality of life is an ephemeral and difficult-to-quantify concept. It cannot be directly measured but must be estimated by subjective judgments elicited by rating scales or questionnaires. Many questionnaires and rating scales have been designed to measure health-related quality of life, but they differ greatly in format, focus, and content, making it difficult or impossible to compare findings from one assessment instrument to another.

Measuring Health-Related Quality of Life

The *Satisfaction with Life Scale (SWLS;* Diener, Emmons, Larsen, & Griffin, 1985) is one of the earliest and most widely used generic measures of quality of life. The SWS is very short and very general, consisting of five statements that respondents rate on a 7-point Likert scale that ranges from *strongly disagree* to *strongly agree:*

1. In most ways, my life is close to my ideal.
2. The conditions in my life are excellent.
3. I am satisfied with my life.
4. So far, I have gotten the important things I want in life.
5. If I could live my life over, I would change almost nothing.

Because it is easily and quickly administered, the SWLS is popular. However, its brevity, the general nature of the statements to be rated, and the high intercorrelations among responses make it of little use in evaluating outcome, measuring respondents' opinions about specific aspects of quality of life, or tracking changes in perceived quality of life.

Likert scales were developed by Rensis Likert, an American social scientist, in 1932. Likert scales are psychometric scales commonly used to measure personal feelings and attitudes. Likert scales usually contain five, seven, or nine statements such as *strongly agree, agree, neither agree nor disagree, disagree,* and *strongly disagree.* However, Likert scale responses may be biased by respondents' reluctance to use the extreme ends of the scale, their desire to favorably portray themselves, their desire to appear normal, or their desire to please the interviewer.

The *Sickness Impact Profile (SIP;* Gilson, Gilson, Bertner, & associates, 1975; Bergner, Bobbitt, Carter, & associates, 1981) is one of the earliest detailed instruments for measuring health-related quality of life. The SIP consists of 136 statements such as *I get dressed only with someone's help.* The statements relate to experiences in two general domains—*physical abilities* (ambulation, mobility, self-care, and movement) and *psychosocial activities* (social interaction, communication, alertness, emotion, sleep and rest, eating, home management, recreation, and employment). The SIP has been widely used in medicine and related disciplines to assess patients' quality of life. Its major disadvantage is its length—the SIP takes about 30 minutes to administer to patients who do not have cognitive, communicative, or intellectual impairments.

Several shortened versions of the SIP have been developed, including a generic 68-item version called the *Sickness Impact Profile–68 (SIP-68;* de Bruin, Diederiks, de Witte, & associates, 1994). The SIP-68 assesses quality of life in six domains:

- Somatic autonomy (e.g., *I stand up only with someone's help.*)
- Mobility (e.g., *I walk shorter distances or stop to rest often.*)
- Psychic autonomy and communication (e.g., *I have difficulty reasoning and solving problems, for example, making plans, making decisions, learning new things.*)
- Social behavior (e.g., *I am doing fewer social activities with groups of people.*)

- Emotional stability (e.g., *I often act irritable toward those around me.*)
- Mobility range (e.g., *I stay at home most of the time.*)

A 30-item version of the SIP, called the *Stroke-Adapted 30-Item Version of the Sickness Impact Profile (SA-SIP30*; van Straten, de Haan, Limburg, & associates, 1997) was designed to assess stroke survivors' quality of life. The SA-SIP30 elicits patient ratings in eight domains (body care and movement, social interaction, mobility, communication, emotional behavior, household management, alertness, ambulation). The SA-SIP30, like the SIP and the SIP-68, gives greater weight to physical issues and mobility than to social behavior, communication, or emotional issues.

Another stroke-related quality-of-life measure was developed from interviews with 34 stroke survivors plus review of other health-related quality-of-life measures. The *Stroke-specific Quality of Life Scale (SS-QOL*; Williams, Weinberger, Harris, & associates, 1999) is a 49-item scale that assesses quality of life in 12 domains known to be of concern to stroke survivors (mobility, energy, upper extremity function, work/productivity, mood, self-care, social roles, family roles, vision, language, thinking, personality). Items in the SS-QOL are a mix of statements (e.g., *I wasn't interested in other people or activities.*) and questions (e.g., *Did you have trouble understanding what other people said?*) phrased in past tense. Ratings for items are made using 5-point Likert scales.

Hilari, Bing, Lamping, and Smith (2003) modified the SS-QOL to make it more sensitive to aphasic adults who may have difficulty understanding scale items or expressing their responses. Their first scale, called the *Stroke and Aphasia Quality of Life Scale—56 (SAQOL-56)* consisted of the 49 items from the SS-QOL plus 7 items added to increase the SAQOL's sensitivity to problems created by aphasia. Analysis of aphasic adults' responses to the SAQOL-56 scale failed to support its 12-domain structure, leading the authors to create a 39-

item, 4-domain version called the *Stroke and Aphasia Quality of Life Scale—39 (SAQOL-39)*. The SAQOL-39 contains 17 items related to physical problems, 4 items related to energy, 11 items related to psychosocial issues, and 7 items related to communication. Although the SAQOL-39 has acceptable test-retest reliability and construct validity, it may lack sensitivity to cognitive-communicative and psychosocial problems because of the large numbers of items devoted to physical problems and energy.

In 1995 the United States Centers for Disease Control and Prevention (CDC) and the WHO each released instruments for assessing health-related quality of life as part of programs for tracking population trends and measuring progress in improving health-related quality of life.

The CDC measure is called the *Centers for Disease Control and Prevention Health-Related Quality-of-Life 14-Item Measure (CDC HRQOL-14*; U.S. Public Health Service, Centers for Disease Control and Prevention, 1995). (Developers of quality-of-life measures seem to delight in wordy titles with many hyphens.) As its title suggests, the CDC HRQOL-14 contains 14 items. The items are grouped into 3 modules—a *Healthy Days Core Module* (4 items), an *Activity Limitations Module* (5 items), and a *Healthy Days Symptoms Module* (4 items). The first item (in the core module) asks *Would you say that your general health is: excellent - very good - fair - poor?* The remaining items ask respondents to estimate how many days during the past 30 days they experienced poor physical or mental health:

- How many days during the past 30 days was your physical health not good?
- During the past 30 days, for about how many days have you felt sad, blue, or depressed?

Or it asks them to answer yes/no questions about health-related conditions:

- Do you need the help of other persons in handling your routine needs such as everyday household chores, doing necessary business, shopping, or getting around for other purposes?

The CDC HRQOL-14 is used primarily for tracking quality of life at the national and state levels to identify disparities among geographic, socioeconomic, cultural, or ethnic groups; to track population trends; and to measure progress toward increasing quality of life and years of healthy life for the U.S. population. It is not well-suited for measuring the effects of intervention on an individual's quality of life or for tracking changes in an individual's feelings about quality of life.

In 1995 the WHO released its own quality-of-life measure, called the WHOQOL-100. The WHOQOL-100 contains 100 Likert scale items representing six domains:

- Physical health (energy, discomfort, sleep)
- Psychological health (body image, feelings, self esteem, thinking, learning, memory, concentration)
- Independence (mobility, activities of daily life, medication, capacity for work)
- Social relations (personal relationships, social support, sexual activity)
- Environment (finances, personal freedom, safety/security, access to healthcare, home, recreation, transportation)
- Spirituality (religion, beliefs)

Three years later the WHO released a shorter, more practical version of the WHOQOL-100, called the *WHOQOL-BREF* (World Health Organization, 1998). The WHOQOL-BREF begins with two Likert scale items related to general health and quality of life, followed by 26 items representing four domains—physical health, psychological health, social relationships, and environmental influences (Table 6-5).

Since its release the WHOQOL-BREF has been used to assess quality of life of persons affected by many health conditions, including stroke, cancer, heart disease, kidney disease, arthritis, HIV/AIDS, spinal cord injury, deafness, aphasia, traumatic brain injury, schizophrenia, panic disorder, obsessive-compulsive disorder, and depression.

Limitations of Generic Measures of Health-Related Quality of Life

Enthusiasm for measuring the effects of cognitive and communicative impairments on quality of life currently exceeds practitioners' ability to measure it reliably. The situation has not changed much from nearly 20 years ago, when Paul Ellwood, a physician, wrote:

> Still, major questions surround attempts to measure the impact of medical care on the quality of life; these involve reliability, sensitivity, specificity, and whether patients' subjective opinions about well-being can be treated as objectively as direct pathophysiologic observations. The interpretation of outcomes is further complicated by the need to make adjustments for comorbidity and the intensity and stage of the patient's illness—a far from trivial undertaking. (Ellwood, 1988)

Comorbidity: the presence of a health condition or disease process that is concomitant with, but unrelated to, another health condition or disease process (e.g., a stroke patient who also is affected by arthritis). Many neurologic conditions and diseases are comorbid with other health conditions. For example, stroke patients often have heart disease, hypertension, or diabetes as comorbid conditions. The presence of comorbid conditions complicates conclusions about the relationship between quality of life and individual health conditions. Quality-of-life ratings by a diabetic person who has had a stroke that causes aphasia and hemiplegia are likely to be less positive than ratings by a person who has had a stroke and is aphasic but has no other major health issues.

Unlike rating scales such as the *Functional Communication Profile* or the *Functional Independence Measure,* which may be completed by a person familiar with the patient, rating scales and questionnaires for estimating quality of life usually are completed by the person to whom the rating scale or questionnaire

TABLE 6-5	Items in the WHOQOL-BREF	
Domain	**Item**	**Scale**
Overall quality of life	How would you rate your quality of life?	VP – VG
Overall health	How satisfied are you with your health?	VD – VS
Physical	To what extent do you feel that physical pain prevents you from doing what you need to do?	NAA – AEA
	How much do you need any medical treatment to function in your daily life?	NAA – AEA
	Do you have enough energy for everyday life?	NAA – CMP
	How well are you able to get around?	NAA – CMP
	How satisfied are you with your sleep?	VD – VS
	How satisfied are you with your ability to perform your daily living activities?	VD – VS
	How satisfied are you with your capacity for work?	VD – VS
Psychological	How much do you enjoy life?	NAA – AEA
	To what extent do you feel your life to be meaningful?	NAA – AEA
	How well are you able to concentrate?	NAA – EXT
	Are you able to accept your bodily appearance?	NAA – CMP
	How satisfied are you with yourself?	VD – VS
	How often do you have negative feelings such as blue mood, despair, anxiety, depression?	NV – ALW
Social	How satisfied are you with your personal relationships?	VD – VS
	How satisfied are you with your sex life?	VD – VS
	How satisfied are you with the support you get from your friends?	VD – VS
Environmental	How safe do you feel in your daily life?	NAA – EXT
	How healthy is your physical environment?	NAA – EXT
	Have you enough money to meet your needs?	NAA – CMP
	How available to you is the information you need in your day-to-day life?	NAA – CMP
	To what extent do you have the opportunity for leisure activities?	NAA – CMP
	How satisfied are you with the conditions of your living space?	NAA – CMP
	How satisfied are you with your access to health services?	VD – VS
	How satisfied are you with your transport?	VD – VS

From World Health Organization (WHO). (2004). *World Health Organization quality of life (WHOQOL) assessment.* Geneva, Switzerland: WHO.

NOTE: Responses to all items are on a 5-point Likert scale.

VP – VG, Very poor – very good; *NAA – AEA,* not at all – an extreme amount; *NAA – CMP,* not at all - completely; *NAA – EXT,* not at all — extremely; *NV – ALW,* never — always; *VD – VS,* very dissatisfied - very satisfied.

applies because responses represent that person's personal feelings and attitudes, which cannot be fully known or appreciated by another. Obtaining quality-of-life ratings from brain-injured adults is complicated by the potential effects of problems with comprehension, attention, judgment, and self-perception that often accompany brain injury. Such problems may prevent many brain-injured adults (especially those with the most serious impairments) from adequately or reliably responding to questionnaires and rating scales about quality of life. Hilari, Bing, Lamping, and Smith (2003), for example, reported that 17% of aphasic adults who agreed to complete the SA-QOL were unable to do so.

Proxies (persons who provide ratings on behalf of persons who are unable to do so) sometimes have been used as a substitute for a brain-injured person's own ratings. Ratings by proxies may not, however, provide an accurate sense of brain-injured persons' judgments about quality of life, especially when the judgments reflect personal feelings and attitudes.

The WHOQOL Group (1994) divided questions that ask for a person's perception of quality of life into three categories:

1. Items that ask for specific information about functioning (e.g., *How many hours did you sleep last night?*)
2. Items that ask for global evaluations of functioning (e.g., *How well do you sleep?*)
3. Items that ask for highly personalized evaluations of functioning (e.g., *How satisfied are you with your sleep?*)

Someone who is familiar with a brain-injured person may provide reasonably dependable estimates of the person's functioning for items in the first two categories because these categories ask for information that is accessible to an observer. Items in the third category, however, reflect personal feelings and attitudes known only by the person to whom the items relate. The use of proxies for persons who cannot complete a quality-of-life assessment may be reasonable for items that ask for specific

information about functioning or global evaluations of functioning but may not be valid for items that ask for highly personalized evaluations of functioning.

Most items in generic health-related quality-of-life assessments ask for global evaluations of functioning, as in the following examples, to which a proxy familiar with the person who is the subject of the assessment might give reasonably dependable responses:

I go out less to visit other people.
I make more mistakes than usual.
I often act irritable to those around me.
I do not take care of personal or household affairs.
I laugh or cry suddenly.

Some items in generic health-related quality-of-life assessments sample personal feelings and attitudes less likely to be known by a proxy:

How positive do you feel about the future?
How much do feelings of depression bother you?
How satisfied are you with your ability to make decisions?
To what extent do you feel your life to be meaningful?

(The WHOQOL assessments are an exception to the customary global-evaluation-of-functioning bias of quality-of-life assessments because almost all of the items in them relate to personalized evaluations of functioning.)

The boundary between global evaluations and personalized evaluations of functioning can be blurry. Changes in how an item is worded can move an item from one category to another. For example, a global-evaluation item such as *I rarely visit with friends* becomes a personalized-evaluation item if it is reworded as *I visit with friends less often than I would like.* Personalized-evaluation items tend to relate to mood, emotion, hope, discouragement, and other subjective personal feelings and often are phrased as questions: *How much confidence do you have in yourself?* or *To what extent do you feel your life to be meaningful?* Global-evaluation items tend to be phrased as statements and portray observable phenomena.

Assessing some severely impaired brain-injured persons' quality of life may require the use of proxies. Although a proxy may guess at how the brain-injured person would respond to personalized-evaluation items, those responses are likely to be less true to the brain-injured person's actual feelings than the proxy's responses to global-evaluation items. Although proxy measures are less than perfect, their use may be necessary when a person with severe cognitive-communicative impairments cannot adequately respond to a quality-of-life assessment. Because severe cognitive-communicative impairments are likely to have substantial negative effects on quality of life, indirect estimates, although imprecise, are nevertheless important for designing an intervention program and documenting its effects.

Measuring Quality of Communicative Life

Most existing quality-of-life assessments do not contain enough items related to communication, cognition, and social relationships to make them sensitive measures of the effects of cognitive-communicative problems on quality of life. Generic health-related quality-of-life measures do not address in any detail specific areas of dysfunction likely to be associated with brain injury such as language comprehension, memory, and attention, making them unsuited for measuring the outcome of cognitive-communicative intervention with brain-injured adults or for tracking the effects of cognitive-communicative intervention on quality of life.

Worrall and Holland (2003) addressed the need for improved quality-of-life measures for severely aphasic adults. Their words apply equally to other adults who have sustained severe brain injuries.

> Quality of life for people with severe and global aphasia is a major challenge. Creative study on how to obtain the opinions of these people is required. Methods of factoring out other variables such as depression and premorbid factors, as well as age-related concerns such as retirement, sensory and cognitive impairments,

and social isolation have not been studied. Perhaps the most important issue is how to cast treatment in ways to maximize quality of life post-aphasia. Examples of interventions that directly and indirectly address quality of life are required as well as high levels of evidence for their effectiveness. (p. 332)

In response to the need for quality-of-life measures sensitive to cognitive-communicative disturbances, ASHA supported development and publication of the *Quality of Communication Life Scale* (*QCL*; Paul, Frattali, Holland, & associates, 2004) designed to permit persons who have significant language impairments to rate their quality of communicative life. The QCL consists of 17 statements about communicative aspects of quality of life (e.g., *I like to talk to people. People understand me when I talk.*) and participation in life (e.g., *My role in the family is the same. I make my own decisions.*), plus one item related to overall quality of life (e.g., *In general, my quality of life is good.*). The statements are short and grammatically simple to minimize the effects of impaired reading comprehension. To minimize the potential effects of cognitive-communicative impairments on the validity of respondents' ratings, respondents rate each statement by making a mark on a simple visual analogue scale (Figure 6-3). A clinician is present as the patient completes the QCL and provides assistance if necessary (i.e., reads statements for the patient or helps the patient mark the scales).

The QCL was field-tested at 10 sites in the United States; 86 brain-injured adults participated. Of the participants, 71% were aphasic, 16% had cognitive-communicative impairments, and 13% were dysarthric. (A group of patients with dementia was included in a preliminary test of the ASHA-QCL, but their responses were not reliable, so dementia patients were not included in the field test.) Participants completed the QCL in an average of 15 minutes (the range was from 5 to 45 minutes). Of the participants, 36% completed the QCL without assistance; 43% needed items read to them by

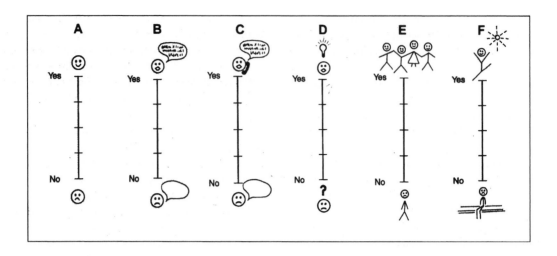

Figure 6-3 ■ Visual analogue scales used in the *Quality of Communication Life Scale (QCL)*. The form of the scale for an item depends on the nature of the item. Examples of items for each of these analogue scales are: **(A)** *I like myself.* **(B)** *I like to talk with people.* **(C)** *I use the telephone.* **(D)** *People understand me when I talk.* **(E)** *My role in the family is the same.* **(F)** *I get out of the house and do things* (such as sports, dinner, shows, parties). (From Paul, D.R., Frattalli, C.M, Holland, A.L., & associates. [2004]. *Quality of communication life scale.* Bethesda, MD: American Speech-Language-Hearing Association.)

the clinician; 5% needed help marking the scales; and 16% needed items read to them plus help marking the scales. The results of the field test led its authors to conclude the following:

> Based on the results of this study, it appears that the QCL is a valid measure of the quality of communication life as a distinct, but related, aspect of general quality of life. The data indicate that the QCL is valid for use with adults with neurogenic communication disorders (i.e., aphasia resulting from left-hemisphere stroke, cognitive-communicative disorder secondary to traumatic brain injury or right-hemisphere stroke, and dysarthria due to an acquired condition or progressive neurological disease), regardless of their age, education level, race/ethnicity, severity or time post-onset. (p. 19)

The QCL is a useful supplement to measures of cognitive-communicative impairment and functional communication. The QCL yields information about the effects of cognitive-communicative disorders on social relationships, communication interactions, work, education, leisure, and overall quality of life. Its design permits persons with significant language impairments to complete the rating scale, thereby reducing the need for proxy respondents and ensuring that ratings represent the person's actual feelings about quality of life and personal well-being. Because it focuses on communication, the QCL provides more detail about communication quality of life and greater sensitivity to change in respondents' ratings of communication quality of life than any other existing quality-of-life measure.

The Role of Impairment-Level Assessment

The contemporary emphasis on functional communication and quality of life, including quality of communicative life, should not obscure the continuing relevance of impairment-level assessment to intervention with brain-injured adults. As Frattalli (1998) commented, impairment-level assessment still has a place alongside activities-level and participation-level assessment in clinical and research practice. Impairment-level measures enable a clinician to identify a brain-injured person's cognitive-communicative disabilities and to design intervention programs that account for the brain-injured person's unique strengths, weaknesses, and needs.

Activities-level assessments enable clinicians to assess a brain-injured person's daily life cognitive-communicative strengths, weaknesses, and needs. Participation-level assessments enable clinicians to assess the effects of a brain-injured person's impairments on the person's social, psychologic, and emotional well-being and quality of life. The mix of impairment-level, activities-level, and participation-level assessment will differ across brain-injured persons, depending on each person's unique pattern of strengths, weaknesses, and needs. Finding the appropriate mix for a given brain-injured person requires skill, judgment, patience, and carefully chosen and carefully administered measures.

GENERAL CONCEPTS 6-2

- Publication of the ICF and the appearance of social approaches to clinical intervention with brain-injured adults have broadened the focus of measurement to include *quality of life.*
- Many rating scales for estimating quality of life have been published, including some designed for stroke patients and one designed for stroke patients who are aphasic.
- Estimates of quality of life are based on subjective ratings made by the disabled person or a family member or close associate. Most rating scales for estimating quality of life are generic measures, and most are not sensitive to the effects of cognitive-communicative impairments on quality of life.
- The United States Centers for Disease Control and Prevention (CDC) have published a quality-of-life scale designed for tracking quality of life at national and state levels to track population trends in quality of life and to evaluate progress toward increasing quality of life for the U.S. population.

- The WHO has published two quality-of-life measures, the *WHOQOL-100* and the shorter *WHOQOL-BREF*, used to quantify quality of life for persons who are affected by many different health conditions and who live in many parts of the world.
- The validity of the use of proxy respondents to estimate quality of life for brain-injured persons who cannot themselves complete quality-of-life ratings has not been established. Responses of proxies to global-evaluation rating-scale items are likely to better represent the rated person's judgments than do responses of proxies to items that assess the rated person's personal feelings and attitudes.
- The *Communication Quality of Life Scale (QCL)* is designed to permit its completion by persons who have significant language impairments.
- Impairment-level, activities-level, and participation-level assessments all have a place in assessing the communicative abilities of brain-injured adults.

THOUGHT QUESTIONS

Question 6-1 You administer a standardized aphasia test, a measure of functional communication, and a quality-of-life scale to two patients with left-hemisphere strokes. Both are male, 63 years old, have 12th-grade education, are retired, married with a living spouse, and have two children who are married and live in different cities. Their performances on the standardized aphasia test (75th percentile for aphasic adults) and their performances on the measure of functional communication (80th percentile) are equivalent, but their ratings of quality of life differ markedly. One rates his overall quality of life as 6.3 on a 7-point scale; the other rates his quality of life as 4.2 on the same 7-point scale. What variables do you think may explain the differences in perceived quality of life?

Question 6-2 The 16 items in the *Communicative Effectiveness Index* (see Table 6-4) span a range of complexity from basic behaviors such as getting attention to more complex behaviors such as following changing topics in conversations. How would you order the 16 items, from basic to complex? Are there gaps or discontinuities in the communicative spacing of items?

The Context for Treatment of Cognitive-Communicative Disorders

> *There is no room for rigidity in clinical practice. Both patient and clinician are part of the therapeutic process and interact in a complex manner. If the method leaves the patient behind, or if the patient outstrips the method, the method must be altered. When an urgent problem arises, the method must be put aside. The clinician must have room to explore, to feel out a need, and use the moment. (Hildred Schuell)*

THE TREATMENT TEAM

Contemporary patient care is structured around the treatment team. When a patient's care is managed by a treatment team, the responsibility rests with a team rather than with one person or with independently operating professionals, although one member of the team (sometimes a physician, often a case manager) has primary responsibility for coordinating the team's activities. Which professions are represented on a patient's treatment team depends on the nature of the patient's physical and medical problems. The treatment team for a patient with chronic obstructive pulmonary disease might include a pulmonary physician, a cardiologist, a respiratory therapist, an occupational therapist, a nurse, and a social worker. The treatment team for a stroke patient might include a neurologist, a nurse, a speech-language pathologist, a neuropsychologist, a physical therapist, an occupational therapist, a dietitian, and a social worker. Each member of a team has primary responsibility for a given aspect of the patient's care, but responsibilities often overlap. Consequently, planning, coordination, and communication among team members is crucial if treatment is to be efficient and effective.

> Case managers are health professionals who have specialized training and experience in clinical and financial aspects of healthcare; knowledge of patient-care resources; ability to manage, negotiate, and collaborate with multidisciplinary groups; and ability to interact and collaborate with patients and families to ensure that the goals of patients' plans of care are reached. Case managers are often nurses or social workers with specialized training in case management.

Speech-language pathologists who participate in the care of brain-injured adults are likely to serve on teams with an assortment of other professionals. Although one cannot always predict who will be on a given patient's treatment team, speech-language pathologists who work with brain-injured adults often serve on teams with the following professionals.

Neurologists

Neurologists have primary responsibility for the medical care of patients with brain injury or other nervous system pathology. Their role in patient care is described in Chapter 2, and it will not be repeated here.

Physiatrists

Physiatrists (rehabilitation medicine physicians) have primary medical responsibility for patients admitted to rehabilitation wards. They help physically disabled patients regain the use of impaired muscles, and when restitution of function is not possible, they help the patient compensate for the muscular impairments. Physiatrists examine the patient, determine the patient's medical and rehabilitation needs, design comprehensive rehabilitation programs, and oversee the activities of physical, occupational, corrective, vocational, and recreation therapists.

Physical Therapists

Physical therapists evaluate muscle strength and range of limb movement. Under the supervision of a physiatrist, they also carry out programs to help patients retain or regain muscle strength and limb movement. When a patient is confined to bed, a physical therapist may see the patient at bedside and teach her or him how to turn over in bed, sit up, and transfer from the bed to a chair or wheelchair. Physical therapists carry out passive range-of-movement exercises in which bedbound patients' limbs are moved and their muscles are stretched to prevent *contractures* (permanent shortening of muscles resulting from paralysis) and to preserve muscle strength and tone. Other physical therapy activities take place in the physical therapy clinic and include muscle strengthening and range-of-movement activities; teaching patients how to transfer to and from a wheelchair; how to use braces, canes, and crutches; and how to get dressed. If a patient is about to be discharged home or to a nursing home, the physical therapist may help the family or nursing home staff prepare the living environment for the special needs of the patient and may provide the patient with exercise programs to be done at home.

Occupational Therapists

Occupational therapists help patients regain abilities necessary for activities of daily living such as cooking, dressing, and grooming. Although both occupational and physical therapists work on muscle strengthening, occupational therapists usually work on muscles with activities that resemble those of daily living. A patient who needs to strengthen hand and arm muscles might sand boards, saw wood, or weave on a loom. A patient with visuospatial impairments might perform craft activities requiring eye-hand coordination. An important part of occupational therapists' responsibilities is to help the patient resume daily life activities such as cooking, cleaning, and making beds. Occupational therapists teach compensatory strategies, provide special tools and appliances, and modify standard tools and appliances to help patients compensate for their impairments. Occupational therapists also help patients develop leisure activities and hobbies, and they sometimes test and treat patients for sensorimotor and visuospatial disorders. Because occupational therapists often deal with visual perception, reading, and writing, speech-language pathologists often collaborate with them on managing those aspects of a patient's needs.

Vocational Therapists

Vocational therapists provide vocational testing and evaluation. They administer work-aptitude tests and real or simulated on-the-job evaluations to determine if a patient can go back to work. Vocational therapists sometimes arrange work placements or modify a patient's work environment and responsibilities to enable the patient to perform work assignments successfully.

Corrective Therapists

Corrective therapists are responsible for ambulation training. They collaborate with physical and occupational therapists to help the patient regain the strength, balance, and endurance needed for walking, and they may teach the patient how to use crutches and canes and how to climb and descend stairs.

Recreation Therapists

Recreation therapists provide therapeutic recreational activities (usually arts and crafts) and may get the patient started in leisure activities that the patient may continue after discharge.

Neuropsychologists

Neuropsychologists administer tests of cognitive functions (e.g., attention, memory, mental flexibility, intellect) that may help the team discriminate between psychiatric and neurologic conditions, distinguish between different neurologic conditions, or predict the course of a patient's recovery. Neuropsychologists provide the treatment team with information about the patient's adjustment to disabilities and her or his present and probable future cognitive and behavioral abilities and limitations. Neuropsychologists help to plan and carry out a plan of care for the patient and may have primary responsibility for assessing the effects of treatment on the patient's cognitive abilities. Neuropsychologists often collaborate closely with speech-language pathologists to assess brain-injured patients' cognitive and communicative status, with the neuropsychologist taking the lead in evaluating cognitive functions such as perception, attention, and memory, and the speech-language pathologist taking primary responsibility for evaluating communicative and linguistic abilities.

Clinical Psychologists

Clinical psychologists administer and interpret tests of intelligence, cognition, and personality and provide the team with information about the patient's intellectual, cognitive, and emotional state. A clinical psychologist may help the patient and family deal with the emotional and psychological effects of the patient's brain injury. When a patient is depressed or anxious, the clinical psychologist may help the patient and family understand and cope with the feelings.

Psychiatrists

Some brain-injured patients develop symptoms of depression, psychosis, neurosis, or other personality aberrations. For these patients a psychiatrist may provide diagnosis, referral, and treatment (especially when medications to control a patient's psychiatric symptoms are appropriate).

Dietitians

Dietitians evaluate patients' nutritional needs and recommend dietary adjustments to correct nutritional deficiencies. Dietitians work with the team to ensure that the patient's food and liquid intake are sufficient to meet nutritional and hydration needs. Dietitians often collaborate with speech-language pathologists to set up special diets and feeding programs for patients with *dysphagia* (impaired swallowing), caused by neurologic or structural damage that disrupts the mechanics of chewing and swallowing.

Speech-Language Pathologists

Speech-language pathologists provide assessment, treatment, and referral services for cognitive-communicative disorders and related impairments. Speech-language pathologists often play a prominent part on treatment teams for brain-injured patients with cognitive-communicative disorders because they are experienced in communicating with such patients. The speech-language pathologist's work with communicatively impaired patients often touches on the needs and concerns of the patient and family, which the speech-language pathologist may communicate to the team.

Social Workers

Social workers coordinate communication between medical facility staff and the patient and family. They also keep families informed about treatment and discharge plans. They suggest, initiate, and coordinate referrals to medical, financial, and social service agencies. They provide patients and families with information about nursing homes, county and state medical and family services, and other social and community resources to help them adjust to altered financial, vocational, and social conditions. Social workers ensure that physicians' orders for wheelchairs and other prosthetic appliances are carried out, and they may make arrangements for programs such as Meals on Wheels or public health nurse visits to the patient's home. Social workers coordinate evaluations of legal competence for patients whose competence is questionable and make referrals to psychologic and mental health services, chemical dependency programs, Social Security or Department of Veterans Affairs (VA) counselors, financial advisors, vocational counselors, or family and marriage counselors. Social workers play a key role in coordinating interactions among the medical facility staff, the patient, the patient's family, and community and state agencies. Social workers help the patient and family adjust to changed lifestyles and ensure that the patient's posthospital placement represents the needs, wishes, and current circumstances of the patient and the family.

Team meetings at which team members review the patient's progress, revise or add to the plan of care, and plan for discharge are held periodically (usually weekly). By maximizing communication among members of the team and by delegating important components of care to team members who are professionally qualified to assume responsibility for those components, the treatment team approach improves the quality and efficiency of patient care by ensuring that a comprehensive treatment plan addressing all important aspects of the patient's care is created and followed.

CANDIDACY FOR TREATMENT

The process of deciding a patient's candidacy for treatment of a neurogenic cognitive-communicative disorder has received little attention in the literature, perhaps because of the number and complexity of variables affecting the process and the subjective nature of the decisions. Although there are no unequivocal criteria with which to separate the good treatment candidates from the poor ones, several patient-related variables are fairly dependable indicators of a brain-injured patient's potential response to treatment.

Patient Variables

Brain Injury. The severity and location of a patient's brain injury are perhaps the most important indicators of his or her potential response to treatment. The greater the brain damage and the more it affects areas of the brain involved in cognition and communication, the less likely it is that a patient will recover cognitive-communicative abilities, with or without treatment. The size and location of a patient's brain injury can be estimated directly from laboratory measures (e.g., computerized tomography or magnetic resonance imaging scans) or indirectly from behavioral measures (e.g., tests of speech, language, memory, and cognition). However, the relationship between lesion size, lesion location, and behavioral deficits may be weak immediately following brain injury, when temporary physiologic alterations (e.g., reduction of cerebral blood flow, neurotransmitter release, cerebral edema, and diaschisis) are present. For this reason, clinicians may choose to wait several weeks before deciding that a patient's brain injury is too severe to warrant treatment of the patient's cognitive-communicative impairments.

Medical and Physical Status. A patient's medical and physical status frequently affects decisions about treatment. Very ill, very depressed, or very weak patients often do not get enough benefit from treatment to justify its cost. Patients who cannot sit up and attend to treatment for at least 15 minutes may not be strong enough to tolerate intensive treatment, and the clinician may elect to forgo treatment or at least to defer it until the patient recovers sufficient health and strength to gainfully participate in treatment activities.

Motivation. Often a patient's motivation to recover has strong effects on the outcome of treatment. Some highly motivated and resourceful patients benefit from treatment in spite of severe impairments. Some unmotivated or unconcerned patients fail to benefit from treatment even though their impairments are relatively mild. A patient's life situation also may affect the outcome of treatment. A supportive, motivated, and caring family usually enhances the effect of treatment, but a nonsupportive family may compromise it.

Trial Treatment

Clinicians often resolve their doubts about the appropriateness of treatment for questionable treatment candidates by offering a few sessions of trial treatment. If the patient responds well to the trial treatment, treatment continues; if the patient responds poorly to the trial treatment, it is discontinued.

If free to do so, and if given unlimited professional and financial resources, most clinicians would offer trial treatment to all questionable treatment candidates to minimize the chance of missing a good treatment candidate. However, healthcare providers face restrictions on who receives treatment and how much the treatment costs. Limitations on resources require that treatment be provided to those who are likely to receive the greatest benefit at the least cost and that decisions about who receives treatment must be made quickly. This means that identifying the patients who are likely to benefit most from treatment, and doing so in a limited amount of time, has become an increasingly important part of the clinician's responsibilities. The issues of how benefit is defined and of what constitutes a reasonable cost-benefit ratio are complex, and, as in the tale of the blind men and the elephant, one's attitude depends greatly on the direction from which one looks at the problem. The issue is one that every clinician must eventually face, although few feel they have satisfactorily resolved it.

Not every patient who may profit from treatment wants it. Patients have the right to refuse treatment, even if a clinician feels that treatment would directly benefit the patient and indirectly benefit the patient's family. If a patient understands the nature of his or her cognitive-communicative impairments, the poten-tial personal and social effects of the impairments, and the nature and potential benefits of treatment, but refuses treatment, the patient's refusal must be accepted. If a patient is confused, intellectually impaired, or otherwise not competent to make decisions about treatment, family members or others with the right to represent the patient may decide for the patient.

HOW CLINICIANS DECIDE WHAT TO TREAT

A clinician's decisions regarding what to treat come from his or her intuitions about the nature of the patient's communicative impairment, the clinician's attitudes about the nature and purpose of therapy, and the clinician's previous clinical successes and failures. There are no rules and few guiding principles, but a few general approaches to deciding what to treat have been described in the literature. Two are impairment-level approaches, and two are activity-participation level approaches.

The history of intervention with brain-injured adults is primarily a history of intervention at the impairment level. Traditional models of intervention reflect the origins of intervention in medical contexts, wherein intervention typically followed the medical care sequence of assessment, diagnosis, treatment, and discharge (Simmons-Mackie, 2000). During the 1980s the focus of intervention began to shift from correcting or compensating for impairments to maximizing communicative success in real life contexts, as funding agencies began requiring that clinicians assess patients' existing functional abilities, develop explicit functional goals, and document progress toward the goals. Publication of the ICIDH and the ICIDH-2 by the World Health Organization provided a terminologic and conceptual foundation for a patient needs–based approach to intervention, and the focus of intervention began to shift from treating patients' *impairments* (e.g., attention, memory, language comprehension, language expression) to enhancing clients' success in *activities* of daily living and reducing or removing barriers to clients' *participation* in social, community, and cultural aspects of daily life.

Many proponents of a social model of intervention reject *aphasic patient* in favor of *aphasic client* as designation for a person who is aphasic.

Impairment Level Approaches

Relative Level of Impairment. Perhaps the most common impairment level approach to treatment planning is the *relative level of impairment approach,* in which the patient's performance on various tests is analyzed to identify peaks and valleys in the patient's performance profile. These peaks and valleys are given special attention in treatment. Clinicians sometimes choose to treat in the *valleys* (areas of relative impairment), but they are more likely to treat at the *peaks* (areas of least impairment). The relative level of impairment approach has been most clearly explicated with reference to aphasia, but the principles apply equally well to treatment of patients with other cognitive-communicative impairments.

Porch (1981b) described a relative level of impairment approach based on variability in patients' performance within and across subtests of the *Porch Index of Communicative Ability (PICA).* Porch calls his measure of across-subtest variability the *high-low gap.* The high-low gap is calculated on the 18 subtests of the PICA. The average for the 9 subtests with the highest scores and the average for the 9 subtests with the lowest scores are calculated. The difference between the two averages is the *high-low gap.* According to Porch the high-low gap represents, in part, the amount of change that can be expected from treatment. Porch recommends that treatment focus on processes represented by tasks in which patients exhibit slight to moderate impairments. As a patient's

performance in the first-treated tasks reaches normalcy, the focus of treatment shifts to a new set of tasks in which the patient exhibits slight to moderate impairments. When the high-low gap is closed (a difference at or near zero), Porch suggests that the patient may have achieved maximum treatment benefits.

Porch also recommends consideration of what he calls *intrasubtest variability (ISV)* when clinicians make decisions about treatment. He defines *ISV* as the number of different scores within a subtest. A 10-item PICA subtest in which a patient receives 8 scores of *13* (with the PICA 16-category scoring system) and 2 scores of *15* would have low ISV, whereas a subtest in which a patient's 10 responses included scores of *7, 9, 10, 13,* and *15* would have large ISV. According to Porch, ISV is related to a patient's potential for change in the task represented by the subtest, with greater potential for change on subtests with high ISV than on subtests with low ISV. According to Porch, ISV decreases as the patient approaches the limits of his or her recovery potential.

Fundamental Processes. In the *fundamental processes approach* to treatment, clinicians attempt to identify impairments in underlying processes that are thought to contribute to several related linguistic, cognitive, or communicative abilities. Clinicians then focus treatment on those processes, assuming that improving a process also improves the abilities that depend on the process. For example, Schuell, Jenkins, and Jimenez-Pabon (1964) considered impaired auditory comprehension a central problem in aphasia and believed that improved auditory comprehension generalizes to other language abilities. Clinicians who agree with Schuell and associates carefully test auditory comprehension and make auditory comprehension disabilities the focus of treatment, expecting that as auditory comprehension improves, so will general linguistic and communicative abilities.

Gardner, Brownell, Wapner, and Michelow (1983) and Myers (1991) have suggested that impaired capacity to make inferences is a central problem for many right hemisphere–damaged persons. Those who subscribe to this view might focus treatment on making inferences, expecting that as inference-making improves, so will related abilities.

Some practitioners believe that attentional impairments are a common problem for patients with traumatic brain injuries. They focus treatment on reducing attentional impairments because they believe that improving attention will improve other attention-related skills.

Activity-Participation Approaches

Activity-participation approaches to intervention (sometimes called *functional approaches*) consider communication a social phenomenon and view the purpose of intervention as enhancement of communicative success in everyday life. Intervention at the *activity* level is designed to help brain-injured persons succeed in targeted daily life activities (e.g., understanding spoken messages, maintaining eye contact in conversations, using the telephone) in which performance is affected by one or more underlying impairments. Intervention at the *participation* level is designed to help brain-injured persons succeed in life situations (e.g., initiating and maintaining social relationships, using public transportation, finding and using community services) in which participation is affected either by the person's underlying impairments or by societal conditions that facilitate or hinder the person's participation. Activity-participation approaches often combine client-specific training in coping and problem-solving (activity-level intervention) with public information and education about brain injury and its effects on communication (participation-level intervention).

Most clinicians combine elements of these approaches, and most consider *functionality* (the relevance of a skill, process, or ability to a client's daily life) when deciding on a treatment approach. Some clients may be best served by intervention at the impairment level (e.g., a client for whom reading comprehension is an important daily life activity); some may merit intervention at the activity level (e.g., a client who wishes to manage his or her financial affairs); and some may profit from intervention at the participation level (e.g., a client who may return to work, given compensatory modifications in the workplace). Sometimes intervention at one level affects a client's competence at another level. For example, improving an aphasic person's compromised word retrieval (an impairment) may make it possible for him or her to order a meal at a restaurant (an activity) or to perform volunteer work at a community center (participation).

GENERAL CHARACTERISTICS OF INTERVENTION

Impairment Level

Treatment sessions at the impairment level tend to have a consistent format. Most begin with a short interval of conversation between the clinician and the patient (the *opening*). The clinician uses the opening to evaluate the patient's performance relative to previous sessions, to estimate the extent to which treated behaviors are generalizing to conversational interactions, and to appraise the patient's mood and energy level. The opening gives the patient time to settle in, get comfortable, and get problems and concerns out of the way. The opening also helps establish and maintain rapport between the patient and the clinician.

The opening leads into a short interval of work on easy tasks in which the patient's performance is nearly error-free *(accommodation)*. *Accommodation tasks* are tasks the patient has mastered in previous sessions. Accommodation tasks get the patient into the sequence and timing of treatment procedures and provide her or him with a warm-up for the more difficult tasks that follow *(goal-directed work)*.

Goal-directed work is the heart of impairment level treatment sessions. Tasks become more challenging and focus on specific treatment objectives. The clinician instructs, explains, delivers treatment stimuli, provides feedback, and records the patient's performance. The patient works at or near maximum capacity in each treatment task. The interaction between the clinician and the patient is governed by the treatment plan—the clinician's contributions and the patient's responses are task-directed. Except for transitions between tasks, there is little purely social interaction.

Some treatment approaches make extensive use of conversational interactions to provide patients with directed experiences in activities resembling those a patient will encounter in daily life. Although the activities resemble conversations, they are in fact goal-directed because the clinician carefully structures the activities to focus on specific skills and conversational behaviors.

Clinicians often follow the work segment with some work on a few familiar tasks in which the patient is highly successful *(cool-down)*.

Many clinicians end treatment sessions with a short interval of conversation about the session, plans for the next session, and other topics of common interest (the *closing*).

Activity-Participation Level

Treatment sessions at the activity-participation level usually have a less-structured, less-prescriptive format. Early sessions may be devoted to clinician-patient collaboration to determine the patient's communicative needs and agree on the goals of intervention. Later sessions may focus on collaboration to devise and implement strategies, measure progress, modify goals, and prepare the patient for life after intervention. The clinician acts as guide or coach rather than as leader or teacher, and the patient (and significant others) play an active part in decisions about the nature, timing, and duration of intervention. However, the general format of individual sessions often resembles the format of impairment level treatment sessions.

GENERAL CONCEPTS 7-1

- Speech-language pathologists who work in medical facilities often serve on treatment teams with other professionals. The treatment team is responsible for planning, implementing, and evaluating a patient's care while the patient is in a medical facility.
- Treatment teams for brain-injured adults often include some or all of the following members:
  - A neurologist, responsible for the medical care of brain-injured patients
  - A physiatrist, responsible for the medical care of patients on rehabilitation wards
  - A physical therapist, responsible for increasing patients' muscle strength and range of movement
- An occupational therapist, responsible for helping patients regain competence in activities of daily life
- A vocational therapist, responsible for vocational evaluation and training
- A corrective therapist, responsible for ambulation training
- A recreation therapist, responsible for therapeutic recreational activities
- A neuropsychologist, responsible for evaluating patients' cognitive functions
- A clinical psychologist, responsible for evaluating patients' intelligence, cognition, and personality
- A psychiatrist, responsible for evaluating and treating patients' personality aberrations

Continued

- A dietitian, responsible for evaluating patients' nutritional needs and for adjusting diets to compensate for impaired swallowing or to correct nutritional deficiencies
- A speech-language pathologist, responsible for evaluating and treating patients' cognitive-communicative or swallowing disabilities
- A social worker, responsible for coordinating and integrating medical care with patients' and families' needs and for helping patients and families find and use social and community resources
- Several variables may affect the probability that a cognitive-communicatively impaired patient will benefit from treatment, including the nature and severity of the brain injury, the patient's medical and physical status, and the patient's motivation and enthusiasm. A few sessions of trial treatment may provide the most dependable indicator of a patient's response to treatment.
- Impairment level approaches to treatment include the *relative level of impairment approach* and the *fundamental processes approach.*
  - Clinicians who use the *relative level of impairment* approach to treatment choose treatment activities based on a patient's test performance. Sometimes clinicians treat in areas of minimal impairment *(peaks).* Less often, clinicians choose to treat in areas of greatest impairment *(valleys).*

- Clinicians who use the *fundamental processes* approach to treatment choose treatment activities to stimulate processes that they believe underlie several related linguistic or communicative abilities.
- Clinicians who use the *functional abilities* approach to treatment choose treatment activities that target abilities they believe are important in patients' daily life communication.
- Activity-participation approaches to treatment may train patients to perform specific activities (e.g., using the telephone, reading the newspaper) or prepare patients for participation in daily living experiences (e.g., maintaining social relationships, using community services).
- Treatment sessions for communicatively impaired adults usually begin with general conversation *(opening),* which leads into work on familiar tasks in which the patient has high success rates *(accommodation).* *Goal-directed work* follows with challenging tasks, focused on specific treatment objectives. A short *cool-down* segment with easy tasks and general patient success follows goal-directed work. A brief interval of conversation *(closing)* ends the session.
- Treatment sessions at the activity-participation level of intervention are usually less structured and less prescriptive than are treatment sessions at the impairment level of intervention.

ADJUSTING TREATMENT TO THE PATIENT

After more than a century of study, treatment of adults with cognitive-communicative impairments remains as much art as science. Hundreds of data-based studies of cognitive-communicative impairments have been published, but only a

fraction are directly relevant to treatment. Many treatment procedures have been described in the literature, but most are little more than descriptions of the procedures, with anecdotes or the authors' opinions substituting for empiric evidence of effectiveness. As a consequence, most decisions about how to approach a given patient's cognitive-communicative anomalies rely more on the clinician's experience and intuition than on empiric evidence.

Beginning clinicians are not, however, condemned to trial and error as their only guide as they accumulate experiences and nurture intuitions that will eventually culminate in clinical expertise. There are regularities in how adults with neurogenic cognitive-communicative impairments respond to manipulations of the clinical environment, and most patients with a particular pattern of impairments respond to the manipulations in predictable ways, although idiosyncratic responses are common. For example, the performance of most brain-injured adults is adversely affected by noisy or distraction-loaded environments, but a few may tolerate noisy and distracting conditions surprisingly well.

Task Difficulty

Most who write about treatment of brain-injured adults agree that treatment tasks should challenge but not overwhelm the patient. The quality of a patient's responses provides a dependable (although subjective) indicator of task difficulty. If the difficulty of a task is well below the level of a patient's abilities, all or nearly all responses are prompt and accurate. As a task becomes more challenging, the patient's responses become hesitant, tentative, or delayed, and false starts, revisions, self-corrections, and a few uncorrected errors appear. As a task becomes even more challenging, uncorrected errors predominate, but cues or repetition of the stimulus by the clinician may elicit correct responses. When the task becomes overwhelming, strings of uncorrected errors appear and cues or repetition of stimuli are of little help.

Not everyone agrees on the precise level of difficulty to which treatment tasks should be adjusted. Porch (1981b) recommends that treatment begin at levels where patients make no outright errors but produce combinations of immediate and correct responses, delayed but correct responses, self-corrected errors, distorted responses, or responses that are corrected after prompting by the clinician. He also declares that clinicians should not change tasks or response criteria until every patient response is immediate and correct, because responses trained to less-than-perfect levels deteriorate in real life situations or in more difficult treatment tasks.

Porch's position, although logically reasonable, may not be appropriate for every brain-injured patient in every treatment task. Brain-injured patients differ in their tolerance for errors just as they differ in many other ways. Some fret and fuss over every misstep, whereas others remain serene in the face of repeated failure. Sensitive clinicians take such patient characteristics into account when deciding how hard to push a patient. For the hypersensitive patient who is troubled by every mistake, the clinician may pitch treatment so that immediate, correct responses greatly outnumber responses of lesser quality. For the patient who is constructively challenged by failure, the clinician may permit greater proportions of delayed, self-corrected, and prompted responses and even some uncorrected errors.

Another reason for structuring treatment tasks to control the frequency of error responses is that an error response on one trial often increases the probability of errors on subsequent trials. Brookshire (1972) found that when aphasic patients made an error in a picture-naming task, they had a strong tendency to misname following items, even when those items were ordinarily easy for them to name. Brookshire (1976) later found the same effect in a sentence comprehension task, and Brookshire, Nicholas, Redmond, and Krueger (1979) found a similar effect in videotaped aphasia treatment sessions. All three studies showed that when a patient made an error on one trial, the probability of errors on subsequent trials went up significantly. Strings of error responses proved to be especially disruptive to performance. When strings of error responses occurred, the probability of a correct response diminished with each error in the string, so that by the time three or four consecutive errors had occurred, the probability of a correct response on the next trial was near zero unless the task was made easier or response requirements were loosened.

As a general rule, it is a good idea to limit most brain-injured patients' percentage of un-corrected error responses to no more than 10% to 15% of all responses. However, clinicians and patients can sometimes tolerate higher error rates if the patient moves closer to the intended response with each attempt. Rosenbek and associates (1989) comment that a stimulus may be adequate even if it does not elicit a correct response if it leads to problem-solving or if a series of incorrect responses moves in the direction of adequacy. However, if there is no improvement across sequences of off-target responses (especially if the patient emits the *same* response on every trial), the patient is not learning much beyond what it feels like to fail, and the clinician should make the task easier.

For the mythical average patient, I try to keep patient performance between 60% and 80% immediate and correct responses during the beginning of a given task and I increase the difficulty of the task when immediate, correct responses exceed 90% to 95% over two or three administrations of the task. If less than 10% of the average patient's responses are delayed or self-corrected across many trials, I usually increase task difficulty, unless the patient is near the end of treatment and her or his performance is plateauing. For these patients I may stay with treatment tasks until all responses are immediate and correct to give the patient extended experience in tasks calling for sus-tained effort at maximum performance levels, to give the patient a strong sense of what success-ful performance at this level of effort feels like, and to build the patient's confidence in her or his ability to handle situations that call for this level of performance.

Resource Allocation

Most adults with brain injury have perceptual, attentional, cognitive, and performance abnor-malities that compromise their ability to per-ceive and discriminate sensory input, diminish the flexibility and efficiency of their cognitive processes, and compromise the speed and accu-racy of their responses to stimulation. Clini-cians who work with brain-injured adults must understand how these impairments may affect a patient's performance during intervention. For-tunately, there are many ways in which clinicians can manipulate the character of intervention to lessen the effects of these perceptual, atten-tional, cognitive, and performance abnormalities.

Because mental processes are internal, they cannot be directly manipulated. Clinicians may, however, manipulate the workload associated with mental processes by manipulating the character of task stimuli and by changing the nature of the responses expected from the patient. Stimulus manipulations permit clini-cians to regulate the workload associated with perception, discrimination, and interpretation of task stimuli. Changing the specifications for responses permits clinicians to regulate the work-load associated with formulation and produc-tion of responses. Knowing which characteris-tics of the procedures to manipulate requires that the clinician have an idea of why the patient is having trouble. If the clinician knows the *why*, the *how* becomes more apparent.

The concept of resource allocation serves as a useful guide in adjusting the difficulty of inter-vention procedures. As described in Chapter 4, the basic concept of resource allocation is that human brains have a limited amount of process-ing resources available for carrying out mental operations. Any mental operation depends on resources from the pool. Complex mental oper-ations require more resources than simple men-tal operations, and if several mental operations are simultaneously active, each draws resources from the pool. If the demand for resources exceeds the capacity of the pool, performance suffers.

We expect performance to be normal when a brain-injured adult performs tasks in which the need for processing resources is less than the resources in the pool. As the complexity of tasks pulls more resources from the pool, performance begins to deteriorate and becomes progressively worse as the need for resources reaches and exceeds those available. Importantly, if some elements of the tasks are simplified, thereby lessening the need for resources, the person's performance improves. The following example shows how this works.

> A brain-injured aphasic patient who has a visuoperceptual impairment is asked to point to black-and-white line drawings of objects when the clinician describes them by function (e.g., *Point to the one used for writing and erasing*). After 10 trials he has made 8 errors. When the clinician pauses after the tenth trial, the patient complains that he is having trouble making out what the drawings represent. The clinician trades the drawings for colored photographs and does 10 more trials. The patient makes only 2 errors.

This patient had trouble with two components of the task—auditory comprehension and visual perception of the drawings. In resource-allocation terms, the patient's aphasia and visuoperceptual problems combined to create a need for resources that exceeded the resources available. By changing the stimuli from line drawings to more realistic colored photographs, the clinician reduced the complexity of the visual processing component of the task, freeing resources that could be redirected to auditory comprehension, which then improved. If the treatment focus had been on perception and recognition of line drawings, the clinician could have facilitated the patient's identification of the line drawings by reducing the difficulty of the auditory comprehension aspects of the task, thereby freeing resources for visual processing.

This *quid pro quo* (one thing in return for another) characteristic of resource allocation has implications for clinicians working with brain-injured adults. The general principle is that clinicians can focus treatment on a targeted process by controlling the processing load associated with incidental task variables that are not related to the treatment objectives. This is what happened in the preceding example, when the clinician facilitated the patient's comprehension (the targeted process) by lowering the processing load associated with perceiving the visual stimuli (an incidental task variable). Resource-allocation concepts help to sensitize clinicians to the unintended effects of incidental task variables when they design treatment tasks. Clinicians who are aware of these effects can control for them, ensuring that treatment tasks focus on the intended processes and are not complicated by processing demands associated with incidental task variables.

Stimulus Manipulations

Clinicians may adjust the difficulty of treatment tasks by manipulating several characteristics of task stimuli to keep the patient working at an optimum level of task difficulty without overwhelming him or her. Clinicians manipulate the mental effort required to perceive, discriminate, and interpret task stimuli by adjusting their *intensity and salience, clarity and intelligibility, redundancy and contextual support,* or *novelty and interest value.*

Intensity and Salience. Increasing the intensity or salience of stimuli helps brain-injured patients who otherwise have difficulty perceiving, attending to, or discriminating them. *Intensity,* as used here, refers to the perceived magnitude or strength of a stimulus. *Salience* refers to the perceived prominence or conspicuousness of a stimulus, or how clearly it stands out from its surroundings. In some ways intensity and salience are related, because making a stimulus more intense (e.g., louder, brighter, larger) usually makes it more salient. However, intensity and salience differ in that intensity is a property of the stimulus, whereas salience expresses a relationship between the stimulus and its surroundings. A loud auditory stimulus presented in a noisy environment may be less salient than a soft auditory stimulus presented in quiet surroundings. A brightly colored visual stimulus presented against a brightly colored background may be less salient than a stimulus with more subdued colors presented against a colorless background.

> Stars in the night sky are easier to see when viewed in rural areas than in urban areas, where city lights raise the level of foreground illumination. The stars are more salient in darker night skies, even though their intensity does not change.

Increasing the intensity or salience of treatment stimuli can help brain-injured patients whose impaired perceptual or attentional processes compromise their perception, recognition, or comprehension of the stimuli. For example, a patient with problems focusing and maintaining attention in the presence of distracting or competing stimuli may perform poorly in structured conversations when a radio is playing in the background. The mental effort required to attend to the conversation and ignore the radio uses processing resources. If resources are diverted from other processes (e.g., comprehension) to shore up attention, attention gets better, and the processes from which the resources are diverted get worse (e.g., the patient attends, but fails to comprehend). If conversational partners increase the intensity of their contributions (e.g., by talking louder, moving in closer, adding gesture) or increase the salience of what they say (e.g., by turning down the radio or moving away from it) the patient's conversational performance improves because the resources no longer needed to overcome the distracting effects of the background noise can be redirected to comprehension and other conversational operations.

> Conversational partners often raise their voices when they talk with brain-injured persons, even though the brain-injured person can hear normally loud speech perfectly well. Many brain-injured persons complain that this is a common (and very annoying) occurrence.

Clinicians sometimes increase the salience of treatment stimuli by presenting them in more than one stimulus modality (most commonly auditory plus visual, as when a clinician simultaneously says the name of an object and shows the patient a picture of it). Several studies have reported slight to moderate improvements in brain-injured adults' performance with multimodality stimulation (Gardiner & Brookshire, 1972; Halpern, 1965; Lambrecht & Marshall, 1983). However, in the studies reporting positive effects of multimodality stimulation for groups of brain-injured adults, the effects, although statistically significant, were not strong, and not all of the participants in the groups exhibited the effects. This suggests that clinicians will know if multimodality stimulation will help a given patient only by trying it and observing its effects on the patient's performance.

> Variability in the effects of a manipulation on the performance of individual participants is common in group studies involving manipulations of treatment stimuli. Although some manipulations seem to have relatively consistent effects across participants, exceptions are common. Consequently, clinicians typically verify the effects of a manipulation by trying it with the patient.

Clarity and Intelligibility. Unclear or ambiguous stimuli are notoriously difficult for brain-injured adults to perceive, discriminate, or interpret. The negative effects of lack of clarity often surface when treatment stimuli are line drawings representing common objects or situations. For patients with visual processing impairments, line drawings that seem unambiguous to the clinician may be ambiguous to the patient. For example, brain-injured adults have a tendency to misperceive the drawing of a harmonica in the Boston Naming Test (Kaplan, Goodglass, & Weintraub, 2001) as a building or a factory (Figure 7-1).

Mills, Knox, Juola, and Salmon (1979) studied the effects of what they called *stimulus uncertainty* as aphasic adults named line drawings of

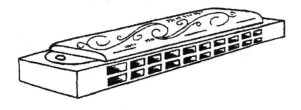

Figure 7-1 ■ An example of a stimulus that sometimes proves ambiguous for brain-injured adults with visual perceptual impairments, who often misidentify it as a building or factory. (From Kaplan, E., Goodglass, H., & Weintraub, S. [2001]. *The Boston Naming Test.* Philadelphia: Lippincott Williams & Wilkins, now owned by Pro-Ed [Austin, Texas].)

common objects. The measure of uncertainty was the number of different names a group of normal adults gave to a drawing. The more different names the normal adults gave a drawing, the higher the drawing's uncertainty. When Mills and associates had a group of non–brain-injured adults and a group of aphasic adults name the drawings, both groups took longer to name drawings with high uncertainty and were more likely to misname them, but the aphasic adults were more strongly affected by stimulus uncertainty than the normal adults. Mills and associates recommended that item uncertainty be added to the list of variables that affect the speed and accuracy of aphasic adults' naming performance.

The operational definition of *uncertainty* provided by Mills and associates provides a way for clinicians or investigators to determine uncertainty values for stimuli used in clinical activities or research.

Redundancy and Context. The words *redundancy* and *context* denote similar and sometimes overlapping concepts. *Redundancy* refers to the presence of information in a stimulus beyond that needed to specify the target response under ideal conditions. For example,

a clinician doing an auditory comprehension drill might increase the redundancy of a command such as *Show me the small red cup.* by saying *I want you to show me a* cup *that is* red *and* small. *Show me the* small red cup. Stimulus redundancy usually improves the performance of brain-injured patients. For example, some patients perform poorly on point-to tasks in which they must point to objects named by the clinician (e.g., *Point to the cup.*), but perform better if the clinician increases the redundancy of the commands by asking the patient to point to objects described by function (e.g., *Point to the one you drink coffee from.*), although the latter command is longer and syntactically more complex. Repetition, paraphrase, and multimodality stimulation are common ways of adding redundancy to task stimuli. (These manipulations no doubt also add salience to the stimuli.)

Some brain-injured patients cannot handle the added information when task stimuli are made more redundant. They seem to have difficulty separating what is important from what is unimportant or redundant. The only way to find out who will profit from redundancy and who will not is to try adding redundancy on a few trials and see what happens.

Context refers to backgrounds or settings that provide information about a stimulus not found in the stimulus itself. For example, a clinician doing an auditory comprehension drill with cups of different sizes and colors might provide contextual support by changing the array of response choices from a group of cups arranged in a row to a group in which each cup is portrayed in its usual location in a place setting.

The context in which responses are elicited often has potent effects on brain-injured patients' response accuracy. One of the most striking characteristics of the behavior of brain-injured adults is that responses that are difficult or impossible in one context can be surprisingly easy in another. Many brain-injured adults say more and say it better when they participate in natural communicative interactions than when they must talk in artificial situations (as when a clinician says *Tell me all the things you can do with a spoon*). Similar effects of context on performance are seen in listening, reading, and writing. The major exceptions are distractible or impulsive right hemisphere–damaged or traumatically brain-injured patients and some aphasic patients who cannot handle unstructured natural situations as well as they handle structured situations in which distractions are minimized and the focus of the interaction is carefully controlled.

Experienced clinicians working one-on-one with brain-injured adults are careful to keep treatment sessions orderly and predictable. They keep instructions and directions concise but complete. They carefully select task stimuli and keep them consistent from trial to trial. They keep the pace of stimulus delivery and responses constant across treatment tasks. They minimize distractions, background noise, and intrusions.

The downside to such orderliness is that patients who perform flawlessly in such supportive contexts often have trouble when they leave the treatment room and have to deal with less well-controlled daily life events. Clinicians may help patients learn to deal with less-structured daily life events by reducing the orderliness and predictability of treatment tasks. For example, when a patient's auditory comprehension reaches normal levels in the clinician's quiet office, the clinician may add background noise or move the activity into a noisy commons room to give the patient practice at comprehending in noisy environments such as those the patient may face in daily life. In addition to building the patient's tolerance for noise, such replication of the elements of daily life environments helps to transfer skills learned in the clinic to daily life by letting the patient practice the skills in situations like those likely to be encountered outside the sheltered clinic environment.

Novelty and Interest Value. The novelty and interest value of treatment stimuli often affect brain-injured patients' performance, although the effect may be subtle, causing clinicians to overlook these characteristics when they select treatment stimuli. Most brain-injured patients attend, comprehend, and respond more accurately and with less effort to novel or personally interesting materials than to materials that lack novelty or interest value, which, unfortunately, are common in many treatment activities. A patient who gives single-word utterances when obliged to talk about cups, spoons, keys, and combs may produce full sentences when asked to talk about family, hobbies, or profession. A patient who struggles to comprehend *Show me the white cup.* may make sense of longer and more complex personally relevant utterances such as *Tell me what the weather was like on the day you got married.*

Faber and Aten (1979) experimentally demonstrated the effects of novelty and interest value on aphasic adults' connected speech. Aphasic adults were instructed to say what they could see in response to drawings that depicted common objects in their normal state and in a broken or altered state (e.g., a shirt with a torn sleeve, a pair of eyeglasses with a broken lens) (Figure 7-2). The aphasic adults produced

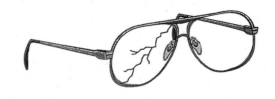

Figure 7-2 ■ An example of how stimulus novelty may be increased by altering the appearance of familiar objects. When shown this drawing without a broken lens, an aphasic patient who was asked to describe this picture said *That's glasses. A pair of glasses.* Later, when asked to talk about the drawing shown here, he said *That's a pair of glasses, but one side is broken. The glass there—the lens—it's broken. Somebody must have dropped 'em on the floor.*

significantly more appropriate words and significantly longer utterances when they talked about the drawings of broken or altered objects than when they talked about the drawings of intact objects.

The apparent pointlessness of many activities used in treatment of brain-injured adults is a common problem. Clinicians should be mindful that pragmatically unnatural activities may not accurately portray a patient's true abilities and may impede generalization of what is acquired in the clinic to daily life. It is not unusual for a brain-injured patient to ask a clinician, *Why am I doing this?* If the clinician does not have a ready answer, reconsideration of the activity may be appropriate.

An item in the 1980 edition of *Communicative Abilities in Daily Living (CADL;* Holland, 1980) illustrates the striking effects of novelty on brain-injured adults' attention and comprehension. The item is contained in a role-playing section of CADL, in which the clinician plays the role of a physician who is giving the patient instructions on lifestyle. The clinician says, *Okay, Mr./Ms. _____ , before our next visit I want you to smoke three packs of cigarettes and drink a bottle of gin a day. Okay?* Few brain-injured patients fail to do a double-take in response to this item. Most express disbelief and ask for clarification. *(What? You want me to smoke and drink? Are you kidding?)*

Cues. Experienced clinicians are careful to maintain consistency in stimuli and how stimuli are presented throughout a treatment activity, but when a patient has trouble, the clinician deviates from the routine. The clinician may intervene to help a struggling patient produce the word *pen* by saying *It starts with "puh."* or *It rhymes with ten.* or *It has ink, and you write with it.* Such clinician behaviors are called *cues*—hints given by a clinician when a patient is having difficulty getting a response out. Cues lead the patient in the direction of a target response without giving the response away. Strategic use of cues gives clinicians control

over the pace of a treatment activity and enables them to adjust the processing load associated with a treatment activity. More importantly, cues give the clinician a dependable way to get the patient back on track when she or he is momentarily defeated by a treatment item. Cues also give clinicians a tool with which to break up strings of error responses and to keep error rates under control.

Response Manipulations

Manipulating the characteristics of responses expected from patients is another way in which clinicians control the difficulty of treatment activities. Clinicians lower the workload associated with formulation and production of responses by reducing the length and complexity of responses, by making responses more natural, by making responses more redundant, or by allowing patients more time to respond.

Length and Complexity. Length and complexity tend to interact in that longer responses also tend to be more complex, but each can be manipulated separately. For example, the number of words in a sentence *(length)* may be manipulated independently of the sentence's syntactic structure *(complexity)*. The length of responses is usually measured by how many units they contain (e.g., syllables or words), or, less often, how much time it takes the patient to perform the responses. The complexity of responses can be defined in many ways, most of which are more subjective than counting units or measuring time. Complexity may be defined *motorically* (the number of different articulatory movements per word or per unit of time), *linguistically* (the number of syntactic operations needed to determine the meaning of a sentence), or *cognitively* (the presumed amount of abstraction or inference needed to produce an appropriate response to a spoken message).

As a general rule, increasing the length or complexity of responses increases their appetite for processing resources, and if resources are in short supply, increasing response length or response complexity leads to worsened patient performance. It is important to understand that the effects of response complexity may not be limited to the adequacy of the responses themselves but may extend back to input processes such as perception, discrimination, and comprehension, depending on how the patient attempts to compensate for resource shortfall.

Familiarity and Meaningfulness. The familiarity and meaningfulness of responses is determined by the frequency with which a patient has performed the responses in the past. Highly practiced and socially meaningful responses (e.g., social greetings and farewells) are almost always easier for brain-injured adults than less-practiced responses produced in unusual contexts (e.g., naming objects or pictures). Many brain-injured patients who can say little else can get out highly practiced social verbalizations such as *hello* and *goodbye* in appropriate contexts.

The effects of familiarity go beyond speech. Brain-injured patients with language comprehension impairments usually comprehend personally relevant material (e.g., questions about home and family) better than impersonal material (e.g., questions about the relative sizes of butterflies and seagulls). Brain-injured patients with impaired vocabulary are typically more successful at accessing frequently occurring words such as *house* or *table* than infrequently occurring words such as *scholar* or *piccolo*.

Delay. Many brain-injured adults have impairments in immediate memory that make it difficult for them to maintain information or action plans in memory for more than a few seconds. One consequence is that the patient's performance deteriorates when the clinician imposes delay between presentation of treatment stimuli and the time at which the patient may respond. Patients whose responses to spoken commands are quick and accurate when they are permitted to respond immediately may falter and stumble if they must wait 5 or 10 seconds before responding. Patients who

flawlessly repeat phrases under no-delay conditions may stumble, struggle, and grope when forced to retain the model in memory for 5 or 10 seconds before producing it.

Delay is not always a stumbling block for brain-injured patients. Sometimes imposing (or permitting) delays between stimuli and responses improves a brain-injured patient's performance rather than hurting it. Most brain-injured adults suffer from slow cognitive processing. They need more time to retrieve the words they need to express their ideas, to combine words into meaningful strings, to recognize complex or unfamiliar stimuli, and to deduce the meaning of incoming messages. Most brain-injured adults are excruciatingly aware of their slow responses and feel compelled to get responses out as quickly as possible. Encouraging these patients to respond quickly adds to their problems. Teaching them to resist the tyranny of the clock usually helps.

Some brain-injured patients try to compensate for their immediate memory problems by responding before the memory traces of the stimulus have time to decay. In treatment activities they may respond before the clinician has finished instructing or providing a stimulus. This strategy rarely works and often makes things worse because the patient misses the information-bearing elements of the stimulus that are given after they have begun their response. Imposing short delays between stimuli and responses usually improves the performance of such hyper-responsive patients.

Although it is not always obvious which patients will be hurt by response delay and which will be helped by it, the following general guidelines may help. When a patient's immediate memory is impaired and a treatment task makes demands on immediate memory, imposing response delay usually adds to the patient's troubles. When a patient's internal processing is slow or inefficient and the treatment task calls on the slow or inefficient processes, permitting response delays may help the patient.

What does a skilled clinician do when a patient has impaired immediate memory plus slow or inefficient internal processes? If the clinician's purpose is to target immediate memory, the clinician might take slow processing out of the picture by slowing the rate at which stimuli are presented while enforcing a delay between delivery of the stimulus and the time at which the patient is permitted to respond. If the clinician's purpose is to target the slow processing, the clinician might minimize memory demands by permitting the patient to respond immediately but speed up the rate at which stimuli are presented to put the appropriate load on processing speed and efficiency.

Response Redundancy. Response redundancy usually enhances patients' performance. Redundancy comes in two forms. Elements may be repeated within responses or across trials.

Within-response redundancy is a prominent feature of many speech-articulation drills in which a patient is asked to produce strings of words in which the same articulatory positions are repeated in elements of each string (e.g., baby, bible, bobbin, beanbag). *Across-trials redundancy* is common in tasks in which some characteristics of the patient's responses are the same from trial to trial (e.g., the pointing or gesturing responses called for on every trial of some auditory comprehension tasks). The ultimate redundancy between task stimuli and the patient's responses happens when the clinician and patient produce responses in unison. One step down in redundancy are *repetition tasks* in which the patient's responses are direct copies of the clinician's productions, produced immediately after the clinician's productions.

GENERAL CONCEPTS 7-2

- Clinicians usually adjust the difficulty of treatment activities for brain-injured adults so that patients are challenged but not overwhelmed. This means that patients' responses include a mix of immediate and correct responses, delayed responses, and self-corrected responses with scattered errors.

- Tasks in which 60% to 70% of a patient's responses are immediate and correct are appropriate for many brain-injured patients. When 90% or more of a patient's responses are immediate and correct, the difficulty of the task may be increased.

- *Resource-allocation models* of cognition assume that every human has a finite amount of cognitive resources available for cognitive processes. If the resources needed for active cognitive processes exceed the supply, performance deteriorates.

- Resource-allocation models of cognition assume that brain injury diminishes the available pool of processing resources. Brain-

- injured adults are thought to be more sensitive to cognitive processing workload than non–brain-injured adults.

- *Cues* provide a dependable way for clinicians to help patients correct or recover from error responses. Clinicians often provide cues in impromptu, trial-by-trial fashion to help patients who are struggling with a specific item in a treatment task.

- Clinicians may adjust the difficulty of treatment tasks by manipulating stimulus aspects such as *intensity and salience, clarity and intelligibility, redundancy and contextual support,* or the *novelty and interest value* of task stimuli.

- Clinicians also may adjust the difficulty of treatment tasks by manipulating response requirements such as response length and complexity, the familiarity and naturalness of responses, response delay, or the redundancy of responses required from patients.

INSTRUCTIONS AND FEEDBACK

Clinicians organize and regulate brain-injured patients' performance in treatment activities (and also in assessment) by *instructing* and *providing feedback*. *Instructions* tell the patient what to do in an upcoming activity. *Feedback* tells the patient how they did on a treatment trial or a collection of trials. Although there is some functional overlap between instructions and feedback, each serves a different purpose. Clinicians who keep the purposes straight keep treatment activities focused and running smoothly. Clinicians who give feedback when they should be instructing or instruct when they should be giving feedback confuse the patient and compromise the effectiveness of treatment.

Instructions

Instructions are the lead-in to treatment activities. They tell patients what they will be doing and (sometimes) why they will be doing it. Good instructions are clear and concise. They are delivered at a rate the patient can handle. They use language the patient can understand. They provide everything the patient needs to know, but no more. Many beginning clinicians (and some experienced ones) overdo instructions by providing more information than the patient needs or by unnecessarily repeating or paraphrasing instructions until the patient is confused. Instructional excess can be avoided or at least minimized by monitoring the patient's apparent understanding and by checking with the patient to see if they understand. Most brain-injured patients, including those with severe impairments, indicate understanding or confusion by facial expression, gesture (especially head nods), and demeanor. Clinicians who attend to these sometimes subtle signs tend not to stray into instructional excess.

Experienced clinicians know that some demonstration and a few practice trials can take the place of much verbal instruction and are a good way to check a patient's understanding of instructions. The clinician begins with a concise explanation of the upcoming activity, demon-strates the expected responses, and gives a few practice trials to see if the patient has gotten the point. If the patient's performance on the practice trials shows that he or she knows what is expected, the clinician moves into the treatment activity. If the patient's performance shows that he or she does not know what is expected, the clinician explains and demonstrates again, guided by what the patient did during the practice trials (Box 7-1).

Box 7-1	*Instruction and Demonstration in a New Treatment Activity*

A clinician is starting a new treatment activity with Mrs. Adair, an aphasic woman with a moderate language comprehension impairment and serious word-retrieval difficulties, both of which cause her great concern.

Clinician: Okay Mrs. Adair, now we'll be doing something different.

The clinician alerts Mrs. Adair to the upcoming change and gives her some time to make the needed mental adjustments.

Clinician: I'm going to show you some pictures, one at a time. They're pictures of things you have in your kitchen at home, and they're the same ones you've been naming for me.

The materials are familiar to Mrs. Adair and relevant to her daily life. The clinician relates the new activity to one with which Mrs. Adair has had experience.

Clinician: I know that you can name them, because you got all their names right last time and this time. Now let's see what else you can say about them.

The clinician tells Mrs. Adair the purpose of the new activity and provides her with time to process and make mental adjustments.

Clinician: Here's what I want you to do. I want you to tell me what you do with each one as I show it to you.

The clinician highlights the upcoming instruction with an alerting phrase.

Clinician: Are you ready?

The clinician monitors Mrs. Adair's facial expression, eye movements, and other indicators of her understanding and readiness. Mrs. Adair

Box 7-1	*Instruction and Demonstration in a New Treatment Activity—cont'd*

nods, and the clinician puts a picture of a broom on the table.

Clinician: See this one? Tell me what you do with it.

The clinician provides a lead-in question to highlight the request.

Mrs. Adair: Broom.

Clinician: No, that's not what I had in mind. Tell me what you do with it.

Mrs. Adair: Sweep.

Clinician: Fine! Here's another one.

The clinician puts down a picture of a food mixer.

Mrs. Adair: Mixer.

Clinician: No, that's not what I'm looking for. Tell me what you do with it. I'll show you what I mean.

The clinician turns over the next card—a picture of a knife.

Clinician: This is something I'd use to cut things up. I'd cut with a knife. See what I mean? I didn't name it. I told you what I do with it. Now you try one. Remember, tell me what you do with it.

The clinician turns over a card—a picture of a kettle.

Mrs. Adair: Well, it's a kettle—and I'd boil potatoes or make a stew in it.

Clinician: Great! That's perfect! Let's do another one...

Several things about the clinician's behavior with Mrs. Adair are noteworthy. The clinician uses repetition, paraphrase, and lead-in phrases liberally to highlight important information and to give Mrs. Adair extra processing time. She asks Mrs. Adair if she is ready before beginning the first trial. For experienced clinicians this behavior is so routine as to be almost automatic. Often this is not true for beginners, who move too fast and present stimuli before the patient is ready. When Mrs. Adair responds to the first practice item with its name, the clinician gives her appropriate feedback, does not correct her, and repeats the instruction. When Mrs. Adair continues to name on the second practice trial,

the clinician adds demonstration to repetition of the task instructions, at which point Mrs. Adair responds appropriately.

Mrs. Adair's clinician combines instruction and explanation with response-contingent feedback to coach her into a new treatment activity with minimum fuss. When Mrs. Adair's responses to the first two practice items are not what the clinician intends, the clinician combines negative feedback *(no)* with explanation *(that's not what I had in mind)* that elaborates on the feedback and also helps to soften its hard edges. Importantly, the clinician does not correct Mrs. Adair's unacceptable responses (e.g., *No, you sweep with a broom.* or *No, you mix food with a mixer.*) because the problem is not with the rightness of Mrs. Adair's responses but with her understanding of the new activity or her ability to change her response set from naming to describing function. After two practice trials in which feedback and explanation fail to elicit the intended responses, the clinician moves on to demonstration combined with explanation. The switch in tactics succeeds, and the clinician and patient continue to the new activity.

Knowing when to provide feedback; knowing what kind of feedback to provide; and knowing how to combine feedback, explanation, and demonstration are important clinical skills. When clinicians choose to deliver feedback, it is important that they observe important distinctions between *incentive feedback* and *information feedback*.

Incentive Feedback

Incentive feedback can maintain or eliminate behaviors whose only purpose is to elicit or avoid the feedback. If the feedback stops, the behavior stops. Food pellets that drop into a hopper when a pigeon pecks a key are incentive feedback (sometimes called *positive reinforcement*) that keeps the pigeon pecking the key. Quarters that drop down the chute of a slot machine are incentive feedback that keeps the tourist from South Dakota putting coins in and pulling the lever. Disconnect the key from the pellet dispenser, and the pigeon loses interest in the key. Program the slot machine to keep the tourist's coins and return none, and the tourist eventually stops putting coins in and pulling the lever.

The power of incentive feedback over behavior depends strongly on the subject's real or apparent state of deprivation for the feedback stimulus. Feed the pigeon until it is no longer hungry, and it loses interest in pecking the key. Give the tourist $4 million, a new BMW, and a ticket to Tahiti, and the tourist loses interest in putting coins in the machine and pulling its lever.

Increasing the magnitude of incentive feedback or increasing the participant's level of deprivation often increases the feedback's effect on behavior, at least within certain ranges. Increase the payoff on the pecking key or the slot machine, and their users respond faster and stay at it longer (unless the payoff is large enough to reduce the subjects' deprivation levels).

Incentive feedback is most useful in the clinic when the objective is to change the frequency of a behavior that the patient can do but doesn't do enough, such as making eye contact with listeners, or does too often, such as shouting at doctors and nurses. Many different stimuli can serve as incentive feedback, and what works as an incentive for one person may not for another. Some stimuli, such as food (to hungry people), water (to thirsty people), electric shocks (to most), and loud noise (except for patrons of rock concerts) seem intrinsically rewarding or punishing—they serve as reward or punishment for most of the adult population. Other stimuli are less intrinsically rewarding or punishing, and they work for smaller segments of the population. Verbal approval and reproof, for example, are not intrinsically rewarding or punishing, but they have rewarding and punishing properties for some individuals.

Information Feedback

Information feedback tells the recipient about the appropriateness, correctness, or accuracy of responses. Information feedback comes in many forms: a tracing on an oscilloscope, a smiley face drawn on a page of spelling words, a smile and spoken *good*. Incentive feedback can also function as information feedback, as when a traumatically brain-injured patient gets an M&M candy contingent on each successful detection of a target in a visual monitoring task. Information feedback need not possess incentive characteristics to be effective in regulating the performance of many brain-injured adults—those who want to get better and for whom the payoff is not in the feedback but in the improved performance that comes with progress in treatment. For these patients it is the information about the appropriateness, correctness, or accuracy of the behaviors leading to the feedback that is important. The incentive properties are an added attraction.

There are no specific rules for how and when feedback should be delivered in treatment of brain-injured adults because patients differ in their need for feedback, and clinicians differ in their preferences with regard to what kind of feedback to deliver and when to deliver it. However, the following comments may help beginning clinicians get at least a general sense of how feedback functions in treatment activities.

Incentive feedback does not play an important part in treatment of most mildly to minimally impaired brain-injured adults because they want to get better and will do what is needed without added incentives. For these patients, recovery is the incentive. Severely impaired, depressed, agitated, or confused patients who do not recognize progress in treatment activities or who are not rewarded by progress may need incentive feedback. Traumatically brain-injured patients in the early stages of recovery often need incentive feedback. They have little tolerance for tasks that require mental or physical effort, so incentives may be the only way to get these patients to work and to keep them on task. Incentive feedback may also be useful for patients in the late stages of dementia, when social rewards and penalties no longer function to maintain or change behavior.

Clinician Comments

Most experienced clinicians sprinkle positive comments such as *You're doing great!* or *That was the best you've ever done!* throughout treatment sessions. Brain-injured adults, like the rest of us, appreciate encouragement when they are working hard. Although such comments do not qualify as feedback because they are not contingent upon responses, they contribute to patient motivation and help to maintain performance in difficult tasks, and they make treatment sessions tolerable and sometimes enjoyable.

Stoicheff (1960) experimentally demonstrated the effects of clinicians' comments on brain-injured adults' performances. She studied three groups of aphasic adults who performed picture-naming and word-reading tasks in three instructional conditions. Those in one group heard encouraging comments such as *I'm very pleased with what you have been able to do today.* or *I expect that you will do very well today.* Those in another group received discouraging instructions such as *As I expected, you did even more poorly this time than last time* or *This seems to be harder for you each time instead of easier.* Those in a third group received neutral instructions such as *We'll be working on different things today.* and neutral feedback such as *Here is the next one.*

Stoicheff also gave positive feedback (e.g., *Good!* or *You're doing fine!*) to the *encouragement group* and negative feedback (e.g., *You missed that one!* or *That's wrong.*) to the *discouragement group.* After three sessions, the performance of the group that received discouraging comments and negative feedback was, not surprisingly, significantly worse than that of the group that received encouraging comments and positive feedback. The performance of the group that received neutral comments and neutral feedback fell between that of the other two groups. Stoicheff commented that participants who had received discouraging comments and negative feedback were withdrawn, tense, and hostile by the end of the third session, whereas participants receiving encouraging comments and positive feedback were spontaneous, friendly, and smiling.

At the end of the study, Stoicheff explained to the participants that they had been in a study, and reassured those in the discouragement and neutral groups to counteract any detrimental effects of their treatment on subsequent performance. It is unlikely that Stoicheff could have done this study today because of rules requiring that subjects be told, in advance, about the purposes and general conduct of any study in which they participate. I think it unlikely that participants in the discouragement group would welcome Stoicheff as their full-time clinician.

How Clinicians Use Feedback

Many clinicians tend to avoid negative feedback, perhaps because they do not wish to discourage patients. Brookshire and associates (1977) evaluated clinicians' use of feedback in 40 videotaped sessions of aphasia treatment and found that clinicians were biased toward positive feedback—the clinicians appearing in the videotapes gave positive feedback for more than 60% of acceptable responses but gave negative feedback for only about 10% of unacceptable patient responses. They were as likely to provide positive feedback as to provide negative feedback for unacceptable responses (Figure 7-3).

It is not clear why clinicians have an apparent aversion to negative feedback. Perhaps they wish to avoid discouraging their patients, as Stoicheff did with her negative instructions and comments. However, it is important to remember that Stoicheff's negative instructions and comments were not contingent on poor performance. It is not surprising that her subjects were tense and hostile following three sessions of negative instructions and criticism unrelated to their performance. Brain-injured adults, like the rest of us, are likely to be irritated by gratuitous negative commentary from another, but few are so sensitive that they cannot deal with

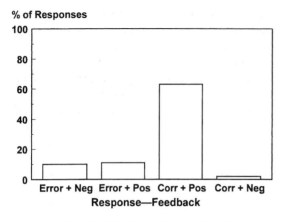

% of Responses

Figure 7-3 ■ Percentage of aphasic adults' error responses receiving negative feedback *(error + neg)*, percentage of aphasic adults' error responses receiving positive feedback *(error + pos)*, percentage of aphasic adults' acceptable responses receiving positive feedback *(corr + pos)*, and percentage of aphasic adults' acceptable responses receiving negative feedback *(corr + neg)*. (Data from Brookshire, R.H., Krueger, K., Nicholas, L., & Cicciarelli [1977]. Analysis of clinician-patient interactions in aphasia treatment. In R. H. Brookshire [Ed.], *Clinical Aphasiology Conference Proceedings* [pp. 181-187]. Minneapolis: BRK Publishers.)

negative feedback if it is delivered contingent on off-target responses and if the overall mood created by the clinician is supportive and reassuring.

It is true, however, that most clinicians (including me) deliver positive feedback at full strength but deliver negative feedback in diluted form. One seldom hears clinicians say *wrong, no,* or *That's not right.* in response to inaccurate patient responses. They are more likely to say *close* or *not quite,* and they sometimes sweeten the dose by blending it with weak positive feedback, as in *good try, but that's not quite it.* Clinicians' positive feedback tends to be more emphatic. Exclamations such as *good!, great!, super!,* or *wonderful!* are commonly heard in treatment sessions. By manipulating the strength

of positive and negative feedback in this way, clinicians may put more emphasis on the positive aspects of a patient's performance, contribute to a patient's self-confidence, and maintain an encouraging and supportive atmosphere.

As the patient and clinician become familiar with each other and with treatment activities, feedback often becomes subtle. When a treatment activity has settled into a consistent pace and rhythm in which the clinician's delivery of stimuli and the patient's responses have fallen into a regular temporal pattern, the clinician need only disrupt the pattern by withholding delivery of a stimulus for a few seconds to signal to the patient that a response was off-target. Similarly, clinicians who acknowledge on-target responses with a consistent head-nod need only withhold it to signal that a response was not satisfactory. Most moderately impaired to mildly impaired brain-injured patients quickly become attuned to these subtle cues, but those with more severe impairments may need more conspicuous feedback, and they may need it after every response, rather than intermittently.

A patient's familiarity with a treatment task also affects the nature and timing of feedback delivered by experienced clinicians. Patients often profit from feedback for every response when new treatment tasks are introduced and the patient is busy determining the point of the task and discovering the criteria the clinician uses to decide what constitutes an on-target response. Consequently, at the beginning of new treatment tasks, feedback schedules tend to be nearly continuous (feedback after every response), and feedback stimuli tend to be more overt and more intense. As a patient gains experience with the task, feedback becomes intermittent, and feedback stimuli often become more subtle.

Delivering overt feedback contingent on every response is rarely necessary once a treatment activity is a familiar routine with a consistent pace. Then, intermittent positive feedback for most on-target responses plus negative feedback for off-target responses is usually sufficient.

If the patient knows when responses are off-target, negative feedback may also be delivered intermittently. Feedback schedules in which every patient response gets overt feedback soon become tiresome for clinicians and patients, and the effectiveness of the feedback diminishes. As noted previously, however, most clinicians provide subtle indications of response acceptability even when they do not provide overt feedback, so in this sense it might be said that most clinicians provide some form of feedback for almost every patient response.

Keeping the purposes of *feedback* separate from the purposes of *instruction* is important. *Feedback* signals to the patient whether responses are acceptable and is distributed throughout treatment activities. *Instructions* come at the beginning of treatment tasks and tell the patient what to do. If a patient's poor performance is caused by misunderstanding or incomplete understanding, the clinician gives more instruction. If a patient's poor performance represents impaired formulation or production, the clinician provides information feedback regarding how or why the response was off-target. Providing negative feedback when deficient performance is caused by the patient's misunderstanding or incomplete understanding of task instructions is a procedural error on the part of the clinician, as is providing instruction when the patient already understands the task but makes off-target responses because of impaired formulation or production.

Comparison of Impairment Level and Activity-Participation Level Intervention

The procedures described in the preceding sections pertain directly to impairment level treatment in which carefully selected stimuli are presented, responses are elicited, and feedback is delivered based on the acceptability of the patient's responses. Although manipulating stimuli and responses, providing instruction, and delivering feedback are key elements of impairment level intervention, they also per-

tain to intervention at activity and participation levels. Although intervention at the activity and participation levels may be less pedagogic, the effects of task difficulty, stimulus characteristics, and response expectations cannot be ignored. Acquisition and perfection of strategies at the activity and participation levels depend on the same principles of learning as facilitation of underlying processes at the impairment level of intervention.

Although principles of learning apply equally to impairment level and activity-participation level treatment, there are some general differences between them, reflecting how the purposes of intervention are conceptualized. Intervention at the activity and participation levels differs from intervention at the impairment level not so much in the procedures used as in the goals of intervention. Whereas the goal of impairment level intervention may be stimulating, repairing, or compensating for impairments in underlying cognitive and communicative processes, the goal of intervention at the activity and participation levels is to help clients maximize daily life communicative success in domains relevant to clients' needs and desires. (Impairment level intervention may, however, indirectly enhance a client's competence and participation in activities of daily living.)

The goals of intervention at activity and participation levels are based not so much on the results of standardized objective testing as on consultation with the client, a significant other, or both, often supplemented with information from rating scales or questionnaires. Estimates of progress and outcome are likewise based not so much on changes on objective standardized tests as on changes in subjective judgments elicited by rating scales or questionnaires.

Worrall (1995) summarized the stages of intervention at the activity and participation levels of disablement as follows:
- Determining the client's everyday communicative needs
- Collaborative goal-setting

- Organizing goals in order of importance to the client
- Observing and rating the client's performance in everyday communication activities
- Constructing a profile of the client's communicative performance in everyday activities
- Implementing intervention and reassessing goals
- Measuring outcome

Individualized assessment of each client's unique communicative needs and wishes provides the starting point for intervention at the activity and participation levels of disablement. The clinician, client, and significant others collaborate to develop a list of the client's most important communicative needs and wishes and rank the items according to their importance to the client. Assessment of the client's communicative strengths and weaknesses in natural settings follows, to identify the client's successful and unsuccessful communicative strategies. The results of the assessment are used to construct a profile of the client's communicative strengths and weaknesses, keyed to the list of communicative needs and wishes.

Intervention continues the collaborative relationship between the client and the clinician. The client and the clinician collaborate to select targets for intervention and to design, evaluate, modify, and replace strategies (if necessary) for enhancing successful information exchange and social interaction. Strategies are selected, constructed, tried, and refined, emphasizing strategies that enhance participation, capitalize on the client's strengths, are easily maintained, and are socially appropriate. Creativity and flexibility in selection, application, and revision of strategies are emphasized. Damico (1992) summarizes principles underlying activities-participation level intervention as follows:

- Interactions are client focused. The clinician does not control topics, activities, or timing of events but elaborates on the client's contributions.

- Activities are natural and meaningful to the client.
- Feedback is natural and situationally appropriate; rather than responding to the client's performance with feedback such as *good* or *not quite,* the clinician responds with natural conversational behaviors such as maintaining the topic, elaborating on the client's contributions, or asking for clarification.
- The client and the clinician work toward agreed-upon specific goals such as improving the client's ability to elaborate on topics or increasing the rate of conversational participation.

Progress toward the goals of activities-participation level intervention is usually assessed with qualitative measures—subjective judgments by the client, clinician, and significant others and rating scales or questionnaires. Worrall (2000) emphasizes the importance of client-based outcome measures that are relevant and meaningful to the client. She recommends *goal-attainment scaling* (Kiresuk & Sherman, 1968) for focusing outcome measures on the specific targets of intervention. In *goal-attainment scaling,* goals are agreed upon by the clinician and the client, and outcome is measured using a 5-point Likert scale with scores ranging from +2 to –2:

- Most favorable outcome (+2)
- Better than expected outcome (+1)
- Expected outcome (0)
- Less than expected outcome (–1)
- Least favorable outcome (–2)

Worrall comments that goal-attainment scaling is appropriate for measuring outcome regardless of the model of intervention used because the goals are patient-specific and the measure of outcome is based on the patient's specific needs.

Some differences between impairment level intervention and activity-participation level intervention are structural (e.g., the location of treatment/intervention), and some differences are procedural (e.g., the timing and duration of intervention).

Impairment level treatment usually takes place at a medical center or clinic. Activity-participation level interventions (especially the first few sessions) often take place at a medical center or clinic but may be held in natural contexts (e.g., the patient's home, a restaurant, a store, or an office). Impairment level treatment typically spans a shorter time and is more intensive than activity-participation level treatment. Sessions in impairment level treatment tend to be closely spaced and last for a few weeks, after which the patient is discharged. Activity-participation level intervention sessions are usually more widely spaced, consisting of periodic meetings in which the patient and the clinician devise, test, and perfect strategies. Coaching and support may continue for months or years, often with no formal end to intervention. Some key differences between impairment level and activity-participation level intervention are summarized in Table 7-1.

TABLE 7-1	General Differences Between Impairment-Level and Activity-Participation Approaches to Treatment of Brain-Injured Adults	
Function	Impairment-Level Approaches	Activity-Level and Participation-Level Approaches
Location of intervention	Clinic or treatment facility	Natural contexts
Role of clinician	Director, manager	Collaborator, guide, coach
Derivation of goals	Based on results of assessment and diagnostic decisions.	Based on collaborative assessment of client's needs and desires.
Decision-making	Clinician selects processes or abilities to restore or repair, sometimes with input from the patient.	Clinician and client select targets for intervention.
Focus of intervention	Restoration, repair, or circumvention of defective processes and functions.	Successful and fulfilling daily-life performance and participation.
Measures of efficacy	Quantitative measures of change on standardized tests.	Qualitative measures based on direct observation of client in daily-life activities or on client's or associate's ratings,
Methods	Stimulation, facilitation of defective processes and functions, compensation for functions that cannot be restored or repaired.	Client/clinician collaboration to identify client's wants and needs and to design and implement strategies to satisfy the wants and needs. Guided practice and coaching.
Measures of progress	Quantitative measures of accuracy, responsiveness, promptness, and efficiency of responses.	Qualitative reports of success, satisfaction, participation in daily life experiences.
Temporal characteristics	Intensive, closely spaced treatment sessions with discharge based on results of quantitative assessment, usually within weeks.	Periodic collaborative meetings to devise, modify, and apply strategies. Coaching and support may continue for months or years, often with no formal discharge.

Based on Lyon, J. G. (1992). Communication use and participation in life for adults with aphasia in natural settings: The scope of the problem. *American Journal of Speech-Language Pathology, 1,* 7-14.

GENERAL CONCEPTS 7-3

- Appropriate use of instructions and feedback is an important clinical skill. *Instructions* tell patients what is expected of them. *Feedback* tells a patient how they did on a particular trial or series of trials.
- *Incentive feedback* entails delivery of consequences that are intrinsically rewarding or punishing. *Information feedback* entails delivery of consequences that give the individual qualitative information about how a response or series of responses relates to the target responses. Incentive feedback is not needed by most brain-injured patients.
- Many clinicians favor positive feedback over negative feedback. They may deliver negative feedback in attenuated form (e.g., *Not quite...*) or soften it with mild positive feedback (e.g., *Nice try, but...*).

- Many brain-injured patients are attuned to subtle forms of feedback conveyed by a clinician's body language, vocal inflection, and timing in delivery of stimuli or feedback.
- *General encouragement* (positive comments that may or may not be contingent on certain responses) helps clinicians keep treatment activities pleasant and rewarding for the patient.
- Activity-participation level approaches to treatment tend to be less structured and less prescriptive than impairment level approaches. They tend to focus on patients' wishes and daily life needs rather than specific cognitive or linguistic processes or behaviors.

RECORDING AND CHARTING PERFORMANCE

Documenting what goes on in treatment by keeping organized and accurate records of patients' performances is an important clinical responsibility. Accurate records permit clinicians to establish stable baseline levels of performance to measure the effects of treatment. Sensitive measures of changes in a patient's performance during treatment give clinicians information they can use to modify treatment procedures or to introduce new procedures to maximize treatment effectiveness. Good record-keeping contributes to the orderliness and efficiency of treatment because accurate and efficient recording of a patient's performance is impossible if the treatment is not orderly and easily described. Finally, healthcare accrediting agencies and those who pay for speech-language pathology services require that clinicians keep accurate and objective records

of patients' performances and the effects of treatment.

There is a trade-off between simplicity and completeness when clinicians record and chart patient performance. Simple scoring systems are easy to use and usually are reliable. Complex scoring systems are harder to use and are less likely to be reliable. Simple scoring systems (e.g., correct/incorrect) may not be sensitive to small but important changes in performance. Complex systems may capture small changes in performance but may not be clinically practical if they are so elaborate and intrusive that they disrupt the rhythm of treatment, compromise the naturalness of the interaction between the clinician and the patient, and divert the attention of the patient and the clinician from the primary objectives of treatment.

Record-keeping methods cover a range of complexity and sophistication, from simple forms devised by individual clinicians to standardized methods marketed commercially.

Both personal and commercial record-keeping methods provide a way of labeling or describing the treatment activity, space for listing treatment stimuli (usually trial-by-trial), and space for entering the patient's responses to treatment stimuli. Figure 7-4 shows an example of a personalized record sheet for a treatment session in which the clinician has recorded a patient's responses to 10 test stimuli across 3 trials in each of 6 treatment activities.

LaPointe's (1991) *Base 10 Programmed Stimulation* is an example of a commercially marketed system for task specification and response recording that formalizes the personalized record-keeping systems used by many clinicians. In Base 10 Programmed Stimulation, scores for patients' responses to treatment stimuli are entered on a response form (Figure 7-5), where the clinician records information about the treatment task, target performance criteria, the scoring system used, and the stimuli presented. The response form also provides a graph on which a patient's performance can be charted over several treatment sessions.

In most didactic treatment tasks (e.g., pointing to pictures named by the clinician or writing words dictated by the clinician), the clinician controls the rate at which stimuli are delivered—the clinician does not deliver the stimulus for a new trial until the patient's response to the last trial has been scored. It is easy for the clinician to score every patient response as it occurs in such highly structured activities *(continuous scoring)*. The situation is different in less structured treatment tasks such as conversations, in which target behaviors occur unpredictably and the clinician no longer controls the rate at which scorable responses occur. In such tasks, target responses may occur so rapidly that the clinician cannot write a score for every response without falling behind. In these situations the clinician has two options— *off-line continuous scoring* or *on-line intermittent scoring*.

In *off-line continuous scoring* the clinician records the treatment activity on audiotape or videotape and does the scoring later, stopping and rewinding the tape as necessary to score every response. The advantage of off-line scoring is that every response can be scored without the need for the clinician to hurry transcription and scoring to keep up. There are some disadvantages to off-line scoring. It requires the use of videotape or audiotape recording equipment, which may not always be available. When recording equipment is available, its presence in the testing or treatment session may distract the patient or make the patient uneasy or tense. The time it takes to do off-line scoring may make it impractical for clinicians with busy schedules and pressing demands on their time.

On-line intermittent scoring provides an alternative to off-line scoring. When clinicians score responses intermittently they score a percentage of patient responses rather than scoring every response. Intermittent scoring makes it possible for clinicians to score rapidly occurring responses on-line. (Intermittent scoring also can be used with off-line scoring.) Various formalized procedures for intermittent scoring have been described, but most clinicians simply try to score as many responses as they comfortably can. They score the first occurrence of a target response, taking as much time as they need to decide on a score and enter it on a record form, ignoring any scorable responses that occur in the meantime. Then they look for the next scorable response, score it, and go on to the next response. The proportion of a patient's responses that gets scored depends on the complexity of the scoring system and the rate at which responses occur. Complex scoring systems and fast response rates reduce the proportion of responses that gets scored.

There is no absolute proportion of responses that must be scored to generate an accurate representation of patient performance in a treatment task. Clinicians using intermittent scoring can usually score at least half of most patients' responses. Brookshire, Nicholas, and Krueger (1978) reported that scoring only 20% of responses yielded records that deviated from

Patient: J. Smith			Date: 7/12/07			Clinician: M. Johnson											
Task	Name			Point by name			Point by function			Imitation			Sentence completion			Point by two's		
Trial	1	2	3	1	2	3	1	2	3	1	2	3	1	2	3	1	2	3
Stimulus																		
Pencil	15	13	15	13	15	15	13	15	15	15	15	15	15	15	13	13	13	15
Bell	15	15	15	15	15	13	13	13	15	15	15	15	13	13	15	13	15	13
Comb	13	15	13	13	13	10	13	9	10	15	13	15	13	15	15	15	15	15
Knife	15	15	15	13	13	13	15	15	15	13	15	13	15	14	14	13	10	15
Flag	15	15	15	15	15	15	15	15	13	13	15	15	15	15	15	9	13	15
Book	15	15	15	5	15	15	13	15	15	15	10	15	14	14	14	13	15	13
Horn	13	15	15	10	15	15	10	15	15	15	15	15	15	15	15	13	13	15
Lamp	15	15	15	15	15	15	15	13	15	15	15	15	15	15	15	15	15	9
Brush	10	15	15	13	15	15	15	15	15	15	15	13	15	15	15	10	15	15
Candle	15	15	15	13	15	15	15	15	13	15	15	15	13	13	15	15	10	15
Mean score	14.6			13.7			13.9			14.5			14.4			13.4		

Figure 7-4 ■ A record sheet for recording patient performance in treatment tasks. Treatment stimuli are listed in the left-hand column, and treatment tasks are listed across the top. The clinician administered three consecutive trials that elicited 30 patient responses within each treatment task.

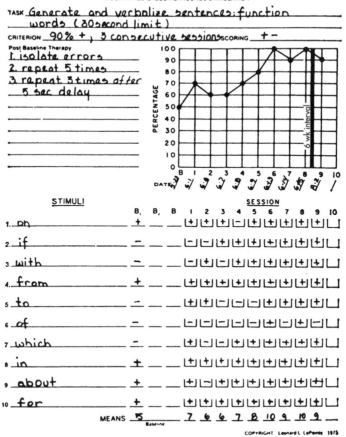

Figure 7-5 ■ The Base 10 Programmed Stimulation task specification and response recording form. The task is described at the top left, the treatment stimuli are described at the bottom left, and the patient's responses are recorded on the bottom right. The columns labeled *B* are for entering the patient's scores in baseline conditions before treatment begins. (From LaPointe, L.L. [1991]. *Base 10 Response Forms and Revised Manual: Performances and Treatment Measurement System.* Clifton Park, NY: Singular/Thomson Delmar Learning. Copyright Leonard L. LaPointe, 1975.)

patients' actual performance by less than 10%, provided that the sample was distributed across the treatment activity. Therefore, scoring half of all responses almost certainly will yield accurate representations of a patient's performance if the scored responses are fairly evenly distributed across the task.

MEASURING THE EFFECTS OF TREATMENT

Measuring patient performance across time permits clinicians to establish baselines against which the effects of treatment can be measured and permits clinicians to describe changes in a patient's performance as treatment progresses.

Establishing pretreatment baselines is particularly important for patients who may be neurologically recovering, because a patient's improvement on a communicative or cognitive task during treatment may reflect the effects of treatment, the effects of spontaneous recovery, or a combination of the two.

Although physiologic recovery is the most obvious and well-known source of spontaneous improvement in brain-injured patient's communicative and cognitive abilities, these abilities may also improve as a patient learns to cope with and compensate for the effects of their neurologic condition. Many patients with central nervous system injury find ways to lessen the behavioral, cognitive, or communicative consequences of their injuries, either on their own or with help from family or friends. Like spontaneous physiologic recovery, these spontaneous behavioral compensations are most likely in the first weeks or months postinjury.

Clinicians providing treatment to patients who may be experiencing spontaneous recovery may choose from several procedures to ensure that treatment, and not some other variable, accounts for changes observed during a treatment program. Consider, for illustrative purposes, Mrs. Benchley, a fictional patient. She is 63 years old and is 1 month postonset of aphasia caused by a thrombotic stroke. The results of testing suggest that Mrs. Benchley may benefit from treatment of auditory comprehension, so the clinician enrolls her in a treatment program designed to enhance her auditory comprehension. Now let us examine the ways in which the clinician might measure the effects of the treatment program.

The simplest way to separate the effects of treatment from the effects of spontaneous recovery is called the *baseline-treatment design*. In a baseline-treatment design the patient's performance on tasks like those to be used in treatment is measured several times before treatment begins *(baseline condition)*. Then

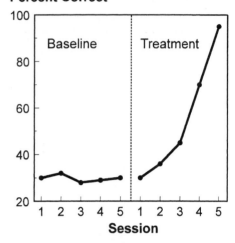

Figure 7-6 ■ A baseline-treatment design. The behavior to be treated is measured several times in succession before treatment begins. Changes in the rate of behavior change from baseline to treatment provide evidence regarding the effects of treatment.

the patient's performance is measured while treatment is provided, and the change (if any) in the patient's performance is measured. Figure 7-6 shows how this might work. Mrs. Benchley's performance in baseline is stable at approximately 30% correct responses across five baseline measurements. When treatment is provided, Mrs. Benchley's performance improves dramatically. After five treatment sessions her performance has improved to approximately 95% correct responses. That Mrs. Benchley's performance is stable and unchanging until treatment begins suggests that treatment, and not some other variable, accounts for her improved performance.

The clinician may not be out of the proverbial woods, however, because the results do not ensure that treatment is the only possible cause of Mrs. Benchley's improved performance. Perhaps a change in an incidental variable related to the onset of treatment such as

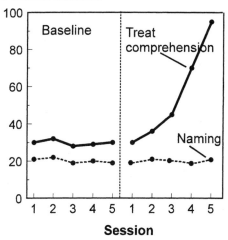

Percent Correct

Figure 7-7 ■ A multiple-baseline design. Two or more behaviors are measured under baseline conditions, then one of the behaviors is treated. If the treated behavior changes and the other behaviors do not change, an effect of treatment is assumed.

Mrs. Benchley's belief that treatment will help, the effects of general stimulation associated with treatment, or increased confidence on Mrs. Benchley's part is the true reason for her improvement.

Multiple-baseline designs were developed to deal with such issues. In multiple-baseline designs two or more behaviors are periodically measured in baseline condition. Then the behaviors are tracked as treatment is applied to one of the behaviors. If the treated behavior changes and the untreated behaviors do not, a treatment effect is assumed. Figure 7-7 shows how a clinician might specify the source of Mrs. Benchley's improved auditory comprehension by measuring a second, untreated behavior (in this case, naming) during the baseline and treatment phases. Figure 7-7 shows that Mrs. Benchley's naming performance does not change during baseline or during auditory comprehension treatment, whereas auditory compre-

hension, stable during baseline, improves during treatment, making it unlikely that changes in Mrs. Benchley's emotional state or spontaneous improvement in her cognitive or communicative skills are responsible for her improved comprehension performance.

A somewhat more complex but more powerful multiple-baseline design is called *crossover design.* In crossover design two or more behaviors are measured several times in baseline. Then one behavior is treated while the other behaviors continue in baseline. After the first behavior has been treated for a predetermined time (usually determined by a criterion such as percent of correct responses per block of *n* trials), treatment of that behavior ends, and treatment moves on to one of the other behaviors. The first behavior now returns to baseline condition, in which it is periodically measured but not treated.

To illustrate how crossover designs work, I have designed a crossover treatment plan for Mrs. Benchley. The clinician measures the effects of treatment on three categories of language behavior—auditory comprehension, naming, and spelling. The clinician chose these behaviors because she does not expect much generalization of treatment from one behavior to another, permitting her to see treatment effects uncontaminated by generalization. The clinician establishes 90% correct responses per block of 20 trials as the criterion for ending one treatment phase and beginning another.

Figure 7-8 shows that all three behaviors are stable across five baseline sessions. Then the clinician treats auditory comprehension, keeping naming and spelling in baseline. Mrs. Benchley reaches criterion in the auditory comprehension treatment phase in five sessions, and treatment shifts to naming, with auditory comprehension and spelling in baseline. Mrs. Benchley reaches criterion in naming treatment in five sessions, and her auditory comprehension performance continues to show the effects of treatment. The clinician shifts attention to spelling, with auditory comprehension

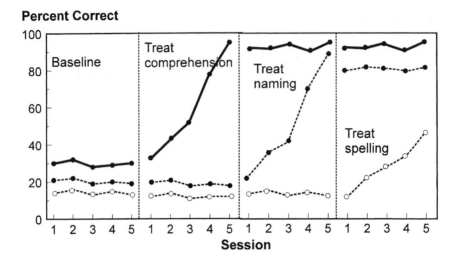

Figure 7-8 ■ A crossover design. Two or more behaviors are measured under baseline conditions, then the behaviors are treated sequentially. If treated behaviors change when treatment is applied but untreated behaviors do not, an effect of treatment is assumed.

and naming in baseline. Auditory comprehension and naming continue to show the effects of treatment while spelling is treated. Mrs. Benchley's spelling performance improves but does not reach criterion in five sessions, so the clinician will probably schedule more sessions of spelling treatment.

The results shown in Figure 7-8 provide compelling evidence for the effects of three different treatments on three categories of Mrs. Benchley's language behavior. All behaviors were stable in baseline conditions both before and after they were treated, each improved when it was treated, and each stabilized when treatment addressed a different behavior. Neither spontaneous recovery nor any other general effect can explain the results in Figure 7-8. Mrs. Benchley's performance can be explained only by the discrete effects of the three treatments administered.

Let's discuss one more design, and then we can let Mrs. Benchley rest. The design is called

changing-criterion design. Changing-criterion design is useful for tracking a patient's performance when stimuli or response requirements change during treatment. In changing-criterion design a target behavior is observed under baseline conditions to ensure that it is stable when not treated. A treatment program is designed in which criterion performance levels are specified, and treatment stimuli or response requirements are systematically changed when a treated behavior reaches the criterion level. We return to Mrs. Benchley's auditory comprehension treatment program to illustrate how changing-criterion designs work (Figure 7-9).

Mrs. Benchley's ability to carry out gestural responses to one-step, two-step, and three-step spoken instructions is measured in baseline condition (Phase 1) for three sessions. Her performance is stable, and her performance on one-step instructions is better than her performance on two-step and three-step instructions (see Figure 7-9). In Phase 2 Mrs. Benchley participates

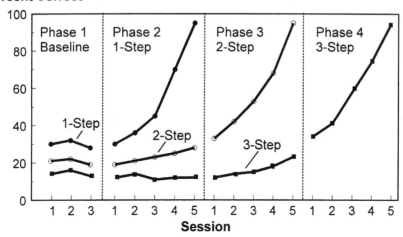

Figure 7-9 ■ A changing-criterion design. A patient's performance at several levels of task difficulty are measured under baseline conditions, then the behaviors are treated, beginning with the easiest level and progressing to the most difficult level. If behaviors representing the treated level change but behaviors representing other levels do not, an effect of treatment is assumed. (Generalization of improved performance from a treated level to an untreated higher level often occurs, as is seen in Phase 2 and Phase 3.)

in drills with one-step spoken instructions (e.g., *Give me the small pencil.*). Her performance on two-step and three-step instructions is measured periodically while one-step instructions are treated. Her performance on one-step instructions improves, and she reaches criterion in five sessions, ending Phase 2. In Phase 3, two-step instructions (e.g., *Touch the blue comb and pick up the red cup.*) are the treatment focus, and Mrs. Benchley's performance is measured periodically. Mrs. Benchley reaches criterion in Phase 3 in five sessions. Phase 4 treatment with three-step instructions (e.g., *Touch the small pencil, point to the white cup, and give me the large key.*) follows. Mrs. Benchley's performance improves, and she reaches criterion in five sessions. The pattern of change in Mrs. Benchley's performance supports the effectiveness of the treatment program in improving her ability to follow instructions of increasing length.

Mrs. Benchley's performance on the baseline measures in Phase 2 and Phase 3 suggests that giving Mrs. Benchley practice with instructions of one length improved her comprehension of longer instructions. Mrs. Benchley's performance on two-step commands improved slightly when one-step commands were treated, and her performance on three-step commands improved slightly when two-step commands were treated (see Figure 7-9). Such generalization across levels is common in treatment with a changing-criterion design and helps prepare a patient for the move from one level of complexity to the next.

Several other single-case design procedures are available. Most are elaborations on the designs described here. The interested reader may wish to consult a general source for single-case design such as Barlow and Herson (1984), Kazdin (1982), or Kratchowill (1978).

GENERAL CONCEPTS 7-4

- Structured procedures for specifying treatment tasks and recording patients' responses to task stimuli are an important part of treatment regimens for communicatively impaired adults.
- *On-line scoring* of responses is practical when response rate and complexity permit responses to be easily scored and recorded. If response rate or complexity make on-line scoring impractical, clinicians may choose to do *off-line scoring* or *sampling*.
- In *baseline-treatment designs* a patient's performance in areas targeted for treatment is measured on several occasions before treatment begins. Changes in performance from baseline to treatment are considered treatment effects. Baseline-treatment designs do not rule out the effects of variables other

than treatment on a patient's change in performance.
- In *multiple-baseline designs* two or more behaviors are measured in baseline sessions and are measured again periodically while one of the behaviors is treated. If the treated behavior changes and the untreated behaviors do not, a treatment effect is assumed.
- In *crossover designs* two or more behaviors are measured in baseline sessions. Then the behaviors are treated one after another. Changes in a behavior coinciding with treatment are considered treatment effects.
- In *changing-criterion designs* a target behavior is measured in baseline sessions, then undergoes treatment in which stimuli or response requirements change as the patient reaches predetermined performance criteria.

ENHANCING GENERALIZATION

Treatment of cognitive-communicative disorders is not successful if changes achieved in the clinic do not extend to the patient's daily life. Although most clinicians recognize that extension of treatment gains to daily life is important, until the 1970s most speech-language pathologists seemed to operate largely on the *train and hope principle* (Stokes & Baer, 1977), in which generalization of treatment effects from the clinic to outside contexts was hoped for, but neither actively pursued nor objectively measured. It is probably true that most speech-language pathologists (at least the better ones) either target communicative behaviors that are relevant to the patient's daily life environment or target underlying processes that are assumed to enhance daily life communicative behavior, but many do not pursue generalization in a systematic way, nor do they measure it carefully.

In the 1970s psychologists and behavior analysts began to address the problem of

extending changes obtained in a training facility to outside environments. A literature on generalization developed, and procedures for enhancing generalization gradually made their way into the clinical literature. These procedures generally resemble those articulated by Stokes and Baer (1977), the first of which (train and hope) has been described. The others consist of the following eight procedures.

Generalization Procedures

Using Natural Maintaining Contingencies. Stokes and Baer see this as *the most dependable of all generalization programming mechanisms* (p. 353). The easiest way to make use of natural contingencies is to target behaviors that naturally elicit favorable consequences in the patient's daily life environment. For example, Thompson and Byrne (1984) trained patients with Broca's aphasia to produce various social conventions such as greetings and farewells, expecting that the patients' uses of such social conventions would be reinforced naturally by others in daily life.

Sometimes natural contingencies are not present in the patient's daily life environment or are not consistent enough to maintain behavior. Then it may be necessary to modify the patient's daily life environment so that the targeted behaviors receive enough pay-off to maintain them. For example, consider a brain-injured patient who learned to produce one-word and two-word requests in the clinic but communicated at home with grunts and gestures, by which he usually succeeded in getting family members to do what he wanted. The clinician taught family members to respond only to spoken requests and to ignore or delay responses to grunts and gestures unaccompanied by speech. This change in the patient's daily life environment soon brought the patient's clinic-learned spoken requests into his home environment, after which natural contingencies maintained them, both in the home and in the patient's interactions with other listeners.

Training Sufficient Exemplars. Exemplar is technical jargon with various meanings. As used here, it means, roughly, *pattern of behavior.* One way of training sufficient exemplars is to train a behavior in enough different settings that the behavior generalizes to all settings in which the behavior is desired. Once the behavior is established dependably in one context, training is extended systematically to other contexts one or two at a time, with the expectation that at some point the behavior will generalize to all contexts of interest. Using social conventions as an example, one might first train social conventions in the clinic, then extend the training to other rooms, to other interactants, and to the patient's home or other community settings, expecting that at some point the patient's use of social conventions will generalize to all relevant communicative contexts.

Exemplar, as used here, seems to me to be fuzzy technical jargon. *Exemplar* has three related dictionary definitions, none of which fit this usage:

(1) something worthy of imitation; a model; (2) an ideal that serves as a pattern; an archetype; (3) a copy, as of a book. *Exemplar* comes from the same root word as *example* and *exemplary.*

Another way of training sufficient exemplars is to train enough different representatives of a class of responses to ensure that a class of responses, rather than a specific response (or subset of responses), generalizes. Using social conventions as an example, one might train several social conventions of a given kind (e.g., several different greetings) with the expectation that increasing the frequency of greetings might naturally lead to increases in the frequency of other conventions such as questions (*How are you?*) and self-disclosures (*I am fine.*).

Loose Training. In *loose training* the clinician permits stimulus conditions, response requirements, and reinforcement contingencies to vary (within limits) to increase generalization across responses within a response class and to increase generalization from the training environment to other environments. Loose training attempts to prevent responses from being tightly bound to specific contexts, which can happen when treatment conditions are carefully controlled (as in many impairment level treatment activities). In loose training a variety of stimuli are used to elicit targeted responses, sometimes in different situational contexts; a range of responses within a predefined response class is considered acceptable, and response contingencies vary both in kind and in schedule.

Loose training is not unsystematic. Specific response classes are targeted. Eliciting stimuli, and situational contexts are planned in advance. Response contingencies and their schedule are predefined. Well-done loose training is as carefully thought out and as carefully controlled as more traditional structured treatment procedures.

Thompson and Byrne (1984) used loose training to train several aphasic adults to use social conventions. They first established the social conventions by asking the aphasic adults to imitate their production of the conventions. Then they systematically extended the eliciting stimuli to (a) requests by the clinician (e.g., *Tell me hello.*); (b) naturalistic prompts given by the clinician (e.g., the clinician said *hello* and waited for a response from the patient); and (c) role-playing situations structured to resemble natural conversations. Verbal feedback (e.g., *nice job*) was provided contingent upon responses, and the schedule of feedback was gradually attenuated from feedback for every response in the early stages of training to a variable schedule (feedback for an average of one response in four) in the later stages. Thompson and Byrne reported that loose training increased their patients' production of social conventions and that the increased production of social conventions generalized to novel social interactions.

Sequential Modification. In *sequential modification* generalization across contexts is obtained by carrying out training in every context to which generalization is desired. Sequential modification may be practical for brain-injured adults when a communicative behavior is appropriate or important in only a few contexts or when there are only a few contexts in which the brain-injured person will be communicating, and it is practical to carry out training in each context. It is usually difficult, however, to identify all potential communicative contexts for a given brain-injured person, and it is almost always impractical in terms of time and resources to carry out training in every context. Consequently, sequential modification usually has limited usefulness in treating cognitive-communicative impairments (except for some patients with restricted communication environments, such as patients who are confined at home or in a nursing home or patients who have contact with only a few others, with communication limited to a small range of topics).

Using Indiscriminable Contingencies. Stokes and Baer suggest that generalization to settings outside the treatment setting is enhanced if the response contingencies in treatment are altered gradually to make them more like those that can be expected in natural settings. These alterations may include (1) changing the schedule of contingencies from continuous (for every response) to intermittent (for every *nth* response) to intermittent and variable (for every *nth* response on the average, but varying around the average); (2) inserting delays between responses and their contingencies; and (3) choosing contingencies that resemble those expected in natural settings. Many clinicians routinely include such alterations in contingencies in their treatment procedures to increase the likelihood of generalization to natural contexts. Making contingencies indiscriminable also is an important part of other techniques, such as loose training.

Programming Common Stimuli. *Programming common stimuli* means that the context in which behavior is trained is purposely made to resemble the context(s) to which the behavior is to generalize (the *target context*). Programming common stimuli manipulates stimulus control to enhance generalization across contexts. *Stimulus control* refers to how stimuli or stimulus complexes govern the occurrence of behavior. A pigeon reinforced with food pellets for pecking a key when a green light is on soon pecks the key only when the green light is on. The pigeon has learned to *discriminate* the reinforcement condition from the nonreinforcement condition. A clinician might incorporate stimuli from a patient's daily life environment into training to extend stimulus control to the patient's daily life environment, expecting that when the patient encounters the stimuli in daily life, she or he will be more likely to perform the trained behavior. The greater the similarity between the training environment and daily life, the more likely it is that the trained behavior(s) will generalize to daily life. The extent to which the training environment and the target environment resemble each other usually is decided subjectively. In most cases certain key elements (such as eliciting stimuli, surroundings, and sometimes people) are selected to resemble elements in the target environment. As is true for alterations in contingencies, programming common stimuli can be incorporated into any treatment approach to increase the likelihood of generalization to natural contexts.

Mediating Generalization. Mediation refers to the elicitation of one response by another response. Mnemonic devices are one example of mediation. One attaches easily remembered verbal labels (the *mnemonic devices*) to difficult-to-remember material and uses the mnemonic devices to retrieve the material (as in rhymes for remembering the names of the cranial nerves). In mediated generalization, easier responses are used to elicit more difficult responses. For example, a brain-injured person might be taught to retrieve words by imagining their visual images. Most of the literature on mediated generalization has studied verbal mediation, but verbal mediation may be inappropriate for many brain-injured adults who have cognitive-communicative impairments. However, verbal mediation is sometimes useful in treatment programs for persons with right-hemisphere syndrome or traumatic brain injuries.

Training Generalization. Sometimes patients spontaneously generalize during treatment activities. For example, a patient who is working on improving syntax in written work may begin using better syntax in spoken utterances. These spontaneous generalizations might themselves be targeted for reinforcement, and reinforcement contingencies might be modified gradually so that such responses receive a greater proportion of reinforcement than rote responses to training stimuli.

Social Validation

Social validation is a procedure for evaluating generalization of skills or behaviors acquired in treatment to a person's daily life. Social validation attempts to determine whether a patient is better in a real world sense than he or she was before treatment. Social validation can be accomplished in two ways (Kazdin, 1982). One way is to compare the socially relevant behav-

ior of the person receiving treatment with the behavior of a normal group of peers. The greater the progression toward normalcy, the more clinically significant is the change in behavior. The other way is to obtain subjective evaluations of the behaviors of interest from persons in the patient's natural environment. Although clinicians have for years carried out informal social validation by soliciting family members' opinions about how a patient is communicating at home, structured procedures for socially validating the effects of treatment have only recently been described.

Doyle, Goldstein, and Bourgeois (1987) trained four adults with Broca's aphasia to produce sentences with various syntactic forms as they described pictures. All improved on measures of accuracy, grammaticality, and utterance length. Doyle and associates then evaluated the social validity of the improvements by playing audiotape recordings of the picture descriptions to five judges who did not know the aphasic speakers and knew nothing about the study. Some of the recordings were made before treatment began, and others were made after treatment had ended. They were arranged so that pretreatment and posttreatment samples occurred in random order. The judges were asked to state whether each sample was *adequate* or *inadequate.* Despite the aphasic adults' improved accuracy, grammaticality, and utterance length during treatment, the social validation procedure produced no general increase in judgments of adequacy. The treatment was effective but did not have social validity.

Thompson and Byrne (1984) used a peer group comparison method to assess the social validity of changes in the use of social conventions such as greetings, farewells, and introductions by their aphasic participants. They had each aphasic participant engage in a conversational interaction with a normal adult whom the aphasic participant had not met before. Then they compared the aphasic participants' use of social conventions with that of the normal adults. Before treatment, the aphasic participants' use of social conventions lagged far behind the normal adults, but by the end of treatment the aphasic participants had essentially caught up with the normal adults.

Social validation in speech-language pathology is in its infancy, but it promises to become an increasingly important aspect of management as structured, reliable procedures for assessing and quantifying social validity are created, improved, and validated and as assessment of clinical results focuses more and more on changes in patients' daily life communicative competence.

CONCLUSION

Contemporary beliefs and attitudes about the purpose of health-related intervention are having profound effects on the nature, timing, and intensity of intervention. Intervention with brain-injured adults is moving from its traditional focus on impairments toward greater emphasis on successful participation in activities of daily living. Economics are a strong driving force behind this changing focus, but economic concerns must not replace clinical expertise and clinicians' judgment regarding what is best for their patients. Some brain-injured patients are best served by intervention that targets impairments. Others are best served by intervention that targets successful performance in daily life activities or enables meaningful participation in those activities. Impairment level intervention, activity level intervention, and participation level intervention all have legitimate places in rehabilitation of brain-injured adults. Many brain-injured adults will best be served by a blending of the three. Others may best be served by intervention focused on a single level. Decisions about the best combination of approaches for a particular patient must come from a clinician's professional judgment in combination with the wishes and needs of the patient, the patient's family, and others concerned with the quality of the patient's daily life.

GENERAL CONCEPTS 7-5

- Clinicians may promote generalization of treatment effects to a patient's daily life environment by:
  - Targeting behaviors that will be naturally rewarded in the daily life environment
  - Training in several settings in which generalization is desired
  - Training in all settings in which generalization is desired
  - Allowing training conditions to vary within limits
  - Altering the training environment, task stimuli, or response contingencies to make them increasingly similar to daily life
  - Rewarding patients' spontaneous generalization of clinic-acquired skills or behaviors to daily life

- *Social validation* is a way of evaluating the daily life significance of changes created by treatment. One approach to social validation is to measure how a patient's performance relates to normal performance. Another approach is to recruit observers to make subjective comparisons of samples of pretreatment and posttreatment behaviors without knowing which samples are pretreatment and which are posttreatment.
- Decisions about the best combination of impairment level, activity level, and participation level treatment must come from a clinician's judgment in combination with the wishes and needs of the patient and the patient's family.

THOUGHT QUESTIONS

Question 7-1 What weaknesses do you see in strict *treat the peaks* or *treat the valleys* approaches to selecting treatment activities?

Question 7-2 An administrative directive declares: *To ensure functional outcomes of speech and language treatment for brain-injured adults, henceforth all treatment activities must simulate daily life communicative interactions.* You are asked to respond. What would you say?

Question 7-3 Consider the following interaction between a clinician and an aphasic patient:

Clinician: Now I'll say a word and I want you to give me a word that means the opposite. Here's the first word: *up.*
Patient: Up. Up the road.
Clinician: No. Give me a word that means the opposite. So if I say *up,* you say *down.* OK, try this one: *white.*
Patient: White. White as snow.
Clinician: No. I want you to give me the opposite. For *white* that would be *black.* Do you understand?
Patient: Black. Black as coal.
Clinician: No, when I say a word, you say its opposite—its antonym. If I say *white,* you say *black.* Let's try another one. What's the opposite of *in?*

What problems do you see represented in this interaction? What would you do to improve it?

Question 7-4 Consider the following interaction between a clinician and a patient:

Clinician: Tell me the name of this one. [shows a drawing of a book]
Patient: Writer.
Clinician: No. That's not it. It's a book. Say *book.*
Patient: Book.
Clinician: Good! Now here's another one. [shows a drawing of a chair]
Patient: Sitter.
Clinician: No. It's a chair. Say *chair.*
Patient: Chair.
Clinician: Fine! How about this one? [shows a picture of a spoon]
Patient: Coffee.
Clinician: No, it's not coffee; it's a spoon. Say *spoon.*
Patient: Spoon.

What do you think of this interaction? Would you do anything differently?

Neuroanatomic Explanations of Aphasia and Related Disorders

Brain, *n. An apparatus with which we think that we think. (Ambrose Bierce: The Devil's Dictionary).*

THE LOCALIZATIONISTS

Neuroanatomic explanations of aphasia are based on models developed during the nineteenth century by European neuroanatomists who, in addition to arguing fiercely among themselves about who was right, began the sometimes haphazard process of finding out which parts of the brain do what. The grist for the neuroanatomists' mill was provided by the brains of patients who had died following stroke or head trauma. The neuroranatomists, most of whom were physicians, laboriously accumulated information about brain-behavior relationships as they recorded their patients' symptoms, and when the patients eventually died, they dissected the deceased patients' brains to find out which parts had been damaged. When damage in a region of the brain produced a given pattern of impairment, it seemed reasonable to assign the impaired functions to the damaged region *(localization of function).*

The localizationist effort received its first major push from Franz Gall, a Viennese physician who in the early 1800s established what he called the science of *phrenology.* Gall published elaborate maps of the brain in which various human faculties such as bravery, honesty, and love were assigned to specific brain regions (Figure 8-1). Gall believed that brain regions responsible for unusually well developed faculties were themselves unusually well developed and that manipulation of the skull could enhance mental faculties. He reasoned that hyperdeveloped brain regions pressed outward on the skull, creating bumps and ridges that a skilled practitioner could analyze, thereby determining the individual's unique pattern of talents and weaknesses.

Gall's methods were naturalistic and, by today's standards, naive. Gall obtained the evidence for his conclusions from observing friends, family members, and others, as well as his patients. *Phrenology* fell into scientific disre-

pute in the late 1830s but remained popular in England and the United States until the late 1800s. Today phrenologic maps are venerable curiosities, found primarily in treatises on the history of neurology and in advertisements for neurologic books and journals.

> Gall assigned responsibility for language to the frontal lobes because several of his acquaintances with unusually well developed verbal skills had protruding foreheads and bulging eyes.

Localizationist models specific to aphasia began with the work of Paul Broca, a French neurologist who in the 1860s published a series of papers in which he asserted that loss of *articulate speech* is caused by damage in the posterior inferior frontal lobe of the left hemisphere.

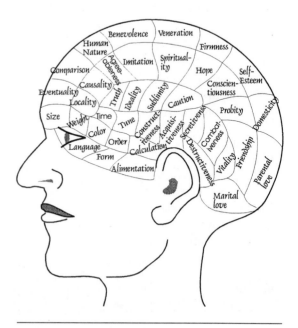

Figure 8-1 ■ A phrenologic diagram, showing the sites of various human faculties in the brain.

Localizationist models of aphasia got a boost in 1874 when Karl Wernicke, a young German neuropsychiatrist, published a description of what he called *sensory aphasia,* caused by lesions in the posterior temporal lobe. In subsequent publications Wernicke went on to construct an elaborate (for the time) account of the relationships between language functions and brain regions—an account that has survived in modified form in contemporary neuroanatomic models of aphasia.

The localizationists did not have the stage to themselves. A vociferous group of *antilocalizationists* was active both in the clinics and in the medical literature of the time. The antilocalizationists asserted that the brain operates as an integrated whole, and they considered absurd the localizationists' obsession with fractionating mental activity and assigning it to various brain regions. The published work of Marie Jean-Pierre Flourens, a contemporary of Gall's, is considered by many to represent the beginning of the antilocalizationist movement. Flourens's beliefs subsequently were built on by others in the late nineteenth and early twentieth centuries, including John Hughlings Jackson and Henry Head, British neurologists, and Pierre Marie, a French neurologist. The antilocalizationists had a point, but they had relatively little effect on the neurologic establishment, partly because the new localizationists were right somewhat more often than they were wrong and partly because localization provided neurologists with a reasonably reliable way of telling what part of a patient's brain had been damaged without having to take the brain out and look at it.

LANGUAGE AND CEREBRAL DOMINANCE

One of the earliest assertions of the localizationists was that the left hemispheres of right-handed adults is responsible for language. This assertion had its beginnings in Broca's case reports and was reinforced by repeated observations of language disturbances following left-hemisphere damage in right-handers. Based on a scattering of case reports (and, no doubt, on logic and a desire for symmetry), it became generally accepted that left-handers' brains were mirror images of right-handers' brains; that is, that the right hemispheres of left-handers' brains carried the language load.

The *mirror-image* concept began to fall apart in the 1950s when published reports (Goodglass & Quadfasel, 1954; Penfield & Roberts, 1959) began suggesting that left-handers who became aphasic seemed not to have heard of the localizationists' assertions, because at least half of these aphasic left-handers had damage only in the left hemisphere. Russell and Espir (1961) studied a group of 58 left-handed adults with traumatic brain injuries. According to the mirror-image theory, the left-handers with right-hemisphere damage should have language impairments, and the left-handers with left-hemisphere damage should have intact language. Contrary to the mirror-image hypothesis, 36% of the left-handers with left-hemisphere damage had significant language impairments, whereas only 13% of the left-handers with right-hemisphere damage had language impairments.

The mirror-image belief was pushed further into disrepute by results reported by Milner (1975). Milner injected sodium amytal (an anesthetic) into the carotid arteries of a group of left-handed adults. The injections anesthetized the brain hemisphere on the side of the injection. The person undergoing amytal testing loses the ability to speak when the language-competent hemisphere is anesthetized. Only 18% of Milner's left-handers stopped talking when their right hemispheres were anesthetized, whereas 69% stopped talking when their left hemispheres were given the drug. When either hemisphere was anesthetized, 13% lost speech, suggesting that their brain hemispheres shared language responsibilities. The results of a retrospective study by Naeser and Borod (1986) supported Milner's findings. They reviewed the medical records of 31 left-handed aphasic adults. Only 4 (13%) had right-hemisphere brain damage.

It seems clear that most adults, regardless of handedness, depend on the left hemisphere for language, because the left hemisphere is dominant for speech and language in approximately 85% of adults. However, left-handers' brains may be more flexible than right-handers' brains about which hemisphere develops language responsibilities. Left-handers who become aphasic seem to have less severe aphasia and to recover language better than their right-handed counterparts, regardless of which hemisphere is affected (Glonig & associates, 1969; Goodglass, 1993; Luria, 1970). Milner's (1975) finding that 13% of left-handed adults became aphasic when either hemisphere was anesthetized provides additional support for the notion that left-handers' brains are less constrained than those of right-handers when it comes to which hemisphere takes care of language.

The question of whether we are born with one hemisphere specialized for language has not been answered, although indirect evidence suggests that we are not. Studies of children and adolescents who sustain brain damage suggest that left-hemisphere specialization for language develops as we mature and that it is not complete before adulthood. A child born with a nonfunctional left hemisphere usually develops normal language, unless the child's right hemisphere also is damaged, and a child or adolescent who becomes aphasic almost always recovers far more language than does an adult with comparable damage. The brain's ability to reassign functions served by damaged tissue diminishes with age. The older a patient is at the time of brain injury, the more severe the persisting consequences of the injury are likely to be (Lenneberg, 1967; Osgood & Miron, 1963).

The brain's potential for reassigning to a different brain region functions that are lost when brain tissue is damaged is called *cerebral plasticity.* Children's brains are said to be more plastic than adults' brains because brain injuries that would cause lasting impairments in adults often leave children with little or no permanent impairment.

THE PERISYLVIAN REGION AND LANGUAGE

Connectionist explanations of language emphasize the importance of the region surrounding the Sylvian fissure (called the *perisylvian region*) in the left hemisphere. Permanent damage anywhere in the perisylvian region in the left hemisphere of adult brains almost always causes language impairment (except for the approximate 15% of left-handers whose right hemisphere is responsible for speech and language).

Many contemporary descriptions of aphasia syndromes use *left hemisphere* instead of the technically more accurate but tedious *language-dominant hemisphere.*

The perisylvian region in the left frontal lobe (sometimes called *the anterior language zone*) plays an important part in planning and performing expressive language actions (speech, writing, and perhaps gesture). The perisylvian region in the left temporal lobe and the left parietal lobe (sometimes called the *posterior language zone*) is important for comprehending and recalling linguistic information and for formulating linguistic messages with appropriate syntactic structure and semantic content.

The heart of the anterior language zone is the posterior inferior frontal lobe, just in front of the primary motor cortex—a region of the cortex called *Broca's area* (Figure 8-2), named after Paul Broca, the French neurologist who first described its role in speech. Broca's area is next to the primary motor cortex, that is responsible for the muscles used to produce speech. Sometimes Broca's area is called the *motor speech area* because of its presumed role in planning and organizing speech movements. *Broca's aphasia* is a major consequence of damage in Broca's area.

The heart of the posterior language zone is *Wernicke's area* (sometimes called the *auditory association cortex*) (see Figure 8-2). Wernicke's

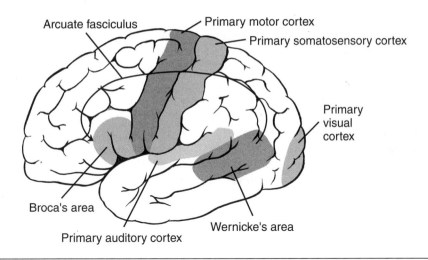

Figure 8-2 ■ Important cortical regions and connecting pathways in connectionist explanations of how the brain produces language.

area is so named because the German neuropsychiatrist Karl Wernicke first described in print an aphasia syndrome caused by temporal lobe damage. Wernicke's area is considered important for storage and retrieval of the mental representations of words and word meanings and for knowledge and retrieval of grammatic and linguistic rules. Damage in Wernicke's area often causes *Wernicke's aphasia.*

Wernicke's area tends to wander around the temporal lobe depending on who localizes it, but most brain mappers place it in the posterior superior left temporal lobe.

Wernicke's area receives a large part of its input from the *primary auditory cortex* (also called the *gyrus of Heschl*) on the top surface of each temporal lobe, in the Sylvian fissure (see Figure 8-2). The two primary auditory cortices are responsible for perception and discrimination of auditory stimuli. The auditory cortex in each brain hemisphere receives information from both ears, although the contralateral ear has a slight advantage.

Destruction of the primary auditory cortex in one hemisphere does not cause lasting deafness, only mild hearing loss (usually in the contralateral ear), and occasionally it causes some difficulty localizing sounds. Destruction of the primary auditory cortex in both hemispheres causes *cortical deafness,* in which the patient initially loses all auditory sensitivity. For some patients with bilateral destruction of the auditory cortex, some hearing sensitivity slowly returns, and the patient's pure tone audiogram may even reach normal. However, perception of speech and other complex auditory stimuli almost always remains profoundly impaired (Jerger & associates, 1969).

Wernicke's area communicates with Broca's area and other frontal regions of the brain by way of the *arcuate fasciculus,* a band of nerve fibers connecting the mid temporal lobe to lower regions of the frontal lobe via the parietal lobe (see Figure 8-2). The arcuate fasciculus is thought to be the primary route by which linguistic messages formulated in Wernicke's area reach Broca's area.

The region in and around the *angular gyrus,* at the junction of the temporal, parietal, and occipital lobes, is considered important for processes involved in reading and writing. Damage to this region usually produces severe impairments in reading (called *alexia*) and severe writing impairments (called *agraphia*).

HOW THE BRAIN PERFORMS LANGUAGE

The connectionist model provides a metaphor for describing how the language-dominant hemisphere makes sense of incoming verbal messages and formulates, plans, and executes verbal and gestural responses. The connectionist model depicts the brain's processing of language as resembling a telephone system, in which various centers send messages here and there over a system of interconnected circuits.

> We know that the brain does not work like a telephone system, and we know that the connectionist model is simplistic and in some respects inaccurate. Nevertheless, the model is a convenient metaphor for what actually happens, and it provides a practical way for students to get a general sense of how damage in the brain yields fairly predictable impairments of language and behavior.

Comprehension of Speech

To explore how the connectionist model works, I have invented a fictional normal adult I have named Norman. According to the connectionist model, when someone talks to Norman, the message goes from Norman's ears via ascending fibers to the primary auditory cortex in his temporal lobes. The auditory cortices encode the acoustic information and send the encoded message off to Wernicke's area in Norman's left hemisphere. (The information from the auditory cortex in the right hemisphere gets to Wernicke's area by way of fibers crossing in the posterior corpus callosum.)

When Wernicke's area recognizes the message as speech, it sorts through its store of semantic representations to find meanings for the words. When it has located the word mean-

ings, it consults its book of syntactic rules to determine the relationships among the words. Then it constructs a representation of the message's overall meaning. Norman's brain (perhaps regions in his right hemisphere) evaluates the situation to determine if the literal meaning of the sentence actually represents the speaker's intent. (Some sentences, such as *Can you open the window?*, are implied requests and are not meant to be interpreted literally. A *yes* or *no* response usually wouldn't be appropriate.) When Wernicke's area has deduced the sentence's meaning and knows whether the message should be interpreted literally or figuratively, it sends instructions to other parts of Norman's brain regarding how he should respond—for example, talk, write, gesture, or open the window.

Comprehension of Printed Materials

When Norman reads printed materials, the process resembles that for comprehension of speech, except that Norman's visual cortex is the first stop for information coming in from his eyes. The visual cortex encodes the information in a form that Wernicke's area can understand and sends it to Wernicke's area. (Information from the visual cortex in Norman's right hemisphere gets to Wernicke's area via fibers passing through the posterior corpus callosum.) From Wernicke's area onward, the process resembles what happens when Norman listens to spoken language. Wernicke's area constructs a representation of the message's meaning and sends the relevant information to the parts of Norman's brain that are to be involved in the response.

Spontaneous Speech

When Norman speaks a sentence spontaneously, Wernicke's area retrieves from the central lexicon the words needed to express the message and constructs a sentence that complies with phonologic, syntactic, and semantic rules. Wernicke's area then sends the neurally coded sentence forward by way of the arcuate fasciculus to Broca's area. Broca's area translates the code into an action plan and sends the plan off to the primary motor cortex. The primary motor cortex puts the finishing touches on the message and sends it down via the pyramidal system to the cranial nerves, which set the speech muscles into motion. As the speech muscles produce the message, Wernicke's area monitors it to ensure that what it sent is what Norman actually says. If it is not, Wernicke's area shifts the system into repair mode.

Repetition

According to the connectionist model, repetition of words, phrases, and sentences tests the entire language circuit from the primary auditory cortex through the motor cortex for speech. Suppose Norman is asked to repeat a phrase such as *Nelson Rockefeller drives a Lincoln Continental.* (a favorite of neurologists for testing speech repetition). The first stop in the brain is Norman's primary auditory cortex, where the phrase is perceived and translated into a neural code that Wernicke's area will understand. Then the coded message is sent to Wernicke's area, where the meaning of the message (that Norman should say *Nelson Rockefeller drives a Lincoln Continental.*) is extracted. Wernicke's area codes the sentence in a form that Broca's area can work with and sends it off via the arcuate fasciculus. When the message arrives at Broca's area, Broca's area recodes the phrase into an articulatory plan for the speech muscles and sends it to the primary motor cortex. The primary motor cortex sends the message down pyramidal fibers to the cranial nerves, which move the speech muscles. Wernicke's area monitors the output and initiates corrective routines if necessary.

Oral Reading

If Norman is asked to read printed material aloud, processes similar to those involved in speech repetition take place once the message has reached Wernicke's area, but Wernicke's area gets the message from the visual cortex rather than the auditory cortex.

Writing

When Norman writes a message, Wernicke's area formulates a message containing the appropriate words in syntactically acceptable order, gets the spelling right, and sends it via the arcuate fasciculus to the premotor cortex for Norman's hand and arm, which sets up the appropriate movement plans and sends them to the motor cortex. Norman's eyes and Wernicke's area collaborate to monitor what he writes. If Wernicke's area is not satisfied, Norman may erase, revise, correct spelling errors, or make other repairs.

Gestural Responses to Spoken Commands

When Norman is asked to make gestural responses to spoken requests (e.g., *Show me how you wave good-bye.*), the neural processes are similar to those for speech, except that the information from Wernicke's area is sent forward to the premotor cortex for Norman's hand and arm, just above Broca's area, rather than to Broca's area. If the gestural response is to be carried out by Norman's right hand (contralateral to his left hemisphere), the message goes from Wernicke's area to the premotor cortex in Norman's left hemisphere, then to the motor cortex in the same hemisphere, which sends the message to Norman's right hand. If the response is to be carried out by Norman's left hand and arm (on the same side as his left hemisphere), the message goes from Wernicke's area to the premotor cortex in the left hemisphere, from whence it is sent via the corpus callosum to the motor cortex in the right hemisphere and then down the corticospinal tract to Norman's left hand. The premotor cortex in Norman's left hemisphere apparently plans volitional movements for both sides of his body.

PATTERNS OF LANGUAGE IMPAIRMENT

The connectionist model relates damage in certain brain regions to distinctive patterns of speech, language, and motor-planning disorders. Some of these patterns are caused by destruction of important centers such as Broca's area or Wernicke's area, and others are caused by damage in pathways that connect the centers, such as the arcuate fasciculus. Those who classify aphasic patients into connectionist syndromes rely heavily on relationships among *speech fluency, paraphasia, repetition,* and *language comprehension.*

Speech fluency is an important concept for understanding the connectionist model, because classic aphasia syndromes can be separated into two types based on speech fluency, which in the connectionist model means the *prosodic* and *melodic* characteristics of speech. Patients with *nonfluent aphasia* typically have damage in the front half of the language-dominant hemisphere, anterior to the central sulcus (fissure of Rolando). They speak slowly and with great effort, pausing between syllables and words. Their speech has a measured, machinelike quality, owing to diminished or absent intonation and stress patterns.

Patients with *fluent aphasia* typically have damage posterior to the central sulcus in the language-dominant hemisphere. They speak smoothly and with little effort. They manipulate speech rate, intonation, and emphatic stress in much the same way as normal speakers do.

Over the years, the labels *fluent* and *nonfluent* have acquired meaning that goes beyond the mechanics of speech to syntax, grammar, and semantic content.

Fluent aphasic patients have normal or near normal speech rates and use a variety of different grammatical constructions; function words and grammatical inflections are present and usually syntactically appropriate. Intonation patterns are present and usually appropriate. Nonfluent aphasic patients have slow and labored speech. The variety of grammatical constructions is often restricted, and intonation may be reduced or absent; function words and grammatical affixes may be omitted, and patients may rely a lot on nouns. (Howard & Hatfield, 1987, p. 147)

Paraphasia is another important concept in connectionist models of aphasia. *Paraphasia* can be loosely defined as speech errors produced by a person with aphasia. (The circularity of this definition has not affected its durability in the literature.) Two kinds of paraphasia have been described, although there is some confusion about which speech errors qualify as paraphasia. *Literal paraphasias* (sometimes called *phonemic paraphasias*) are phonologic errors in which incorrect sounds replace correct sounds, as when an aphasic person says *shooshbruss* for *toothbrush* or in which sounds within words are transposed, as when an aphasic person says *tevilision* for *television*. *Verbal paraphasias* (sometimes called *semantic paraphasias*) are errors in which an incorrect word (usually semantically related to the target) unintentionally is substituted for the target word, as when an aphasic person says *door* for *window* or *knife* for *fork*.

Goodglass, Kaplan, and Barresi (2001) divided verbal paraphasia into three categories. *Semantic paraphasias* are substitutions of semantically related words for target words, as in *father* for *mother*. *Unrelated paraphasias* are substitutions in which the substituted words have no clear relationship to target words, as in *cigarette* for *motorcycle*. *Perseverative paraphasias* are substitutions in which a previously used word is substituted for a target word, such as when an aphasic patient who has correctly named a comb subsequently calls a fork a *toothbrush*, and a key *comb*. Goodglass, Barresi, and Kaplan make an exception for intentional one word *circumlocutions* (deliberate use of a substitute word for a word that a patient cannot retrieve) because paraphasias are unintentional substitutions. (The reliability of this distinction seems questionable. It is not easy to tell when an aphasic person's substitutions are unintentional or deliberate. The concept, however, has merit.)

According to Canter (1973), the term *literal paraphasia* denotes a pattern of articulatory errors, and he asserted that individual articulatory errors are not necessarily paraphasic—

especially those made by dysarthric persons. According to Canter, the diagnostician must consider not only the form of speech errors, but the context in which they occur to tell if the errors truly are literal paraphasias. When an aphasic person makes articulatory errors in a context of fluent, effortless speech, they are likely to be literal paraphasias. When articulatory errors are embedded in a context of nonfluent and effortful articulatory posturing, they are likely to represent the phonetic dissolution associated with motor-planning impairments *(apraxia of speech).*

APHASIA CAUSED BY DESTRUCTION OF CORTICAL CENTERS FOR LANGUAGE

Three of the most common connectionist aphasia syndromes (Broca's aphasia, Wernicke's aphasia, and global aphasia) are caused by damage in the central region of the language-dominant hemisphere, served by the middle cerebral artery. Occlusion of the anterior branch of the middle cerebral artery often causes Broca's aphasia; occlusion of the posterior branch often causes Wernicke's aphasia; occlusion of the main trunk of the middle cerebral artery usually causes global aphasia.

Broca's Aphasia

As noted earlier, Broca's aphasia is caused by damage in Broca's area. Broca's area makes up the lower part of the *premotor cortex,* a strip of cortex just anterior to the primary motor cortex. Broca's area is adjacent to the primary motor cortex for the speech muscles, so it is in a geographically prime location for planning speech movements. Broca's area also is close to the primary motor cortex for the face, hand, and arm. Descending pyramidal tract fibers pass under Broca's area. For this reason patients with Broca's aphasia usually have right-sided hemiparesis or hemiplegia. Broca's aphasia sometimes goes by other names, such as *expressive aphasia, motor aphasia,* or *anterior aphasia.*

Patients with Broca's aphasia are nonfluent. They speak as if the motor plans for speech have gone awry. Words come out singly or in groups of two or three, separated by abnormally long pauses. Multisyllabic words may be produced syllable by syllable with abnormal pauses between syllables. Misarticulations are common, with distortion of consonants and vowels (a phenomenon called *phonetic dissolution*). Patients with Broca's aphasia are laconic. Utterances consist primarily of content words (nouns, verbs, and an occasional adjective, but rarely adverbs). Function words (conjunctions, articles, and prepositions) are infrequent, leading some writers to describe their speech as *agrammatic* or *telegraphic.*

> The word *and,* however, is prevalent in the speech of most patients with Broca's aphasia. The word typically serves as a general purpose connector to give a sense of continuity to strings of sentence fragments.

The following is what a patient with Broca's aphasia said when she was asked to describe the *cookie theft* picture from the *Boston Diagnostic Aphasia Examination—Third Edition* (Goodglass, Kaplan, & Barressi, 2001; see Figure 5-19):

> uh...mother and dad...no...mother...and and disses...uh...runnin over...and waduh...and floor...and they ...uh...wipin disses...and...uh... two kids...uh...stool...and cookie...cookie jar... uh...and uh ...cabinet and stool...uh...tippin over ...and...uh...bad...and somebody...uh...somebody gonna get huht.

The content of written materials produced by patients with Broca's aphasia resembles the content of their speech—strings of content words, often connected by the word *and.* Patients with Broca's aphasia rarely write in cursive form. Letters within words are distorted and clumsily formed (perhaps because patients with Broca's aphasia are writing with their

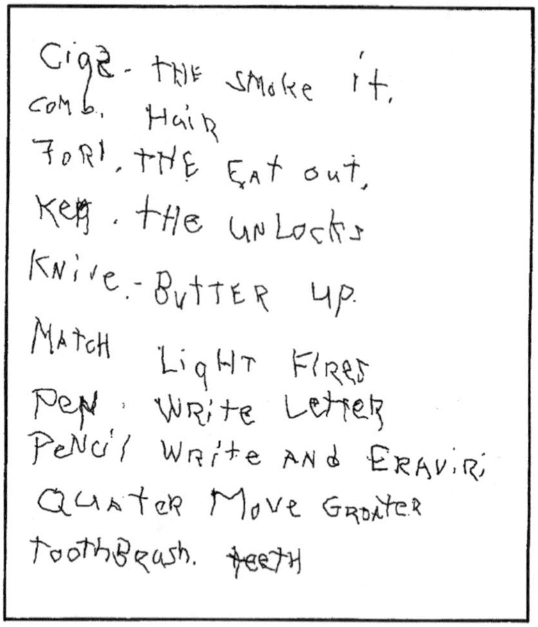

Cig2 - tHE smoke it,
comb. Hair
7oRl, tHE Eat out,
key. tHe unLocks
Knife. - ButTER up.
MatcH   LiqHT Fires
PeN . WRite Letter
PeNcil WRite ANd ERaviri
Quater Move Gronter
tootHBrush. teeTH

Figure 8-3 ■ A sample of writing produced by a patient with Broca's aphasia.

nonpreferred hand because of hemiplegia). Omissions of letters are common. Sentences are written with great effort and often slant downward across the page. Figure 8-3 shows a sample of writing from a patient with Broca's aphasia who is describing in writing what one does with the 10 test objects (cigarette, comb, fork, key, knife, match, pen, pencil, quarter, and toothbrush) from the *Porch Index of Communicative Ability* (Porch, 1981a).

Patients with Broca's aphasia comprehend spoken and written language better than they speak or write, although they are slow readers, and careful testing almost always reveals subtle impairment of both reading and listening comprehension. Their self-monitoring usually is well preserved. Patients with Broca's aphasia typically are aware of their physical and communicative impairments and often become upset by failed communication attempts, sometimes to the point of emotional outbursts. When

patients with Broca's aphasia make errors in speech or writing or are unsuccessful in communicating, they typically repeat or attempt repairs. Patients with Broca's aphasia are cooperative and task-oriented in testing and treatment activities. They remember treatment procedures and goals from day to day and may spontaneously generalize skills and strategies acquired in treatment to their daily life environment.

Wernicke's Aphasia

Like Broca's aphasia, Wernicke's aphasia has several aliases, including *sensory aphasia, receptive aphasia*, and *posterior aphasia*. Wernicke's aphasia typically is caused by damage in the temporal lobe of the language-dominant hemisphere. One of the most striking language characteristics of patients with Wernicke's aphasia is their impaired comprehension of spoken or printed verbal materials. Patients with severe Wernicke's aphasia fail to comprehend even simple spoken or written verbal materials, although some may get a smattering of what is said in conversations. Patients with mild or moderate Wernicke's aphasia usually get the overall point of conversations but miss the specifics.

Patients with Wernicke's aphasia often exhibit dissociations between the sound or sight of words and their meanings, and in extreme cases, may be unable to discriminate between phonologically valid nonwords (e.g., *spome*) and real words (e.g., *spoon*). Their language comprehension may be compromised by blurring of semantic distinctions among words, rendering them unable to appreciate differences between words with related meanings (e.g., *happy* versus *joyful*) and causing some patients with Wernicke's aphasia to lose their sense of semantic typicality (e.g., whether *carrot* is a more typical vegetable than *artichoke*).

Evidence of Wernicke's aphasic patients' confusion about semantic typicality comes from tests in which they must make typicality judgments about printed words. Their confusion does not extend to daily life.

fun fact

Patients with Wernicke's aphasia do not confuse real carrots and real artichokes when it comes time to peel, cook, or eat them.

The semantic impairments of patients with Wernicke's aphasia are exacerbated by impaired short-term retention and recall of verbal materials. Patients with Wernicke's aphasia perform poorly on tests of short-term memory in which they must repeat strings of numbers or recall word lists. When asked to perform sequences of manipulative or gestural responses to spoken or printed commands (e.g., *put the pencil beside the spoon and put the quarter beside the box*), their performance rapidly deteriorates as commands become longer.

In contrast with the slow, laborious, and halting speech of patients with Broca's aphasia, patients with Wernicke's aphasia talk smoothly, effortlessly, and usually copiously. (Wernicke's aphasia is a *fluent* aphasia.) Patients with Wernicke's aphasia can produce long, syntactically well-formed sentences with normal intonation and stress patterns, although they may pause and muddle about when experiencing word retrieval difficulties, which are common. That the mechanics of speech are preserved in Wernicke's aphasia does not mean, however, that patients with Wernicke's aphasia have no difficulty communicating by talking. Their connected speech may be littered with *verbal paraphasias* (substitution of one word for another), *occasional literal paraphasias* (substitution or transposition of sounds within words), and *neologisms* (nonwords such as *carabis*). The speech pattern of patients with mild to moderate Wernicke's aphasia sometimes is called *paragrammatism:*

Clinician: Tell me about where you live.
Patient: Well, it's a meender place and it has two...two of them. For dreaming and pinding after supper. And up and down. Four of down and three of up...

Patients with severe Wernicke's aphasia may produce *jargon*—strings of neologisms with a sprinkling of connecting words:

Clinician: What's the weather like today?
Patient: Fully under the jimjam and on the altigrabber.

Patients with severe Wernicke's aphasia often produce strings in which major content words are replaced by neologisms but in which the *connectives* (articles, conjunctions, and prepositions) are real words, as in the preceding speech sample. The strings also seem syntactically well formed (Goodglass, 1993). Wernicke's aphasic patients with word retrieval impairments may produce what is called *empty speech,* substituting general words such as *thing* or *stuff* or pronouns without referents for more specific words.

A patient with moderate Wernicke's aphasia was attempting to explain what he had done on a shopping trip the previous day. He concluded with, *I went down to the thing to do the other one and she was only the last there, so I never did.*

Some Wernicke's aphasic patients talk around missing words—a behavior called *circumlocution.*

A patient with moderate Wernicke's aphasia was attempting to tell the examiner what she had had for breakfast that morning. Unable to come up with the needed words, she circumlocuted to get her intended meaning across:

This morning for...that meal...the first thing this morning...what I ate...I dined on...chickens, but little...and pig...pork...hen fruit and some bacon, I guess.

The ease with which Wernicke's aphasic patients produce speech, their circumlocution, and their deficient self-monitoring may contribute to their well-known inclination to run on when they talk—a phenomenon called *press of speech* or *logorrhea:*

Clinician: Tell me what you do with a comb.
Patient: What do I do with a comb...what I do with a comb. Well, a comb is a utensil or some such thing that can be used for arranging and rearranging the hair on the

head both by men and by women. One could also make music with it by putting a piece of paper behind it and blowing through it. Sometimes it could be used in art—in sculpture, for example, to make a series of lines in soft clay. It's usually made of plastic and usually black, although it comes in other colors. It is carried in the pocket until it's needed, when it is taken out and used, then put back in the pocket. Is that what you had in mind?

The handwriting of patients with Wernicke's aphasia usually resembles their speech. They write effortlessly with well-formed letters. Most write in cursive form. Although their handwriting, like their speech, may be mechanically normal, their handwriting, like their speech, is deficient in content. Patients who produce verbal paraphasias in speech produce them in writing. Patients who speak neologistically write neologistically. (But the letters in neologistic words usually are grouped in clusters that are consistent with letter groupings for real words.) Patients with press of speech when they talk usually exhibit press of writing when they write.

Figure 8-4 shows a writing sample generated by a Wernicke's aphasic patient with mild aphasia describing what one does with the 10 test items from the *Porch Index of Communicative Ability* (Porch, 1981a).

Most patients with Wernicke's aphasia are alert, attentive, and task-oriented. Those with mild Wernicke's aphasia are aware of their errors (at least most of them), the content of their speech is semantically appropriate, and they generally follow conversational rules such as those governing turn-taking.

Patients with moderate Wernicke's aphasia rarely notice errors or attempt repairs. They are attentive and cooperative in testing and treatment but may stray from the task unless the clinician intervenes to keep them on track. In conversations, patients with moderate Wernicke's aphasia tend to wander off on verbal tangents and may talk at length about unrelated or trivial topics.

Patients with severe Wernicke's aphasia usually are attentive, but their profound comprehension impairments greatly interfere with their performance of all but the simplest verbal tasks. They are oblivious to errors and communication failure but appear sensitive to the basic rules governing conversational interactions. They acknowledge and attend to their conversational partner and respect turn-taking rules, although once they get the conversational floor they tend to talk excessively, tangentially, and sometimes neologistically.

Patients with Wernicke's aphasia usually show less outward concern about their communication impairments than do patients with Broca's aphasia. Part of their unconcern may relate to their lack of awareness, but many who do recognize errors and understand that they have communication impairments are remarkably complacent and unconcerned about them.

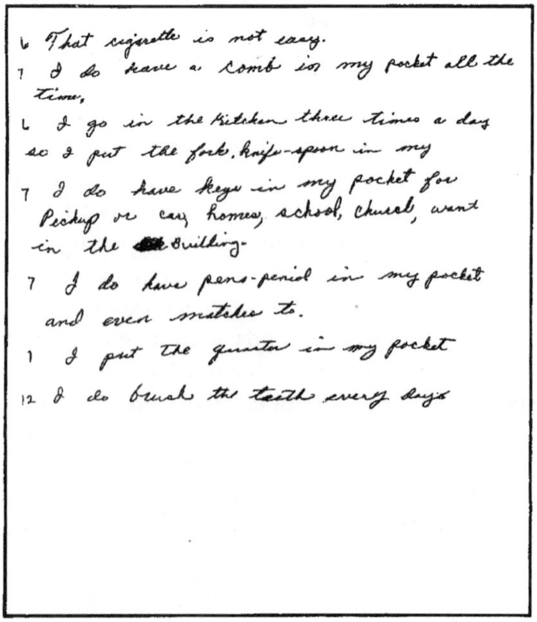
6 That cigarette is not easy.
7 I do have a comb in my pocket all the time,
6 I go in the Kitchen three times a day so I put the fork, knife-spoon in my
7 I do have keys in my pocket for Pickup or car, homes, school, church, want in the building.
7 I do have pens-penciel in my pocket and even matches to.
1 I put the quarter in my pocket
12 I do brush the teeth every days

Figure 8-4 ■ A sample of writing produced by a patient with Wernicke's aphasia.

Because Wernicke's area is not close to the motor cortex, few patients with Wernicke's aphasia are hemiparetic or hemiplegic, unless the lesion responsible for the aphasia extends into the frontal lobe or affects descending pyramidal tracts (in which case the aphasia might be more appropriately labeled as *global aphasia*). However, fibers in the optic tract pass under Wernicke's area on their way to the visual cortex. Lesions extending deep into the temporal lobe often destroy these fibers, causing contralateral visual field blindness (described in Chapter 2).

Global Aphasia

As mentioned earlier, global aphasia most often follows occlusion of the trunk of the middle cerebral artery, causing massive damage throughout the perisylvian region. However, a few cases of global aphasia have been reported in which either Wernicke's area or Broca's area is spared (Basso & associates, 1985; Vignolo & associates, 1986), and global aphasia also has been reported following subcortical damage in the thalamus and basal ganglia (Naeser & associates, 1982).

Occlusion of the trunk of the middle cerebral artery has enormous effects on the patient. Globally aphasic patients invariably exhibit severe impairments in all language functions. Most cannot perform even the simplest tests of listening comprehension, and most cannot reliably answer simple yes-no questions, although some may respond to conversations in a way that suggests that they get at least a rudimentary sense of what is said.

Some globally aphasic patients who do not respond appropriately to any other spoken materials may respond appropriately to *whole body commands* such as *stand up, turn around, lie down,* and so forth. The reason for this phenomenon is not clear, but Albert, Goodglass, Helm, and associates (1981) suggest that it may be attributable to right-hemisphere participation in responses to such commands.

Few globally aphasic patients can read even simple words, and their reading of sentences or longer printed materials is invariably nonfunctional. The speech of globally aphasic patients is severely limited, consisting of a few single words, stereotypical utterances (e.g., *kakie-kakie-kakie*), overlearned phrases (e.g., *how-dee-do*), or expletives. Over time, some globally aphasic patients become proficient at communicating in a limited way with a combination of intoned stereotypic utterances, gesture, and facial expression, but verbal communication remains largely nonfunctional.

Most globally aphasic patients are attentive, alert, task-oriented, and socially appropriate (which helps to differentiate the globally aphasic patient from the confused or demented patient). They usually can perform nonverbal tasks (e.g., matching objects or pictures, matching pictures to objects) satisfactorily, and some may perform normally or nearly so on nonverbal (performance) tests of intellect. Globally aphasic patients occasionally comprehend questions related to personally relevant information fairly well compared with their universally poor comprehension of other spoken material. Some globally aphasic patients reliably answer spoken yes-no questions about family, personal information, and recent experiences but respond at chance levels to all other kinds of spoken materials (Goodglass, Kaplan, & Barresi, 2001).

APHASIA CAUSED BY DAMAGE TO ASSOCIATION FIBER TRACTS

Several aphasia syndromes are caused by damage in association fiber tracts between Wernicke's area and Broca's area or by damage to tracts that connect Wernicke's area and Broca's area to the rest of the brain. In *conduction aphasia* the pathway connecting (language-competent) Wernicke's area to (speech-competent) Broca's area is affected. In the *transcortical aphasias*, pathways connecting the perisylvian region with other regions of the brain are affected. The brain damage producing these aphasia syndromes may involve the cortex but always extends beneath the cortex to affect association fiber tracts.

Conduction Aphasia

Conduction aphasia typically is caused by lesions in the upper temporal lobe, lower parietal lobe, or insula—lesions that damage the arcuate fasciculus but spare Wernicke's area and Broca's area. The defining behavioral characteristics of conduction aphasia are grossly impaired repetition and relatively preserved language comprehension. Language comprehension is preserved in conduction aphasia because the primary auditory cortex and Wernicke's area are spared.

That comprehension is *preserved* does not mean that conduction aphasic patients' comprehension is *intact.* They typically exhibit mild to moderate comprehension impairments. The point is that their ability to repeat phrases and sentences is strikingly worse than their ability to comprehend the same phrases and sentences.

Patients with conduction aphasia have extraordinary difficulty repeating what they hear because of poor communication between Wernicke's area and Broca's area. Multisyllabic words create more problems for conduction aphasic patients than do monosyllabic words. Long and phonologically complex words tie most patients with conduction aphasia into verbal knots.

Clinician: Now I want you to say some words after me. Say *boy.*

Patient: Boy.

Clinician: *Home.*

Patient: Home.

Clinician: *Seventy-nine.*

Patient: Ninety-seven. No...sevinty-sine... seventy-nice...

Clinician: Let's try another one. Say *refrigerator.*

Patient: Frigilator...no. But how about...fre-rigilator...no...frigaliterlater...aahh! I can't say it!

Patients with conduction aphasia speak fluently (speech rate, intonation, and stress patterns are normal), but their speech contains many literal paraphasias and some verbal paraphasias. Their spontaneous speech is better than their repetition, although literal paraphasias and pauses related to word retrieval difficulties are common. Patients with conduction aphasia have difficulty reading aloud because oral reading, like repetition, depends on communication between Wernicke's area and Broca's area. Conduction aphasic patients' problems with oral reading do not extend to their reading comprehension, which, like their auditory comprehension, usually is relatively good.

Conduction aphasic patients' handwriting typically is well-formed and legible, but self-formulated writing and writing to dictation usually contain spelling errors and transpositions of letters, syllables, and words. Just as they are better at saying what they think than repeating what they hear, they can write self-formulated material better than they can write what is said to them.

Conduction aphasic patients are alert, attentive, and task-oriented. They are aware of errors in speech and writing and attempt repairs. Conduction aphasic patients often seem surprised by their speech miscues, and comments to that effect are not unusual (e.g., *Why can't I say that? What's going on here?*) produced normally and without conscious effort. Their first attempts at correcting speech errors often are unsuccessful, and long strings of unsuccessful repair attempts are common, with the patient getting further and further from the target until she or he throws in the towel or the examiner supplies the target word or words, as in the following example in which a patient with conduction aphasia is trying to say the word *circus:*

It's a kriskus. ... No, that's not right, but it's near. ... Sirsis ... No. ...This is very strange that I can't say this word. ... How about kirsis? ... No. ... I'll have to bye that. Kriskus? For some reason I can't say it right now. But I'm close. Kirsis?

No... I'll have to bye that because I can't think of the word. I can think of the word, but I can't say it. That's it. ... Kirsis?

Transcortical Aphasia

Transcortical aphasia (sometimes called *isolation syndrome*) is caused by dominant-hemisphere brain damage that spares the central region (Wernicke's area, Broca's area, and the arcuate fasciculus) but disconnects (isolates) all or parts of the central region from the rest of the brain. Because association fibers are compromised in the transcortical aphasias, Lichtheim (1885) called what we know as transcortical aphasia *commissural dysphasia* or *white matter dysphasia*. The disconnection causing transcortical aphasias usually is created by damage in the border zone (watershed region) surrounding the perisylvian cortex.

Preserved repetition is a defining characteristic of the transcortical aphasias. Because Wernicke's area, Broca's area, and the arcuate fasciculus are spared, repetition of spoken words, phrases, and sentences is preserved, although other language functions may be substantially compromised. Three kinds of transcortical aphasia have been described in the literature. They are *transcortical motor aphasia, transcortical sensory aphasia,* and *mixed transcortical aphasia.*

Transcortical Motor Aphasia. The classic neurologic cause of *transcortical motor aphasia* is damage in the anterior superior frontal lobe in the language-dominant hemisphere. The defining characteristics of transcortical motor aphasia are markedly reduced speech output, good repetition, and good auditory comprehension. The reduced speech output of transcortical motor aphasic patients seems to be a consequence of anterior frontal lobe dysfunction. The anterior frontal lobes are important for initiation and maintenance of purposeful activity. It follows, then, that patients with damage in the anterior frontal lobe of the language-dominant hemisphere are likely to have problems initiating and maintaining speech. Luria (1966) called what we know as transcortical motor aphasia

dynamic aphasia and called its behavioral manifestation *pathologic inertia*. Right hemiparesis (or less frequently right hemiplegia) may accompany transcortical motor aphasia caused by large anterior frontal lobe lesions extending into the posterior frontal lobe. Wernicke's area is not affected in transcortical motor aphasia, so patients with transcortical motor aphasia comprehend language relatively well. The arcuate fasciculus is spared in transcortical motor aphasia, so patients with transcortical motor aphasia are good at repeating what they hear and are good at reading aloud.

Although they are attentive, task-oriented, and cooperative, patients with transcortical motor aphasia are poor conversationalists, content to sit quietly while the conversational partner carries the communicative burden. When it is their turn to speak, they usually produce a perfunctory word or two and turn responsibility back to the conversational partner. In highly structured interactions with highly predicable content, patients with transcortical motor aphasia often respond fluently and without delay. A surprising characteristic of patients with transcortical motor aphasia is how well they repeat phrases or sentences once they get started. Once started, these patients can repeat long and complex phrases and sentences fluently and without error, as in the following example.

A patient with transcortical motor aphasia was asked what kind of work he did. After a long delay he responded with the word *bakery* and lapsed into silence. Repeated requests by the examiner to tell more elicited only the word *bakery,* then *Minneapolis* following delays of 10 to 20 seconds. When the examiner subsequently tested the patient's repetition, the patient fluently repeated after the examiner the following sentence without delay: *Before I had my stroke I worked in a bakery in Minneapolis, Minnesota.*

Transcortical Sensory Aphasia. Transcortical sensory aphasia (sometimes called *posterior isolation syndrome*), like transcortical motor aphasia, is caused by brain damage that spares Wernicke's area, the arcuate fasciculus, and Broca's area. The brain damage responsible for transcortical sensory aphasia typically affects the watershed region of the upper parietal lobe in the language-dominant hemisphere. Patients with transcortical sensory aphasia, like those with transcortical motor aphasia, do well when asked to repeat phrases or sentences. Unlike patients with transcortical motor aphasia, those with transcortical sensory aphasia speak without having to be cajoled by their conversational partner, and some seem compelled to repeat what they hear even when instructed not to do so (a phenomenon called *echolalia*). In an examination they tend to repeat the instructions or the examiner's requests before responding. In conversations they may include all or part of what the conversational partner says in their responses to the partner:

Clinician: Does the sun rise in the west?

Patient: Does the sun rise in the west? The sun rises in the west...in the west...the sun rises...Yes...I think the sun does rise in the west...yes the sun rises in the west.

Because the brain damage that produces transcortical sensory aphasia isolates Wernicke's area from much of the rest of the brain, patients with transcortical sensory aphasia always have major impairments in comprehension of spoken and written language. In some respects patients with transcortical sensory aphasia resemble patients with Wernicke's aphasia. They speak fluently, but their speech is semantically empty and verbal paraphasias are common.

Most patients with transcortical sensory aphasia are unaware of their errors and do not attempt to self-correct. However, they usually do not exhibit press of speech, as many Wernicke's aphasic patients do, and their excellent repetition clearly differentiates them from patients with Wernicke's aphasia. A striking characteristic of patients with transcortical sensory aphasia is their ability to repeat or read aloud material that they do not comprehend. They may be at a loss when asked to perform even simple manipulations in response to spoken instructions, but

they can flawlessly repeat long and complex instructions.

A patient with transcortical sensory aphasia was befuddled by simple commands such as *Pick up the pencil,* but without hesitation repeated after the examiner *Put the comb beside the matches, point to the quarter, and give me the spoon.*

Because the brain damage that produces transcortical sensory aphasia involves the parieto-occipital-temporal junction and isolates Wernicke's area from the visual cortex, transcortical sensory aphasic patients invariably have severely impaired reading comprehension, although oral reading is preserved.

Mixed Transcortical Aphasia. This rare syndrome sometimes is called *isolation of the speech area* (Geschwind, Quadfasel, & Segarra, 1968). Patients with *mixed transcortical aphasia* retain their ability to repeat what is said to them in the presence of profound impairment of all other communicative abilities. The prototypical patient with isolation of the speech area "is nonfluent (in fact does not speak at all unless spoken to), does not comprehend spoken language, cannot name, cannot read or write, but can repeat what is said by the examiner" (Benson, 1979b, p. 46). These patients often have a striking tendency to repeat, in parrot-like fashion, what is said to them, and if the examiner says the first few words of familiar songs or rhymes, these patients often complete the phrase and may go on to provide one or more following lines:

Clinician: Hello, Mrs. Fenton.

Patient: Mrs. Fenton. Yes.

Clinician: How are you doing today?

Patient: How are you doing today?

Clinician: I'm very fine, thank you. How are you doing?

Patient: I'm very fine, thank you.

Clinician: My name is Mary. I'll be working with you today.

Patient: My name is Mary. I'm working today.

Mixed transcortical aphasia is a result of damage that spares Broca's area, Wernicke's area, and the arcuate fasciculus but isolates those areas from other brain regions. The most frequent cause of mixed transcortical aphasia is stenosis (partial occlusion) of the internal carotid artery, which reduces the volume of blood reaching the watershed region in the language-dominant hemisphere. Mixed transcortical aphasia sometimes follows cerebral hypoxia, severe cerebral swelling, or multiple embolic strokes that affect the peripheral branches of the middle cerebral artery.

Anomic Aphasia

Whether *anomic aphasia* exists as a separate syndrome is not clear (Albert & associates, 1981). Goodglass (1993) comments, "Of all the aphasia subtypes, anomic aphasia is the one that appears as a result of diverse causes and as a result of lesion sites that are remote from each other" (p. 214). The label *anomic aphasia* usually is applied to patients whose only obvious symptom is impaired word retrieval in speech and writing. Anomic aphasic patients' spontaneous speech is fluent and grammatically correct but marred by word retrieval failures. The word retrieval failures lead to unusual pauses, circumlocution, and substitution of nonspecific words for missing specific words. Careful testing usually reveals that patients with anomic aphasia have subtle comprehension impairments, sometimes accompanied by other mild language impairments:

Clinician: Do you have children?
Patient: I have a son and two daughters.
Clinician: Tell me about them.
Patient: My son...Paul, he works in a...he works at...in the ... that thing...but not TV. At the...I don't know...I know, but...At the *Register*...the *Register.* It's a paper...a news...newspaper. Paul is a...he goes out, and he talks to people. He does...he does...I guess you'd say he does interviews. People, you know. On the street and wherever...

Goodglass (1993) described four varieties of aphasia in which anomia appears in relative isolation. According to Goodglass, patients with *frontal anomia* represent mild versions of transcortical motor aphasia. The major characteristic of patients with frontal anomia is the remarkable degree to which their word retrieval improves if the examiner provides the first sound of the target word. Patients with *anomia of the angular gyrus region* speak fluently but with many word retrieval failures. The phenomenon that sets this syndrome apart from the other anomic syndromes is intermittent occasions on which the patient fails to retrieve a word and fails to recognize it when it is supplied by the examiner. Patients with anomia of the angular gyrus often exhibit *alienation of word meaning*—repeating a word over and over without recognition. According to Goodglass (1993), anomia of the angular gyrus may be a mild form of transcortical sensory aphasia:

Clinician: Tell me what the *word* apple means.
Patient: Apple...apple...apple. Is that the word?
Clinician: Yes. Apple.
Patient: You mean apple? A-P-P-L-E? [spells aloud]
Clinician: Yes. Apple. A-P-P-L-E.
Patient: I should know what it means, but I really don't...
Clinician: Think about a fruit that you might put in a pie.
Patient: Oh! Apple! It's round and red, and it grows on trees, and you put it in a pie!

Patients with *anomia of the inferior temporal gyrus* have severe word retrieval problems but speak fluently and grammatically and have near normal reading, writing, and, presumably (although Goodglass does not mention it) near normal auditory comprehension. Patients with *anomia as an expression of residual aphasia* probably represent the most common anomic syndrome. These are patients who have passed through a more severe form of another aphasia syndrome and have recovered nearly normal language function but continue to exhibit mild to moderate word retrieval impairments. Goodglass, Kaplan, and Barresi

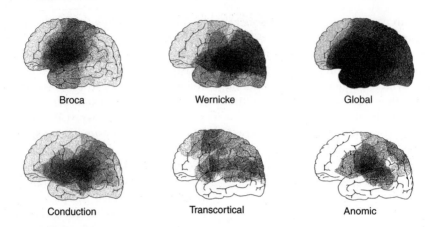

Figure 8-5 ■ Composite brain scans showing the distribution of lesions that produced Broca's, Wernicke's, global, conduction, transcortical motor, and anomic aphasias. (From Kertesz, A., Lesk, D., McCabe, P. [1977]. Isotope localization of infarcts in aphasia. *Archives of Neurology, 34,* 590-601.)

(2001) recommend the label *residual aphasia* rather than *anomia* for these patients.

It is not clear if Goodglass's anomic aphasia syndromes are unique syndromes or if they simply represent milder versions of other aphasia syndromes, which seems likely. Anomia certainly is not a localizing phenomenon. As Goodglass notes, it can occur with damage in many different regions of the brain and in combination with a variety of other aphasic symptoms.

Figure 8-5 shows composite brain scans of groups of aphasic patients who exhibited Broca's, Wernicke's, global, conduction, transcortical motor, and anomic aphasia. Figure 8-6 shows the proportions of patients exhibiting various aphasia syndromes in a group of 444 patients seen in the Aphasia Research Center at the Boston Veterans Administration Medical Center during a 10-year period (Benson, 1979a). Table 8-1 summarizes the important characteristics of the connectionist aphasia syndromes.

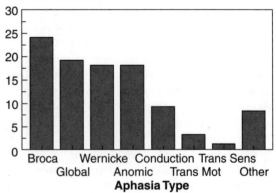

Figure 8-6 ■ Proportions of patients exhibiting various aphasia syndromes in a group of 444 aphasic adults seen in the Aphasia Research Center, Boston Veterans Administration Medical Center. (Data from Benson, D. F. [1979]. *Aphasia, alexia, and agraphia.* New York: Churchill-Livingstone.)

TABLE 8-1   Characteristics of Connectionist Aphasia Syndromes

Aphasia Syndrome	Lesion Location	Fluency	Speech	Word Retrieval	Repetition	Comprehension
Broca	Posterior inferior frontal lobe	Nonfluent, telegraphic	Phonetic dissolution*	Fair but misarticulated	Labored, misarticulated, telegraphic	Fair to good
Wernicke	Posterior superior temporal lobe	Fluent, empty	Verbal (semantic) paraphasia	Poor, with verbal paraphasias	Fluent, verbal paraphasia; grossly restricted retention span	Poor
Conduction	Parietal lobe	Fluent, sensical	Literal (phonemic) paraphasia	Fair, with literal paraphasias	Fluent, literal paraphasia; some restriction of retention span	Fair to good
Anomic	Temporal, parietal lobe	Fluent, sensical	Verbal (semantic) paraphasia	Fair, with verbal paraphasias	Good	Fair to good
Transcortical motor (anterior isolation syndrome)	Anterior, superior frontal lobe	Fluent, sparse†	Variable	Variable, with delays in initiation	Good, but delays in initiation	Good
Transcortical sensory (posterior isolation syndrome)	Posterior, superior parietal lobe	Fluent, empty	Variable	Poor	Good	Poor
Global	Large, perisylvian	Nonfluent	Literal, verbal paraphasia; verbal stereotypies	Poor	Poor, literal, verbal paraphasia; grossly restricted retention span	Poor

*Phonetic dissolution: distortion of consonants (and sometimes vowels); a result of disrupted articulatory programming (apraxia of speech). In contrast, literal paraphasia involves substitution of a correctly articulated but inappropriate sound for another.
†Sparse but with unusual delays in initiation. Utterances tend to be one or two words long.

GENERAL CONCEPTS 8-1

- Localizationist models of aphasia began in the early 1800s. The observations of Paul Broca and Karl Wernicke laid the foundation for contemporary connectionist models of aphasia and related disorders.
- For most adults the left brain hemisphere has major responsibility for speech and language. This relationship is stronger for right-handers than for left-handers. Nearly 100% of right-handed adults are left hemisphere–dominant for speech and language, compared with about 85% of left-handed adults. The *perisylvian region* in the central region of the language-dominant hemisphere serves many important speech and language functions.
- *Broca's area,* in the posterior inferior frontal lobe of the language-dominant hemisphere, plays an important part in organizing movement sequences for the speech muscles.
- *Wernicke's area,* in the temporal lobe of the language-dominant hemisphere, plays an important part in language comprehension and in rule-governed aspects of language.
- The *arcuate fasciculus,* a band of nerve fibers connecting Wernicke's area to Broca's area, is thought to provide a communicative link between Wernicke's and Broca's areas.
- *Paraphasias* are errors in spoken or written word production. *Verbal paraphasia* (sometimes called *semantic paraphasia*) denotes substitution of one word for another (e.g., *table* for *chair*). *Literal paraphasia* (sometimes called *phonemic paraphasia*) denotes substitution or transposition of sounds in words (e.g., *dirthday tarpi* for *birthday party*).
- *Broca's aphasia* is caused by damage in the posterior inferior region of the frontal lobe in the language-dominant hemisphere. Patients with Broca's aphasia speak slowly and with great effort, and they often omit function words (*agrammatism* or *telegraphic speech*). Patients with Broca's aphasia usually comprehend language better than they speak it or write it.
- *Wernicke's aphasia* is caused by damage in the central or posterior regions of the temporal lobe in the language-dominant hemisphere. Patients with Wernicke's aphasia typically have problems comprehending spoken and written language. They speak effortlessly and with essentially normal rate. However, their speech may contain paraphasias and word retrieval failures.
- *Global aphasia* is caused by massive damage in the perisylvian region of the language-dominant hemisphere. Patients with global aphasia have profound impairment of all speech, language, and comprehension, although some may say a few common words and phrases, and some may get a rudimentary sense of simple conversations.
- *Conduction aphasia* is caused by damage in the parietal lobe of the language-dominant hemisphere, affecting transmission of information from Wernicke's area to Broca's area by way of the arcuate fasciculus. Patients with conduction aphasia typically have fairly good language comprehension but grossly impaired repetition. They speak fluently but with literal paraphasias.
- *Preserved repetition* is a defining characteristic of *transcortical aphasia* (sometimes called *isolation syndrome*).
- *Transcortical motor aphasia* is caused by damage in the watershed region of the anterior frontal lobe in the language-dominant hemisphere. Patients with transcortical motor aphasia have markedly reduced speech output, good repetition, and good listening comprehension.

- *Transcortical sensory aphasia* is caused by damage in the parietal watershed region of the language-dominant hemisphere. Patients with transcortical sensory aphasia speak effortlessly, but many are echolalic. They have few problems repeating what is said to them but have profoundly impaired language comprehension.

- It is not clear whether *anomic aphasia* represents a distinct aphasia syndrome or is simply a milder version of other aphasia syndromes. The primary characteristics of anomic aphasia are impaired word retrieval in speech and writing with relative preservation of other speech and language functions.

RELATED DISORDERS

Nonlinguistic disorders sometimes occur in combination with the linguistic disorders characterizing aphasia syndromes. *Disconnection syndromes* appear when the language-competent brain hemisphere is isolated from its nonlinguistic partner. *Visual field blindness* often accompanies aphasia caused by temporal lobe or parietal lobe damage. *Apraxia* often appears in combination with aphasia caused by frontal lobe damage. A variety of perceptual impairments called *agnosias* may follow damage in cortical association areas.

Callosal Disconnection Syndromes

Callosal disconnection syndromes appear when nerve fiber tracts connecting the brain hemispheres are damaged or destroyed. *Complete disconnection syndromes* usually are created by neurosurgeons who cut the connections between the hemispheres (a procedure called *commissurotomy*) to keep epileptic seizures originating in one hemisphere from spreading across the corpus callosum to the other hemisphere. The most common causes of *partial disconnection syndromes* are occlusions of the anterior or posterior cerebral arteries, which provide most of the blood supply to the corpus callosum. Partial disconnection syndromes occasionally are caused by tumors growing into the corpus callosum or putting pressure on it.

For simplicity I have limited the following description of disconnection syndromes to right-handed persons. Although there are few published reports of disconnection syndromes in left-handed persons, it seems reasonable that left-handed persons with right-hemisphere language would exhibit similar impairments but as mirror images to the impairments of right-handed persons.

Occlusion of the anterior cerebral artery may produce *anterior disconnection syndrome*. Right-handed patients with anterior disconnection syndrome exhibit an unusual collection of symptoms caused by isolation of the right-hemisphere somatosensory and motor cortex from the language-competent left hemisphere. Patients with anterior disconnection syndrome cannot accurately respond to verbal commands asking for responses by the left hand (a condition called *unilateral limb apraxia*). The right hemisphere (which controls the left hand) is cut off from the meaning of the commands, which is stuck in the left hemisphere. Patients with anterior disconnection syndrome also cannot name or talk about objects held out of sight in the left hand, because sensory information from the left hand goes to the mute right hemisphere. These patients easily name and talk about objects held out of sight in the right hand, because the sensory information goes to the language-competent left hemisphere. Some patients with anterior disconnection syndrome who cannot name, describe, or talk about objects palpated with the left hand may provide a few bits of rudimentary description (e.g., *It's small. It's long and thin. It's soft and not very heavy.*).

If a patient with anterior disconnection syndrome is blindfolded, given objects to palpate in one hand, then is asked to choose the palpated objects from a group, they choose correctly when a palpated object and the choice objects are palpated with the same hand, but not when the test object is palpated with one hand and the choice objects are palpated with the other. This differential performance happens because the sensory information from the hand that palpated the object cannot cross the corpus callosum to tell the other hand what to search for. Patients with anterior disconnection syndrome can draw, demonstrate the function of, or choose an unseen palpated object from a group, provided they use the hand with which they palpated the object.

Right-handers with anterior disconnection syndrome can name objects held out of sight in the right hand. (The tactile information goes to the language-competent left hemisphere.) If they are allowed to name the objects they hold, they can choose the correct matches with either hand, because both hemispheres have heard the spoken names. Likewise if they can sneak a peek at the test objects from under the blindfold, they can choose the correct objects with either hand because the visual information gets to both hemispheres.

Occlusion of the posterior cerebral artery may produce *posterior disconnection syndrome.* The most common impairments of patients with posterior disconnection syndrome are visual abnormalities attributable to isolation of the visual cortex from the language-competent left hemisphere, caused by destruction of visual fibers crossing in the posterior corpus callosum. These patients' visual abnormalities are measurable only by special testing in which printed words or pictures are flashed

into the eyes in such a way that the image goes only to the right hemisphere. A patient with posterior disconnection syndrome can report seeing words or pictures flashed into the right hemisphere but cannot name them, talk about them, or write about them. If the patient is allowed to choose a picture that has been flashed into the right hemisphere from among several pictures, the patient can choose the correct picture with the left hand but not the with the right hand. If printed commands calling for arm or hand movements are flashed into the right hemisphere, the patient cannot carry out the commands. If the commands are flashed into the left hemisphere, the patient responds correctly with the right hand but not the left.

Patients with *complete disconnection syndrome* (sometimes called *split-brain syndrome*) exhibit a combination of anterior and posterior disconnection syndromes. Patients with complete disconnection syndrome, like patients with anterior disconnection syndrome, are unable to name objects held out of sight in the left hand. They also exhibit visual impairments like those of patients with posterior disconnection syndrome, wherein the patient cannot verbalize about visual stimuli restricted to the right hemisphere. Because there is no communication between the brain hemispheres to coordinate behavior, patients' hands sometimes behave independently and inconsistently (e.g., one hand is buttoning the patient's shirt while the other is unbuttoning it, or one hand is putting items in a drawer while the other is taking them out). Patients will sometimes slap or grab the misbehaving hand in an attempt to control it. Patients who experience such conflict between the hands often comment that the aberrant hand does not belong to them (called *alien hand syndrome*).

Patients with anterior callosal disconnection sometimes experience alien hand syndrome, but not as often as do patients with complete callosal disconnection.

Commisurotomized patients do not ordinarily encounter situations outside the clinic or laboratory that restrict stimulus input to one hemisphere. They appear normal to family and friends, and their cognitive and communicative functions usually are essentially normal. Signs of disconnection appear only when tests designed to identify callosal disconnection are given.

Commisssurotomies are performed in only a few centers and are reserved for patients with intractable seizures that have not responded to less dramatic intervention. Because their disconnected brain hemispheres provide neuropsychologists and neurophysiologists with such fascinating insights into hemispheric functions, commissurotimized individuals are in such great demand as study participants that some have retained agents to negotiate fees with interested investigators.

Patients with posterior disconnection syndrome sometimes have an unusual reading impairment called *alexia without agraphia* (also known as *occipital alexia* or *pure word blindness*). Patients who have alexia without agraphia have "...a serious inability to read contrasted with an almost uncanny preservation of writing ability" (Benson, 1979a, p. 110). These patients may write personal letters or long and grammatically accurate narrative paragraphs, but they are mystified when asked to read what they have written. Some patients who have alexia without agraphia may retain the ability to read and comprehend a few highly familiar words (e.g., their names and the cities and states where they live). Patients who have alexia without agraphia experience great difficulty copying written material but can spell aloud, and they instantly recognize words spelled aloud by the examiner. Some can read slowly and may make sense of printed materials by reading individual letter names aloud and identifying the words by oral spelling, which gets the information to the brain through the ears rather than through the eyes.

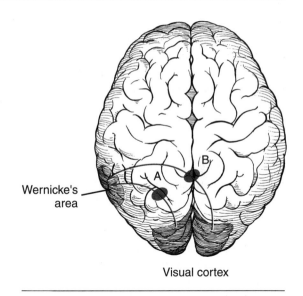

Wernicke's area

Visual cortex

Figure 8-7 ■ How brain damage produces alexia without agraphia. The visual cortices in both hemispheres are isolated from Wernicke's areas by a lesion that destroys the left visual cortex or disconnects the left visual cortex from Wernicke's area *(A)* and a second lesion that cuts the visual fibers crossing through the corpus callosum from the right visual cortex *(B)*.

The presence of alexia without agraphia is evidence of a complex lesion (or a combination of lesions) that destroys the left visual cortex and interrupts exchange of information between the brain hemispheres via the posterior corpus callosum (Figure 8-7). The left hemisphere cannot see the material, and visual information from the language-incompetent right hemisphere (which can see the material) cannot reach the language-competent left hemisphere. The patient can write, because the connections between Wernicke's area (which formulates verbal messages) and the anterior motor planning and motor control regions (which do the writing) are intact. Patients with posterior disconnection syndrome do not exhibit the tactile disconnection symptoms seen in anterior disconnection syndrome. They can name, describe, and talk about or write about unseen objects palpated with either hand. Because the left visual cortex is no longer functioning, patients with alexia without agraphia invariably have right homonymous hemianopia. Strokes affecting the posterior cerebral artery are the most common cause of alexia without agraphia. Tumors and arteriovenous malformations are less common causes.

Alexia with agraphia (sometimes called *parieto-temporal alexia*) often appears following damage in the vicinity of the angular gyrus, at the posterior end of the Sylvian fissure. The damage isolates the visual cortex from Wernicke's area and isolates Wernicke's area from anterior motor planning and motor control regions. Visual information obtained from printed materials cannot be communicated either to Wernicke's area or from Wernicke's area to the anterior motor regions, leaving the patient unable either to read orally or silently or to write. In contrast with patients who have alexia without agraphia, patients who have alexia with agraphia cannot identify words spelled aloud by the examiner. They can copy printed materials much better than they can write words to dictation, but most are unable to translate material from cursive to printed form or from printed to cursive form. Alexia with agraphia is seen in many aphasia syndromes. It rarely occurs in isolation.

Visual Field Blindness

Patients with superior temporal lobe or low parietal lobe damage often are blind in all or parts of the contralateral visual field. This condition is called *visual field blindness*. (See Chapter 2 for more on how lesions in the visual system cause perceptual problems.) Because the visual fibers travel through the inferior parietal lobes and the superior temporal lobes on their way to the visual cortex, many patients with Wernicke's aphasia or conduction aphasia experience visual field blindness. Patients with anterior aphasia (Broca's aphasia, transcortical

motor aphasia) rarely have visual field blindness, and visual field blindness is unusual for patients with transcortical sensory aphasia because lesions in the watershed regions of the brain usually do not affect visual fibers. Visual field blindness appearing in combination with transcortical sensory aphasia usually is in the lower quadrant of the contralateral visual field *(inferior quadrantanopsia).* Patients with global aphasia often experience contralateral visual field blindness because of massive temporal lobe and parietal lobe damage.

APRAXIA

Characteristics of Apraxia

Apraxia (from a Greek word meaning *unable to do*) is a label for several syndromes characterized by difficulty carrying out volitional movement sequences in the absence of sensory loss or paralysis sufficient to explain the difficulty. Apraxia often accompanies aphasia, especially aphasia caused by damage in the frontal lobe or anterior parietal lobe.

John Hughlings Jackson (1866) first described in print the behavioral manifestations of apraxia. Jackson described several patients who were unable to perform certain skilled movements even though the muscles required for the movements were neither weak nor incoordinated. Most writers credit Heyman Steinthal, a German physician, with the first published use (in 1871) of the term *apraxia*. Hugo Liepmann, also a German physician, in 1900 published the first model explaining the neuroanatomical basis for apraxia. Liepmann's model has survived with minor modifications until contemporary times. Liepmann described two apraxia syndromes in his 1900 paper, calling them *ideational apraxia* and *ideomotor apraxia.*

Ideational Apraxia

Liepmann characterized *ideational apraxia* as disruption of the concepts or ideas needed to understand the use of objects. Persons with ideational apraxia are unable to carry out movement sequences that lead to a given result, such as putting a key in a lock, filling a pipe with tobacco, or folding a letter, putting it in an envelope, and sealing the envelope. Patients with ideational apraxia seem not to grasp the overall intent of everyday goal-directed movements. Individual movements are motorically normal but appear in the wrong order and produce the wrong results. (For example, a patient puts a match instead of tobacco into the bowl of his pipe, or a patient inserts an envelope into the folds of a letter instead of putting the letter in the envelope.) Kertesz (1979) defined ideational apraxia as follows:

> ...a defect of purposeful movements, where the ideational project or plan appeared to be disordered, although engrams for individual movements were considered to be intact. Instead of accomplishing the desired object, a false one is realized. The patient puts the match into his mouth in trying to light a cigarette, tries to drink from a cup by leaning over or under it, etc. Here, the whole series of actions is impaired due to the conceptual disturbance. (p. 234)

Liepmann attributed ideational apraxia to damage in the left parietal lobe, but more recent studies of patients with apparent ideational apraxia suggest that ideational apraxia typically is associated with diffuse brain damage and is especially common in patients with dementia, in which case it may reflect confusion or attentional impairments rather than a motoric impairment.

Because ideational apraxia is a conceptual impairment, it is a bilateral phenomenon: it affects movements of both right-sided and left-sided limbs. The fuzziness of the concept of ideational apraxia has contributed to confusion about its nature and its neuroanatomic roots. Some contemporary writers declare that the label *ideational apraxia* should be abandoned because the behaviors to which it refers reflect cognitive or conceptual impairment rather than impaired motor control.

Ideomotor Apraxia

Ideomotor apraxia refers to disruption of the motor plans needed to demonstrate volitional actions—disruptions that cannot be accounted for by weakness, paralysis, sensory loss, or incoordination of the muscles required to perform the actions. According to Goodglass (1993):

> Elementary movements are adequately coordinated, but the motor plan for the intended action appears to be absent, inadequately formulated, or else poorly related to the patient's actual movement. (p. 195)

Ideomotor apraxia becomes evident when a patient is asked to perform an everyday series of movements with arm and hand (e.g., *Show me how you wave good-bye.*) or with orofacial structures (e.g., *Show me how you blow dust off a shelf.*).

As noted, the motoric impairments of patients with ideomotor apraxia are not caused by weakness, paralysis, or incoordination of muscles. Apraxic patients who cannot demonstrate a set of movements in response to the examiner's request typically can perform the movements flawlessly in real life contexts. For example, an apraxic patient who cannot wave good-bye when the examiner requests the movements during testing may effortlessly wave good-bye 10 minutes later as she or he leaves the testing room.

Providing objects for the apraxic patient's use in demonstrating a series of movements also helps. A patient who cannot demonstrate the use of scissors in response to the examiner's requests may produce a fluent and flawless demonstration when given a pair of scissors and a piece of paper to cut. A patient who is at a loss when asked to pantomime blowing out a match will infallibly blow out an actual lighted match held by the examiner. Apraxic complications rarely occur in daily life, where contextual support for everyday movement sequences is strong, which explains why most apraxic patients are unaware of apraxia until it is revealed during testing.

The presence of ideomotor apraxia is an almost certain sign of damage in the central zone of the language-dominant brain hemisphere. From 30% to 60% of right-handed patients with left-hemisphere damage exhibit ideomotor apraxia (DeRenzi, 1989; Kertesz, Ferro, & Shewan, 1984; Liepmann, 1908), but less than 10% of right-handed patients with right-hemisphere damage are apraxic (DeRenzi, 1989). Ideomotor apraxia is strongly related to language. Nonaphasic left hemisphere–damaged patients are less likely to be apraxic than aphasic left hemisphere–damaged patients, and patients with severe aphasia are twice as likely to be apraxic as are patients with mild to moderate aphasia (Liepmann, 1908; Kertesz, Ferro, & Shewan, 1984).

From Liepmann's time until the 1970s, the presence of apraxia was taken as evidence for damage in the premotor cortex, which is regarded as the center for motor planning. Geschwind (1975) added to Liepmann's model by suggesting that apraxia may be caused by damage in the left hemisphere that disconnects the premotor cortex from posterior parietal and temporal areas. Geschwind's connectionist model of apraxia describes a process in which apraxia follows damage to fibers passing under the parietal lobe, isolating the premotor cortex from Wernicke's area. The cortical motor planning region is intact but unable to respond to verbal commands, because the information from Wernicke's area regarding what the examiner has requested is not available.

Buckingham (1979) described a model of apraxia resembling Geschwind's model, but he added that apraxias caused by damage in the premotor cortex and apraxias caused by damage in the parietal lobe can be differentiated by eliciting movements nonverbally (e.g., showing the patient a picture or modeling the movements). According to Buckingham, patients with apraxia caused by damage in the premotor area are apraxic regardless of how the movements are elicited because the motor-planning region is damaged, whereas patients with parietal lobe

damage are apraxic when the movements are requested verbally but not when they are elicited nonverbally, because nonverbal elicitation eliminates the premotor cortex's dependence on information from Wernicke's area.

Ideomotor apraxia may be expressed in disturbed limb movements (a condition called *limb apraxia*) or in movements of orofacial structures (a condition called *buccofacial apraxia*). Patients with limb apraxia cannot pantomime everyday sequences of arm and hand movements in response to spoken requests such as *Show me how you wave good-bye., Show me how you flip a coin.,* or *Show me how you thumb a ride.* When patients with limb apraxia respond to such requests, they typically place the arm and hand in the approximate spatial location for the movements but fail to perform the fine-grained wrist, hand, and finger-flexion movements required for accurate rendition. The result is a stiff, boardlike approximation to the requested movements. The boardlike appearance of apraxic patients' limb movements during testing reflects the tendency for *distal* (away from the torso) muscle groups to be more severely apraxic than *proximal* (near the torso) muscle groups. When patients with limb apraxia perform movement sequences requiring shoulder, elbow, wrist, and finger movements, shoulder and elbow movements appear more nearly normal than wrist and finger movements. For this reason, test items requiring wrist and finger movements (e.g., flipping a coin or winding a watch) are more sensitive to the presence of limb apraxia than test items requiring shoulder and elbow movements (e.g., saluting or drinking from a glass).

Limb apraxia almost always affects arms and hands on both sides of the body, although apraxia in the right arm and hand may not be observable if that arm and hand are paralyzed as a consequence of left-hemisphere brain injury. (Liepmann called this left-sided apraxia *sympathetic apraxia*.) Unilateral apraxia of the left arm and hand may, however, be caused by brain injury that prevents transmission of motor

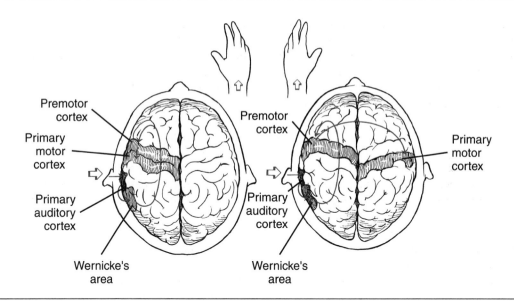

Figure 8-8 ■ A connectionist explanation for limb apraxia. The spoken command requesting a limb movement is perceived by the primary auditory cortex, comprehended by Wernicke's area, and sent by way of the arcuate fasciculus to the premotor cortex for the hand, where a plan for the movement is formulated. The premotor cortex sends the plan to the motor cortex for execution. If the movement is to be carried out by the right hand, the plan is sent to the motor cortex in the left hemisphere. If the movement is to be carried out by the left hand, the plan is sent across the corpus callosum to the motor cortex in the right hemisphere.

control information across the corpus callosum from the left hemisphere to the right hemisphere (a condition called *callosal apraxia*).

Successful performance during a limb apraxia test requires the functional adequacy of four brain regions: (1) *Wernicke's area,* where the meaning of the examiner's requests is deduced; (2) the *lower parietal lobe,* through which information from Wernicke's area is relayed to (3) the *premotor cortex,* which sets up a motor plan to be executed by (4) the *motor cortex.*

If the movements are to be accomplished with the right hand and arm, the motor plan is sent to the adjacent left-hemisphere motor cortex, but if the movements are to be accomplished with the left hand and arm, the motor plan is sent across the corpus callosum to the right-hemisphere motor cortex (Figure 8-8).

Destruction of Wernicke's area prevents the patient from comprehending the meaning of the examiner's requests. The patient fails to execute the movement with either limb because of impaired comprehension, not because of apraxia. Damage in the parietal lobe prevents communication between Wernicke's area and the premotor cortex, leaving the patient bilaterally apraxic. Damage affecting the motor control centers in the premotor cortex also leaves the patient bilaterally apraxic. Unilateral apraxia of the left arm and hand occurs if connections between Wernicke's area and the premotor cortex in the left hemisphere are functional and if damage in the corpus callosum prevents information comprehended by the left hemisphere from reaching the motor cortex in the right hemisphere.

Patients with *buccofacial apraxia* (sometimes called *oral nonverbal apraxia*) are unable to pantomime sequences of movements that require lip positioning, blowing, sucking, or sniffing (e.g., whistling, sucking up through a straw, or sniffing a flower). Buccofacial apraxia and limb apraxia usually appear together, although either can appear by itself. Buccofacial apraxia is common in patients with Broca's aphasia. DeRenzi, Pieczuro, and Vignolo (1966) diagnosed buccofacial apraxia in 90% of patients with Broca's aphasia.

Misuses of the Apraxia Label

The *apraxia* label has been at times carelessly used, causing confusion about what apraxia is and what causes it.

> Apraxia is one of the most consistently misused terms in medical literature. Most of the types of apraxia currently described by medical and paramedical workers (e.g., verbal, constructional, dressing) represent fixed motor or visuospatial disturbances and should not be defined by the term *apraxia* any more than a hemiplegia should. Despite the widespread misuse of apraxia to denote many types of motor performance failure, the presence of motor apraxia in individuals with aphasia is almost routinely overlooked. (Benson, 1979a, p. 172)

The two most commonly misused apraxia labels are *dressing apraxia* and *constructional apraxia,* neither of which represents impaired control of volitional movements. Patients with so-called *dressing apraxia* have difficulty getting into articles of clothing. They may put articles of clothing on backward, upside-down, or inside-out and may attempt to put their arms through trouser legs or their legs through shirt or blouse sleeves. Dressing apraxia usually is a consequence of nondominant-hemisphere brain damage and probably represents a combination of disturbed body image, disturbed appreciation of the body's relationship to surrounding space, or inattention to one side of the body and one side of extrapersonal space. So-called dressing

apraxia clearly is not a problem with control of volitional movements. The patient's movements during attempted dressing are normal in rate, amplitude, direction, and coordination.

Constructional apraxia is a descriptive label for deficient performance on tests that require the person tested to copy geometric designs or simple drawings, construct simple designs with blocks or sticks, or assemble cut-up representations of everyday objects. The hand and arm movements of patients with compromised constructional abilities are effortless and coordinated, but the drawings or designs they produce are distorted, fragmented, or incomplete. The poor quality of these patients' constructions is believed to be the result of disturbed visuospatial skills such as distinguishing figures from backgrounds, appreciating spatial relationships, and attending to visual space. The label *constructional apraxia* now is fading into disuse, replaced by the more apt *constructional impairment.*

Apraxia of Speech

The label *apraxia of speech* first appeared in the literature in the late 1800s and early 1900s as part of a syndrome called *oral apraxia.* During the first half of the twentieth century, writers began separating apraxic speech movements from apraxic nonspeech movements, and labels such as *apraxic dysarthria, peripheral motor aphasia, articulatory dysarthria,* and *apraxia of vocal expression* appeared in the literature. Darley (1969) settled on the label *apraxia of speech,* and since then speech-language pathologists and many others have used this label for a collection of articulatory impairments, described by Darley, Aronson, and Brown (1975):

> Apraxia of speech is a distinct motor speech disorder distinguishable from the dysarthrias (speech disorders due to impaired innervation of speech musculature) and aphasia (a language disorder due to impairment of the brain mechanism for decoding and encoding the symbol system used in spoken and written

communication). Apraxia of speech is a disorder of motor speech programming manifested primarily by errors in articulation and secondarily by compensatory alterations of prosody. The speaker shows reduced efficiency in accomplishing the oral postures necessary for phoneme production and the sequences of those postures for production of words. The disorder is frequently associated with aphasia but may also occur in isolation. Oral (nonspeech) apraxia may cooccur. (p 267)

Apraxia of speech (sometimes called *verbal apraxia*) resembles other forms of ideomotor apraxia in several ways. It is not caused by weakness, paralysis, or sensory loss in the speech muscles. Unplanned, automatic speech is much less clumsy and effortful than speech requested by an examiner. Speech elicited by natural contexts is less effortful and sounds more nearly normal than speech elicited in artificial contexts (such as a typical speech evaluation). Apraxia of speech is discussed in greater detail in Chapter 13.

AGNOSIA

Agnosia is a generic label for a group of perceptual impairments in which patients fail to recognize stimuli in a sensory modality (e.g., vision, hearing), although perception in the affected modality is preserved. Patients with *visual agnosia* do not recognize objects visually even though they can see (which they can prove by matching identical objects or forms) and even though they are familiar with the visually unrecognized objects (which they can prove by recognizing them when they feel them or hear the sounds they make). Visual agnosia characteristically is caused by damage (usually bilateral) in the occipital lobes, in the posterior parietal lobes, or in the fiber tracts connecting the visual cortex to other areas in the brain. Visual agnosias often are incomplete, intermittent, and inconsistent, and patients with visual agnosias usually function reasonably well in daily life. Because they can see, they do not bump into things and

grope their way about, and they usually recognize and respond appropriately to familiar visual cues in their daily life environment.

Patients with *auditory agnosia* do not appreciate the meaning of sounds, despite adequate hearing acuity. Patients with auditory agnosia respond to sound by turning toward its source, and they are startled by loud sounds. However, they cannot match an object with the sound it makes, even though they recognize the object when it is shown to them. Auditory agnosia, like visual agnosia, may be incomplete or intermittent. Auditory agnosia suggests damage (usually bilateral) in the auditory association cortex. Patients with auditory agnosia may sporadically respond appropriately to sounds or may respond appropriately to certain sounds or categories of sounds.

Patients who have brain damage that isolates Wernicke's area from the auditory cortex in both hemispheres sometimes exhibit a syndrome called *auditory-verbal agnosia* (or *pure word deafness*). *Auditory-verbal agnosia* is a rare phenomenon in which comprehension of speech is severely impaired, although other language skills (reading, writing, and speaking) are retained. Patients with auditory-verbal agnosia fail to appreciate the meaning of spoken words but respond appropriately to nonverbal sounds such as ringing telephones or sirens. They attend to people who speak to them, but they do not understand the meaning of what others say even though they comprehend the same information in printed or written form. Patients with auditory-verbal agnosia often respond to speech as if their native language is unknown to them. However, their speech usually is appropriate in content and form.

Patients with *tactile agnosia* do not recognize objects by touch although their tactile perception is intact. They do recognize the objects if they see them, smell them, or hear the sounds they make. Tactile agnosia usually is a result of parietal lobe damage that isolates the somatosensory cortex from other parts of the brain. Patients with tactile agnosia can report touch, pinprick, and other simple stimulations of the cutaneous receptors in the hands but cannot name, describe, talk about, or demonstrate the use of objects palpated with the hands even though they may recognize basic characteristics such as size, shape, or weight. Patients with tactile agnosia can draw or demonstrate the shape and size of palpated objects, and they can choose matching objects from a group of objects when vision is blocked. The term *astereognosis* is a synonym for tactile agnosia, but sometimes it is used erroneously in a broader sense to denote loss of tactile recognition when tactile sensation is diminished or lost.

Prevalence of Agnosia

True modality-specific agnosia is rare, despite its frequent mention in the literature. Some cases of agnosia reported in the literature may not be true agnosias but may represent perceptual impairments, comprehension impairments, cognitive impairments, or psychogenic symptoms. In deciding on a diagnosis of agnosia, the clinician must exclude several alternative explanations:

- Sensory deficits that interfere with perception in the affected modality; a diagnosis of agnosia requires that sensory function in the affected modality be adequate for perception
- Comprehension disorders that prevent the patient from understanding what is required in a test for agnosia
- Expressive disturbances that prevent the patient from verbally identifying test stimuli
- Unfamiliarity with test stimuli that prevents the patient from relating the stimuli to knowledge and previous experience; unfamiliarity does not explain the agnosia if the patient recognizes the stimuli in another modality

---

GENERAL CONCEPTS 8-2

- *Callosal disconnection syndromes* are caused by destruction of nerve fibers in the corpus callosum—destruction that prevents communication between the brain hemispheres.
- Right-handed patients with *anterior disconnection syndrome* cannot name, describe, write about, or talk about unseen objects palpated with the left hand, because sensory information from the left hand cannot reach the language-competent left hemisphere.
- Right-handed patients with *posterior disconnection syndrome* cannot verbally respond to visual information that is presented only to the right hemisphere. Some patients with posterior disconnection syndrome have *alexia without agraphia,* in which reading is grossly impaired but spontaneous writing and copying are preserved.

- Patients with *complete disconnection syndrome* (also called *split-brain syndrome*) exhibit impairments that combine the impairments caused by anterior and posterior disconnection syndromes. Some may experience *alien hand syndrome.*
- Patients with posterior temporal lobe damage or low parietal lobe damage often experience contralateral visual field blindness.
- *Apraxia* denotes difficulty in carrying out sequences of volitional movements in the absence of weakness, paralysis, sensory loss, or incoordination in the muscles used for the movements.
- *Ideational apraxia* denotes the loss of the ideas needed to understand and demonstrate the use of objects. Ideational apraxia is not considered a true apraxia by some contemporary writers.

GENERAL CONCEPTS 8-2—cont'd

- *Ideomotor apraxia* denotes disruption of the motor plans needed to demonstrate actions. Ideomotor apraxia is more common than is ideational apraxia.
- *Buccofacial apraxia, limb apraxia,* and *apraxia of speech* are forms of ideomotor apraxia.
- Diagnosis of ideomotor apraxia requires that alternative explanations for the movement disorder be eliminated. Alternative explanations include weakness or paralysis, sensory loss, incoordination, and comprehension impairment.

- *Apraxia of speech* (or *verbal apraxia*) is characterized by variable articulatory errors and trial-and-error articulatory groping in a context of slow and effortful speech.
- *Agnosia* denotes a condition in which patients fail to recognize otherwise familiar stimuli in a sensory modality even though basic perception in that modality is preserved. *Visual agnosia, auditory agnosia,* and *tactile agnosia (astereognosis)* are the three basic agnosia syndromes described in the literature.

LIMITATIONS OF CONNECTIONISTIC EXPLANATIONS OF APHASIA AND RELATED DISORDERS

With the advent of brain-imaging technology such as computerized tomography (CT), magnetic resonance imaging (MRI), positron-emission tomography (PET), and single-photon emission computed tomography (SPECT), cerebral damage came to be localized with greater accuracy and in greater detail than ever before (except, of course, for postmortem examination of patients' brains). The use of brain-imaging technology has created new insights into the relationships between brain damage and aphasia syndromes. Numerous reports on the relationships between aphasia and lesions located and measured with brain-imaging technology have appeared in the literature during the last 2 decades. These reports have led to several modifications to the classic concepts of the relationships between brain damage and aphasia syndromes. Two of the most important are:

- Damage confined to Broca's area or Wernicke's area usually does not produce chronic Broca's or Wernicke's aphasia.

- Aphasia may be caused by damage deep in the brain, below the perisylvian cortex and its association fibers.

Several reports have suggested that lesions confined to Broca's area or Wernicke's area do not produce persisting Broca's aphasia or Wernicke's aphasia. Mohr, Pessin, Finkelstein, and associates (1978) studied 22 cases of aphasia in which the site and extent of brain damage was documented and reviewed 83 published reports in which the brains of aphasic patients came to autopsy. They concluded that lesions confined to Broca's area do not produce chronic Broca's aphasia but produce transitory mutism progressing to rapidly resolving articulatory targeting and sequencing impairments (apraxia of speech), with no significant persisting impairments in language. According to Mohr and associates, lesions must extend beyond Broca's area to produce persisting Broca's aphasia. Knopman, Selnes, Niccum, and associates (1983) published similar findings. They reported that patients with lesions confined to Broca's area exhibit transient nonfluent speech without persisting Broca's aphasia. According to Knopman and associates, persisting Broca's aphasia requires a lesion extending from Broca's area into the primary motor cortex or the parietal lobe.

Similar doubts have been raised concerning the relationship between damage confined to Wernicke's area and chronic Wernicke's aphasia. Selnes, Knopman, Niccum, and associates (1983) measured recovery of language by 39 aphasic adults with single left-hemisphere lesions. They tested the patients' language comprehension once a month for 5 months. Patients with damage confined to Wernicke's area recovered near-normal language comprehension. Patients with persisting severe language comprehension deficits characteristically had damage extending beyond Wernicke's area into the inferior parietal lobe.

Selnes, Knopman, Niccum, and associates (1985) later reported that the most striking persisting consequence of damage confined to Wernicke's area is impaired repetition. They studied 10 patients who were judged to have Wernicke's aphasia at 1 month postonset. At 6 months postonset, 8 of the 10 were subsequently judged to have conduction aphasia. They had poor speech repetition and relatively good (although not normal) comprehension.

Classical connectionist models attribute aphasia to damage in key regions of the cerebral cortex or in fibers connecting one key region to another. The classic models disregard the possibility of aphasia resulting from deep subcortical damage. However, it is now apparent that right-handed patients with damage in the left basal ganglia or left thalamus can become aphasic (Alexander & Lo Verme, 1980; Cappa & Vignolo, 1979; Mohr, Walters, & Duncan, 1975; Naeser & associates, 1982; Ojemann, 1975; and others).

Naeser, Alexander, Helm-Estabrooks, and associates (1982) studied nine cases of aphasia caused by damage in and around the left basal ganglia and reported three subcortical aphasia syndromes, based on the front-to-back location of damage. Patients with an *anterior syndrome* (caused by damage in the internal capsule, the lenticular nucleus, and extending into anterior white matter) exhibited hemiplegia, slow, dysarthric speech with good phrase length and prosody, good comprehension; good repetition, poor oral reading and writing, and poor confrontation naming.

Patients with a *posterior syndrome* (caused by damage in the putamen and internal capsule, extending into posterior white matter) exhibited hemiplegia, fluent speech without dysarthria, poor comprehension, good single-word repetition, poor sentence repetition, impaired reading and writing, and poor confrontation naming. (The posterior syndrome resembles Wernicke's aphasia except for the presence of hemiplegia in the subcortical syndrome.) Cappa, Cavalotti, Guidotti, and associates (1983) also described an anterior syndrome and a posterior syndrome similar to those described by Naeser and associates.

Robin and Schienberg (1990) reported speech and language impairments in 10 right-handed aphasic patients with damage in the left basal ganglia. Four spoke fluently, five were nonfluent, and one was initially fluent but became nonfluent. One fluent patient had severe language impairment and jargon speech output, and three had mild impairments of auditory comprehension plus literal and verbal paraphasias in their speech. Naming was moderately impaired in all four. Three of the five nonfluent patients had severe (global) aphasia; two had moderately severe aphasia. Four of the five exhibited signs of apraxia of speech, dysarthria, or both.

Aphasia caused by lesions in the left thalamus has been described in several published reports, and the role of the thalamus in language has received considerable attention (Mohr, Walters, & Duncan, 1975; Ojemann, 1975; Cappa & Vignolo, 1979; and others). Patients with aphasia caused by thalamic lesions almost always are hemiplegic because of damage to pyramidal-tract fibers passing through the internal capsule. Patients with thalamic aphasia often have difficulty initiating spontaneous speech, but when they get started they speak fluently with normal rate and prosody, although literal paraphasias, verbal paraphasias, neologisms, and word retrieval failures are common. *Hypophonia* (weak voice) is common. Naming usually is mildly to moderately impaired. Auditory and reading comprehension usually are minimally impaired. Patients with left thalamic damage tend to be perseverative, and their performance tends to fluctuate from task to task and from moment to moment.

Murdoch (1990) has commented that aphasia syndromes resulting from thalamic lesions resemble transcortical motor aphasia in that repetition and comprehension tend to be preserved, but self-initiated speech tends to be reduced. According to Murdoch, the language impairments of patients with left subcortical damage usually are mild, and patients with subcortical aphasia have a better prognosis for recovery than patients with aphasia caused by cortical damage. Damasio, Damasio, Rizzo, and associates (1982) and Mateer and Ojemann (1983), among others, have commented that subcortical aphasia usually spontaneously resolves within a few weeks or months. Robin and Schienberg reported, however, that three patients with thalamic damage experienced persisting aphasia 2 years after onset. Robin and Schienberg commented:

> ...assuming that aphasia accompanying a subcortical lesion may be transient may have negative consequences. Until we began to study these patients, our medical staff frequently counseled patients that their "speech" would get better on its own. Consequently, referrals were not made, and many patients went untreated. (p. 99)

Although aphasia syndromes follow subcortical damage, it is not clear that the damaged subcortical structures are directly involved in language. In many of the patients studied, damage was not confined to subcortical structures but extended to the cortex. Dewitt, Grek, Buonanno, and associates (1985) asserted that MRI scans of patients with subcortical aphasias usually reveal involvement of cortical tissue not shown by CT scans. Metter, Riege, Hanson, and associates (1983) reported that PET studies of patients with subcortical aphasia almost always reveal decreased cortical metabolism in areas of the left hemisphere without observable structural damage. Alexander, Naeser, and Palumbo (1987) studied 18 patients with only subcortical damage and retrospectively reviewed the cases of 61 more. They reported that damage confined to the thalamus does not cause persisting aphasia but may cause mild word retrieval impairments. They suggested that subcortical lesions causing aphasia must involve deep nerve fiber tracts connecting subcortical regions with one another or nerve fiber tracts connecting subcortical regions to cortical regions. At this time it is not clear if the basal ganglia and the thalamus are directly responsible for some aspects of language, or if the two regions produce language impairment by disrupting communication to, from, or between cortical language areas.

THE EXPLANATORY POWER OF CONNECTIONIST MODELS

Despite the seeming objectivity of connectionist explanations of aphasia, they do not and probably cannot provide a complete explanation of brain-behavior relationships. As Jackson (1866) pointed out, symptoms appearing after brain damage identify the brain location in which damage produces a *symptom* and do not necessarily identify the location in the brain of the underlying *function* or *process* to which the symptom relates. Kertesz (1979) extends Jackson's assertion, saying "Only lesions causing impairments are localizable, not the impairment itself" (p. 142).

When symptoms are produced not by destruction of functional regions of cortex but by destruction of association fibers, localizationist interpretations are likely to go astray. For example, damage in the left hemisphere at the parieto-occipital-temporal junction (the angular gyrus region) is known to cause reading impairments. From this evidence a strict localizationist might conclude that the parieto-occipital-junction in the left hemisphere is a center for reading. The conclusion would be neurophysiologically naive, because reading is a complex process that requires the participation of several brain regions. Reading impairments and damage in the region of the angular gyrus of the left hemisphere may occur together because damage there disrupts communication between the visual cortex and Wernicke's area, not because the angular gyrus region is a center for reading. Few would argue that the lesions producing transcortical motor aphasia do so by destroying a center for initiation of speech, but most would agree that these patients' reticence is caused by isolation of regions responsible for speech from regions responsible for activation and arousal.

According to Goodglass (1993), connectionist syndromes represent "the result of modal tendencies for the functional organization of language in adult human brains" (p. 218). Goodglass believes that adult human brains are to some extent *hard wired,* but as an individual matures, the individual's brain develops its own most efficient neural organization for carrying out the processes involved in language. According to Goodglass, there are common (modal) patterns of brain organization toward which brains gravitate (presumably these common patterns are the result of the hard wiring). These modal patterns produce enough consistency in brain organization to make connectionistic explanations of brain-behavior relationships useful. However, according to Goodglass, individual differences in how the brain has organized itself for language may be superimposed on these modal patterns, producing exceptions, contradictions, or incomplete representations of the classic connectionist aphasia syndromes in individual patients.

Because of these individual differences, connectionist explanations of aphasia work better for groups than for individuals. If a large group of right-handed adults with left temporal lobe damage were to be tested, the overall pattern of performance would almost certainly match the classic pattern for Wernicke's aphasia. Comprehension would be impaired, paraphasic speech errors (especially verbal paraphasias) and vague and indefinite words would be common, and the group would use more words than necessary to communicate a given amount of information. However, there would undoubtedly be some in the group who produced few or no paraphasic errors, some who produced few vague and indefinite words, some who did not exhibit press of speech, and perhaps a few whose comprehension was relatively good.

The uncertainty of connectionist models increases not only as one moves from groups of aphasic patients to individuals, but as one moves from global characteristics (such as speech fluency) to more specific aspects of language (e.g., word retrieval failure). The fuzziness of connectionist models with regard to specifics is apparent when aphasia test batteries designed expressly to classify aphasic patients into connectionist syndromes prove unable to classify unambiguously from 15% (Poeck, 1983) to 40% (Benson, 1979) or up to 80% (Goodglass & Kaplan, 1983) of patients into classic connectionist syndromes based on their language behaviors.

Despite these shortcomings, connectionist aphasia syndromes and their terminology are useful to the clinician who wishes to communicate efficiently or to venture a guess about the location and severity of a patient's brain damage from a patient's neurologic abnormalities. Goodglass (1993) has commented that classic patterns of Wernicke's or Broca's aphasia usually point unambiguously to damage in the temporal lobe (in the case of Wernicke's aphasia) or the posterior inferior frontal lobe (in the case of Broca's aphasia), but when the classic patterns are mixed or incomplete, predicting the location of the brain damage underlying the symptoms becomes uncertain. Often those who use the connectionist model will be surprised by patients who do not fit the model, but their predictions will be supported by enough patients who do fit the model to make it a convenient tool.

The connectionist model is in many respects a fiction, but it remains a useful one for the speech-language pathologist who wishes to understand the basic relationships between symptoms of aphasia and their source in the nervous system. The speech-language pathologist who understands the relationships between connectionist aphasia syndromes and various patterns of language impairments can use the presence of a connectionist aphasia syndrome to help them plan assessment of the patient's communication impairments. In addition, knowledge of the connectionist model helps speech-language pathologists communicate with neurologists and other professionals who make referrals and talk in the language of the model.

GENERAL CONCEPTS 8-3

- Contemporary evidence suggests that brain injury must extend beyond Broca's area to cause persisting Broca's aphasia and must extend beyond Wernicke's area to cause persisting Wernicke's aphasia.
- Patients with brain injury deep in the subcortical regions of the language-dominant hemisphere may become aphasic. It is not clear whether their aphasia is caused by damage to deep brain structures serving language, by disruption of neural communica-

tion between deep brain structures and the cortex, or by extension of damage from deep brain structures into the cortex.
- Connectionist models of aphasia are better at describing brain-behavior relationships for groups of patients than for predicting an individual patient's aphasic symptoms. Connnectionist models predict global symptoms such as speech fluency better than they predict specific impairments such as word retrieval failure.

THOUGHT QUESTIONS

Question 8-1 A patient exhibits no paralysis of either hand or arm but exhibits unilateral limb apraxia of the right hand and arm. Is this what one would expect? Speculate as to the location of the neuropathology that might yield such a pattern of signs.

Question 8-2 An examiner wishes to test a right-handed aphasic patient without hemiplegia for limb apraxia. She points to the patient's right arm and says, *With that arm, show me how you wave good-bye.* After the patient responds, she points to the patient's left arm and says, *With that arm, show me how you wave good-bye.* What is the potential problem with this way of testing?

Question 8-3 A right-handed stroke patient with presumed alexia without agraphia and no other neurologic signs has intact visual fields. The patient has no previous history of neurologic problems. Is this possible?

Question 8-4 What nonlanguage problems would you expect in a right-handed patient who has conduction aphasia?

Question 8-5 What nonlanguage problems would you expect in a right-handed patient who has transcortical motor aphasia? In a right-handed patient who has transcortical sensory aphasia?

CHAPTER 9

Treatment of Aphasia and Related Disorders

Aphasic patients need help with all aspects of their changing and evolving condition during recovery. Some of the problems are manifest concurrently with the linguistic problems; others persist or may become expressed as the aphasic patient comes to appreciate the full reality of his or her condition. A few are able to manage most of the problems by themselves. Most require help from others. (Eisenson [1974]. Adult aphasia. 2nd ed. Englewood Cliffs, NJ: Prentice Hall.)

This chapter describes in a general way how clinicians go about treating adults with aphasia and related communicative disorders. The concepts and procedures described in this chapter relate directly to treatment of aphasia and also relate, although less directly, to treatment of other cognitive-communicative disorders. The chapter begins with an overarching concern—is what speech-language pathologists do in treatment of aphasic adults worth doing?

PROCESS-ORIENTED TREATMENT

Treatment for aphasia had its origins in medical settings in which intervention typically progressed from diagnosis to treatment to discharge. Clinicians who provided treatment for aphasic conditions at that time had backgrounds in education, psychology, and linguistics. The combination yielded a pedagogic approach to treatment that had as its goal the reeducation, reorganization, or restimulation of language processes. From the 1940s to the late 1970s, aphasia treatment customarily relied on didactic methods in which aphasic patients participated in drills designed to reactivate language processes. The general objective of such didactic treatment was to help aphasic adults become better communicators by improving the linguistic and grammatic quality of their communication. Process-oriented treatment predominated in clinical aphasiology from the 1940s to the 1970s, when functional approaches to aphasia treatment appeared, and in the 1980s the concepts of social participation and quality of life began to affect intervention. In the next several sections I will describe some characteristics of process-oriented treatment. Then I will do the same for functional and social approaches to intervention.

Effectiveness of Process-Oriented Treatment

The value of process-oriented treatment for aphasic adults' communicative disorders has been a source of controversy for many years. The skeptics (mostly neurologists and others in the medical profession) doubted that treatment provided benefits beyond those attributable to neurologic recovery. The believers (mostly speech-language pathologists, aphasic patients, and aphasic patients' families) were convinced that treatment provided benefits that could not be explained away by neurologic recovery.

The Evidence. A retrospective study by Butfield and Zangwill (1946) was one of the first to address the issue, although their primary purpose was to describe the time-course of recovery from aphasia. Butfield and Zangwill reviewed the records of 70 aphasic patients, all of whom had received treatment for their aphasia. The number of treatment sessions the patients received was not controlled, and it ranged from 5 to 290. Butfield and Zangwill's outcome measure was a 3-category rating scale—much improved, improved, or unchanged.

They concluded that treatment was beneficial because 3 to 6 times as many patients were "*improved*" or "*much improved*" than were "*unchanged*" at the end of treatment. Although good news to speech-language pathologists, the quality of the evidence is not impressive. Participants included stroke patients, tumor patients, patients with traumatic brain injuries, and several other kinds of brain injury patients. The treatment procedures were described only in general terms. The outcome measure was subjective, insensitive, and of questionable reliability. It was a reasonable effort for its time, but Butfield and Zangwill's study falls far short of contemporary standards for scientific precision and control.

Vignolo (1964) followed with a retrospective study of the records of 69 aphasic patients, each of whom had received treatment and had been tested at least twice with at least 40 days between the 2 tests. Vignolo's outcome measure was a 3-category subjective rating—unchanged, improved, or recovered. Of the participants who received treatment, 70% improved or recovered, whereas 56% of the participants who were not treated recovered, and the effects of treatment were stronger for participants who began treatment at least 6 months after onset. Vignolo found that spontaneous recovery added to treatment effects in the first 6 months after onset— the difference between treated and untreated participants was smaller for participants treated in the first 6 months postonset than for participants treated 6 months or more after onset. Vignolo also suggested that treatment for patients who are more than 6 months post-onset is most effective if it is continued for at least 6 months. Vignolo's study, like that of Butfield and Zangqwill, was reasonable for its time but does not meet contemporary standards for precision and control.

A study by Sarno, Silverman, and Sands (1970) provided grist for the skeptics' mill. Sarno and her associates placed severely aphasic patients into one of three groups: traditional treatment, programmed instruction treatment, or no treatment. Each participant received from 7 to 46 hours of treatment (the average was 28 hours). There were no significant differences among the groups at the end of treatment, leading Sarno and her associates to conclude that "severe aphasic stroke patients do not benefit from therapy" (p. 621). However, they also commented, "The fact that speech therapy of either type did not affect language recovery in this study is no doubt related to the severity of their aphasia" (p. 621).

Despite its popularity with the skeptics, the Sarno study provided no convincing evidence for or against the value of treatment for aphasia. The study included only patients who were severely aphasic, and severely aphasic patients are known to be notoriously unresponsive to treatment. Programmed instruction treatment, though in vogue at the time, was essentially abandoned in favor of other approaches to treatment within a few years, presumably because those who used it were disappointed in its results. Several outcome measures (e.g., writing, connected speech) may have been inappropriate for severely aphasic patients, who are unlikely to improve in these higher-level abilities. The Sarno study was a well-intentioned attempt to get at an important question in aphasiology, but its results tell us nothing about aphasia treatment in general and little about treatment of severely aphasic adults.

Basso, Capitani, and Vignolo (1979) provided fresh ammunition for the backers of aphasia treatment. Basso and her associates retrospectively compared the effect of "stimulation" treatment for a group of 162 aphasic patients with the effect of no treatment for a group of 119 aphasic patients. The outcome measure was the number of patients who improved or did not improve on tests of auditory comprehension, reading, speech, and writing. A significantly greater percentage of patients who received treatment improved compared with patients who received no treatment, and the

effects of treatment were stronger for patients with severe aphasia than for patients with moderate aphasia. Basso and associates concluded that treatment had a highly significant positive effect on recovery from aphasia and that early treatment was better than later treatment. The Basso study was well designed and executed. Its major weakness is that the no-treatment group was made up of aphasic persons who did not receive treatment because they lived too far from the clinic, had no transportation, were unwilling to participate, or declined treatment for similar reasons, rather than being randomly assigned to the no-treatment group.

In the first randomized trial of aphasia treatment, Wertz, Collins, Weiss, and associates (1981) prospectively studied the effects of individual treatment and group treatment for aphasic adults. Participants were carefully selected, reliable outcome measures were chosen, and the nature of treatment was well controlled. Each participant was tested with a comprehensive battery of tests at intake and at 15, 26, 37, and 48 weeks after intake. Both groups improved significantly between intake and each subsequent test, with few significant differences between the groups at any test point. Wertz and his associates asserted that both treatments were efficacious, because both groups continued to improve beyond 24 weeks post-onset—when spontaneous neurologic recovery is assumed to be complete. Because no untreated control group was included, Wertz and his associates could make no claims regarding the benefits of treatment versus no treatment.

Lincoln, Mulloy, Jones, and associates (1984) weighed in on the side of the skeptics with an 87-patient prospective study of the effects of aphasia treatment. The control group comprised 74 patients who received no treatment. Patients were tested at 4 weeks after onset, 10 weeks after onset (when treated patients entered treatment), 22 weeks after onset, and 44 weeks after onset. There were no significant differences between groups at any test point, leading the authors to conclude that "speech therapy does not improve language abilities any more than was achieved by spontaneous recovery" (p. 1199). Unfortunately for the authors' conclusions, serious flaws in design and execution seriously compromise the value of their results. Participants were not screened to exclude those with multiple lesions or with cognitive, emotional, or physical impairments that would diminish their response to treatment. Few treated patients received the prescribed amount of treatment. Of the patients, 48% received less than half of the prescribed 48 treatment sessions, and about 75% of the patients would be considered drop-outs in a well-designed study. Wertz, Deal, Holland, Kurtzke, and Weiss (1986) subsequently commented, "The results indicated that when one does not treat patients who may or may not be aphasic, those patients do not improve" (p. 31).

Shewan and Kertesz (1984) added to the confidence of those who believe in the efficacy of treatment with the results of a prospective study in which they assigned aphasic adults to language-oriented treatment, stimulation-facilitation treatment, unstructured treatment, or no treatment. Each patient was tested with the *Western Aphasia Battery (WAB)* at 2 to 4 weeks after onset and at 3, 6, and 12 months after the first test. There were no significant differences in the amount of improvement on the WAB among the groups at the 6-month test point, which Shewan and Kertesz attributed to the strong effects of spontaneous recovery. When the change in WAB performance from the first test to the 12-month test was measured, however, each of the three treated groups had improved significantly more than the untreated group. Shewan and Kertesz concluded that treatment administered by trained speech-language pathologists is efficacious.

Wertz, Weiss, Aten, and associates (1986) provided more good news for believers in aphasia treatment with the results of a study of clinic treatment, home treatment, and deferred treat-ment. The clinic treatment group received 8 to 10 hours of treatment provided by a speech-language pathologist each week for 12 weeks, followed by 12 weeks of no treatment but periodic testing. The home treatment group received treatment from a family member or friend in the patient's home who was supervised by a speech-language pathologist. The home treatment group, like the clinic treatment group, received 8 to 10 hours of treatment per week for 12 weeks followed by 12 weeks of no treatment with periodic testing. The deferred treatment group was tested but not treated for 12 weeks, followed by 8 to 10 hours of treatment provided by a speech-language pathologist each week for 12 weeks. At 12 weeks the clinic treatment group had made significantly greater improvement on the criterion measure—the overall percentile score on the *Porch Index of Communicative Ability (PICA*; Porch, 1981a)—than either of the other two groups. At 24 weeks the deferred-treatment group had caught up with the other two groups; there were no significant differences among the groups at the 24-week test (Figure 9-1).

Poeck, Huber, and Willmes (1989) also concluded that aphasia treatment is efficacious, based on the results of a well-designed study in which they provided 6 to 8 weeks of intensive treatment to 68 aphasic adults. A control group of 92 aphasic adults received no treatment but were tested on the same schedule as the treated group. Both the treated group and the untreated group improved significantly on measures of speech and language, but those who received treatment improved significantly more than those who did not, even when the effects of spontaneous recovery were accounted for.

In addition to group studies of the effects of aphasia treatment, a number of well-designed single-case design studies (e.g., Boser, Weinrich, & McCall, 2000; Kearns and Salmon, 1984; Murray & Heather, 2001; Thompson & Byrne, 1984) show that individualized treatment programs produce meaningful changes in targeted

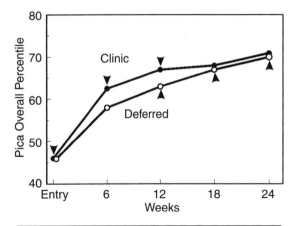

Figure 9-1 ■ Change in PICA overall percentile for participants in the Clinic Treatment group and the Deferred Treatment group from entry in the study to 6, 12, 18, and 24 weeks after entry. The arrows denote times at which participants received treatment. (Data from Wertz, R.T., Weiss, D.G., Aten, J.L., and associates. [1986]. A comparison of clinic, home, and deferred language treatment for aphasia: A VA cooperative study. *Archives of Neurology, 43,* 653-658.)

aspects of individual aphasic patients' performance and that generalization of the changes to patients' daily life environments can be obtained. Thompson and Byrne, for example, trained two adults with Broca's aphasia to use social conventions (greetings, self-disclosures, and questions) in conversations. Training progressed from traditional clinician-patient treatment to role playing in simulated daily life situations. Generalization of participants' use of social conventions to conversations with unfamiliar partners was assessed. Training resulted in increased use of social conventions by both aphasic participants, and both participants generalized their use of greetings and self-disclosures (but not questions) to conversations with unfamiliar partners.

Robey (1998) and Robey, Schultz, Crawford, and associates (1999) have reported results from two meta-analyses of treatment literature in aphasia. Meta-analysis is a statistical procedure for finding converging evidence in a group of independent studies—in this case, evidence related to treatment efficacy in studies of aphasia treatment. Robey and associates' results suggest that recovery of communication by treated aphasic adults is approximately twice that of untreated aphasic adults when treatment begins in the first month after onset of aphasia, with a smaller, but statistically significant, benefit for aphasic adults whose treatment begins after the first month following onset.

Conclusion. The evidence from group and single-case studies clearly supports the efficacy of process-oriented treatment for aphasia, provided several conditions are met:

- Treatment is delivered or directed by qualified professionals.
- Patients with irreversible aphasia are excluded.
- The content, intensity, duration, and timing of treatment are appropriate for those receiving treatment.
- Sensitive and reliable measures are used to track changes in performance.

This does not mean, however, that speech-language pathologists are off the effectiveness hook, because the emphasis has shifted from *efficacy* (whether treatment yields a significant change on one or more tests) to *effectiveness* (whether treatment causes meaningful changes in daily life communication performance). When the concepts of efficacy and effectiveness are separated, it becomes clear that most existing studies of aphasia treatment are efficacy studies—their measures of the effects of treatment are changes on one or more tests of communication ability. Consequently, the evidence supports the *efficacy* of aphasia treatment but not necessarily its *effectiveness.* The issue of effectiveness has now taken center stage, and investigators are at work developing measures of treatment effectiveness and planning studies to determine if aphasia treatment is effective as well as efficacious.

Holland (1996) asserted that changes on standardized language tests do, in fact, reflect changes in functional communication, because the standardized measures are significantly correlated with functional performance. The validity of Holland's assertion depends on the strength of the correlation. A significant correlation does not necessarily mean that the correlated phenomena are strongly related—it simply means that the coefficient of correlation is significantly greater than zero. Holland presumably based her assertion on correlations of .84 and .93 between aphasic patients' performance on *Communicative Activities of Daily Living* (*CADL*; Holland, 1980), considered a measure of functional communication, and performance on two standardized language assessment batteries. Correlations of this magnitude suggest that performance on the standardized language assessment batteries is a relatively strong indicator of functional communication as measured by CADL.

The Timing of Intervention

Another issue that has bedeviled clinical aphasiology relates to the timing of intervention; is treatment begun a month or more after onset of aphasia as efficacious (or effective) as treatment begun soon after a patient becomes aphasic? Studies of early versus late intervention yield equivocal results. Several investigators report that delaying treatment by 2 months or more after the onset of aphasia has significant negative effects on patients' eventual recovery (Butfield & Zangwill, 1946; Sands, Sarno, & Shankweiler, 1969; Vignolo, 1964; Wepman, 1951). Vignolo (1964), for example, studied the recovery of 69 aphasic patients. Some received treatment, and some did not. Vignolo concluded that it is important that treatment begin while physiologic recovery is most rapid. "Only the period which extends from 2 to 6 months after the onset of aphasia seems to provide a ground where intrinsic capacity for recovery can be highly enhanced by the intervention of planned training" (p. 366).

Poeck and associates (1989) reported that neither age nor time after onset of aphasia significantly affected aphasic adults' recovery of language. However, time after onset appeared to affect the magnitude of patients' response to treatment. Of those who began treatment within the first 4 months after onset of aphasia, 78% improved significantly on a standardized aphasia test, whereas 46% of those who began treatment from 4 to 12 months after onset improved significantly on the same test even when subjects' test scores were corrected for the effects of spontaneous neurologic recovery. The results of Robey's (1998) meta-analysis of 21 aphasia treatment studies also suggested that treatment begun in the first few weeks after onset of aphasia produces greater improvement than treatment begun after that time.

Others have concluded that delaying treatment has no major effects on outcome. Wertz and associates (1986) concluded that delaying treatment for 12 weeks had no irreversible effects on aphasic patients' eventual overall PICA scores, because the performance of patients who received treatment after a 12-week delay approximated the scores of patients who received treatment upon entry into the study. As this is written, we do not know if delaying treatment has important or irreversible effects on aphasic adults' recovery of communicative abilities, because group studies have reached conflicting conclusions, and single-case studies have not addressed the question.

If delaying treatment were to have few or no significant effects on patient's scores on standardized tests of language and communication (the criterion used in published studies), it may not be legitimate to conclude that delaying treatment has no negative effects on the patient or the patient's family. Clinicians do more than treat specific speech and language behaviors in the first weeks following the onset of a patient's aphasia. They help patients and patients' families prepare for participation in life. They educate patients and families about the causes of aphasia and provide them with strategies for dealing with communication breakdown. They make referrals to other disciplines and help the patient and family make use of community resources. They provide reassurance, advice, and support as the patient and the family come to grips with the changes in lifestyle produced by the patient's physical, medical, and communicative disabilities.

Education, counseling, and support may not affect an aphasic patient's scores on standardized tests, yet they are important to patients and families immediately after onset of aphasia. Therefore, even if delaying treatment does not affect test scores, it cannot be said that clinicians have little to contribute to aphasic patients during the first 10 or 12 weeks after onset that cannot just as well be done later. It may be that delaying treatment is not fatal to aphasic adults' recovery of communicative abilities as measured with standardized tests, but it seems likely that delaying or eliminating counseling, education, and support during the first weeks after the patient becomes aphasic may have important and irreversible negative effects on the patient and the patient's family.

Contemporary third-party payers' restrictions on the duration and intensity of treatment and the current emphasis on expanding aphasic persons' participation in everyday life and enhancing aphasic persons' quality of life add to the importance of early intervention. Clinicians may no longer have the option of waiting until aphasic patients are neurologically stable before intervening, and dozens or hundreds of impairment level treatment sessions may no longer be possible.

The data on the relationships between the time at which intervention begins and the effects of intervention come from studies of process-oriented treatment in which patients' specific linguistic and communicative impairments were the focus of intervention. Anecdotal evidence suggests that social approaches to intervention that enhance chronically aphasic persons' access to and participation in activities of daily life have meaningful positive effects even when they begin months or years after the onset of aphasia. I discuss social approaches to intervention later in this chapter.

Candidacy for Treatment

Not all adults with aphasia receive process-oriented treatment for their aphasia, and not all should. Some have such mild impairments that spontaneous neurologic recovery leaves them with no significant linguistic or communicative impairments. Some are too ill or too weak to tolerate treatment. Some are so severely impaired that existing process-oriented treatment approaches offer no hope of linguistic recovery sufficient to justify the cost of treatment. Some who would otherwise be candidates for treatment refuse it. And, regrettably, some who are treatment candidates do not have the money or the insurance coverage to pay for it. Patient refusal and financial coverage are not under the clinician's control, so the clinician's decision to offer treatment usually depends on the clinician's best guess as to whether treatment will produce improvements in the patient's communication sufficient to justify its cost.

As we will see later in this chapter, many severely aphasic persons may be helped by socially oriented interventions that teach aphasic persons and their communicative partners strategies and techniques for enhancing interpersonal communication and social interaction.

Schuell (1965) described the test performance of a group of aphasic adults who exhibited what she called *irreversible aphasic syndrome*, which she characterized as "almost complete loss of functional language skills in all modalities" (p. 14). According to Schuell, patients with irreversible aphasic syndrome cannot reliably point to common objects named by the examiner, cannot follow simple spoken directions, cannot read aloud nor comprehend simple printed sentences, cannot name objects or give simple biographic information, and cannot write simple words, either spontaneously or to dictation. A few can match some simple words to pictures, some produce a few automatic and overlearned speech responses such as counting or profanity, and some can copy simple drawings. Schuell commented that a few patients with irreversible aphasic syndrome make limited gains in auditory comprehension, but she asserted that none recover functional language in any modality.

Presumably Schuell was referring to verbal language (auditory comprehension, reading, speaking, and writing) and not gestural communication, body language, or other nonverbal means of communication, which often are retained by patients with severe aphasia and which may enable success in communicating with familiar conversation partners.

What Schuell calls *irreversible aphasic syndrome* others call *global aphasia.* Collins (1991) characterizes global aphasia as follows:

Global aphasia is a severe, acquired impairment of communicative ability across all language modalities, and often no single communicative modality is strikingly better than another. Visual nonverbal problem-solving abilities are often severely depressed as well and are usually compatible with language performance. It [global aphasia] usually results from extensive damage to the language zones of the left hemisphere but may result from smaller, subcortical lesions. (p. 6)

Goodglass and Kaplan (1983) likewise characterized global aphasia as loss of almost all verbal communication:

In global aphasia, all aspects of language are so severely impaired that there is no longer a distinctive pattern of preserved versus impaired

components. It is only articulation that is sometimes well preserved in the few words or stereotyped utterances that are preserved. Global aphasics sometimes produce stereotyped utterances that may consist of real or nonsense words. Some patients produce a continuous output of syllables that employ a limited set of vowel-consonant combinations that make no sense, even though they are uttered with expressive intonation...Auditory comprehension of conversation concerning material of immediate personal relevance may appear fairly good in comparison to the patient's poor performance on all the formal auditory comprehension subtests. (p. 97)

The foregoing descriptions are remarkably consistent. They portray the globally aphasic adult as one who has limited comprehension of personally relevant spoken language but little usable expressive language beyond a few stereotyped utterances.

The healing effects of time apparently have little effect on the language abilities of most patients who remain globally aphasic beyond the first month or so after onset. Studies by Brust, Shafer, Richter, and Bruun (1976); Kertesz and McCabe (1977); and Prins, Snow, and Wagenaar (1978) suggest a grim prognosis for most patients who remain globally aphasic at one month or more after onset.

Brust and associates reviewed the medical records of 177 aphasic stroke patients. Of those who were diagnosed as globally aphasic at onset, 75% remained globally aphasic 1 month to 3 months later. Kertesz and McCabe reported that 83% of patients who were globally aphasic at 1 month after onset remained globally aphasic at 1 year after onset. Prins, Snow, and Wagenaar found that 80% of patients who were globally aphasic at 3 months after onset remained globally aphasic at 1 year after onset.

Collins (1991) reminds us, however, that global aphasia can be *acute, evolving,* or *chronic.* According to Collins, many aphasic patients are globally aphasic at onset and immediately thereafter. Those with *acute global aphasia* evolve to less severe forms within the first week or so after onset. Those with *evolving global aphasia* are globally aphasic at onset, but over a period of months or years slowly evolve to less severe forms of aphasia (usually Broca's aphasia with coexisting agrammatism). Those with *chronic global aphasia* experience profound communicative disabilities for the rest of their lives.

There seems little doubt that the presence of global aphasia in a neurologically recovered patient is an ominous prognostic sign for recovery of functional language. Only about one in five achieve some functional use of language, and most of those who do regain some functional language remain markedly aphasic, with functional verbal communication limited to communication of basic needs, and comprehension limited to bits and pieces of simple conversational interactions on highly familiar topics.

I will use the appellation *"neurologically recovered"* to denote patients for whom physiologic recovery is essentially complete. For most patients with occlusive strokes, physiologic recovery is essentially complete within 4 to 6 weeks, although slow improvement beyond that time is common. For patients with hemorrhagic strokes and for those with traumatic brain injuries, physiologic recovery may last longer, but it usually is essentially complete within 3 to 6 months.

Not surprisingly, globally aphasic patients perform poorly on language test batteries. Their overall test performance places them well below the 25th percentile for aphasic adults (usually around the 10th to 15th percentile), and their performance across subtests is consistently poor, with no subtest or group of subtests yielding strikingly better performance than others. Figure 9-2 summarizes the performance of a globally aphasic patient on the PICA. The patient makes no intelligible, accurate stimulus-related responses on any subtest except Subtest X (pointing to objects by name), Subtest VIII (matching pictures to objects), and Subtest XI (matching objects to objects).

Universally poor performance across all subtests in language test batteries is one sign of global aphasia. In addition to their poor performance on all tests of speaking, listening, comprehension, reading, and writing, globally aphasic patients typically exhibit other signs of severe impairment that may become evident before formal testing begins—when the clinician interviews the patient or during screening tests of communication, memory, and cognition.

Verbal stereotypies—repetitive, stereotypical utterances (e.g., *me-me-me-me, oh boy-oh boy-oh boy-oh boy*) are common in the speech of patients with global aphasia, and verbal stereotypies may be the only spontaneous speech produced by some globally aphasic patients. Some patients with severe Wernicke's aphasia also produce verbal stereotypies, but the stereotypies alternate with or occur within words, phrases, or sentences that convey meaning, although the meaning may not be appropriate to the context.

Globally aphasic patients often cannot match identical common objects (e.g., forks, pencils, or keys) or cannot match common objects to pictures—tasks that patients with less severe aphasia easily accomplish. Failure to match objects to identical objects or objects to their pictorial representations is considered by some practitioners to be a sign of bilateral brain damage.

Aphasic patients with posterior brain injury and visual impairments caused by damage in the visual cortex or visual association regions may fail visual matching tests. These patients have great difficulty in tasks that depend on visual input, but their performance improves in tasks in which visual input is not crucial.

Globally aphasic patients often have unreliable yes-no responses. Many cannot reliably indicate (or learn to indicate) *yes* and *no* by speech, gesture, head nod, or pointing to cards showing words or symbols representing *yes* and *no*. Most

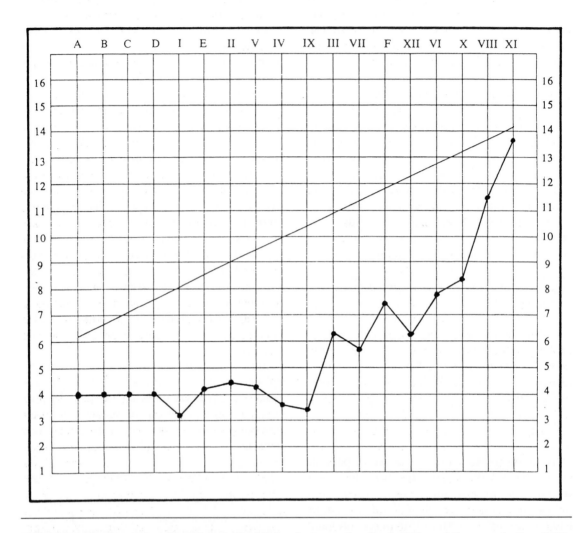

Figure 9-2 ■ Performance of an adult with global aphasia on the *Porch Index of Communicative Ability* (*PICA*; Porch, 1981a). The subtests are arranged from left to right in approximate order of difficulty. The patient makes no intelligible responses (represented by PICA scores of 5 or below) in the 10 most difficult subtests. The patient makes intelligible but inaccurate responses (represented by PICA scores of 6 or 7) on the next 5 less difficult subtests. The patient makes accurate but prompted or delayed responses on the 3 easiest subtests— pointing to test objects by name (X), matching pictures to objects (VIII), and matching identical objects (XI).

aphasic patients who are not globally aphasic can acquire reliable yes-no responses to simple nonverbal stimuli in a single session, but many globally aphasic patients seem unable to grasp the concepts of *yes* and *no* or are unable to match the concepts with the appropriate gesture or with the words *yes* and *no.*

Globally aphasic patients often produce jargon and meaningless speech without self-correction. Some globally aphasic patients' spontaneous speech consists primarily of jargon (nonwords such as *kalimfropper*) or meaningless strings of true words (e.g., *that's Sheila's aunt in a full subscription*) uttered uncritically whenever the patient is moved to speak. Patients with severe Wernicke's aphasia or severe transcortical sensory aphasia also produce jargon and meaningless word strings, but as mentioned previously, these patients also produce some words, phrases, or sentences that convey meaning, although the meaning may not be appropriate to the context.

Process-oriented treatment options for patients with chronic global aphasia are limited. Globally aphasic patients do not become competent language users as speakers, listeners, readers, or writers, no matter how tenaciously the clinician tries. Globally aphasic patients' daily life communicative success and quality of life may be enhanced by intervention with modest goals and having a reasonable probability of success, such as those recommended by Collins (1991), who comments that they should be minimal goals for all globally aphasic patients. I have arranged Collins's goals in what I consider to be descending order of importance:

- Provide the patient with consistent and reliable *yes* and *no* responses in structured situations.
- Provide the patient with a set of simple, unequivocal gestures, which may include gestures to express *yes* and *no.*
- Ensure that the patient can convey a small, basic set of communicative intentions in one or a combination of modalities.

- Improve the patient's auditory comprehension to permit comprehension of one-step commands (e.g., *hand me the pencil*) in controlled situations with contextual cues.
- Improve the patient's writing of a few simple important daily life words.
- Improve the patient's drawing to permit simple unequivocal messages.

Not every globally aphasic patient may reach all of these goals. Some may rely on gestures rather than speech to express basic needs. Some with artistic talent may communicate by drawing. Some may write words they cannot say. Which goals are attainable depend on each patient's abilities, needs, motivation, and life situation. The clinician, patient, and caregivers must collaborate to choose appropriate goals and to devise treatment procedures. Some globally aphasic persons may profit from programs designed to provide severely aphasic persons and their conversational partners with skills and strategies to increase aphasic persons' access to and participation in daily life communicative interactions. I describe these programs later in this chapter.

Focus and Progression

Aphasia test batteries typically partition communication among traditional verbal processes (listening, speaking, reading, and writing) and provide tasks that test various input and output modalities (auditory, visual, and sometimes tactile input; oral, gestural, and graphic output). Such partitioning of communication can prove attractive to novice clinicians who are searching for a rationale to guide treatment, but it may entice them into *treat-to-the-test treatment,* in which the clinician identifies tests in which a patient's performance is deficient and constructs treatment tasks that imitate the content and structure of the tests.

The clinician who treats to the test may distribute treatment tasks across processes or modalities to increase the generality of treatment and may select tasks in which the patient's performance is somewhat deficient but not completely erroneous to ensure that treatment tasks are at an appropriate level of difficulty. If a simple treat-to-the-test approach is to be effective (which means that it has positive effects on the patient's daily life communication), the tasks in the test that guides treatment must represent processes or skills that operate in the patient's daily life. If they do not, the treatment may improve a patient's test scores but have little effect on her or his daily life communication. (The treatment is efficacious, but not effective.)

A more sophisticated version of the treat-to-the-test approach is the *selective treat-to-the-test approach.* Clinicians using this approach consider deficient performance in some tests more important than deficient performance in other tests. For example, those who believe that impaired auditory comprehension is a central problem in aphasia pay particular attention to patients' performance on tests of auditory comprehension and design treatment to mimic the auditory comprehension tests on which a patient's performance is deficient. The selective treat-to-the-test approach assigns greater importance to some tests than others based on some underlying rationale, but the tasks included in treatment resemble the tests which led to their inclusion in the treatment program.

Clinicians who believe that impaired auditory comprehension is a central problem in aphasia often enroll their aphasic patients in auditory comprehension drills in which the patient must carry out gestural responses to the clinician's spoken commands. Some mimic the *Token Test* by asking the patient to point to or manipulate colored geometric forms (a tedious business for patient and clinician). Others ask the patient to point to or manipulate picture cards or pictures of objects in response to spoken commands (e.g., *Point to the spotted dog, the red book, and the fat man.*).

The major problem with treat-to-the-test approaches is that the tasks in aphasia test batteries may have little to do with patients'

daily life communication needs. Treat-to-the-test approaches run the risk of wasting the clinician's and the patient's time, energy, and resources on treatment tasks that have little or no positive effect on the patient's life beyond escalation of the patient's test scores (an escalation which often proves temporary—when treatment stops, the patient's test scores decline).

The *treat-underlying-processes approach* orients clinicians toward underlying cognitive processes that are assumed to be responsible for a patient's impaired test performance. Most clinicians and investigators agree that aphasia is not a loss of vocabulary or linguistic rules, but is caused by impairments in processes necessary for comprehending, formulating, and producing spoken and written language. For example, comprehension impairments in aphasia may be caused by reduced speed and efficiency in attaching meaning to words rather than by loss of word meanings. Impaired naming may be caused by reduced speed, efficiency, or accuracy of word retrieval rather than by loss of vocabulary. Speech production problems may be caused by disruptions of word retrieval or phonologic selection and sequencing rather than by loss of words or syntactic rules.

Clinicians who believe that aphasia represents a reduction in the speed and efficiency of processes underlying language focus process-oriented treatment on *reactivating* or *restimulating* language processes, rather than focusing on *teaching* specific responses (Schuell, Jenkins, & Jimenez-Pabon, 1964). For example, if an aphasic patient has impaired reading, the clinician might attempt to determine whether the problem is related to one or more of the following:

- Eye movements and visual search
- Single-word comprehension
- Use of syntactic rules
- Ability to deduce main ideas, make inferences, or draw conclusions
- Storage and recall of information gained from printed materials

After a deficient process is identified, treatment focuses on the process. One of the major advantages of a process-directed approach to treatment is that stimulating a general process may affect several specific communicative abilities that depend on the process. For example, improving a patient's auditory retention span by means of *point to drills* may improve a patient's comprehension of spoken sentences and discourse and may enhance reading comprehension, because both auditory comprehension and reading comprehension depend on retention of verbal information in immediate memory.

Schuell, Jenkins, and Jimenez-Pabon (1964) offered the following principles for stimulating disrupted processes in aphasia:

- Provide repetitive sensory stimulation.
- Provide intensive auditory stimulation, but combine auditory and visual stimulation to maximize patients' responses.
- Ensure that treatment stimuli are strong enough to get into the patient's brain via compromised sensory systems.
- Ensure that treatment stimuli are strong enough to get and hold the patient's attention.
- Ensure that every stimulus elicits a response.
- Elicit responses—do not force them; if stimulation is adequate, responses follow.
- Stimulate, rather than correct; error responses do not appear if stimulation is adequate.

Schuell, Jenkins, and Jimenez-Pabon comment that the clinician's role is not to teach, but to communicate with the patient and to stimulate disrupted processes to function maximally.

Goals

> *The primary objective in treatment of aphasia is to increase communication. What the aphasic patient wants is to recover enough language to get on with his life. (Schuell, Jenkins, & Jimenez-Pabon, 1964, p. 333)*

As Schuell and her associates suggest, complete recovery of language and communication is not an option for most aphasic adults. Most will be left with persisting language and communicative impairments. Process-oriented treatment may, however, accelerate aphasic adults' recovery of language and communication. When recovery stops, process-oriented, function-oriented, or social-oriented treatment may help aphasic adults compensate for residual impairments. The objective of aphasia treatment, whether process, function, or social in orientation, is to help aphasic adults be effective communicators and participants in life despite residual language and communicative impairments.

GENERAL CONCEPTS 9-1

- Early group studies of the effectiveness of process-oriented treatment for aphasia yielded conflicting results. Recent and better designed studies suggest that treatment of aphasia in adults is efficacious provided that:
  - The treatment is delivered by qualified personnel.
  - Patients with irreversible aphasia are excluded.
  - The intensity, content, duration, and timing are appropriate for the recipients.
- Sensitive and reliable measures are used to document the effects of treatment.
- Single-case design studies show that specific treatment procedures provide meaningful changes in targeted skills and that generalization of changes to patients' daily lives may be obtained.

Continued

GENERAL CONCEPTS 9-1—cont'd

- Early intervention (within a few weeks of the onset of aphasia) appears to be somewhat more efficacious than late intervention.
- The primary objective of aphasia treatment is to improve aphasic adults' daily life communication, not simply to change their test scores.
- Some aphasic adults may not be candidates for process-oriented treatment, including those who are too ill or too weak, those who are too severely aphasic, and those who elect not to participate in treatment.
- Globally aphasic adults have severely impaired comprehension and little expressive language beyond stereotypic utterances. Individuals who are globally aphasic at 1 month or more after onset are likely to remain globally aphasic for the rest of their lives.
- The two most common generic approaches to process-oriented treatment are:

- The *treat-to-the-test approach* (or the *selective-treat-to-the-test approach*), in which treatment tasks resemble the tests used to measure the aphasic patient's impairments
- The *treat-underlying-processes approach*, in which treatment tasks focus on cognitive processes that underlie several communicative skills
- Clinicians who believe that aphasia represents reduced speed and efficiency of underlying language processes focus treatment on *reactivating* or *restimulating* the processes.
- Contemporary process-oriented aphasia treatment philosophies consider *functionality* (the daily life utility of skills) and *generalization* (transfer of skills learned in the clinic to a patient's daily life) when designing and implementing treatment.

Auditory Comprehension

Listening Comprehension and Memory.

Listening comprehension and memory cannot be separated. Listeners cannot comprehend spoken language unless they can retain it in memory long enough to carry out the processes needed to deduce its meaning, and they must retain the mental representation of its meaning long enough to respond. That listening comprehension and memory are related is clear. However, the relationships between memory and listening comprehension have not yet been well described.

The exact role of memory in aphasic adults' comprehension impairments is not well understood. Most aphasic adults have impairments in short-term verbal memory that interfere with comprehension and recall of spoken or printed language In fact, Schuell, Jenkins, and Jimenez-

Pabon (1964) identified impaired short-term retention and recall as a defining characteristic of adult aphasia. There is little doubt that short-term verbal memory impairments affect comprehension of single-sentence messages such as those in the *Token Test* (De Renzi & Vignolo, 1962) and other tests of single-sentence comprehension in which test takers must comprehend and retain unrelated sentences such as, *Touch the large yellow square and the small green circle.* or *The thin girl with a bow in her hair chases the small black dog with no collar.* Aphasic adults' performance on such tests has been shown to correlate strongly with their performance on tests of short-term memory (Lesser, 1976; Martin & Feher, 1990).

Short-term memory impairment apparently does not account for aphasic adults' problems in comprehending syntactically complex sentences (e.g., *The dog the cat chased was white.*). Non-aphasic adults with impaired short-term memory usually have little difficulty with comprehension of such sentences (Vallar & Baddeley, 1984), and aphasic adults' performance on tests of short-term memory is not meaningfully related to their performance on tests that assess comprehension of syntactically complex sentences (Martin & Feher, 1990). That aphasic adults comprehend longer sentences such as *The man was greeted by his wife, and he was smoking a pipe.* better than shorter but syntactically more complex sentences such as *The man greeted by his wife was smoking a pipe.* (Goodglass & associates, 1979) also suggests that short-term memory does not fully explain aphasic adults' difficulties with syntactically complex sentences.

Normal listeners retain the syntactic form of spoken sentences in short-term memory, but syntactic information is lost within a few minutes unless the sentence is rehearsed. When the information in a sentence is passed into long-term memory, its meaning is retained, but its syntactic structure is lost. A normal listener who hears the sentence *The white rabbit was chased by the brown dog.* and after 30 minutes or so hears the sentence *The brown dog chased the white rabbit.* may claim to have previously heard the latter sentence, even though the syntactic structures differ. The person remembers the meaning of the sentence and not its syntactic structure.

Models of Auditory Comprehension. Schuell, Jenkins, and Jimenez-Pabon (1964) considered impaired auditory comprehension and constricted auditory retention span central problems in aphasia. Since that time, treating auditory comprehension impairments has had special status for many clinicians who believe that improving auditory comprehension is the most efficient way to improve aphasic adults' general language competence. The validity of this belief has not been experimentally confirmed, but treatment of auditory comprehension impairments continues to occupy a prominent place in many approaches to aphasia treatment.

For many years auditory comprehension was thought to proceed through a series of stages in which listeners analyzed the phonemic content of utterances, combined the phonemes into representations of words, retrieved the meanings of the words, determined the relationships among the words, and constructed a mental representation for the meaning of the utterances. Such models of comprehension eventually became known as *bottom-up models*, because listeners start with the physical characteristics of the message and work their way up through levels of increasing complexity until the meaning of the utterance becomes apparent.

During the 1960s and 1970s models of comprehension were developed in which listeners' knowledge and expectations played a central part in comprehension of spoken and printed language. These models were built on the idea that comprehension is not simply the result of a series of computations by which listeners deduce the meaning of what they hear. For listeners in natural situations, the words seem only to provide a starting point from which listeners guess a speaker's intent, construct presuppositions, develop expectations, decide what is important, and relate what is heard to what is already known. These models of comprehension became known as *top-down models*, because they assumed that listeners begin with general expectations of what a speaker is likely to say, use their general knowledge to support or refute their expectations, and resort to lower-level linguistic analyses only when higher-level processes leave the speaker's meaning in doubt.

Listeners seem to use lexical and syntactic processes primarily to establish what the speaker is talking about and to identify how the speaker's message relates to what the speaker has previously said. These lexical and syntactic processes are sometimes called *text-based processes* because they depend on the words and syntax of what is said, in contrast with *knowledge-based* or *heuristic processes* in which the listener invokes general knowledge, intuition, and guessing to deduce the meaning of spoken language.

Text-based processes require more mental effort than knowledge-based (heuristic) processes. Heuristic processes lighten workload by allowing a listener to deduce a speaker's general meaning and intent without resorting to continuous word-by-word lexical and syntactic analysis. Normal listeners usually emphasize heuristic processes over text-based processes and resort to text-based processes only when forced to so do by the absence of extralinguistic sources of information, by unusual vocabulary, or by complex syntax.

Scripts often make an important contribution to heuristic processes. Scripts are mental representations of familiar daily life situations in which certain events typically occur and occur in a typical order. Consider, for example, a speaker who says to a friend *Let me tell you about the party I went to last night.* The listener with party-going experience can call upon knowledge of what typically happens at parties to construct a set of expectations about what took place at the party. Once the listener has activated a mental party script, expectations of what the speaker is likely to convey come into play:

- A number of people were there.
- Food and drink were served.
- There was a host or hostess.
- The party was at the host or hostess's home.
- Social conversations took place.

Normal listeners use such mental representations to organize information from discourse and to form expectations of what is likely to be conveyed in a sample of discourse (Adams & Collins, 1979; Bower, Black, & Turner, 1979; and others). Armus, Brookshire, and Nicholas (1989) have shown that adults with mild to moderate aphasia retain knowledge of scripts for common

situations and they have suggested that preserved script knowledge may at least partially account for some aphasic adults' good comprehension of spoken discourse in the face of substantially impaired performance on tests of single-sentence comprehension.

Script knowledge apparently does not help aphasic adults with poor single-word comprehension who also have poor comprehension of spoken sentences and spoken discourse. For them, treatment focused on single-word comprehension is a logical starting place.

Single-Word Comprehension. The prototypical treatment for impaired single-word comprehension is a *pointing drill* in which the clinician places an array of pictures or (less frequently) objects before the patient and asks the patient to point to each item as it is named. The clinician manipulates the difficulty of the task by manipulating the familiarity or abstractness of the stimulus words.

Most clinicians put the stimulus word at the end of a short carrier phrase, as in *"Point to the _____."* or *"Show me the _____."* Although the clinician's utterances are technically sentences, the redundancy of the carrier phrase makes it irrelevant to successful performance.

Single-word comprehension drills are appropriate for patients with severe comprehension impairments who cannot comprehend phrase-length or sentence-length materials. Single-word comprehension drills serve as a starting point for drills in which the length, information density, and complexity of the treatment stimuli increase as the patient's comprehension improves.

Single-word comprehension drills are not appropriate for patients who can comprehend short phrases or sentences but have mild to moderate single-word comprehension impairments. These patients' single-word comprehension impairments usually relate to low-frequency words, which are not common in daily life. The context in which words occur often gives strong hints about their meanings, and the aphasic listener who can make use of context to deduce the meaning of words he or she does not comprehend is unlikely to have much difficulty comprehending most daily life spoken language, even when it contains some low-frequency words.

A small number of patients with mild or moderate aphasia experience remarkable difficulties in attaching meanings to words they hear or read. They behave (usually intermittently) as if they do not know the meanings of spoken or printed words, even when the words are common in the language. Their performance is not word-specific. Sometimes they comprehend a word, and at other times they do not. Sometimes they behave as if they are hearing words from a foreign language. They may repeat an unrecognized word over and over and may even spell the word while attempting to associate it with a meaning. When given a clue to the meaning of an unrecognized word (such as a synonym or an antonym), they often recognize the word, as happens in the following interaction:

Clinician: Tell me what the word *wagon* means.

Patient: Wagon...wagon. It seems like I...but I can't...What was the word again?

Clinician: Wagon. Have you heard this word before? Wagon.

Patient: Wagon...wagon.......wagon. I should know...I think I've heard it before, but... wagon.........wagon................wagon. Huh! I guess I don't know it.

Clinician: O.K., here's a hint. It has something to do with moving things from place to place, like a load of rocks. It might be found on a farm. It might be used with a horse...

Patient: Oh! Wagon! It's a thing with wheels, and you'd maybe use a horse or a donkey or even a goat to pull it around. Like a cart. Like don't put the cart before the horse.

Clinician: What does *"don't put the cart before the horse"* mean?

Patient: Well it means the cart goes behind the horse, or don't get ahead of yourself.

Treatment for patients with impaired single-word comprehension usually consists of drills in which they match spoken words to pictures or give definitions, synonyms, or antonyms for spoken words. If such drills do not lead to improved single-word comprehension, these patients' single-word comprehension may be treated indirectly by working on short-term auditory memory and sentence comprehension or by teaching them to use context to arrive at the meaning of unrecognized words.

Understanding Spoken Sentences. Impaired sentence comprehension is commonly targeted in process-oriented treatment programs for aphasic adults, not only because it seems important in daily life, but also because of the central role played by auditory comprehension in some models of aphasia. Treatment to improve comprehension of spoken sentences typically consists of drills in which patients answer questions, follow directions, or verify the meaning of sentences.

Answering Questions. The questions in *question-answering drills* can be either yes-no questions to which patients can respond with spoken or gestural indicators of *yes* or *no,* or open-ended questions that call for longer and more complex responses.

Yes-no questions may call upon general knowledge (e.g., *Is Mason City the capital of Iowa?*), verbal retention span (e.g., *Can you buy stamps, envelopes, and money orders at the post office?*), semantic discriminations (e.g., *Do you brush teeth with a comb?*), phonemic discriminations (e.g., *Do you wear a shirt and pie?*), syntactic analysis (e.g., *Do you wear feet on your shoes?*), or semantic relationships (e.g., *Is a banana a vegetable?*).

Yes-no questions commonly are used for treating severely impaired patients who cannot produce enough speech to answer open-ended questions. Most of these patients can indicate *yes* and *no* either verbally, by head movements, or by pointing to words or symbols signifying *yes* and *no,* making yes-no questions a reasonable treatment procedure.

Open-ended questions such as *Why do people put locks on their doors?* permit clinicians to sample a greater variety of information and permit greater flexibility in the structure of the questions than is possible with yes-no questions, but their validity as comprehension training items is reduced by the need for patients to formulate and produce longer verbal responses. Because of this, clinicians often use open-ended questions as vehicles for work on word retrieval and speech formulation, rather than as items in comprehension drills.

Following Spoken Directions. Treatment tasks in which patients follow spoken directions are an important component of many clinicians' repertoires. *Spoken-direction tasks* require patients to perform sequential pointing or manipulative responses in response to directions spoken by the clinician, as in *Put the spoon beside the pencil, put the quarter beside the comb, and give me the key.* In spoken-direction drills the length and complexity of the directions are controlled so that the patient works at a level that challenges but does not overwhelm. As the patient's comprehension improves, treatment follows a hierarchy of increasingly longer and/or syntactically complex sentences such as the hierarchy described by Kearns and Hubbard (1977), who measured the average difficulty of 13 levels of spoken directions for a group of 10 aphasic adults. The group's average scores on a 16-point scale are given in parentheses (Box 9-1).

Kearns and Hubbard's 13-level hierarchy may be useful for setting up a hierarchy of task difficulty for individual patients, although the hierarchy for a given patient may not match Kearns and Hubbard's, which was based on group average performance. Consequently, clinicians may have to personalize a hierarchy for individual patients by assessing their performance at various levels in the hierarchy and selecting the level at which the patient's performance has the appropriate proportions of correct, nearly correct, and incorrect responses.

Spoken-direction drills primarily target patients' verbal retention span. Many clinicians believe that if an aphasic patient's verbal retention span improves, the patient's general language comprehension also will improve. No empiric evidence supports that assumption, and evidence from studies of normal language comprehension suggest that comprehending language in natural situations does not depend strongly on verbal retention span. Given that most utterances in daily life conversations occur in context, are less than eight words long (Goldman-Eisler, 1968), and are not as informationally dense as the sentences in verbal retention span drills, improving aphasic patients' verbal retention span beyond six- to eight-word moderately redundant utterances may have weaker effects on daily life comprehension than many clinicians believe.

This does not mean, however, that spoken-direction drills may not indirectly improve daily life comprehension by improving the operation of processes that support comprehension. One likely candidate for such a supporting role is attention. Successful performance on spoken-direction drills requires that the patient focus and maintain attention throughout each spoken direction. Patients who cannot quickly focus attention tend to miss information at the beginning of the directions, and those who cannot maintain attention lose information at the end of the directions. Therefore it seems reasonable that spoken-direction drills may enhance auditory comprehension for some patients by enhancing attentional skills that support comprehension.

Sentence Verification. In *sentence verification drills* the patient hears spoken sentences and makes judgments about the relationship of each sentence to one or more pictures. In one form (called *yes-no*), the clinician shows the patient a picture and says a sentence which may or may not match the picture. The patient indicates whether the picture accurately portrays the meaning of the sentence. Each sentence

Box 9-1	*Kearns and Hubbard's (1977) 13-Level Hierarchy**

- Point to one common object by name. (*Point to the pencil.* 14.30)
- Point to one common object by function. (*Point to the one you write with.* 14.02)
- Point in sequence to two common objects by function. (*Show me the one you write with and the one you lock a door with.* 12.90)
- Point in sequence to two common objects by name. (*Point to the pencil and the key.* 12.67)
- Point to one object spelled by the examiner. (*Point to the p-e-n-c-i-l.* 12.51)
- Point to one object described by the examiner with three descriptors. (*Which one is white, plastic, and has bristles?* 12.23)
- Follow one-verb instructions. (*Pick up the pen.* 12.05)
- Point in sequence to three common objects by name. (*Show me the spoon, the pencil, and the dime.* 10.74)
- Point in sequence to three common objects by function. (*Point to the one you write with, the one you lock a door with, and the one you spend.* 10.72)
- Carry out two-object location instructions. (*Put the pen in front of the knife.* 10.20)
- Carry out, in sequence, two-verb instructions. (*Point to the knife and turn over the fork.* 9.77)
- Carry out, in sequence, two-verb instructions with time constraint. (*Before you pick up the knife, hand me the fork.* 8.60)
- Carry out three-verb instructions. (*Point to the knife, turn over the fork, and hand me the pencil.* 7.53)

Data from Kearns, K., Hubbard, D.J. (1977). A comparison of audience comprehension tasks. In R.H. Brookshire (Ed.), *Clinical aphasiology conference proceedings*, (pp. 32-45). Minneapolis: BRK Publishers.
*Average scores on a 16-point scale are given in parentheses. Differences of less than 0.5-point may not be clinically meaningful.

usually is presented several nonconsecutive times, sometimes with a picture that matches the sentence's meaning and sometimes with a foil. The foil pictures usually are chosen to contrast with the stimulus sentence in specified ways (e.g., differing from the stimulus sentence in subject, verb, or object, as in Figure 9-3).

In a second form of sentence verification (called *multiple choice*), each time the clinician says a sentence, he or she shows the patient a page containing several pictures, one of which portrays the meaning of the sentence (Figure 9-4). The foil pictures usually contrast with the stimulus sentence in specified ways, as described above. The patient points to the picture that represents the meaning of the sentence.

In most sentence-verification drills, foil pictures have systematic relationships to target pictures. Figure 9-4 shows a set of four pictures that might accompany the sentence *The man is hugging the woman.* To respond correctly, listeners have to perceive subject, object, or verb mismatches between foil pictures and the stimulus sentence. The difficulty of such an item for aphasic listeners depends primarily on the semantic closeness of the foils to the target. *The man is chasing the dog.* as a foil for Figure 9-4 would be easily identified as a foil by most aphasic adults, whereas *The girl is hugging the man* would mislead many.

Task-Switching Activities. Many aphasic adults are tripped up in conversational interactions in which they must maintain a sense of the overall purpose or theme of a conversation while simultaneously dealing with changes in topics, speakers, or conversational roles. *Task-switching drills* can help these patients. Task-switching drills are sentence-comprehension drills in which the form of the stimulus sentences and the nature of the responses expected from the patient change unpredictably from trial to trial, as in the following sequence:
Pick up the spoon.
Point to the black one.

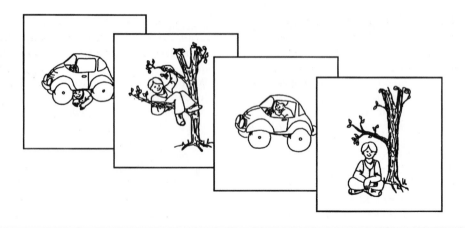

Figure 9-3 ■ Response cards that might be used in a sentence verification drill for the sentence *The boy is in the tree.* These four cards would be mixed with other cards, and the clinician would say the sentence whenever one of these cards came up.

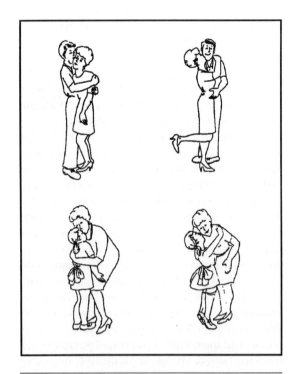

Figure 9-4 ■ A sentence-to-picture match-to-sample response card that might be shown as the clinician says *The man is hugging the woman.*

Which one do you drink from?
Does Thursday come after Wednesday?
Make a fist and blink three times.
Put the key in the cup.
Is your name Fred?

The drill continues in this way.

Discourse Comprehension. When planning treatment for patients with impaired discourse comprehension, it is important to remember that the traditional concept of comprehension skills as progressing from words to sentences to texts (bottom-up processing) is inappropriate. Words and sentences in discourse are easier to comprehend than words and sentences in isolation. When sentences occur in discourse, comprehension depends more on their relationship to the overall theme of the discourse and the degree to which the discourse relates to a listener's knowledge and experience than on the length or syntactic complexity of the sentences.

The difficulty of a discourse comprehension task is determined not only by the content and structure of the discourse, but by what listeners are asked to comprehend and remember from the discourse. If listeners are asked to comprehend and remember only the main ideas and the overall point of the discourse, they do better than if asked to remember details. If listeners are asked to comprehend and remember only directly stated information, they do better than if asked to comprehend and remember implied information.

Most adults with mild to moderate aphasia are likely to have retained at least some of their discourse comprehension ability. Most should get the main ideas if the discourse is well-structured and unambiguous. Most should be able to construct the major inferences suggested by the discourse, especially inferences that relate to the main ideas or overall theme. However, the comprehension of patients with mild to moderate aphasia suffers when discourse is not well-structured with clearly identified main ideas and an obvious topic or theme, or if the information is outside their experience.

The typical format for discourse comprehension treatment is for the clinician to read aloud or play a recording of a sample of discourse, after which the patient answers questions about information in the discourse. The questions typically are yes-no questions such as those in the *Discourse Comprehension Test* (Brookshire & Nicholas, 1993; previously described). Yes-no questions (e.g., *Did the women put up a sign at a shopping center?*) typically are used, because they minimize the effects of patients' memory and speech-production impairments on their discourse comprehension.

Yes-no questions test patients' *recognition,* rather than their *recall* of information from discourse. To move patients toward recall, yet keep memory, speech formulation, and speech production demands under control, yes-no questions can be replaced by *sentence completion items,* in which patients complete sentence fragments provided by the clinician, as in *The women put up a sign at* _____. For patients who can handle the limited formulation and speech production demands, sentence completion places more demands on recall of information from discourse than do yes-no questions.

Open-ended questions (e.g., *What did the women do to advertise their garage sale?*) provide fewer clues about the answer, but they require greater competence in speech formulation and production than yes-no questions or sentence completion items. For patients who can handle the speech-production demands, open-ended questions are more flexible and more challenging than yes-no questions or sentence completion items.

Retelling, in which patients recount as much as they can remember from a sample of discourse, requires patients to retrieve and produce information from memory without help from the content of the clinician's questions. Retelling provides the strongest indicator of patients' ability to comprehend, store, and retrieve information from discourse. However, speech formulation and production impairments may masquerade as comprehension impairments, making retelling inappropriate for treating comprehension in patients with limited speech.

Stimulus Manipulations in Treating Discourse Comprehension. Clinicians may regulate the difficulty of discourse comprehension tasks by manipulating several variables.

Familiarity. Treatment typically begins with material familiar to the patient. Familiar material permits patients to use their existing knowledge to help them comprehend discourse. As a patient's comprehension of familiar material improves, the clinician may gradually introduce less familiar material, forcing the patient to depend less on existing knowledge and more on the content of the discourse itself.

Many familiar situations and routines (e.g., going to a restaurant, buying groceries, or taking a plane trip) can be represented by scripts. As previously described, *scripts* are mental devices by which individuals organize knowledge of common situations. They permit individuals to formulate expectations of which events are likely to occur in a situation and the order in which they are likely to occur. Armus and associates suggested that aphasic adults' knowledge of scripts be exploited to facilitate their comprehension of discourse by:

- Teaching patients and their families that some daily life spoken discourse is predictable, based on what the listener already knows of the topic or situation being discussed
- Having patients practice identifying scripts that underlie samples of discourse
- Asking patients to predict what is likely to happen next in samples of discourse representing scripts

Length. Treatment usually begins with short samples of discourse and progresses to longer ones. The samples should be long enough, however, to permit the patient to develop a sense of their overall theme and to identify the main ideas (100 to 200 words). As the patient's comprehension improves, the length of the discourse increases.

Redundancy, Cohesion, and Coherence. Treatment typically begins with samples of discourse in which repetition, paraphrase, and elaboration create redundancy and high levels of cohesion and coherence. Redundancy, cohesion, and coherence establish relationships among ideas and help the listener determine the topic and identify the main ideas. Redundancy, cohesion, and coherence also permit patients to substitute less effortful heuristic processes for more effortful lexical and syntactic processes as they listen to discourse. As the patient's comprehension improves, materials with less redundancy, cohesion, and coherence gradually may be introduced to increase the patient's ability to deal with less redundant and less coherent discourse.

Salience. Treatment begins with material in which the main ideas are easily identified, and the focus of treatment is on identification of main ideas. As the patient's comprehension improves, the focus progresses to comprehension of details.

Directness. Treatment begins with materials in which the important information is stated rather than implied, and questions relate to information present in verbatim form in the discourse. As the patient's comprehension improves, questions that require simple inferences are introduced, followed by questions requiring more complex inferences.

Speech Rate. For those whose comprehension declines when materials are spoken at normal or fast rates, the rate at which discourse is presented may be slowed by placing pauses at strategic locations. As the patient's comprehension of slowly spoken material improves, the rate at which discourse is presented may be increased gradually, until the patient is working with materials spoken at a normal rate.

Pauses after main ideas may help to highlight the main ideas and may provide the listener with extra processing time for comprehending the main ideas and storing them in memory.

Nicholas and Brookshire (1986) suggested that increasing the salience or redundancy of information in discourse and stating information more directly are more dependable ways to improve aphasic listeners' comprehension of discourse than is slowing the rate at which it is spoken, because not all aphasic adults are helped by slow speech rate. However, they recommended that clinicians still advise those who communicate with aphasic patients to speak slowly, because negative effects of slow speech rate are rare, and some aphasic listeners do benefit from slow speech rate. Nicholas and Brookshire also recommended that if a clinician intends to manipulate speech rate in treatment of aphasic adults' comprehension impairments, the clinician should pretest the patient to determine how that patient is affected by the manipulation.

Reading Comprehension

Aphasic adults almost always have impaired reading comprehension, and their reading comprehension usually is more impaired than their auditory comprehension. Aphasic adults face several problems when confronted with printed texts. Many aphasic adults read slowly, misperceive letters and words, and rely on laborious word-by-word analysis to decode complex syntax. Aphasic readers' impairments of semantic and syntactic processes cause them to misinterpret individual textual elements and prevent them from appreciating the overall meaning of printed language. Aphasic readers' impaired short-term retention may prevent them from establishing the overall topic of printed materials or, having established the topic, may cause them to lose it along the way. Given the multiplicity of obstacles, it should not be surprising that reading comprehension is a major problem for most aphasic adults and that only those with mild aphasia become recreational readers.

Processes in Reading

Word Recognition. Recognizing and attaching meanings to words begins the process of comprehending printed texts. Word recognition quickly becomes automatic for normal readers as they become skilled at reading. Skilled readers do not read sentences or texts word by word unless the material is complex or contains many unfamiliar words. Only unskilled readers rely on word-by-word reading.

Readers deduce the meaning of individual printed words in any of three ways:

- In *whole-word reading,* the reader recognizes words as units and does not analyze letters or letter strings within words. Whole-word reading requires that words be in the reader's reading vocabulary.
- In *phonemic analysis,* the reader segments words into letters or letter combinations, translates the letters or letter combinations

into the sounds they represent, blends the sound representations together, and identifies the word represented by the sequence of sounds. Word recognition by phonemic analysis requires that the unfamiliar word be in the reader's listening vocabulary, but not necessarily in the reader's reading vocabulary.

- In *word recognition by context,* the reader uses the meaning of the context in which a word appears to guess its meaning. Recognition by context does not require that the unfamiliar word be in the reader's reading or listening vocabulary.

Skilled readers read most words as whole words, and they use phonemic analysis and recognition by context only when they encounter unfamiliar words. When these methods fail, the reader may look up a word in a dictionary.

Syntactic Analysis. Syntactic analysis is the primary way in which readers deduce relationships among words. Syntactic analysis presupposes knowledge of syntactic rules and recognition of syntactic structures and allows readers to combine word strings into units of meaning that can be stored in long-term memory. Failure to perform syntactic analysis overloads the reader's short-term memory, and errors in syntactic analysis lead to miscomprehension of sentence meanings. An important difference between failure to recognize a word and failure to recognize a syntactic structure is that readers usually know when they fail to recognize a word but may be unaware when they fail to recognize a syntactic structure.

At one time there was general acceptance of the idea that if a reader could translate letters into their corresponding words, they could comprehend printed texts. This assumption is no longer considered valid, because it neglects the role of syntactic processes in reading. Reading depends on syntactic processes more than listening does. In listening, syntactic information may be conveyed by a speaker's pauses, intonation, and emphatic stress, as well as by word order and syntactic markers. In reading, the reader depends completely on word order and

syntactic markers to deduce syntactic structure. Most printed texts also are more formal in style than spoken discourse, making them syntactically more complex than spoken discourse.

Semantic Mapping. *Semantic mapping* is a process by which readers relate a writer's intended meanings to their own knowledge and experience. Semantic mapping is the stage at which a text can be said to make sense to a reader. In semantic mapping the ideas conveyed by a text are organized into a meaningful whole, and the overall meaning of the text is integrated into memory. A reader's failure to organize the information in a text leads to confusion about which elements of the text are important and which are unimportant, and may contribute to difficulty in getting the information into memory and later retrieving it. A reader's failure to relate meanings from texts to existing knowledge leads to problems in appreciating the true meanings of metaphor, idioms, and figurative language.

Most of the top-down processes that contribute to comprehension of spoken discourse also contribute to comprehension of printed texts. Readers, like listeners, use the lexical content and syntactic structure of printed texts to identify relationships among units of information. From there they go on to use general knowledge and intuition to determine a text's overall meaning. Readers, like listeners, use heuristic processes to bypass continuous word-by-word lexical and syntactic analysis when permitted to do so by the structure and content of printed texts. Readers, like listeners, often emphasize heuristic processes over text-based processes and may rely on text-based processes only when pushed to do so by unfamiliar subject matter, complex syntax, ambiguity, or uncertainty.

Surface Dyslexia and Deep Dyslexia. Two patterns of word-reading impairment—called *surface dyslexia* and *deep dyslexia* (Marshall & Newcombe, 1973)—sometimes accompany aphasia. The concepts of surface dyslexia and deep dyslexia are based on a model of reading that postulates two routes from the visual form

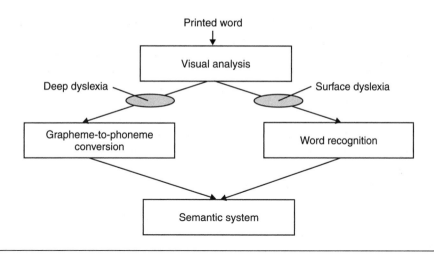

Figure 9-5 ■ A schematic diagram showing impaired processes responsible for surface dyslexia and deep dyslexia. In *surface dyslexia* the direct route from the printed stimulus to semantic representations is unavailable, and the patient must depend on the indirect route (grapheme-to-phoneme conversion). In *deep dyslexia* the grapheme-to-phoneme conversion route is unavailable, and the patient must depend on whole-word reading.

of words to the mental representations of word meanings. Readers who use the *direct (lexical) route* access the mental representations of words directly, based on the visual form of the words—*whole-word reading*. Readers who use the *indirect (phonologic) route* access the mental representations of words indirectly, by converting printed letters into their phonologic equivalents *(phonemic analysis)* and accessing meaning via these internal phonologic representations (Figure 9-5).

Individuals with *surface dyslexia* have lost or are impaired in the direct (lexical) route and depend on the indirect (phonologic) route, which requires letter-by-letter decoding to deduce the meaning of printed words. Individuals with surface dyslexia read regularly spelled words (such as *keep* and *banana*) or phonologically legitimate nonwords (such as *tobada*) accurately, but they misread irregularly spelled words by regularizing their pronunciation (e.g., *neighbor* may be read as *negbor*). Because analysis is letter-by-letter, long words

take readers with surface dyslexia longer to identify than short words.

Individuals with *deep dyslexia* have lost or are impaired in the indirect (phonologic) route and depend on the direct (whole-word) route to deduce the meaning of printed words. These patients misread phonologically legitimate non-words like *tobada,* and their misreadings of real words represent semantic errors (e.g., reading *chair* as *table*). Individuals with deep dyslexia may substitute morphologically related or visually similar words for target words (such as *steal* for *stealth, wise* for *wisdom*). Individuals with deep dyslexia have more difficulty reading *closed-class (function) words* (articles, conjunctions, and prepositions) than *open class (content) words* (nouns, verbs, adjectives, and adverbs). Semantically supportive context often helps these individuals recognize words they otherwise fail to recognize.

The various forms of acquired dyslexia have received much attention from investigators who are interested in how the brain recognizes printed words and connects the visual images of words to their semantic representations. The models of the reading process constructed by these investigators provide a systematic approach to differential diagnosis of acquired reading impairments. Nevertheless, it is important to keep in mind that descriptions of acquired dyslexia focus on single-word recognition, whereas reading comprehension (at least for normal readers) is largely a top-down process. Consequently, the effects of word recognition impairments, as typified in the various forms of acquired dyslexia, may not be as striking when the individual is reading texts as when he or she is reading single words. It seems likely that mild to moderate word recognition impairment would not dramatically affect a reader's comprehension of printed texts, if semantic and syntactic contexts give them clues to the identity of words that are not recognized in isolation.

Treating Neurogenic Reading Impairments. Treating a brain-injured adult's reading impairment often begins with what Webb (1990) calls a *literacy history.* The literacy history comes from the patient, family members, caregivers, associates, or a combination of sources. The literacy history tells the clinician how much reading the patient did before becoming aphasic, identifies reading topics of special interest to the patient, and gives the clinician a sense of the patient's level of reading competence before the onset of aphasia.

The clinician considers the patient's literacy history, current reading skills, and potential for recovery of reading to decide how (or whether) to make reading a focus of treatment. Patients for whom reading was a significant part of daily life, who have the necessary visuoperceptual and language abilities, and who are motivated to regain reading are the best candidates for treatment of reading. Patients who were nonfunctional readers before they became aphasic will not become functional readers with treatment, and there is little point in attempting to make recreational readers of patients who were

not interested in reading before they became aphasic.

Treatment of aphasic adults' reading impairments usually is most successful for patients with mild to moderate aphasia who were functional readers before the onset of aphasia. Patients with severe aphasia usually are more concerned with improving their speech production and enhancing their listening comprehension than with improving their reading. Few patients with chronic severe aphasia regain functional reading of newspapers, books, magazines, or other printed texts. However, severely aphasic patients and less severely aphasic patients who were not recreational readers before they became aphasic may benefit from acquiring what have been called *survival reading skills* (Rosenbek, LaPointe, & Wertz, 1989; Webb, 1990).

Survival Reading Skills. Survival reading skills are the skills needed to read materials commonly encountered in daily life, such as signs, labels, bills, checkbook registers, addresses, telephone listings, and menus. The first step in teaching or reactivating survival reading skills is to determine which daily life reading activities are most important to the patient. Rosenbek, LaPointe, and Wertz (1989) suggest that clinicians ask aphasic patients and family members to make two lists. One list specifies the materials the patient most wants to be able to read, and the other identifies materials the patient wishes to be able to read but can do without. A list produced by one of Rosenbek and associates' patients is shown in Table 9-1. Treatment focused on the materials in the two lists, beginning with the items in the *most important* list, and when the patient could sight-read those items, treatment progressed to the second list.

Parr (1992) compiled a similar but more generic list by asking 50 non-brain-injured British adults to make a list of daily life reading activities and to rate how important each activity was. Parr then calculated an index of importance for the group by multiplying the number

TABLE 9-1	Aphasic Adults' Responses About Reading Habits

Most Want to Read	Want to Read but Could Do Without
Mail	Messages
Checkbook	Signs
Medicine labels	Newspapers
Maps	Magazines
Phone book	TV Guide
Elevator	Menus
Calendar	Bible
Product labels	Playing cards

From Rosenbek, J.C., LaPointe, L.L., Wertz, R.T. (1989). *Aphasia: A clinical approach.* Boston: Little, Brown and Company.

TABLE 9-2	Reading Activities Ranked for Importance by a Group of Non–Brain-Damaged British Adults

Activity	Index of Importance
Personal letters	188
Bills	171
Forms	168
Official letters	162
Advertisements	144
Phone numbers	140
Newspaper	136
Television listings	131
Books	130
Bank statement	130
Address book	125
Dosage instructions for medications	130
Personal letters	118
Menus	107

Data from Parr, S. (1992). Everyday reading and writing practices of normal adults: Implications for aphasia assessment. *Aphasiology, 6,* 273-283.

of individuals who listed an activity by its average rating of importance. Table 9-2 shows Parr's ranked list.

Lists such as these provide a useful beginning point for the clinician who wishes to help an aphasic patient regain functional reading. The clinician cannot assume, however, that an individual's needs will match those of groups of individuals who contributed to such lists. A patient with no bank account is unlikely to consider reading bank statements or checkbook registers important, and a patient who has no television is unlikely to be very concerned with reading television program listings. Consequently, the clinician must devise an individualized list of important daily life reading activities for each patient by asking the patient and family members to generate and rank a list of reading activities. Treatment can begin with the highest-ranked activities and progress down the list as functional reading is achieved for each activity.

Functional reading for categories of everyday materials such as those in Tables 9-1 and 9-2 depends on the patient's acquisition of a sight-reading vocabulary of commonly occurring words for each category. A core sight-reading vocabulary for the instructions on medicine

labels might contain only 15 or 20 words, whereas a core sight-reading vocabulary for advertisements in newspapers and magazines might contain several hundred words. When a sight-reading vocabulary has been selected, the clinician may test the patient to determine which words the patient cannot presently sight read. The problem words may then be incorporated into treatment activities.

Drills in which the patient reads aloud core vocabulary words from flash cards are a popular way to train sight-reading of core vocabulary words. Flash-card drills give patients intensive sight-reading practice but may not be the most efficient way to promote sight-reading of vocabulary in daily life, because training sight-reading of free-standing vocabulary words deprives the patient of contextual cues that may enhance word recognition. For example, the meaning of *tablet* is more readily apparent in *Take one tablet by mouth twice a day.* than when printed on a flash card. Furthermore, generalization to daily life is more likely if a patient acquires sight-reading vocabulary with natural materials.

Several computer-based programs to enhance sight-reading for daily life vocabulary have been designed. Such programs may prove useful in providing patients with intensive sight-reading drills without requiring the clinician's full-time participation (Katz & Nagy, 1983; Major & Wilson, 1985; Weiner, 1983; and others). However, information about their effectiveness is limited to a few case reports.

Treating Mild to Moderate Reading Impairments.

Treatment of patients with mild to moderate reading impairment typically begins with a literacy history, followed by standardized tests to measure the patient's reading vocabulary, sentence comprehension, and paragraph comprehension. Clinicians typically measure both the patient's *reading capacity* (the level of vocabulary and complexity that the patient can comprehend) and the patient's *reading rate* (how quickly the patient can progress through a text with acceptable comprehension). Reading test scores often are defined by grade level. *Grade level* quantifies the difficulty of the reading materials in terms of the school grade at which average students can comprehend them. Most newspapers, popular books, and magazines are at Grade 5 or Grade 6 in reading difficulty. Consequently, those reading at fifth to sixth grade level or above are likely to comprehend most daily life reading materials (Chall, 1983).

Comprehension of Printed Words.

As noted earlier, many patients with acquired reading impairments have difficulty recognizing and assigning meaning to printed words. Problems in comprehending printed words can arise from several sources.

Many aphasic adults exhibit *deep dyslexia.* They struggle with phonemic analysis of printed words because they do not recognize words in whole-word form, cannot convert the printed letters into their phonologic equivalents, and cannot blend the individual sounds into sound patterns for words. These patients' printed-word recognition may be improved by exercises in which they:

- Orally sound out words and nonwords that have one-to-one grapheme-to-phoneme correspondence
- Discriminate between words with similar phonologic structure (e.g., *cabbage/cottage*)
- Supply missing letters to complete regularly spelled partial words (e.g., *ban_na, anniver__ry*)

Some aphasic adults have visual impairments that interfere with their perception of printed letters and words. They confuse words that look alike and may confuse letters with similar appearance (such as *b/c/d, m/w/n,* and *e/f/k*). These patients may be helped by exercises in which they discriminate between visually similar words (e.g., *taxes/taxies, hear/clear*) or identify transposed or reversed letters within words (e.g., *birhtday, gadren*). Such single-word discrimination drills may not be needed if a patient can read and comprehend printed sentences, because the context provided by the sentences may nullify the effects of the patient's word-level misperceptions on comprehension of the sentences.

Though annoying to patients, scattered visual misperceptions may not seriously interfere with patients' comprehension of printed texts, because the semantic and syntactic context provided by the texts diminish the frequency of misperceptions, and when misperceptions do occur, context may permit patients to recognize and repair the misperceptions. A reader who confuses *p* and *d* may misread the word *pen* as *den* when shown the word in isolation but may read it correctly in a sentence (e.g., *A pen is used to sign important documents.*). For these patients the primary effects of scattered visual misperceptions are annoyance and slow reading rate. However, if misperceptions are very frequent or if a patient's reading vocabulary and sentence comprehension skills are marginal, visual misperceptions may have more important effects.

Sometimes patients are given practice in identifying inverted or reversed letters in isolation. For some patients this is a necessary preliminary to identifying them in context. However, the clinician should move into contextual stimuli as soon as possible.

Some aphasic patients can translate printed words into phonemic representations but are unable to attach meaning to the representations. They may repeat a troublesome word over and over but fail to deduce its meaning:

> Conventional...conventional...I should know this word. I've seen it before. I'm thinking *"easy to get at"* but that's not it...conventional...I'll need help on this one.

These patients may become better readers if they are taught to use context to deduce word meanings. Vocabulary drills and word-association exercises also may help these patients read better.

These patients usually have similar problems recognizing spoken words. Treating auditory comprehension in tandem with reading comprehension may be appropriate for these patients.

Comprehension of Printed Sentences.

Aphasic readers' comprehension of printed sentences is influenced by many of the same variables that affect their comprehension of spoken sentences, discussed previously (length, syntactic complexity, redundancy, etc.). Most aphasic patients' reading comprehension is worse than their comprehension of equivalent spoken materials. Many have difficulty converting printed words into their phonemic representations—a process that is important in reading but not in listening. The syntactic structure of printed texts tends to be more complex than that of spoken discourse, creating problems for many aphasic adults. Aphasic readers tend to overlook or misread function words such as *to, but,* and *by,* causing them to confuse or mis-

interpret the meaning of printed sentences. Printed sentences have less extralinguistic support than spoken sentences. When a listener fails to comprehend a spoken sentence, the speaker may repeat, paraphrase, or simplify. The speaker's pauses, intonation, stress, reiteration, paraphrasing, and gestures support listening comprehension. The time of day, the location of the interaction, the speaker's identity, and other situational characteristics of spoken interactions also reduce the listener's dependence on the linguistic content of the speaker's utterances.

Reading comprehension, like auditory comprehension, is largely a top-down process for competent readers. Competent readers use context to establish topic, infer the meaning of unfamiliar or unrecognized words, and bypass laborious syntactic analysis. Brain-injured patients who can read at the sentence level may comprehend sentences in paragraph contexts better than sentences in isolation, although their reading rate may be slow and their comprehension of details less than perfect.

Treatment with isolated sentences may be appropriate for some mildly impaired readers who have trouble with syntax in printed sentences. These patients' reading comprehension may be enhanced by drills in which they are asked to interpret sentences with troublesome syntactic structures, such as passive (e.g., *The woman was hugged by the man.*), center-embedded (e.g., *The dog the boy chased ran into the street.*) and comparative (e.g., *The policeman was shorter than the burglar.*). Sentence comprehension drills are appropriate for mildly impaired readers whose primary complaint is failure to appreciate the meaning of syntactically complex sentences due to impaired heuristic (top-down) processes, but whose word recognition, vocabulary, appreciation of text structure, and retention of information are reasonably well preserved.

Reading drills with free-standing sentences also are appropriate for patients whose comprehension of printed texts is so poor that the beneficial effects of context cannot operate. Improving the rate and accuracy with which these patients read and comprehend individual sentences may diminish their workload enough to permit the effects of context to come into play.

Numerous workbooks containing sentence-level reading exercises appropriate for aphasic adults are on the market.

Some require the patient to complete sentences with words missing:

For breakfast, John likes bacon and _____.

Others require the patient to choose a target word from a list of foils:

Brush is to teeth as comb is to _____.

ear   hair   brush   rooster

Some require the patient to rearrange scrambled words into a sentence:

school is day most happy last the time for of a students

Some are *match-to-sample tasks* in which a printed sentence is presented together with several pictures, one of which matches the printed sentence, as in Figure 9-6.

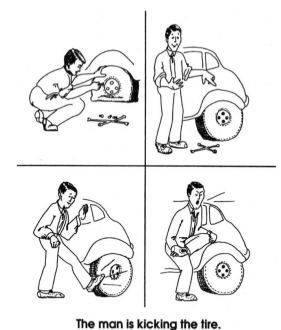

The man is kicking the tire.

Figure 9-6 ■ A response card for reading comprehension of the sentence *The man is kicking the tire.*

Scrambled-word sentences may challenge even patients with very mild impairments. Some non-brain-damaged readers may find longer scrambled-word sentences a challenge. Creating a sentence from scrambled words requires knowledge of syntactic rules, analytic skills, attention, and good short-term memory.

Most patients who can read and comprehend at least some information from printed texts should be working with printed texts that challenge them. Reading passages should be selected so that the patient can, at minimum, determine the overall topic of the passage, get most of the main ideas, and get at least some of the details. Clinicians can adjust the difficulty of reading materials by manipulating many of the variables that affect comprehension of spoken discourse (familiarity, length, redundancy, cohesion, coherence, salience, abstractness, and directness), plus variables that have a wider range in reading materials than in spoken discourse (vocabulary and syntactic complexity).

Stimulus Manipulations in Reading Treatment

Familiarity. The familiarity of reading material has strong effects on how easily a reader comprehends the material. Familiar material helps readers establish context, separate main ideas from details, and relate what they are reading to what they already know. Clinicians can exploit the effects of familiarity in treatment by using reading material that relates to a patient's knowledge, experience, and interests. As the patient's reading proficiency increases, less familiar material may be introduced to increase demands on lexical and semantic analysis, reasoning, intuition, and the ability to organize and retain information from texts.

Length. Making reading passages longer increases their difficulty, provided the passages are made longer by adding new information and not by restating or paraphrasing old information. Increasing a passage's length by restating or paraphrasing information may actually diminish passage difficulty by increasing the redundancy of the material and making its topic more obvious. Making passages shorter does not always make them easier. When a passage is drastically shortened, it becomes more difficult for the reader to develop a sense of its topic and theme and to employ context-based processes that permit top-down processing.

There is no absolute limit below which reading passages are too short to permit efficient use of top-down processes, because a passage's suitability for top-down processing depends on its structure as well as its length. As a general rule, passages less than about 100 words are likely to be too short to permit efficient use of top-down processes by most aphasic adults. Webb (1990) comments that it takes average readers at least 200 words to develop a sense of the overall meaning of reading passages. She suggests that reading passages used in treating aphasic adults' reading should be longer—averaging about 500 words. However, 500-word passages may be too long for aphasic adults who have impaired retention and memory.

Redundancy, Salience, and Directness. As is true for spoken discourse, redundancy (from repetition, elaboration, and paraphrase) in printed material makes it easier for readers to establish the overall sense of the material, organize it in memory, and recall its content. Repetition, elaboration, and paraphrase also contribute to the cohesion and coherence of printed material in the same way they contribute to the cohesion and coherence of information in spoken discourse (discussed previously).

Salience and directness affect aphasic readers in the same way that they affect aphasic listeners' comprehension of spoken discourse. Aphasic readers, like non-brain-damaged readers, are better at comprehending and remembering main ideas than details, and aphasic readers, like non-brain-damaged readers, com-

prehend and remember stated information better than implied information.

Vocabulary. Increasing the number of uncommon words in a reading passage makes it more difficult to read. Fortunately for readers with limited vocabulary, newspapers, magazines, books, and similar materials written for the general public do not contain many uncommon words. According to Hayes (1989), 75% of the words in typical books for adult readers are within the 1000 most frequent words in English, and 88% are within the 5000 most frequent English words. Table 9-3 provides frequency-of-occurrence estimates for various reading materials in the United States. If a patient's goal is recreational reading, Hayes's data suggest that it makes little sense to burden them with materials containing many uncommon words, because only specialized works contain many uncommon words.

Syntactic Complexity. The syntactic complexity of reading materials affects their reading difficulty, and, as noted earlier, aphasic adults often are tripped up by complex syntax. Fortunately most newspapers, magazines, and books are written with uncomplicated syntax. (The primary exceptions are some editorial and

TABLE 9-3	Percent of Words That Are within the 500, 1000, 5000, and 10,000 Most Frequent English Words for Various Reading Materials			
	Percentage of Words in the First:			
Material	500	1,000	5,000	10,000
Preschool books	73	81	94	97
Children's books	72	79	92	96
Comic books	68	75	89	93
Adult books	69	75	88	93
Popular magazines	62	69	85	91
Science abstracts	46	52	70	78

Data from Hayes, D.P. (1989). *Guide to the lexical analysis of texts.* (Tech. Rep. Series 89-96). Ithaca, NY: Cornell University Department of Sociology.

opinion pieces in newspapers or magazines and some novels.) Most recreational readers are unlikely to encounter syntactically complex materials, and when they do, context may permit them to substitute heuristic, top-down strategies for more laborious syntactic analysis. A reader who can cope with passive sentences (e.g., *The cat was chased by the dog.*), cleft-object sentences (e.g., *It was the cat that the dog chased.*), dative sentences (e.g., *The banker gave the money to the robber.*), and conjoined sentences (e.g., *The dog barked at the cat and chased the rabbit.*) should be able to handle the syntax of most commonly available reading materials, even when top-down processes cannot be substituted for syntactic analysis.

Readability Formulas. Readability formulas attempt to quantify reading difficulty by measuring specific characteristics of printed texts and assigning a reading grade level to the result. Several dozen readability formulas have been published (see Klare, 1984 for descriptions of the major formulas). Most readability formulas consider sentence length and vocabulary difficulty. Some count the number of long words (e.g., words of three or more syllables). Some consider grammatical characteristics such as number of prepositional phrases per 100 words. The most widely used formulas calculate readability by estimating syntactic complexity and vocabulary difficulty. These formulas estimate syntactic complexity by the average number of words per sentence, and they estimate vocabulary difficulty either by the average number of syllables per word or the number of low-frequency words in the passage.

A few readability formulas use *cloze procedures* to measure readability. Readers are given printed texts with words missing and are instructed to fill in the missing words. The readability of the text is based on the number of errors readers make when they fill in the missing words.

Although there is some variability in how readability formulas predict reading difficulty, no one procedure stands out as particularly accu-

rate, so clinicians who wish to estimate the reading difficulty of printed materials might choose an easily calculated formula such as the *Dale-Chall Formula* (Dale & Chall, 1948) the *Flesch Reading Ease Formula* (Flesch, 1948), or the *Fog Index* (Gunning, 1952).

The Dale-Chall Formula is based on the average number of words per sentence and the number of words not in a 4000-word list of words known by most fourth grade readers. The Flesch formula is calculated using the average number of words per sentence and average word length in syllables. The Fog Index, in addition to having one of the more interesting names, is easy to calculate. It is based on the average number of words per sentence and the number of words three or more syllables long.

It takes from 10 to 20 minutes to calculate readability for a 100- to 200-word text with even the simplest readability formulas. Some readability procedures have been computerized to lessen the time required to get a readability estimate, but the computerized procedures require that the text first be typed into an appropriately formatted computer text file, which may take longer than hand calculation.

Clinicians often bypass the time and effort of readability estimation by using commercially prepared materials with known readability, specified as a reading grade level. If their content is suitable for adult readers, these materials provide a convenient way for clinicians to obtain materials of predetermined reading difficulty for use in treatment of adults with reading impairments.

Commercial Reading Programs. Commercial reading programs may be a good source of materials for treating brain-injured patients' reading impairments. *Basal readers* are commonly used to teach reading comprehension in elementary schools. Basal readers provide an integrated approach to reading instruction, with teachers' manuals, stories for students to read, and workbook exercises for students to complete. Most basal readers focus on specific reading and comprehension skills, but the number and type of skills differ from one basal reading program to another, and materials are not specific to any skill or subset of skills.

Objectives-oriented reading programs target specific reading skills such as *getting main ideas* or *using context* at several levels of reading difficulty and provide tests for measuring an individual's performance in each skill. Objectives-oriented programs differ in the number and kinds of skills addressed, and the reading levels for which they are appropriate. Most are designed for elementary-school use (Grades 1 through 6), so some may be inappropriate for use with adults because of their juvenile content. The *Specific Skills Series* of remedial reading materials (Boning, 1990), described in Chapter 5, is an objectives-oriented program that may prove useful for treating aphasic adults' reading impairments.

Rosenshine (1980) divided the skills addressed by objectives-oriented reading programs into three categories: *locating details* (recognizing, paraphrasing, and matching specific information), *simple inferential skills* (understanding words in context, recognizing sequences of events, recognizing cause-and-effect relationships, comparing and contrasting), and *complex inferential skills* (recognizing main ideas or topics, drawing conclusions, predicting outcomes).

Carver (1973) has commented that only skills such as those subsumed under *locating details* (above) are truly reading skills. He asserts that skills such as those subsumed under *simple* or *complex inferential skills* are not specific to reading but represent general reasoning ability. The implication is that if they represent general reasoning skills, one would not work on these skills only in reading (or that working on them in reading might enhance performance on other activities that call upon reasoning skills).

Treatment of aphasic patients' reading disabilities usually relies heavily on homework. Patients may work on reading assignments at home and bring the completed assignments to the clinic, where the clinician goes over the completed work, discusses errors with the patient, and provides instruction and practice with new materials. Sometimes work on auditory comprehension is carried on simultaneously with work on reading to enhance generalization between the two skills.

GENERAL CONCEPTS 9-3

- Reading comprehension is a synergistic process, combining *word recognition*, *syntactic analysis*, and *semantic mapping*.
- *Surface dyslexia* and *deep dyslexia* are two patterns of reading impairment sometimes exhibited by brain-injured adults. Readers with *surface dyslexia* must use *phonologic analysis* to identify problem words. Readers with *deep dyslexia* must use *whole-word recognition* to identify problem words.
- Obtaining a *literary history* often is the first step in designing a program to treat acquired reading impairments.
- Aphasic adults who will not become recreational readers usually benefit from acquiring *survival reading skills,* which permit them to read simple everyday materials such as signs, bills, and medication instructions.
- *Word recognition drills* may be appropriate for patients who cannot read at the sentence level and who exhibit signs of either surface dyslexia or deep dyslexia.
- Most patients who can read sentences should be working with sentences or paragraphs in treatment, to permit top-down processes to operate.
- Patients who can comprehend simple texts generally should be working with texts that challenge their reading skills via manipulation of familiarity, length, redundancy, cohesion, coherence, salience, directness, vocabulary, and syntactic complexity.

Continued

- *Readability formulas* are a way to measure the reading difficulty of printed texts. Most readability formulas calculate reading grade levels based on vocabulary difficulty and sentence length.
- Commercial reading programs (*basal readers* and *objectives-oriented reading programs*) are a useful source of materials for clinicians who work with reading-impaired adults.

Speech Production

Aphasic adults tend to be more troubled by impairments in speaking than by impairments in reading, writing, or listening comprehension, and aphasic adults' speech has important effects on how they are regarded by others in daily life. Accordingly, most speech-language pathologists give treatment of speech production an important place in their plans for aphasic adults. Which aspects of speech production get treated and how much speech production is emphasized relative to other communication modalities depends, of course, on the nature and severity of the patient's communication impairments. For patients who can produce few, if any, volitional words, drills requiring them to produce single words may be appropriate. For patients with some volitional speech, the emphasis may be on efficient and accurate production of phrases, sentences, or discourse.

Volitional Speech

Sentence Completion Tasks. Sentence completion tasks can help get volitional speech from patients who on their own can produce little more than automatisms and stereotypic utterances. The clinician says a sentence in which the final word or the final few words are missing, and the patient supplies the missing word or words. Highly constrained sentences containing word combinations that are common in daily life (e.g., *a cup of* _____) are the strongest facilitators of volitional speech. When a patient's responses to such highly constrained sentences are quick and accurate, treatment can move on to less-constrained sentences (e.g., *Put a stamp on the* _____ or *We wear shoes on our* _____). Stimulus sentences in which the missing elements are not constrained (e.g., *Today Joe bought a* _____ .) do not elicit specific target words but may be incorporated into the late stages of sentence completion treatment tasks to put more emphasis on volitional vocabulary search, word retrieval, and speech production.

Completing phrases or sentences representing overlearned everyday expressions is almost always easier for aphasic speakers than confrontation naming (Barton, Maruszewski, & Urrea, 1969; Podraza & Darley, 1977; Wyke & Holgate, 1973) or providing words in response to definitions given by the clinician (Barton & associates, 1969; Goodglass & Stuss, 1979). Highly constrained sentence completion tasks can be used to facilitate confrontation naming. That is, a clinician might elicit a set of object names with highly constrained sentence completion stimuli, then follow with confrontation naming of the same objects. Confrontation naming usually improves when it follows sentence completion.

Unfortunately the facilitating effects of sentence completion on confrontation naming are not very durable (Kremin, 1993). If the clinician waits a day or two and retests the patient's confrontation naming of items previously facilitated by sentence completion, they usually find that the patient's confrontation naming has returned to baseline. Less-constrained sentence completion items seem to have somewhat more durable effects. According to Kremin (1993):

> "The deblocking of a word via an automatic expression, although immediately very effective, leaves but a faint trace over time. On the other hand, the active search for a word

within the semantico-syntactic framework of a neutral sentence induces less immediate success but guarantees nonetheless the same level of performance on naming tasks after 24 hours." (p. 271)

It seems apparent that highly constrained sentence completion tasks are best used as stepping-stones to tasks in which volitional vocabulary search and word retrieval are required. If a patient cannot move from sentence completion to volitional word retrieval and speech production, sentence completion tasks are dead ends and probably should be abandoned.

Word and Phrase Repetition. Word and phrase repetition provides a somewhat less powerful but fairly dependable way to get volitional speech from patients who produce little or no volitional speech in less constrained contexts. Repetition drills are common in treatment for patients with articulatory selection and sequencing impairments (apraxia of speech) and for patients with weakness, paralysis, or incoordination of muscle groups involved in speech (dysarthria). For these patients, the emphasis is on the mechanics of speech production. The use of repetition drills for dysarthric patients is discussed in Chapter 13.

Word and phrase repetition tasks sometimes may be used early in treatment programs when the ultimate goal is to enhance processes such as word retrieval and sentence formulation. Repetition drills are used to get the patient started. Then the repetition drills are gradually replaced by activities that require vocabulary search and word retrieval, such as naming drills.

Confrontation Naming Drills. These drills require patients to name pictures (usually) or objects (sometimes) designated by the clinician. Confrontation naming drills can be used to move patients away from rote production of words and phrases toward more purposeful retrieval, encoding, and production of words and phrases. However, confrontation naming drills as an end in themselves may provide little

lasting benefit to patients. Brookshire (1975) trained 10 aphasic adults to name pictures of common objects. Their naming improved within training sessions, but there was no evidence that the improvements carried over to the next day, and there was no generalization of improved naming from trained items to untrained items within training sessions.

Naming objects or pictures is not a very useful behavior, unless one is a child learning the names of things or an adult learning a new language. If the to-be-named item is present, naming it usually is unnecessary and often inappropriate, because its presence creates shared knowledge between speaker and listener, making its name redundant. An aphasic patient who wishes to communicate the name of an object or picture that is present in the environment can do so by pointing instead of naming. Consequently naming drills, like sentence completion and repetition drills, are best thought of as stepping-stones to more advanced and functional speech communication.

Cueing Hierarchies. Clinicians have known for decades that aphasic adults' retrieval and production of single words can be facilitated if the clinician provides prompts or cues to lead the patient in the direction of the target words. Weigl (1968) described what he called a "*deblocking*" approach to treatment, in which brain-injured patients' inadequate responses to stimuli in one modality were facilitated by prestimulating the patient with cues delivered in another modality. For example, a clinician might provide the sound an object makes or a semantically related word prior to showing the patient a picture to be named. Those who use deblocking assume that prestimulation primes the patient's response to the target stimulus.

Podraza and Darley (1977) studied the effects of four kinds of prestimulation on aphasic adults' picture naming: (1) prestimulation with the first sound of the name plus a neutral vowel (e.g., *buh* followed by a picture of a bee); (2) prestimulation with an open-ended sentence (e.g., *I got stung by a bumble___*); (3) prestimulation with the target word plus two unrelated foils (e.g., *line, bee, goat*); and (4) prestimulation with three semantically related words (e.g., *sting, honey, hive*).

Podraza and Darley reported that three kinds of prestimulation (first sound plus neutral vowel, open-ended sentence, and target word plus two foils) facilitated naming performance with no clear differences among the three. Prestimulation with three semantically related foils worsened participants' naming performance rather than helping it. The pattern of facilitation differed across participants, leading Podraza and Darley to conclude:

> "The emergence of a slightly different hierarchy of effectiveness for each of the participants in the study suggests that the use of these techniques or any other technique in language therapy must be based on a hierarchy determined individually for each patient." (p. 681)

Podraza and Darley's procedures differ from those described by Weigl and his associates and, except for the open-ended sentence condition, differ from deblocking procedures typically used in the clinic. Prestimulating with the target word plus several unrelated words seems strange, because stimulation with the target word alone would be more effective in eliciting the target name. However, this changes the picture-naming task into a word-repetition task, which should be easy for most aphasic adults. That prestimulation with semantically related words worsened aphasic adults' naming performance is not surprising, given that aphasic adults' errors in confrontation-naming tasks often are semantically related to the target words, as Podraza and Darley mention.

Not all cues have equal effects on aphasic adults' naming. Over the years, numerous studies of the relative power of various cues have been reported (Barton, Maruszewski, & Urrea, 1969; Love & Webb, 1977; Pease & Goodglass, 1978; Weidner & Jinks, 1983), and several

cueing hierarchies for clinical use have been proposed (Brown, 1972; Davis, 1993, Linebaugh & Lehner, 1977). Pease and Goodglass (1978) asked aphasic adults to name each of 174 pictures of common objects. When participants failed to name an item, they were prompted with one of five cues:

1. First sound/syllable (*"It starts with* kuh. or *"It starts with* kof.)
2. Sentence completion (*"Pour me a cup of ___."*)
3. Rhyme (*"It rhymes with toffee."*)
4. Function/location (*"You drink it at breakfast."*)
5. Superordinate (*"It's something you drink."*)

The participants' success rates following each kind of cue were tabulated. The results are shown in Figure 9-7. The pattern of cue effectiveness was similar for participants with anomic aphasia, Broca's aphasia, and Wernicke's aphasia, although the magnitude of the effects differed across groups. Providing the first sound or syllable was most effective, followed in order by sentence completion, rhyme, location/function, and superordinate cues.

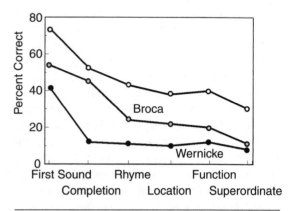

Figure 9-7 ■ Effectiveness of cues in eliciting correct picture-naming responses from adults with anomic, Broca's, or Wernicke's aphasia. (Data from Pease, D.M., Goodglass, H. [1978]. The effects of cueing on picture naming in aphasia. *Cortex, 14,* 178-189.)

Adding cues studied by others to Pease and Goodglass's list produces the following hierarchy, with cues arranged in approximate order of decreasing power:

- Imitation *("Say _____.")*
- First sound or first syllable
- Sentence completion
- Word spelled aloud
- Rhyme
- Synonym/antonym
- Function/location
- Superordinate

Standard hierarchies such as this give clinicians a general idea of what to expect on the average from a group of aphasic patients, but exceptions for individual patients are common. Therefore clinicians typically do a test run to determine the best cueing hierarchy for any given patient. They place the patient in a naming task, and when the patient misnames or fails to name a target item, the clinician provides a cue and observes its effect on the patient's naming. Some clinicians begin with the potentially most powerful cues and move down the hierarchy to less powerful cues until a cue consistently fails to elicit target names. Others begin with the potentially least powerful cues and move up the hierarchy until a cue consistently elicits target names. The frequency with which each cue elicits target words is then used to arrange the cues into a personalized hierarchy for the patient.

A patient's cueing hierarchy is used in word-retrieval tasks as follows. When the patient fails to retrieve a target word, the clinician provides the least powerful cue in the hierarchy. If this cue elicits an accurate response, the patient and clinician move on to the next item. If the cue does not elicit an accurate response, the clinician delivers the next more powerful cue. This continues until a cue elicits an accurate response. When the patient produces the target word in response to a cue, the clinician reverses course through the hierarchy and presents the next less powerful cue, continuing until the patient either makes an error or makes accurate responses to all cues. If the patient makes it all the way through the hierarchy with accurate responses, the patient and clinician move on. If the patient makes an error somewhere along the way, the clinician once again reverses course and delivers progressively more powerful cues until the patient responds accurately, at which time the clinician and patient move on to the next item. This ensures that the patient's final attempt at naming an item is successful.

When word-retrieval drills yield a corpus of words that the patient can dependably produce, treatment procedures may be modified to diminish the patient's reliance on clinician-supplied cues and substitute patient-generated cues or retrieval strategies. For example, patients whose word retrieval has been facilitated by rhyming cues may be trained to think of rhymes on their own, and patients whose word retrieval is facilitated by synonyms or an antonyms may be trained to think of synonyms or antonyms on their own. If patients' gestures help them produce the words they want, their use of gesture may be encouraged or trained.

Word Retrieval Failure. What aphasic adults do when they fail to retrieve a word sometimes gives a clinician clues to the nature of the patient's word retrieval troubles and may suggest strategies the patient may be using to cope with word retrieval failure. Marshall (1976) studied the spontaneous speech of 18 aphasic adults to determine what they did in response to word retrieval failures. He described five such coping behaviors—*delay, semantic association, phonetic association, description,* and *generalization:*

- In *delay* the patient produces a filled or unfilled pause or "some stalling tactic to let the listener know they did not want to be interrupted and needed more time to produce the word" (p. 446).
- In *semantic association* the patient produces one or more words that are semantically related to the target word, including antonyms (front/back), class membership (fruit/banana), part-whole relationship (foot/

toe), or serial relationship (Sunday/Monday/Tuesday).

- In *phonetic association* the patient produces words that are phonologically similar to the target word (hamper/clamper/camper).
- In *description* the patient describes characteristics of the target (*"It's round and red and it grows on trees—it's an apple."*).
- In *generalization* the patient produces general words and phrases without specific meaning (*It's one of those things. It's a thing that I know. It's a spider.*).

Marshall reported that semantic association was the most frequently occurring behavior, followed by description, generalization, delay, and phonetic association.

Marshall evaluated the apparent success of these behaviors by calculating the percentage of times each behavior led to the target word. Delay was followed by successful production of the target word about 90% of the time. Semantic association and phonetic association preceded correct production of the target about 55% of the time. Description and generalization were followed by their intended targets only 35% and 17% of the time, respectively (Figure 9-8).

It is tempting to assume a cause-effect relationship between behaviors preceding successful production of target words and the subsequent production of the target words. Although some of the behaviors described by Marshall may represent purposeful strategies on the part of aphasic speakers, some or all may be the outward manifestations of an aphasic person's attempts to cope with word retrieval gone awry. This is a crucial difference, because if the behaviors represent strategies, one might wish to encourage the patients to engage in those that have the greatest success. If the behaviors are signs of unsuccessful retrieval strategies, one would probably not wish to increase their frequency and might even search for ways to eliminate them, because they may diminish communicative efficiency.

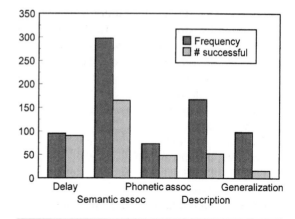

Figure 9-8 ■ Frequency of behaviors associated with aphasic adults' word retrieval failures and the number of times each behavior preceded successful word retrieval. (Data from Marshall, R.C. [1976]. Word retrieval behavior of aphasic adults. *Journal of Speech and Hearing Disorders, 41,* 444-451.)

The behaviors Marshall describes may reflect simply how close patients are to the target word. Patients who delay and then produce the target may be on the verge of retrieving the target word at the beginning of the delay (the *tip of the tongue phenomenon*). Delay was the most "successful" behavior. Semantic and phonetic association behaviors suggest that the patient has some information about the word, but not enough to retrieve the word. Semantic and phonetic association were moderately successful. Generalization and description suggest that the patient has failed to retrieve much beyond the semantic flavor of the word. Generalization and description were least likely to precede successful production of target words.

Enhancing Word Retrieval in Speech.
Rosenbek and associates (1989) described a three-part program for enhancing aphasic adults' word retrieval in connected speech. The program begins with diagnosis, moves on to

strategy development and practice in controlled environments, and ends with the patient's internalization of strategies and generalization of strategy use across words and environments. The following program is modeled on that of Rosenbek and associates.

Part 1: Diagnosis. Diagnosis involves two activities:

1. Generating a list of words and semantic categories (e.g., foodstuffs, tools, personal care items) that are especially important to the patient and family
2. Obtaining baseline measures of the patient's successful and unsuccessful word retrieval strategies

The clinician interviews the patient and one or more family members to develop a list of important words representing several semantic categories. The clinician also observes the patient in unstructured interactions and in structured drill activities to determine how reliably the patient produces various categories of words (with special attention to those on the list), to identify strategies the patient may be using to cope with word retrieval failure, and to get a sense of which strategies work and which do not.

Part 2: Strategy Development and Practice. In this part of the program the patient receives structured practice to expand and strengthen word retrieval strategies. If the patient is using strategies that facilitate word retrieval, their use is reinforced. If the patient has few or no successful strategies, the clinician and patient work together to develop some. The primary vehicle for strategy development is the patient's use of self-cueing (such as saying a related word, a rhyme, or the first sound of a word). The patient practices the strategies in controlled drill activities using words from the patient's list of important words. When retrieval of a word has been strengthened, the clinician may introduce other forms of the word. For example, if the patient's retrieval of the word *chair* has been stabilized, practice with words such as *armchair, chairman, wheelchair, easy chair,* or *high chair* may follow. Rosenbek and associates caution against introducing semantically related prompts (such as *table* or *couch* for *chair*), noting that semantically related words often interfere with retrieval of the previously stabilized target words.

As previously noted, Podraza and Darley (1977) found that prestimulating with semantically related words worsened aphasic adults' word retrieval.

Part 3: Stabilization and Generalization. In this part of the program the focus is on helping the patient extend effective word retrieval strategies to environments beyond the clinic and on moving the patient's word retrieval toward normalcy by replacing overt self-cueing strategies with covert ones. The emphasis is on self-correction and self-cueing by the patient and on extension of improved word retrieval from the tightly controlled elicitation conditions typical of the clinic to the less predictable conditions typical of daily life.

Activities to strengthen word associations and enhance semantic representations may be incorporated into this phase of treatment. The patient may be asked to:

- Provide synonyms, antonyms, or rhymes for words presented by the clinician
- Provide lists of words that are in categories specified by the clinician
- Provide words to fill in blanks in sentences or narratives
- Separate printed semantically related words from unrelated words
- Produce lists of words or word combinations with a common root (e.g., *wash, washer, washcloth, washing machine, car wash*)

As the patient's internal semantic associations and organization move toward normalcy, it is assumed that the patient's word retrieval will improve, diminishing the need for strategies to volitionally evoke words the patient wishes to say.

Sentence Production. Sentence-length utterances can be elicited in several ways. The simplest way is *sentence imitation drill* in which the clinician says a sentence, and the patient repeats it. Sentence imitation drills are most commonly used to increase articulatory accuracy for patients with motor speech impairments or motor programming impairments. They sometimes are used to increase auditory retention span for patients with aphasia. Sentence-imitation drills sometimes follow word-repetition drills for patients with speech production impairments. Imitation gets them talking. Then treatment moves them on to more difficult (and more natural) sentence production tasks.

Repetition-elaboration drills are used to move patients from repetition to less constrained responses. In repetition-elaboration drills, the clinician asks questions designed to elicit formulaic, stereotypical responses typical of those in social encounters and conversations:

Clinician: "How are you?"
Patient: "Fine. And how are you?"
Clinician: "What do you like for breakfast?"
Patient: "Bacon and eggs. What do you like for breakfast?"

Story completion drills elicit responses that are less constrained than those in repetition-elaboration drills. In story completion the clinician provides a two- or three-sentence narrative and asks the patient to provide a phrase or sentence to complete it:

Clinician: "It's ten o'clock, and my children are still up. I want them to go to bed. So I say to them ...."
Patient: "Go to bed."

Helm-Estabrooks (1982) developed a program for eliciting such utterances from aphasic adults, called the *Helm Elicited Language Program for Syntax Stimulation (HELPSS)*.

Question-answer drills further diminish response constraints. The clinician asks questions related to the patient's experiences, opinions, or general knowledge. The patient responds with a phrase or sentence:

Clinician: "What did you do last evening?"
Patient: "Watched TV and went to bed."
Clinician: "What's the most important difference between cats and dogs?"
Patient: "You don't have to walk a cat."

In *story elaboration drills* the clinician tells a short story and follows with a series of questions designed to elicit a phrase or sentence:

Clinician: "Fred and Ethyl decided to go out for dinner to celebrate Ethyl's birthday. They drove across town to a fancy restaurant and had a nice meal. When the bill came, Fred reached for his wallet, only to discover that it was not there. What do you think Fred and Ethyl did next?"
Patient: "Maybe Ethyl paid the bill, if she had any money."
Clinician: "Where do you think Fred left his wallet?"
Patient: "At the bar, I suppose."

Story elaboration calls on several processes in addition to sentence formulation and production. The patient must comprehend the stories and retain the information long enough to respond. The patient also must call on general knowledge, make inferences, and foresee consequences to formulate a response that is consistent with the story.

Picture-story elaboration drills are similar to story elaboration, except that instead of telling the patient a story, the clinician shows the patient a picture depicting a situation with a salient theme and a predictable outcome (as in Figure 9-9) or a series of pictures depicting a sequence of events. Then the clinician asks the patient a series of questions to elicit phrase-length or sentence-length responses.

The clinician might ask the following questions about Figure 9-9:

"What's the occasion?"
"Why is the boy crying?"
"What do you think will happen next?"

In *sentence construction drills* the clinician provides a spoken or printed word, phrase, or two or more related words and asks the patient to produce a sentence containing the words:

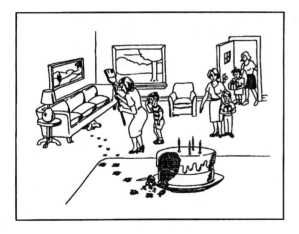

Figure 9-9 ■ A picture that might be used to elicit connected speech. The picture has a central theme and a predictable outcome and suggests events that happened before the events portrayed.

Clinician: "Give me a sentence containing the word *boy.*"

Patient: "The boy is happy."

Clinician: "Give me a sentence containing the words *man, drink,* and *coffee.*"

Patient: "Man, I like to drink coffee."

Sentence construction drills permit considerable flexibility in manipulating task difficulty. When the eliciting stimulus is a single word, task difficulty depends primarily on the part of speech and the frequency in English of the stimulus word. Nouns usually are easiest for aphasic adults (and the rest of us) to incorporate into a sentence, followed by verbs, pronouns, adjectives, adverbs, and function words. (It is easier to construct a sentence with the word *man* than it is to construct a sentence with the word *before.*) Frequently occurring concrete words make sentence production easier for most aphasic adults. When aphasic patients have to combine several words into a sentence, providing the words in noun-verb or noun-verb-noun order facilitates performance, because the order of the words in the stimulus matches the subject-verb or subject-verb-object order of the two most common sentence structures. Scrambling the order of the words in the stimulus increases task difficulty by requiring the patient to rearrange the words to create a syntactically correct sentence. Providing stimuli that represent common word combinations (e.g., *a piece of pie*) or express commonly encountered relationships (e.g., *man-drink-coffee*) makes the task easier for most aphasic patients.

Sentence production tasks can sometimes entice clinicians into thinking that grammaticality is what they and the patient should be seeking, when for most patients, communication, not grammaticality, is the answer. Ungrammatic utterances often do an adequate job of communicating an aphasic speaker's thoughts, wishes, and intentions. The patient who responds to *What did you do last evening?* with *TV... bed... sleep* has successfully (though not elegantly) communicated the essentials. Clinicians who insist on grammatic utterances run the risk of wasting their time and wasting the patient's time and energy. The principal exceptions are some high-level aphasic patients who, with a reasonable amount of coaching, are capable of speaking both informatively and grammatically.

Connected Speech

Connected speech is a generic label for speech in which a person produces several utterances in response to a stimulus, topic, or event. The utterances may be continuous, on a common topic, and not separated either by introduction of a new stimulus or by the contributions of another speaker *(monologue),* or the utterances may be separated by questions, comments, or contributions from another speaker *(conversation, interview).* Monologues are more commonly used in process-oriented testing and treatment than conversation and interview, perhaps because monologues provide better control over the content and form of patients' responses and are easier to quantify.

Conversations are the focus of several functional-social approaches to intervention (discussed later in this chapter). Measuring aphasic persons' conversational behaviors is an important part of these interventions.

Picture Description. Picture description is one way of eliciting monologues. In *picture description,* target sentences are not constrained, and the patient has free choice of the kinds of sentences produced plus considerable latitude in word choice. However, the nature of the picture or pictures used to elicit descriptions may affect both the amount and kind of verbalizations elicited from the patient. Familiar occurrences or situations elicit more verbalization than unfamiliar ones. Pictures that suggest a *past* (events leading up to the situation or event depicted) and a *future* (events following the situation or event depicted) encourage those who describe them to go beyond the content of the pictures and talk about preceding and

following events. Pictures depicting static situations often elicit *enumeration* (naming items in the picture), whereas pictures depicting dynamic interactions usually elicit more elaborate descriptions. Figure 9-10 shows two pictures. The one on the left is more likely to elicit enumeration than the one on the right. When a non-brain-damaged adult described the left-hand picture, she said, *Well there's a small stream running through a meadow, some toadstools or mushrooms in the foreground.* When she described the right-hand picture, she said, *There's an old man and his dog, probably in a park, because the man is sitting on a park bench, and there are squirrels around. The man is feeding popcorn or peanuts to the squirrels—I can't tell which. The dog is sitting by the bench wagging his tail. I wonder why he's not chasing the squirrels. That's a natural thing for dogs to do, you know.*

Correia, Brookshire, and Nicholas (1990) empirically demonstrated that static speech elicitation pictures tend to elicit enumeration from aphasic adults. They had aphasic adults

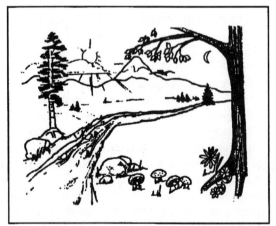 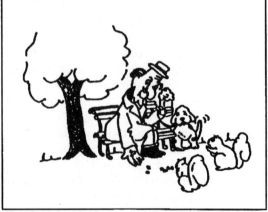

Figure 9-10 ■ Two pictures that might be used to elicit connected speech. The picture on the left is more likely to elicit enumeration than the picture on the right. (Courtesy Howard E. Gardner, Ph.D.)

describe the speech elicitation pictures from the *Boston Diagnostic Aphasia Examination* (*BDAE*; Goodglass & Kaplan, 1983), the WAB, and the *Minnesota Test for Differential Diagnosis of Aphasia* (*MTDDA*; Schuell, 1972) (see Figure 5-19). The aphasic speakers' responses to the static WAB and MTDDA pictures contained greater percentages of enumerations (42% and 45% respectively) than their responses to the more dynamic BDAE picture (38%), but only the difference between the WAB picture and the BDAE picture was statistically significant.

Even non-brain-damaged adults produce fewer storylike narratives when they talk about the MTDDA picture than when they talk about the BDAE picture. Box 9-2 contains a transcript of what a graduate student said when asked to describe each picture.

Prompted Story Telling. *Prompted story telling* elicits stories by means of sequences of pictures that represent events in a story (Figure 9-11). The amount of speech a picture sequence elicits depends on the number of incidents in

Box 9-2	*A Graduate Student Describes the MTDDA Picture and the BDAE Picture*

The MTDDA Picture

There's a house with a mailbox. The name on the mailbox is J. Smith. There's also a man flying a kite. There's another kite caught in a tree. There's a dog looking at the man. There's a woman pointing to the kite in the tree. There's a duck on a small pond. There's a house with smoke coming out of the chimney. That's about it.

The BDAE Picture

There's a woman standing at a sink drying dishes. The water is on and running onto the floor, but she doesn't seem to notice. There are two kids behind the woman—probably the woman's son and daughter. The boy is standing on a stool which is gonna tip over. He's in the act of getting—of stealing cookies from a cookie jar there in the cupboard. The stool is tipping, and he's gonna land on the floor. His sister is reaching up to get a cookie from him. The mother is completely oblivious to all that's going on. She's either asleep or on drugs.

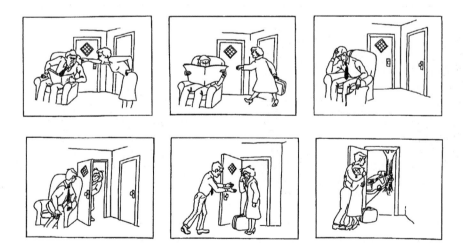

Figure 9-11 ▪ A picture sequence that might be used to elicit prompted story telling in treatment activities.

the sequence, with more incidents generating longer speech samples. The picture sequence shown in Figure 9-11 elicited, on the average, slightly more than 80 words from aphasic speakers, but the range was substantial (23 words for a nonfluent aphasic speaker to 164 words for a fluent aphasic speaker).

Procedural Discourse. *Procedural discourse* is connected speech made in response to requests such as *Tell me how you make scrambled eggs.* When non-brain-damaged adults describe procedures such as making scrambled eggs, writing and mailing a letter, and doing dishes by hand, they produce from 75 to 125 words per procedure, depending on the procedure (with more complex procedures eliciting longer samples). The range for aphasic speakers is great. Some nonfluent aphasic speakers may generate 25 to 30 words per procedure, and some fluent aphasic speakers may generate nearly 300.

Procedural discourse usually is not syntactically complex. Ulatowska, Doyel, Freedman-Stern, and associates (1983) evaluated procedural descriptions produced by nonaphasic adults and aphasic adults, and they found that neither group produced many syntactically complex sentences. They commented that procedural descriptions do not require syntactically complex language, so even many patients with relatively severe aphasia produce syntactically adequate procedural descriptions (excepting, of course, those with Broca's aphasia, who speak agrammatically).

Conversation. *Conversation* sometimes is used to elicit speech from aphasic patients in treatment activities. However, many of these interactions do not resemble natural conversations, because the clinician does most of the talking, and the patient's responses do not go beyond providing what the clinician requests, making the interaction more of an interview than a conversation, as in the following sample:

Clinician: "What kind of work did you do before your stroke?"

Patient: "Foreman."

Clinician: "A foreman. What company did you work for?"

Patient: "Amurcan."

Clinician: "Amurcan? Do you mean American? American what?"

Patient: "Amurican Freight."

Clinician: "American Freight. Is that a trucking company?"

Patient: "Yeah."

Clinician: "And you were a foreman. What kinds of workers did you supervise?"

Patient: "Dock."

Clinician: "People on the dock?"

Patient: "Yeah."

Clinician: "And what kind of jobs did they do?"

Patient: "Oh… most ever'thing."

Unless carefully structured with pragmatic principles about conversational interactions firmly in place, such clinician-patient interactions may not be very effective in eliciting connected speech from the patient. They are more appropriately employed when the objective is to improve the patient's conversational behaviors (such as turn-taking, eye contact, and topic maintenance).

GENERAL CONCEPTS 9-4

- *Sentence completion drills* may increase volitional speech for patients whose spontaneous speech is limited to automatic stereotypic utterances.

- *Confrontation-naming drills* are popular with clinicians but may not produce lasting effects or improve patients' daily life communication.

- *Cueing hierarchies* permit clinicians to manipulate the power of stimuli used to facilitate aphasic patients' performance in word retrieval drills.

- Behaviors associated with word retrieval failure may represent strategies used by a patient to retrieve words or may simply reflect a patient's unplanned response to word retrieval failure.

GENERAL CONCEPTS 9-4—cont'd

- *Sentence production drills* often proceed from tasks in which patients' responses are highly constrained (imitation, story completion) to open-ended tasks in which patients have considerable latitude in the nature of their responses (story elaboration, sentence construction).

- *Connected-speech drills* often proceed from tasks in which patients' responses are constrained (picture description) to less constrained tasks (prompted story telling, procedural discourse, conversation).

Writing

Many of the same cognitive processes used to produce spoken messages are used to produce written messages. It is only at the production stage that speaking and writing appreciably differ. Writers, unlike speakers, need a sense of how to spell. Writing requires enough visual-motor coordination and limb strength to produce written letters. Writers need better syntax than speakers, because speakers can compensate for deficient syntax by providing prosodic clues to meanings, but writers do not have this option. Written style is more formal and more grammatically complex than spoken style. It should not be surprising that aphasic adults almost always write less well than they speak.

Aphasic patients' writing resembles their speech. Fluent speakers tend to be fluent writers. They write in cursive, produce well-shaped letters, and maintain horizontal and equally spaced writing lines. Nonfluent speakers tend to be nonfluent writers (partly because they are using their nonpreferred hand). They produce distorted letters, and their lines are uneven in contour and spacing. Nonfluent writers usually print rather than write in cursive. Agrammatic speakers are likely to be agrammatic writers, and aphasic speakers who generate "*empty*" (devoid of meaning) speech are likely to generate "empty" written materials (Figure 9-12).

Most aphasic adults have disabilities in spelling and syntax that make it difficult or impossible for them to communicate effectively by writing. Consequently, most writing treatment programs for aphasic adults focus on spelling, syntax, and grammar, using didactic procedures and relying heavily on homework. Sometimes commercially available spelling and writing workbooks are used. Teaching written spelling and syntax to aphasic adults may be an exception to the general assumption that treatment involves *stimulation* or *reactivation*

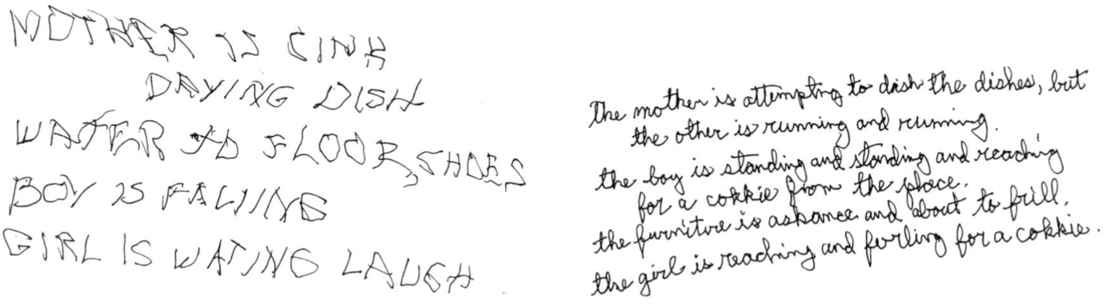

Figure 9-12 ■ Written responses produced by an aphasic adult with Broca's aphasia *(left)* and an aphasic adult with fluent aphasia *(right)* as they described the *cookie theft* picture from the *Boston Diagnostic Aphasia Examination*. (Goodglass, Kaplan, and Barresi [2001].)

rather than *teaching*. In most cases, procedures used in teaching aphasic adults to spell and write do not differ from those used to teach beginning writers.

It may be fortunate that most aphasic adults do not really need advanced writing skills in daily life. If an aphasic adult can write short notes, fill out forms, and write checks, she or he may get by in most daily life environments. Consequently, treatment programs that can get aphasic writers to this level are likely to be sufficient for many. Writing one's name is no doubt the most frequent single daily life writing act and often is the first treatment objective for patients who cannot write. Fortunately, writing one's name is highly automatized. Adults with severe aphasia often can write their name when they can write nothing else.

Most of the linguistic variables that affect how easy it is to produce spoken sentences (length, word frequency, syntactic complexity, and so on) also affect how easy it is to write them. Context affects aphasic persons' writing in the same way that it affects their speaking. If part of a sentence is provided, and patients have only to complete the sentence, success rates are higher than if they have to produce the same words without contextual support. *Cloze procedures,* in which single words are deleted from printed passages, sometimes help patients get started. Most aphasic patients write single words better when they can fill in blanks in a sentence or paragraph than when they have to write them in isolation.

Survival Writing Skills. The concept of *survival writing skills* is a useful guide to treatment for patients with severely impaired writing. The clinician and the patient (and sometimes family members) make a list of things that the patient would most like to be able to write. Treatment is structured to develop a core writing vocabulary and enough syntactic skills to enable the patient to perform the writing tasks on the list. The following list of writing skills was produced by a woman with moderately severe Broca's aphasia. The skills are listed in order of importance to the patient, from most important (top) to least important (bottom).

- Signing forms (which she could do)
- Writing shopping lists
- Writing checks
- Writing notes in greeting cards
- Writing personal letters

Treatment began with shopping lists. The patient brought several favorite recipes to each clinic appointment, and the patient and the clinician used the recipes to make up a list of ingredients needed to prepare the recipes. The words in the ingredient list were incorporated into spelling drills, and the patient practiced writing problem words at home. The patient also brought utility bills and check registers to clinic sessions. The patient and clinician used the bills and check registers to make up a list of words needed to write the checks. The words in the list were incorporated into check writing drills, and the patient practiced writing problem words at home. When treatment moved on to note and letter writing, similar procedures were used to identify words the patient often misspelled when writing personal notes and letters. The word lists thus obtained were incorporated into spelling drills and spelling homework.

Two principles governing treatment in general also are relevant to treating impaired writing: (1) exploit context whenever possible and (2) begin treatment at a level at which the patient is challenged but not overwhelmed.

It is unusual for an aphasic adult's treatment program to concentrate exclusively on writing. Treatment of writing impairments usually is an adjunct to other treatment, with considerable reliance on homework for the writing part of the program. If the clinician plans carefully, treatment of writing impairments can be coordinated with other treatment activities to create maximum generalization from writing to other communicative abilities, from other communicative abilities to writing, and from the clinic to daily life.

Spelling. Intelligible writing requires reasonably good spelling. Aphasic patients are universally poor spellers. The severity of a patient's spelling troubles almost always parallels the severity of the patient's aphasia. Patients with severe aphasia rarely write or spell well enough to become functional writers. Most patients with moderate aphasia can write comprehensible simple sentences, short notes, and personal letters, but frequent spelling errors make some words unintelligible, and errors in syntax make some sentences unfathomable even to resourceful readers. Most patients with mild aphasia can write more complex sentences and longer texts, but frequent spelling errors may annoy both the patient and those who read what the patient has written. Figure 9-13 shows a moderately aphasic person's performance when asked to write the function of each of the ten test objects from the PICA.

Computer-assisted spelling drills may be helpful to clinicians and patients who are working on spelling. A few such programs have been devised for aphasic adults (Katz & Nagy, 1984; Katz, Wertz, Davidoff, Schubitowski, & Devitt, 1989; Seron, Deloche, Mouolard, & Rouselle, 1980). Computer-based spelling programs designed for children also may be useful, although the juvenile themes of some programs may offend aphasic adults. Contemporary word processing software can be of immense help to aphasic adults (and nonaphasic adults, too) who spell well enough to get close to the correct spelling of problem words. Most of these programs highlight misspelled words and some provide a drop-down window in which the correct spellings of possible alternatives are given. (The word processing program I used to write this chapter gave *possible* and *possibly* as alternatives for *possilbe*, which I mistyped.) Many contemporary word processing programs also include style checking software, which may help aphasic adults identify syntactic miscues in sentences and text. Spell checking and style checking programs may be beneficial to higher-level aphasic adults who are at least mediocre spellers and who can write sentences with at least fair syntax.

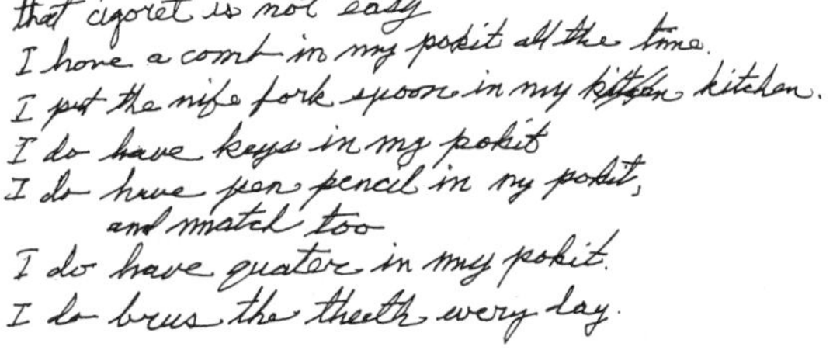

Figure 9-13 ■ Written responses produced by an aphasic adult in response to the command "*Write here what you do with each of these.*" ("*these*" being the 10 stimulus objects in the *Porch Index of Communicative Ability;* Porch, 1981a.)

GENERAL CONCEPTS 9-5

- Most of the linguistic variables that affect how easy it is for aphasic persons to produce spoken sentences (length, syntactic complexity, etc.) affect how easy it is for aphasic persons to write them.
- Aphasic patients with grossly impaired writing may benefit from acquiring *survival writing skills* that enable them to sign forms, make lists, write checks, and do similar writing tasks.
- Aphasic patients who need more than survival writing skills may benefit from structured programs that progress from letter (*grapheme*) writing and word writing to sentence and paragraph writing.
- Published programs for treating aphasic persons' writing impairments usually must be modified to fit the needs of aphasic individuals.
- Commercially published spelling workbooks and computer-based spelling programs are suitable for many aphasic persons for whom work on spelling is an appropriate treatment focus.

FUNCTIONAL AND SOCIAL APPROACHES TO INTERVENTION

Until the late 1970s intervention to address aphasic adults' communicative disabilities focused on treatment of linguistic impairments (e.g., listening comprehension, word retrieval, reading, speech production). Impairment level intervention was structured around the traditional medical progression of diagnosis, treatment, and discharge. An aphasic person's communicative impairments were measured (usually with standardized tests), treatment to reduce the impairments or to provide the patient with strategies to compensate for the impairments was provided, and the patient was discharged when the goals of treatment (defined as change in the level of impairment) had been achieved.

During the late 1970s and throughout the 1980s, many clinicians began to move away from traditional linguistically oriented, didactic treatment toward treatment that emphasized functional communication in natural contexts— a trend that has continued to the present. Holland (1977) observed that traditional didactic treatment approaches tend to focus on linguistic correctness and propositional accuracy:

> ...by means of activities such as matching, naming, and helping aphasics to comprehend utterances defined by their linguistic structure, instead of their likelihood of being heard in everyday communication....Most therapy is disproportionately centered on the propositionality of an utterance, not on its communicative value. (p. 171)

Holland went on to recommend that treatment focus on *communicative competence*—a person's use of language in naturalistic contexts, now commonly referred to as *functional communication.*

Functional communication treatment programs downplay traditional didactic drills and emphasize communication in natural contexts.

Clinicians and patients might act out daily life situations such as making a purchase in a department store, calling for information about airline schedules, and the like. Patients are encouraged or taught to communicate nonverbally (e.g., with gestures and facial expression) and to enhance their comprehension of what others say by using the information provided by others' gestures and facial expressions and by the situational contexts in which communication takes place. Functional approaches to intervention recognize that aphasic persons need not be perfect speakers or perfect listeners to communicate adequately.

Some functional approaches to intervention provide aphasic persons with strategies and techniques to enhance their success in daily life communicative interactions. Others focus training on actual or potential partners of aphasic persons, teaching them ways in which they can enhance the aphasic person's success and sense of accomplishment in daily life communicative interactions.

Following the World Health Organization's publication of the ICIDH and ICIDH-2, the concept of functional communication, which until then had focused primarily on improving aphasic persons' communicative competence in activities of daily life, was broadened to include the social aspects of communication, including access to and participation in cultural and social activities of daily living. Several new labels (e.g., *social approaches, life participation approaches*) were coined to characterize the treatment approaches representing this broadened concept of functionality. Social models of intervention expand the focus of communication from its *transactional function* (i.e., exchange of information) to include its *interactional function* (i.e., establishing and maintaining social relationships). Social approaches to intervention recognize that aphasia often has lifelong consequences for the aphasic person and the aphasic person's family, and that helping the aphasic person regain personal autonomy and a sense of self-worth are important goals of intervention.

For all the benefit that has accrued from what we have learned about aphasia, and all the good that has been derived from our treatment for people confronting aphasia, nothing *"cures"* its underlying pathology or its functional and psychosocial consequences or eliminates the necessity of overhauling most of the primary

domains of daily life. Furthermore, this perpetual state of interference in the living of life is not restricted to the person with aphasia, but rather affects the well-being of everyone who depended upon that person for their own daily sustenance, partnership, or companionship." (Lyon & Shadden, 2001, p. 297)

According to Simmons-Mackie (2001), social approaches to aphasia are structured according to nine basic principles (Box 9-3).

Box 9-3	*Nine Principles of Social Approaches to Aphasia*

1. *Information exchange and social relationships are complementary goals of communication.* Communication entails exchange of information (its *transactional* function) but also permits individuals to maintain personal identity and sense of self, fulfill emotional needs, connect with others, and permit membership in groups (its *interactional* function).
2. *Communication takes place within authentic, relevant, and natural contexts.* Intervention should respect the fact that purposes, roles, and intentions change during interactions in natural communicative contexts.
3. *Communication is dynamic, flexible, and multidimensional.* Linguistically less-than-perfect communication may result in effective information exchange while simultaneously fulfilling the individual's personal and social needs.
4. *Communication is collaborative.* Intervention should focus on the collaborative, interactional aspects of communication. The communication skills and behaviors of those around the aphasic person are important, as well as the communication skills and behaviors of the aphasic person.
5. *Intervention should focus on natural interaction, particularly on conversation.* Conversation is for most adults the central element in daily life communication. Improving the aphasic person's ability to participate in natural conversa-

tions contributes to the aphasic person's sense of self and personal well-being.
6. *Intervention should consider the personal and social consequences of aphasia.* There is great variability in how individuals respond to the presence of aphasia. Some adaptations may be successful, appropriate, and palatable to an aphasic person in one situation but not in another.
7. *Intervention should emphasize adaptations to communicative impairments.* Intervention should emphasize the positive aspects of life with aphasia by focusing on the aphasic person's successful adaptations to the consequences of aphasia and by exploiting the aphasic person's retained abilities. Intervention also should include the adaptation of society to the person with aphasia.
8. *Intervention should consider the perspective of those affected by aphasia.* Clinicians should refrain from deciding what an aphasic person needs but structure intervention to respect the perceptions, attitudes, and needs of those who are affected by the presence of aphasia (family members and associates as well as the aphasic person).
9. *Intervention should include qualitative as well as quantitative measures.* Qualitative and descriptive measures, rather than quantitative impairment level measures, best capture the subjective experiences of persons affected by aphasia.

Based on Simmons-Mackie, N. (2001). Social approaches to aphasia intervention. In R. Chapey (Ed.) *Language intervention strategies in aphasia and related neurogenic communication disorders* (4th ed.). Philadelphia: Lippincott Williams & Wilkins (pp. 246-268).

Interventions Designed for Aphasic Persons

Functionally oriented approaches designed for aphasic persons provide an aphasic person with general strategies or skills (e.g., cueing strategies for word retrieval, visualization strategies for written spelling, turn-taking strategies in conversations) that can be used in a variety of daily life contexts. Intervention sessions simulate daily life situations, and the aphasic person is trained to use a targeted strategy or skill in several related situations, with the expectation that the strategy or skill will generalize to related but untrained daily life situations. Most are designed to enhance or highlight aphasic persons' competence in conversations or conversation-like interactions, often with a specific conversational partner.

Promoting Aphasics' Communicative Effectiveness (PACE; Davis & Wilcox, 1985) was one of the first intervention programs designed specifically to target functional communication in situations that simulated daily life communicative interactions. PACE is based on four general principles (Davis, 2000):

- *The clinician and patient exchange new information.* The clinician does not know the probable content of the patient's communication when the patient begins her or his communication turn.
- *The clinician and patient participate equally as senders and receivers of messages.* Communication turns alternate between clinician and patient.
- *The patient has free choice of communicative modes used to convey a message.* The patient may use gesture, drawing, writing, or any other means to communicate the content of messages. The clinician does not dictate the patient's mode of communication.
- *The clinician's feedback is based on the patient's success in conveying messages.* The clinician does not label the patient's communicative attempts as adequate or deficient but responds as conversational part-

ners normally would—by asking questions, agreeing, paraphrasing, etc.

In the standard format for a PACE session, a pack of message cards is placed face-down between the patient and the clinician. The message cards may contain pictures, words, phrases, sentences, short narratives, or anything that provides a practical medium for information exchange between the patient and the clinician. The patient and the clinician alternate turns in which the person whose turn it is draws a card from the pack and, without showing it to the other participant, attempts to convey the content of the message on the card to the other participant, using any communicative mode that contributes to message transmission. The clinician may model communicative behaviors the patient could use but is not using to enhance communication. The clinician does not directly train communicative behaviors or dictate the patient's choice of communicative behaviors. (However, the clinician may first teach a patient to use specific communicative strategies, then use PACE to train the patient to incorporate them into communicative interactions.)

Conversational coaching (Holland, 1991; Hopper, Holland, & Rewega, 2002) teaches conversation partners to use verbal or nonverbal strategies to improve conversational interactions. One form of conversational coaching (Holland, 1991) focuses on the aphasic person. The clinician provides the aphasic person with a short script that is written at a level that is slightly too difficult for her or him to produce. The aphasic person practices producing the script, and the clinician suggests ways in which the aphasic person might communicate the content of the script and guides her or him in practicing the script. Then the aphasic person communicates the script to a new listener who does not know the content of the script (usually a family member). As the aphasic person communicates the script to the new listener, the clinician may remind the aphasic person what she or he needs to do to communicate the important information in the script.

Another form of conversational coaching (Hopper, Holland, & Rewega, 2002) teaches an aphasic person and a conversational partner techniques for enhancing conversations. First the clinician and the aphasic person watch 2- to 3-minute videotaped segments of humorous, adventurous, or dangerous real-life events extracted from commercial television programs. Then the aphasic person is recorded on videotape as he or she attempts to communicate the gist of the videotaped segment to someone who has not seen it (usually the aphasic person's spouse or another family member). The aphasic person and the patient's conversational partner are told to "communicate as they normally would." Later the clinician watches the videotape of the interaction and develops a small set of verbal and nonverbal strategies that may facilitate communication. Then the clinician, the aphasic person, and the partner watch the videotape together. The clinician highlights successful communicative behaviors and suggests communicative strategies (for both the aphasic person and the communicative partner) that would enhance communication. Guided practice in incorporating the strategies into conversational interactions between the aphasic person and the conversational partner follows.

Some functionally oriented intervention approaches are designed to provide the aphasic person with strategies or skills that are specific to certain daily life activities (e.g., using the telephone, ordering in a restaurant, writing personal letters). Intervention sessions simulate specific daily life situations, and the aphasic person is trained to use specific strategies or is helped to develop specific skills that ensure success in the targeted situation. Although generalization to activities other than those trained may occur, such generalization typically is not formally addressed in these approaches.

Hopper and Holland (1998) described a functionally oriented intervention of the latter type called *situation-specific training* to enable aphasic adults to summon help from emergency response agencies. They described situation-specific training as "therapy in which the goal is to teach a small set of specific responses related to a functional situation, such as ordering food in a restaurant or writing a check" (p. 933). Hopper and Holland noted that situation-specific training differs from what they called *process-based approaches,* which they characterized as "training strategies and responses to be applied to a wide range of situations or behaviors" (p. 933). Hopper and Holland taught two aphasic adults to use a telephone to communicate pictured emergency situations (e.g., someone drowning in a pool, a house on fire). At the end of training, both aphasic adults could dial the emergency number (911) and communicate information about what was happening in the simulated emergencies. One participant generalized the training to untrained emergency pictures; the other had to be taught responses to the untrained pictures. Hopper and Holland concluded that the training program was effective, produced some generalization, and had lasting effects at 4 weeks after treatment ended. They advocated situation-specific training for tasks that are relevant to the patient and are ranked according to their importance and potential effect on the patient's life, noting that the training can be accomplished in a few sessions, and that the effects of training appear durable—the effects of training were apparent 4 weeks after training ended.

Interventions Designed for Communication Partners of Aphasic Persons

Several functionally oriented approaches to intervention depart from tradition by focusing on the conversational partners of aphasic persons rather than on the aphasic person. The conversational partners are taught techniques that help them support and enhance the communicative competence of their aphasic conversational partner. The concept underlying communication partners is that conversation is a collaborative activity in which the behavior of each conversational partner affects the other. Consequently, when conversational partners of aphasic persons use techniques for facilitating the aphasic person's use of preserved cognitive abilities and social knowledge, the conversational interaction is enhanced, the aphasic person's social participation increases, and the aphasic person's confidence and sense of self-worth grows.

> In conversations with those with aphasia, the conversational partner can be viewed as being jointly responsible for maintaining the integrity of the conversational process. (Kagan & associates, 2001, p. 625)

Lyon (1989, 1992) described a program called *communication partners* in which volunteers from the community are recruited and trained to serve as communication partners for adults who have moderate to severe aphasia. The communication partners are trained to help aphasic adults select, plan, and undertake daily life activities of their own choosing, either at home or in community settings. An aphasic adult, the aphasic adult's primary caregiver, and a communication partner make up a communicative triad. The communication partners are trained and supervised by speech-language pathologists as the triads devise and test communication and participation strategies in mock-ups of real life situations and settings. When the strategies have been perfected, the triads try them out in natural daily life settings. Strategies and settings are selected by the aphasic participant to reflect aspects of daily life participation that are important to the aphasic participant—ordering in a restaurant, making purchases in stores, visiting friends, and so on. The communication partner supports the aphasic person and the caregiver with advice and

encouragement and may accompany the aphasic person in selected activities until the aphasic person has the confidence and skills needed for self-sufficient participation.

Lyon and associates (1997) evaluated the effects of communication partners' intervention on aphasic persons' participation in communicative activities in daily life and on their psychosocial well-being. Pretreatment and posttreatment assessments suggested significant positive changes in both characteristics. Importantly, the aphasic persons continued to engage in their activities of choice after communication partner support ended.

Supported conversation (*SCA;* Kagan, 1998), like Lyon's communication partners program, is designed to enhance and expand aphasic persons' participation in daily life communicative interactions. These goals are accomplished by training family members or volunteers to provide aphasic participants with controlled experiences in conversational interactions. Supported conversation is intended for aphasic persons with severe language impairments because, as Kagan (1998) comments:

> First, this is the group generally requiring the full range of SCA techniques (in contrast to moderate and mild aphasia where less support is required); and second, conversation partners need to discover that it is possible to have conversations with severely aphasic adults who are often excluded from participating in programmes, both traditional and nontraditional, because their aphasia is regarded as 'too severe'. (p 819)

Kagan (1998) comments that supported conversation is similar in intent to Lyon's communication partners approach in that both approaches seek to increase aphasic persons' confidence in communication and participation, and much of the work in both approaches is done with partners of aphasic persons. Those who provide supported conversation for aphasic persons are trained in a 1-day workshop that introduces the philosophy of supported conversation, provides information about aphasia, shows participants ways to acknowledge the competence of aphasic persons, shows participants ways to reveal aphasic persons' competence, and provides role-play experience in which the instructor assumes the role of an aphasic person in conversational interactions with participants.

> Kagan cautions her readers that work with conversation partners should be considered an addition to, and not a replacement for, working to enhance the communicative effectiveness of the aphasic partners.

Kagan, Black, Duchan, and associates (2001) reported the results of a study to determine if supported conversation training improved the conversational skills of volunteers, and, if it does, whether the improvements affected the communicative success of their aphasic conversation partners. The results suggested affirmative answers to both questions, although the changes in aphasic partners' communicative success were not strongly correlated with changes in the conversational skills of the volunteers.

Socially oriented interventions to increase aphasic persons' access to and participation in daily life communicative interactions have considerable promise for making a meaningful difference in the lives of aphasic persons, their families, and their associates. As this is written, those who design and implement these interventions are defining and refining the goals of intervention; are developing, testing, and improving intervention procedures; and are creating measures that capture the qualitative effects of the interventions. Compelling evidence for the effectiveness of these interventions awaits systematic and controlled investigation. As Marshall (1998) has commented:

> Providing the quantitative and qualitative research which shows that these endeavors improve the quality of life for those who are aphasic will require a lot of work. (p. 815)

GENERAL CONCEPTS 9-6

- Until the late 1970s interventions for treatment of aphasia focused on linguistic impairments, but in the 1960s and 1970s the focus began to shift to the functional and social aspects of communication.
- Social models of intervention expand the focus of communication from its *transactional* function (i.e., exchange of information) to include its *interactional* function (i.e., establishing and maintaining social relationships). Social approaches to intervention recognize that aphasia has lifelong consequences for the aphasic person and the aphasic person's family.
- Social models of intervention consider communication a collaborative process between conversational partners and focus intervention on natural interactions, particularly conversation in authentic, natural contexts.
- Some functionally oriented interventions are designed to provide aphasic persons with strategies or skills (such as cueing strategies for word retrieval) that can be used in a variety of daily life contexts.
- PACE (*Promoting Aphasics' Communicative Effectiveness*) is based on four principles that are representative of most functionally oriented interventions for aphasia: (1) the clinician and patient exchange new information, (2) the clinician and patient participate equally as senders and receivers of messages, (3) the patient has free choice

Continued

of communicative modes used to convey messages, and (4) the clinician's feedback is based on the patient's success in conveying messages.

- *Conversational coaching* provides aphasic persons and conversational partners with verbal or nonverbal strategies to improve conversational interactions. *Situation-specific training* teaches aphasic persons to communicate important information in specific daily life situations.

- Some functionally oriented approaches to intervention focus on the conversational partners of aphasic persons. Conversational partners are trained to support and enhance the communicative success of aphasic conversational partners. Lyon's *conversational partners* program and Kagan's *supported conversation* program are examples of such interventions.

- Although socially oriented approaches to intervention have promise for enhancing the quality of life for aphasic persons and their conversational partners, compelling evidence for their effectiveness awaits sensitive and reliable measures of their effectiveness and replicable descriptions of their methods.

GROUP TREATMENT FOR APHASIC ADULTS

History

Group treatment for aphasic adults became an important clinical concern during and after World War II, with the arrival in military hospitals of large numbers of veterans with head injuries. Only a few trained professionals were available to treat head-injured veterans, and group treatment permitted clinicians to provide treatment to large numbers of them.

Although those who treated these brain-injured veterans called them aphasic, almost all the injured veterans had sustained traumatic brain injuries from bullets, shrapnel, or blows to the head. Of 696 "aphasic" patients seen in one army medical center, 681 had sustained traumatic brain injuries from external sources (Wepman, 1951). Their average age was 26 years. Contemporary practitioners would not call young patients with traumatic brain injuries *aphasic*. The cognitive-communicative impairments exhibited by individuals with traumatic brain injuries differ strikingly from those exhibited by patients with stroke (the primary cause of aphasia). Treatment objectives, treatment procedures, and patterns of recovery also differ between individuals who have experienced traumatic brain injuries and those who have experienced strokes.

One objective of the early group treatment programs was to "reeducate" brain-injured veterans by means of drill activities focused on speech, reading, writing, and mathematics. Psychotherapy and social and recreational activities provided additional psychological and emotional support (Wepman, 1951). Few, if any, reliable tests were available to measure the effects of treatment, and practitioners typically provided testimonials, rather than data, about the effectiveness of their treatment programs.

We have felt it [treatment of brain-injured veterans] worthwhile. Some of the results are measurable enough; others show simply in the healthier and happier attitudes of those who leave us. We feel that we can conclude that we have been able to hasten the process of reeducation; that we have pushed it far beyond the level usually obtained by the patient allowed to drift his own way without guidance. (Sheehan, 1945, p. 153)

Group treatment for aphasic adults became popular in the 1950s and remained so until the early 1960s. Objectives typically included reducing group members' communicative impairments and providing social and psychologic support (Agranowitz & associates, 1954; Aronson, Shatin, & Cook, 1956; Backus & Dunn, 1952; Bloom, 1962; Corbin, 1951; and others).

> In the group situation it is possible to recreate and structure everyday situations with appropriate verbal behavior, which was not only well established in the repertoire of the individual previous to his injury, but which occurs with great frequency in his daily immediate experience. Further, it is possible to reduce such verbal behavior to specific situational language units which can be structured and repeatedly reinforced in the learning environment. (Bloom, 1962, p. 13)

During the 1960s and 1970s, the clinical emphasis in aphasia shifted away from group treatment and toward clinician-patient treatment dyads. Those who wrote about aphasia advocated individual treatment and considered group treatment a sometimes useful adjunct to individual treatment.

> We would argue that individual therapy and group therapy are entirely different classes of events, serve different purposes, and should not be confused. The clinician needs to judge when and how to facilitate a response, and when to give the patient time to produce one independently. He needs to adapt materials to individual needs and interests at successive stages of recovery. In short, treatment for aphasia must constantly be dovetailed to patient response. There are no mass methods, and none are possible. What reaches or helps one patient at one point in time loses another. For

these reasons, we are unable to have confidence in group therapy as a basic method of treatment for aphasia...group therapy is wasteful, and sometimes deleterious, if used as a substitute for individual treatment. (Schuell, Jenkins, & Jimenez-Pabon, 1964, pp. 343, 344)

> Group therapy...may be justified as an adjunct to individual therapy, providing that the adjunctive values can be achieved better in a group setting than on an individual basis and better in a "structured" arrangement than in some other informal social situation. (Eisenson, 1974, p. 234)

> We believe that one clinician and one aphasic person are the heart of successful treatment. ...Groups replace individual treatment only if a patient has never responded or has stopped responding in individual work, but wants to continue treatment. (Rosenbek, LaPointe, & Wertz, 1989, p. 184)

During the 1980s and 1990s, cost containment became a prominent focus in healthcare, and shortened hospital lengths of stay and restrictions on reimbursement for patient-care services contributed to speech-language pathologists' renewed interest in treatment groups for aphasic adults. Treatment groups became a way of maintaining the integrity of treatment in the face of declining reimbursement from those who pay for patients' healthcare.

> We feel that it [group treatment] contributes in a very positive manner to the total rehabilitative process and is a solution to the "chronic stroke patient" syndrome. Group programs such as these are cost effective, both in dollars and in improved quality of life, because they integrate the patient into existing family and community structures. This reduces hospital dependency and focuses on health rather than disability. (West, 1981, p. 151, 152)

Some clinicians who had been pushed into group treatment by reimbursement considerations became convinced not only that group treatment could lead to meaningful changes in aphasic adults' communicative ability, but that group treatment might actually be superior to individual treatment in creating meaningful changes in aphasic adults' daily life communicative competence.

> There was a time in the not-too-distant past when I [ALH] believed that group treatment was a useful adjunct to individual treatment for chronically aphasic adults. I have changed my mind. I now believe that individual treatment is a useful adjunct to group treatment for such patients. (Holland & Ross, 1999, p. 116)

Purposes of Aphasia Groups

Group activities for aphasic adults historically have served multiple purposes. Some groups were organized to provide emotional and psychological support to aphasic persons and family members. Some were organized to provide a more natural environment for aphasic persons' communication practice. Some were organized to help aphasic persons prepare for reentry into familial, social, and community roles. The purposes of group activities were not always clearly defined, and combinations of purposes were common. Kearns and Simmons (1985) surveyed 91 Veterans Administration Medical Centers to find out what kinds of group activities they offered to aphasic persons. Most respondents (84%) reported that the primary goal of their group activities was language stimulation. However, many respondents reported other goals—emotional support (59%), carryover (47%), and socialization (45%), and multiple goals were common.

Family Support Groups. Support groups for family members or caregivers (usually the spouses of aphasic persons) have been a part of clinical aphasiology since the 1940s. Family support groups provide information to participants about the nature of aphasia and its effects on the aphasic person and his or her family. They permit participants to express feelings, share reactions, and discuss changes in family roles caused by the presence of aphasia. They

help participants cope with the effects of aphasia on the family's social life and recreation. They facilitate exploration and discussion of attitudes toward rehabilitation and expectations of outcome. They provide opportunities for cooperative problem-solving. They provide strategies by which family members may improve communication between themselves and their aphasic family member. They help family members find and practice ways to promote the aphasic person's independence and self-sufficiency.

Family support groups typically offer activities such as:

- Group discussions in which members ask questions, exchange ideas and information, express attitudes, and discuss problems associated with aphasia and stroke
- Cooperative problem-solving, in which participants help each other devise strategies for dealing with personal and familial issues created by the presence of aphasia in the family
- Role playing and group discussions in which participants act out typical problem situations and interactions
- Lectures, demonstrations, or discussions by resource persons about problems related to stroke and aphasia

Psychosocial Groups. Psychosocial groups typically are made up of aphasic persons. Their primary purpose is "to foster the development of emotional and psychological bonds that help members cope with the consequences of aphasia" (Kearns, 1994, p. 305). Psychosocial groups provide a supportive context in which aphasic participants may express feelings and get help in identifying and coping with the psychological and emotional effects of aphasia. Psychosocial groups provide participants with social contact and interaction with other aphasic adults who may be facing similar emotional, psychological, and social issues. Psychosocial groups are designed to increase aphasic participants' self-esteem and capacity for independence and to increase aphasic participants' motivation for social interaction and the confidence with which they communicate.

Psychosocial group activities may include:

- Discussions in which participants express feelings and attitudes about personal, familial, or social issues
- Cooperative problem-solving in which the group helps individual participants analyze and find solutions to interpersonal and lifestyle issues and problems
- Role playing in which participants act out daily life encounters, interactions, or situations
- Group activities such as games, competitions, field trips, sightseeing excursions, or attendance at theater or sporting events

Language Stimulation Groups. Language stimulation groups provide controlled experiences in communication in an environment in which participants can try out new behaviors or new ways of communicating. Group treatment sessions may offer participants a more natural communication environment than individual treatment sessions, but an environment that is better controlled and less threatening than everyday social interactions. Activities for language stimulation groups typically are more clinician-controlled and task-oriented than psychosocial group activities. The group leader (typically a speech-language pathologist) structures group activities so that each group member receives stimulation appropriate to her or his abilities and so that what happens in the group is consistent with the therapeutic objectives for each group member. Group activities range from didactic activities such as those typically seen in individual treatment, to relatively free-form conversational interactions, with emphasis on communication among group members, who are expected to apply skills and strategies they have acquired in individual treatment.

Life Participation Groups. During the last decade, the philosophy underlying group treatment for aphasic persons has begun to reflect the World Health Organization's restructuring of the concepts of impairment, disability, handicap, participation in life, and quality of life. Group interventions to address aphasic persons'

social and interpersonal communicative needs and to enhance aphasic persons' quality of life were developed at several centers in Europe, Canada, and the United States. These interventions, which I will call *life participation groups,* are structured to help aphasic participants establish rewarding personal lifestyles and renew participation in family and community activities. Life participation groups provide training and practice with strategies and problem-solving that enhance the aphasic person's confidence, independence, and competence in daily life. Life participation groups may have several objectives:

- To help aphasic persons, families, and associates develop and implement strategies to restore the aphasic person's participation in social, community, and cultural activities
- To help aphasic persons discover and use appropriate social and community resources
- To help aphasic persons, families, and associates accept persisting changes in the aphasic person's physical, cognitive, and communicative abilities
- To advocate for cultural and social changes to enhance aphasic persons' personal well-being and quality of life

Kagan and associates (Kagan & Cohen-Schneider, 1999; Kagan & Dailey, 1993) described a comprehensive volunteer-based life participation program in which aphasic participants progress from an *introductory group* stressing psychosocial support in a context of free-flowing conversation, to a *community aphasia program* in which participants can choose from a variety of groups, including special-interest groups (cooking, music, etc.), skill-building groups (reading, writing, etc.), family support groups, or generic conversation groups.

Kagan and her associates recruit volunteers from the community and train them to serve as conversational partners, group leaders, and group facilitators so that they can rate participants' performance, deal with participants' feelings of grief and loss, and monitor and facilitate group evolution. The volunteers also are trained in conversational techniques "…that will help them better reveal the competence of those with aphasia" (Kagan, Black, Duchan, Simmons-Mackie, & Square, 2001, p. 625). Participants in the life participation program (aphasic persons, family members, and other concerned individuals) progress through a pre-planned sequence of activities. In the initial group sessions, participants and trained volunteers share personal information and tell their stories. These activities lead into group sessions in which the volunteers help group members discuss and better understand the nature of aphasia and its consequences for aphasic persons and their families. Following these educational sessions, the focus is on improving participants' communicative competence. Volunteers help participants devise, practice, and perfect strategies for successful communication. As the group moves toward closure, the focus shifts to establishing personal goals and planning for a productive life following the group experiences. In the final sessions, participants evaluate the effectiveness of the group, assess their personal progress, and prepare for leaving the group. Many aphasic participants then join community aphasia programs in which they explore special interests, enhance skills, or participate in social activities. Kagan and Cohen-Schneider (1999) comment that by the time aphasic participants have completed the program, they have become "…people who hold themselves differently, show genuine attachment to a new community of friends, and are beginning to see some kind of future for themselves" (p. 106).

Walker-Batson, Curtis, Smith, and Ford (1999) described a life participation program called *Lifelink*—a weekly half-day program for aphasic adults, designed to facilitate community reentry and "participation in life." The program begins with individual treatment for each participant and progresses to community outings for groups of participants. Psychosocial support groups, led by a social worker, are provided for program participants and family members. Individual treatment is designed to (a) reestablish as much language as possible by systematic treatment, (b) establish at least one efficient modality for communication, and (c) prepare the aphasic person for success in group and community interactions. A personalized packet of material (vocabulary lists, outlines, pictures, articles, activities, etc.) is prepared for each aphasic person to use in individual and group treatment activities.

Lifelink group sessions begin with a review to ensure that all participants are aware of the group's overall goals and to ensure that each participant has established personal goals. Group members may participate in conversations related to personal experiences (e.g., activities, vacations, children), clinician-led discussions of current events, or theme-related group activities (discussions, debates, role-play activities, problem-solving exercises).

Bernstein-Ellis and Elman (2007) described a comprehensive group communication treatment program offered by the Aphasia Center of California (ACC). The ACC program was organized partly in response to "…the urgent need to develop a viable, effective model for providing aphasia treatment in view of changes in health care provision and reimbursement… Although we still valued individual treatment for aphasia, we were forced to consider lower cost and efficacious options for meeting the needs of our clients" (p. 74). The program is based on two assumptions—that aphasia is a chronic condition, and that people with chronic aphasia deserve the same ongoing management as other chronic health-related conditions. The primary treatment goals of the program are to (a) enhance communication skills and (b) maximize the psychosocial well-being and quality of life for persons affected by aphasia.

> A group composed of adults with aphasia needs to progress beyond an emphasis on linguistic changes to adaptations that have a positive impact on members' quality of life. (Bernstein-Ellis & Elman, 2007, p. 88)

The ACC program focuses intervention on several aspects of aphasic persons' lives, skills, and experiences:

- *Member and family education.* Aphasic participants and their families are provided with information about aphasia by means of publications, videotapes, stroke support groups, and an ACC newsletter.
- *Personal goals.* The program emphasizes awareness of each participant's personal goals and his or her progress toward those goals.
- *Expanding participation and conversational practice.* Group interactions are designed to help participants connect with each other, gain confidence, and strengthen personal identity. Topics and themes of group interactions are based on the interests of group members, but discussions are allowed to follow unplanned conversational paths that the group finds more interesting and more conversationally productive.
- *Developing and enhancing effective communicative strategies.* The focus of interactions is on successful exchange of content rather than linguistic accuracy. A variety of strategies for successful exchange of information are modeled by clinicians and group members (e.g., gestures, drawing, personalized notebooks, maps, newspapers).
- *Increasing skills at conversational initiation.* Group interactions focus on both the initiator and the responder roles in communication to enhance each group member's ability to enter and direct discussion. A clinician may act as facilitator and moderator, but the primary responsibility for the content and direction of discussion rests with the group.
- *Encouraging conversational cross-talk.* Exchanges among group members (cross-talk) are encouraged. Group members are encouraged to comment on, ask questions about, or elaborate on contributions by other members of the group.

Bernstein-Ellis and Elman acknowledge the challenge of documenting progress in an atmosphere of limited resources and restrictions on services—a challenge intensified by the scarcity of assessment tools that provide meaningful qualitative information about aphasic persons' real life communicative adequacy and quality of life.

Efficacy of Group Treatment for Aphasia

The results of several studies of group treatment for aphasic adults conducted in the 1980s and 1990s supported the efficacy of group treatment for aphasic adults (as group treatment was characterized at the time). Wertz and associates (1981) experimentally evaluated the efficacy of individual and group treatment for aphasic adults in a multiple-facility cooperative study. Aphasic patients in individual treatment *(Group A)* received 8 hours of clinician-directed treatment each week for 44 weeks. Patients in group treatment *(Group B)* received 8 hours of group treatment and group recreational activities each week for 44 weeks. With minor exceptions, both groups made significant improvement on speech and language measures between 4 weeks after onset (when they entered treatment) and tests at the end of 11, 22, 33, and 44 weeks of treatment. There were few significant differences between the two groups on any test occasion, although Group A almost always performed somewhat better than Group B (Figure 9-14). Both groups improved significantly between 26 and 48 weeks after onset (after 22 to 44 weeks of treatment, when, according to Wertz and associates, spontaneous recovery should no longer be taking place).

Wertz and associates concluded that both individual and group treatment of the kind provided in their study were efficacious:

> Our results indicate that individual treatment may be slightly superior to group treatment. However, the improvement displayed by our group-treated patients and the cost-effective advantages of group therapy should prompt speech-language pathologists to consider it for at least part of an aphasic patient's care. (p. 592)

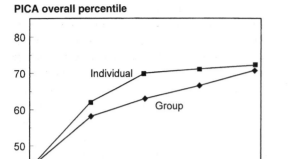

PICA overall percentile

Figure 9-14 ■ Change in *Porch Index of Communicative Ability* (Porch, 1981a) overall percentile scores for participants who received individual treatment and for participants who received group treatment from intake into the study (4 weeks after onset of aphasia) to 15, 26, 37, and 48 weeks after onset.

In a study reported by Aten, Caligiuri, and Holland (1982) seven adults with chronic nonfluent aphasia received 2 hours of group treatment weekly. Treatment was directed toward improving the aphasic participants' functional communication by participation in simulated daily life activities such as shopping; giving and following directions; giving personal information; reading signs, labels, and posters; and expressing ideas. Aten and associates reported little change in participants' scores on the PICA but significant improvement on the CADL measure.

Holland and Beeson (1999) reported outcome data for 40 aphasic adults who joined aphasia treatment groups at various times after onset, ranging from 3 months to 14 years. (The average was 2.8 years.) Each had participated in an aphasia group for at least one year, and each participant was tested yearly with the WAB. Fifteen of the 40 participants made significant improvement, as measured by a gain of at least 5

points in the WAB aphasia quotient (AQ), 23 made no significant change in WAB AQ, and 2 significantly declined in WAB AQ. Holland and Beeson concluded that their results were encouraging "…in that more than one-third of our group members showed continued measurable language improvement during a period when they would be considered to have chronic aphasia" (p. 83).

> We do not know, however, what percentage of these patients would have improved without participating in a group, because Holland and Beeson had no control group with which to compare the group that participated in the treatment groups.

Elman and Bernstein-Ellis (1999) evaluated the effects of group treatment ranging from 7 months to 336 months in duration on the communicative performance of 24 adults with chronic aphasia. Elman and Bernstein-Ellis randomly assigned participants to an *immediate-treatment group* or a *deferred-treatment group*. The immediate-treatment group received 5 hours of group treatment per week for 4 months. Treatment began as soon as participants were enrolled in the study. Group treatment focused on increasing participation in conversations and communicating information by whatever means possible.

The deferred-treatment group received immediate assessment but did not begin group treatment until the immediate-treatment group had completed its 4 months of treatment. To control for the effects of social contact, each participant in the deferred-treatment group attended 3 or more hours of social group activities of their choice (e.g., movement classes, art groups, church activities, support groups) while they waited for their 4 months of group communication treatment.

Several outcome measures, including a shortened version of the Porch Index of Communicative Ability (*SPICA*; Disimoni, Keith, &

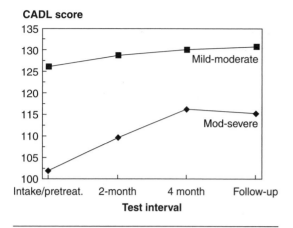

CADL score

Mild-moderate

Mod-severe

Intake/pretreat. 2-month 4 month Follow-up

Test interval

Figure 9-15 ■ *Communicative Abilities of Daily Living (CADL;* Holland, 1980) scores for aphasic participants with mild-to-moderate aphasia and participants with moderate-to-severe aphasia at intake, after 2 months and 4 months of treatment, and at follow-up (4 to 6 weeks after treatment ended). (Data from Elman, R.J., Bernstein-Ellis, E. [1999]. The efficacy of group communication treatment in adults with chronic aphasia. *Journal of Speech, Language, and Hearing Research, 42,* 411-419.)

Darley, 1980), the WAB, and CADL were administered at intake, after 2 and 4 months of treatment, and 4 to 6 weeks following cessation of treatment. The delayed-treatment group was also tested when they began group treatment. The test scores of the immediate-treatment group were significantly higher after 4 months of treatment than those of the delayed-treatment group (which had received only social stimulation). The delayed-treatment group did not change significantly on any measure from intake until the time at which they began group treatment, but after 4 months of delayed treatment, their SPICA overall scores and their WAB AQ had significantly increased. Both groups maintained their improved test performance on follow-up testing after 4 to 6 weeks of no treatment. The CADL scores of participants with moderate-to-severe aphasia significantly increased after 2

and 4 months of group treatment, but the CADL scores of participants with mild-to-moderate aphasia did not, perhaps due to a ceiling effect for the less severely aphasic participants (Figure 9-15). Elman and Bernstein-Ellis concluded that their treatment was efficacious: "The present study demonstrated that 5 hours per week of group communication treatment over 2- and 4-months duration provided efficacious treatment for adults with chronic aphasia" (p. 417).

Elman (1999) subsequently concluded a review of studies of the efficacy of group treatment for aphasia with the following statement:

What is encouraging about the research done to date is the growing consensus that group communication treatment holds real promise as a treatment method. Given the rapidly changing health care reimbursement environment, including the emergence and dominance of a managed care model, group communication treatment for individuals appears to provide an effective and economical option for delivering neurogenic communication treatment. (Elman, 1999, p. 6)

There is at this time no compelling evidence to support the superiority of group treatment over individual treatment, or vice-versa. It is clear that at least some group treatment approaches significantly improve aphasic adults' communicative skills and daily life communicative competence. It is not clear that group treatment does this better than individual treatment, and it is not clear whether some combination of individual and group treatment might not be better than either approach by itself.

Although empiric evidence supports the efficacy of group treatment for aphasic adults, much work remains. Additional data-based research is needed to establish the efficacy of group treatment for aphasic adults, to determine which aspects of group treatment are responsible for any treatment effects observed, to formulate and test new approaches to group treatment, and to evaluate the effects of multiple-component group treatment programs. The benefits of family support groups, psychosocial groups, and life participation groups for aphasic adults and family members are at this time largely undocumented, except for what Kearns (1994) calls *"advocacy reports"*—reports that assert the clinical value of aphasia groups without clearly describing treatment procedures or presenting data to support their claims. Data-based evidence for the effectiveness and efficiency of such groups is badly needed, as is development of reliable measurement instruments that permit objective assessment of outcomes that until now have been described using subjective measures of undocumented reliability and validity.

GENERAL CONCEPTS 9-7

- Groups for aphasic adults may serve several purposes, either singly or in combination. Common purposes include family support, psychosocial support, language stimulation, and life participation.
- Group treatment for aphasic adults became important after World War II, to meet the needs of large numbers of head-injured veterans.
- In the 1960s and 1970s group treatment fell out of favor, usually replaced by one-to-one, didactic treatment activities.
- In the 1980s and 1990s group treatment regained popularity as concerns about cost containment and functional communication intensified.
- Life participation groups usually have several goals:
  - To help aphasic persons and concerned others restore the aphasic person's participation in social, community, and cultural activities
  - To help aphasic persons discover and use appropriate social and community resources

- To help aphasic persons and concerned others accept persisting changes in the aphasic person's physical, cognitive, and communicative abilities
- To advocate for cultural and social changes to enhance aphasic persons' personal well-being and quality of life
- Several studies have shown that group treatment improves communicative abilities of adults with chronic aphasia. A few studies suggest that group treatment may be appropriate for adults in earlier stages of recovery from aphasia.
- Research is needed to measure the effects of well-defined group treatments to determine which aspects of a group treatment are responsible for observed treatment effects, to formulate and test new approaches to group treatment, and to evaluate the effects of multiple-component group treatment programs on aphasic persons' personal well-being and quality of life.

THOUGHT QUESTIONS

Question 9-1 A speech-language pathologist has completed his assessment of Mr. Murphy, an aphasic man, and is preparing to begin treatment of Mr. Murphy's comprehension impairments. Mr. Murphy's performance on spoken yes-no questions places him at the 25th percentile for aphasic adults. His performance on following spoken directions and sentence verification comprehension tests places him at the 76th percentile for aphasic adults. What potential reasons do you see for the disparities in Mr. Murphy's test performance? What might the disparities suggest to you regarding treatment?

Question 9-2 You plan to begin treatment for Ms. Snyder, who is aphasic following a left-hemisphere stroke 2 months ago. Test results indicate that she has severe apraxia of speech and agrammatism, but listening comprehension and reading comprehension are relatively well preserved. You and Ms. Snyder agree that treatment will focus on improving her speech. The following transcript represents her description of the *cookie theft* picture (Figure 5-19):

Uh...uh...uh......moman....um........disses.........
but....no...uh...uh...and...and...waduh...um...
floah.......and...and...and...um...kidz......and...
and...and...er....skool...no......spool....but.....but
....skool.....and...and.....and.....tookies....no....
but......turkies.....no......and...and...kookus...um
....and...um....fall.

Her description of the cookie theft picture is a good representation of her speech in daily life activities. What do you see as the most debilitating problems? What would you work on to make the greatest changes in Ms. Snyder's daily life communicative competence?

Question 9-3 The following speech samples represent transcripts of Mrs. Bloom and Mr. Jones talking about the "birthday party" picture. They are typed without punctuation. The number of dots indicate the relative durations of pauses.

Mrs. Bloom produces the following speech sample (she produces 105 words per minute):

and..um..what do you call it....but I guess the cat got into it and..uh he's hiding under the sitter and the mother is gonna......trying to get him out of there...and he cleaned up the rug and..uh the rest of the birthday cake...those ones there...children...boys and girls...are arriving and it's....um not too good a deal I'd say

Mr. Jones produces the following speech sample (he produces 40 words per minute):

um...um...uh.....cake..and..um..and..and dog .....dog ate cake..and..and...trouble..... mom is mad....and..and..um..um..kid is crying...and.. and...neighbors.....neighbors is coming

If you were to work with Mrs. Bloom and Mr. Jones to improve their speech, on what aspects of their speech would you focus your treatment?

Question 9-4 Mr. Osborne is moderately aphasic and wishes to regain enough reading ability for recreational reading (newspapers, magazines, novels). You evaluate his reading and find that his major problem is missing or misreading function words. His reading vocabulary and word recognition skills are relatively well preserved. How might you go about improving his reading comprehension?

Right Hemisphere Syndrome

The right brain has nothing to do with language. (C. Mirallie, 1896)

HISTORICAL OVERVIEW

Until the mid 1800s neuroanatomists believed that the human brain was functionally and physically symmetrical. Then in 1836 Marc Dax, an obscure general practitioner in the wine-producing region of southern France, read a paper at a regional meeting of physicians. In the paper Dax asserted that "memory for words" resides in the left brain hemisphere of right-handers. Dax died a year later, and his paper was generally ignored by the medical community. Then 25 years later, Paul Broca, a French surgeon and amateur anthropologist, described eight patients with language disturbance secondary to brain injury, all of whom had injuries in the left brain hemisphere. In his report Broca proclaimed that the left hemisphere of right-handers is responsible for articulate speech:

> I have been struck by the fact that in my first aphemics [*persons with motor aphasia*] the lesion lay, not only in the same part of the brain, but always on the same side—the left.

Within the next few years Broca's claims were widely circulated, and the dominance of the left hemisphere for language became widely accepted.

Marc Dax's son, Gustave, also a physician, spent many years trying to force the medical community to recognize his father's precedence, claiming that Broca and others had ignored the senior Dax's 1836 report. He had little success, and Broca's place in the history of neurology was never seriously threatened.

During the last half of the nineteenth century a consensus developed among physicians and neuroanatomists that the left hemisphere dominated intellectual and cognitive processes, whereas the right hemisphere dominated perceptual and motor processes. In 1874 John Hughlings Jackson, a British neurologist, summarized contemporary thought by asserting that language belonged to the left hemisphere and that visual recognition, discrimination, and recall belonged to the right hemisphere. Jackson speculated that the right hemisphere might participate in simple automatic language behaviors, but he assigned creative use of language to the left hemisphere.

There is nothing to show that the right brain has any specific language function as indicated by Hughlings Jackson and more recent investigators. (Weisenburg & McBride, 1935, p. 104)

During the next half century, the right hemisphere's contribution to cognition and intellect

was largely neglected, as investigators who were fascinated by Broca's findings concentrated on exploring the organization of language in the left hemisphere. It was not until the twentieth century that investigators began to explore the organization and function of the right hemisphere in any organized way.

The two world wars (1914-1917, 1941-1945) provided new insights into brain functions as physicians, psychologists, and others studied how missile wounds to the brains of battle-wounded veterans affected their behavior and cognition. These clinical studies provided an intriguing picture of how the two brain hemispheres collaborate in intellectual, cognitive, and behavioral activities, and the concept of independently functioning brain hemispheres was replaced with the concept of collaborative hemispheres, each hemisphere contributing to cognition and behavior in unique ways. Patients with left-hemisphere brain injuries were characterized as socially appropriate but impaired in comprehension and production of language, whereas patients with right-hemisphere brain injuries were characterized as socially inappropriate but with intact comprehension and production of language.

Understanding of the right hemisphere's responsibilities got a boost in the 1960s, when neurosurgeons began surgically disconnecting the two hemispheres by cutting the corpus callosum to control otherwise intractable seizures (a procedure called *commissurotomy*). Commissurotomized patients, who now had brain hemispheres that could be tested independently, enabled investigators to describe more explicitly the unique capabilities of the right hemisphere.

Procedures that made it possible to direct stimulus input to a single hemisphere in neurologically intact adults were devised. The concept of hemispheric specialization gradually changed as investigators found that the two hemispheres appeared to operate in fundamentally different ways. Writers began to describe the left hemisphere as rational, analytic, and specialized for processing sequential, time-related material. They described the right hemisphere as intuitive, holistic, and specialized for processing nonlinear, spatially distributed arrays of information. Because auditory information comes in time-ordered sequences (syllables in a word, words in a sentence), the left hemisphere was thought to have greater responsibility for auditory events; because visual information often comes in multidimensional arrays (pictures, scenes, faces), the right hemisphere was thought to have greater responsibility for visual events. The concept of the right hemisphere as linguistically naive now is changing as contemporary studies of normal, right-hemisphere-injured, and commissurotomized adults suggest that the right hemisphere possesses at least some rudimentary linguistic abilities (Joanette, Goulet, & Hannequin, 1990).

> Zaidel (1978) concluded that the adult right hemisphere possesses grammatical competence equivalent to that of a 5-year-old child.

Contemporary neural network models of hemispheric specialization are moving away from the appealing but simplistic concept of isolated and specialized brain hemispheres to emphasize the ways in which the hemispheres collaborate to accomplish mental functions and to produce and regulate behavior. Although what is known about the right hemisphere is largely descriptive, with little sense of cause and effect, investigators slowly are becoming more sophisticated about its role in communication, cognition, and behavior.

> Statements about hemispheric specialization may be misleading unless the qualifier *"in right-handed adults"* is added. Few writers add the qualifier, and I will not belabor the reader with it. However, the reader should keep it in mind whenever reading descriptions of right-hemisphere brain-injured adults.

The label *nondominant hemisphere* has replaced *right hemisphere* in many contemporary writings about hemispheric specialization. I have chosen to retain the older label, because almost all investigation of nondominant brain hemisphere functions have studied adults who have right-hemisphere brain injuries. Consequently, *right hemisphere* seems to me the more accurate appellation, at least until studies of left-hemisphere functions in right-hemisphere-dominant adults are published.

Regardless of how one chooses to explain the right hemisphere's contribution to cognition and behavior, it is clear that only about half of adults who sustain right-hemisphere brain injury develop communication impairments (Joanette, Lecours, Lamoureux, & Lepage, 1983). The variables contributing to communication impairments following right-hemisphere brain injury are not well understood, although Joanette and associates suggest that patients with cortical lesions, a history of familial left-handedness, and low education levels are the most likely candidates.

BEHAVIORAL AND COGNITIVE SYMPTOMS OF RIGHT-HEMISPHERE BRAIN INJURY

Descriptions of the perceptual, cognitive, and behavioral consequences of right-hemisphere brain injury *(nondominant-hemisphere brain injury)* usually describe a stereotypic collection of impairments that, by implication, is exhibited by all adults with right-hemisphere brain injury. Adults with right-hemisphere brain injury are characterized as:

- Insensitive to others, preoccupied with self
- Oblivious to social conventions
- Unaware of or inattentive to their physical and mental limitations
- Verbose, tangential, and rambling in speech
- Insensitive to the meaning of abstract or implied material
- Unable to grasp the overall significance or meaning of complex events

Some adults with right-hemisphere brain injury are characterized as behaviorally passive:

- Unresponsive to social or environmental stimuli
- Use short utterances that lack emotional inflection
- Have difficulty maintaining attention for more than a few seconds

Writers who describe the typical adult with right-hemisphere brain injury often do not mention that many adults with right-hemisphere brain injury do not exhibit the stereotypic collection of impairments, and writers often pay little attention to variability in symptoms among right-hemisphere-injured adults, although it is well known that not all have the same cognitive or communicative impairments.

Group studies of adults with right-hemisphere brain injury contribute to misconceptions about the universality of stereotypic patterns of impairment by reporting results for heterogeneous groups in which the location and severity of participants' brain injuries have not been controlled for or reported. Group studies typically report the average performance of groups and do not report how well individual participants conform to the group average. Most group studies of adults with right-hemisphere brain injuries do not include a control group with left-hemisphere injuries—a requirement if the effects of right-hemisphere brain injury are to be differentiated from the general effects of brain injury. (The same can be said for many studies of left-hemisphere brain injury.)

Group studies of right-hemisphere-injured adults tend to include disproportionately large numbers of participants who have frontal lobe injuries. Right-hemisphere-injured adults who have posterior lesions usually are not paralyzed and are discharged from the hospital within a few days of admission, leaving the patients who have anterior brain injuries and left-sided paralysis and who are in need of physical therapy to be recruited by investigators looking for participants. Individuals with posterior

right-hemisphere brain injury who do make it into studies are likely to be within a few days of onset, when their impairments may represent the acute effects of cerebral swelling, diaschisis, and neurotransmitter release in addition to the potentially chronic effects of right-hemisphere brain injury.

McDonald (1993) pointed out striking similarities between the communicative and cognitive impairments of groups of patients with frontal lobe injuries and the communicative and cognitive impairments of groups with right-hemisphere brain injury. McDonald comments that these similarities arise, at least in part, from the inclusion of large proportions of patients with frontal lobe injuries in groups with right-hemisphere brain injuries. Brownell and associates (2000) agree: "The catalogue of linguistic and cognitive impairments observed in RHD [right-hemisphere-damaged] patients could be substituted, usually without notice, into any review article on prefrontal impairments" (p. 321).

Tompkins (1995) alluded to the heterogeneity of symptoms in right-hemisphere-injured adults.

One of the most important things to remember about adults with RHD [right-hemisphere damage] is one of the most important characteristics of any "category" of people; they are quite heterogeneous. Not all patients will have communicative impairments. Those who do will not have all symptoms, and individual patients will display different patterns of behavior. Complicating things further, it can be quite difficult to specify "disordered" status, because normative information is almost nonexistent for abilities and performance broken down by age, education, socioeconomic status, and cultural variables. It is part of the clinical challenge in working with brain-damaged individuals to identify the presence and absence of the deficits that result from neurologic insult, as well as those that are not necessarily due to the brain injury. (pp. 15-16)

The physical, behavioral, and cognitive abnormalities generated by right-hemisphere brain injury, like those generated by injury to the left hemisphere, depend on the location and magnitude of the injury, but as noted previously, our understanding of these relationships is imperfect. Although relationships between right-hemisphere brain injury and specific patterns of impairment have yet to be specified, many right-hemisphere-injured adults do exhibit distinctive cognitive and behavioral abnormalities. Some of the most striking affect perception and attention.

Perceptual Impairments

Neglect. Neglect (often called *hemispatial neglect*, sometimes called *unilateral spatial neglect*) refers to a condition in which affected individuals fail to respond to stimuli on the side of the body opposite the side of brain injury. (To make reading easier I will, in what follows, refer simply to *neglect*.) Left neglect is a common consequence of right-hemisphere brain injuries, although not every person with right-hemisphere brain injury experiences neglect.

At this time we do not have dependable statistics regarding the neuroanatomical location of lesions responsible for left neglect, the proportion of patients with right-hemisphere brain injuries who exhibit neglect, or the frequency of neglect in patients with left-hemisphere brain injuries. Differences in how neglect has been measured, inconsistent and incomplete specification of sites and extents of brain injuries, variability in study group sizes, and variability in time after onset at which assessments were carried out all contribute to variability in results, making the demographic characteristics of neglect uncertain. The literature does, however, permit a few general statements about the demography of neglect.

Neglect may be caused by injury in either brain hemisphere but is more frequent, more severe and more persistent following right-hemisphere brain injury. Neglect has been reported in from one third to more than four fifths of adults with right-hemisphere brain injuries, but in less than one fourth of adults

with left-hemisphere brain injuries (Appelros & associates, 2002; Kinsella & Ford, 1985; Marotta & associates, 2003; Sunderland & associates, 1987; Warlow & associates, 1996). Bowen and associates (1999) for example, reviewed the results of 17 studies comparing the incidence of neglect in persons with right-hemisphere brain injuries to that of persons with left-hemisphere brain injuries. Of the participants with right-hemisphere brain injuries, 43% had neglect, versus 21% of participants with left-hemisphere brain injuries.

Neglect may follow injury in several regions of the right hemisphere, but it is most common and most severe after right parietal lobe injury (Cherney & Halper, 2001; Marotta & associates, 2003; Mesulam, 1982a; Watson & Heilman, 1979), especially following injuries in the posterior and inferior right parietal lobe. Vallar and Perani (1986), for example, found that 89% of a group of patients with left neglect had injuries in the right parietal lobe. Neglect occasionally follows subcortical injury (most often in the thalamus and basal ganglia), but the incidence of subcortical neglect is much lower than that of cortical neglect (Ferro, Kertesz, & Black, 1987; Rafal & Posner, 1987; Vallar & Perani, 1986; Watson & Heilman, 1979; and others).

Persons with left neglect sometimes are partially or completely blind in the left visual field, but individuals with intact visual fields may nevertheless have neglect. The true incidence of visual field blindness in individuals with left neglect is not known because of differences in methodology among studies. Cassidy and associates (1999) reported that two thirds of a group of 44 persons with left neglect also had left visual field blindness. Jehkonen and associates (2000) reported that 28% of a sample of 56 persons with left neglect had left-side visual field blindness. Ferber and Karnath (2001) reported left visual field blindness in 23% of a sample of 35 persons with left neglect. Mattingley and associates (2004) reported the presence of visual field blindness in 53% of a sample of 25 persons with left neglect. Although left neglect and partial or complete left visual field blindness often cooccur, the literature suggests that from about one quarter to one half of persons with left neglect have intact visual fields.

Whether the presence of visual field deficits increases the severity of neglect is an open question. Doricchi and Angelelli (1999) and Toth and Kirk (2002) reported that neglect patients with hemianopia made more errors in line bisection than patients without hemianopia. Ferber and Karnath (1999), on the other hand, found no significant relationship between the presence of visual field deficits and the severity of neglect. Halligan, Marshall, and Wade (1990) concluded that visual field deficits "do not exacerbate neglect" (p. 491). Clearly, the presence of left visual field blindness does not cause left neglect, although it may make it worse.

Neglect usually improves or resolves in the days and weeks after brain injury. Cassidy, Lewis, and Gray (1998) reported that three fourths of patients with left neglect at 1 week after stroke had recovered from their neglect 3 months later. Jehkonen and associates (2000) reported neglect in 28% of 56 right-hemisphere-injured patients evaluated at 10 days poststroke. At 12 months after stroke, 7% still had neglect. Cherney and Halper (2001) studied patterns of recovery from left neglect in a group of 14 adults with right-hemisphere brain injuries and neglect, and 8 exhibited what Cherney and Halper called *persistent neglect*—they exhibited neglect 6 to 9 months after initial testing. The other 6 exhibited what Cherney and Halper called *transient neglect,* scoring within the normal range on tests of neglect 6 to 9 months after initial testing. Cherney and Halper commented that neither initial severity of neglect nor location of brain injury predicted the persistence of neglect.

Several studies have suggested that unilateral spatial neglect is associated with poor long-term functional recovery (Appelros & associates, 2002; Buxbaum & associates, 2004; Gillen, Tennen, & McKee, 2005: Jehkonnen & associ-

ates, 2000; Katz & associates, 1999; Pederson & associates, 1997). Jehkonnen and associates (2000) measured neglect and rated the daily life functional status of 50 stroke patients at 3, 6, and 12 months poststroke. They reported that the presence of neglect was a "powerful predictor of poor functional recovery" (p. 200), especially for older patients. Appelros and associates (2002) reported similar findings and commented that the relationship between neglect and poor functional recovery cannot be explained by greater overall severity of impairment in neglect patients. The results of these studies suggest that treatment to reduce neglect may be needed to improve daily life functional outcome for persons with right-hemisphere brain injuries and left neglect, at least for those whose neglect does not resolve within a few days or weeks after onset.

Cherney and Halper (2001) commented that identifying patients with transient versus persistent neglect would help with the timing of treatment and with allocation of clinical resources—perhaps treatment would not be necessary for patients with transient neglect, because they would recover without treatment.

Right-hemisphere-injured adults with left neglect may not respond to touch on the left side of the body or attend to visual or auditory stimuli in left-sided space. If asked to point to the midline of their body with their eyes closed, they typically point too far to the right. If asked to explore a group of objects on a table with their eyes closed, they find the objects on the right but miss those on the left. If asked to copy drawings or to draw figures, objects, or scenes from memory, they typically leave out left-side details. If asked to read printed materials, they may read only the words on the right side of the page and complain that the material makes no sense.

Box 10-1 is a transcript of a patient with right-hemisphere brain injury and left neglect

Box 10-1	Transcript of a Patient with Right-Hemisphere Brain Injury and Left Neglect

Stimulus Story

Fred and Ben were cousins who decided to go into business together painting houses. They put an ad in the paper and then spent all day Sunday getting their supplies organized. The next day, a woman named Mrs. Foster called and offered them their first job. She told them that she needed her house painted before Saturday because she wanted it to look nice for her daughter's wedding. Fred and Ben promised to work quickly and have the house painted by Thursday. They also offered to do the job at a reduced price because Mrs. Foster was their first customer. Mrs. Foster was pleased with their offer and told them to start painting whenever they were ready. Early the next morning, the men arrived at the Foster's house and immediately went to work. By three o'clock they had finished the front of the house and were painting the trim on the upstairs windows. Then a man walked around the corner of the house and asked them what they were doing there. "Oh, you must be Mr. Foster," Ben responded. "I guess your wife forgot to tell you that she hired us to paint the house." The man frowned and replied, "But my name is Nelson. The Fosters live next door."

Transcript

(Patient comments and Clinician responses are in italics.)

The patient begins: ...went into business painting houses. They put an ad getting their supplies organized... The next day... *Is this supposed to make sense?*

Clinician: *It should. Keep reading, and we'll see if we can figure it out.*

Patient: *Well, all right. Should I start over?*

Clinician: *No, just keep reading from where you stopped.*

Patient: *Well, now I don't remember where I was.*

Clinician: *I think you had just finished reading this...The next day...*

Patient: *Okay...* The next day a woman told them that she needed her house to look nice for her daughter's wedding. Fred and Ben...the house painted by Thursda...*Now it's not making sense again. What's going on here?*

Clinician: *Why not just keep reading and see what happens?*

Patient: *Well...* They offered to do the job and Mrs. Foster was pleased with their offer. Early the next morning the men had finished the front and walked around the corner. Oh you must be Mr. Foster, Ben responded. The man frowned and said the Foster's live next door.

Clinician: *Well, what did you think of that?*

Patient: *I guess it's a story, but it doesn't make much sense. It could have been written a lot clearer.*

who was asked to read a story from the *Discourse Comprehension Test* (Brookshire & Nicholas, 1993).

The patient fails to include words on the left side of the page, but when what he reads is grammatically and semantically unnatural, he realizes that something is wrong. However, he attributes the problem to the printed material rather than to his reading. As he reads he adjusts his starting place from line to line to maximize the grammaticality and meaningfulness of what he reads, but when the adjustment requires moving more than a few words, he gets lost. As he progresses through the passage, he begins changing words in the text to make it meaningful. When he finishes, he knows that something was wrong in what he read, but he continues to believe that the problem is the material, rather than his reading.

Persons with left neglect may produce neglect-related errors when reading single words as well as text. They may miss left-side letters (e.g., reading *mistake* as *take*) or leave out the left half of compound words (e.g., reading *blackboard* as *board*). When what they see does not yield a true word, they may substitute or add letters to make a word (e.g., reading *chain* as *train* and *fearless* as *careless*). Longer words are more likely to be read incorrectly than are shorter words.

> Interestingly, when persons with left neglect substitute letters at the beginning of a word, their substitutions tend to contain the same number of letters as the part of the target word that was substituted for, perhaps suggesting low-level awareness of the missed letters (Myers, 1999).

Persons with left neglect typically use only the right side of the page when they write words, sentences, or text, and they displace successive lines of text to the right, giving margins a stair-step look. The lines of writing they produce often slant upward from left to right. Persons with left neglect often leave out words (especially on the left) and omit letters (especially at the beginnings of words). They may add extra lines and strokes to printed letters. Figure 10-1 shows a writing sample produced by a right-hemisphere-injured patient who described in writing the 10 test objects from the *Porch Index of Communicative Ability* (*PICA*; Porch, 1981a).

In daily life, individuals with left neglect often bump into objects on the left, and those in wheelchairs sometimes get trapped against the left side of doorways or other obstructions because they do not perceive the obstruction and seem unaware of the obstruction even when trapped. Some individuals with left neglect attend to stimuli in their left hemispace if reminded, but if left to their own devices, they bump into left-side obstructions and show other signs of inattention, such as using only right-side pockets in clothing or the right-side drawers and shelves of dressers, cupboards, and bureaus.

Mild neglect may be detectable only with *simultaneous stimulation,* in which brief stim-

uli (such as flashes of light, gentle touches, or pinpricks) are presented simultaneously on both sides of the body. Individuals with mild neglect (sometimes called *hemispatial inattention*) do not perceive stimuli on the left when both sides are stimulated, but they perceive the stimuli when only the left side is stimulated.

Myers (1999) summarized common signs of left neglect:

- Failure to respond to people, sounds, and objects to the left of the body's midline
- Attending only to the right in self-care activities (e.g., dressing, shaving)
- Failure to move or attend to the left arm and leg
- Bumping into walls and doorways on the left
- Reading only the right-side parts of printed materials
- Displacing writing to the right side of the page
- Diminished awareness of physical and cognitive impairments
- Disinterest and lack of participation in rehabilitation

Neglect often affects right-hemisphere-injured adults' use and placement of their arms and legs. Persons with left neglect often fail to use their left arm and leg to their full potential, although neurologic examination yields no evidence of left-sided weakness or sensory loss—a condition called *motor neglect.* When questioned, these individuals may claim that the left-side limbs are dead, useless, or do not belong to them. Wheelchair-bound persons with left neglect sometimes let their left arm hang down beside the wheel of the wheelchair, risking injury to their fingers or hand. They also may let their left foot drag, unless someone puts it on the footrest for them.

Left hemispatial neglect is not simply a perceptual or motor impairment. Clinical reports and experimental studies suggest that left neglect is related to disrupted mental representations of external space, diminished ability to direct attention to left-sided space, or both. There are several accounts in the literature of

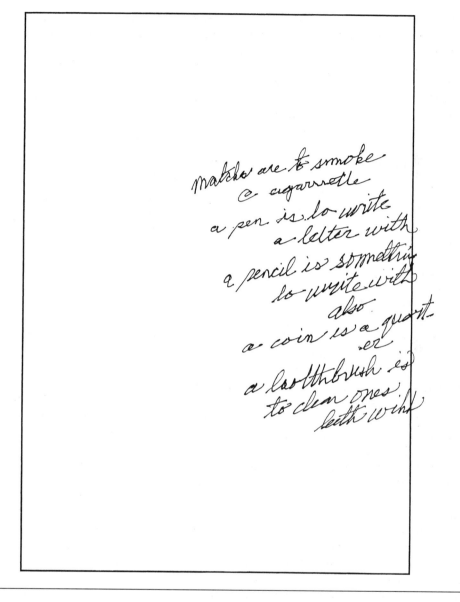

Figure 10-1 ■ A writing sample produced by a patient with right-hemisphere brain injury. The patient is describing in writing the 10 objects from the *Porch Index of Communicative Ability* (Porch, 1981a). The patient neglects the left-side test objects. The patient writes in cursive form, but what he writes is shifted rightward and sometimes crosses the right-side margin line. The patient begins writing part-way down the page, and his written lines slant upward on the right. Several words contain extra strokes, and the patient fails to cross several *t*'s (especially on the left).

right-hemisphere-injured adults who describe familiar spaces by describing only right-sided space or by describing right-sided space in greater detail than left-sided space. A right-hemisphere-injured woman who was asked to describe her home while mentally walking through it from front to back provided an elaborate description of rooms on the right but ignored rooms on the left. When asked to describe the same living space while mentally walking through it from back to front, she described rooms on the previously neglected side and ignored those now on her mental left side.

Bisiach and Luzzati (1987) asked several Italian right hemisphere–damaged residents of Milan with left neglect to describe the Piazza del Duomo, Milan's central square, while facing the cathedral from across the square. The patients described only the buildings on their mental right. When asked to describe the square while mentally standing on the cathedral steps, they described the previously ignored buildings and did not mention the buildings they had previously described.

Several theories have been proposed to explain neglect. *Representational theories* (Bisiach & associates, 1979, 1981, 1996) suggest that neglect is caused by disturbed mental representation of external space. That is, one's mental concept of extrapersonal space fails to include all or part of left-side space. Representational theories can explain the omission of left-side information when adults with neglect are asked to describe familiar scenes from memory. *Arousal theories* (Heilman, Schwartz, & Watson, 1978; Watson, Miller, & Heilman, 1978; and others) propose that right-hemisphere-injured individuals are less responsive to stimuli in neglected space. *Attentional engagement theories* (Arguin & Bub, 1993) propose that individuals with neglect have difficulty shifting attention to stimuli in neglected space, and *attentional disengagement theories* (Posner, Walker, Friederich, & Rafal, 1987) propose that

stimuli in nonneglected space capture and hold the individual's attention, preventing him or her from shifting attention to stimuli on the neglected side.

Individuals with right-hemisphere brain injury and left neglect often exhibit signs of engagement/ disengagement in everyday life. When sitting quietly, these individuals often lean toward the right and turn their head to the right, regardless of the surrounding environment. If sitting next to a blank wall on the right, they lean toward and stare at the wall rather than attending to what is happening in the world away from the wall.

Support for attentional theories of neglect comes from studies showing positive effects of cueing, in which individuals with neglect are instructed to attend to left-sided space, and from studies showing that individuals with neglect tend to neglect the left side of *ipsilesional* space. (That is, they exhibit reduced sensitivity to visual stimuli in the left half of visual displays presented in the right visual field.) However, Hornak (1992) and Karnath and Fetter (1995) reported that left neglect patients exhibited a rightward attentional bias as they searched for (nonexistent) targets in a darkened room, findings not consistent with attentional engagement or disengagement theories.

Neglect has traditionally been considered a contralateral phenomenon—that all stimuli in the visual half-field contralateral to the side of the brain injury are ignored. Recent studies have suggested, however, that neglect may not be constant across the entire contralateral visual field and that neglect may affect the ipsilateral visual field, although to a lesser degree than it affects the contralateral visual field. As Taylor (2003) commented:

Definitions of neglect...suggest that all stimuli on the side contralateral to the brain lesion are ignored. This may not be the case; it may be more realistic to imagine the visual field as a gradient with stimuli in the extreme contralateral side having a higher probability of being

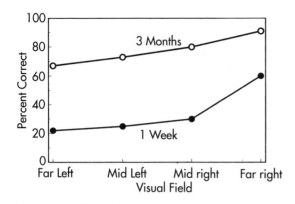

Figure 10-2 ■ Change in letter-cancellation scores across four quadrants of the visual fields at 1 week after onset and at 3 months after onset for 27 patients with visuospatial neglect. At 1 week after onset, neglect extended into the far right visual field. At 3 months after onset, little neglect was evident in the far right visual field but gradually increased from right to left. (Data from Cassidy, T.P., Lewis, S., & Gray, C.S. (1998). Recovery from visuospatial neglect in stroke patients. *Journal of Neurology, Neurosurgery and Psychiatry, 64,* 555-557.

ignored, and stimuli closer to the midline having a lower probability of being ignored. In a person with severe neglect the unattended area may be large, but in a person with mild neglect this area may be relatively small, or only be obvious under certain circumstances. (p. 67)

Cassidy, Lewis, and Gray (1998) used 3 line-cancellation tests to measure neglect across left and right visual fields in 27 patients with left neglect tested within 1 week of a right-hemisphere stroke and retested 1, 2, or 3 months later. When tested at 1 week poststroke, the group made errors across both left and right visual fields, with gradually improving performance from the far-left to the far-right visual fields (Figure 10-2). At 3 months poststroke, cancellation test performance across all 4 quadrants of the visual field had improved substantially, with the greatest improvement in the far-right quadrant (Figure 10-2).

Denial of Illness. Denial of illness *(anosognosia)* is a common behavioral consequence of right-hemisphere brain injury, especially when individuals have right parietal lobe injury. Denial of illness spans a range of severity. Some individuals with right-hemisphere brain injury acknowledge but are indifferent to impairments. Some acknowledge impairments but underestimate their severity and minimize their effects, as did the right-hemisphere-injured individual with dense left hemiplegia who asserted that his paralyzed left arm and leg were just a little weak and gave him problems only when he attempted to climb stairs. Those with the most extreme denial disavow the existence of major disabilities such as paralysis, sensory loss, and visual field blindness, and some even deny ownership of their hemiplegic limbs, as did the woman who complained of waking and finding a stranger's leg in bed with her. These individuals may claim to perform activities that are beyond their physical abilities, as did the patient with left-sided paralysis who claimed to be training for a speed-skating competition. Less overt patterns of denial are common among right-hemisphere-injured adults, who may ignore errors and confabulate, argue, and justify their mistakes when someone calls attention to them, as did the woman who said, *Well of course it doesn't make sense! You didn't tell me it had to make sense!* when questioned about a sentence she had written.

Constructional Impairment. Many brain-injured adults perform poorly when they are asked to draw or copy geometric designs, create designs with colored blocks, copy two-dimensional stick figures, or reproduce three-dimensional constructions using wooden blocks. Deficient performance on such tasks in the absence of perceptual or motor impairments is called *constructional impairment* (sometimes erroneously called *constructional apraxia*).

Apraxia is a disorder in which planning and execution of volitional sequential movements are disrupted. *Constructional impairments* represent visuospatial, perceptual, and organizational impairments rather than motor planning impairments.

Constructional impairments appear after injury in either brain hemisphere, but are more frequent and more severe after right-hemisphere injury, especially following injuries in the right parietal lobe or the right parieto-occipital region. Adults with left-hemisphere brain injury also make errors on constructional tests, and counting errors does not discriminate between individuals with left-hemisphere brain injury and individuals with right-hemisphere brain injury (Gainotti & Tiacci, 1970). Adults with right-hemisphere injury and adults with left-hemisphere injury do not, however, make the same kinds of errors.

Adults with right-hemisphere brain injuries tend to respond quickly and impulsively. They make frequent errors and try to correct them by adding more lines to their drawings or by aimlessly rearranging stick or block designs. They often leave out details on the left side of drawings or constructions, and those with severe neglect often leave out everything in left-side visual space. When they copy drawings, they add extra lines, rotate and fragment the drawings, and render three-dimensional drawings in two dimensions. Their drawings look fragmented, disorganized, and crowded, and they often are displaced to the right side of the page.

Whereas adults who have right-hemisphere brain injuries are impulsive, adults who have left-hemisphere brain injuries are cautious. Adults with left-hemisphere injuries respond slowly, with false starts, hesitations, and self-corrections, but they usually do not make mistakes that must be corrected by starting over. They simplify figures or constructions and produce drawings in which proportions and dimensionality are accurate, but angles and lines are distorted. Their drawings look incomplete and clumsy, but they are coherent. Adults with left-hemisphere brain injuries benefit from having a model to copy, whereas those with right-hemisphere injuries do not (Hecaen & Assal, 1970). Many of these differences are apparent in Figure 10-3, which shows a set of figures copied by an adult with left-hemisphere brain injury, and the same set of figures copied by an adult with right-hemisphere brain injury.

Topographic Impairment. Topographic impairment (sometimes called *topological disorientation*) denotes a condition in which the affected person has difficulty orienting to extrapersonal space. Individuals with topographic impairment have difficulty following familiar routes, reading maps, giving directions, and performing other tasks that depend on internal

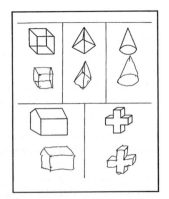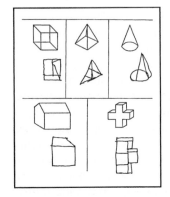

Figure 10-3 ■ Performance on a figure-copying test by a patient with left-hemisphere brain injury *(left)* and a patient with right-hemisphere brain injury *(right)*.

representations of external space. Topographic impairments are a common consequence of right-hemisphere brain injury. Myers (1994) has suggested that at least some of right-hemisphere-injured adults' problems in this domain may arise from failure to recognize familiar landmarks or to learn new landmarks, because they fail to attend to visual cues. Some individuals with topographic impairment compensate for the impairment by talking themselves through a sequence of directions. One right-hemisphere-injured patient reported that he found his way back to his room by talking himself through the following sequence:

I go to the end of the hall and look both ways. I find the hall with the window at the end. I go down that hall. The first door past the nurses' station is my room.

Right-hemisphere-injured adults' ability to talk themselves through a route sets them apart from individuals with disorientation and confusion, who also get lost easily but have no idea where they are or how they got there.

Geographic Disorientation. Geographic disorientation is less common than topographic impairment, but the two often occur together (Tompkins, 1995). Individuals with *geographic disorientation* recognize at least the general nature of their surroundings but are mistaken about where they are. (A patient at a medical center in Minnesota believed that he was at a medical center in South Africa. Another patient at the same medical center believed that he was at a school in South Dakota.) Geographic disorientation is distinct from orientation to time and person. Individuals with geographic disorientation know the day, month, and year, and they know who they are and have at least a general sense of the identity of those around them, but they are confused about where they are. The reasons for geographic disorientation are unknown. Geographic disorientation may arise from the affected individual's inability to

construct a mental representation of geographic locations based on cues available from their immediate surroundings (Tompkins, 1995).

Many hospitalized adults, non-brain-injured as well as brain-injured, lose track of what day it is after several days in the hospital, because there are few reminders of what day it is in most hospitals. Most hospitalized adults do, however, know where they are geographically.

Reduplicative Paramnesia. An unusual disturbance called *reduplicative paramnesia* occasionally follows right-hemisphere brain injury. Individuals with reduplicative paramnesia believe in the existence of duplicate persons, places, body parts, or events. One patient with reduplicative paramnesia claimed that there were two identical hospitals in his home city, another claimed to have two left legs, and a third claimed that she was living with two identical husbands. The causes of reduplicative paramnesia are not known, but its presence may be related to disturbed spatial perception and impaired visual memory. Reduplicative paramnesia is strongly related to injury in the right brain hemisphere, but a more precise localization in the right hemisphere has not been suggested.

Visuoperceptual Impairments. Right-hemisphere-injured adults typically have little difficulty identifying real objects or recognizing pictures or drawings of objects when they are portrayed naturalistically, in prototypic views. Visuoperceptual impairments become apparent when right-hemisphere-injured adults are asked to identify objects, pictures, or drawings that are incomplete, distorted, or otherwise changed from their traditional prototypic form (Myers, 1994). They have difficulty identifying line drawings of objects when one drawing is superimposed on another, and they often fail to recognize familiar objects depicted in incomplete or fragmented form, shown in unusual orientation, or depicted with unusual size relationships, as

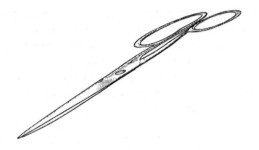

Figure 10-4 ▪ A drawing of a common object depicted in an unusual orientation. Patients with right-hemisphere brain injury often find it difficult to identify drawings that depict familiar objects in unusual orientations, with unusual size relationships, or in distorted form.

in Figure 10-4. Right-hemisphere-injured adults' visuospatial impairments seem less perceptual than organizational—they have no difficulty describing the visual characteristics of the stimuli they fail to recognize. When visual stimuli are simple, clear, and unambiguous, right-hemisphere-injured adults usually respond normally, but when the stimuli are incomplete, degraded, or distorted, right-hemisphere-injured adults are inclined to misinterpret them.

Facial Recognition Deficits. Some adults with right-hemisphere brain injury are unable to recognize otherwise familiar persons by their facial features. They also perform poorly on other tasks that depend on perception and integration of facial features, such as identifying famous people from photographs and choosing previously seen pictures of people from a group containing a mix of previously seen pictures and previously unseen foils. This facial recognition impairment is called *prosopagnosia*, (from the Greek words for *face* and *knowledge*). Facial recognition deficits sometimes affect perception of cartoons and line-drawn faces as well as actual faces and photographs, and they may extend beyond human faces—for example, a

bird watcher who no longer recognized different species of birds and a farmer who no longer recognized his cows, following right-hemisphere strokes (Albert & associates, 1981). Individuals who fail to recognize others by their facial features usually recognize them when they speak or exhibit other features such as clothing, hair color and style, body type, or gait.

> Presumably the birdwatcher could still tell different birds by their songs, and perhaps the farmer could tell his cows apart by the sound of their voices, their coloring, or the way they walked.

Some individuals with prosopagnosia have difficulty telling male faces from female faces, old faces from young faces, or human faces from animal faces. Prosopagnosia often follows posterior right-hemisphere brain injury (Hecaen & Angelergues, 1962; Warrington & James, 1967; Whitely & Warrington, 1977), but persisting prosopagnosia may require bilateral injury (Albert & associates, 1981; Cohn, Neumann, & Wood, 1977; Damasio, 1985; Damasio & Damasio, 1983; Meadows, 1974). Prosopagnosia is not caused by impaired visuospatial perception (McKeever & Dixon, 1981) or inability to recognize facially portrayed emotion (Cicone, Wapner, & Gardner, 1980; Ley & Bryden, 1979). A few right-hemisphere-injured patients with prosopagnosia claim that one or more relatives and friends have been abducted and replaced by impostors who are exact doubles of the missing persons—a condition called *Capgras syndrome.*

> Capgras syndrome was first described in 1923 by Jean Marie Joseph Capgras, a French psychiatrist. The imposter usually is a key figure in the affected person's life—if married, the spouse. Sometimes persons with Capgras syndrome perceive themselves as their own double. Occasionally the delusion extends to inanimate objects such as personal possessions and furniture. Capgras syndrome

is associated with several conditions affecting the brain, including psychosis, traumatic brain injury, substance abuse, dementia, and posterior right-hemisphere brain injury. The affected person usually is aware that their perceptions are abnormal but is convinced of their accuracy.

Recognition and Expression of Emotion

Our experience of emotion is a product of the limbic system, but our appreciation of others' emotions and our expression of our own emotions appear to be regulated in large part by the right hemisphere in right-handed adults (Tucker & Frederick, 1989). Right-hemisphere-injured adults often appear not to recognize the emotional tone of others' facial expressions and tone of voice and do not use facial expression and tone of voice to express their own emotions. The source of these impairments is unknown, but they may represent failure to appreciate prosodic cues to emotion in others' speech, failure to appreciate the emotional implications of facial expressions, or failure to appreciate the emotional tone associated with stereotypic emotional situations such as weddings or funerals.

The limbic system includes phylogenetically old portions of the cerebral cortex, subcortical structures, and pathways connecting them to the diencephalon and brain stem. The functions of the limbic system are related to survival of the individual and continuation of the species, including eating behavior, aggression, expression of emotion, and endocrinal aspects of the sexual response.

Many right-hemisphere-injured adults do not seem to appreciate the significance of prosodic indicators of emotion provided by vocal pitch and intonation. Whether this deficit actually represents an underlying disturbance of emotional competence is not clear. There is some evidence that right-hemisphere-injured adults'

insensitivity to prosodic indicators of emotion is caused by failure to perceive, discriminate, and process the acoustic information related to pitch and intonation patterns, rather than by failure to attach emotional significance to accurately perceived pitch and intonation patterns. Patients who fail to attach appropriate meanings to prosodic indicators of emotion nevertheless can identify upward and downward vocal intonation patterns (Robin, Tranel, & Damasio, 1990).

Many investigators have reported that adults with right-hemisphere brain injury fail to correctly interpret facial expressions indicative of emotion (Blonder, Bowers, & Heilman, 1991; Cicone, Wapner, & Gardner, 1980; DeKosky, Heilman, Bowers, & Valenstein, 1980; and others). Right-hemisphere-injured adults' interpretation of facial expression typically has been tested by presenting still photographs of people producing static representations of feigned emotions. Because movement cues to the expressions are not available, identification of the emotions portrayed in the photographs depends completely on analysis of visuospatial information (e.g., narrowed eyes, downward curvature of the mouth). Because adults with right-hemisphere brain injury have difficulty analyzing visuospatial information and integrating individual features into a composite whole, it may be that what seems to be a problem in interpreting facial expression actually reflects an underlying impairment in the analysis and integration of visuospatial information (Myers, 1999).

Myers (1999) has commented that patients with right-hemisphere brain injury rarely complain about impaired recognition of facial expressions, perhaps because they are unaware of it.

Several studies have reported that adults with right-hemisphere brain injury perform poorly when asked to match the emotional tone of short stories to pictured scenes (Cicone, Wapner, &

Gardner, 1980), identify emotions portrayed in pictured scenes (Bloom, Borod, Obler, & Gerstman, 1992; Cancelliere & Kertesz, 1990), or identify emotions portrayed in spoken sentences (Blonder, Bowers, & Heilman, 1991). However, some contradictory evidence has been reported. Tompkins and Flowers (1985) reported that adults with right-hemisphere brain injury performed comparably to adults with left-hemisphere brain injury when asked to identify the emotions conveyed by spoken sentences. Myers (1994) has asserted that determining the emotional tone of situations, sentences, and narratives requires that individuals recognize that emotional tone is present, discriminate cues that signal emotions, and integrate the cues into an overall representation of an emotion—all of which characteristically are problems for adults with right-hemisphere brain injury.

In summary, many adults with right-hemisphere brain injury appear to have diminished appreciation of emotions conveyed by speech prosody, facial expression, narratives, or pictorial representations, at least when they are asked to identify the emotional tone of such materials presented in a test environment. It is not clear, however, that abnormal performance on these tasks actually reflects impaired appreciation of emotions and not impairment of some other cognitive process or processes. Regardless of the underlying reasons, many adults with right hemisphere injuries seem deficient in recognizing and expressing emotion in daily life interactions. They seem insensitive to emotional tones conveyed by others' facial expression and tone of voice, and when they do assign emotional significance to spoken materials, facial expressions, body language, or situations, they often assign the wrong emotion.

Attentional Impairments

Attentional impairments are common in brain-injured adults, and adults with right-

hemisphere brain injury are no exception. It may be that many of the surface manifestations of right-hemisphere brain injury represent, at least in part, disturbances of underlying attentional processes. Many adults with right-hemisphere brain injury have difficulty focusing, maintaining, and shifting attention. These impairments make it difficult or impossible for right-hemisphere-injured adults to maintain focus in treatment activities. Attentional impairments also complicate right-hemisphere-injured adults' daily lives, making it difficult for them to determine the overall meaning of situations and events, separate what is important from what is not, identify relationships among elements of information, maintain appropriate patterns of interactions with conversational partners, and maintain coherence in speech and writing.

Attention no doubt represents the interaction of several cognitive processes, and some investigators have divided attentional processes into multiple components that they believe represent different underlying skills. Adults with right-hemisphere brain injury may exhibit impairments in some or all of these attentional processes. (See Chapter 4 for discussion of these attentional processes.)

- *Arousal*—physiologic and behavioral readiness to respond
- *Vigilance*—ongoing sensitivity to stimulation
- *Orienting*—direction of attention toward a stimulus
- *Sustained attention*—maintenance of attention over time
- *Selective attention* (sometimes called *focused attention*)—maintenance of attention in the presence of competing or distracting stimuli or attending to individual stimuli within an array
- *Alternating attention*—moving attention from stimulus to stimulus in response to changing task requirements or changing intentions
- *Divided attention*—performing more than one activity at the same time.

GENERAL CONCEPTS 10-1

- Contemporary theories of hemispheric function depict the left hemisphere as better at processing sequential, time-related material suitable for linear processing and depict the right hemisphere as better at processing nonlinear, spatially distributed arrays.

- About one half of adults with right-hemisphere injury develop significant communicative impairments. Right-hemisphere-damaged adults with cortical lesions, a family history of left handedness, and low education levels are most likely to develop communicative impairments.

- Patients with right-hemisphere brain injury are described in the literature as insensitive to others and preoccupied with self; oblivious to social conventions; unconcerned about physical and mental impairments; verbose, tangential, and rambling in speech; insensitive to the meaning of implied or abstract material; and unable to grasp the overall significance of complex events.

- Some patients with right-hemisphere brain injury are behaviorally passive, seem emotionally flat, and have problems maintaining attention.

- The literature on right-hemisphere brain injury is biased toward patients with anterior right-hemisphere injuries because they are likely to be hospitalized longer than patients with posterior right-hemisphere injuries and thus are available to investigators who study the right hemisphere.

- *Left hemispatial neglect* is a common consequence of right-hemisphere brain injuries. Visual field blindness does not cause neglect, although patients with left hemispatial neglect often have left homonymous hemianopia. Neglect often resolves in the days and weeks after brain injury.

- Several theories have been offered to explain neglect. *Representational theories* suggest that neglect is caused by disturbed mental representation of external space. *Arousal theories* propose that right-hemisphere-damaged adults are less sensitive to stimuli in neglected space. *Attentional engagement theories* propose that right-hemisphere-damaged adults have difficulty directing attention to neglected space. *Attentional disengagement theories* propose that right-hemisphere-damaged adults' attention is caught and held by stimuli in nonneglected space.

- Denial of illness *(anosognosia)* is a common behavioral consequence of right-hemisphere brain injury. Patients with anosognosia deny or minimize physical, cognitive, or communicative impairments.

- *Constructional impairment* (inability to draw or copy geometric designs) is a common consequence of right-hemisphere brain injury.

- *Topographic impairment* and *geographic disorientation* sometimes follow right-hemisphere brain injury. Patients with topographic impairment appear to have distorted internal representations of external space. Patients with geographic disorientation confuse the geographic location of familiar people, places, or things, perhaps because of difficulty inferring location from cues provided by the patient's surroundings.

- *Visuoperceptual impairments* (difficulty recognizing objects, pictures, or drawings presented in unusual formats) and *prosopagnosia* (facial recognition deficits) are common consequences of right-hemisphere brain injuries. These impairments may represent failure to integrate elements of visual information into a coherent representation of the perceived stimulus.

Continued

GENERAL CONCEPTS 10-1—cont'd

- Some patients with right-hemisphere brain injuries appear insensitive to the emotional tone of facial expression, body language, situations, and verbal materials. Some fail to communicate emotional tone by speech prosody, facial expression, and body language. It is not clear if these impairments are truly emotional in nature and not the result of impairment in some other cognitive processes.
- Attentional impairments are common following right-hemisphere brain injury. The impairments may affect arousal, vigilance, orienting, sustained attention, selective attention, alternating attention, or divided attention.

COMMUNICATIVE IMPAIRMENTS ASSOCIATED WITH RIGHT-HEMISPHERE BRAIN INJURY

In addition to perceptual, affective, and attentional impairments, many adults with right-hemisphere brain injury have communicative impairments that make it difficult for them to communicate emotion, express themselves coherently and efficiently, comprehend humor, sarcasm, and nonliteral material, and behave appropriately in conversations.

Diminished Speech Prosody

The speech of many right-hemisphere-injured adults lacks normal variability in pitch and loudness, making their speech monotonous and seemingly devoid of emotion. Many also have reduced spontaneity and variety in nonverbal movements that typically accompany speech (e.g., head nod and gestures). Although prosodic disturbances are most obvious in right-hemisphere-injured adults' expression of emotion, they frequently affect their nonemotional utterances as well. These prosodic disturbances include:

- Slower-than-normal speech rate, with uniform spacing between sounds, syllables, and words, giving speech a robotlike quality

- Reduced emphatic stress in phrases and sentences. (e.g., *George* wrecked Linda's car, versus George wrecked *Linda's* car).
- Diminished pitch variability, leading to restricted intonation and failure to distinguish between questions (upward pitch change) and assertions (downward pitch change)

It is not clear which right-hemisphere-injured adults are most likely to have prosodically flattened speech. Bryden and Ley (1983) and Shapiro and Danley (1985) attributed this phenomenon to injury in the right frontal lobe. Colsher, Cooper, and Graff-Radford (1987) claimed that adults with right-hemisphere frontal lobe injury have essentially normal variability in vocal pitch. Myers (1994) and Tompkins (1995) comment that some right-hemisphere-injured adults' reduced speech prosody may be caused by muscle weakness *(dysarthria)* rather than by an underlying affective impairment. Tompkins also reminded her readers that diminished speech prosody sometimes follows brain injury outside the right hemisphere.

Some right-hemisphere-injured adults seem aware that their voice does not communicate their emotional state, and they compensate by communicating emotion with propositional speech, such as the right-hemisphere-injured adult who, in the middle of a challenging treatment activity, said to the clinician (in a monotone), *You don't seem to realize it, so I guess I have to tell you that I'm tired of doing this.* That some right-hemisphere-injured adults verbally compensate for their lack of vocal prosody suggests that prosodic deficiencies do not necessarily signify an underlying affective impairment. It is true, however, that many of the same individuals who fail to communicate emotion via speech prosody also fail to appreciate emotions conveyed by others' speech prosody and facial expression, lending credence to the assumption that they have an underlying affective impairment.

Anomalous Content and Organization of Connected Speech

One of the most striking communicative impairments of right-hemisphere-injured adults is their excessive, confabulatory, and sometimes inappropriate connected speech. These anomalies become apparent when right-hemisphere-injured adults perform narrative production tasks wherein they tell or retell stories in response to pictures, picture sequences, or stories told to them by another. The speech they produce under these conditions has been described as *excessive* and *rambling* (Gardner, Brownell, Wapner, & Michelow, 1983); *repetitive* and *irrelevant* (Tompkins & Flowers, 1985); and *tangential, digressive,* and *inefficient* (Myers, 1994). They use more words but produce less information than either non-brain-injured adults or adults with left-hemisphere brain injury (Diggs & Basili, 1987; Myers, 1979; Rivers & Love, 1980). Their narratives are fragmented, lack cohesion, and do not have an overall theme or point, because they tend to focus on incidental details, fail to establish relationships among events, insert tangential comments, and permit personal experiences and opinions to intrude into their narratives. The transcript in Figure 10-5 shows several of these characteristics.

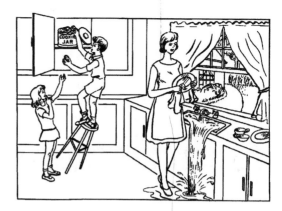

Well, this is a scene in a house. It looks like a fine spring day. The window is open. I guess it's not Minnesota, or the flies and mosquitoes would be coming in. Outside I see a tree and another window. Looks like the neighbors have their windows closed. There's a woman near the window wearing what appears to be an inexpensive pair of shoes. She's holding something that looks like a plate. On the counter there, there's a hat and two caps that look like they would fit on a child's head. The woman is looking out the window, and the water's on, and it's running on the floor. Looks like she needs to call the plumber. *(Clinician: "Is there anything over here?" Points to left side of picture.)* Well, I see two people... children... a boy and a girl. The boy is getting cookies from the cupboard and the girl is laughing and waving. There's also a stool. Perhaps the boy is stealing cookies and perhaps the girl...or the stool is going to fall. There's a window beside the cookie jar, but it doesn't have any curtains.

Figure 10-5 ■ A right-hemisphere-injured patient's description of the *Cookie Theft* picture from the *Boston Diagnostic Aphasia Examination.* (Drawing from Goodglass H., Kaplan E., and Barresi B. [2001]. *The Assessment of aphasia and related disorders* [3rd ed.]. Philadelphia: Lippincott, Williams and Wilkins, now owned by Pro-Ed [Austin, Texas].)

The patient begins by making three inferences. One is correct and relevant *(the scene is in a house),* the other two are potentially correct but irrelevant *(it looks like a spring day; it must not be Minnesota).* The patient then continues to enumerate elements on the right side of the drawing, with occasional interjection of irrelevant comments. After misinterpreting the plate and two cups shown on the counter as a hat and two caps (but inferring from their size that they must be for children), the patient begins to appreciate the problem with the overflowing sink. When the clinician directs the patient to the left side of the drawing, the patient begins by enumerating pictured elements, then eventually arrives at the appropriate interpretation. He ends by misinterpreting a cupboard door as a window, but correctly perceives that the "window" has no curtains. This patient's narrative contains many characteristics of right-hemisphere syndrome. He focuses on the right-hand side of the picture. He begins by enumerating pictured elements and slowly develops interpretations expressing relationships among the elements. He adds irrelevant and tangential comments. He misinterprets visual information. He makes inferences that may be consistent with his interpretation of visual information or underlying relationships but are inconsistent with the true sense of what is portrayed.

Impaired Comprehension of Narratives and Conversations

Adults with aphasia comprehend discourse better than their performance on tests of single-sentence comprehension suggests that they should, but the converse seems true for most adults with right-hemisphere brain injury (Brownell, 1988). Right-hemisphere-injured adults' impairments in discourse comprehension reflect many of the same underlying disabilities that compromise their production of narratives and undermine their ability to get along in daily life—insensitivity to relationships among events, failure to judge the appropriateness of events or situations, and premature assumptions based on incomplete analysis of events and situations.

Many adults with right-hemisphere brain injury have particular difficulty comprehending implied meanings in narratives and conversations (Brownell, Potter, Bihrle, & Gardner, 1986) and are seemingly unable to get beyond

literal interpretations of what they hear or read. They interpret idiomatic expressions, figures of speech, and metaphors literally. They fail to identify incongruous, irrelevant, or absurd statements, and offer confabulatory or bizarre reasons for accepting them as true. They are unable to judge the appropriateness of facts, situations, or characterizations in stories or conversations, and they cannot extract morals from stories. These deficiencies in discourse comprehension carry over into their comprehension of conversations, where they

> ...often seem to lack a full understanding of the context of an utterance, the presuppositions entailed, the affective tone, or the point of a conversational exchange. They appear to have difficulties in processing abstract sentences, in reasoning logically, and in maintaining a coherent stream of thought. (Gardner & associates, 1983, p. 172)

Myers (1999) echoes Gardner and associates' description. She comments that right-hemisphere-injured adults respond to conversations in piecemeal fashion without making connections between related items of information and fail to appreciate situational variables that denote the nature of a conversation.

Right-hemisphere-injured adults' difficulties with nonliteral language are not always complete. Sometimes they fail to appreciate nonliteral meanings in one context, but get them in another. For example, some right-hemisphere-injured adults who cannot select pictures representing the implied meanings of nonliteral statements can explain them orally; some who cannot choose the best punch lines for printed jokes nevertheless choose endings that are surprising; and some who do not choose the appropriate printed responses to indirect requests such as *Can you open the door?* respond appropriately to their nonliteral meaning in daily life (Tompkins, 1995). Some who misperceive or misinterpret elements of narratives in test situations perceive and interpret similar elements appropriately when narratives occur in daily life situations with more contextual support. Like adults with left-hemisphere injuries, those with right-hemisphere brain injury tend to perform better in natural situations that provide situational context than in testing or treatment activities that limit context.

Brownell, Potter, Bihrle, and Gardner (1986) have suggested that right-hemisphere-injured adults actually do make inferences suggested by discourse, but that their inferences are premature and incorrect. According to Brownell and associates, these individuals are trapped by spur-of-the-moment erroneous inferences and are unable to reject or revise them when subsequent material shows the inferences to be incorrect. The problem seems not to be that these individuals cannot make inferences, but that they are too readily led into inappropriate inferences from which they cannot escape.

Results reported by Nicholas and Brookshire (1995b) support Brownell and associates' suggestion that right-hemisphere-injured adults can make inferences. Nicholas and Brookshire evaluated the Discourse Comprehension Test performance of 20 adults with right-hemisphere brain injury. The group of right-hemisphere-injured adults correctly answered 80% of the questions that required inferences based on information given in short narratives. The right-hemisphere-injured adults performed as well on questions related to implied information as either aphasic adults with left-hemisphere injuries or traumatically brain-injured adults.

Tompkins and her associates offer a *suppression-deficit hypothesis* to explain right-hemisphere-injured adults' inability to escape from inappropriate inferences in discourse comprehension (Tompkins, Baumgaertner, Lehman, & Fossett, 1997; Tompkins & Lehman, 1998; Tompkins, Lehman, Baumgaertner, Fossett, & Vance, 1996; Tompkins, Lehman-Blake, Baumgaertner, & Fassbinder, 2001). The suppression-deficit hypothesis assumes (1) that right-hemisphere-injured adults activate multiple

meanings when they interpret materials that are conducive to multiple interpretations and (2) that right-hemisphere-injured adults are impaired in their ability to suppress interpretations that are initially activated but later prove irrelevant or incompatible. "RHD [right-hemisphere-damaged] patients do generate inferences and hold on too long to those that become inappropriate to a final, integrated interpretation" (Tompkins & Lehman, 1998, p. 41).

> Tompkins's suppression-deficit hypothesis seems to have implications similar to Brownell and associates' *"trap"* hypothesis, although couched in different terminology.

Tompkins and Lehman (1998) offer the results of several studies of right-hemisphere-injured adults' performance in online language processing tasks as support for a suppression-deficit hypothesis. However, a study by Tompkins and associates (2001) failed to confirm the existence of a suppression deficit specific to right-hemisphere-injured adults. Under the conditions of the study, both normal elderly adults and adults with right-hemisphere brain injury failed to suppress initial inferences that subsequently were shown to be inappropriate. As this is written, the suppression deficit hypothesis awaits definitive confirmation.

> A suppression-deficit hypothesis could conceivably explain other prototypical right-hemisphere-injury impairments such as impulsivity; tangential speech, social inappropriateness, and difficulty with idioms, metaphor and humor, although Tompkins and her associates make no such claims.

Brownell and his associates have related right-hemisphere-injured adults' problems in comprehending discourse to impaired *theory of mind* (Brownell & Friedman, 2001; Brownell, Griffin, Winner, Friedman, & Happe, 2000;

Happe, Brownell, & Winner, 1999; Winner, Brownell, Happe, Blum, & Pincus, 1998). *Theory of mind* denotes the ability to appreciate "the contents of other people's minds—their beliefs and emotions—to understand their actions and utterances" (Brownell & Friedman, 2001, p. 197). Brownell and associates base their assertions concerning adults with right-hemisphere brain injury on the results of several studies in which right-hemisphere-injured adults performed tasks in which they were asked to distinguish lies from jokes (Winner, Brownell, Happe, Blum, & Pincus, 1998); evaluate speakers' choice of terms with which to refer to people who were not present (Brownell, Pincus, Blum, Rehak, & Winner, 1997); or comprehend stories that depend on appreciating story participants' beliefs (Happe, Brownell, & Winner, 1999). According to Brownell and associates, accurate performance in these tasks requires that those doing the tasks appreciate others' mental states, emotions, knowledge, and beliefs.

Right-hemisphere-injured adults as a group performed poorly on tasks that presumably depended on theory of mind, whereas their performance on tasks that required comprehension of material that did not presumably depend on theory of mind approximated the performance of normal elderly adults. The results led Brownell and associates to consider impaired theory of mind a possible explanation for other characteristic signs of right-hemisphere brain injury such as anosognosia:

> It may be fruitful to think of acquired RHD [right-hemisphere damage] as (in some cases) a syndrome of impaired theory of mind. (Happe, Brownell, & Winner, 1999, p. 230)

Group performance did not, however, always represent the performance of individuals in the groups:

> Not all of our RHD patients were equally impaired; a few were not measurably impaired

at all. Somewhat more surprising is that some control subjects consistently performed poorly. An impaired ability to conceptualize others' mental states may thus be a nonspecific marker for various conditions, including but not limited to focal right-hemisphere brain injury. (Winner, Brownell, Happe, Blum, & Pincus, 1998, p. 101)

Although a theory-of-mind explanation for right-hemisphere-injured adults' impairments may be intuitively appealing, definitive evidence for a central role in right-hemisphere-injured adults' impairments is not currently available. The studies that identified apparent theory-of-mind impairments in right-hemisphere-injured adults relied on metalinguistic tasks in which participants make interpretations or judgments about printed or spoken situations or vignettes after the fact. Studies have not consistently shown theory-of-mind impairments when right-hemisphere-injured adults are called on to exercise theory of mind in natural situations. Tompkins and Lehman (1998) have commented that in metalinguistic tasks:

> "...the mental effort and conscious awareness of stimulus properties that are required by these kinds of tasks render them inappropriate for assessing the relatively automatic operations that are integral to language processing and other aspects of cognitive functioning." (p. 31)

It is not clear that right-hemisphere-injured adults' differential performance on theory-of-mind tasks versus non-theory-of-mind tasks uniquely depends on theory of mind, because the tasks in which right-hemisphere-injured adults exhibit theory-of-mind impairments appear to require more effortful cognitive processing than non-theory-of-mind tasks. What appears to be impaired theory of mind actually may reflect the increased processing demands of theory-of-mind tasks relative to control (non-theory-of-mind) tasks.

In Winner and associates (1998), right-hemisphere-injured adults and normal controls listened to short stories that ended either with an ironic joke or a lie by one character. Participants in the study answered questions about story characters' mental states. First-order mental states represented one character's knowledge (X knows…). Second-order mental states represented one character's knowledge of what another character knew (X knows that Y knows…). Right-hemisphere-injured adults' appreciation of first-order mental states approximated that of the control group, but their appreciation of second-order mental states was significantly impaired. Winner and associates attributed the right-hemisphere-injured adults' impaired performance to impaired theory of mind. However, inferring second-order mental states seems a more demanding task in terms of processing workload, making the source of the right-hemisphere-injured adults' impaired performance questionable.

Pragmatic Impairments

Pragmatic impairments affect the social and interactional aspects of language, such as turn-taking, topic maintenance, social conventions, and eye contact. Pragmatic impairments are common consequences of right-hemisphere brain injury. Many right-hemisphere-injured adults begin and end conversations abruptly, are poor at maintaining eye contact with conversational partners, talk excessively and without regard for their listener, have difficulty staying on topic, interject irrelevant, tangential, and inappropriate comments into conversations, and fail to make needed conversational repairs. Many right-hemisphere-injured adults also are insensitive to rules governing conversational turn-taking, especially those related to yielding the floor to conversational partners.

Clinician: Well, Mr. Spencer, what are you planning to do this afternoon?

Patient: Well, I have OT [occupational therapy].

Clinician: What are you doing in OT?

Patient: Yesterday they were having us bake a cake…from a mix in a box…white cake with pink icing. It looked awful, and it tasted worse.

Clinician: Why were you baking a cake?

Patient: It wasn't just me. There were a couple or three other people in on it. I don't have the foggiest why they were there or what planet they came from. How come you're wearing that scarf around your neck? Are you cold?

Clinician: No, it's what you call a fashion accessory. It adds some color. Do you like it?

Patient: Maybe if you were sitting on a horse.

Not all right-hemisphere-injured adults are pragmatically inappropriate in conversations. Prutting and Kirchner (1987) evaluated the conversational behavior of right-hemisphere-injured adults while they engaged in a 15-minute conversation with another adult. They tabulated the occurrence of 30 categories of appropriate or inappropriate conversational behaviors. As a group, the right-hemisphere-injured adults failed to maintain adequate eye contact, produced speech with diminished emotional tone, were slow in responding to the conversational partner's utterances, deviated from conversational topics, and talked too much. However, not all exhibited this pattern. Of the nine right-hemisphere-injured participants, two had violations in only one category (eye contact), whereas one subject had violations in 13 of the 30 categories. Prutting and Kirchner's results at the group level are consistent with descriptions of right-hemisphere-injured adults' conversational behavior found in the literature, but it is clear that not all adults with right-hemisphere brain injury fit the stereotypic pattern.

Kennedy, Strand, Burton, and Peterson (1994) evaluated 12 right-hemisphere-injured adults' conversational behaviors as the brain-injured adults conversed with non-brain-injured adults. Kennedy and associates divided the conversational behaviors into two categories, one representing *topic-related skills* (introducing, maintaining, elaborating on, and terminating topics) and the other representing *turn-taking skills* (making assertions, requesting information or action, communicating emotion, acknowledging the other's contributions, and committing to a future action).

The two groups did not differ significantly in topic-related skills, but they differed in turn-taking. The right-hemisphere-injured group made significantly more assertions than the non-brain-injured group, but they also made significantly fewer requests for information. The right-hemisphere-injured group took more conversational turns but said fewer words in each turn (which Kennedy and associates said may be why they took more turns). Kennedy and associates commented that several right-hemisphere-injured participants spent most of their turns talking about themselves and rarely asked their conversational partners for information. They also commented that some right-hemisphere-injured participants introduced new topics after their conversational partner had indicated the conversation was over, suggesting that they were insensitive to their conversational partner's intent.

Clinician: I've really enjoyed talking with you. Perhaps we can do this again someday soon.

Patient: And tonight I'm going to the football game with my brother.

There was great variability among the right-hemisphere-injured participants, with some participants exhibiting severely impaired conversational skills, and others appearing essentially normal, leading Kennedy and associates to comment that right-hemisphere-injured adults' premorbid conversational style should be considered when evaluating their postmorbid conversational skills.

The results reported by Kennedy and her associates and by Prutting and Kirchner show that not all adults with right-hemisphere injuries have significant pragmatic impairments, and they also show that those who are pragmatically impaired do not necessarily exhibit the same impairments. Consequently, treatment of right-hemisphere-injured adults' pragmatic impairments must be based on careful analysis of the performance of individuals.

> This could be said for all aspects of communication and related skills for all categories of brain-injured adults.

TESTS FOR ASSESSING ADULTS WITH RIGHT-HEMISPHERE BRAIN INJURY

Objective assessment of right-hemisphere-injured adults' linguistic, cognitive, and communicative abilities received little attention before the mid 1970s and remains less sophisticated than assessment of aphasic adults, which has been going on for more than 50 years. At the time this is written, four standardized procedures for evaluation of adults with right-hemisphere brain injury have been published, and several nonstandardized procedures have been described.

Standardized Procedures

The *Right Hemisphere Language Battery—Second Edition* (*RHLB-2*; Bryan, 1995) is a comprehensive test battery for evaluating right-hemisphere-injured adults. It contains seven subtests:

1. The *metaphor picture subtest* assesses comprehension of spoken metaphors such as *under the weather* or *keep it under your hat*. The patient chooses a picture representing the metaphor from a set of four pictures.

2. The *written metaphor subtest* assesses comprehension of similar metaphors in printed form. The patient chooses a sentence expressing the meaning of a printed metaphor from a set of three sentences.

3. The *comprehension of inferred meaning* subtest assesses appreciation of implied meanings expressed by three short printed narratives.

4. The *appreciation of humor subtest* assesses the patient's ability to choose the correct humorous punch line for jokes printed on cards with four possible punch lines.

5. The *lexical semantic subtest* is a subtest for matching spoken words to pictures, in which the patient points to pictures named by the

examiner. The pictures are presented with foils having functional, semantic, phonologic, or visual similarities to the target picture.

6. In the *production of emphatic stress subtest* the examiner reads the first clause of a two-clause sentence aloud, and the patient reads the second, which is designed to elicit certain patterns of emphatic stress (e.g., the clinician says, *He sold the **large** car and ...*" The patient responds, *...bought a **small** one.*)

7. The *discourse analysis rating* permits the examiner to rate a patient's cumulative performance during the test, when in conversation with the examiner, and when describing a picture. Ratings are assigned in 11 categories (e.g., humor, variety, turn-taking).

The RHLB-2 provides a reasonably comprehensive look at the major communicative functions likely to be affected by right-hemisphere brain injury. However, Tompkins (1995) asserted that the RHLB-2 has several deficiencies in reliability and validity, and an inadequate normative sample. (The RHLB-2 was standardized on 30 adults with vascular right-hemisphere brain injuries, 10 adults with nonvascular right-hemisphere brain injuries, 30 adults with vascular left-hemisphere brain injuries, 10 adults with nonvascular left-hemisphere injuries, and 30 neurologically normal adults.)

The *Mini Inventory of Right Brain Injury—Second Edition* (*MIRBI-2*; Pimental & Knight, 2000) is a standardized test that, according to the authors, can be used to identify the presence of right-hemisphere brain injury and determine its severity, identify the strengths and weaknesses of right-hemisphere-injured adults, guide treatment, and document progress.

The MIRBI-2 contains 35 test items divided among 10 categories:

- Visual scanning (2 items)
- Integrity of gnosis (finger identification, tactile perception, 2-point tactile discrimination; 3 items)
- Integrity of body image, including neglect (1 item)
- Reading and writing (5 items)

- Serial 7s (e.g., subtracting 7 from 100, subtracting 7 from the remainder; 1 item)
- Clock drawing (1 item)
- Affective language (repeating sentences with happy intonation and sad intonation; 2 items)
- Appreciation of humor, incongruities, absurdities, figurative language (8 items)
- Similarities (8 items)
- Affect, general behavior, impulsivity, distractibility, and eye contact (observation and rating by examiner; 4 items)

The test manual contains sections on administration, scoring, and test interpretation, and a summary of MIRBI-2 results for 30 adults with right-hemisphere brain injury, 13 adults with left-hemisphere brain injury, and 30 non-brain-injured adults. Correlations between MIRBI-2 scores and age, education, and time after onset are reported. Comparisons of overall MIRBI-2 scores and scores on each item are reported for the 3 groups. Sections on the reliability and validity of the MIRBI-2 are also included.

The MIRBI-2 is a short test. Because it contains only 35 items spread across 10 categories, the MIRBI-2 seems best used as a screening test to identify individuals who may have communication impairments that may be assessed in greater detail by additional testing.

The *Rehabilitation Institute of Chicago Evaluation of Communicative Problems in Right-Hemisphere Dysfunction–Revised* (*RICE-R*; Halper, Cherney, Burns, & Mogil, 1996) includes:

- An interview with the patient
- Observation of the patient in interactions with family members and hospital staff
- Ratings of attention, eye contact, awareness of illness, and orientation to place, time, and person
- Ratings of facial expression, speech intonation, and topic maintenance in conversation
- Four tests of visual scanning and tracking
- Ratings of written expression
- A scale for rating pragmatic communication skills
- A story-retelling task
- A metaphoric language test

Cut-off scores for assigning a severity rating to an individual's level of impairment are provided for each subtest. The RICE-R is standardized on 40 right-hemisphere-injured adults and 36 non-brain-injured adults.

The *Burns Brief Inventory of Communication and Cognition (BICC;* Burns, 1997) contains a section for assessing cognitive-communicative dysfunction in adults who have right-hemisphere brain injuries. BICC items in the right-hemisphere section assess performance in three domains: *attention* (e.g., visual scanning), *visuospatial and construction* (e.g., clock drawing), and *communication* (e.g., explaining idioms). The right-hemisphere section of the BICC takes about 30 minutes to administer and can be administered at bedside. A patient's test performance can be plotted on a grid to identify patients who are unlikely to improve rapidly in treatment (severe deficits), patients who are likely to profit from treatment (moderate deficits), patients who are unlikely to need immediate treatment (mild deficits), and patients who are not impaired (no errors).

Nonstandardized Procedures

The *Evanston Northwestern Healthcare—Right Hemisphere Screen (ENH-RHS;* Schneider, Buth, Eisenberg, & associates, 1999) is primarily intended to determine if patients who have right-hemisphere brain damage require additional assessment, and, if so, which areas need additional assessment. The ENH-RHS permits assessment of cognitive-communicative abilities in eight domains:

1. Orientation to person, place, and time (e.g., name, location, day of the week)
2. Selective attention (e.g., counting backwards from 30 by 3s; patient follows clinician instructions such as *When I tap my finger once, you tap twice.*)
3. Divided attention (patient draws a house while answering simple questions)
4. Memory (e.g., digit span, digits backwards, delayed recall of a word list, delayed recall of paragraphs, recall of biographical information,

and recall of information from remote memory, such as *Where is the Statue of Liberty?*)
5. Sequencing (putting the steps in taking a shower or making scrambled eggs in order)
6. Abstract verbal reasoning and problem solving
   - Auditory comprehension of complex sentences (e.g., *Is your father's mother your aunt?*)
   - Verbal absurdities (e.g., *The coffee was so sweet, I added some sugar.*)
   - Problem solving (e.g., *What would you do if you fell down at home and could not get up?*)
   - Causes (e.g., *Give me two reasons why electricity might go out in your house.*)
   - Consequences (e.g., *What could happen if you forget to turn off the stove before you leave the house?*)
   - Explaining proverbs (e.g., *What does* don't cry over spilled milk *mean?*)
   - Convergent thinking (e.g., *Tell me what these words have in common: coffee, tea, soda.*)
   - Similarities and differences (e.g., *How are a typewriter and a computer alike?*)
   - Dual meanings of words (e.g., *Give me two meanings for the word* bat.)
   - Exclusion (e.g., *Listen to the following words and tell me which one doesn't belong and why: Arizona, Florida, Chicago, Georgia, Texas.*)
7. Numerical reasoning and calculation
   - Simple numerical calculations with or without a calculator
   - Oral problems (e.g., *How much is 10% tax on $65?*)
   - Checkbook entry and balancing
8. Visuospatial skills
   - Clock drawing
   - Scanning and tracking (finding designated letters in a line of letters, finding designated words in sentences)
   - Following written directions (e.g., *Draw two large circles next to each other. Draw a line under both circles.*)

The ENH-RHS is designed to give clinicians a comprehensive picture of cognitive-communicative impairments likely to be experienced by persons with right-hemisphere brain injury. The ENH-RHS may not be practical for quick bedside screening because of its length and the many materials needed for writing and drawing tasks. However, clinicians could shorten the ENH-RHS by administering selected items to identify areas in which a patient is having problems, then test later with more items in the problem areas.

Gordon and associates (1984) described an extensive nonstandardized protocol for evaluation of adults with right-hemisphere brain injury. The protocol provides for assessment of:

- Visual scanning and visual inattention (neglect and visuospatial abilities)
- Activities of daily living skills (arithmetic, reading, and copying)
- Sensorimotor integration (tactile perception, estimation of body midline, and manual dexterity)
- Visual integration (face recognition, visual assembly, figure-ground discrimination, and copying geometric forms)
- Higher cognitive and perceptual functions (verbal and performance subtests from the *Wechsler Adult Intelligence Scale*)
- Linguistic and cognitive flexibility (analogies, auditory comprehension, generative naming, and logical memory)
- Affective state (comprehension of affect, plus depression and mood rating made by the examiner)

Gordon and associates (1984) tested 385 right-hemisphere-injured adults with their protocol, but the number of participants tested differed across subtests. Gordon and associates provide numerous statistics for each subtest. For many subtests the data are subdivided according to patient variables such as age, education, or presence of visual field deficit. Although not standardized, the protocol describes materials and procedures for numerous tests of linguistic, cognitive, perceptual, and affective functions, and it provides a large corpus of data about how adults with right-hemisphere brain injury perform on those tests. It should prove useful to clinicians who are looking for assessment materials or need information about how adults with right-hemisphere brain injury perform on tests such as those in the protocol. The protocol includes some standardized tests as subtests, many of which have been revised since the Gordon and associates report, so the norms provided will not be usable with current versions of the standardized tests (Tompkins, 1995).

Adamovich and Brooks (1981) described a procedure for evaluating the communicative deficits of adults with right-hemisphere brain injury. Their procedure includes tests of auditory comprehension, oral expression, and reading from the *Boston Diagnostic Aphasia Examination* (*BDAE*; Goodglass & Kaplan, 1983); the *Revised Token Test* (McNeil & Prescott, 1978); the *Hooper Visual Organization Test* (Hooper, 1983); the *Boston Naming Test* (*BNT*; Kaplan, Goodglass, & Weintraub, 2001); the *Word Fluency Task* (Borkowski, Benton, & Spreen, 1967); and portions of the verbal absurdities, verbal opposites, and likenesses and differences subtests of the *Detroit Tests of Learning Aptitude—Second Edition* (Hammill, 1985).

The Adamovich and Brooks procedures are unstandardized, do not have adequate norms, and do not have documented reliability or validity. However, they may prove useful as a source of materials and ideas for locally constructed protocols for evaluation of adults with right-hemisphere brain injury.

Tests of Pragmatic Abilities

Right-hemisphere-injured adults' pragmatic abilities typically are assessed with rating scales, not all of which were designed for use with right-hemisphere-injured adults. The RHLB-2 and the RICE-R each contain short scales for rating pragmatic behaviors. The RHLB-2 provides a scale for rating discourse that addresses several categories of pragmatic behavior:

- Supportive routines (e.g., greetings, farewells, thanks)
- Assertive routines (e.g., complaining, demanding, criticizing)

- Formality (formality of language and behavior)
- Turn-taking (taking and yielding the conversational "floor")
- Meshing (pace, timing, and pauses)

The RICE-R scale provides for rating 12 pragmatic behaviors divided among four categories:

1. Nonverbal communication (intonation, facial expression, eye contact, gestures, and movements)
2. Conversational skills (initiation, turn-taking, and verbosity)
3. Use of linguistic context (topic maintenance and presupposition)
4. Referencing skills (organization and completeness of a narrative)

The RHLB-2's coverage of truly pragmatic behaviors is limited. The scale in the RICE-R has enough detail to make it useful as a screening measure or as a quick assessment of changes in pragmatic behaviors as a consequence of treatment.

The *Pragmatic Protocol* (Prutting & Kirchner, 1987), although not designed specifically for adults with right-hemisphere brain injury, permits assessment of conversational behaviors that are likely to be affected by right-hemisphere brain injury.

The *Communicative Effectiveness Index* (*CETI*; Lomas & associates, 1989) is a rating scale for assessing severely aphasic adults' functional communication. The CETI may be useful for rating severely impaired right-hemisphere-injured adults' functional communication, but would not be sensitive to the communicative aberrations of right-hemisphere-injured adults with mild to moderate impairments. The Pragmatic Protocol and the CETI are described in Chapter 5.

Communication Activities in Daily Living—Second Edition (*CADL-2*; Holland, Frattali, & Fromm, 1998), like the CETI, was designed to assess aphasic adults' functional communication, but it may be used to assess the communicative effectiveness of adults with right-hemisphere brain injury. Because CADL-2 samples communicative behavior in a number of contexts other than conversational inter-

actions, using it together with a conversationally oriented instrument such as the Pragmatic Protocol may provide a more comprehensive picture of right-hemisphere-injured adults' pragmatic strengths and weaknesses than use of either instrument by itself. CADL-2 is described in Chapter 6.

Tests of Visual and Spatial Perception, Attention, and Organization

Adults with right-hemisphere brain injury often have difficulty in tasks requiring perception of complex visual stimuli and appreciation of spatial relationships. These difficulties appear to reflect attentional and integrational impairments, such as inattention to visual stimuli (especially on the side contralateral to the patient's brain injury), diminished ability to perceive or discriminate complex stimuli, and inability to integrate or synthesize individual elements of complex visual stimuli into a meaningful whole. Consequently, tests of visual attention and organization are an important part of the assessment protocol for adults who may have right-hemisphere brain injury.

Most tests for visual inattention (neglect) are paper-and-pencil tests. *Cancellation tests* are the most common. The patient is asked to mark, circle, or cross out lines, letters, or symbols (e.g., stars, crosses) printed at various locations on a printed page. Individuals with neglect tend to miss stimuli opposite to the side of their brain injury. Albert's (1973) *Test of Visual Neglect* is typical. The patient is given a sheet of paper on which short lines have been drawn in random locations and is asked to cross out each line. A variation on these simple cancellation tests is provided by the *Bells Test* (Gauthier, Dehaut, & Joanette, 1989). In the Bells Test, the test taker is required to circle drawings of bells that are scattered across the page and interspersed with drawings of other objects. Because test takers must selectively circle only the drawings of bells, the Bells Test is more difficult than straight cancellation tasks and may be a more sensitive

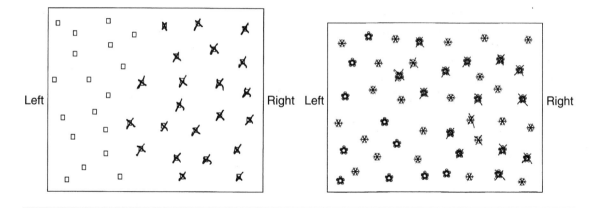

Figure 10-6 ■ A simple cancellation test for neglect *(left)* and a more complex one *(right)* completed by a patient with right-hemisphere brain injury. The patient was instructed to cross out all the boxes on the page on the left and to cross out only the flowers on the page on the right. The patient shows evidence of neglect on both tests. The patient also erroneously crossed out several snowflakes on the page on the right.

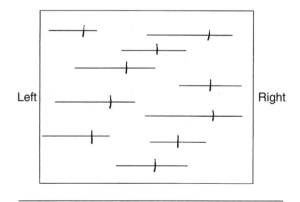

Figure 10-7 ■ A right-hemisphere-injured patient's performance on a line bisection test. The patient's line bisection marks are displaced to the right, toward nonneglected space.

Line bisection tests are another way to test for visual neglect. The patient is given a page on which several horizontal lines of different lengths are printed, and she or he draws a slash on each line to divide it into two equal halves. Individuals with neglect tend to divide the lines so that the segment in the neglected visual field is longer than the segment in the intact field— the bisecting line is displaced into the non-neglected half of the visual field, as in Figure 10-7. Displacement of the patient's dividing mark toward the nonneglected half-field tends to increase as lines move farther into the neglected visual field.

Myers (1999) suggests that the lines in line bisection tasks should be about 1 inch (2.5 cm) long. According to Myers, shorter lines are too easy to bisect, and longer lines create too much variability in non-brain-injured adults' line bisection performance to make them a reasonable test for right-hemisphere-injured adults.

test of inattention than straight cancellation tasks (Gauthier & associates, 1989).

Figure 10-6 *(left)* shows a simple cancellation test in which a patient with left neglect was asked to cross out small squares. Figure 10-6 *(right)* shows a more complex cancellation test in which a patient with left neglect was asked to cross out flowers and ignore snowflakes.

Copying and drawing tests are yet another way to test for visual neglect. The patient is given a drawing to copy. Often the drawing

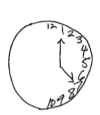 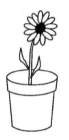 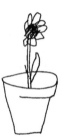

Figure 10-8 ■ A clock face drawn from memory and a flower copied by a patient with right-hemisphere brain injury and neglect.

is of a symmetrical object with (more-or-less) mirror image properties on each side of the midline (e.g., a clock face, a daisy, or a human figure). Individuals with neglect tend to leave out details on the side of the drawing contralateral to their brain injury (Figure 10-8). Myers (1999) recommends that drawings used to test neglect should have a midline with an equal number of objects on each side of the midline and an equal number of lines on the left and right sides of each object.

In *drawing from memory tests* the patient is asked to draw familiar objects or simple scenes from memory. Individuals with neglect tend to leave out details on the side of the drawing contralateral to their brain injury (Figure 10-9).

Scanning tests are another way to test for visual neglect. The patient is given a page on which a horizontal array of numbers, letters, or (less frequently) objects is printed, and the patient is asked to circle or cross out every occurrence of a target item (e.g., all occurrences of the letter *B* in a line of randomly arranged alphabet letters). Scanning tests resemble cancellation tests, except that in scanning tests the stimuli are in horizontal linear arrays rather than random arrays, and in scanning tests there are more distractors (stimuli not to be marked).

Horner, Massey, Woodruff, Chase, and Dawson (1989) suggested that it may take more than one test of neglect to identify neglect in many right-hemisphere-injured adults' test performance.

They administered tests of line bisection, drawing from memory, copying simple drawings, reading, and writing to 106 adults with right-hemisphere brain injury and reported that no single test identified the presence of neglect in all who had neglect.

Myers (1999) concurs, and she recommends that combinations of neglect tests be administered to ensure that if neglect is present it will be detected. She also suggests that a patient's combined score on several tests of neglect may

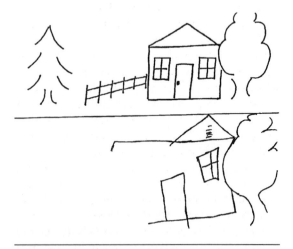

Figure 10-9 ■ A scene copied by a patient with right-hemisphere brain injury and neglect. The stimulus drawing is on top, and the patient's reproduction is on the bottom. (Courtesy of Penelope Myers, Ph.D.)

give the best estimate of the overall severity of neglect. Myers recommends the following combination of tasks for assessing neglect:

- A simple cancellation task
- Copying a drawing
- Drawing from memory (e.g., a clock, a human figure)
- Line bisection

Myers recommends calculating a left-right ratio for each test. The ratio is calculated by dividing the number of elements missed in the left half of visual space by the number of elements missed in the right half of visual space. According to Myers, ratios greater than 1.0 denote the presence of left neglect, with larger ratios denoting more severe neglect.

The *Behavioural Inattention Test* (*BIT*; Wilson, Cockburn, & Halligan, 1987) is a standardized test battery for assessing neglect. It is unique among neglect tests in its inclusion of subtests to assess performance in daily life activities that might be affected by neglect (e.g., reading maps, dialing telephones, or reading menus and newspaper articles), in addition to traditional paper-and-pencil tests. The BIT includes six "conventional" paper-and-pencil subtests (line crossing, letter cancellation, star cancellation, figure and shape copying, line bisection, and representational drawing) and nine "behavioral" subtests (picture scanning, telephone dialing, menu reading, article reading, map reading, address and sentence copying, coin sorting, card sorting, telling time, and setting time). The BIT was normed on 54 adults with right-hemisphere strokes, 26 adults with left-hemisphere strokes, and 50 non-brain-damaged adults.

Several studies have attempted to determine which neglect tests are most sensitive to the presence of neglect. Jehkonen and associates (2000) reported little difference in sensitivity between the conventional and behavioral sections of the BIT. Each identified about the same proportion of persons with neglect in a group of adults with right-hemisphere brain injuries. (However, a few exhibited neglect in the conventional section but not in the behavioral sec-

tion, and a few others exhibited neglect in the behavioral section but not in the conventional section.)

Letter cancellation and star cancellation appear to be the most sensitive individual BIT subtests. Halligan, Marshall, and Wade (1989) found star cancellation to be the most sensitive BIT subtest. Performance on star cancellation correctly identified all patients whose overall BIT score fell below that of a non-brain-injured control group. Halligan, Wilson, and Cockburn (1990) reported that letter cancellation and star cancellation correctly identified 74% of neglect patients with no false positives. They commented that "letter and star cancellation offer an adequate yet brief screening test for determining which patients might benefit from administration of the complete test battery" (p. 99). Cherney and Halper (2001) noted that the behavioral subtests in the BIT take about 45 minutes to administer, whereas the conventional subtests (that include letter cancellation and star cancellation) take about 10 minutes to administer (Figure 10-10). They commented: "With the current constraints placed on the time that can be spent evaluating patients, the practicing clinician may need to administer only the conventional subtests to identify neglect" (p. 590).

Ferber and Karnath (2001) found that three cancellation tests (bells, letters, and stars) were more sensitive to neglect than a line-crossing test. They reported that bell cancellation or letter cancellation tests missed about 6% of persons with neglect, whereas the line-crossing test missed about 30%. (Ferber and Karnath defined neglect as missing at least 15% of items in four cancellation tasks.)

Mattingly and associates (1994) proposed a *greyscales task* as a measure of attentional bias following unilateral brain injury. The task requires participants to judge which of two mirror-image brightness gradients appears darker. One gradient is shaded from black to white; the other is shaded in reverse (Figure 10-11). Mattingley and associates (2004)

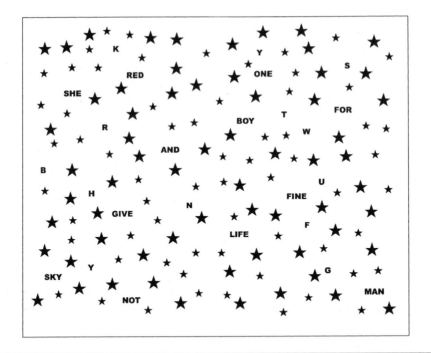

Figure 10-10 ■ A cancellation task similar to the star cancellation task in the *Behavioural Inattention Test* (Wilson, Cockburn, & Halligan, 1987). The test taker is instructed to cross out all the large stars or all the small stars.

reported that the greyscales task is a sensitive measure of attentional bias (e.g., inattention, neglect) in vision and recommend it as an easily administered and efficient way of quantifying attentional bias in studies of recovery and rehabilitation following stroke.

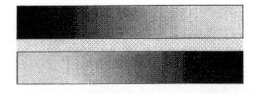

Figure 10-11 ■ Sample stimuli from the greyscales task. The two bars are the same in overall brightness. (From Mattingly, J.B., Berberovic, N., Corben, L., et al. [2004]. The greyscales task: A perceptual measure of attentional bias following unilateral hemispheric damage. *Neuropsychologia, 42,* 387-394.)

Tests of Component Attentional Processes

Although attentional processes implicitly are tested in many of the tests previously described, clinicians sometimes supplement them with tests that assess specific attentional processes in more detail. These supplemental tests may include tests of visual or auditory sustained attention, selective attention, alternating attention, or divided attention. These tests of attention are described in Chapter 4.

Tests of Visual Organization

Tests of visual organization may require the patient to identify drawings of objects with missing elements, identify drawings of fragmented objects, or discriminate pictured objects

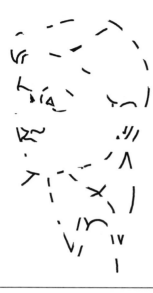

Figure 10-12 ■ An example of an incomplete-figures test item.

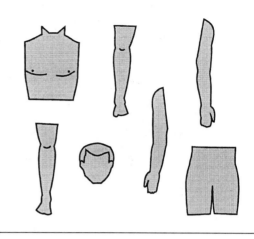

Figure 10-13 ■ An example of an object assembly test item. The components of the figure are made of heavy paperboard or fiberboard. The test taker assembles them as he or she would assemble a jigsaw puzzle.

from a background. Figure 10-12 shows an example of a test item with missing elements. Figure 10-13 shows an example of a drawing in which a common object has been fragmented and the parts rearranged to disguise their identity.

Tests with fragmented stimuli usually are more sensitive to visual organization impairments than tests with incomplete stimuli (Lezak, 1995). The *Object Assembly* subtest of the *Wechsler Adult Intelligence Scale (WAIS;* Wechsler, 1981) requires identification of fragmented visual stimuli, as does the Hooper Visual Organization Test. In the WAIS Object Assembly subtest, the patient is given cut-up pressboard figures of familiar objects (a human figure, a human head in profile, a hand, or an elephant) and is asked to assemble them. In the Hooper test, the patient is presented with a series of pictures depicting cut-up line drawings of common objects and is asked to say or write the name of the object depicted in each item.

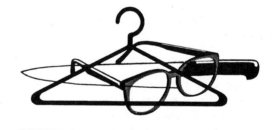

Figure 10-14 ■ An example of an overlapping figures test item.

Visual figure-ground tests contain stimuli in which test figures are embedded in more complex figures (as in the *Hidden Figures Test;* Thurstone, 1944), stimuli in which test figures overlap (Poppelreuter, 1917), stimuli in which lines are drawn over test figures, or stimuli in which test figures are partially occluded by masks (Luria, 1965). Figures 10-14, 10-15, and 10-16 are examples of items in visual figure-ground tests.

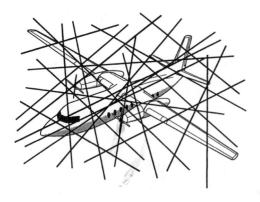

Figure 10-15 ■ An example of a figure-ground test item in which lines have been drawn over the test stimulus.

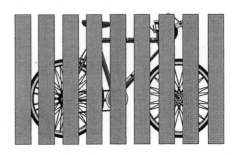

Figure 10-16 ■ An example of a figure-ground test item in which the test stimulus is partially occluded by a mask.

GENERAL CONCEPTS 10-2

- Several communicative impairments may follow right-hemisphere brain injury:
  - Diminished speech prosody and reductions in movements that accompany speech
  - Excessive, confabulatory, tangential, and sometimes inappropriate connected speech
  - Impaired comprehension of narratives and conversations attributable to insensitivity to relationships, premature assumptions, failing to judge the appropriateness of events and situations, and failing to appreciate implied meanings
  - Pragmatic impairments related to turn-taking, topic maintenance, social conventions, and eye contact
- Brownell and his associates suggest that right-hemisphere-injured patients' difficulties in comprehending discourse arise because they make spur-of-the-moment incorrect inferences and cannot abandon them when subsequent information shows the inferences to be erroneous.
- Tompkins and her associates have offered a *suppression deficit hypothesis,* which sug-

gests that right-hemisphere-damaged adults cannot suppress initially activated assumptions or inferences that are later shown to be inappropriate or irrelevant, to account for right-hemisphere-damaged adults' impaired discourse comprehension.
- Brownell and his associates have suggested that right-hemisphere-damaged adults' impaired discourse comprehension may be caused by impaired *theory of mind*—the ability to appreciate the content of other people's minds (their knowledge, intents, and emotions).
- Several standardized and nonstandardized tests for measuring cognitive and communicative impairments of patients with right-hemisphere brain injury are available and may provide an overview of a right-hemisphere-damaged patient's communicative and cognitive strengths and weaknesses. Detailed assessment often requires administration of supplemental tests of pragmatics, communication, visuospatial abilities, and attention.

GENERAL CONCEPTS 10-2—cont'd

- Right-hemisphere-damaged adults' pragmatic abilities typically are assessed with rating scales. Some rating scales are part of larger test batteries for assessing right-hemisphere-damaged adults such as the *Right Hemisphere Language Battery* or the *Rehabilitation Institute of Chicago Evaluation of Communicative Problems in Right-Hemisphere Dysfunction*. Others are free-standing rating scales such as the *Pragmatic Protocol* or the *Communicative Effectiveness Index*, which are not designed exclusively for right-hemisphere-damaged adults.
- The presence and severity of neglect may be assessed with cancellation tests, line bisection tests, copying and drawing tests, or scanning tests. A combination of several tests may be required to detect subtle signs of neglect.
- The *Behavioural Inattention Test* is designed to measure the effects of neglect on everyday activities.
- Comprehensive assessment of right-hemisphere-damaged adults' attentional abilities requires assessment of sustained attention, selective attention, alternating attention, and divided attention.
- Right-hemisphere-damaged adults' visual organization may be assessed with tests that require them to identify incomplete or fragmented visual stimuli or to discriminate visual stimuli from a background.

INTERVENTION

We know less about clinical intervention with right-hemisphere-injured adults than we do about intervention with left-hemisphere-injured (aphasic) adults, in part because the communication impairments of right-hemisphere-injured adults largely were unrecognized and untreated until about 20 years ago, and in part because focal right-hemisphere brain injury produces more diffuse effects than focal left-hemisphere injury. Consequently, identifiable and treatable right-hemisphere syndromes are not as well described as left-hemisphere aphasic syndromes.

Within the last few years a treatment literature on right-hemisphere-injured adults has begun to develop, although most is anecdote and opinion, without much empiric support. Nevertheless, we now know that many right-hemisphere-injured adults exhibit communicative impairments that can be objectively described and that treatment can help at least some of them. However, there are several major differences between right-hemisphere-injured adults and left-hemisphere-injured aphasic adults that affect both the nature of treatment and its probable outcome. These differences largely are attributable to the fact that left-hemisphere brain injury tends to produce focal effects on specific linguistic and communicative abilities, whereas right-hemisphere brain injury tends to produce diffuse effects that are not readily reducible to specific linguistic or communicative abilities.

Communicative impairments of adults with left-hemisphere injuries are relatively discrete and can be classified and quantified with reasonable reliability, because the communicative missteps of adults with left-hemisphere injuries are obvious and can be counted (e.g., misnaming pictures, missing the last two parts of a three-part command). The relationships between left-hemisphere-injured adults' performance on diagnostic tests and underlying cognitive or linguistic impairments tend to be straightforward (e.g., the relationship between errors on tests of confrontation naming and impaired word retrieval).

In contrast, the communicative impairments of adults with right-hemisphere brain injury are less discrete and tend to be less amenable to simple counts of errors, because they represent more diffuse failures, such as treating serious situations as humorous or failing to follow conversational rules. The relationships between right-hemisphere-injured adults' performance on diagnostic tests and underlying cognitive or linguistic impairments are less straightforward and require more assumptions (e.g., the relationship between misinterpretation of idioms or metaphors and failure to make inferences).

Criteria for what constitutes normal performance are better defined for the impairments of adults with left-hemisphere brain injury and aphasia than for adults with right-hemisphere brain injury. Reasonably comprehensive and valid norms for communicative abilities such as listening comprehension, reading comprehension, vocabulary, naming, and speech production (likely to be affected by left-hemisphere brain injury) are available, but similar norms are not available for most of the cognitive and communicative abilities likely to be affected by right-hemisphere brain injury. The clinician's intuition, judgment, and consultation with patient, family, and caregivers often replace standardized norms in determining what is "normal" for a particular patient when the focus is on pragmatic appropriateness, conversational style, appreciation of nonliteral material, and the like.

Treatment of right-hemisphere-injured adults' communication impairments may target a variety of deficits affecting receptive and expressive aspects of communication—difficulty organizing and synthesizing information, difficulty separating what is important from what is not, inability to use contextual cues to ascertain meanings, interpreting figurative language literally, overpersonalization, reduced sensitivity to pragmatic or extralinguistic aspects of communication, or tangentiality and excessive detail in speech. Right-hemisphere-injured adults' communicative impairments often are magnified by cognitive and behavioral abnormalities such as denial of illness, indifference to or denial of impairments, distractibility, inattention, impulsivity, or impaired reasoning and problem-solving.

Cognitive and Behavioral Abnormalities

Denial of Impairments. Denial of physical, cognitive, or communicative impairments can be an important obstacle to the success of intervention with right-hemisphere-injured adults. Many adults with right-hemisphere brain injury seem insensitive to the presence of impairments or minimize their severity. Most become less oblivious to impairments as they recover neurologically, but some remain indifferent or oblivious for months or years, putting them at risk when denial combines with poor judgment about daily life activities such as driving, hunting, or solo trekking.

Most right-hemisphere-injured adults are compliant and willingly participate in treatment programs, although their participation is likely to be more passive than active. If asked to participate in making decisions about the content and focus of treatment, they often talk a good game but fail in follow-through. They tend to not do more than is specifically required. Homework assignments may be neglected unless someone provides supervision and direction. When confronted with their failure to carry out assignments, they may confabulate or offer implausible reasons for not doing the assignments, as in the following interaction.

A right-hemisphere-injured patient is taking a written spelling test. The clinician gets the patient started and watches as the patient completes the first 10 of 30 items in the test:

Clinician: You're doing fine, Mrs. Perkins. Do you think you can finish by yourself?

Patient: Of course I can. This is not really very hard, after all.

Clinician: O.K. I'll come back in about 10 minutes and see how you're doing.

(Leaves; 10 minutes later the clinician returns and looks at the test.)

Clinician: What happened? You're still on number 10.

Patient: Well, for goodness sake. You left, you know.

Clinician: But you said you could finish by yourself.

Patient: When you left, you didn't say anything about me going on. So I assumed that we'd finished this. Are we finished, or not?

Tompkins (1995) asserts that right-hemisphere-injured adults who are unaware of poor performance and unconcerned about impairments are poor treatment candidates, and recommends that treatment be deferred until denial resolves. Tompkins suggests that the clinician may establish baselines, identify impairments, and select potential treatment approaches while waiting for denial to resolve. For patients who are neurologically recovered but who remain indifferent to impairments, Tompkins recommends simplifying treatment goals, modifying the patient's living environment to limit the negative effects of indifference, and teaching compensatory strategies to family members and associates.

Clinicians may structure treatment activities to compensate for the effects of denial by keeping activities highly structured, clearly defining treatment goals, and communicating treatment goals to the patient and family. Indifference sometimes can be treated indirectly in the context of activities directed toward other goals, by giving the patient immediate feedback after erroneous or inappropriate responses, by supportively challenging the patient when she or he denies errors, and by improving the patient's self-monitoring, first in highly structured activities and later in less structured activities.

Clinicians may directly work on indifference by having the patient (or the patient and family) collaborate in making a list of the patient's strengths and weaknesses. Entries in the list then may be selected for attention in treatment. Videotaping treatment activities and reviewing them with the patient may improve a patient's awareness of errors and inappropriate responses. For patients with extreme denial, the clinician and patient may watch and talk about videotapes of social interactions or staged interactions in which one participant makes errors or inappropriate responses resembling those made by the patient. When the patient becomes adept at identifying errors and inappropriate responses in the behavior of others, videotapes in which the patient is a participant may be introduced.

Many right-hemisphere-injured adults who deny their own errors are quick to spot errors when others make them.

Finally, a few words of caution. Many right-hemisphere-injured adults can, with help, make lists of mistakes and inappropriate behaviors, talk constructively about the lists, and even identify errors and inappropriate responses in carefully structured treatment activities, then fail to anticipate them or do anything about them either in less structured treatment activities or in daily life. The transition from identifying and talking about erroneous or inappropriate responses to doing something about them may be arduous, requiring carefully programmed generalization procedures and the active participation of the patient's family and daily life associates. Family members and caregivers must play active roles in treatment programs for patients with denial to ensure that the patient, caregivers, and family understand the relationship between treatment activities and goals, to ensure that homework assignments are completed, and to facilitate transfer of treatment gains from the clinic to the patient's daily life.

Attentional Impairments and Distractibility. Tompkins (1995) commented that attentional impairments may cause or exacerbate communication problems for individuals with right-hemisphere brain injury. According to Tompkins, *sustained attention* is crucial for comprehension and production of discourse, and *selective attention* is crucial for making sense of printed texts, establishing referential relationships, and making inferences. Tompkins comments that attention is important in daily life for keeping track of plots in movies and television shows, revising misinterpretations, and resisting distractions. She suggests that working on attentional processes may provide a greater clinical payoff than working on their surface behavioral manifestations.

Treatment of attentional impairments takes many forms, ranging from paper-and-pencil or computer-presented attention drills to activities requiring patients to focus and maintain attention in natural contexts. A sampling of these activities follows.

Sustained Attention. Drills to improve sustained attention range from paper-and-pencil tasks such as letter cancellation and mazes to vigilance drills that require the patient to monitor a visual display or strings of auditory stimuli and signal when a target stimulus occurs. The easiest visual and auditory sustained attention tasks are those in which a single target stimulus appears against a constant background. Increasing the time between stimuli, making the intervals between stimuli less predictable, and increasing the overall duration of the task make sustained attention tasks more difficult.

Auditory sustained attention may be addressed by drills in which the patient listens for designated targets in lists of letters, numbers, or words read aloud by the clinician and signals each time he or she hears a target. The difficulty of such tasks may be adjusted by manipulating the number of items between targets, manipulating the frequency with which targets occur, or manipulating the acoustic or semantic similarity between target and non-target stimuli.

The *starry night task* (Rizzo & Robin, 1990) is a computerized visual sustained attention task that permits adjustment across a wide range of task difficulty. A pattern of dots that resembles a starry night sky appears on the monitor screen within which dots appear and disappear unpredictably. The patient presses a key when he or she sees a dot appear or disappear. The computer keeps a record of hits, misses, and reaction times. The density of the dots, the rate at which they appear or disappear, and the duration of the task can be adjusted to manipulate task difficulty.

Paper-and-pencil sustained attention tasks are less challenging than computerized tasks, because paper-and-pencil tasks do not require a constant level of sustained attention. Patients can minimize errors by slowing down or stopping when attention lags and resuming the task when attention recovers. This strategy diminishes errors but adds to the time it takes the patient to finish the task.

Patients with attentional impairments often do well at the beginning of sustained-attention tasks, but performance deteriorates as the task progresses and the load on sustained attention increases.

Selective Attention. Treatment of selective attention typically relies on drills in which the patient performs sustained-attention tasks in the presence of competing or distracting stimuli—for example, performing a sustained-attention task with a tape recording of distracting sounds (e.g., conversations, popular music) playing in the background. Distractors that the patient is likely to encounter in daily life (e.g., conversations, commercials, announcements) may enhance generalization of improved selective attention to the patient's daily life.

Tasks such as the Stroop task (see Chapter 4) in which a patient must inhibit a habitual or automatic response in favor of a clinician-defined response (e.g., reading aloud color words printed in colors that conflict with the words, telling the size of the words *large* and *small* printed in type sizes that conflict with the words) are more difficult selective-attention tasks that may be useful for patients who have moderately impaired selective attention, but these tasks may be too difficult for patients with more severe impairments.

Alternating Attention. Almost any sustained-attention task can be modified to make an alternating attention task by periodically changing stimulus characteristics or response requirements. For example, a patient might practice shifting attention from one conversational partner to another in recorded conversational interactions. Alternating-attention tasks also can be created by combining two tasks and alternately switching between them. For example, a patient might alternate between a paper-and-pencil sustained-attention task and a conversational interaction. Alternating-attention tasks also can be created by periodically changing response requirements. For example, a patient might alternate between adding and subtracting strings of numbers spoken by the clinician as the clinician says *add* or *subtract*.

Divided Attention. Tompkins (1995) commented that one objective of divided-attention treatment for patients with right-hemisphere brain injury is to give them training in volitional allocation of mental resources. According to Tompkins such training is necessary, because some patients with right-hemisphere brain injury cannot tell which aspects of a task are most important and should get the most attention. Tompkins recommends training such patients to analyze tasks and decide which aspects are most important, then to practice volitional allocation of attention in the tasks. Executive function tasks such as those in the *Six Elements Test,* the *Behavioural Assessment of Disexecutive Function Test,* the *Multiple Errands Task,* and the *Executive Route-Finding Task* (see Chapter 4) may prove useful in training right-hemisphere-injured adults in task analysis and allocation of resources.

There is no strong empiric evidence that right-hemisphere-injured adults' improved performance on attention drills generalizes to everyday contexts, although anecdotal reports suggest that such generalization occurs, at least for some. Clinicians may enhance generalization by working on attention in contexts similar to those the patient will encounter in daily life. Group sessions may provide a naturalistic context for such work. Group participants may engage in conversational interactions in which they must maintain eye contact, stay on topic, respond appropriately to changes in topic, and get and retain a reasonable amount of specific information. As group members become adept at meeting their personal goals in group activities, noise, movement, or interruptions may be introduced to simulate intrusions of daily life and to increase participants' ability to resist the effects of such intrusions.

Impulsivity. Impulsivity compromises many right-hemisphere-injured patients' performance in treatment and complicates their daily life. A treatment session with a right-hemisphere-injured patient can be trying for the clinician. The patient responds before the clinician finishes delivering task instructions or stimuli, interrupts with tangential and irrelevant comments, begins tasks before he or she understands what is expected, and stops working before completing assignments. Daily life can be trying for families and caregivers of a right-hemisphere-injured patient. The patient fails to anticipate the demands and risks of common daily life activities, takes on tasks and enters situations that are beyond his or her abilities, starts but fails to complete projects, engages in socially inappropriate behavior, and misconstrues messages, events, and situations.

Treatment of impulsivity can be arduous. Some right-hemisphere-injured patients' impulsiveness may be inhibited by providing distinctive *stop* and *go* signals (e.g., a signal light, the clinician's hand gestures). A patient may be taught to monitor a clinician-controlled signal light as an indicator of when they are permitted to respond. When the patient's responses are controlled by the light, the clinician may substitute hand gestures to signify *stop* and *go*. When the patient's impulsive responses are controlled by the hand gestures, the clinician may substitute head shakes and head nods as *stop* and *go* signals. As the clinician's head movements gain control of the patient's impulsive responses, the head movements may be replaced by patient self-cueing.

Impaired Reasoning and Problem-Solving.
Right-hemisphere-injured patients' impaired
reasoning and problem-solving can have important effects on the course and outcome of treatment. Right-hemisphere-injured patients tend
to get lost in the details of activities and lose
track of general goals and objectives. They
are poor at anticipating when a task is likely to
give them trouble, and when they get into trouble, their responses are likely to be impulsive,
inappropriate, and ineffective. These patients'
impaired reasoning and problem-solving makes
them of little help to the clinician in deciding on
treatment objectives and choosing the ways in
which the objectives are to be reached.

Treatment of reasoning and problem-solving
impairments may require structured practice in
a variety of tasks requiring reasoning, foresight,
and problem-solving (e.g., role-playing activities
in which problem-solving skills are needed,
such as getting a refund for defective merchan-
dise); proposing solutions to problems posed by
the clinician (e.g., *You are at a shopping mall
and you come upon a 3-year-old boy standing
alone and crying. What would you do?*);
and planning activities such as vacations, field
trips, and picnics. A prescriptive and structured
approach to problem-solving such as the following may help right-hemisphere-injured patients
get started:

- Identify the problem
- Think of several possible solutions
- Evaluate the feasibility and potential conse-
  quences of each solution
- Choose the best solution
- Apply it
- Evaluate the results

With extended practice, some right-
hemisphere-injured patients can move away
from such a highly structured and prescriptive
problem-solving strategy toward a less formal
and less laborious strategy, but few progress
to the point at which problem-solving becomes
automatic and instinctive.

Communicative Impairments

Affective Communication and Prosody.
Some persons who have right-hemisphere brain
injuries do not comprehend or communicate
emotion conveyed by speech, facial expression,
and body language. Several attempts to treat
these affective impairments have been reported
in the literature. Impaired comprehension of
emotion typically is treated by showing patients
pictures of faces expressing various emotions or
playing tape-recorded voices expressing various
emotions and training patients to identify the
emotions portrayed. Expression of emotion typically is addressed by having the patient imitate
the clinician's tone of voice, facial expression,
and body language as the clinician portrays various emotions. The clinician's models gradually
are faded and replaced by (1) photographs of
faces portraying emotions or (2) cards on which
the names of emotions are printed.

Leon, Rosenbek, Crucian, and associates
(2005) reported a single-case design study of
two treatments (*imitative treatment* and *cognitive-linguistic treatment*) for expressive aprosodia. Both treatments followed a six-step cueing
procedure in which maximal cueing was provided in the first step and systematically diminished in following steps. In the first steps of
imitative treatment the clinician read aloud sentences conveying a targeted emotion, and the
patient attempted to say the sentence using
the same emotional tone of voice. In later steps,
the clinician's model was gradually faded until the
patient independently produced sentences with
the appropriate emotional tone of voice. In the
first step of *cognitive-linguistic treatment* the
patient was given cards on which were printed
an emotion name, the vocal characteristics of
that emotional tone of voice, and a picture of a
face showing the emotion. Then the clinician
trained the patient to produce designated emotions based on the information on the cards. In
later steps the cards gradually were removed
until the patient produced the emotions without reference to the cards.

Three participants who exhibited expressive aprosodia following right-hemisphere strokes were trained on nine sentences (three each of happy, sad, and angry). All three showed positive effects of both treatments, with no generalization to sentences conveying an untreated emotion (fear). The authors suggested that additional study of expressive aprosodia with more participants is needed to determine the relative effects of imitative and cognitive-linguistic treatment, the relationship of expressive aprosodia to receptive impairments, and the ecologic validity of the two treatments. They also commented that the results are the first empiric evidence that affective aprosodia may be amenable to behavioral treatment.

Reading. Visual neglect is a common treatment target for right-hemisphere-injured patients, because neglect compromises their ability to read and comprehend printed materials in daily life. Several procedures for getting patients with left neglect to attend to the left side of printed texts (called *scanning training*) have been described in the literature. Most employ markers such as colored vertical lines, colored dots, or rulers placed at the left margin of printed material. Patients are instructed when they begin to read a line of text to scan leftward until they see the marker. Sometimes patients are instructed to keep one finger on the marker and to scan back to it when beginning each line of text. Patients' reliance on the markers gradually is reduced by making the markers less salient and by eventually substituting the patient's monitoring of whether the material makes sense for the external markers.

Scanning training using visual cues or patient-initiated reminders has had limited success in getting patients to generalize the training to daily life. Patients usually learn to scan to the left in training but fail to incorporate scanning into daily life activities. However, Pizzamiglio, Antonucci, Judica, and associates (1992) trained patients who had neglect to look to the left as they engaged in daily life activities such as read-ing, writing, and eating. Following training, Pizzamiglio and associates' patients as a group improved their leftward scanning in daily life, although some participants failed to generalize the effects of the training.

Diller and Weinberg (1977) described a treatment program for training persons with visual neglect to scan both sides of visual space. Participants practiced activities such as visually tracking a moving target across both visual fields, detecting flashing lights at various locations in both visual fields, letter cancellation across both visual fields, and reading printed paragraphs projected on a wall to span both visual fields. Diller and Weinberg's program was designed to make patients aware of their neglect, induce them to search for visual stimuli systematically, and to make visual scanning automatic by massed repetition.

Stanton and associates (1981) described a comprehensive approach to treating neglect in reading. Their program includes several tasks designed to enhance patients' awareness of and attention to neglected space. In one task, patients match printed letters, numbers, and words from a column in the right visual field to numbers, letters, and words printed in a column in the left visual field. In another task they read aloud printed sentences. The first sentences are in large print with large blank spaces between sentences. The print size and spacing between words gradually are reduced until the patient is reading single-spaced small-print sentences. In another task, patients read printed paragraphs aloud, progressing from paragraphs printed in large letters with double spacing between lines to standard books, magazines, and newspapers, some in double-column format.

Stanton and associates use verbal cues to remind patients to attend to the left side of materials. They begin by instructing the patient (e.g., *Tell yourself out loud—look to the left.*) at the end of each line, and progress to patient-initiated verbal cues (e.g., training the patient to vocalize or subvocalize *look to the left* at the end of each line). As the patient becomes adept at attending to left-side space, she or he is trained to think *look to the left* instead of saying it aloud. Stanton and associates recommend that clinicians take advantage of right-hemisphere-injured patients' good verbal skills by having them ask themselves, *Does that make sense?* at the end of each sentence or periodically while they read.

Myers (1999) comments that visual cues on the left are of little use if the patient's gaze is fixed to the right. She recommends the use of *process-oriented tasks* to mobilize volitional attention and to stimulate unconscious perception of leftward information. Myers suggests that the most effective techniques for treating neglect are those in which patients internalize the need to look to the left rather than depending on external cues or self-cueing. The materials and tasks in process-oriented training simulate materials and tasks the patient is likely to encounter in daily life, and the emphasis is on increasing the patient's attention to left hemispace with materials that encourage leftward search.

Myers and Mackisack (1990) describe one such procedure. The procedure is built around two techniques, called *edgeness* and *bookness*. The *edgeness technique* requires the use of a work space (a rectangular board or grid) with a raised border. First the patient becomes familiar with the spatial boundaries of the work space by tracing its perimeter with a finger. Then the clinician distributes colored cubes about the work space. The patient is told how many cubes are on the work space and that she or he is to find and remove all of them. The clinician does not tell the patient where to look, but simply encourages her or him to continue until all the cubes are found and removed. The difficulty of the task is determined by the number of cubes (increasing their number increases difficulty), their placement (placing more cubes in neglected space increases difficulty), and the presence of foils (adding cubes of different colors, only one of which is to

be removed, increases difficulty). To extend improved scanning from this task to other tasks, Myers and Mackisack suggest that patients be encouraged to extend the edgeness technique to other tasks by tracing the boundaries of other common work surfaces such as writing tablets and books.

The *bookness technique* resembles the edgeness technique but is specific to reading. First the patient orally describes a closed book placed at his or her visual midline, then traces its perimeter with a finger. Next the patient opens and describes the book while tracing its perimeter. Next the patient carries out activities printed in the book, beginning with matching tasks that require the patient to match stimuli on the left and right pages of the book. The patient traces the perimeter of the book before each trial. The clinician increases the difficulty of the reading tasks by increasing the number of stimuli and adding foils. As the patient's attention to the left side of the book improves, the requirement that the patient trace the perimeter of the book fades.

Myers (1994) claims two advantages for the edgeness and bookness techniques. First, they teach the patient to search to the left without external cues, which increases the likelihood of generalization to other tasks. Second, they maximize the patient's overall level of attention, which may generalize to other treatment tasks.

Myers (1999) suggests that manipulating the meaningfulness of the right and left sides of printed materials may help neglect patients attend to the left side of the materials. To encourage leftward search, information that permits interpretation of printed materials should be distributed from left to right so that the patient must attend to the left side to make sense of the material. This means that lists of single words should be controlled so that reading only the right half of the words does not yield a real word. Words such as *cavalry, lemonade,* and *conversation* encourage leftward search; words such as *pancake, everything,* and *sunset* do not.

The characteristics of printed sentences may be manipulated in similar fashion to encourage leftward search. A sentence such as: *George hid the key to his aunt's house under a rock.* does not yield a complete sentence without the information provided by the words on the left. In contrast, a sentence such as: *When she saw the rattlesnake in the garage, Emma screamed and ran to the phone to call 911.* yields a complete sentence without the eight words on the left. (Long sentences make it more likely that a patient with neglect will see only right-side words.)

Myers (1999) also suggests that stimulus arrays in which items are physically linked are more likely to encourage leftward search than stimulus arrays in which items are separate. Linked or overlapping geometric figures (Figure 10-17, *B*) are more likely to encourage leftward search than are geometric figures with space between them (Figure 10-17, *A*). Geometric figures whose physical characteristics (e.g., size, color, orientation) create a consistent left-to-right pattern encourage leftward search to complete the pattern (Figure 10-17, *C*). Human or animal figures that are physically connected (e.g., one person handing something to another) are more likely to encourage leftward search than figures with space between them (Figure 10-17, *D*).

Several writers have suggested that neglect patients' performance on tests of left neglect may be improved by requiring them to perform left-limb movements in left hemispace before tests of neglect are administered (Halligan, Manning, & Marshall, 1991; Joanette, Brouchon, Cauthier, & Samson, 1986). Several explanations have been offered for this phenomenon, including increased activation of the right hemisphere, visual cueing toward left hemispace, and motor cueing toward left hemispace. At present no one knows how long the facilitating effects of left-limb movements last, or whether they affect neglect in tasks other than those used to test neglect. Myers (1999) suggests priming attention to left hemispace by requiring

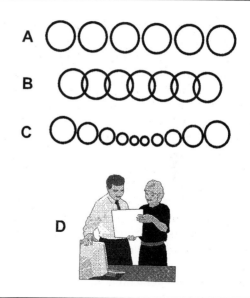

Figure 10-17 ■ Geometric figures in which connected elements (**B**) are more likely to encourage leftward search than figures with unconnected elements (**A**). Geometric figures that form a left-to-right pattern (**C**) also encourage leftward search. Human or animal figures that overlap or interact (**D**) encourage leftward search.

that the patient perform purposeful left-limb movements such as tracing the border of the workspace with the left hand, moving the left arm up and down, or tapping with the left foot before starting tasks requiring attention to left hemispace. Robertson and North (1993) have asserted, however, that passive limb movements have no effect on neglect. Many patients with right-hemisphere brain injury have paralyzed left limbs, making it impossible to prime attention to left hemispace by means of left-limb movements.

Improving right-hemisphere-injured adults' level of overall attention is thought by some writers to have positive effects on their neglect. Myers (1994) suggests that treatment for neglect include tasks to increase right-hemisphere-injured patients' level of arousal, their capacity to sustain attention, and their capacity to selectively attend to some stimuli while ignoring others. Many models of neglect give a prominent role to attentional abnormalities. Therefore, indirectly treating neglect by directly treating attention seems reasonable, but the relationship between attention and neglect awaits empiric verification.

Pragmatics. Most who write about treating right-hemisphere-injured patients' pragmatic impairments recommend enlisting their preserved verbal skills. Treatment of pragmatic impairments often requires clinician coaching and clinician-patient strategy development alternating with structured practice. Videotapes of structured practice may provide feedback to patients regarding their pragmatic behavior in conversational interactions and may serve as a record of patients' progress or lack thereof in increasing their pragmatic appropriateness. Such treatment often progresses as follows.

At the beginning of treatment, one or more 15- to 20-minute conversations between the patient and another person (the clinician or someone chosen by the clinician and patient) are recorded on videotape. These videotapes provide baseline measures of the patient's conversational behaviors.

After the baseline videotapes are made, the clinician leads the patient through a short general discussion of language pragmatics, focusing on what language pragmatics are and how pragmatic behaviors function to maintain and regulate communication. The clinician and patient view several videotapes of conversations not involving the patient (e.g., television talk shows, excerpts from movies, or videotapes made for this purpose). As they view the videotapes, they evaluate the occurrence and appropriateness of pragmatic behaviors, with special attention to violations of pragmatic rules and social conventions, (e.g., interruptions, tangentiality, and monopolizing the conversation).

When the patient can reliably identify violations of pragmatic rules and social conventions in these videotapes, the clinician and patient view the baseline videotape(s) and identify the patient's appropriate and inappropriate pragmatic behaviors and his or her adherence to or violations of social conventions. Then they select behaviors to be addressed in treatment. They formulate immediate and long-term goals and set up a plan for reaching the goals. The plan usually includes structured conversational interactions between the patient and clinician in which the patient practices agreed-on strategies for improving a targeted behavior, alternating with videotaped conversational interactions in which the patient uses the strategies either with the clinician or with others. These videotapes provide the patient with documentation of progress and provide the clinician and patient with indications of behaviors that should be attended to in the next phase of treatment. The process is repeated for successive behaviors until all behaviors selected for treatment have been addressed. Group training sessions in which patients practice communicative strategies in conversational interactions with others consolidate the strategies and facilitate generalization to daily life.

Eye contact, turn-taking, and topic maintenance are frequent targets for treatment because they often are problematic for patients with right-hemisphere brain injury, and improving them can strongly affect right-hemisphere-injured patients' conversational appropriateness. Increasing a patient's eye contact may require only that the clinician say *look at me* at appropriate times in treatment interactions. When the patient responds consistently to the clinician's spoken cues, the cues may be faded and replaced with patient self-cues. Giving the patient specific points at which to make eye contact may be helpful if the patient has difficulty making the transition from clinician cues to self-cues. Teaching the patient to make eye contact when he or she begins and ends each utterance, then extending eye contact to the beginning and end of the conversational partner's utterances may provide a structured way for patients to maintain reasonably appropriate eye contact in conversations.

Teaching right-hemisphere-injured patients to follow conversational turn-taking rules may be approached in stepwise fashion. The clinician explains turn-taking rules and talks about how conversational participants know when to take or yield conversational turns. Then the clinician and the patient engage in structured practice in which the patient concentrates on turn-taking without being concerned about other aspects of communication such as message formulation or inferential reasoning. The structured practice may include (1) watching videotapes of conversational interactions (such as television talk shows) and discussing how the participants knew when to talk and when to let the other person talk; (2) preparing a script for a conversational interaction with appropriate conversational turns, videotaping it, then critiquing it; and (3) videotaping a free conversation, viewing it, and identifying appropriate and inappropriate turn-taking behavior. When the patient begins to exhibit reasonably good appreciation of normal turn-taking, turn-taking may be incorporated into other treatment activities, free conversation with the clinician, and group activities with other patients.

Teaching right-hemisphere-injured patients to maintain conversational topics usually requires some instruction and much structured practice. The instruction involves pointing out to the patient that conversations usually have a central theme or topic that lasts through several conversational turns and that certain behaviors mark topic shifts, and convincing the patient that he or she strays from the topic during conversations. Structured practice may involve activities such as (1) identifying topics in printed materials such as newspaper or magazine articles; (2) watching videotapes of conversational interactions and identifying topics, identifying when the topic changes, and discussing how the topic change was brought about by the participants; (3) engaging in structured conversations with the clinician while maintaining a specified topic for a given length of time or a given number of conversational turns; and (4) practicing topic maintenance in group conversations with other patients.

Treatment approaches designed to enhance aphasic adults' success in conversational interactions such as *Promoting Aphasics' Communicative Effectiveness* (*PACE*; Davis & Wilcox, 1985) and *Conversational Coaching* (Holland, 1991; Hopper, Holland, & Rewega, 2002) may prove useful in work with persons who have right-hemisphere brain injuries, if the procedures are modified to take advantage of right-hemisphere-injured adults' preserved language, to focus on the interactional aspects of conversations, and to increase the patient's appreciation of the nonliteral aspects of conversational partners' speech and behavior. (See Chapter 9 for descriptions of PACE and conversational coaching.) Some of what appear to be pragmatic impairments, such as failure to observe social conventions, failure to appreciate a speaker's implied intent, verbosity, tangentiality, and inappropriate responses to figurative language, actually may represent problems in attending to subtle cues, organizing and interpreting complex information, or making inferences. These impairments may be more effectively and efficiently treated, at least in the initial stages of treatment, by treating the underlying cognitive impairments rather than by working on conversational interactions. In later stages of treatment, direct work on conversational interactions may be appropriate.

Resource Allocation and Right-Hemisphere Brain Injury

Tompkins (1995) has proposed that many right-hemisphere-injured patients' impairments and behavioral aberrations can be explained by limitations on the availability of mental resources. She notes that right-hemisphere-injured patients' performance varies with the processing demands placed on cognitive resources, that right-hemisphere-injured patients can use context to facilitate problematic performance, that right-hemisphere-injured patients' performance in conditions of high processing load covaries with their functional working memory, and that right-hemisphere-injured patients' partially correct performance is consistent with limitations in processing resources.

Tompkins cautions that a resource allocation explanation of right-hemisphere-injured patients' performance "can be made to fit almost any outcome, and, as such, runs the risk of explaining nothing" (p. 85). She recommends that investigators test specific predictions to validate (or disprove) resource allocation as an explanation of right-hemisphere-injured adults' cognitive and behavioral aberrations.

Joanette and Goulet (1994) offered a hypothesis similar to that of Tompkins, namely that right-hemisphere-injured patients' performance may be governed by task complexity—the more complex the task, the more difficulty right-hemisphere-injured patients have with it. Task complexity and resource allocation explanations of right-hemisphere-injured patients' impairments may offer equivalent explanations using different labels, because more complex tasks should require more cognitive resources and vice versa. Both explanations await experimental validation, and it remains to be seen if resource allocation and task complexity actually represent different concepts.

Inference Failure and Right-Hemisphere Brain Injury

Myers (1991) has asserted that many right-hemisphere-injured patients' communicative impairments can be accounted for by a central impairment in making inferences. She called this impairment *inference failure*. According to Myers, inference "requires an interaction between two types of recognition—the recognition of key elements and the recognition of their relationship to one another and to other contextual cues" (p. 4). According to Myers, a general failure to go beyond the superficial meaning of events or situations to their deeper (implied) meanings may explain right-hemisphere-injured patients' tendency to interpret metaphor, humor, idioms, and indirect requests literally, their pragmatic deficits in conversations, their impaired expression of emotion, their impulsivity, their denial of illness, their facial recognition deficits, their verbose, tangential, and inefficient speech, and their failure to produce integrated stories and descriptions.

If Myers is correct, treatment of right-hemisphere-injured patients' communicative impairments might focus on teaching them to make inferences. As their ability to make inferences improves, the surface impairments that depended on making inferences should improve. Tompkins (1995) comments, however, that Myers's explanation is "underspecified," that other impairments may masquerade as inference failure, and that inference failure may be related to a more general concept—that of *mental effort*. Myers's hypothesis has yet to be validated, but if the existence of inference failure as a central process were to be confirmed, clinicians would have a promising alternative to current treatment-by-symptom approaches for remediating right-hemisphere-injured patients' communicative impairments.

As noted earlier, Brownell and associates (1986) have reported that right-hemisphere-injured adults make inferences but make the wrong ones based on their initial surface interpretations, and they fail to revise their initial inferences based on subsequent information. The transcript of a right-hemisphere-injured adult earlier in this chapter is striking not so much because the patient failed to make inferences, but because he made incorrect ones. These findings somewhat weaken Myers's arguments for inference failure as a general explanation for right-hemisphere-injured adults' impairments. One might argue that training patients with right-hemisphere brain injuries to evaluate the plausibility of their first inferences and to modify them according to the situation would be a more profitable approach than teaching them to make inferences.

The following short list of tasks contains examples of activities that would be appropriate for teaching patients to make inferences or to revise faulty inferences.

Activation of Alternative Meanings. The patient is shown printed *homonyms* (words that are spelled and pronounced alike but have two or more meanings; e.g., *fair, pen, park*) and is asked to provide two meanings for each word. The patient is shown printed sentences that have two or more interpretations (e.g., *Fred was surprised when he saw the fork in the road. A broken leg kept Sue from sitting in the chair.*) and is asked to provide two meanings for each sentence.

The patient categorizes items according to similarities and differences or class membership (e.g., telling why scissors and a saw are alike, listing things that one might find at a picnic, naming ferocious animals). The patient analyzes familial relationships (e.g., *How is your son's uncle related to you?*). The patient generates lists of divergent functions (e.g., all the ways in which one could use a brick).

Divergent tasks may exacerbate some patients' tendency toward tangentiality. If carefully controlled, divergent tasks may provide ways of working on tangentiality. If not carefully controlled, they may reinforce it.

Appreciation of Humor. The patient is given a cartoon minus its caption, and she or he chooses the humorous caption from a set containing a humorous caption and nonhumorous foils. The patient is given a printed joke minus its punch line, and she or he chooses the humorous punch line from a set containing a humorous punch line and nonhumorous foils:

The quack was selling a potion which he claimed would make men live to a great age. He claimed he himself was hale and hearty and over 300 years old. "Is he really as old as that?" asked a listener of the youthful assistant. "I can't say," replied the assistant.

"I don't know how old he is." *(Nonhumorous ending)*

"I've only worked for him 100 years." *(Humorous ending)*

"There are over 300 days in a year." *(Non sequitur)*

(From Molloy, R., Brownell, H.H., & Gardner, H. [1991]. Discourse comprehension by right-hemisphere stroke patients: Deficits of prediction and revision. In Y. Joanette & H. Brownell [Eds.]. *Discourse ability and brain damage: Theoretical and empirical perspectives.* New York: Springer-Verlag, pp. 113-130.)

Appreciation of the Implied Meanings of Metaphors and Idioms. The patient hears or reads a common metaphor or idiomatic expression, then chooses the correct interpretation from a group containing the correct interpretation plus foils that include a literal interpretation of the metaphor or idiom:

Frank didn't go to work because he felt *under the weather.*
Frank got caught in the rain. *(Literal interpretation)*
Frank felt ill. *(Correct idiomatic interpretation)*
Frank was afraid of storms. *(Related response)*
Frank lived in the city. *(Unrelated response)*

Identification of Verbal and Pictorial Absurdities. The patient is shown pictures containing absurd or unlikely relationships (e.g., a rabbit chasing a dog), identifies the absurd or unlikely relationships, and explains why they are absurd or unlikely. The patient listens to or reads a narrative in which there are absurd or inconsistent statements, identifies the absurd or inconsistent statements, and explains why they are absurd or inconsistent:

Mrs. Ensley took her daughter Hannah to the doctor. She said to the doctor, "I brought her in because she's had a fever for two days and has been coughing and sneezing. *I think her shoes are too tight.*"

Comprehension of Discourse. The patient listens to or reads short samples of discourse, answers questions testing implied information, and tells the main point or moral for the discourse. The patient listens to or reads a story, then retells it by paraphrasing and interpreting it rather than repeating it verbatim. The presence of main ideas and the presence of implied information in the retellings is evaluated to determine the extent to which the patient organizes information from the story and makes the appropriate inferences.

Small-Step Treatment

One way of dealing with right-hemisphere-injured patients' stimulus boundedness and impaired inferencing is to make the steps between treatment levels small. Making the steps small and minimizing changes in stimuli and responses between levels helps right-hemisphere-injured patients by diminishing the need for them to make inferences and change response sets. Yorkston's (1981) description of a program to teach a right-hemisphere-injured patient to transfer from his wheelchair to his bed underscores the need for small-step transitions for some patients with right-hemisphere brain injury. Yorkston began with a seven-step procedure that proved completely beyond the patient's capacity. She then expanded it to 17 steps, then 27 steps, and eventually added the self-cue *Have you finished this step?* at the end of each step before the patient eventually learned to transfer. Yorkston cautioned that clinicians should never assume that a right-hemisphere-injured patient will make logical transitions from one step to another, and she commented that, "Rarely, if ever, does one err in the direction of breaking a task into too many steps" (p. 283).

Generalization

Generalization of improved performance from level to level within treatment tasks, from one treatment task to another, and from treatment tasks to the patient's daily life is an important issue for right-hemisphere-injured patients, their

clinicians, and their families. As a group, right-hemisphere-injured adults tend not to spontaneously generalize responses or strategies from one context to another. Their progress through successive levels of treatment may be slowed by failure to apply skills and strategies learned at one level to the next level. Transitions between treatment tasks may be compromised by the patient's failure to generalize what is learned in one task to related tasks. Finally (and perhaps most importantly), generalization of gains made in the clinic to the patient's daily life may be compromised by the patient's failure to apply what is learned in the clinic to daily life interactions. Successful treatment of right-hemisphere-injured adults requires that clinicians give careful attention to procedures for enhancing generalization, both within treatment and from treatment to daily life.

Generalization within Treatment. The generalization procedures described in Chapter 7 provide some methods by which clinicians can build generalization into their treatment procedures for right-hemisphere-injured patients. These procedures may be modified or elaborated on as needed to account for the behavioral and cognitive impairments exhibited by right-hemisphere-injured patients (e.g., impaired attention, impaired inferencing, impulsiveness, indifference). Because of right-hemisphere-injured patients' behavioral and cognitive impairments, generalization procedures for them tend to be more prescriptive and more carefully structured than generalization procedures for patients with left-hemisphere injury.

Generalization from task to task within treatment activities can be enhanced by making the source task (the one in which the patient has learned a set of responses or a strategy) resemble the target task (the one to which generalization is intended). Similarity between tasks can be manipulated by adjusting the task stimuli, the responses required in the task, or the context in which the task is presented (e.g., paper-and-pencil versus computer presentation). Requiring new responses to new stimuli in a new context maximizes between-task differences and works against generalization, whereas maintaining consistency of stimuli, responses, and context minimizes between-task differences and increases the probability that learning will generalize. (For related information, see *programming common stimuli* in Chapter 7.)

Loose training (see Chapter 7) is another way in which clinicians can enhance right-hemisphere-injured patients' generalization across tasks. By allowing stimulus conditions, response requirements, and reinforcement contingencies to vary within a controlled range, the clinician prevents the patient's performance from becoming too tightly bound to a restricted set of conditions and also increases the probability that learned responses and strategies will transfer across treatment tasks.

Many clinicians routinely begin treatment in a task under tightly controlled conditions, and when the new learning has stabilized, gradually loosen the training conditions, regardless of the source and nature of a patient's cognitive or communicative impairments.

Generalization from Treatment to Daily Life. Right-hemisphere-injured patients' tendency not to generalize from task to task or from level to level within tasks in the clinic is mirrored in their tendency not to generalize what they acquire in the clinic to outside environments. However, clinicians are not powerless. Tompkins (1995) identifies several ways in which clinicians can ensure or enhance generalization across settings:

1. *Provide enough training trials to consolidate and stabilize responses so that patients can produce them in novel or stressful contexts.*

   Responses or strategies requiring attention and high-level volitional control tend not to generalize from the context in which they are acquired to other contexts. If given careful coaching, some patients with right-hemisphere brain injury may eventually make such generalizations, but few spontaneously

generalize learned behaviors and strategies from one context to another. Clinicians usually must make responses and strategies overlearned and automatic to ensure that they generalize from treatment to daily life.

2. *Train a variety of related responses (e.g., eye contact, turn-taking, and relevance in conversations) rather than single responses.*

   This resembles loose training. The idea behind this principle is that training several related responses provides the patient with alternatives when the primary response is not available, and it creates a network of associations that raises the overall probability of appropriate responses in the target contexts.

3. *Train responses and strategies in a variety of tasks and present the tasks in a variety of contexts (e.g., role-playing, simulated natural environments, and natural environments).*

   This principle incorporates elements of programming common stimuli and sequential modification (see Chapter 7). Training responses or strategies in a variety of tasks helps to stabilize and consolidate responses and diminishes the patient's reliance on the exact conditions under which responses are acquired. Presenting treatment tasks in a variety of contexts increases the patient's tolerance for changes in context and increases the probability that the treated responses or strategies will generalize from the treatment setting to other settings.

4. *Incorporate aspects of the target environment (e.g., topics, stimuli, contingencies, people, situations) into treatment activities.*

   This principle is related to the preceding one and speaks more directly to how clinicians enhance generalization from clinic activities to the patient's daily life environment. Topics, situations, response contingencies, and sometimes people can be recruited from the patient's daily life environment and incorporated into treatment activities. Their presence in treatment activities imbues them with power to elicit, maintain, and control the patient's strategies.

5. *Train self-instruction and verbal mediation.*

Self-instruction and verbal mediation can be important adjuncts to other generalization procedures for patients with right-hemisphere brain injury. Clinicians can exploit right-hemisphere-injured patients' preserved verbal skills by teaching them self-instructional or self-cueing strategies that are (overtly or covertly) verbally mediated (e.g., a patient with neglect might be taught to compensate while reading by saying or thinking, *Look to the left at the beginning of every line of text.*)

6. *Enlist the help of family members, friends, and caregivers.*

Family, friends, and caregivers can be a powerful force for generalization of behaviors and strategies from the clinic to the patient's daily life. In many respects family, friends, and caregivers can function as sur-

rogate clinicians by manipulating stimuli, arranging situations, and managing response contingencies under the direction of the speech-language pathologist. Family, friends, and caregivers also can monitor the patient's daily life performance and provide the clinician with information about how much generalization actually is taking place.

Generalization is one of the most challenging components of treatment for clinicians who work with right-hemisphere-injured adults. Unless generalization is specifically targeted and systematically trained, what the right-hemisphere-injured patient learns in the clinic is likely to stay there. Fortunately, procedures to enhance and ensure generalization are available, and their systematic application can help to ensure that improvements in right-hemisphere-injured adults' communication transfer to their daily life.

GENERAL CONCEPTS 10-3

- Left-hemisphere damage tends to produce focal impairments that may be quantified relatively easily, whereas right-hemisphere damage tends to produce diffuse impairments that are less amenable to quantification.
- Treatment of right-hemisphere-damaged patients' cognitive and communicative impairments may be complicated by one or more of several cognitive and behavioral abnormalities:
  - Denial and indifference, which sometimes may be amenable to direct or indirect intervention
  - Attentional impairments and distractibility, which may be treated with paper-and-pencil or computer-based tasks that target sustained attention, selective attention, alternating attention, or divided attention
  - Impulsivity, which may be treated with external stop and go signals that are pro-

  gressively shaped into patient-generated self-cues
  - Impaired reasoning and problem-solving, which may be treated with structured activities such as role-playing and prescriptive problem-solving strategies
  - Diminished affect and vocal prosody, which may be treated by imitation training, cognitive/linguistic training, or a combination of the two
  - Neglect in reading, which may be treated by external cues to the left side of printed materials, by treatment activities that heighten patients' awareness of left hemispace, or by treatment activities that enhance general attentional processes
  - Pragmatic impairments, which may be treated by calling on right-hemisphere-damaged adults' intact verbal skills together with coaching and structured practice with compensatory strategies.

GENERAL CONCEPTS 10-3—cont'd

- Some right-hemisphere-damaged adults' apparent pragmatic impairments may actually represent problems in attending to subtle cues, problems in making inferences, or problems organizing and interpreting complex information.
- Tompkins has suggested that many of the cognitive, communicative, and behavioral abnormalities exhibited by patients with right-hemisphere brain injuries are caused by limitations in the resources required to carry out the mental operations required in tasks that are sensitive to right-hemisphere brain injury. Joanette and Goulet offer a similar explanation, phrased in terms of task complexity.
- Myers has suggested that a central impairment called *inference failure* causes many right-hemisphere-damaged patients' communicative and cognitive impairments, and she recommends that treatment focus on enhancing right-hemisphere-damaged patients' ability to make inferences. Impairments in constructing inferences may be treated by activities in which patients provide alternative meanings for words and sentences, choose humorous punch lines for jokes,

interpret idioms and metaphors, or identify verbal or pictorial absurdities.

- Generalization is a crucial issue for patients with right-hemisphere damage, because they tend not to spontaneously generalize new learning from the clinic to daily life, from one task to another, or from level to level within treatment tasks. Consequently, procedures to enhance and maintain generalization are an important part of treatment for most patients with right-hemisphere brain damage.
- Tompkins has suggested several ways to enhance right-hemisphere-damaged adults' generalization of behavior across settings:
  - Provide enough training trials to consolidate and stabilize responses
  - Train a variety of related responses
  - Train responses across a variety of tasks and contexts
  - Incorporate aspects of the target environment into treatment
  - Train self-instruction and verbal mediation
  - Involve right-hemisphere-damaged adults' family members, friends, and caregivers in treatment

THOUGHT QUESTIONS

Question 10-1 Fred Bicep is a 26-year-old man who experienced sudden headache and left-side arm and leg weakness shortly after bench-pressing 350 pounds at his fitness center. He was taken to his local hospital's emergency room, where the examining physician recorded the following findings:

Alert and cooperative, but seemed confused

Complains of severe headache

Speech intelligible, but rambling and incoherent

Left-side hemiparesis, arm greater than leg

Exaggerated reflexes, left arm and leg; plantar extensor reflex (Babinski), left

Left homonymous hemianopia

Left neglect

What do you think caused Fred's signs and symptoms? What do you think the physician will do after she finishes examining Fred? What would you predict regarding Fred's potential course of recovery?

Question 10-2 Sophia Snyder, a right-handed woman with right-hemisphere damage and moderately severe left hemispatial neglect, is shown the three arrays (A, B, C) several times each, in random order, and is asked to point to the squares in each array. What pattern of responses would you expect from Ms. Snyder in this task? Which squares would you expect her to consistently identify? Which ones would you expect her to consistently miss? Are there squares that you would expect her to identify only part of the time? What do you think would happen if you gave her a large number of trials (50 or more) with these stimuli (presented in random order) in one session?

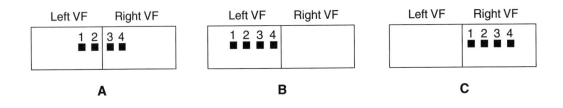

Question 10-3 Consider the following excerpt from an interview with Glenda Glindon, a hospitalized 67-year-old right-handed woman who is 3 days after onset of a stroke in the posterior branch of the middle cerebral artery in her right brain hemisphere:

Clinician: What brings you to the hospital?
Patient: Well, they say I'm having trouble walking.
Clinician: Why is that?
Patient: I guess I'm having trouble with my legs. They put me in physical therapy every day.
Clinician: Why are you in physical therapy? What kind of trouble are you having with your legs?
Patient: They say it's my left leg.
Clinician: What happened to your left leg?
Patient: They say it's not working because I had a stroke, but I don't know about that.
Clinician: Are you having any other problems?
Patient: Just being in this place and putting up with all the doctors.

What behavioral characteristics of right-hemisphere brain injury are reflected in the interview? What does the interview suggest regarding potential issues that might arise during evaluation and treatment of this patient? (Assume that reimbursement issues and access to the patient will not be problems. Someone will pay for reasonable services, and the patient will be available to you for assessment and treatment.)

Question 10-4 You receive a referral on Mr. Blanding, a 51-year-old right-handed man who had a posterior right-hemisphere stroke 3 days ago. The referring neurologist asks you to evaluate the patient to determine if Mr. Blanding is a candidate for cognitive-communicative therapy. If you determine that he is a candidate for such treatment, Mr. Blanding will be transferred to a long-term care ward for the duration of the treatment, up to 6 weeks. If you determine that he is not a treatment candidate, he will be discharged to his home in northern Minnesota in 2 days. (He lives in a small town in a rural area. Treatment there is not an option.) You can schedule Mr. Blanding for no more than 4 hours of testing in the next 2 days.

What tests would you administer? You do not have access to a "right-hemisphere test battery" such as those described in the textbook. You must choose individual tests that address specific impairments. Consider how you can fit your selections into a 4-hour period, and choose tests that are most likely to indicate Mr. Blanding's potential as a treatment candidate.

Question 10-5 How would the risks for an individual with left neglect who elects to drive an automobile in England differ from those for an individual with left neglect who elects to drive an automobile in the United States?

Traumatic Brain Injury

Brain damage is a family affair. (Muriel Lezak)

Traumatic brain injuries are the result of abrupt external forces acting on the skull and the brain, as when a moving object such as a bullet, club, or baseball strikes the head, or the moving head strikes a stationary object such as an automobile dashboard, tree, or sidewalk. Injuries in which the skull is fractured or perforated and the meninges are torn are called *penetrating head injuries.* Injuries in which the skull and meninges remain intact are called *closed-head injuries.* Penetrating injuries usually are caused by missile wounds or blows to the head by sharp objects. Closed-head injuries usually are caused by motor-vehicle accidents or falls.

INCIDENCE AND PREVALENCE OF TRAUMATIC BRAIN INJURIES

Traumatic brain injury is a significant social, economic, and medical problem in contemporary society. About 1.4 million United States residents receive medical attention for traumatic brain injuries each year (Langlois & associates, 2004). The incidence of traumatic brain injury in the U.S. is about 4 times the incidence of breast cancer and about 34 times the number of new cases of HIV/AIDS (Centers for Disease Control and Prevention, National Center for Injury Prevention and Control, 2001).

About one in four persons who experience traumatic brain injuries are hospitalized (300,000 per year). Of those hospitalized, about one in six die from their injuries. Of those who survive hospitalization, about one in three are left with permanent disabilities (Figure 11-1). Bushnik and associates (2003) estimate that there are about 5.3 million survivors of traumatic brain injury in the United States who are living with permanent disabilities related to their brain injuries.

Estimates of the incidence of traumatic brain injury vary widely, ranging from 95 per 100,000 (Centers for Disease Control and Pre-

vention, 1997) to 200 per 100,000 (Kraus, 1993; Rosenthal & associates, 1990). The reported incidence of traumatic brain injury has declined in the past decade, perhaps because of declining rates of hospitalization for less severe brain injuries and newer counting methods that focus on hospitalized cases and cases ending in death. The precise incidence of traumatic brain injury in the United States is not known, primarily because some persons who experience mild head injuries do not seek medical attention. If only persons who receive treatment for traumatic brain injury are counted, the incidence is likely to be about 100 per 100,000 per year. If the count includes an estimate of persons injured but not counted, the incidence may be as high as 250 per 100,000 per year.

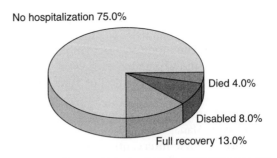

Figure 11-1 ■ Outcome for adults who sustain traumatic brain injuries in the United States. Of those who sustain injury, 25% are hospitalized. Of those who are hospitalized, about 4% die before leaving the hospital, about 8% leave the hospital with permanent communicative or cognitive disabilities, and about 13% recover with no substantial communicative or cognitive disabilities (although many will exhibit subtle impairments with careful testing). (Based on data reported by Thurman, D.J., Alverson, C.A., Dunn, K.A., & associates. [1999]. Traumatic brain injury in the United States: A public health perspective. *Journal of Head Trauma Rehabilitation, 14,* 602-615.)

Most traumatic brain injuries (about 90% in the U.S.) are closed-head injuries caused by falls, motor-vehicle accidents, and assaults. Falls account for slightly more than one-fourth of all traumatic brain injuries (Figure 11-2). Motor-vehicle accidents and assaults account for about one fifth and one tenth, respectively. About one third of traumatic brain injuries have other causes (e.g., injuries from participation in contact sports, work-related injuries).

More males than females experience traumatic brain injuries, especially for young adults. For young adults between 15 and 25 years old, about twice as many males as females experience traumatic brain injuries (Figure 11-3). Traumatic brain injury is the leading cause of neurologic disability in persons under the age of 50 (Finlayson & Garner, 1994).

Toddlers and older adults are more likely to experience traumatic brain injuries than the general population, although they are less likely to experience them than young adults (Finlayson & Garner, 1994). Falls account for most traumatic brain injuries in toddlers and the very old, whereas motor-vehicle accidents account for most traumatic brain injuries in young adults (Finlayson & Garner, 1994; Van Houten & associates, 1994).

RISK FACTORS

Several variables other than age and sex affect the probability of traumatic brain injury. One of the most striking is substance abuse. About half (40% to 60%) of patients admitted to hospitals with traumatic brain injuries are intoxicated when admitted (Brismar, Engstrom, & Rydberg, 1983; Rutherford, 1977). Motor-vehicle accidents, falls, and assaults (in that order) cause most intoxicated adults' traumatic brain injuries. Many assault-related injuries are related to the use of alcohol or drugs by the aggressor, the victim, or both (Giles & Clark-Wilson, 1993). Hillbom and Holm (1986) estimate that the incidence of brain injury in alcoholic adults is two to four times greater than the incidence of brain injury in the general population. Alcohol intoxication is a major contributor to fatalities in motor-vehicle accidents, especially for younger

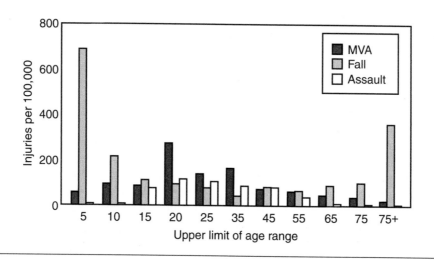

Figure 11-2 ■ Traumatic-brain-injury rates for injuries caused by motor-vehicle accidents (MVAs), falls, and assaults, by age (United States 2004). (Data from National Center for Injury Prevention and Control. [2006]. *Web-based injury statistics query and reporting system (WISQARS)*. Atlanta: National Center for Injury Prevention and Control.)

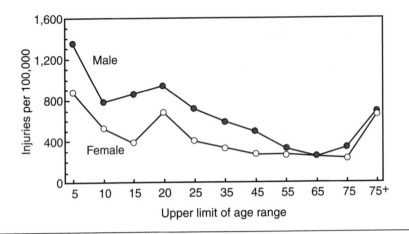

Figure 11-3 ■ Average annual traumatic-brain-injury related rates for emergency department visits, hospitalizations, and deaths by age and sex (United States, 1995-2001). (From Langlois, J.A., Rutland-Brown, W., & Thomas, K.E. (2004). *Traumatic brain injury in the United States: Emergency department visits, hospitalizations, and deaths.* Atlanta: Centers for Disease Control and Prevention, National Center for Injury Prevention and Control.)

drivers. Drivers 16 to 44 years old are 3 to 4 times more likely to be legally intoxicated at the time of a fatal accident than drivers 45 years old and older (Figure 11-4). Male drivers involved in fatal accidents are twice as likely to be intoxicated as female drivers.

School adjustment and social history also affect the probability of traumatic brain injury. Haas, Cope, and Hall (1987) reported that 50% of a large group of severely brain-injured patients had a history of poor academic performance (i.e., failure in two or more subjects, diagnosed learning disability, or school dropout). Giles and Clark-Wilson (1993) comment that poor academic performance may be related to underlying neurologic impairments causing distractibility, attentional impairments, low frustration tolerance, impulsivity, rebelliousness, egocentrism, sociopathic behavior, and substance abuse, all of which increase the probability of head injuries.

Socioeconomic status also is related to the incidence of traumatic brain injury. Individ-

uals with low income, especially those who live in areas with high population density (central cities), have a higher probability of traumatic brain injury (primarily from assaults and falls) than do individuals with higher income who live in areas of low population density (Macniven, 1994).

The divorce rate for traumatically brain-injured adults in the United States is approximately four times the rate of divorce in the general U.S. population (Kerr, Kay, & Lassman, 1971). However, the high divorce rate for traumatically brain-injured adults may itself be related to other variables such as substance abuse, social maladjustment, and maladaptive personality, and may not reflect the effects of brain injury *per se*.

The relationship of personality to traumatic brain injury has received a fair amount of attention. The general conclusion is that *Type A personalities* (characterized by competitiveness, impulsivity, belligerence, and hostility) are more likely to experience traumatic brain injuries

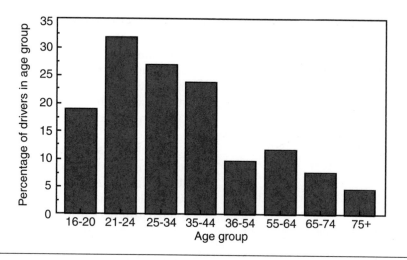

Figure 11-4 ■ Percentage of drivers with blood alcohol content 0.08 or higher (legally intoxicated in 50 U.S. states) who were involved in fatal motor-vehicle accidents in 2003. (Data from National Highway Traffic Safety Administration [2006]. *Traffic Safety Facts*, Washington, D.C.)

than are *Type B personalities* (characterized by cooperativeness, deliberateness, and helpfulness) (Evans, Palsane, & Carrere, 1987).

A history of traumatic brain injury increases the probability of additional traumatic brain injuries. The probability of a second traumatic brain injury is three times greater for individuals who have a previous traumatic brain injury than for the general population. The probability of a third traumatic brain injury for an individual who has had two traumatic brain injuries is eight times greater than the probability of traumatic brain injury for an individual with no previous brain injury (Annegers & associates, 1980).

Participation in high-risk sports also increases the risk of traumatic brain injury. Professional and amateur boxers have a particularly high rate of diffuse brain injury, with gradually increasing impairment throughout the boxer's career, presumably because of repeated mild brain trauma—a condition called *dementia pugilistica.* Motorcycling, bicycling, snowmobiling, and rock climbing are associated with increased risk of brain injury, although wearing appropriate safety helmets significantly diminishes the risk of head injury.

Bicycle riders wearing helmets have an 88% reduction in risk of traumatic brain injury (Thompson, Rivara, & Thompson, 1989), and comparable reductions in injury are no doubt associated with helmet use in other sporting activities in which participants' heads receive sudden acceleration or deceleration, strike unyielding surfaces, or are struck by moving objects.

Although each of these variables affects the probability of traumatic brain injury, interactions among variables are certain, making it difficult or impossible to isolate the effect of any single variable. For example, alcohol and drug abuse are related to socioeconomic status, school adjustment, educational achievement, and personality variables, and each of the latter variables is likely to interact with one or more of the others, making it impossible to estimate the amount by which the presence of any single variable increases the probability of brain injury. It seems clear, however, that multiple risk factors add to the probability that an individual will experience a head injury.

Most young head-injured adults are unmarried, unemployed males of low socioeconomic status (Barber & Webster, 1974).

PATHOPHYSIOLOGY OF TRAUMATIC BRAIN INJURY

Information about what happens inside the skull during traumatic brain injury comes from two sources—studies of the brains of animals with laboratory-induced brain injuries and studies of the brains of humans who have succumbed to brain injuries. Because the human brains available for study belong to patients who die from their injuries, most of what we know about traumatic brain injury comes from patients who have died from severe brain injuries. Consequently, the neuropathology of mild or moderate traumatic brain injury is based more on extrapolation and intuition than on empiric evidence.

Penetrating Brain Injuries

Most penetrating brain injuries are caused by missiles (e.g., bullets, artillery shell fragments). Some are caused by blunt instruments (e.g., clubs, baseball bats), and a few are caused by falls in which the head strikes a sharp object.

The amount and nature of brain damage caused by missiles depends on the velocity of the missile. High-velocity missiles (e.g., rifle bullets, military projectiles) cause more physical damage to cranial contents than low-velocity missiles. High-velocity missiles perforate the skull and tunnel through the brain before exiting through the skull opposite the point of entry. Their high kinetic energy creates a pressure wave with explosive effects on the skull and brain, destroying tissue on both sides of the projectile's track and causing diffuse bleeding

and tissue disruption throughout the brain and brain stem. The missile carries foreign material (hair, skin, and bone fragments) into the brain, increasing the risk of infection. High-velocity missile wounds to the brain almost always are fatal, usually within minutes to hours after injury (Grafman & Salazar, 1987).

Low-velocity missile wounds (e.g., bullets from handguns, shrapnel) are less often fatal, but nevertheless are dangerous. Low-velocity missiles perforate the skull and brain, causing tissue destruction adjacent to the missile's track. Foreign material carried into the brain increases the risk of infection. If the missile has enough velocity to strike the skull opposite the point of entry, it may ricochet and cause additional brain injury opposite of the entry point.

Some low-velocity impacts (e.g., being struck on the head with a club or striking the head on a table edge in a fall) may cause penetrating injuries if the force of the impact is concentrated in a small area. Such low-velocity impacts may fracture the skull. If the fracture is severe, bone fragments may be pushed into the brain beneath the fracture. Brain tissue beneath the impact site may be cut, torn, and bruised. Damage to the brain following low-velocity impacts may be surprisingly slight, because most of the energy of the blow to the head is spent in fracturing the skull and comparatively little is transmitted to the brain.

Between 20% and 40% of low-velocity penetrating injuries cause the patient's death (Grafman & Salazar, 1987), although mortality is greater (up to 90%) for penetrating injuries caused by handguns. If the patient survives the first day after a penetrating brain injury, infection, bleeding, and increased intracranial pressure caused by swelling of the brain become important threats to the patient's survival. Penetrating injuries affecting the brain stem usually are fatal because of damage to the structures that regulate respiration, heart rate, blood pressure, and other vital functions.

Adults who survive penetrating head injuries and their physiologic consequences almost always are left with physical, cognitive, and linguistic impairments. These impairments (except for those caused by high-velocity missiles) usually are focal rather than diffuse, and they reflect the loss of functions served by the damaged brain tissue.

Nonpenetrating Brain Injuries

In *nonpenetrating brain injuries* (or *closed-head trauma*) the meninges remain intact, and foreign substances do not enter the brain. Nonpenetrating injuries can be divided into two general categories: *nonacceleration injuries* and *acceleration injuries. Nonacceleration injuries* (sometimes called *fixed-head trauma*) are produced when the restrained head is struck by a moving object. *Acceleration injuries* (sometimes called *moving-head trauma*) are produced when the unrestrained head is struck by a moving object or when the moving head strikes a stationary object. Acceleration injuries also occur when the rapidly moving head abruptly changes direction without striking a surface, as in whiplash injuries in motor-vehicle accidents.

Nonacceleration Injuries. Nonacceleration injuries usually cause less severe brain injuries than do acceleration injuries. Blows to a moveable head are up to 20 times more devastating than blows to a fixed head (Pang, 1989). The primary consequences of nonacceleration injuries are related to deformation of the skull by the impact of the object striking the skull. The skull is slightly elastic, so a blow to the head deforms the skull at the point of impact and drives the skull inward, causing localized damage to the meninges and brain cortex at the point of impact—damage called *impression trauma* (Figure 11-5). (It is not clear if impression trauma is caused by the impact of the depressed skull against the brain or by negative pressure that develops when the skull snaps back to its original shape.)

If a nonacceleration injury is caused by a slow-moving object with a large surface area, the skull may be forced from its customary oval shape to a more nearly circular shape (a condition called *ellipsoidal deformation;* see Figure 11-5). The change in shape increases the skull's volume because circular containers have more volume than ovoid containers. The increased volume reduces the pressure in the cranial vault, with the greatest pressure reduction in the regions closest to the skull. As a result, tissues deep in the brain (the corpus callosum and basal ganglia) expand outward into regions of less pressure. The expansion stretches and shears brain tissues and blood vessels, causing bleeding and swelling inside the brain.

Some nonacceleration injuries fracture the skull. Fractures at the base of the skull are more dangerous than fractures higher up, because basal skull fractures may damage cranial nerves or the carotid arteries, endangering the patient's life. Any skull fracture is dangerous if the meninges beneath the fracture are torn, because of bleeding from damaged meningeal blood vessels and the potential for infection. At one time the severity of closed-head injuries was measured by whether or not the skull was fractured. However, it is now clear that the presence or absence of skull fracture does not predict the severity of brain damage.

Acceleration Injuries. When traumatic brain injury is caused by sudden acceleration or deceleration of the head, the brain and brain stem often suffer diffuse damage caused by their movement inside the skull. The movement is caused by inertial forces generated either when the head is moving rapidly through space and comes to a sudden stop (as when it strikes the floor after a fall) or when the head is at rest and is suddenly accelerated (as when it is struck by a blunt object). Acceleration injuries take two forms, depending on the direction from which the head is struck.

Linear acceleration injuries occur when the head is struck by a force aligned with the center axis of the head (see Figure 11-5). Resting bodies tend to stay at rest because of inertia. Therefore the stationary head resists acceleration, but in

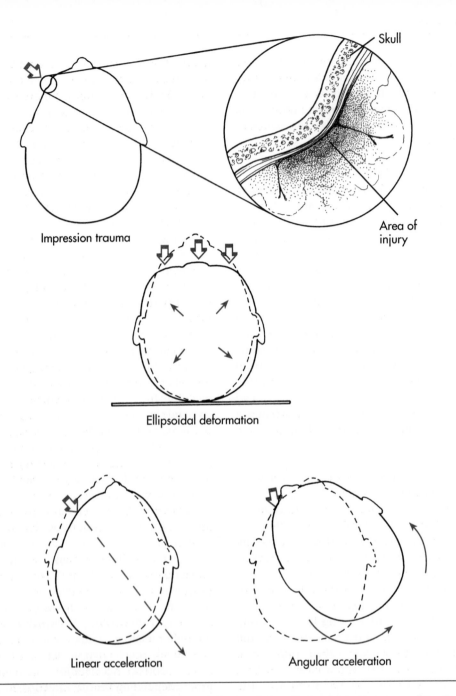

Skull

Impression trauma

Area of injury

Ellipsoidal deformation

Linear acceleration

Angular acceleration

Figure 11-5 ■ Physical consequences of blows to the head. *Impression trauma* is caused by blunt force applied to a small area of the skull. The skull is depressed at the point of impact with consequent injury to meninges and brain tissue beneath the point of impact. *Ellipsoidal deformation* is caused by blunt force applied to a large area on the restrained head. The skull is forced from its usual ellipsoidal shape to a more nearly circular shape. *Linear acceleration* of the skull and its contents is caused by blunt force applied on a line through the central axis of the unrestrained head. *Angular acceleration* of the skull and its contents is caused by blunt force applied at an angle to the central axis of the unrestrained head, causing the head to rotate away from the point of impact.

a few milliseconds the head begins to move away from the point of impact. The brain, however, has its own resting inertia. It remains motionless for a few milliseconds after the head begins to move. This inertial lag compresses the brain against the inside of the skull at the point of impact, causing bruises and abrasions on the surface of the brain. Such injuries are called *coup injuries* (*coup* is a French word pronounced *coo*, which means *blow* or *impact*).

The brain, now compressed against the skull, rebounds and accelerates to match the rate at which the head is moving. Within a few milliseconds, however, the head abruptly stops moving, either because it strikes an object or because of the tethering action of the vertebrae and neck muscles. The momentum of the brain keeps it in motion for a few more milliseconds, and it becomes compressed against the skull opposite the point of impact, causing bruises and abrasions opposite to the blow that started the head moving. These opposite-side injuries are called *contrecoup* (pronounced *contra-coo*) injuries. Coup and contrecoup brain injuries are a salient characteristic of linear-acceleration injuries.

The same physical processes operate when the head is moving at a constant rate of speed in a linear path and is suddenly stopped. *Shaken-baby syndrome* (also called *shaken-impact syndrome*) is the medical label for a collection of brain injuries in infants and toddlers caused by violent shaking (usually intentional, by an angry caregiver). The combination of violent shaking and the child's weak neck muscles cause the child's head to bounce to and fro, causing diffuse acceleration injuries to the child's fragile brain tissue. Whiplash injuries in motor-vehicle accidents, in which the head does not strike a surface but is snapped back and forth, also may cause linear-acceleration injuries to the brain.

Coup and contrecoup injuries cause focal damage to the meninges and brain tissue where the brain is compressed against the skull. The combination of coup and contrecoup injuries is called *translational trauma* (Teasdale & Men-

delow, 1984). Translational trauma occurs only with linear acceleration and deceleration of the head. Translational trauma is more likely following blows to the front or back of the head than blows to the side of the head, because the space between the brain and the skull (the *epidural space*) is greater at the front and back than at the sides. Consequently, the potential for linear brain movement inside the skull is greater when the head moves front-to-back than when it moves side-to-side.

Angular acceleration injuries are caused by blows that strike the head off-center, causing it to rotate and move at an angle away from the point of impact (see Figure 11-5). The brain's inertia keeps it at rest when the head begins to move. The mismatch in rotational acceleration creates twisting forces in axial structures (the midbrain, basal ganglia, brain stem, and cerebellum). Within a few milliseconds the brain begins to rotate in the same direction as the head. When the head has reached the limit of its range of movement, the tethering action of the vertebrae and the neck muscles causes it to rebound in the opposite direction. The brain, however, continues its rotation for a few additional milliseconds, causing a second episode of twisting forces concentrated in axial structures. (The twisting in the second episode moves in the opposite direction from that in the first episode.)

Twisting and shearing forces tend to be concentrated at the boundaries between gray matter (soft supportive tissue) and white matter (firm fiber tracts). Consequently, tissue damage, bleeding, and swelling affect major nerve fiber tracts in the internal capsule, corpus callosum, and brain stem. Angular acceleration of the head and rotational injury to the brain usually produce more severe brain injuries than linear acceleration of the head, wherein cranial contents are not subjected to twisting forces (Ommaya, Grubb, & Naumann, 1971).

Cranial nerve injuries are common following acceleration injuries to the brain. Front-to-back acceleration injuries (e.g., falling and striking the back of the head) may stretch and tear the olfactory nerve (CN 1) leading to loss of the sense of smell *(anosmia)*. Injuries to nerves controlling the extraocular muscles (CN 3, CN 4, CN 6) may compromise eye movements and cause double vision *(diplopia)* because of misalignment of the eyes. Injury to CN 8 may cause ringing or buzzing in the ears *(tinnitus)* or vertigo. Forces created by acceleration may stretch nerve-cell axons throughout the brain and brain stem—a condition called *diffuse axonal injury*. Diffuse axonal injury is common in acceleration injuries and is assumed to be responsible for many diffuse cognitive and behavioral impairments after such injuries.

Diffuse brain damage also may be caused by other conditions, such as cerebral anoxia or bacterial or viral infection, but the damage affects nerve cell bodies, not just their axons.

The forces causing axonal injuries stretch nerve axons rather than tearing them. Two to three hours after injury, the stretched axons swell, and in the next several hours (sometimes up to 24) the axons separate. The disconnected axonal segments then deteriorate, a process that may not be complete until 2 days after injury. Axonal degeneration is a diffuse process, affecting some axons in a region of injury and leaving others untouched, creating a spotty pattern of *deafferentation* (loss of input to a neuron from other neurons). This means that neurons in the region of injury may lose only part of their synaptic inputs from other neurons.

Intact axon terminals adjacent to regions of limited deafferentation may send fibers into the regions of deafferentation—a process called *collateral sprouting* or *dendritic proliferation*. This repair process may at least partially explain physiologic recovery in patients with mild to moderate traumatic brain injury. (Patients with severe traumatic brain injuries may have lost too many axons to permit meaningful recovery related to reafferentation.)

Severe diffuse axonal injury may lead to *vegetative state,* in which a patient has sleep-wake cycles but makes no purposeful movements, does not talk, does not follow instructions, and does not track visual stimuli. Vegetative state is a sign of severe diffuse damage to cortical and subcortical tissues with relative sparing of the brain stem.

Abrasions and contusions on the undersides of the brain hemispheres are common in acceleration injuries to the brain. The walls and roof of the cranial vault are smooth, but the floor is uneven and has sharp edges, especially under the frontal lobes (Figure 11-6).

As the brain moves in the skull during acceleration and deceleration, it scrapes along these sharp edges, abrading and lacerating the bottom surfaces of the frontal lobes and the anterior temporal lobes. The parietal lobes, occipital lobes, and the convexities of the frontal lobes usually are spared such injuries, because the inner surface of the cranial vault in those regions is smooth and featureless (Figure 11-7).

Traumatic Hemorrhage. Cuts, bruises, twisting, and shearing forces in the brain cause bleeding *(hemorrhages)* and accumulations of blood *(hematomas)*. *Epidural hematomas* are accumulations of blood between the dura mater and the skull. Most epidural hematomas are caused by skull fractures that lacerate arterial channels in the bone. Most epidural hematomas (90%) are a result of skull fracture (Teasdale & Mendelow, 1984). Automobile accidents are the most common cause of epidural hematomas, but some follow trivial events such as falls and sports injuries. About 20% to 30% of patients with epidural hematomas die as a consequence of their head injuries. Mortality from epidural hematoma is strongly related to whether the bleeding is from an artery (death in about 85% of cases) or a vein (death in about 15% of cases). Arterial bleeding usually is marked by massive hemorrhage, with symptoms progressing rapidly, often culminating in death within a few hours. Venous bleeding usually follows a less dramatic course, with slow progression of symptoms.

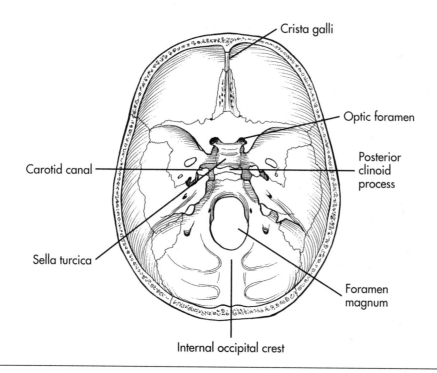

Figure 11-6 ■ The floor of the skull. The crista galli, the clinoid process, and the sella turcica are ridges in the skull floor. These and other prominences on the skull floor contribute to contusions and abrasions on the bottom surface of the brain in acceleration injuries.

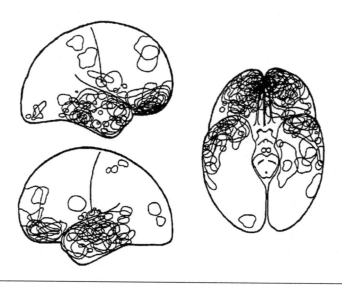

Figure 11-7 ■ The location of brain contusions in a series of 40 traumatically brain-injured adults. The most frequent location for contusions is the bottom surface of the frontal lobes, followed by the bottom surface of the anterior temporal lobes. (From Courville, C.B. [1937]. *Pathology of the central nervous system*. Mountain View, CA: Pacific.)

Small venous hemorrhages may ooze blood so slowly that they produce no overt symptoms, and the bleeding may be detected only with imaging scans of the head during routine evaluation of a patient.

The magnitude of the symptoms caused by epidural hemorrhages depends to some extent on the location of the hemorrhage. Bleeding into the posterior inferior epidural space can cause compression of the brain stem, leading to respiratory distress, decreased heart rate, and increased blood pressure. Bleeding into the frontal and superior epidural space is likely to be less serious because centers for vital functions are far away and there is more epidural space to accommodate the hematoma before it begins to displace brain structures. The most common treatment for an epidural hematoma is surgical removal, which usually is practical because of the hematoma's location just beneath the skull.

Subdural hematomas are accumulations of blood beneath the dura mater, above the arachnoid. Subdural hematomas are twice as common and twice as deadly as epidural hematomas, with 60% or greater overall mortality. Motor-vehicle accidents are the most common cause of subdural hematoma. Most subdural hematomas are caused by laceration of veins rather than arteries—most commonly injury to bridging veins that travel from the cerebral cortex to the dura mater. Acute subdural hematomas usually develop within a few hours and almost always appear within a week of the injury. If not controlled, the combination of increasing pressure and displacement of brain tissue by the expanding hematoma may lead to coma and death within a few hours. Surgical removal is the most common treatment for acute subdural hematomas.

Chronic subdural hematomas are common in older patients and in patients with long-term alcoholism, both of whom have increased risk of falling and "usually have some degree of brain atrophy with a resultant increase in the size of

the subdural space" (Friedman, 1983, p. 10). Often the injury that precipitates the hematoma seems trivial (e.g., a person falls and bumps her or his head). The hemorrhage gradually fills the subdural space. Eventually the hematoma may reach a size at which it produces symptoms that wax and wane. Surgical evacuation of subdural hematomas was the treatment of choice for many years, but mortality was high. In the last decade a more conservative procedure has replaced surgery. A catheter is inserted into the hematoma through an opening in the skull, and the fluid is drained away.

Subarachnoid hematomas, caused by rupture of pial vessels within the subarachnoid space, are a common consequence of traumatic brain injuries and often are associated with subdural hemorrhages. Rapid accumulation of blood from massive subarachnoid hemorrhages typically causes severe headache and rapid neurologic deterioration, with death as a common outcome. Slowly accumulating blood in the subarachnoid space has less ominous consequences. Patients with slowly developing subarachnoid hematomas may go for years without overt symptoms. Little is known about the long-range consequences of such slowly progressing hematomas, although they are known to contribute to *cerebral vasospasm* (discussed later in this chapter).

Intracerebral hematomas are caused by the rupture of blood vessels inside the brain *(intracerebral hemorrhage)*. Intracerebral hemorrhages usually develop in subcortical white matter, the basal ganglia, and the brain stem. Occasionally a large intracerebral hematoma bleeds into the ventricles, creating a secondary subarachnoid hematoma, usually with devastating effects on the patient. A pattern of multiple small intracerebral hemorrhages sometimes occurs in combination with diffuse axonal injury caused by translational trauma—a combination that often leads to coma and death of the patient (Adams, Graham, Scott, and associates, 1980).

Secondary Consequences of Traumatic Brain Injury

The foregoing consequences of traumatic brain injury are the result of the forces exerted on the brain at the time of injury. For this reason they are sometimes called *primary consequences*. They are caused by the mechanical effects of compression, stretching, shearing, abrasion, and laceration of the brain and meninges. These primary consequences of brain injury usually are followed by *secondary consequences*, which represent the brain's physiologic response to trauma or to the failure of other somatic functions (e.g., cardiac output or pulmonary function). Secondary consequences often are more devastating than primary consequences. Although no statistics are available, it is likely that more patients with traumatic brain injuries die from the secondary consequences of their injuries than from the physical damage to the brain suffered at the time of the accident. (Death rates from traumatic brain injuries are highest in the first 3 days, with 50% to 75% of deaths occurring within 72 hours.)

Cerebral Edema. Accumulation of fluid is the brain's generic response to a wide variety of conditions (e.g., trauma, anoxia, infection, inflammation). Fluid may accumulate between the brain and the skull, in the ventricles, or in brain tissues, causing tissues to swell—a condition called *cerebral edema.* Cerebral edema almost always develops around the primary site of the brain injury, but it may also appear far from the primary injury site. Cerebral edema is a common consequence of diffuse injuries such as those caused by translational trauma, and is an important cause of increased intracranial pressure. The effects of cerebral edema on intracranial pressure usually become significant within 4 to 6 hours after injury and peak in 24 to 36 hours.

Traumatic Hydrocephalus. Swelling of brain tissues (especially in midbrain regions) sometimes compresses the passages through which cerebrospinal fluid (CSF) circulates among the ventricles and into the subarachnoid space. The trapped CSF exerts pressure on the walls of the ventricles, causing the ventricles to expand. As the ventricles expand, brain tissues are compressed and intracranial pressure rises.

Elevated Intracranial Pressure. Perhaps the most dramatic (and deadly) consequence of traumatic brain injury is pressure buildup inside the skull. Heightened pressure inside the skull usually is a consequence of cerebral edema, traumatic hydrocephalus, or hemorrhage. Elevated intracranial pressure compresses and displaces brain tissues, causing increasing neurologic impairment as pressure increases. Elevated intracranial pressure is the most frequent cause of death from traumatic brain injury. Therefore, monitoring and controlling intracranial pressure is a primary concern in medical management of traumatically brain-injured persons.

The brain is remarkably tolerant of modest increases in pressure, provided the pressure is distributed equally throughout the cranial vault. Traumatic brain injuries, however, create pressure gradients in which pressure is greatest at and around the site of the injury and decreases with increasing distance from the injury. The pressure gradients push brain tissues away from regions of high pressure into regions of low pressure. Brain tissues are distorted, stretched, compressed, and forced against partitions in the skull, usually with ominous consequences, because the brain is as intolerant of displacement and distortion as it is tolerant of moderate increments in generalized intracranial pressure.

The most dangerous consequence of regional increases in intracranial pressure is *herniation,* in which brain tissue is pushed around rigid partitions in the cranial vault or extruded through cranial orifices. Herniation is discussed in Chapter 1.

Prolonged high levels of intracranial pressure inevitably cause irreversible brain damage, often culminating in coma and death. Fortunately, intracranial pressure can be medically managed. The patient may be hyperventilated to increase blood oxygen levels. Increased blood oxygen causes cerebral arteries to constrict, decreases cerebral blood volume, and provides at least a temporary reduction in intracranial pressure. *Steroids* (antiinflammatory medications) may be administered to reduce cerebral swelling. The patient's body temperature may be lowered *(hypothermia)* to diminish brain swelling. *Diuretics* (medications that increase the body's excretion of fluids) may be administered. If these treatments are unsuccessful, the patient may be put into a barbiturate coma to decrease cerebral metabolism and constrict cerebral blood vessels. If less radical measures fail, surgical removal of swollen brain tissue may be necessary.

Ischemic Brain Damage. Most traumatically brain-injured patients sustain at least some ischemic brain damage in addition to the damage caused by tissue destruction, swelling, and tissue displacement. Graham, Adams, and Doyle (1978) reported ischemic damage in 91% of a group of patients who had died of head injuries. Ischemic brain damage in traumatic brain injury may have several sources. Physical injury to the heart and lungs may compromise respiratory and cardiac output, leading to diminished blood oxygenation and reduced blood supply to the brain. Elevated intracranial pressure may squeeze blood vessels and reduce the volume of blood reaching the brain. Cerebral vasospasm (discussed in the next section) may decrease the carrying capacity of the cerebral vessels, especially when cardiac output is reduced.

Cerebral ischemia and its effects are far more prominent in patients with severe head injuries than in patients with mild to moderately severe head injuries, but it seems likely that some patients with moderate head injuries (and perhaps a few with mild head injuries) may be affected in subtle ways by brain ischemia. The distribution of damage from ischemia varies, but damage is most common in the basal ganglia and surrounding structures and in the watershed cortical regions adjacent to the distributions of the three major cerebral arteries

(regions where small-diameter arteries resist blood flow).

Cerebral vasospasm (contraction of the muscular layer surrounding blood vessels) occurs in 15% to 20% of head injuries. Cortical arteries that are inflamed by the presence of blood from a subarachnoid hemorrhage most frequently are affected, although any artery may be affected (especially if it is in or near the primary injury). Cerebral vasospasm also may be caused by injury to control centers that regulate dilation and constriction of cerebral arteries or by stimulation of cerebral blood vessels by chemical or metabolic disruptions. Cerebral vasospasm alone rarely is responsible for major neurologic complications. However, when vasospasm is inflicted on a system already compromised by other consequences of brain injury, it may contribute to significant worsening of a patient's condition.

Alterations in the Blood-Brain Barrier. In addition to the tissue destruction, neural disorganization, and vascular changes previously described, traumatic brain injury also induces changes in the blood-brain barrier (Povlishock & associates, 1978). The *blood-brain barrier* normally regulates the movement of substances from the blood into the tissues of the brain. Brain injury may disrupt this regulation, allowing normally excluded substances (proteins, neurotransmitter chemicals) to enter brain tissue. More severe brain injuries are more likely to disrupt the blood-brain barrier than are less severe injuries. (This relationship between the severity of injury and the magnitude of secondary consequences is, of course, true for all secondary consequences.) The passage of normally excluded substances into the brain may contribute to accumulation of fluid and swelling of brain tissues (cerebral edema).

Severity of Brain Injury and Physiologic Consequences

Not surprisingly, the nature and severity of neuropathology caused by traumatic brain injury determines the nature and severity of a patient's symptoms and also determines, in large part, the extent of a patient's recovery. The least severe head injuries are called *concussions*. The Academy of Neurology defines *concussion* as *physiologic injury to the brain without evidence of structural alteration*. More than a dozen scales for rating the severity of concussions have been published in the last decade (most with professional athletes in mind). The American Academy of Neurology (1997) suggested a three-level scale for rating the severity of concussion:

- *Grade 1:* Transient confusion, no loss of consciousness; concussion symptoms or mental status abnormalities resolve in less than 15 minutes
- *Grade 2:* Transient confusion, no loss of consciousness; concussion symptoms or mental status abnormalities last more than 15 minutes
- *Grade 3:* Any loss of consciousness, whether brief (seconds) or prolonged (minutes)

For many years practitioners assumed that concussion caused no long-term effects on mental processes, but recent studies have shown that this is not true. High school athletes who experience Grade 1 concussions may experience memory impairments and other signs of cognitive impairment for up to 6 days after their injuries (Maroon & associates, 2000).

Concussion comes from a Latin word which means *to shake violently.*

As many of 30% of persons who experience concussion develop *postconcussive syndrome (PCS),* in which physical, psychological, and cognitive effects of brain injury (e.g., headache, nausea, vomiting, memory loss, dizziness, double vision, blurred vision, emotional lability, sleep disturbances) persist for weeks or months after what appears at onset to be a typical concussion. PCS usually lasts from 2 to 4 months, with symptoms peaking about 4 to 6 weeks after injury, although sometimes symptoms may last 1 year or longer. PCS is more frequent and more severe in children than in adults.

Patients who experience concussions are assumed not to have lasting physiologic injury to the brain. Patients who have persisting mild impairments of memory and cognition typically have damaged axons scattered throughout the brain. Relatively good physiologic recovery usually occurs, no doubt aided by *neuroplasticity* (collateral axonal sprouting, dendritic proliferation).

Patients with moderate traumatic brain injury have diffuse axonal damage spread throughout the brain and brain stem. Lacerations and contusions on the surface of the brain, primarily in the inferior temporal and frontal lobes, destroy brain tissue, creating focal lesions. Lacerated and torn blood vessels leak, creating hematomas. Neuroplasticity usually contributes to moderate amounts of physiologic recovery for patients with moderate traumatic brain injury.

Patients with severe traumatic brain injury typically have extensive axonal damage throughout the brain and brain stem. Hemorrhages are common and may be life-threatening. Vascular ischemic changes are common in the first few days following injury. Hypotension from blood loss or from compromised autoregulation of blood pressure may add to brain ischemia. Hypoxia from pulmonary obstruction or hypoventilation may further diminish the brain's oxygen supply. Neuroplasticity typically contributes little to physiologic recovery, because the density of axonal damage throughout the brain precludes the important beneficial effects of collateral axonal sprouting and dendritic proliferation.

The primary and secondary physical consequences of traumatic brain injury are important determinants of traumatically brain-injured patients' eventual level of recovery, but they are not the only determinants. Patient variables such as age, gender, and personal history also affect recovery, although their influence is not as strong as that of physical consequences. In the following section we consider how some of these variables relate to recovery from traumatic brain injury and to each other.

GENERAL CONCEPTS 11-1

- Traumatic head injuries are a significant social, economic, and medical problem in contemporary society. About 1.4 million U.S. residents per year experience head injuries. An estimated 5 million U.S. residents are living with permanent disabilities caused by head injuries.
- The probability of traumatic head injury is higher for young adults and elderly persons than for the remainder of the U.S. population. Young male adults are particularly likely to experience head injuries, usually caused by motor-vehicle accidents.
- Substance abuse is one of the major risk factors for traumatic head injury in the U.S. Other risk factors include school adjustment and social history, socioeconomic status, personality, a history of head injury, and participation in high-risk sports.
- Traumatic head injuries can be classified as *penetrating* or *nonpenetrating,* depending on whether the skull is fractured or perforated and the meninges are torn or cut. Most *penetrating brain injuries* (in which the skull and meninges are compromised) are caused by *missiles* (bullets or other projectiles).
- Nonpenetrating *(closed-head)* injuries are more common than penetrating head injuries. Most closed-head injuries are caused by motor-vehicle accidents.
- Closed-head injuries may occur when the restrained head is struck by a moving object *(fixed-head injury* or *nonacceleration injury)* or when the moving head strikes a stationary object or abruptly changes direction *(moving-head injury* or *acceleration injury).* Acceleration injuries usually produce more severe brain trauma than nonacceleration injuries.
- *Linear acceleration injuries* are caused by sudden acceleration of the head by a force that moves through the midline of the head.

Angular acceleration injuries are caused by sudden deflection and rotation of the head by a force that strikes the head at an angle.
- *Coup* and *contrecoup brain trauma* are most common following linear acceleration of the head, and *rotational trauma* is most common following angular acceleration. Angular acceleration usually produces more severe brain trauma than does linear acceleration.
- Both linear acceleration and angular acceleration cause stretching and shearing of brain tissues, which in turn cause *diffuse axonal injury* within the brain. Movement of the brain within the cranial vault causes *abrasions* and *lacerations* on the surface of the brain.
- Movement and deformation of the brain within the cranial vault may cause bleeding *(traumatic hemorrhage)* within the brain *(intracerebral hemorrhage)* or on the surface of the brain *(extracerebral hemorrhage).* Extracerebral hemorrhages may be *epidural, subdural,* or *subarachnoid hemorrhages.*
- Cerebral swelling *(edema)* is an important secondary consequence of traumatic brain injury. Cerebral swelling can cause *traumatic hydrocephalus* or *elevated intracranial pressure.* Elevated intracranial pressure is an important cause of death within the first hours after brain injury. Death often occurs because of *herniation,* in which brain tissues are pushed against cranial partitions or through openings in the skull by localized regions of increased pressure within the cranial vault.
- Head trauma often causes disruption of blood supply to the brain, may disrupt autoregulation of blood pressure, and may cause cerebral vasospasm, all of which may contribute to *brain ischemia* (insufficient oxygen supply to brain tissues).

PROGNOSTIC INDICATORS IN TRAUMATIC BRAIN INJURY

Duration of Coma

Not surprisingly, patients who have severe brain injuries recover less well than patients with milder injuries. This relationship has been recognized for more than 100 years. Investigators have worked not so much to confirm the relationship between severity of brain injury and outcome as to find reliable indicators of severity that do not require postmortem examination of the brain.

One of the most reliable indirect indicators of severity of brain injury is the magnitude and duration of alterations in consciousness (Macniven, 1994). Deeper and longer-lasting unconsciousness (coma) is associated with poorer eventual recovery (Carlsson, Svardsudd, & Welin, 1987; Gilchrist & Wilkinson, 1979; Jennett & associates, 1977; Ruesch, 1944; and others). Katz and Alexander (1994) reported outcomes based on length of coma for 119 traumatic-brain-injury patients with diffuse axonal injury. Outcomes were progressively worse as the duration of coma increased (Figure 11-8).

Until the 1970s, investigators' understanding of the relationship between the magnitude and duration of altered consciousness and outcome was compromised, because different investigators measured the level and duration of unconsciousness in different ways and used different measures of outcome, which prevented comparisons across studies. Then, in the early 1970s, investigators began to develop standardized measures of consciousness and outcome.

Teasdale and Jennett (1974) helped bring uniformity to how levels of consciousness are measured by introducing the *Glasgow Coma Scale (GCS),* which provided a consistent way of rating a patient's level of consciousness based on eye opening, verbal responses, and motor

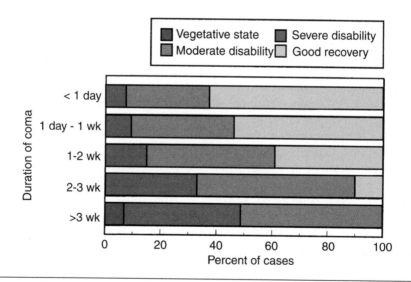

Figure 11-8 ■ The relationship between the duration of coma following severe traumatic brain injury and eventual recovery. Longer durations of coma are associated with poorer eventual recovery. (Data from Katz, D.I., Alexander, M.P. [1994]. Traumatic brain injury. In D.C. Good, J.R. Couch. *Handbook of neurorehabilitation* [pp. 493-549]. New York: Dekker. Data normalized by author.)

TABLE 11-1	The Glasgow Coma Scale (GCS)	
Category of Behavior	Description	Value
Eye Opening	Opens eyes spontaneously	4
	Opens eyes on request	3
	Opens eyes in response to pain	2
	Does not open eyes	1
Motor Responses	Obeys requests to move	6
	Pushes painful stimulation away	5
	Moves limb away from painful stimulus	4
	Abnormal (decorticate*) response to pain	3
	Abnormal (decerebrate[†]) response to pain	2
	Makes no motor response	1
Verbal Responses	Converses and is oriented	5
	Confusion or disoriented speech	4
	Utters intelligible words, but does not make sense	3
	Produces unintelligible sounds	2
	Makes no sound	1

From Teasdale, G., Jennett, B. (1974). Assessment of coma and impaired consciousness. *Lancet, 2,* 81-84.

*Decorticate: flexion of the arm at the elbow, adduction of the shoulder, extension of the leg and ankle.

[†]Decerebrate: extension of the arm at the elbow, internal rotation of shoulder and forearm, leg extension. Both conditions suggest severe brain dysfunction.

responses observed during the immediate post-injury period (Table 11-1). To arrive at a GCS score, the examiner determines the patient's highest level of eye-opening, motor behavior, and verbal responses and then sums the scores for the three levels. GCS scores can range from 3 to 15, and *coma* is operationally defined as a GCS score of 8 or less (Eisenberg & Weiner, 1987). Practitioners routinely divide patients into three levels of severity based on GCS score. Scores of 3 to 8 denote *severe head injury;* scores of 9 to 12 denote *moderate head injury;* and scores of 13 to 15 denote *mild head injury.*

> A normal adult would score 15 on the Glasgow Coma Scale, but the GCS rating follows a known head injury; hence 15 = mild head injury.

Initial GCS scores have been shown to predict traumatically brain-injured patients' even-tual recovery, if the patient is assessed during the early stages of recovery but long enough after injury that non-neurologic contributors to the patient's impairments (e.g., alcohol intoxication) have dissipated (Bowers & Marshall, 1980; Jennett & associates, 1976; Katz, 1992; Langfitt, 1978; and others). Most studies of the relationship between GCS scores and outcome have used the GCS score at 6 hours after injury as the reference value for predicting outcome.

The *Glasgow Coma Scale* has acceptable test-retest and interexaminer reliability, but it is insensitive, because a wide range of behaviors must be reduced to a small number of possible scores. Apparently, experience with the GCS counts—experienced users are more reliable than inexperienced users (Rowley & Fielding, 1991). Because no exceptions are made for untestable categories of behavior, the GCS may overestimate the severity of impairment for some patients, such as patients who are verbally competent but cannot talk because of intubation, patients with facial injuries whose eyes are swollen shut, or patients with paralyzed or immobilized limbs for whom motor responses are difficult or impossible. The timing of assessment also can affect the predictive reliability of the GCS. Some patients with traumatic brain injuries are alert and clear-headed in the first few hours after injury and then deteriorate, so GCS scores obtained at the standard 6 hours after injury may give an unduly optimistic estimate of recovery for these patients.

Some practitioners adjust GCS scores for patients who cannot speak because they are intubated. They are evaluated only for eye opening and motor response, and the letter *T* is appended to the score to indicate that the patient was intubated. The maximum GCS score for intubated patients is 10T, and the minimum score for these patients is 2T.

The GCS has been shown to predict recovery best for patients at the two ends of the severity continuum—patients who eventually "die or walk away" (Segatore & Way, 1992). For traumatically brain-injured patients at middle severity ranges (the patients for whom clinicians typically are most concerned with predicting recovery) the GCS may not predict patients' eventual level of independence (Segatore & Way, 1992; Shatz & Chute, 1995).

The *Comprehensive Level of Consciousness Scale* (*CLOCS*; Stanczak & associates, 1984) was designed to compensate for some of the deficiencies of the Glasgow Coma Scale by assessing a broader range of responses. The CLOCS provides for ratings of posture, resting eye position, spontaneous eye opening, ocular movements, pupillary reflexes, motor functioning, responsiveness, and communicative effort. Behaviors in these eight categories are subjectively rated using 5-point to 9-point scales.

The CLOCS is more sensitive to subtle changes in patients' responsiveness than the Glasgow Coma Scale. Stanczak and associates (1984) have shown that CLOCS scores at discharge from the hospital reliably predict traumatically brain-injured patients' recovery. Although the CLOCS is a more sensitive instrument, it takes longer than the Glasgow Coma Scale to administer and score. Consequently, the GCS remains the most widely used measure for assessing traumatically brain-injured patients' level of consciousness in the immediate post-injury period. Table 11-2 shows how *eye opening, responsiveness,* and *communication* are rated with scales such as the CLOCS.

Duration of Posttraumatic Amnesia

The duration of *posttraumatic amnesia* (the time following coma during which the patient is unable to store new information and experiences in memory) has been considered an indirect indicator of the severity of brain injury and a fair predictor of outcome. Several studies have shown that the duration of posttraumatic amnesia is inversely related to a patient's eventual level of recovery from traumatic brain injury (Bond, 1976; Dikman & associates, 1995; Levin & associates, 1979; Katz, 1992; and others). Katz (1992) reported GCS outcome scores for 114 patients who had diffuse axonal injury. Posttraumatic amnesia lasting less than 2 weeks was associated with good recovery in 80% of cases, whereas no patient with posttraumatic amnesia lasting longer than 12 weeks made a good recovery.

In the late 1970s investigators began to question the reliability of retrospective estimates of posttraumatic amnesia, and subjective estimates of posttraumatic amnesia were largely abandoned in favor of standardized procedures to permit more sensitive and reliable estimates.

The *Galveston Orientation and Amnesia Test* (*GOAT*; Levin, O'Donnell, & Grossman, 1979) was designed to track recovery of orientation and memory for traumatically brain-injured patients who are emerging from coma (Table 11-3). The GOAT consists of 10 questions with which to

TABLE 11-2	**Scales for Rating Eye Opening, Responsiveness, and Communication**

Eye Opening

5   The patient's eyes are open during normal waking times.
4   The patient opens eyes on request.
3   The patient opens eyes in response to mild stimulation.
2   The patient opens eyes in response to moderate stimulation.
1   The patient opens eyes only in response to noxious stimulation.
0   The patient does not open eyes volitionally or to stimulation.

Alertness, Responsiveness

5   The patient is awake and alert during normal waking hours. When asleep, the patient wakens to mild or
      moderate stimuli and attends to the source of stimulation.
4   The patient sleeps or is somnolent during normal waking hours. The patient responds to mild or
      moderate stimulation but returns to sleep or somnolence when stimulation ends.
3   The patient is comatose and is aroused only by noxious stimulation. Responses are oriented to the
      source of stimulation but arousal lasts only as long as stimulation continues.
2   The patient is comatose and is aroused only by noxious stimulation. Responses to stimulation are
      primitive and are not oriented to the source of stimulation (e.g., limb withdrawal, facial grimacing,
      vocalization).
1   The patient is comatose and is aroused only by noxious stimulation. Responses to stimulation are
      generalized and unfocused (e.g., limb flexion, disorganized movement).
0   The patient does not respond to stimulation.

Communication

5   The patient communicates thoughts, needs, and desires by means of speech, writing, or gesturing.
      Maintains eye contact and comprehends most spoken language and meaningful gestures.
4   The patient communicates simple information by simple motor responses (e.g., head movements, eye
      blinks, finger movements). Maintains eye contact and comprehends most spoken language and
      meaningful gestures.
3   The patient attempts to communicate by speech, writing, or gestural communicative behavior that is
      intelligible but confused, disoriented, stereotypic, or perseverative. Eye contact is intermittently
      appropriate. Comprehension and retention of spoken language is moderately to severely impaired.
2   The patient produces unintelligible vocalizations or meaningless gestures when spoken to.
      Comprehension and retention of spoken language is severely impaired.
1   The patient vocalizes or grimaces when spoken to. No evidence of comprehension of spoken language.
0   The patient neither vocalizes nor attempts to speak when spoken to.

TABLE 11-3 Galveston Orientation & Amnesia Test (GOAT)	
Question	Point Value
What is your name?	2
When were you born?	4
Where do you live?	4
Where are you now? (City)	5
Where are you now? (Hospital)	5
On what date were you admitted to this hospital?	5
How did you get here?	5
What is the first event you can remember after the injury?	5
Can you describe in detail (e.g., date, time, companions) the first event you can recall after injury?	5
Can you describe the last event you recall before the accident?	5
Can you describe in detail (e.g., date, time, companions) the first event you can recall before the injury?	5
What time is it now?	(A)
What day of the week is it?	(B)
What day of the month is it?	(C)
What is the month?	(D)
What is the year?	(E)

(A) 1 for each ½ hour removed from correct time to maximum of 5
(B) 1 for each day removed from correct one
(C) 1 for each day removed from correct date to maximum of 5
(D) 5 for each month removed from correct one to maximum of 15
(E) 10 for each year removed from correct one to maximum of 30.

From Levin, H.S., O'Donnell, V.M., & Grossman, R.G. (1979). The Galveston orientation and amnesia test: A practical scale to assess cognition after head injury. *Journal of Nervous and Mental Disorders, 167,* 675-684.

assess the patient's ability to remember and produce biographic information (orientation to person), the patient's orientation to place and time, and the patient's memory for events immediately preceding or following injury.

The patient begins the GOAT with 100 points, and points are subtracted for each failed test item. Scores from 80 to 100 are considered average; scores from 66 to 79 are considered borderline; and scores from 0 to 65 are considered impaired. For most traumatically brain-injured patients, orientation to person returns before orientation to place, and orientation to time is last to recover. Scores on the GOAT have been found to correlate with the severity of brain injury as indicated by CT scans and GCS scores (although the correlations are not strong enough to permit predictions of recovery for individual patients), and scores on the GOAT also have been found to correlate with traumatically brain-injured patients' eventual level of recovery and their return to work (Levin, O'Donnell, & Grossman, 1979; Dikman & associates, 1995).

The GOAT is a useful screening test for getting a general idea of a patient's level of cognitive functioning and responsiveness, although orientation is weighted more heavily than

TABLE 11-4	The Glasgow Outcome Scale (GOS)

Rating	Definition
1	**Death.** Includes death clearly attributable to indirect or secondary effects of brain injury, such as pneumonia.
2	**Persistent Vegetative State.** The patient displays sleep-wake cycles but makes no organized responses to stimulation during periods of wakefulness.
3	**Severe Disability (conscious but disabled).** The patient is dependent on others for daily care by reason of mental or physical disabilities, or a combination of both.
4	**Moderate Disability (disabled but independent).** The patient can travel by public transportation and work in a sheltered workshop. The patient may have motor impairment, language impairment, intellectual and/or memory impairment, and personality disruption.
5	**Good Recovery.** The patient resumes normal life but may have minor neurological and psychological impairments. Return to work is not a prerequisite for this rating.

From Jennett, B., Bond, M. (1975). Assessment of outcome after severe brain damage: A practical scale. *Lancet, 1,* 480-484.

amnesia and memory. Because it requires spoken responses, the GOAT may overestimate the severity of impairment for patients with focal damage in regions serving speech and language in addition to the diffuse damage typical of traumatic brain injury.

The GCS and the CLOCS were designed to measure patients' responsiveness in the immediate postinjury period, and the GOAT was designed to measure memory and orientation in the immediate postinjury period. Not surprisingly, practitioners also began using them to predict traumatically brain-injured patients' eventual recovery, but it soon became apparent that these measures did not reliably predict the eventual recovery of individual patients, which (in fairness to their designers) they were not designed to do. These measures were designed to allow investigators to assess the relationship of postinjury responsiveness, memory, and orientation to outcome for groups of patients. They were not intended as a tool to describe the recovery of individual patients.

In 1975, Jennett and Bond proposed a standardized procedure for characterizing recovery in traumatic brain injury, called the *Glasgow*

Outcome Scale (*GOS*; Table 11-4). The GOS has acceptable reliability but may not have sufficient sensitivity to predict small but important differences in outcome. It seems best suited for quantifying gross differences in outcome among traumatically brain-injured persons.

Several attempts to expand the GOS to make it more sensitive have run into problems of unreliability. As a general rule, the more choices judges are given in rating any phenomenon, the less they will agree on their ratings. The simplest way to ensure the reliability of a rating scale is to keep the number of possible ratings small, but rating scales with small numbers of possible ratings tend to be insensitive to small differences in the phenomenon being rated. There is almost always a trade-off between sensitivity and reliability when one develops a rating scale.

The *Rancho Los Amigos Scale of Cognitive Levels* (*RLAS*; Hagen & Malkamus, 1979) was designed to provide a more comprehensive estimate of brain-injured patients' cognitive and behavioral characteristics than previous

TABLE 11-5	The Rancho Los Amigos Scale of Cognitive Levels (RLAS)
Level	**Definition**
1. No Response	No response to pain, touch, sound, or sight
2. Generalized Responses	Inconsistent, nonpurposeful, nonspecific responses to intense stimuli Responds to pain, but response may be delayed
3. Localized Responses	Blinks to strong light, turns toward/away from sound, responds to physical discomfort Inconsistent responses to some commands
4. Confused-Agitated	Alert, very active, with aggressive and/or bizarre behaviors Attention span is short Behavior is nonpurposeful, and patient is disoriented and unaware of present events
5. Confused-Inappropriate	Exhibits gross attention to environment Is highly distractible, requires continual redirection to keep on task Is alert and responds to simple commands Performs previously learned tasks but has great difficulty learning new ones Becomes agitated by too much stimulation May engage in social conversation but with inappropriate verbalizations
6. Confused-Appropriate	Behavior is goal-directed, with assistance Inconsistent orientation to time and place Retention span and recent memory are impaired Consistently follows simple directions
7. Automatic-Appropriate	Performs daily routine in highly familiar environments without confusion, but in an automatic robotlike manner Is oriented to setting, but insight, judgment, and problem-solving are poor
8. Purposeful-Appropriate	Responds appropriately in most situations Can generalize new learning across situations Does not require daily supervision May have poor tolerance for stress and may exhibit some abstract reasoning disabilities

From Hagen, C., Malkamus, D. (1979). *Interaction strategies for language disorders secondary to head trauma.* Paper presented at the annual convention of the American Speech-Language-Hearing Association, Atlanta, GA.

measures. The original RLAS provided a standard set of eight categories to which brain-injured patients could be assigned according to their arousal, responsiveness, restlessness, attention, memory, and executive ability (Table 11-5).

A revised version of the RLAS, the *Rancho Los Amigos Scale of Cognitive Levels—Revised* (*RLAS-R*; Hagen, 1997) added two categories to which patients could be assigned and added seven levels reflecting patients' levels of independence (Box 11-1). Most institutions that were using the 8-level RLAS are now using the 10-level RLAS-R, although some continue to use the RLAS.

Box 11-1	**The Rancho Los Amigos Scale of Cognitive Levels—Revised**

Total Assistance

Level I: No Response

- No observable change in behavior in response to any stimuli, including painful stimuli

Level II: Generalized Response

- Responds to painful stimuli with generalized reflexive movements
- Responds to other stimuli with changes in respiration, gross body movement, or nonpurposeful vocalization; responses may be delayed and do not change according to the type and location of stimulation

Level III: Localized Response

- Withdraws or vocalizes in response to painful stimuli; responds to discomfort by pulling on tubes or restraints
- Blinks in response to bright light, visually follows moving objects
- Turns toward or away from auditory stimuli
- Responses related to type of stimulus
- Inconsistently responds to spoken commands such as "*close your eyes*"
- May respond to some persons (especially family, friends) but not to others

Maximal Assistance

Level IV: Confused, Agitated

- Alert but hyperactive; may try to remove restraints or get out of bed
- May sit up, reach, and walk, but without purpose and not on request
- May shout or scream in response to nonpainful stimuli; shouting or screaming may persist after stimulation ends
- May utter incoherent verbalizations unrelated to activity or environment
- Brief but nonpurposeful intervals of sustained attention; no evidence of short-term memory
- May exhibit aggressive or flight behaviors
- Mood may swing unpredictably from euphoria to hostility
- Does not cooperate with treatment efforts

Level V: Confused, Appropriate, Nonagitated

- Not oriented to person, place, or time
- Alert, not agitated, but may wander purposelessly
- May become agitated in response to stimulation or unexpected changes in environment
- Occasional short intervals of nonpurposeful sustained attention
- Severely impaired recent memory. Confuses past and present
- Uses objects inappropriately unless given direction
- May perform familiar tasks in highly structured situations if cues are provided
- No evidence of problem solving
- Does not learn and retain new information
- Often responds appropriately to simple commands in highly structured situations if cues are provided
- Converses on an automatic level for short intervals in highly structured situations if cues are provided; otherwise verbal behavior is inappropriate and confabulatory

Moderate Assistance

Level VI: Confused, Appropriate

- Inconsistently oriented to person, place, and time
- Unaware of impairments, disabilities, and safety risks
- Attends to highly familiar tasks in nondistracting environments for up to 30 minutes with moderate assistance
- Recalls remote past events; memory for recent events is grossly impaired
- Uses assistive memory aids with maximum assistance
- Problem-solves in structured tasks with moderate assistance
- Carries out familiar tasks (e.g., self-care) with supervision; shows carry-over for relearned familiar tasks
- Learns new tasks with maximum assistance but with little or no carry-over
- Consistently follows simple directions
- Converses appropriately for short intervals in highly structured situations if cues are provided

From Hagen, C. (1997). The *Rancho Los Amigos Scale of Cognitive Levels – Revised*. Unpublished document. (Personal communication from author, 2005.)

| Box 11-1 | *The Rancho Los Amigos Scale of Cognitive Levels—Revised—cont'd* |

Minimal Assistance
Level VII: Automatic, Appropriate

- Consistently oriented to person and place in highly familiar environments; oriented to time with moderate assistance
- Has superficial awareness of personal condition but is unaware of specific impairments and disabilities and the limitations they impose
- Safely performs routine everyday activities with minimal supervision
- Attends to highly familiar tasks in nondistracting environments for at least 30 minutes with minimal assistance
- Initiates and completes familiar everyday routines but with poor memory for what parts of routines have been done
- Judges accuracy and completeness of steps in familiar everyday routines; can modify routines with minimal assistance
- Acquires and retains new learning with minimal assistance
- Unrealistic in planning for future; does not anticipate consequences of decisions or actions; overestimates own abilities
- Unaware of others' needs and feelings; does not recognize socially inappropriate behavior
- Uncooperative and oppositional in social interactions

Standby Assistance
Level VIII: Purposeful, Appropriate

- Consistently oriented to person, place, and time
- Acknowledges impairments and disabilities when they interfere with task completion; requires standby assistance to take corrective action
- Overestimates or underestimates own abilities; may be excessively dependent or independent
- Initiates and completes familiar personal, household, community, work, and leisure routines with minimal assistance
- Independently attends to and completes familiar tasks in distracting environments for up to 1 hour
- Accurately recalls remote past and recent events
- Uses assistive memory devices to recall daily schedule, "to-do" lists, and store important information for later use with standby assistance

- Retains newly learned tasks and activities without assistance
- Anticipates consequences of decisions or actions with minimal assistance
- Acknowledges and responds appropriately to others' feelings and needs with minimal assistance
- May be depressed, irritable, argumentative, self-centered, and easily angered, with low tolerance for frustration
- Recognizes and acknowledges inappropriate social behavior and takes corrective action with minimal assistance

Standby Assistance on Request
Level IX: Purposeful, Appropriate

- Accurately estimates abilities but requires standby assistance to adjust to task requirements
- Moves among and completes tasks for at least 2 consecutive hours without assistance
- Initiates, modifies, and completes familiar personal, household, community, work, and leisure routines without assistance
- Initiates, modifies, and completes unfamiliar personal, household, community, work, and leisure routines with assistance when requested
- Acknowledges impairments and disabilities when they interfere with task completion and takes corrective action
- Requires standby assistance to anticipate a problem and act to avoid it
- Uses assistive memory devices to recall daily schedules and "to-do" lists and to store important information for later use with assistance when requested
- Anticipates consequences of decisions or actions with assistance when requested
- Acknowledges and responds appropriately to others' feelings and needs with standby assistance
- May be depressed and irritable and may have low tolerance for frustration
- Monitors and regulates appropriateness of social behavior with standby assistance

Continued

| **Box 11-1** | *The Rancho Los Amigos Scale of Cognitive Levels—Revised—cont'd* |

Modified Independent

Level X: Purposeful, Appropriate

- Accurately estimates abilities and adjusts to task requirements
- Anticipates effects of impairments and disabilities on completion of daily living tasks; takes action to avoid problems but may need extra time or compensatory strategies
- Works at multiple tasks simultaneously in all environments; may require periodic breaks
- Initiates, modifies, and completes familiar and unfamiliar personal, household, community, work, and leisure routines without assistance; may require extra time, compensatory strategies, or both to complete them

- Independently obtains, creates, and maintains assistive memory devices
- Independently anticipates consequences of decisions or actions but may require extra time or compensatory strategies to select appropriate decisions or actions
- Acknowledges and responds appropriately to others' feelings and needs
- May be periodically depressed
- Irritable with low tolerance for frustration when ill, fatigued, or emotionally stressed
- Consistently appropriate in social interactions

For brevity and ease of reading in the following material, I will use the acronym *RLAS* rather than the cumbersome acronym *RLAS-R* to refer to the Rancho Los Amigos Scale of Cognitive Levels–Revised. When I occasionally refer to the 8-level RLAS, I will tell the reader.

Many clinicians assume that the time-course of individual patients' recovery follows RLAS levels. Many patients do progress through RLAS levels as they recover, but the length of time spent at each level differs among patients. According to Hagen and Malkamus (1979), there is some evidence that the length of time spent at lower RLAS levels is related to eventual outcome—the longer a patient remains at RLAS levels I through IV, the poorer the prognosis for recovery—but substantial errors in prediction can occur. The five highest RLAS levels are more sensitive to language impairments than the five lowest levels. Consequently, higher-level patients with damage in the language-dominant hemisphere tend to be rated somewhat lower than patients with diffuse but symmetric

damage or patients with damage in the non-language-dominant hemisphere.

The *Disability Rating Scale* (*DRS*; Rappoport & associates, 1982) was created to provide a more sensitive measure of progress and to measure a wider range of recovery than the GOS, from which the DRS is derived. The DRS permits observers to rate a patient's level of function in eight areas: eye opening, verbal response, motor response, feeding, toileting, grooming, dependence on others, and employability (Table 11-6). Possible DRS scores range from 0 to 29, with higher scores indicating greater disability.

The DRS is more sensitive to change than the GOS (Hall, Cope, & Rappoport, 1985) and has greater reliability than the (8-level) RLAS (Gouvier & associates, 1987). The DRS, like the GOS, is relatively insensitive to change for patients with mild traumatic brain injuries.

Livingstone and Livingstone (1985) described another procedure for measuring outcome, called the *Glasgow Assessment Schedule* (*GAS*; Table 11-7). The GAS permits users to rate outcome in six domains: physical condition, subjective complaints, personality change, cognitive

TABLE 11-6	The Disability Rating Scale (DRS)	
Category	**Patient Characteristic**	**Rating**
Arousability, awareness, responsivity	Eye opening	0 = spontaneous
		1 = to speech
		2 = to pain
		3 = none
	Communication ability	0 = oriented
		1 = confused
		2 = inappropriate
		3 = incomprehensible
		4 = none
	Motor responses	0 = obeying
		1 = localizing
		2 = withdrawing
		3 = flexing
		4 = extending
		5 = none
Self-care activities	Feeding	0 = complete
		1 = partial
		2 = minimal
		3 = none
	Toileting	0 = complete
		1 = partial
		2 = minimal
		3 = none
	Grooming	0 = complete
		1 = partial
		2 = minimal
		3 = none
Dependence on others	Level of functioning	0 = completely independent
		1 = independent in special environment
		2 = mildly dependent
		3 = moderately dependent
		4 = markedly dependent
		5 = totally dependent
Psychosocial adaptability	Employability	0 = not restricted
		1 = selected jobs
		2 = sheltered workshop (noncompetitive)
		3 = not employable

DRS Total Score	Level of Disability
0	None
1	Mild
2-3	Partial
4-6	Moderate
7-11	Moderately Severe
12-16	Severe
17-21	Extremely Severe
22-24	Vegetative State
25-29	Extreme Vegetative State

From Rappoport, M., Hall, K.M., Hopkins, K., & associates. (1982). Disability rating scale for severe head trauma: Coma to community. *Archives of Physical Medicine and Rehabilitation, 63,* 118-123.

TABLE 11-7	The Glasgow Assessment Schedule (GAS)

Patient Characteristic	Scoring	Patient Characteristic	Scoring
Personality Change		**Cognitive Functioning**	
Emotional lability	a	Immediate recall	a
Irritability	a	2-minute recall	a
Aggressiveness	a	Attention, concentration	a
Other behavioral change	a	Orientation	a
		Current intelligence	a
Subjective Complaints			
Sleep disturbance	a	**Physical Examination**	
Incontinence	a	Dysphasia	a
Family stress	a	Dysarthria	a
Financial problems	a	Abnormal tone: R leg	a
Sexual problems	a	Abnormal tone: L leg	a
Alcohol: excess, poor tolerance	a	Abnormal tone: upper limbs	a
Reduced leisure, sporting activities	a	Walking	a
Headache	a	Cranial nerves	a
Dizziness, loss of balance	a	Seizures	a
Paresthesia	a		
Reduced sense of smell	a	**Activities of Daily Living**	
Reduced hearing	a	Cooking	b
Reduced vision	a	Other domestic tasks	b
		Shopping	b
Occupational Functioning		Traveling	b
Working: same job	0	Personal hygiene	b
Working: similar job	0	Feeding	b
Working: less skilled job	1	Dressing	b
Not working: employable	2	Mobility	b
Not working: not employable	3		

Scoring: a: normal (0), moderate (1), severe (2); **b:** on own (0), with help (1), unable to do (2)

Modified from Livingstone, M.G. & Livingstone, H.M. (1985). The Glasgow Assessment Schedule: Clinical and research assessment of head injury outcome. *International Rehabilitation Medicine, 7,* 145-149.

functioning, occupational functioning, and proficiency in activities of daily living. Overall scores on the GAS range from 0 to 81, with higher scores representing more severe impairment. The DRS and the GAS are more sensitive to changes in performance than the GOS. The DRS now is more widely used than the GAS or the GOS, perhaps because it is shorter and easier to score and interpret.

Rating scales such as those described here were developed to estimate the severity of brain injury and to describe outcome in general terms. Some have been used to estimate population trends. None are sensitive enough for planning intervention for specific individuals or for measuring the effects of intervention. Ylvisaker, Szekeres, and Feeney (2001) comment as follows:

These scales are not intended to be used for planning interventions for specific individuals. Sensitive individualized assessments are needed for this purpose. Furthermore, rating scales are rarely sufficient to measure the effectiveness of intervention in individual cases. For that purpose, there is no substitute for objective documentation of achievement of individualized functional objectives directly related to important personal life goals. (p. 750)

Although the severity of traumatic injury plays the most prominent part in determining patients' eventual recovery, the nature of the injury also plays a part. Focal injuries usually have a better prognosis than diffuse injuries. Neurologic recovery following focal brain injuries proceeds faster and plateaus earlier (but usually at a higher level) than recovery from diffuse injuries (Katz & Alexander, 1994). However, when focal injuries are superimposed on diffuse injuries, the prognosis for recovery suffers (Filley & associates, 1987). The presence of diffuse axonal injury is associated with poor outcome (Uzzell & associates, 1987), as is the presence of secondary brain damage caused by increased intracranial pressure, cerebral edema, anoxia, or hypoxia (Andrews & associates, 1990; Miller & associates, 1978). Patients with diffuse hypoxic injury have a particularly ominous prognosis, especially those who remain comatose for 1 week or more. These unfortunate patients are virtually certain to remain severely disabled for the rest of their lives (Katz, 1992).

Patient-Related Variables

Of several patient-related variables, age is the most important predictor of outcome following traumatic brain injury. Older patients with traumatic brain injuries have higher mortality than younger patients—the mortality of traumatically brain-injured patients age 60 and older is approximately twice that of patients age 20 or younger (Wilson & associates, 1987). Older patients are more likely than younger patients to suffer hemorrhages, and the hemorrhages are likely to be larger (Katz & Alexander, 1994). Older traumatically brain-injured patients recover less rapidly and are more likely to exhibit persisting confusion, attentional impairments, and memory impairments than are younger patients (Jennett & Teasdale, 1981), making older patients more likely than younger patients to remain dependent on caregivers.

Substance abuse also has negative effects on outcome following traumatic brain injury. Alcoholic traumatically brain-injured patients experience longer intervals of coma, lower levels of consciousness after emerging from coma, longer hospitalizations, and greater impairments of memory and verbal learning than nonalcoholic patients (Alfano, 1994). These relationships may be explained, at least in part, by the physiologic consequences of alcohol intoxication at the time of brain injury. Patients who are alcohol-intoxicated at time of injury are more likely to experience cerebral hypoxia, hemorrhage, or cerebral edema than their nonintoxicated counterparts (Alfano, 1994). The effects of substance abuse other than alcohol abuse on recovery from traumatic brain injury have received little empiric study, although presumably chronic drug abuse would have similar negative effects.

Several other patient-related variables have been shown to have minor effects on recovery from traumatic brain injury. Education, intelligence, and socioeconomic status apparently have some effect. Persons with more education, higher intelligence, and higher socioeconomic status seem to recover better than less intelligent individuals or those with lower socioeconomic status. Premorbid personality disorders and emotional disturbances also may negatively affect recovery. Patients with maladaptive personality characteristics and premorbid emotional instability have a somewhat poorer prognosis than those without such disturbances (Humphrey & Oddy, 1981; Rutter, 1981).

The effects of individual patient-related variables on outcome are weak and easily overwhelmed by more potent variables such as the severity and nature of brain injury. Additionally, many patient-related variables are correlated and tend to occur in combination (e.g., low intelligence, low socioeconomic status, and substance abuse), making determination of the effects of individual variables intimidating if not impossible. Finally, even the most dependable prognostic variables are best at predicting average outcomes for groups of patients and are less reliable when applied to individuals. Experienced clinicians give the greatest prognostic weight to the most robust indicators (severity and nature of brain injury), but they recognize that outcome for individual patients may not replicate group findings, even for the most robust indicators.

Clinicians must be cautious in applying group findings to individual patients. Idiosyncratic personal characteristics often play an important part in recovery from brain injury. Persons with a history of motivation, perseverance, and personal achievement may experience better outcomes than group estimates suggest that they should. Persons with a history of underachievement and apathy toward personal accomplishment may experience poorer outcomes than group estimates suggest that they should. Persons with strong support systems may exceed expectations. Persons with weak support systems may fall below expectations. These personal characteristics and many others often confound predictions based on rating scales or group findings. The effects of these personal characteristics may be discovered only by evaluating the brain-injured person's history and support systems and by observing his or her response to the challenges and rewards associated with recovery.

BEHAVIORAL AND COGNITIVE RECOVERY

The general pattern of recovery following traumatic brain injury is one of improvement, but the pattern differs from that seen after strokes. Recovery from strokes typically decreases gradually as time postonset progresses, with rapid recovery immediately after onset and diminishing thereafter. Recovery from traumatic brain injuries often follows a stair-step pattern in which intervals of little or no change alternate with intervals of rapid improvement. The rela-tionship between the severity of patients' impairments in the first few weeks after onset and their permanent level of impairment is much stronger for vascular accidents than it is for traumatic brain injury, making it more difficult to predict traumatically brain-injured patients' permanent level of impairment in the first weeks after onset than it is to make the same prediction for vascular patients.

Traumatically brain-injured patients typically progress through a fairly predictable sequence of stages during recovery. When a patient's brain injury is moderate to severe, the patient invariably loses consciousness immediately after the accident. The interval of unconsciousness may last from a few seconds to weeks or, rarely, months. Return to consciousness begins a period of undifferentiated activity. The patient is awake but responds indiscriminately and purposelessly to the environment, is hyper-responsive to stimulation, and is agitated and irritable. Repetitive stereotyped movements (e.g., rocking, thrashing) are common, as are striking out, shouting, biting, and emotional lability. The patient does not maintain attention for more than a few seconds. The patient's level of arousal fluctuates from moment to moment. As recovery continues, the patient becomes more lucid, and behavior becomes more purposeful, but restlessness, agitation, and irritability persist (at lower levels).

Eventually the patient becomes oriented to time and place and begins to respond appropriately to simple requests, although attention span is limited and distractibility is high. With the passage of time, the patient begins to perform daily routines with supervision and direction, but judgment, memory, and abstract reasoning remain impaired. With continued recovery, the patient begins to function independently in familiar situations, but problems with memory and abstract reasoning remain. A few patients eventually resume work or school activities, although almost always with subtle but important impairments in memory, abstract reasoning, and tolerance for noise and distractions.

The RLAS (see Box 11-1) provides a convenient way to characterize traumatically brain-injured patients' cognitive and behavioral status at various stages of recovery, although not all spend time at each RLAS level. Some with mild injuries skip early levels or pass through them so quickly that intervention is not an issue. Some with severe brain injuries do not make it to the higher levels. The rate at which patients pass through each level varies across patients. Some linger at a level longer than others, and some pass through levels very rapidly or skip levels entirely. RLAS levels indicate the severity of brain injury; they are not a timetable for recovery. A severely injured patient may be at RLAS Level III at 4 weeks after injury, whereas a less severely injured patient may be at RLAS Level VI at the same time after injury.

The following is a description of behavior associated with the various RLAS levels:

- *Comatose, semi-comatose (RLAS Levels I, II, III).* RLAS Level I, II, and III patients are bedbound, usually in an intensive care unit. Most are comatose or minimally responsive. Many have tubes in place to maintain an open airway, assist breathing, and provide for removal of secretions. Most have intravenous lines and urinary catheters in place. Some have sensors attached to monitor intracranial pressure, heartbeat, and respiration. Some have nasogastric tubes in place for administration of liquid nutrition, and a few have *gastrostomies* (openings into the stomach through which liquid diets are administered). Level I patients are unresponsive. Level II patients are minimally responsive to all external stimulation. Level III patients may respond intermittently and inconsistently to intense stimulation.

- *Confused, agitated (RLAS Level IV).* Patients at RLAS Level IV are awake and responsive, but their responses are inconsistent, unpredictable, and without purpose. RLAS Level IV patients are agitated, restless, impulsive, highly distractible, and have profoundly impaired attention, memory, reasoning, and problem-solving. They are not oriented to person, place, or time; they do not cooperate with caregivers; and they are not sensitive to environmental or social cues that normally regulate behavior.

- *Confused, appropriate, nonagitated (RLAS Level V).* Patients at RLAS Level V are not oriented to person, place, or time, and they are unaware of disabilities. They may perform familiar tasks (e.g., self-care) if structure and supervision are provided. They have little tolerance for stress or frustration, which may precipitate explosive emotional outbursts, including physical aggression. Level V patients can follow simple directions but do not monitor their behavior and do not notice mistakes. They do not learn or retain new information.

- *Confused, appropriate (RLAS Level VI).* Patients at RLAS Level VI are intermittently oriented to person and place but usually are not oriented to time. (Orientation to time seems to be particularly resistant to the effects of recovery.) Memory for remote past events is fair, but recent memory is grossly impaired. Patients at RLAS Level VI may interact purposefully with their environment in highly structured contexts. They may perform familiar tasks (e.g., washing, putting possessions away) with supervision, follow simple directions, and learn simple new tasks, although they usually do not retain new learning.

- *Automatic, appropriate (RLAS Level VII).* Patients at RLAS Level VII are restless, distractible, and impulsive, but not agitated. Most are oriented to person and place and intermittently to time. Most are aware that they have been injured, but they are unaware of the nature of their impairments and do not notice errors and inappropriate responses. RLAS level VII patients usually have substantial impairments in attention, memory, reasoning, judgment, and problem-solving. They may perform everyday routines and familiar tasks in supportive environments and can modify routines with assistance from others. They fatigue easily and their attention span is short, which prevents them from participating meaningfully in tasks that require sustained attention and effort. Most do not attend to or appreciate others' wishes, needs, and feelings and tend to be self-centered and uncooperative in social interactions. They are inconsistently responsive to social cues and often fail to respect basic social conventions. Patients at RLAS level VII are highly controlled by their immediate environment, exhibit little capacity for independent thought or behavior, and generally carry out daily life activities in a robotlike manner. Stressful or challenging situations often provoke these patients into emotional outbursts that are striking in their intensity and are equally striking in how quickly they disappear.

- *Purposeful, appropriate (RLAS Level VIII).* Patients at RLAS Level VIII are oriented to person, place, and time, and they are capable of independent action in familiar environments. They can learn and retain new routines and activities. They initiate and carry out familiar daily life routines with little assistance, and they have moderate success in carrying out well-learned activities in nondistracting environments. Patients at RLAS Level VIII acknowledge impairments but may overestimate or underestimate them. Memory for the recent and remote past is functional for most, and most can use assistive memory devices with minimal assistance. They usually recognize others' wishes, needs, and feelings, and they recognize and modify their own inappropriate social behavior. Patients at RLAS Level VIII are generally cooperative and participate willingly in treatment activities, although many are intermittently depressed, irritable, and have little tolerance for stress or frustration. Patients at RLAS Level VIII typically have mildly to moderately impaired attention and problem-solving skills, and insight, judgment, and problem-solving are problematic. They

often get lost in details and fail to grasp the overall meaning of events. They behave appropriately in most interpersonal interactions, although the content of what they say may not always be appropriate.

- *Purposeful, appropriate (RLAS Level IX).* Patients at RLAS Level IX function adequately in most familiar situations, although occasional assistance from others may be needed. Patients at RLAS Level IX usually recognize their need for assistance and request it when needed. They perform familiar daily routines competently and without assistance, and they can learn and perform unfamiliar routines and activities with assistance on request. Patients at RLAS Level IX usually can resolve typical daily life problems independently, but most do not independently anticipate potential problems or act to avoid them. Most can use assistive prospective memory devices with little or no supervision. Many have intermittent word retrieval failures and low verbal fluency, and most have difficulty with abstraction, implication, and inference. Depression and anger often become prominent for patients at RLAS Level IX, as it becomes clear that complete recovery of premorbid abilities is unlikely or unattainable.

- *Purposeful, appropriate (RLAS Level X).* Patients at RLAS Level X function independently in most activities of daily living. They recognize their limitations and anticipate the effects of limitations on daily life activities. When they anticipate a problem, they usually can avoid it, using compensatory strategies if necessary. Patients at RLAS Level X can plan, initiate, and complete familiar and unfamiliar activities of daily life independently, although they may need extra time, assistive devices, or compensatory strategies, which they usually invoke without assistance. Most can predict the amount of time and effort needed to perform activities of daily living, although time management may be problematic. Most have subtle impairments of attention and memory, although communication and interpersonal skills usually are essentially normal. However, when they are fatigued or feel stressed, their performance may deteriorate, and emotional outbursts may occur. Some may experience periodic episodes of depression. Some patients at RLAS Level X may return to school, work, or assume other preinjury responsibilities, although usually at a reduced level or with alterations to the environment to minimize the effects of the patient's impairments.

Ylvisaker, Szekeres, and Feeney (2001) described three general stages of recovery based on the 1979 version of the RLAS:

- *Early Stage (RLAS Levels 2,3).* The early stage (sometimes called the *coma stimulation stage*) begins with the patient's first generalized responses to environmental stimuli and ends when the patient selectively responds to stimuli (e.g., localizing sound, tracking visual stimuli) and follows simple spoken commands. Patients in the early stage of recovery require intensive, fulltime environmental support.

- *Middle Stage (RLAS Levels 4-6).* At the beginning of this stage, patients are alert and increasingly active but are confused, disoriented, and often agitated. At the end of this stage, patients are oriented and less confused, and their behavior in familiar environments generally is goal-directed. Most have difficulty organizing and executing complex tasks. During this stage, patients require moderate but systematically decreasing levels of environmental support in everyday activities.

- *Late Stage (RLAS Level 7 and beyond).* At the beginning of this stage, patients have "an adequate, though perhaps superficial and fragile orientation to important aspects of life" (Ylvisaker & associates, 2001, p. 752). The RLAS stage the patient eventually reaches is determined by his or her neurologic, cognitive, communicative, and behavioral recovery, which may or may not include functionally disabling cognitive or communicative impair-

ments. Environmental supports for patients at Level 7 and beyond gradually are reduced as the patient becomes increasingly independent and adept at compensating for his or her residual impairments. Intervention focuses on refining skills needed for effective participation in everyday life.

GENERAL CONCEPTS 11-2

- Deeper and longer-lasting unconsciousness *(coma)* following head injury is associated with poorer eventual physical and cognitive recovery.

- The *Glasgow Coma Scale (GCS)* is a popular scale for rating head-injured patients' level of consciousness. GCS scores assigned a few hours after head injury reliably predict head-injured patients' recovery, but GCS scores are too coarse to capture small but important patient characteristics.

- The *Comprehensive Level of Consciousness Scale (CLOCS)* is more sensitive than the GCS because it samples a broader range of responses, but it is not as widely used as the GCS.

- The duration of *posttraumatic amnesia* is an indirect indicator of the severity of brain injury and is inversely related to degree of recovery. The *Galveston Orientation and Amnesia Test (GOAT)* is designed to track recovery of orientation and memory by traumatically brain-injured patients who are emerging from coma.

- The *Glasgow Outcome Scale (GOS)* provides a standardized and reliable procedure for quantifying gross differences in recovery among brain-injured patients.

- The *Disability Rating Scale (DRS)* provides a more sensitive measure of progress and measures a wider range of recovery than the GOS does.

Continued

GENERAL CONCEPTS 11-2—cont'd

- The *Rancho Los Amigos Scale of Cognitive Levels* and the *Rancho Los Amigos Scale-Revised (RLAS-R)* are widely used scales that provide categories to which clinicians can assign brain-injured patients based on the patients' cognitive and behavioral characteristics.
- Age is the most important patient-related variable for predicting recovery from traumatic brain injury. Other patient-related variables include substance abuse, education, intelligence, personality, and socioeconomic status. Many patient-related variables are correlated and occur in combinations.
- Traumatically brain-injured patients typically progress through a fairly predictable sequence of stages as they recover. The Rancho Los Amigos Scales provide reasonably accurate chronologies for this sequence of stages.
- As brain-injured patients progress through the levels of the RLAS their behavior progresses from *unresponsive* to *responsive,* from *agitated* to *nonagitated,* from *confused* to *oriented,* from *inappropriate* to *appropriate,* and from *automatic* to *purposeful.*

ASSESSING ADULTS WITH TRAUMATIC BRAIN INJURIES

Assessing traumatically brain-injured adults is an evolutionary process. As a patient's physical, cognitive, and behavioral abilities change with recovery, what happens in testing also changes. Tests that are appropriate for patients with severe brain injuries in the immediate postinjury period (when confusion and agitation are prominent) may be irrelevant for patients in later stages of recovery or for patients with less severe brain injuries, for whom cognitive impairments are a primary concern.

Level of Consciousness and Responsiveness to Stimulation

For comatose and semicomatose patients, the primary objectives of assessment are to determine the patient's level of consciousness, to get a sense of the nature and severity of the patient's injuries, and to estimate the patient's physical, behavioral, and cognitive recovery between the time of injury and the time of assessment.

Assessment of comatose and semicomatose patients focuses on alertness and responsiveness to stimulation. Rating scales such as the Glasgow Coma Scale or the Glasgow Assessment Schedule provide general estimates of alertness and stimulability, but clinicians usually augment these estimates with direct observation of the patient's alertness and responsiveness to stimulation. During the observation, the clinician documents the frequency and nature of (often subtle) responses to stimulation, such as changes in respiration rate, changes in muscle tone, changes in facial expression, eye-opening, or vocalization. The observation usually assesses the following aspects of the patient's condition:

- How much of the day the patient spends sleeping, what parts of the day the patient typically is awake, and the times of day during which the patient is most alert and responsive
- How easily the patient is aroused from sleep by environmental sounds, verbal commands, light touch, shaking, or painful stimulation (comatose and semicomatose patients who do not respond to neutral or pleasant stimuli often respond to unpleasant or noxious stimuli, usually by some sort of avoidance response, such as limb withdrawal or head aversion)
- Responsiveness to environmental stimuli (e.g., a television or radio playing; people entering and leaving the patient's room; being talked to, touched, or moved by nursing personnel)
- Responsiveness to speech: whether the patient looks toward the speaker, changes

facial expression, attempts to speak, or responds motorically

- Comprehension of simple requests such as *open your eyes* or *look at the ceiling*
- Responsiveness to visual stimulation: whether the patient looks at or visually tracks lights or brightly colored objects moved across the patient's field of vision
- Responsiveness to tactile stimulation: eye opening, movement, or vocalization in response to light touch or stroking (if a patient does not respond to light touch or stroking, the clinician may assess the patient's response to pressure by pinching or squeezing or may assess tactile stimulation using hot, cold, rough, or smooth stimuli)
- Responsiveness to olfactory stimuli: eye opening, movement, or vocalization in response to pleasant odors such as cologne, vanilla extract, or almond extract and unpleasant odors such as garlic, mustard, or rubbing alcohol
- Responsiveness to taste stimuli: eye opening, facial grimacing, movement, or vocalization in response to sweet tastes such as fruit juice or honey or to sour or bitter tastes such as lemon juice or vinegar.

Taste and smell are phylogenetically primitive senses and may elicit responses from severely brain-injured patients when visual and auditory stimuli do not. Patients who have nasogastric tubes that block air from the nostrils and patients who have tracheostomies that limit air movement through the nostrils have diminished sense of smell. Many patients who have experienced traumatic brain injuries have injured olfactory nerves. Olfactory nerve injury is the most common cranial nerve injury in traumatic brain injury.

A few organized protocols for assessing severely impaired patients with traumatic brain injuries have been described in the literature (Ansell & Keenan, 1989; Helm-Estabrooks & Hotz, 1991; Rader & Ellis, 1994; Lippert, Gruner, & Terhaag, 2000; and others). Although they differ in specifics, all provide for assessing arousal, attentiveness, and responses to auditory, visual, tactile, and olfactory stimulation. The information from the assessment of the patient's responsiveness to stimulation serves as a baseline against which the rate and magnitude of the patient's cognitive and behavioral recovery may be measured as the clinician periodically observes and documents the patient's responsiveness.

Orientation

As traumatically brain-injured patients return to consciousness and begin responding to environmental stimuli, most remain profoundly disoriented, confused, and agitated. The primary purpose of assessment for patients at this stage of recovery is to establish baseline measures of orientation and memory. Long or difficult tests of cognition, language, or communication are impossible for these patients because of their behavioral and cognitive impairments. Assessment typically is limited to brief tests that provide a limited sample of performance and that reflect basic communicative and cognitive ability.

Screening tests of orientation, memory, and amnesia such as the *Mini Mental Status Examination (MMSE*; Folstein, Folstein, & McHugh, 1975) or the *Galveston Memory and Orientation Test* (Levin, O'Donnell, & Grossman, 1979) often suffice to track these patients' progress. Performance data obtained with such tests may be supplemented with subjective ratings, using any of several rating scales designed for use with traumatically brain-injured adults. The simplest rating scales (such as the Glasgow Coma Scale), which are intended for frequent ratings (daily or more often) are too insensitive to be of much value for tracking traumatically brain-injured adults' performance at this stage of recovery. Consequently, the clinician usually chooses a more detailed rating scale, such as the Glasgow Assessment Schedule, the Disability Rating Scale, or subsections of the Comprehensive Level of Consciousness Scale to track these patients' recovery.

Orientation (awareness of self and appreciation of how one relates to others or to the environment) is a major problem as a patient emerges from coma. Clinicians customarily divide orientation into orientation for *person* (the patient's knowledge of who he or she is and who others are), *place* (the patient's knowledge of where he or she is), and *time* (what year, month, day, and hour it is, plus a sense of the passage of time). A few standardized procedures for assessing orientation have been reported in the literature, but most clinicians rely on the orientation items from screening examinations of mental status such as the MMSE or the GOAT, plus questions asked during the patient interview.

Most mental status screening examinations contain items that test patients' basic orientation to time and place and their ability to report personal information such as name, age, and marital status. The clinician often supplements the information obtained from standard measures of orientation to place by asking questions to assess concepts of direction and distance— for example, asking the patient to indicate the direction of his or her home from the present location or to estimate the distance between the present location and his or her home. The clinician may assess a patient's sense of time beyond the standard questions relating to day, hour, month, year, and season by asking the patient what time of the day certain events such as meals, group meetings, or visits by family occur. The clinician may test a patient's sense of elapsed time by asking questions such as, *How long have you been in this medical center?* or *How long has it been since your family last came to visit?*

Agitation

Agitation is a common problem for confused and disoriented patients. Agitated bed-bound patients may try to remove tubes and monitoring devices and try to get out of bed. Agitated wheelchair-bound patients may try to remove restraints, unlock wheel brakes, or wheel themselves about with no concern for safety. Ambulatory patients may wander and resist others' attempts to control wandering. Some agitated patients shout or scream spontaneously or in response to stimulation or attempt to strike, kick, or bite persons who come within range. Some may be physically or verbally self-abusive.

The *Agitated Behavior Scale (ABS*; Bogner & associates, 1999) was designed to estimate the nature and extent of agitation in brain-injured patients and to provide an objective means of tracking changes in agitation as brain-injured patients recover. The ABS contains 14 descriptive statements (e.g., *impulsive, impatient, low tolerance for pain or frustration. Explosive and/or unpredictable anger. Restlessness, pacing, excessive movement.*), each of which is assigned one of four ratings: absent, present to a slight degree, present to a moderate degree, present to an extreme degree. Bogner and associates (1999) reported data suggesting that the ABS reliably measures agitated behavior in persons who have traumatic brain injuries. If agitation lessens but aggression remains, measures designed for measuring aggression such as the *Overt Aggression Scale (OAS*; Yudofsky & associates, 1986) may be used to track changes in aggressive behavior. The OAS provides for ratings of aggression in four domains: verbal aggression, physical aggression against self, physical aggression against others, and physical aggression against objects.

Cognitive and Communicative Abilities

As a patient's orientation improves and her or his agitation and confusion diminish, cognitive and communicative impairments become more obvious, and assessment of cognitive and communicative abilities becomes practical. The scope and pattern of testing depends, of course, on each patient's tolerance for testing and each patient's particular pattern of impairments. However, most clinicians assess alertness, attention, memory, visuoperceptual abilities, language and communication, and reasoning and problem solving, with follow-up testing to specify the limits of impairments identified in the initial tests. (Tests mentioned but not described in what follows are described in Chapter 4.)

Attention

Attentional impairments are a universal consequence of traumatic brain injury, and assessment of attention is an important part of intervention for traumatically brain-injured patients. Most traumatically brain-injured patients experience impaired *selective attention*. They are distractible and cannot maintain attention in the face of competing stimuli. They have difficulty discriminating foreground figures from backgrounds and may be distracted by irrelevant aspects of stimuli, such as the border around a picture or irrelevant details in stories or events. They perform poorly on visual figure-ground tests (embedded figures, overlapping figures, masked or occluded figures), and they may have difficulty separating what is important from what is not important in spoken and printed materials.

Impairments in *sustained attention* are not clearly separable from impairments in selective attention, because impaired selective attention is certain to disrupt performance in tasks that require sustained attention. However, some traumatically brain-injured patients perform well on selective-attention tasks but do poorly on tests requiring sustained attention. These patients' performance deteriorates as the time during which they must maintain attention increases. They do poorly in sustained-attention tasks such as trail making, digits backward, backward spelling, oral arithmetic, and challenging vigilance tasks.

Most traumatically brain-injured patients are slow to shift attentional focus from one stimulus to another or from one aspect of a task or situation to another *(alternating attention)*. They perform poorly in tasks in which response requirements change or in which they are required to transfer attentional focus from one characteristic of task stimuli to another. Con-

versational interactions in which speakers and topics quickly change are especially difficult for these patients.

Divided attention tasks are enormously difficult for most traumatically brain-injured patients, who cannot attend simultaneously to two aspects of a task, such as carrying on a conversation while driving an automobile in heavy traffic or listening to broadcast news while baking a cake. The *Brief Test of Attention (BTA*; Schretlin, Bobholtz, & Brandt, 1996) may be used to assess divided attention in patients with mild to moderate impairments of attention. In the BTA, the test taker hears a series of numbers and letters from a tape recording and counts either the numbers or the letters in response to the examiner's commands. The *Paced Auditory Serial Addition Test (PASAT*; Gronwall, 1977) may be used to assess divided attention in patients with mild impairments. The PASAT is too difficult for patients with moderate or severe attentional impairments.

Tests designed to assess functional attention such as the *Test of Everyday Attention (TEA*; Robertson, Ward, Ridgeway, & Nimmo-Smith, 1996) may provide estimates of attentional capacity in simulated daily life activities.

Memory Impairments

Loss of memory for events occurring immediately before and immediately after brain injury is common in traumatically brain-injured adults. Loss of memory for the events immediately preceding injury is called *pretraumatic memory loss*. Loss of memory for the events immediately following injury is called *posttraumatic memory loss*. The concepts of pretraumatic and posttraumatic memory loss were developed by Russell and associates (Russell, 1971; Russell & Espir, 1961; Russell & Nathan, 1946), based on their studies of traumatically brain-injured British armed forces personnel during and after World War II. Russell and his contemporaries called pretraumatic memory loss *retrograde amnesia*, and they called posttraumatic memory loss *anterograde amnesia*. Both sets of

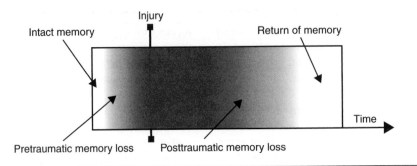

Figure 11-9 ■ A schematic representation of memory loss associated with traumatic brain injury. *Pretraumatic memory loss* is loss of memory for experiences preceding the injury, and *posttraumatic memory loss* is loss of memory for experiences following the injury. Posttraumatic memory loss almost always covers a longer time interval than pretraumatic memory loss.

labels refer to a period of time for which a traumatically brain-injured patient has no recollection of experiences that happened during the period—hence the terms *amnesia* and *memory loss*. Over the years these labels gradually have been replaced by *pretraumatic memory loss* and *posttraumatic memory loss*. However, some contemporary writers still use the original labels.

Pretraumatic memory loss may have two components. Loss of memory for the seconds to minutes immediately preceding brain injury apparently is caused by disruption of neurochemical processes necessary for encoding information in long-term memory. Consequently, events occurring in the seconds to minutes preceding injury do not enter the patient's memory. Loss of memory for hours or days preceding brain injury apparently is caused by disrupted access to information stored in long-term memory prior to the injury. Events occurring hours or days before injury are in memory but cannot be accessed and retrieved. Pretraumatic memory loss usually shrinks as the patient recovers, and most patients eventually recover memory for all but the last few seconds or minutes before their brain injury, presumably because experiences in the last few seconds or minutes never made it into long-term memory (Figure 11-9).

Corkin, Hurt, Twitchell, Franklin, and Yin (1987) reported the duration of pretraumatic memory loss in 121 cases of traumatic brain injury in veterans of the Korean conflict. About one-third of the patients experienced no pretraumatic memory loss, and for most that did, the interval of memory loss was less than 1 hour (Figure 11-10). The duration of pretraumatic memory loss was not significantly related to whether the injuries were penetrating or nonpenetrating. These results are consistent with results reported by Russell and Nathan (1946), who studied the duration of pretraumatic memory loss in 973 traumatically brain-injured survivors of World War II. Of Russell and Nathan's subjects, 86% experienced pretraumatic memory loss, but only 14% experienced loss for time intervals of more than 30 minutes.

Posttraumatic memory loss has been defined as, "inability to retain new information in the minutes, hours, days, or weeks following the injury" (Corkin & associates, 1987, p. 318). Posttraumatic memory loss generally is thought to represent failure to incorporate experiences into long-term memory. Posttraumatic memory loss usually begins at the time of the injury, but some patients may have brief intervals of memory for events that happened immediately after their injury, with loss of memory for events

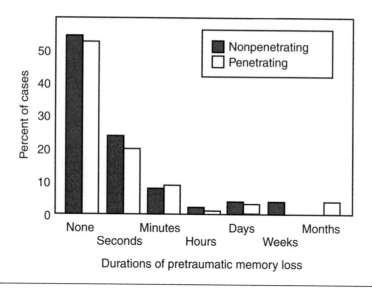

Figure 11-10 ■ The duration of pretraumatic memory loss in 121 cases of penetrating or nonpenetrating traumatic brain injuries from the Korean conflict. (Data from Corkin, S.H., Hurt, R.W., Twitchell, T.E., & associates. [1987]. Consequences of penetrating and nonpenetrating head injury: Posttraumatic amnesia and lasting effects on cognition. In H.S. Levin, J. Grafman, H.M. Eisenberg [Eds.]. *Neurobehavioral recovery from head injury* [pp. 318-329]. New York: Oxford University Press.)

occurring later. Russell's (1971) original definition of posttraumatic memory loss included both the time of coma and the time following it during which a patient fails to remember experiences. Most contemporary writers exclude the time of coma and assume that posttraumatic memory loss coincides roughly with the time of confusion and disorientation following a patient's emergence from coma (Baddelly & associates, 1987).

Most measures of the duration of pretraumatic and posttraumatic memory loss are actually retrospective estimates based on patients' accounts of when they first began remembering experiences after their accidents. There are no standard procedures for obtaining these estimates. Consequently, it seems likely that considerable unaccounted-for variability exists in measures of pretraumatic and posttraumatic memory loss. For example, it is difficult and perhaps impossible to separate what a patient

actually remembers about the time immediately following her or his accident from what family members, staff, or others have told the patient about that period. Even so, there is sufficient consistency of results across studies of pretraumatic and posttraumatic memory loss to give us reasonable confidence about the relative duration and time-course of these memory impairments.

Posttraumatic memory loss almost always lasts longer than pretraumatic memory loss. Figure 11-11 summarizes results reported by Corkin and associates (1987) for Korean conflict survivors. Whereas pretraumatic memory loss rarely spanned more than seconds to minutes, posttraumatic memory loss often spanned days or weeks. Russell (1971) and Jennett (1976) have reported similar results.

As mentioned earlier, the problem in posttraumatic memory loss is getting information into long-term memory. Patients with posttraumatic

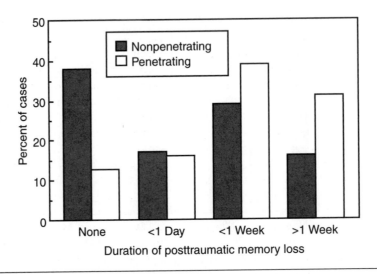

Figure 11-11 ■ The duration of posttraumatic memory loss in 121 cases of penetrating or nonpenetrating traumatic brain injuries from the Korean conflict. (Data from Corkin, S.H., Hurt, R.W., Twitchell, T.E., & associates. [1987]. Consequences of penetrating and nonpenetrating head injury: Posttraumatic amnesia and lasting effects on cognition. In H.S. Levin, J. Grafman, H.M. Eisenberg [Eds.]. *Neurobehavioral recovery from head injury* [pp. 318-329]. New York: Oxford University Press.)

memory loss may participate in conversations, take tests, and carry out activities of daily living but have no subsequent recollection of the experiences. These patients do not remember meetings, conversations, or people from hour to hour or from day to day. Posttraumatic memory loss has far more serious daily life consequences for the patient than pretraumatic memory loss.

According to Lezak (1983), traumatically brain-injured patients are most troubled by posttraumatic memory loss because of its effects on daily life, whereas their lawyers are most troubled by pretraumatic memory loss, because of their client's failure to remember events leading up to the accident.

The duration of posttraumatic memory loss is moderately related to the duration of coma but may be a better predictor of eventual recovery than is duration of coma (Levin, Benton, & Grossman, 1982), with longer posttraumatic

memory loss suggesting greater residual impairments. Patients with posttraumatic memory loss of 1 month or more are likely to have permanent memory deficits, and if posttraumatic memory loss lasts 3 months or more, the patient is likely to have permanent and severe impairments of cognition, learning, and memory (Brooks, 1989; Katz & Alexander, 1994).

Visual Processing

Visual processing impairments are common in the early stages of recovery from traumatic brain injury, although some patients, (especially those with posterior brain injury) continue to have persisting difficulty processing visual information into the middle and late stages of recovery. Patients with visual processing impairments perform poorly on tests that require identification of incomplete, fragmented, or partially occluded visual stimuli or tests that require discrimination of figures from backgrounds in drawings or photographs.

GENERAL CONCEPTS 11-3

- The primary objectives of assessment with comatose and semicomatose patients who have traumatic brain injuries are to estimate the nature and severity of the patients' injury, to evaluate the progression of the patients' status since their time of injury, and to determine their alertness and responsiveness to stimulation.
- Assessment of patients who have returned to consciousness and begun responding to stimuli usually focuses on determining their *orientation* (to person, place, and time) and assessing their *mental status*. The *Galveston Orientation and Amnesia Test (GOAT)* and the *Mini Mental Status Examination (MMSE)* often are used for these purposes.
- Agitation is a common problem for confused and disoriented patients. The *Agitated Behavior Scale (ABS)* may be used to measure and track agitation in brain-injured patients.
- Persons who have experienced traumatic brain injuries often have problems with selective attention, sustained attention, and alternating attention. The *Test of Everyday Attention (TEA)* is designed to evaluate the effects of attentional impairments on daily life.
- Memory impairments of individuals who have traumatic brain injury can be characterized as *pretraumatic memory loss* (loss of memory for events happening before the injury) or *posttraumatic memory loss* (loss of memory for events happening after the injury). Pretraumatic memory loss usually spans a shorter time interval than posttraumatic memory loss, although both tend to shrink as patients recover.
- Visual processing impairments are a common early consequence of brain injury and sometimes become chronic impairments of persons with posterior brain injuries.
- Assessment of executive function is an important management concern for brain-injured patients at RLAS Level V and above.
- The speech of most traumatically brain-injured adults is irrelevant, confabulatory, circumlocutory, tangential, fragmented, and noncohesive but is linguistically acceptable. Most often fail to recognize and follow pragmatic rules and conventions.
- Most traumatically brain-injured adults comprehend well-structured and literal spoken or printed language, but their comprehension deteriorates when they must deal with unstructured material or nonliteral material such as metaphor, humor, or sarcasm.
- Standard aphasia tests are not usually appropriate for assessing traumatically brain-injured adults' language and communication, because they focus on skills that usually are not much affected by traumatic brain injury (e.g., word retrieval, comprehension of literal material) and neglect skills that are affected by traumatic brain injury (e.g., organization of complex information, appreciation of nonliteral meanings, language pragmatics).
- Tests of *receptive vocabulary*, *naming* (especially generative naming), *sentence comprehension*, *discourse comprehension*, *picture description*, and *pragmatic appropriateness* are likely to be appropriate for adults with traumatic brain injury, depending on the severity of their injury.
- Several test batteries for assessing traumatically brain-damaged adults have been published and may be used to identify gross impairments that can be evaluated in greater detail with follow-up tests.
- Subtests of the *Woodcock-Johnson Psychoeducational Battery (WJR)* may be useful for evaluating specific cognitive abilities of higher-level individuals with traumatic brain injuries. Subtests from achievement test batteries such as the *Woodcock-Johnson Tests of Achievement—Revised (WJR-ACH)* or the *Peabody Individual Achievement Test—Revised (PIAT-R)* may also be used to evaluate the performance of higher-level traumatically brain-injured patients, especially those who may return to school.

Executive Function (Abstract Thinking, Reasoning, Problem Solving)

Assessment of executive function usually is not an important management concern for brain-injured patients at RLAS Level IV and below, whose confusion, agitation, and attentional impairments make abstract thinking, reasoning, and problem-solving all but impossible. As patients reach RLAS Level V and above, impairments of executive function no longer are masked by confusion, agitation, and attentional impairments, and assessment of executive function becomes an increasingly important aspect of management. Comprehensive assessment of executive function typically includes tests of abstract thinking, reasoning, and problem-solving, in addition to tests of attention and memory. Assessment of executive function is discussed in Chapter 4.

Language and Communication

Traumatically brain-injured patients at RLAS Level III and below do not communicate verbally beyond incoherent utterances that are devoid of propositional content. Patients at RLAS Level IV may intermittently utter a communicative word or two, but most vocalizations are incoherent and unrelated to the situational context. Most traumatically brain-injured adults at RLAS Level V and above produce speech that is phonologically and syntactically within normal limits. The primary exceptions are those with brain stem, cerebellar, or peripheral nervous system damage who are dysarthric. Assessment of those patients resembles assessment of patients with dysarthria from other causes (see Chapter 13).

Traumatically brain-injured patients at RLAS Level V and above often make errors on tests of confrontation naming, but most errors reflect visual misperceptions or the patient's inability to inhibit competing responses, rather than word-retrieval impairments *per se*. Although traumatically brain-injured persons may experience annoying word-retrieval failures in spontaneous speech, the failures usually do not seriously compromise communication in everyday activities.

Traumatically brain-injured patients at RLAS Levels VI, VII, and VIII speak fluently, with normal speech rate and prosody, but they say more than is needed and stray from the topic. Those at Levels VI and VII produce speech that is (at least) intermittently irrelevant, confabulatory, circumlocutory, tangential, fragmented, and noncohesive, but (usually) linguistically acceptable. Add to this their faulty appreciation and failure to respect pragmatic rules and conventions, and the stereotypic picture of the moderately impaired traumatically brain-injured speaker emerges.

Most traumatically brain-injured adults at RLAS Levels VI, VII, and VIII comprehend what others say if what is said is well-structured and literal, but comprehension suffers when they must follow changes in topic or when the meaning of the material depends on their appreciation of indirect meanings such as metaphor, humor, or sarcasm.

The speech and comprehension of traumatically brain-injured adults has much in common with that of adults with right-hemisphere brain damage. One reason for this commonality may be the large proportions of patients with frontal lobe damage in groups of right-hemisphere-damaged adults, and the high probability that traumatically brain-injured adults will have frontal lobe damage (McDonald, 1993).

Few traumatically brain-injured adults exhibit patterns of language impairment that justify calling them aphasic, although many of those at RLAS Levels VII and above have word-retrieval problems, impaired auditory and reading comprehension for complex materials, and occasional literal or verbal paraphasias. The communication impairments of higher-level patients with traumatic brain injuries usually are secondary consequences of underlying impairments in attention, memory, reasoning, and problem-solving, rather than being linguistic impairments *per se.*

Standard aphasia tests are not well suited for assessing the communicative impairments of traumatically brain-injured adults, because they highlight skills such as word retrieval, syntactic skills, and comprehension of literal material (skills that usually are preserved following traumatic brain injury) and downplay or ignore skills such as organization and integration of complex information and appreciation of non-literal and implied meanings (skills that are likely to be affected by traumatic brain injury). As a result, performance on an aphasia test usually overestimates traumatically brain-injured adults' actual communicative competence.

Ylvisaker and Urbanczyk (1994) describe the reasons that aphasia tests may not be appropriate for traumatically brain-injured patients:

> To the extent that communication is negatively affected by attentional, perceptual, organizational, and executive system dysfunction, language testing by its very nature may compensate for the underlying weakness. For example, the controlled testing environment reduces attentional challenges; clear instructions and well defined tasks help to ensure orientation to task and reduce the effects of cognitive inflexibility; test items that include only relatively small amounts of language compensate for organizational weakness; the deliberate rate at which information is presented compensates for difficulties with speeded performance; the supportive and encouraging manner of the examiner may compensate for an inability to cope with interpersonal stress; and commonly used tests fail to measure the individual's ability to learn new information and skills and to generalize new skills from one setting or task to another. (p. 174)

Ylvisaker and Urbanczyk's last sentence gets the award for the longest sentence in this book.

Ylvisaker and Urbanczyk's comments do not mean that tests used to evaluate aphasic adults have no place in evaluation of adults with traumatic brain injuries. Selective testing of reading, writing, speaking, and listening that focuses on the perceptual and processing impairments likely to be affected by traumatic brain injury may be useful in quantifying traumatically brain-injured persons' language and communicative impairments. Depending on the severity of the patient's brain injury and the pattern of the patient's impairments, some or all of the following tests may be appropriate, provided the patient is cooperative and can attend well enough that the test performance is a valid indication of the patient's true ability and not a consequence of perceptual, attentional, or memory impairment:

- A test of generative naming to assess the patient's ability to produce conceptually related words under time pressure
- A sample of connected speech elicited by picture description or story narration to assess the content, organization, and efficiency of the patient's connected speech
- A sample of conversation in which the appropriateness of pragmatic aspects of the patient's communication may be evaluated. The sample should represent a true conversation, not an interview (sometimes called "*semistructured conversation*)" in which the examiner asks questions and the patient answers them. Such "conversations" do not discriminate traumatically brain-injured adults from adults without brain injuries (Snow, Douglas, & Ponsford, 1995)
- A test of word-finding in sentences or discourse to assess retrieval and production of words in context
- A receptive vocabulary test to estimate usable listening vocabulary
- A test of spoken or printed sentence comprehension to assess short-term auditory retention and comprehension of spoken sentences

- A test of spoken discourse comprehension to assess comprehension of stated and implied main ideas and details from spoken narratives
- A standardized test of reading vocabulary and reading comprehension

Depending on the patient's pattern of communicative impairments, other tests of speech, language, and communication may be appropriate. Tests of written spelling, arithmetic, and higher-level reading comprehension, plus challenging language production tests (such as proverb interpretation) may be appropriate for patients with mild cognitive or communicative impairments. Comprehensive testing of spelling and reading comprehension may be important for high-level patients who may return to school or work. In-depth assessment of pragmatic skills may be important for patients who may return to environments requiring social interaction with others. Comprehensive evaluation of verbal planning and problem-solving may be important for patients who may return to jobs in which those skills are important. For traumatically brain-injured adults with dysarthria, a comprehensive motor-speech examination and a measure of speech intelligibility may be appropriate.

Test Batteries for Evaluation of Traumatically Brain-Injured Adults

Several test batteries for assessing traumatically brain-injured adults' cognition and language have been published, but most have weaknesses in coverage, norms, reliability, or standardization that compromise their value as stand-alone instruments. Some may be useful as screening tests to identify gross impairments, which then can be evaluated in more detail with follow-up tests. Brief descriptions of some of the major test batteries follow and are listed in Box 11-2. Because there is considerable variability in their psychometric properties, potential users should examine a test's validity, reliability, norms,

Box 11-2	Major Test Batteries for Evaluation and Treatment of Traumatically Brain-Injured Adults

Brief Test of Head Injury (BTHI): 31 items

Ross Information Processing Assessment (2nd ed., RIPA-2): 10 subtests

Scales of Cognitive Ability for Traumatic Brain Injury (SCATBI): 41 subtests

Woodcock-Johnson Psychoeducational Battery—Revised (WJR)

Woodcock Johnson Tests of Cognitive Ability—Revised (WJR-COG)
- Standard battery: 7 subtests
- Supplemental battery: 12 supplemental tests

Woodcock-Johnson Tests of Achievement—Revised (WJR-ACH)
- Standard battery: 12 tests
- Supplemental battery: 4 subtests

Peabody Individual Achievement Test—Revised (PIAT-R): 6 subtests

and coverage before adopting it for routine clinical use.

The *Brief Test of Head Injury* (*BTHI*; Helm-Estabrooks & Hotz, 1991) is a screening test for evaluating adults with severe impairments following traumatic brain injury. The BTHI contains 31 items in seven sections: orientation-attention, following commands, linguistic organization, reading comprehension, naming (pictures and objects), immediate, recent, and remote memory, and visuospatial skills. Clinicians may find the BTHI a useful supplement to rating scales such as the RLAS for establishing baseline performance and tracking recovery of severely impaired traumatically brain-injured patients.

The *Ross Information Processing Assessment —Second Edition* (*RIPA-2*; Ross, 1996) contains 10 subtests to assess immediate memory, recent memory, remote memory, spatial orientation, orientation to the environment, recall of information, problem-solving and reasoning, organization of information, and auditory comprehension and retention.

The *Scales of Cognitive Ability for Traumatic Brain Injury* (*SCATBI*; Adamovich & Henderson, 1992) contains 41 subtests divided among five sections: perception and discrimination, orientation, organization (categorization, association, sequencing), recall, and reasoning. The SCATBI has a greater range of item difficulty than most tests for traumatically brain-injured adults. (It contains some items that non-brain-damaged adults are likely to find difficult.) Because of its length (it takes approximately 2 hours to administer the entire SCATBI) and the range of difficulty of test items, clinicians are unlikely to administer the entire test in a single session. However, clinicians may administer individual sections of the SCATBI, because norms are provided for individual sections. The SCATBI appears to be a reasonable general purpose test battery for higher-level traumatically brain-injured adults, although clinicians may wish to supplement information provided by the SCATBI with the results of other tests that provide more detailed information about areas of impairment identified with the SCATBI.

Although not normed on traumatically brain-injured adults, the *Woodcock-Johnson Psychoeducational Battery—Revised* (*WJR*; Woodcock & Johnson, 1989) includes several tests that may be appropriate for assessing specific cognitive abilities of higher-level patients with traumatic brain injuries. The WJR has two components—the *Woodcock-Johnson Tests of Cognitive Ability—Revised* (*WJR-COG*) and the *Woodcock-Johnson Tests of Achievement—Revised* (*WJR-ACH*). The range for most of the subtests in the WJR is from age 2 to adult, and norms are provided for ages 2 to 90. The design and standardization of the WJR permit use of most subtests in isolation. For these reasons, the WJR-COG can provide a set of tests for assessing a broad range of abilities across a wide range of ability levels, and performance of traumatically brain-injured patients can reliably be compared with that of non-brain-damaged individuals of equivalent age.

The WJR-COG tests are divided into two sections (batteries). The standard battery contains seven subtests:

- *Memory for names:* the patient must remember nonsense names for cartoon figures (e.g., *jawl, kiptron*)
- *Sentence recall:* the patient repeats words and sentences, ranging from a one-syllable word to a 33-syllable sentence
- *Visual matching:* the patient searches an array of numbers for a designated target
- *Incomplete words:* the patient identifies spoken words with missing sounds
- *Visual closure:* the patient identifies common objects represented by incomplete drawings or by photographs taken from unusual angles
- *Picture vocabulary:* the patient says the names of pictured items representing a range of English word frequency
- *Analysis-synthesis:* the patient solves puzzle-like problems by applying symbolically represented rules

The supplemental battery of the WJR-COG contains 12 supplemental subtests that relate to the subtests in the standard battery:

- *Visual-auditory learning:* the patient learns real word names for nonrepresentational symbols
- *Memory for words:* the patient recalls word lists ranging from 1 to 8 words
- *Cross-out:* the patient crosses out target symbols in a linear array of targets and foils
- *Sound blending:* the patient identifies fragmented spoken words
- *Picture recognition:* the patient chooses previously seen drawings from an array containing previously seen items and foils
- *Oral vocabulary:* the patient gives synonyms and antonyms for familiar words

- *Concept formation:* the patient learns rules that determine the placement of large and small colored forms
- *Delayed recall—names:* the patient is given a delayed-recall trial (2 to 4 days later) of the *memory for names* subtest in the standard WJR-COG battery
- *Delayed recall—visual/auditory learning:* the patient is given a delayed version of the *visual-auditory learning* subtest
- *Sound patterns:* the patient tells whether pairs of nonsense words are the same or different.
- *Spatial relations:* the patient chooses jigsaw-puzzle–like forms that combine to form a more complex figure
- *Listening comprehension:* the patient provides a missing word to complete a sentence

Achievement test batteries provide another important resource for clinicians who wish to evaluate the performance of higher-level traumatically brain-injured patients in tasks that provide an indication of potential success in school or other activities that depend on mathematics, reading, writing, spelling, and vocabulary skills.

The WJR-ACH is divided into two sections. The standard battery contains 12 tests to assess reading, mathematics, and written language. The supplemental battery contains two reading subtests and two writing subtests.

The *Peabody Individual Achievement Test— Revised* (PIAT-R; Markwardt, 1989) is another test battery from which clinicians may select tests for higher-level brain-injured patients. The PIAT-R contains six subtests:

- *Mathematics:* the patient works out multiple-choice problems ranging from number and symbol recognition to complex algebra and geometry problems
- *Reading recognition:* the patient reads single-letter and word-recognition items, plus items in which the patient reads aloud familiar and unfamiliar printed words
- *Reading comprehension:* the patient chooses from a set of four pictures the one described by a printed sentence

- *Spelling:* a multiple-choice test in which the patient identifies printed letters and words and chooses correctly spelled words from sets containing a correctly spelled word and three incorrect spellings
- *Written expression:* the patient writes a short narrative related to a picture stimulus
- *General information:* a question-answer test of information gained in daily life, reading, or school

The PIAT-R subtests, like the WJR subtests, can be administered and interpreted individually. Subtest scores can be converted into percentile ranks for ages from 5 to 18 years, and into grade equivalents and age equivalents.

INTERVENTION

Cognitive-communicative interventions with traumatically brain-injured adults require the collaboration of many professionals, including physicians, nurses, neuropsychologists, speech-language pathologists, occupational therapists, physical therapists, clinical psychologists, social workers, vocational counselors, and others. The physical, cognitive, and behavioral impairments experienced by traumatically brain-injured patients cross professional boundaries and require a unified, integrated program of intervention that extends from the clinic to the patient's daily environment.

Interdisciplinary collaboration is especially important in the early stages of a patient's recovery, when medical, physical, and behavioral impairments are most severe. According to Kay and Silver (1989):

"Rehabilitation [of traumatically brain-injured patients] must be interdisciplinary in the truest sense of the word. There must be ongoing communication among team members (not just with a central leader), care planning that cuts across disciplines, and coordination by a professional who is an expert in the cognitive and behavioral problems of head-injured persons." (p. 147)

Sensory Stimulation, Orientation

Sensory Stimulation. Intervention with comatose or semicomatose patients consists primarily of sensory stimulation. The primary purposes of intervention are to increase the patient's responsiveness to the environment and to facilitate the patient's return to consciousness.

Comatose: The patient exhibits neither arousal nor awareness of surroundings. The patient's eyes are closed, and the patient shows no evidence of sleep-wake cycles. *Semicomatose* (sometimes called *vegetative state*): The patient has sleep-wake cycles, may open his or her eyes in response to stimulation, and may inconsistently orient to the source of stimulation, but neither comprehends nor produces language or gesture and makes no purposeful motor responses. If vegetative state lasts longer than 1 month it may be called *persistent vegetative state.*

During sensory stimulation (sometimes called *coma stimulation* or *coma arousal therapy*), the patient is repeatedly exposed to auditory, visual, tactile, olfactory, and taste stimuli, usually in several 10- to 15-minute intervals of stimulation each day. The purposes of sensory stimulation are "… to increase the patient's alertness/ arousal and responsiveness to the environment and to prevent sensory deprivation…to facilitate changes in responsiveness such as increased consistency and specificity of response and/or decreased latency of response" (Cherney, Halper, & Miller, 1991, p. 59).

Many practitioners believe that sensory stimulation hastens traumatically brain-injured patients' emergence from coma and increases their eventual level of recovery, but there is no objective evidence to support this belief. Nevertheless, the idea makes intuitive sense, and as Kay and Silver (1989) point out, "It would seem to make sense on rational grounds that it is better to provide regular, gentle sensory input to comatose patients than to let them lie unattended and unstimulated (physically and sensorially) for long periods of time" (p. 149).

Studies of animals provide some indirect evidence for the benefits of sensory stimulation. The studies have shown that animals with experimenter-induced brain damage who are then placed in a stimulating environment recover their ability to learn new behaviors to a greater degree than animals with equivalent brain damage kept in a nonstimulating environment. Other studies have shown that animals raised under conditions of sensory deprivation are less active and have more difficulty learning than do animals raised under normal conditions. (The relevance of the latter research to traumatically brain-injured adults depends on the assumption that their comatose or semi-comatose state causes sensory deprivation.) Lippert, Gruner, and Terhaag (2000) reported changes in autonomic functions (e.g., heart rate, respiration rate) concurrent with stimulation administered to 16 brain-injured patients who were in deep coma. However, the authors did not show that these changes accelerated either the patients' emergence from coma or their eventual level of recovery.

Sensory stimulation is an uncomplicated but labor-intensive procedure, and most adults of average intelligence can learn it in two or three training sessions. Consequently, speech-language pathologists usually collaborate with other caregivers and with relatives or significant others to provide stimulation. The speech-language pathologist may provide controlled stimulation according to a systematic schedule, record the results of stimulation, review records of the patient's response to stimulation to determine if changes in the patient's responsiveness are taking place, and collaborate with other team members in making appropriate changes in the stimulation program.

Relatives and significant others may be better than strangers for administering coma stimulation, because they are familiar to the patient, know the patient's interests, likes, and dislikes, and have access to materials (e.g., photographs and tape recordings) that are meaningful to the patient—characteristics that are believed to increase the effectiveness of stimulation. However, relatives and significant others may misinterpret random movements, spontaneous changes in respiration, or chance vocalizations as responses to stimulation, because they are looking for reassuring signs that the patient will recover.

The following list of general principles reflects the basic philosophy of most contemporary stimulation programs:

- Begin stimulation as soon as possible after the patient enters coma, provided his or her medical condition is stable
- Control the environment to eliminate distractions—close doors and turn the television off before beginning stimulation
- Ensure that the patient is comfortable before beginning stimulation
- Stimulate one modality at a time
- Stimulate acoustic, tactile, olfactory, and kinesthetic senses
- Select meaningful stimuli such as favorite music or the voices of relatives or significant others
- Alternate intervals of no stimulation with intervals of stimulation to prevent habituation and support the patient's sense of the passage of time
- Keep objective observational records of the nature and intensity of the patient's response to each stimulation interval

Acoustic stimulation often is provided by relatives or significant others and may include conversing with the patient about familiar people, places, and events, reading to the patient using literature the patient knows and likes, or playing recordings of the patient's favorite music. Acoustic stimulation also may be provided by patient-care personnel and may include recorded music, radio or television programs, general conversation with the patient, and spoken information about person, place, and time. Most stimulation programs require quiet times between stimulation sessions. The presence of sound from radios, televisions, and background noise are controlled to minimize habituation and to maximize the effects of programmed acoustic stimulation.

Visual stimulation often involves moving lights or brightly colored objects across the patient's field of vision, plus changing the level of illumination in the patient's room to coincide with daytime and nighttime.

Tactile stimulation addresses touch, pressure, and temperature sensations. Light touch, firm pressure, and gentle stroking may be applied to the patient's extremities and face. Warm and cool objects may be applied to or stroked across the patient's extremities and face. The patient's limbs and face may be stroked with rough and smooth or firm and soft textures such as towels, dry or moist sponges, flannel, or burlap.

Olfactory stimulation exposes the patient to a variety of familiar scents, both pleasant (perfume, coffee, flavor extracts) and unpleasant (garlic, mustard, vinegar) for short intervals (e.g., 10 seconds per stimulation).

Kinesthetic stimulation involves moving the patient's limbs (range of motion exercises, flexion and extension) or changing the patient's body positions (tilting the patient's head from side to side, rolling the patient's body from side to side, moving the patient to an upright position with pillows or a tilt table).

Intense stimulation (e.g., bright light, loud sound, intense odors, painful tactile stimulation) may be needed to elicit responses from patients in deep coma. Patients in deep coma may respond to intense stimuli with increased respiration rate, withdrawal, increased muscle tension, grimaces, grunts, or unintelligible vocalizations. As the depth of a patient's coma lessens, the patient's responses become more oriented to the source of stimulation and gradually become less automatic and more purposeful (e.g., reaching for or grasping objects, tracking and fixating visual stimuli, attending to auditory stimuli).

The patient's responses to each stimulation usually are recorded using a rating scale such as the *Rappoport Coma/Near Coma Scale* (Rappoport, Dougherty, & Ketling, 1992) or the *JFK Coma Recovery Scale—Revised* (Kalmar & Giacino, 2005). The JFK scale is shown in Table 11-8.

Orientation. Treatment of confused and agitated patients usually combines environmental control to reduce confusion and disorientation and to control maladaptive behavior; response contingencies to directly manage and modify inappropriate or maladaptive behavior; and (sometimes) pharmacologic management to reduce the patient's agitation and to facilitate new learning or relearning.

Orientation training becomes the focus of intervention as a patient's confusion and agitation diminish, and she or he begins to respond to caregivers and environmental conditions. Orientation training typically relies on environmental prompts placed in the patient's living space, verbal orientation delivered by caregivers, orientation drills, and behavior management.

Environmental prompts used in orientation training take many forms. Signs, notes, appointment calendars, and appointment books may help the patient anticipate upcoming events and assume responsibility for daily routines. Prominently displayed calendars, clocks, and schedules may help orient the patient to time. Maps showing city, state, and facility locations and signs, posters, and pictures identifying significant locations in the treatment facility (e.g., the patient's room, lounges, and dining areas) may orient the patient to place. The patient's room may be identified with the patient's name and photograph next to the door and by prominently placed personal possessions within. Pictures of home and family members in the patient's room and name tags worn by staff may orient the patient to person.

These passive reminders of time, place, and person may be supplemented by overt cues provided by staff and family members. Staff and family members may include references to time,

TABLE 11-8	The JFK Coma Recovery Scale—Revised
Score	**Description**
Auditory Function	
4	Consistent movement to command
3	Reproducible movement to command
2	Localization to sound
1	Auditory startle
0	None
Visual Function	
5	Object recognition
4	Object localization, reaching
3	Visual pursuit
2	Fixation
1	Visual startle
0	None
Motor Function	
6	Functional object use
5	Automatic motor response
4	Object manipulation
3	Localization to noxious stimulation
2	Flexion withdrawal
1	Abnormal posturing
0	None/flaccid
Oromotor/Verbal Function	
3	Intelligible verbalization
2	Vocalization/oral movement
1	Oral reflexive movement
0	None
Communication	
2	Functional, accurate
1	Nonfunctional, intentional
0	None
Arousal	
3	Attention
2	Eye opening without stimulation
1	Eye opening with stimulation
0	Unarousable

From Kalmar, K., Giacino, J.T. (2005). The JFK Coma Recovery Scale—Revised. *Neuropsychological Rehabilitation, 15,* 454-460.

place, and person in routine interactions with the patient and may provide orientation drills to stimulate the patient to acquire and retain a sense of time, place, and person.

Orientation drills come in two basic forms (Cherney, Halper, & Miller, 1991). *Passive orientation drills* are best suited for patients in the immediate postcoma phase of recovery, whose confusion, agitation, and profound attentional and memory impairments make their active participation in structured treatment activities unlikely. The clinician provides instruction, demonstration, prompts, and cues to help the patient understand who they are, what has happened to them, and where they are and to help the patient identify the current hour, day, month, and year.

Passive orientation often is carried out in groups. Group members are asked to repeat orientation information after the clinician, but they are not expected to produce the information without prompts or cues. When group members can repeat orientation information after the clinician, the clinician may train them to verbalize accurate information about person, place, and time in response to prompts or requests. However, the ability to verbalize this information does not mean that the patient has internalized the concepts well enough to incorporate the concepts into daily life activities. That often requires active orientation training.

Active orientation training helps patients incorporate their imperfectly developed sense of person, place, and time into daily life activities. The patient is given responsibility for carrying out daily life activities that depend on internalized concepts of person, place, and time. Passive orientation training usually precedes active orientation training. For example, patients are taught how to tell time (passive orientation) before they are expected to monitor the passage of time or follow appointment schedules (active orientation), and they are taught where they are (passive orientation) before they are expected to find their way around their environment (active orientation).

Environmental control usually is a dependable way to lessen a brain-injured patient's confusion and agitation. Environmental control lessens confusion and agitation by controlling the patient's environment to ensure that it is stable and predictable. Significant events (e.g., therapy appointments, meals, or visits from family members) take place according to a consistent schedule (e.g., at the same time, in the same place, and with the same people every day). As agitation and confusion diminish, controls over the environment gradually are loosened, permitting the patient to take increasing responsibility for daily routines but keeping challenges manageable.

Behavior Management

Behavior management complements orientation training and environmental control by incorporating procedures to increase adaptive behavior or decrease maladaptive behavior. Environmental control facilitates successful performance by reducing or eliminating conditions that agitate or confuse a brain-injured patient and replacing them with conditions that help the patient cope with cognitive limitations and alterations in emotions and personality. Behavior management may manipulate *antecedent stimuli* (stimuli that elicit or maintain certain behaviors) or *response contingencies* (consequences for behaviors).

In Chapter 7, two main categories of feedback were identified. *Incentive feedback* denotes a class of response-contingent stimuli that can maintain or eliminate behaviors whose only function is to elicit or avoid the stimuli. *Information feedback* denotes a class of stimuli that provides information about the appropriateness, correctness, or accuracy of the responses that elicit the stimuli.

Traumatically brain-injured patients who are in the early stages of recovery usually are not affected by intangible consequences (information feedback) such as verbal praise or reproof. Tangible, primary consequences (incentive feedback) typically are needed. Tangible consequences include positive consequences such as sweets, music, touching, massaging, or other pleasurable stimuli, and negative consequences such as noise, bright light, or painful stimuli.

Traumatically brain-injured patients in the early stages of recovery do not meet the conditions under which intangible consequences (information feedback) are effective. They are not internally motivated to get better. Much of their behavior is primitive and unmodulated by cortical control mechanisms. Consequences that depend on interpretation by the cerebral cortex and appreciation of others' intentions and desires are unlikely to affect these patients' behavior.

Four procedures for directly managing behavior by means of manipulation of response contingencies are available to clinicians. In *positive reinforcement,* pleasurable stimuli are delivered contingent on desired responses. In *negative reinforcement,* aversive stimuli are removed contingent on desired responses. In *punishment,* aversive stimuli are delivered contingent on undesired responses. In *extinction,* selected responses elicit neither pleasurable nor aversive stimuli.

When response contingencies are used to modify or maintain the behavior of confused and agitated traumatically brain-injured patients, the stimuli used as response contingencies must have incentive value, and they must be delivered consistently following each occurrence of the target behavior(s). Positive reinforcement can increase the frequency of some target behaviors, provided that the behaviors do not require great effort and do not lead to conditions that the patient finds adverse (such as the clinician asking the patient to repeat or elaborate on a behavior).

Negative reinforcement sometimes can be a powerful tool for modifying the behavior of severely agitated and confused patients, who prefer being left alone to being harassed by the clinician to make effortful responses that have no immediate payoff. Sometimes a clinician may turn a confused and agitated patient's desire to be left alone to clinical advantage by making termination of an activity contingent on the patient's performance. Initially only one or two simple responses are required to terminate the activity (e.g., *If you read this paragraph, I'll go away and leave you alone.*). As treatment proceeds, the clinician gradually changes the criteria so that more responses or more effortful responses are required to end the activity. As the patient's agitation and confusion diminish, treatment activities (and the clinician's presence) usually become less unpleasant to the patient, and response contingencies shift from negative reinforcement to positive reinforcement.

A subtle side effect of such negative reinforcement procedures is that they give severely disabled patients an opportunity to control what happens in their environment—control that is not often afforded patients at this stage of recovery.

Punishment has a limited role in managing the behavior of confused and agitated patients. Physical punishment (e.g., slapping, pinching) is morally and legally impermissible. Milder forms of punishment, such as the sound of a buzzer or loud verbal reproof sometimes may help suppress a confused and agitated patient's inappropriate behavior. However, the suppressive effects of punishment usually are temporary, because the behavior usually reappears as soon as the punishment is discontinued. More durable changes in behavior usually can be obtained by other forms of reinforcement and by controlling the patient's environment to minimize undesirable behavior.

Sometimes caregivers or others unintentionally provide positive reinforcement for undesirable behaviors by paying attention when a patient behaves unacceptably and ignoring the patient at other times. *Extinction* (ensuring that a behavior receives no reinforcement) may help eliminate unacceptable behaviors, especially if extinction is combined with positive reinforcement of alternative behaviors. However, extinction may not be very effective at modifying confused and agitated patients' behavior, because, as noted earlier, these patients may consider being ignored by others a positive consequence rather than a negative one.

The response contingencies used and the schedule on which they are delivered change as a patient recovers. When patients are confused and agitated, only a few important behaviors are treated, response-contingent stimuli have incentive value, and consequences follow every occurrence of the targeted behavior. Negative reinforcement may be an important intervention procedure. As the patient recovers, the number and complexity of behaviors targeted for intervention increase, the emphasis shifts from negative reinforcement to positive reinforcement, and partial reinforcement schedules, in which not every occurrence of the target behavior receives consequences, replace continuous schedules of reinforcement.

Manipulation of antecedent stimuli often has more powerful effects on brain-injured patient's behavior than manipulation of response contingencies. Environmental control (described earlier) manipulates general classes of antecedent stimuli (e.g., schedules, reminders, environmental prompts) to increase the frequency of general classes of adaptive behavior and to decrease the frequency of maladaptive behavior. Specific antecedent stimuli (e.g., verbal prompts, cues) may also be managed to manipulate the frequency of specific behaviors.

Ylvisaker and associates (2001) question the effectiveness of traditional, consequence-based behavior management with persons who have traumatic brain injuries involving the frontal lobes (most do). They summarize the results of several studies done in the 1990s suggesting that the frontal lobes are important for learning and retaining the relationships between antecedent events, response contingencies, and behavior. Several hypotheses have been offered to explain why patients who have frontal lobe injuries do not respond to consequence-based behavior management:

- They do not store the internal markers needed to learn contingencies.
- Their impulsiveness overrides the effects of response-contingent training.
- Impaired working memory prevents them from learning connections between antecedent events and consequences.
- Impaired initiation *(behavioral inertia)* prevents them from performing actions learned by consequence-based intervention.
- Some brain-injured adults (especially younger ones) resist response-contingent training because they react negatively to others' attempts to control them and consider rewards and punishments childlike and offensive.

Ylvisaker and associates (2001) recommend that clinicians who work with brain-injured adults attend to *setting events*—internal states or external conditions that are not specific to a given behavior but which potentially can affect individual behaviors. Internal states include the following:

- *Neurologic states* include positive setting events (e.g., normal neurology) or negative setting events (e.g., seizures, compromised cerebral blood flow, neurochemical imbalances)
- *Physiologic states* include positive setting events (e.g., rested, relaxed, appropriately medicated) and negative setting events (e.g., pain, illness, over-medication, under-medication, motor impairments, sensory impairments)
- *Cognitive states* include positive setting events (e.g., orientation, familiarity of tasks, adequate memory and attention) and negative setting events (e.g., confusion, disorientation, inadequate memory)
- *Emotional states* include positive setting events (e.g., sense of accomplishment, acceptance by others, meaningful roles, sense of personal control) and negative setting events (e.g., anxiety, anger, depression, sense of helplessness, and loss of control)

- *Attitude and belief states* include positive setting events (e.g., belief that tasks are meaningful and can be accomplished) and negative setting events (e.g., belief that tasks are meaningless, demeaning, or impossible) External conditions include the following:
- *Living arrangement:* living in a personally chosen environment without restrictions imposed by others (positive) versus living in a restrictive environment or living with parents after having lived independently (negative)
- *Presence or absence of specific people:* presence of preferred, personally chosen people (positive) versus presence of nonpreferred people or absence of friends (negative).
- *Recent history of interaction:* recent pleasant and productive interactions (positive) versus recent stressful, conflict-producing, or disrespectful interactions (negative)
- *Environmental stresses:* supportive environment, appropriate kinds and levels of stimulation (positive) versus nonsupportive or irritating environment—noise, intrusions, sterile, uncomfortable furnishings (negative)
- *Time of day:* activities conforming to the person's natural sleep-wake cycles and taking place when the person is alert (positive) versus activities that ignore the person's level of alertness and natural cycles (negative)

Ylvisaker and associates distinguish between the traditional *(molecular)* definition of *antecedents* as discrete, measurable stimuli that precede a behavior and increase or decrease its likelihood of occurrence (e.g., cues, warnings, promises) and the setting-events *(molar)* definition of *antecedents* as broad, potentially continuous, often hard-to-measure variables (e.g. internal states, living arrangements) that may increase or decrease the likelihood of positive or negative behavior. Setting events, though remote from a specific instance of behavior, have the potential to affect that behavior in addition to affecting other behaviors that are targets of intervention. Setting events often may have stronger effects on specific behaviors or classes of behaviors than do manipulations of response-contingent antecedent events and consequences, especially for persons with frontal lobe injuries.

Although objective evidence is lacking, it seems reasonable that the relative effectiveness of response-contingent antecedents and consequences versus positive and negative setting events may depend on a patient's overall severity of impairment. Confused, disoriented, and agitated patients may be less responsive to response-contingent antecedents and consequences and may be more affected by positive and negative setting events than patients who are oriented and neither confused nor agitated. Nevertheless, positive and negative setting events seem likely to have important effects on patients across all severity levels. A minimally impaired patient who is ill, depressed, over-medicated, or feeling helpless is likely to respond to intervention worse than a comparably impaired patient who experiences fewer negative setting events. Likewise, positive setting events are likely to have important positive effects on patients across all severity levels.

Pharmacologic Intervention

It is the rare patient who remains drug-free during TBI (traumatic-brain-injury) recovery. Seizures, hypertension, pain, spasticity, and disorders of mood and behavior are frequently encountered and require treatment. Often, the treating clinician has a choice between various medications, some of which may have unintended effects on neuronal recovery. Understanding what these effects might be helps in making appropriate clinical decisions (Phillips, Devier, & Feeney, 2003, p. 351).

Pharmacologic management sometimes is used to reduce brain-injured patients' agitated behavior. Sedative or antipsychotic drugs may be prescribed to reduce agitation when agitation is not controlled by behavior management. Medication may help a patient be less agitated, but it makes many patients lethargic. Finding the dosage at which a patient's agitated behavior is controlled without making the patient too lethargic and sleepy to benefit from intervention requires careful tuning of dosage and medication schedule.

Stimulant drugs may be prescribed to improve a lethargic patient's alertness and attention and to facilitate rehabilitation. (Some stimulants also lessen psychological depression.) Although some studies have shown apparent acceleration of recovery following administration of stimulant drugs, others have shown no meaningful effects. At this time there is no conclusive evidence for their efficacy in facilitating traumatically brain-injured adults' recovery.

Some traumatically brain-injured patients become clinically depressed in the later stages of recovery, usually as a consequence of their experiences with social and vocational dislocation, compromised physical and mental abilities, financial hardship, isolation, and inactivity. Depression also may reflect disruption of brain neurochemistry by brain injury. Antidepressant medications may be prescribed for such patients. However, some antidepressant medications have sedative effects that can compromise cognition and motor performance, making them a questionable choice for depressed patients with brain injuries. Antidepressants (or other medications) that are fatal in overdose should not, of course, be prescribed if a patient has suicidal tendencies.

A few traumatically brain-injured patients develop psychotic conditions (paranoia, delusional states, schizophrenic-like disorders). Antipsychotic medications may be prescribed for these patients. However, most of these medications have undesirable extrapyramidal side effects such as dyskinesia, suppressed volitional movement, and tremor. Therefore, antipsychotic medications should be administered at minimum effective dosage, and patients must be monitored carefully for side effects.

Anticonvulsant medications routinely are prescribed for patients in the acute stages of recovery from traumatic brain injuries, whether or not the patient actually has had a seizure. These medications have several potential side effects, including sedation, depression, motor impairments, and memory impairments. Consequently, anticonvulsants should not be prescribed indiscriminately or continued unnecessarily.

Interest in pharmacologic intervention to improve cognitive functions in traumatically brain-injured patients has grown substantially in the last decade, and there are indications that some psychoactive medications may have beneficial effects on attention, memory, and executive function. Phillips, Devier, and Feeney (2003) commented that the results of studies of pharmacologic intervention for cognitive impairments permit "cautious optimism." They concluded a review of laboratory studies of pharmacologic intervention in brain injury with the following statement:

> Currently the most that can be concluded is that it is possible to promote recovery weeks to months after brain injury. Why some patients and animals show benefit and others do not, and how late after injury this regimen can be initiated to enhance outcome is unknown. The other important aspect is the deleterious effect of some medications administered after brain injury.... The significant results from controlled clinical trials, despite small samples of diverse injuries, are promising and may lead to new options for those in clinical practice responsible for treating those young lives devastated by brain injury. These data at least indicate the potential for intervention long after the time of injury when it is widely believed untreatable. (p. 353)

After reviewing studies of pharmacologic therapies for posttraumatic cognitive impairments, Arciniegas and Silver (2006) offered two primary conclusions: (1) medications that augment cerebral catecholaminergic function may enhance arousal, speed of mental processing, and perhaps attention; and (2) cholinesterase inhibitors may contribute to enhanced memory.

Catecholamines cause physiological changes that prepare the body for physical activity (e.g., increased heart rate, increased blood pressure, increased blood glucose levels). Catecholamine medications include stimulants such as the amphetamines and dopamine. *Cholinesterase inhibitors* increase levels of acetylcholine, a neurotransmitter thought to be involved in attention, memory, and other cognitive processes.

Studies of pharmacologic intervention with traumatically brain-injured adults continue. It seems likely that the next decade will see fruitful applications of existing medications and development of new medications that provide clinically significant benefits to brain-injured adults' physical, cognitive, and psychologic well-being.

Cognitive-Communicative Rehabilitation

The first intervention programs for cognitive-communicative impairments of traumatically brain-injured adults were designed to repair damaged cognitive processes. These intervention programs were not based on any particular theoretic rationale; they assumed that stimulation of impaired mental processes was the key to improving traumatically brain-injured adults' cognitive and communicative competence. Early restorative interventions often used a *teach-to-the-test* approach, in which tests of generic skills (reading, reasoning, and problem-solving) were administered, deficient performance in those skills was identified, and drills to restore or repair the deficient skills were provided. Activities tended to resemble the tests used to identify compromised skills, and treatment often relied on workbooks designed for remedial education in the schools. Sohlberg and Mateer (1989) called this approach to intervention the *general stimulation* approach. In recent years general stimulation approaches to rehabilitation of traumatically brain-injured adults have been largely abandoned in favor of

theory-driven or model-driven approaches, often called *cognitive rehabilitation approaches.*

Cognitive rehabilitation interventions can be divided into two main categories. *Restorative interventions* (remedial) are designed to repair compromised cognitive and communicative processes by means of noncontextual, repetitive, process-specific drills to stimulate, restructure, or rebuild damaged neural networks. (Restorative approaches to intervention sometimes are referred to as *mental muscle-building*.) Restorative approaches seek to promote patients' capacity for independence in daily life by treating specific cognitive processes such as attention, memory, and language. The choice of cognitive processes and the hierarchic arrangement of drills are based on an explicit or implicit theoretic rationale. Improvements in a cognitive process are assumed to create improved performance in a broad range of skills dependent on the process. For example, intervention that improves a patient's sustained attention would be expected to improve the patient's performance in other activities requiring sustained attention. Restorative interventions sometimes are called *component training*, because they focus on individual components of a patient's overall pattern of impairment.

Compensatory interventions (adaptive)—sometimes called *external aids*—lessen the effects of cognitive impairments on daily life activities by providing brain-injured persons with compensatory strategies, by training specific daily life skills, or by modifying the brain-injured person's environment to lessen the negative effects of impairments on daily life success and well-being. Compensatory interventions are designed to improve brain-injured persons' daily life competence and success despite cognitive impairments that make it impossible for them to perform daily life activities as they did prior to injury. Compensatory interventions focus on adaptive behaviors rather than cognitive processes.

Although the distinction between restorative and compensatory approaches is common in the literature, in clinical practice the two approaches are not completely independent (Carney, Chesnut, Maynard, & associates, 1999). Ylvisaker (1998) has argued that compensatory intervention is in fact restorative in that it restores brain-injured persons' capacity for strategic thinking and strategic behavior. Sohlberg and Mateer (2001) comment that the distinction is somewhat blurry, because both approaches require learning, and both depend on repetitive activation of cognitive processes required for learning adaptive behaviors.

Component Training. *Component training* is designed to stimulate and reactivate cognitive and linguistic processes by means of drill activities that usually have little surface similarity to natural contexts. Individual processes (e.g., attention, memory, language, communication) may be treated individually and in a sequence governed either by a theoretic rationale or the clinician's intuitions and preferences. Specific cognitive or linguistic impairments (e.g., attention, memory, problem-solving) are targeted sequentially for intervention, which usually consists of repetitive drills. Those who perform component training assume that as treated cognitive and linguistic processes improve, other skills that depend on the processes also will improve. In this respect, component training has much in common with the *treat underlying processes* approach to aphasia intervention. Component training is the mode of intervention for many confused, nonagitated, and socially appropriate patients.

Attention. Attentional impairments have a prominent place in component training, in part because most traumatically brain-injured adults have attentional impairments, and in part because attention is so important for other cognitive processes.

One of the most well-known and widely used programs for treatment of attentional impairments is *Attention Process Training* (*APT*; Sohlberg & Mateer, 1989; Sohlberg, Johnson, Paule, & associates, 1994). APT is based on Sohlberg and Mateer's five-component model of

attentional processes: *focused attention, sustained attention, selective attention, alternating attention,* and *divided attention.* Sohlberg and associates recommend that training sequentially address sustained attention, selective attention, alternating attention, and divided attention, apparently in the belief that the sequence represents a hierarchy of attentional processes and that focused, selective, and sustained attention are prerequisites for alternating and divided attention.

> According to Sohlberg and Mateer, focused attention usually is disrupted only in the early stages of emergence from coma. Consequently, it is not a concern for most patients who can participate in structured intervention activities.

Sustained attention may be treated with several APT tasks. In *visual cancellation tasks,* the patient scans and crosses out specified targets in visual arrays. In *auditory vigilance tasks,* the patient pushes a button to sound a buzzer whenever she or he hears specified targets. The auditory vigilance tasks range from simple (e.g., *Push the buzzer every time you hear the number 6.*) to complex (e.g., *Push the buzzer every time you hear two months in a row, such that the second month comes just before the first one on the calendar.*). In *serial calculation activities,* patients perform tasks such as backward counting, adding 4 and subtracting 2 from successive numbers, and so on.

Visual selective attention is treated with cancellation tasks such as those used to treat visual sustained attention but in which overlays with distracting designs are placed over the stimuli. Auditory selective attention is treated with audiotapes containing the same stimuli as the APT auditory sustained-attention tasks but with targets presented against a background of distracting noise (e.g., conversations, news broadcasts).

APT provides several response-switching activities to treat alternating attention. In *alternating cancellation tasks,* the patient begins crossing out a specified target, such as all the even numbers in an array of numbers. Then the examiner says *change*, and the patient crosses out all the odd numbers. This continues for several changes in target. In *add-subtract alternation* the patient begins by adding numbers presented in pairs until the examiner says *change*, at which time the patient begins subtracting, and so on, for several changes in direction. In *Strooplike activities*, the words *high*, *mid*, and *low* are printed in high, middle, and low positions on a line. The patient is directed to alternate between reading the words and saying their position on the line. In another Strooplike task, the patient is shown cards on which the words *big* and *little* are printed in large and small letters, and he or she alternates between reading the words and saying the size of the letters in response to the examiner's commands.

Divided attention may be treated with tasks requiring simultaneous attention to two aspects of a single task or with tasks that require simultaneous attention to two different activities. An example of the former is the *card-sort task*, in which the patient sorts playing cards by suit, but cards whose names contain a designated target letter must be turned face-down (e.g., if the target letter is e, all aces, 3s, 5s, 7s, 8s, 9s, 10s, and queens must be turned face down). An example of the latter task is requiring the patient to do a letter cancellation task while simultaneously saying *yes* each time the examiner says the number *5* in a string of randomly arranged spoken numbers.

Evidence for the efficacy of attention process training is mixed. Studies in which the measure of efficacy is improved performance in the trained tasks or in tasks like those used to train attention usually report meaningful positive changes. Studies in which the measure of efficacy is improvement in measures of attention unlike those received in training report mixed results—some report significant changes in performance on untrained measures of attention, and some report no meaningful changes in

attention beyond changes attributable to practice or to neurologic recovery.

Park and Ingles (2001) reported the results of a meta-analysis of 30 studies of attention training. The 30 studies involved 359 participants who received an average of 31 hours of attention training. Park and Ingles divided the training provided into two categories. *Direct retraining* focused directly on attention by providing intensive practice in repetitive, attention-demanding exercises (e.g., attention process training). *Specific-skills training* provided practice in performing a functional skill that required attention (e.g., driving an automobile).

Park and Ingles divided the 30 studies into two categories based on their designs: (1) studies that measured the difference between pretraining and posttraining with no control for practice effects (the measures of outcome were identical to or similar to the tasks used in training), and (2) studies that controlled for practice effects (the measures of outcome did not resemble the tasks used in training). Park and Ingles's major finding was that direct-training studies that did not control for practice effects typically reported large and statistically significant changes in attention from pretraining to posttraining, whereas direct-training studies that controlled for practice effects typically reported small and statistically nonsignificant changes in attention following training.

Park and Ingles concluded that the significant effects of attention training reported in studies that did not control for practice effects were simply the effects of practice in the tasks used to measure outcome and did not represent improvement in attention or attention-related cognitive processes. Specific-skills training, in which participants received practice on the outcome measures (e.g., improved driving) typically yielded large and statistically significant improvements in the trained skill. Park and Ingles concluded that the results from the specific-skills studies "...clearly show that performance on attention-demanding tasks can be improved" (p. 206), whereas "...there is little evidence in the currently reviewed studies to support the efficacy of direct retraining programs" (p. 206).

Palmese and Raskin (2000) reported results that seem not to agree with Park and Ingles's conclusions. Palmese and Raskin reported positive results of APT training for three traumatically brain-injured adults. Each participant received 1 hour of APT training per week for 10 weeks. Seven psychometric tests of attention were administered as training began, when training ended, and, for two participants, 6 weeks after APT training ended. Each participant's performance improved on one or more of the psychometric tests from pretest to posttest, but there was no uniform pattern of improvement across the tests. The two participants tested 6 weeks after APT training improved on the Paced Auditory Serial Retention Test (PASAT) between the posttest and the 6-week follow-up test. The authors concluded that APT training "seemed to improve attention in individuals with MTBI [mild traumatic brain injury] under certain conditions" (p. 545). (Whether the PASAT is sufficiently similar to the tasks in attention process training to compromise its validity as an outcome measure remains an open question; see Chapter 4 for a description of the PASAT.)

Sohlberg, McLaughlin, Parese, and associates (2000) compared the effects of APT with *therapeutic support* (education about brain injury, conversation with a supportive listener, and relaxation training) on several psychometric measures of attention and cognition, as well as patients' and significant others' self-reports of changes. Sohlberg and associates reported that participants who received APT reported more cognitive changes than participants who received therapeutic support and that participants who received APT had greater improvement on the PASAT than participants who received therapeutic support. Sohlberg and associates concluded (A) that their results "provide support for differential effects of therapeutic strategies in the rehabilitation of

patients with acquired brain injury," (B) that APT "seems to improve performance on a wide range of tasks that involve executive functions and attentional control," and (C) "because the tasks used in the APT were different from the neuropsychological tests used to assess cognitive functions, improvement on those tests represents generalization of learning" (p. 670-671).

Cicerone, Dahlberg, Malek, and associates (2005) reviewed five studies of remediation of attention deficits after traumatic brain injury (including that of Sohlberg and associates, 2000). They concluded that training such as that provided by APT (which they called *strategy training*) is effective "in the postacute period of rehabilitation" (p. 1683).

Park and Ingles have asserted that the effects of direct training of attention are practice effects that do not extend beyond the tasks used to train attention or to other similar tasks. Cicerone and associates conclude that direct training of attention is effective "in the postacute period of recovery." Sohlberg and associates claim significant effects of APT on a number of attentional and cognitive abilities. Resolution of these apparently conflicting claims awaits additional carefully designed, data-based research. Data-based research also is needed to determine if either direct-training or specific-skills training provides meaningful improvements in attention in daily life or enhances participation in activities of everyday life. In the meantime, neither direct training nor specific skills training is likely to be abandoned. Carney, Chesnut, Maynard, and associates (1999) concluded a review of 32 published cognitive-rehabilitation studies with the following statement:

> In effectively all of the studies in this review, patients improved. Although group differences were rarely observed, recovery across groups occurred. Until we have done the work necessary to be able to demonstrate what is operating to produce improvement, we are bound to provide the services and care at our disposal for this population of people. (p. 306)

Memory. Memory impairments are a common and stubborn consequence of traumatic brain injury, often persisting for years despite intensive treatment. The pervasiveness of memory impairments following traumatic brain injury, and their resistance to treatment have challenged patients, clinicians, and investigators for decades. In response to that challenge, clinicians and scientists have developed numerous programs for improving traumatically brain-injured adults' memory.

Most of the early memory training programs attempted to restore memory by means of what Sohlberg and Mateer (1989) call the *muscle building* approach to memory rehabilitation. Memory restoration programs use repetitive drills to strengthen and revitalize memory. The drills typically require patients to memorize and recall lists of numbers or words or to read printed texts or listen to spoken narratives and later retell them or answer questions about them.

As personal computers became more common and less expensive, computer-based memory retraining programs were marketed to clinics and individuals. These programs resembled their noncomputerized ancestors in that they focused on drills in which patients practiced remembering letters, numbers, words, pictures, shapes, and stories. They differed from their predecessors in that they controlled stimulus presentation rate and exposure time with great consistency and accuracy; they kept precise records of correct and error responses and of how long it took a patient to respond to each stimulus; and they did not require the presence of a clinician throughout the treatment session. These advantages contributed to a proliferation of computerized memory rehabilitation programs and their incorporation into the activities of clinics throughout the United States and in many other countries.

It gradually became apparent that the payoff of these computerized programs was considerably less than their promise. Articles began to appear in the literature asserting that stimulation approaches to memory rehabilitation in general, and computerized stimulation programs in particular, are of little value for creating meaningful changes in traumatically brain-injured adults' daily life memory performance (Brooks, 1984; Gloag, 1985; Godfrey & Knight, 1985; Hart & Hayden, 1986; Kreutzer & Wehman, 1991; Prigitano & associates, 1984; Robertson, 1990; Schacter, Rich, & Stampp, 1985; and others). As a consequence, stimulation treatment to restore traumatically brain-injured adults' memory has been largely abandoned in favor of compensatory approaches.

However, there are some indications that treating attentional impairments may indirectly facilitate memory (Sohlberg & Mateer, 1989). Cicerone and associates (2005) reviewed 13 published studies of memory remediation. They concluded that the results (A) do not support the use of direct memory training, (B) do support the use of strategy training (internal strategies such a visual imagery and external strategies such as notebooks or diaries) for patients with mild memory impairments, and (C) do support the use of external compensations (e.g., pagers, electronic organizers) for patients with moderate or severe memory impairments.

Most investigators and clinicians agree that memory drills and repetitive practice at encoding, retaining, and recalling specified information are of little value in restoring retrospective memory in persons with traumatic brain injury. There is some evidence, however, that restorative training of prospective memory may have some meaningful benefits. Raskin and Sohlberg (1996) reported that repeated administration of prospective-memory tasks (4 to 6 hours per week for several months) increased the prospective memory abilities of two adults with traumatic brain injuries. The training procedure involved systematically increasing the time between a request to perform an action and the time at which the action was to be performed, with prompts given when an action was not performed at the designated time. Both

---

Box 11-3	**Effects of Brain-Injured Persons' Unawareness on Task Performance**

Estimating Task Performance
- Does not accurately estimate task difficulty
- Does not perceive, recognize, or make use of all aspects of a task or task requirements
- Bases estimates of task performance on prior experience, beliefs, and knowledge, without regard for current level of abilities
- Bases estimates of task performance on what he or she would like to do, rather than what he or she can do

Task Performance
- Begins tasks without planning or setting goals
- Focuses on irrelevant aspects of tasks

- Does not use previous experience and knowledge when performing tasks
- Is uninterested, unconcerned about performance
- Does not monitor adequacy of performance relative to expectations, previous experience, or goals
- Does not recognize errors
- Does not adjust performance when errors occur
- Does not recognize cues for implementation of strategies or cues for changing strategy
- Does not spontaneously initiate strategies
- Does not modify or abandon ineffective strategies
- Does not relate actions or performance to outcome

Data from Fischer, S., Gauggel, S., Trexler, L. (2004). Awareness of activity limitations, goal setting, and rehabilitation outcome in patients with brain injury. *Brain Injury, 18,* 547-562.

---

participants improved their performance on the prospective-memory tasks, and there were indications that improved performance generalized to tasks that resembled daily life prospective-memory tasks. Raskin and Sohlberg did not report whether the participants' daily life prospective memory improved, and they did not report whether improved prospective-memory performance continued after treatment ended.

Awareness. *Unawareness* (absent or limited appreciation of the existence, nature, scope, and effects of physical, emotional, behavioral or cognitive impairments) is a common consequence of traumatic brain injury. Unawareness compromises rehabilitation. Brain-injured persons who are unaware of their impairments are likely to be passive participants in rehabilitation efforts, noncompliant or resistant to intervention, reluctant to learn and use compensatory strategies, and unlikely to use external aids. Traumatically brain-injured adults typically overestimate their cognitive, social, and emotional competence but are more realistic in estimating their physical competence and their competence in performing basic self-care (Fischer, Gauggel, & Trexler, 2004), perhaps because cognitive, social, and

emotional impairments are more abstract than are physical impairments.

Unawareness can affect a brain-injured response to intervention in many ways. Box 11-3 lists some of them.

Several hierarchic models of awareness have been proposed to guide research and intervention, the best known of which is Crossen, Barco, Velozo, and associates' (1989) three-level pyramid model. Crosson and associates' model of awareness has not been empirically verified but has proven popular in brain-injury rehabilitation. The model divides awareness into three hierarchic levels, as follows:

- *Intellectual awareness*—knowledge that a function is impaired
- *Emergent awareness*—ability to recognize impairment-related problems when they occur
- *Anticipatory awareness*—ability to realize that a problem is likely to occur as the result of an impairment

Intellectual awareness forms the base of the pyramid. Anticipatory awareness forms the top. Brain-injured persons may have deficits in one, two, or all three levels of awareness, but the assumption is that lower levels of awareness are prerequisites to higher levels—one would not expect to see a person with intact emergent awareness but no intellectual awareness, or to encounter a person with intact anticipatory awareness but no intellectual or emergent awareness. A patient with intellectual awareness but not emergent awareness may acknowledge the existence of impairments, but fails to recognize errors unless someone points them out. A patient with intellectual and emergent awareness but not anticipatory awareness may acknowledge impairments and recognize errors during a task, but is unable to predict when a task may be difficult and cannot predict her or his overall performance. Many clinicians assume that recovery of awareness progresses from intellectual awareness to emergent awareness to anticipatory awareness, but that progression is not specified by the model.

Prigitano and Klonoff (1998) differentiate between *lack of self-awareness* and *denial*. They describe persons with impaired self-awareness as follows:

- They lack accurate information about themselves and the nature and magnitude of their impairments.
- They are puzzled when given feedback about their behavioral and functional limitations.
- They are cautiously willing or indifferent when asked to work with new information about themselves and their limitations.

Prigitano and Klonoff describe persons with denial as follows:

- They have partial or implicit knowledge about their limitations.
- They resist or become angry when given feedback about their behavioral and functional limitations.
- They actively struggle to work with new information about themselves and their limitations.

Prigitano and Klonoff consider lack of self-awareness a negative symptom—an impairment inflicted by brain injury. They consider denial a positive symptom reflecting "the individual's attempt to cope and make sense of the world

---

Box 11-4	**Items from the Impaired Self-Awareness Scale and the Denial of Disability Scale**

Impaired Self-Awareness Scale

- Patient spontaneously reports few, if any, neuropsychological problems since the onset of their brain insult.
- Patient shows little affective reaction to hearing feedback in the interview that he or she may have more difficulties than what he or she reports.
- Patient does not appear to recognize the interpersonal or social impact of an impairment.
- Patient demonstrates "cognitive perplexity" and/or no emotional reaction when they cannot solve various neuropsychological tasks during testing and/or rehabilitation.

Denial of Disability Scale

- Patient spontaneously reports noticing some change in his or her abilities but has a difficult time defining exactly what those changes are.
- Patient shows a negative affective reaction when given feedback that he or she may be more impaired than he or she reports.
- Patient does not appear perplexed when hearing a relative's or significant other's feedback, but counters their statement with evidence as to why they are incorrect.
- Within the context of neuropsychological examination or rehabilitation, the patient is quick to show a catastrophic reaction when faced with a behavior failure.

Items are scored *yes* (present) or *no* (absent). Items scored *yes* are ranked in severity using a scale of 1 to 10.

Data from Prigitano, G.P. & Klonoff, P.S. (1998). A clinician's rating scale for evaluating impaired self-awareness and denial of disability after brain injury. *Clinical Neuropsychologist, 12,* 56-67.

given past experiences, values, and interpretations of the meaning of the impairment in the individual's social setting" (p. 57). Prigitano and Klonoff developed two rating scales—the *Impaired Self-Awareness Scale* and the *Denial of Disability Scale*. Box 11-4 shows representative items from the two scales.

Prigitano and Klonoff tested the validity and reliability of their scales with two groups of brain-injured patients, 16 whom the authors identified as exhibiting primarily impaired self-awareness, and 17 whom the authors identified as exhibiting primarily denial of disability. They identified three characteristics as most indicative of impaired self-awareness: (1) perplexity about behavioral limitations, (2) apparent lack of information about the self after brain injury, and (3) emotional indifference and bland affect. The impaired-self-awareness group and the denial-of-disability group did not differ in age, education, diagnosis, duration of brain injury, or handedness, but the denial of disability group was primarily male.

In a review of published interventions for improving self-awareness following brain injury, Lucas and Fleming (2005) found that most interventions were restorative rather than compensatory. Lucas and Fleming grouped the components of awareness-enhancing interventions into seven categories (most interventions included combinations of the components):

1. *Education.* Educational components focus on educating patients and their families about the nature of the patient's injury, the resulting impairments, and the functional implications of the impairments. Education often is carried out in groups, which provide nonthreatening environments in which patients can learn about potential difficulties without specifically admitting impairments and in which clinicians can draw attention to discrepancies between patients' self-perceptions and reality.

2. *Clinician-delivered feedback.* Feedback-based components focus on providing specific, timely, consistent, and respectful feedback about performance. Feedback may be given using the *"sandwich technique"*—preceding and following negative feedback with positive feedback. Videotapes may be used to provide feedback, with goal-setting and definition of targeted behaviors prior to viewing

and collaborative review of performance after viewing.

3. *Experiential feedback* (sometimes called *supported risk-taking* or *planned failure*). Experiential feedback components provide experiences that guide a patient to discover her or his own errors instead of relying on feedback from others, often by allowing the patient to experience difficulty in real-life situations. Intervention may involve goal-setting and practice prior to experiences, cueing during the experiences, and review of performance following experiences. Emotional support, counseling, and education are provided when a patient experiences failure.

4. *Behavior therapy.* Behavior therapy components focus on modification of behavior by manipulation of antecedents and consequences. Lucas and Fleming comment that if behavior therapy is confrontational, it may solidify patients' unrealistic beliefs about impairments and competencies. They add that effective behavior therapy requires collaboration between the clinician and the patient. Emotional support, counseling, and education are important components of behavior therapy.

5. *Counseling, support, psychotherapy.* These components often use group meetings to permit patients to observe other patients denying or admitting to impairments, expressing realistic or unrealistic goals, expressing realistic or unrealistic expectations, and responding to feedback constructively or angrily. These interventions are designed to reestablish a sense of meaning in patients' lives and to help patients' form realistic goals.

6. *Strengths/weaknesses lists.* In strengths/weaknesses components the clinician and patient collaborate to identify and make lists of the patient's strengths and weaknesses, to call attention to weaknesses the patient may have overlooked, and to identify areas that may require the use of compensatory strategies or external aids.

7. *Ratings of task performance.* In ratings components, the patient rates himself or herself in specific problem areas (e.g., attention, memory, social interactions). Discussing the ratings with the clinician helps the patient recognize and accept the validity of the impairments. A patient and another (clinician or family member) rate the patient's abilities in specific areas. Agreements and disagreements are discussed by the patient and the clinician. A patient may be asked to predict his or her performance in a task, then evaluate his or her actual performance, after which the patient and clinician may discuss discrepancies between predictions and performance.

Kennedy (2004) reported that brain-injured adults are barely above chance in predicting their memory performance when they make the predictions during or immediately after studying the materials to be remembered. If the predictions are delayed by about 30 seconds, they are much more accurate.

Although Lucas and Fleming concluded that there is little empiric evidence to support the effectiveness of interventions to improve brain-injured adults' self-awareness, they suggested that if awareness training is provided, it should begin with restoration (working to improve patients' self-awareness) followed by compensatory intervention for patients whom restorative intervention has left unaware.

Sohlberg and Mateer (2001) described three approaches to enhancing self-awareness in brain-injured persons—*individual awareness-enhancing programs, caregiver training and education,* and *procedural training and environmental support.* They commented that it is not unusual for all three approaches to be used in self-awareness intervention for a single brain-injured patient. Descriptions of the three approaches follow.

Individual awareness-enhancing programs resemble what Lucas and Fleming called *restorative/facilitative intervention.* Sohlberg and Mateer recommend these programs for patients who exhibit denial or a combination of denial and unawareness but who have at least rudimentary understanding that some of their abilities have changed as a result of brain injury and who have sufficient cognitive capacity to integrate information and experience. Sohlberg and Mateer do not recommend these programs for patients who have severe unawareness and severe cognitive impairments.

Sohlberg and Mateer divide individual awareness-enhancing programs into two components—educational and experiential. In the *educational component,* the patient is provided with personalized information about brain injury, using print materials, videotapes, and audiotapes, participates with the clinician in review of the patient's medical records, and compares his or her own ratings of abilities with ratings of others chosen by the patient. In the *experiential component,* the patient predicts his or her performance in a task, compares his or her actual performance with the prediction, and discusses agreements and disagreements with the clinician. A patient may be trained to track a specific performance or behavior by self-monitoring, may keep logs of performance or behavioral successes and failures, and may record matches or mismatches between goals and accomplishments in specific tasks.

Sohlberg and Mateer consider caregiver training and education an important component of awareness intervention. They comment that, although caregivers may seem unaware of a brain-injured person's impairments because of psychological denial, they may be unaware because they lack information about brain injury and its effects. Sohlberg and Mateer recommend that clinicians explore caregivers' expectations about the goals of intervention (e.g., improving a behavior versus improving insight into self), train caregivers in constructive ways of responding to the brain-injured persons' cognitive and behavioral missteps, and train caregivers to track their behaviors with the brain-injured person and note how the brain-injured person reacts to the caregiver's actions or reactions.

Sohlberg and Mateer reserve *procedural training and environmental support (PTES)* for brain-injured persons who have pervasive unawareness and severe cognitive impairments that preclude benefit from awareness-enhancing intervention. The goal of PTES is to maximize the brain-injured person's daily life function by means of compensatory strategies and environmental management even though the brain-injured person neither acknowledges nor understands her or his limitations. PTES training may include:

- Training automatic use of compensatory strategies or external aids without educating the brain-injured person about why to use them or under what conditions to use them
- Training others in the brain-injured person's environment in specific skills or routines to increase the brain-injured person's level of functioning
- Modifying the brain-injured person's environment to reduce the effects of his or her impairments on daily life functioning (e.g., arranging a workspace so that materials are laid out in the order in which they are used)

Sohlberg and Mateer comment that PTES must be customized for every brain-injured person and every routine. They add that PTES may be effective because it exploits brain-injured persons' preserved procedural memory for learning and retaining behavioral routines without the need for awareness or insight on the part of the brain-injured person.

At present there is little empiric evidence for the effectiveness of interventions for improving self-awareness. As Lucas and Fleming comment:

> The majority of the literature regarding intervention for impaired self-awareness includes treatment recommendations that are not based on evidence of effectiveness. As a relatively new area of rehabilitation, there is little research

into the effectiveness of specific interventions aimed at improving clients' self-awareness after acquired brain injury. (p. 765)

Clearly there is a need for scientifically sound investigation into the effectiveness of awareness training for brain-injured persons. There is particular need for investigation of the effects of awareness training on employability, independent living, and participation in social and leisure activities. The interventions evaluated in such investigations should be described in enough detail to permit replication in laboratories and clinics. Until that time, practitioners will depend on anecdotal assertions regarding effectiveness, which are many and universally positive. It seems likely that some interventions with some brain-injured persons are effective. Specifying which interventions are effective and for which brain-injured persons they are effective awaits systematic investigation.

> *The first step toward change is awareness. The second step is acceptance. (Nathaniel Branden)*

Reasoning and Problem-Solving. Reasoning and problem-solving are a part of almost any treatment activity that a clinician might carry out with traumatically brain-injured adults. Nevertheless, clinicians may focus intervention on restoration of reasoning and problem-solving, usually with paper-and-pencil workbook-like exercises.

Many workbooks and paper-and-pencil programs for treating reasoning and problem-solving have been published. There is no strong evidence that doing such paper-and-pencil activities has any significant effects on traumatically brain-injured patients' ability to reason and solve problems in daily life. Nevertheless, many clinicians use them, usually as homework. Because such exercises may do at least some patients some good and are unlikely to cause harm, their use in treatment seems appropriate, provided clinicians ensure that improved performance on the paper-and-pencil exercises also leads to improved reasoning and problem-solving in daily life activities, and provided that the paper-and-pencil exercises do not take the place of other activities with documented effectiveness.

Few data-based studies of interventions to enhance brain-injured persons' reasoning and problem solving have been published. Cicerone and associates (2005) reviewed 9 studies of interventions for brain-injured adults that included training of reasoning and problem solving. They concluded that the studies provide "limited support" for intervention to enhance problem solving and self-regulation, but they commented that additional research is needed to evaluate the effectiveness of intervention and to identify which aspects of intervention account for any beneficial effects found.

Visual Processing. Traumatically brain-injured persons' visuoperceptual impairments have received less attention than their attention, memory, and language impairments, and for speech-language pathologists, treatment of visual impairments may seem to lie somewhat outside their usual clinical territory. However, as Sohlberg and Mateer (1989) have noted, visual and visuospatial processing are crucial for carrying out activities of daily living, for adequate job performance, and for performing academic and clerical tasks. Consequently, speech-language pathologists may find that reducing visual processing impairments is an important part of the overall plan of care for a traumatically brain-injured patient, especially if the visual processing impairments compromise the adequacy or effectiveness of the patient's communication. Some interventions for visual processing impairments focus on discrimination and recognition of visual stimuli, and others focus on visuospatial processes. Work on discrimination and recognition usually precedes work on visuospatial processes, the rationale being that discrimination and recognition are prerequisites to more complex visuospatial processing.

> Treatment of attention often precedes treatment of visual perception and discrimination and sometimes accompanies it.

Activities to improve visual discrimination and recognition include visual scanning drills in which the patient scans an array of symbols, designs, or pictures to find those that match a target; visual closure tasks in which the patient must identify familiar objects or scenes based on partial information; and visual figure-ground discrimination tasks in which the patient must identify familiar objects or scenes presented on an interfering or distracting background. These tasks sometimes are presented with a time limit to increase the speed and efficiency of the patient's visual processing.

Treatment of visuospatial processing impairments usually incorporates drills that emphasize analysis of spatial relationships. Tasks that require the patient to copy or draw simple or complex geometric figures from memory or to use sticks or blocks to construct duplicates of a model commonly are used in treating visuospatial impairments. These tasks usually are arranged from simple to complex. For example, paper-and-pencil tasks might begin with copying two-dimensional figures, then progress to drawing two-dimensional figures from memory, copying three-dimensional figures, and drawing three-dimensional figures from memory.

Tasks that require the patient to mentally rotate printed visual stimuli (as in Figure 11-12) sometimes are used to treat visuospatial impairments. The tasks are presented in hierarchic fashion. For example, the patient may begin by arranging blocks in a row to replicate a model constructed by the clinician. Then the patient may be required to arrange blocks in several rows with different numbers in each row. Finally, the patient may be required to reproduce complex three-dimensional constructions (Figure 11-13). More naturalistic tasks that require visuospatial processing, such as interpreting maps, floor plans, and flowcharts also may be

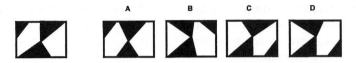

Figure 11-12 ■ A visual rotation test item. The test taker chooses from patterns A through D the one that represents a rotated version of the pattern on the left.

incorporated into interventions for visuospatial impairments.

Language and Communication. As noted earlier, most traumatically brain-injured patients' linguistic and communicative impairments are attributable to underlying impairments in basic cognitive processes such as attention, memory, and executive function (reasoning, abstract thinking, problem-solving).

Attentional impairments can contribute to:
- Poor comprehension of spoken and written verbal materials, especially when the materials are long or complex
- Missing the details in spoken and written material
- Fragmented, disjointed, noncoherent spoken discourse
- Weak or inappropriate topic maintenance and failure to observe turn-taking rules and conventions
- Failure to appreciate and respond appropriately to social cues in conversational interactions

Memory impairments can contribute to:
- Tangentiality, irrelevance, and failure to stay on topic in conversations and writing
- Excessive repetition and redundancy in spoken and written language
- Inability to keep goals, objectives, and strategies for improving communication in mind

Impairments in reasoning and abstract thinking can contribute to:
- Concrete language and inability to appreciate inferences and indirectly stated material
- Inability to appreciate relationships in spoken or written discourse

- Egocentrism in social interactions and inability to appreciate others' points of view

Impairments in problem-solving can contribute to:
- Failure to implement learned strategies to enhance communicative effectiveness
- Inappropriate conversational content and maladaptive interpersonal behaviors

These secondary effects of cognitive impairments on communication may be treated most effectively and efficiently by treating the underlying cognitive impairments, provided such treatment is effective. However, many traumatically brain-injured patients may benefit from direct treatment of communicative impairments. Direct treatment of communicative impairments most often targets the social and interpersonal (pragmatic) aspects of communication. The general objective is to increase the appropriateness, relevance, and efficiency of

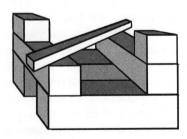

Figure 11-13 ■ A complex block construction test item. The test taker constructs a duplicate of a model constructed from a set of blocks by the examiner.

the patient's participation in conversational interactions, to enhance the patient's ability to follow shifts in topic, and to improve the patient's appreciation of nonliteral aspects of communication.

Traumatically brain-injured patients and patients with right-hemisphere brain damage often exhibit similar impairments in communicative interactions. Both tend to be impulsive and egocentric in interpersonal interactions, to miss nonliteral and implied meanings, to make faulty assumptions based on first impressions, and to be tangential, verbose, circumlocutory, and inappropriate in what they say. Consequently, interventions for traumatically brain-injured patients' impairments in communicative interactions often resemble interventions for patients with right-hemisphere brain damage (discussed in Chapter 10).

Compensatory Training. When component treatment leaves a patient with residual impairments that compromise his or her successful participation in daily life, the focus of intervention shifts to providing the patient with compensatory strategies. *Compensatory strategies* are deliberate, volitional (and sometimes unconventional) behaviors that allow the patient to perform activities that otherwise would be impossible. For example, a traumatically brain-injured college student who cannot take notes fast enough to keep up with lectures may be trained to tape-record the lectures, write down only major points while the lecture is going on, and later use the tape recording to fill in the details. Ylvisaker and Holland (1985) cite four principles of compensatory training:

- Select strategies that fit the patient's strengths and weaknesses
- Train the patient in the use of efficient and effective strategies
- Help the patient control or eliminate inefficient, maladaptive, or escapist strategies
- Guide the patient through practice with the strategies until they become automatic, thereby limiting demands on attention, memory, and other cognitive processes

Not every traumatically brain-injured patient can learn compensatory strategies, and some who learn compensatory strategies in a structured clinic environment do not use them outside the clinic. Ylvisaker and Holland assert that the success of compensatory strategy training depends partly on the patient and partly on the strategy:

- The patient must recognize the existence of impairments that cannot be alleviated by restitution of underlying processes, must be capable of recognizing problems as they occur or, better yet, anticipate problems before they occur, and must be capable of invoking a strategy based on recognition of a present or potential problem situation.
- The strategy must be fitted to the patient's needs, personality, and abilities.
- The strategy must fulfill an obvious and apparent need that personally is felt by the patient. (Teaching a patient a strategy for remembering information from printed texts will be of little use to a patient who is uninterested in reading.)
- The strategy must fit the personal inclinations and attitudes of the patient. (Teaching a shy and unassertive patient strategies that require assertiveness is unlikely to lead to the patient's use of the strategy in daily life.)
- The strategy must be easy enough that the patient can invoke it automatically and effortlessly. (Strategies that require substantial mental effort from the patient are unlikely to be used outside the environment in which they are learned.)

Barco and associates (1991) addressed the problem of matching compensatory strategies to patients by dividing compensatory strategies into four categories, each of which is appropriate for patients at a given level of ability. (The categories reflect the influence of Crosson, Barco, Velozo, and associates' pyramid model of awareness.)

External compensations (changes in the environment initiated by an agent other than the patient) are appropriate for patients who are oriented and responsive but unaware of their impairments and who do not recognize when their impairments cause problems.

Situational compensations (compensatory strategies to be used habitually in all situations in which they might be appropriate) are suitable for patients who are aware of their impairments but do not recognize problems as they occur. The patient routinely invokes the strategy whenever entering the situation and continues it throughout the situation whether or not problems targeted by the strategy occur. For example, a patient who occasionally misses some of the steps in a daily life procedure may use a checklist whenever performing that procedure.

Recognition compensations (compensations implemented when the patient perceives that a problem of a given nature is occurring) are appropriate for patients who recognize problems when they occur but do not anticipate them. For example, a patient may be trained to begin writing down key points whenever they begin to lose the sense of printed materials. Situational and recognition compensations may be identical in content. The difference is that situational compensations are implemented routinely within a specified context, whereas recognition compensations are implemented only when the patient gets into difficulty.

Anticipatory compensations (compensations implemented at the first signs of an impending problem) are appropriate for patients who can anticipate problems before they occur. Anticipatory compensations are flexible and effective, but they require high levels of awareness and problem-solving ability, putting them beyond the reach of many traumatically brain-injured patients.

Time-Pressure Management. Fasotti, Kovacs, Eling, and Brouwer (2000) described a compensatory strategy called *time-pressure management (TPM)* to enable brain-injured persons to cope with slowed information processing in daily life tasks such as driving in traffic, participating in conversations, or preparing meals. Time-pressure management trains brain-injured persons to give themselves enough time to perform daily life tasks by increasing their awareness of impairments and their awareness of the potential effects of impairments on task completion.

TPM is based on task-analysis models developed to describe drivers' decision making during motor-vehicle operation in traffic. The basis of the model is that decision making in complex activities can be arranged in three hierarchic levels—*strategic, tactical,* and *operational.* Time pressure typically is greatest at the operational level (e.g., responding to unexpected developments in heavy traffic), less at the tactical level (e.g., maintaining speed, adjusting following distance, and changing lanes), and least at the strategic level (deciding on the route and time of day for the trip before the trip begins). Importantly, decisions made at the strategic and tactical levels reduce time pressure at the operational level (e.g., if the tactical decision is made to minimize lane changes and adjust speed to conform to traffic flow, time pressure at the operational level is less than if the tactical decision is made to minimize the time spent in transit regardless of traffic conditions).

For brain-injured persons, decisions made at the strategic and tactical levels are less affected by slowed information processing than are decisions made at the operational level. Consequently, brain-injured persons may compensate for poor performance under time pressure by making decisions at the strategic and tactical levels to prevent (strategic level) or minimize (tactical level) time pressure. Fasotti and associates conceptualize TPM for brain-injured persons as a four-stage process:

1. Awareness that one's limitations require planning and organization

2. Accepting and learning time management strategies

3. Learning and practicing strategies for specific situations

4. Routinely employing the strategies in the situations

The brain-injured person is trained to "give herself or himself enough time to do the task" using the following generic routine:

1. Are there two or more things to be done at the same time for which there may not be enough time? If yes, go to Step 2. If no, do the task. (*Purpose:* to recognize potential time pressure in the task at hand)
2. Make a short list of things that can be done before the task begins. (*Purpose:* to prevent time pressure; *level:* strategic)
3. Make an emergency plan describing what to do in case of overwhelming time pressure. (*Purpose:* to deal with time pressure quickly and effectively; *level:* tactical)
4. Use the plan whenever time pressure is sensed. (*Purpose:* to monitor performance and take corrective action when under time pressure; *level:* operational)

Fasotti and associates trained an experimental group of 12 brain-injured adults in TPM and provided "concentration training" to a control group of 10 brain-injured adults. The two groups performed experimental tasks in which they were required to perform under time pressure before beginning training, as training ended, and 6 weeks after training ended. The group trained in TPM significantly increased the number of in-task time-pressure management behaviors after training, whereas the control group did not. The trained group did not increase the frequency of preplanned time-pressure management strategies as a result of training—they relied on procedural level strategies rather than strategic level or tactical level strategies. Fasotti and associates concluded that training brain-injured persons in time-pressure management techniques is appropriate for those in whom mental slowness is prominent.

Memory Strategies, External Aids. Compensating for memory impairments is a major focus of intervention for most traumatically brain-injured patients. Sohlberg and Mateer (1989)

divided strategies with which traumatically brain-injured adults may compensate for impaired memory into two general categories—*internal strategies* and *external aids.*

Training patients to make use of *internal strategies* depends primarily on mnemonic devices or imagery, and they are best suited for facilitating retrospective memory. Most mnemonic devices are verbal. In *verbal chaining strategies,* patients are taught to arrange lists of to-be-remembered items into sentences or short stories to facilitate recall. For example, a patient who has to remember the words *dog, book, rain,* and *bus* might mentally put them into a sentence such as *The dog chewed up the book and ran under the bus to get out of the rain.* In *first-letter mnemonic strategies,* patients are taught to associate the first letters of words to be remembered with words that can be arranged into easy-to-remember sayings, phrases, or rhymes. The mnemonic for remembering the names of the cranial nerves is an example of a first-letter mnemonic strategy.

Sometimes patients may be trained to create a mental image that organizes the words in a to-be-remembered list into a visual scene (e.g., a dog lying under a bus in the rain and chewing on a book) or puts to-be-remembered items in a certain location within an imagined scene. When it comes time to retrieve the item from memory, the patient mentally looks for it in the imagined scene.

Some patients may be able to use *elaborative encoding*—linking new information to related information that is already in memory. Elaborative encoding facilitates retrieval of information from memory by creating associations between multiple bits of information. The associations may create a mental pathway to the desired bit of information. For example, remembering that a person's name is Sam Smith is made more likely if one knows that Sam Smith also is a neurologist who lives in Detroit, drives a 1983 Plymouth, and participates in the Chicago marathon. Elaborative encoding is similar to *grouping* or *chunking,* in which information to be remembered is organized into categories (e.g., novels, biographies, self-help books).

Giles and Clark-Wilson (1993) described a method for helping traumatically brain-injured adults encode, store, and retrieve information from printed materials. They called the method the *PQRST* method (for *preview, question, read, state, test*). First the patient skims the material to learn its general content (preview). Then the patient makes up questions about the central features of the material (question). Then the patient actively reads the material with emphasis on answering the questions (read). Then the patient repeats and rehearses the information from the printed material (state). Finally, the patient evaluates the information to ensure that the questions were satisfactorily answered (test).

Some studies have shown that training traumatically brain-injured adults to use such internal strategies improves their performance on tests of recall (Cermak, 1975; Wilson, 1981; and others), but others have shown that the beneficial effects of training decay rapidly over time and do not generalize to natural situations (Glisky & Schacter, 1986; Lewinsohn, Danaher, & Kikel, 1977; Schacter & Glisky, 1986; and others). Sohlberg and Mateer (1989) point out that most traumatically brain-injured patients do not have sufficient cognitive resources to carry out such internal strategies successfully:

> The utility of internal memory aids for this population should be suspect. These techniques place heavy demands on patients' already deficient cognitive systems; they are thus ineffectual for many persons with significantly compromised intellectual functions. (p. 153)

Parente and DiCesare (1991) also have pointed out that the practical application of internal mnemonic strategies is likely to be limited by traumatically brain-injured patients' general impairments in attention, planning, and encoding, all of which are necessary for successful use of mnemonic strategies. However, step-by-step strategies such as PQRST may be used successfully by some higher-level traumatically brain-injured adults, provided that they write down the results of each step in the strategy before moving on to the next step.

External memory aids are more practical than internal strategies for most traumatically brain-injured adults. External memory aids are particularly well suited for enhancing *prospective memory*—remembering to do things at a given time. External memory aids span a range of sophistication from handwritten notes, calendars, and checklists to electronic organizers that permit the patient to organize, store, and retrieve complex information. External memory aids also may include modifications to the patient's environment (e.g., posted reminders and checklists).

The simplest, cheapest, and easiest-to-use prospective memory aids are calendars, schedules, checklists, and memory notebooks. Carrying a pocket calendar or printed schedule in which appointments and important events are listed may be sufficient for some high-level patients who can remember to carry the calendar or schedule and look at it. However, many traumatically brain-injured patients cannot remember to check the calendar or schedule often enough to prevent missing appointments or other important events. Checklists are helpful for patients who cannot keep track of which tasks they have accomplished and which remain undone, but checklists, like calendars, are of little value if the patient cannot remember to check the checklist. The solution for many of these patients is a signaling device (e.g., an alarm watch) that can be set to sound an alarm at preset times to remind them to check their calendar, schedule, or checklist.

Electronic memory devices may be appropriate for some higher-level traumatically brain-injured adults. *Electronic organizers* (pocket-sized electronic devices for storing and retrieving information), multi-function cell phones, and computer-based personal information managers are more expensive and not as easy to use as calendars, schedules, and checklists, but they provide more power and greater flexibility in storing names, addresses, phone numbers, appointments, and other personal information, and they are more versatile in sounding alarms and displaying reminders at times programmed into the device. (Some of these devices also permit users to print a paper copy of appointment lists or calendars, which may be kept in a notebook.) Programming these devices requires sustained attention, reasoning ability, and problem-solving skills, which means that programming will not be feasible for many traumatically brain-injured patients. However, many who cannot program the devices can use them successfully in daily life, provided someone in the patient's life is available to do the programming.

Kapur, Glisky, and Wilson (2004) recommend that clinicians keep several principles in mind when considering an external memory device for a brain-injured person:

- Consider the brain-injured person's history of memory aid use. Elderly persons may be accustomed to using handwritten materials such a notes, logs, and diaries but may resist using electronic aids. Young persons may consider some aids (e.g., pagers, cell phones) status symbols and welcome their use.
- Involve the brain-injured person in the choice of a memory aid. An aid that is imposed upon a reluctant client is unlikely to be used.
- Involve a caregiver or relative in the process from the beginning. If the aid is complex, this person must be taught to program, maintain, and use it.
- Train the brain-injured person to recognize situations in which a memory aid will be useful, how to choose an aid that will be useful in the particular circumstances, how to motivate herself or himself to use the aid, and how to use the aid effectively.

- Encourage the brain-injured person not only to learn to use the aid but to adapt daily routines and habits to incorporate the aid into daily life activities.

Sohlberg and Mateer (2001) recommend that clinicians perform a systematic assessment of a brain-injured patient's needs when selecting an external memory aid for the patient. This assessment should include the patient, plus family members and caregivers who know the patient, have a sense of the patient's needs, and know the patient's attitudes and personal preferences. Sohlberg and Mateer recommend that the needs assessment consider *organic factors, personal factors, situational factors,* and *historical factors.*

Organic factors reflect the patient's cognitive, learning, and physical capabilities. The system or strategy should be consistent with the patient's ability to learn and remember new skills and with the patient's ability to implement the newly learned skills in appropriate circumstances. The system or strategy should be consistent with the patient's physical abilities. Motor impairments may preclude use of systems requiring legible handwriting or motor dexterity in manipulating, maintaining, and using electronic devices. Visual or auditory impairments may preclude use of systems in which the user must read small print, read characters displayed on a screen, or hear beeps or alarms sounded by electronic devices.

Personal factors reflect the patient's attitudes, preferences, and resources. The system or strategy should capitalize on the patient's spontaneous use of compensatory strategies. Often it is more effective to build on a strategy the patient has used or is using than to teach a new strategy. For example, if a patient has used an electronic organizer, day planner, or pager before being injured, he or she is likely to welcome its use as a compensatory device. Devices should respect the patient's preferences with regard to appearance (color, style, size), mode (paper-and-pencil, electronic, auditory, visual), and functions (checklists, calendars, alarms). Devices must be selected with consideration of the patient's financial resources. Expensive electronic devices may be out of reach for patients with limited resources. (However, clinicians may help patients with limited resources obtain funds for such a device by providing an insurer with a rationale and plan for its use.) Selection of a strategy or device must consider the support available in the patient's environment. If someone in the patient's environment is available, willing, and competent to help the patient learn and use a strategy or device, more complex strategies or devices may be appropriate. If the patient has limited support and is essentially on her or his own to learn to use the strategy or device, a simple system may be needed.

Situational factors reflect the context in which the strategy or device will be used, including the circumstances in which the patient's cognitive impairments interfere with functioning, the consequences of breakdown, and the contexts in which the function served by the strategy or device is not a concern. The strategy or device should enable the patient to be successful in circumstances in which not having the strategy or device would lead to failure and wherein failure has meaningful consequences for the patient's access to and participation in important daily life activities.

Historical factors relate primarily to patients who have been using strategies or devices that have been taught, recommended, or provided by others. Strategies or devices the patient has used successfully may be good choices, whereas strategies or devices the patient has failed to use or has used without success likely are poor choices for the patient's current needs.

An option for patients who cannot manage portable memory devices is *environmental modification*, in which memory props are posted in conspicuous locations in the patient's living environment. For these patients, reminder notes may be posted on mirrors and in other conspicuous places, and schedules of appointments and activities and check-off sheets may be posted in strategic locations to permit the patient to keep track of completed and pending tasks. Cupboards, shelves, and drawers may be labeled according to their contents, and closets and cupboards may be arranged systematically (e.g., items that are used together may be placed adjacent to each other, or items may be arranged alphabetically or by color).

Planning, Problem-Solving. Training in daily life planning and problem-solving typically entails practice, coaching, and role-playing in simulated daily life situations. Patients with severe impairments may practice reasoning and problem-solving in simple, highly structured activities such as planning a meal, planning a trip to a shopping center on public transportation, or balancing a checking account. Patients with less severe impairments may practice problem-solving in less structured and more complex activities such as planning a vacation trip, role-playing the return of a defective item to a store for a refund, or role-playing an employment interview.

Ylvisaker and Feeney (1998) described a general *goal-plan-predict-do-review* routine to help brain-injured persons set reasonable goals for themselves, formulate a workable plan to achieve a goal, predict their performance when using the plan, implement the plan, and review their performance to determine what aspects of the plan worked and what aspects of the plan did not work. *Setting the goal* calls for answering the question: "*What do I want to accomplish?*" *Making the plan* calls for answering three questions: "*How am I going to accomplish my goal?*" "*What materials or equipment will I need?*" and "*What are the steps to be followed?*" Two questions are called for in *prediction*: "*How well will I do?*" and "*How much will I get done?*" *Do* entails carrying out the task while noting problems that arise and coping with problems using trained strategies. *Review* calls for answering four questions: "*How did I do? What worked? What didn't work?* and *What will I do differently next time?*

Ylvisaker and Feeney's *positive everyday routines* (described later) as well as strategies for time-pressure management (described earlier) also appear well suited for interventions to improve planning and problem-solving.

Environmental Compensation. Another way to help traumatically brain-injured adults compensate for residual impairments is to restructure the patient's daily life environment to minimize the effects of the impairments on the patient, family members, and associates. Such restructuring may require physical modifications to the patient's home, school, or work environment to facilitate access and ease of movement (e.g., installation of ramps and modifications of living spaces to accommodate a patient in a wheelchair). Such physical modifications usually are the province of physical and occupational therapists.

Environmental modifications also may entail educating family members, teachers, supervisors, and others to promote constructive attitudes and minimize unrealistic expectations. Such education is especially important for families and associates of traumatically brain-injured patients who have residual cognitive impairments but few or no major physical impairments and who talk and behave much as they did before their injury. Because these patients appear so normal, family members, friends, teachers, and supervisors often expect the patient to perform as competently as before the injury. When the patient does not meet their expectations, these persons may conclude that the patient is uncooperative, unmotivated, stubborn, or acting out of hostility and anger. When this happens, environmental modification may require education of family members about why the patient behaves as he or she does, teaching family members appropriate strategies for interacting with the patient, and helping the patient and family organize the patient's daily life environment to maximize

successful interactions and minimize unsuccessful ones.

Environmental modifications may include:

- Establishing consistent routines and regular schedules for daily life activities
- Instructing family members, friends, and associates in how to facilitate the patient's success in daily life activities
- Limiting or eliminating distractions by keeping radios and televisions turned down and closing doors and windows to reduce noise from outside or from other rooms
- Keeping the patient's possessions in designated places and putting them away when they are not being used
- Organizing the patient's workspace and scheduling work at difficult tasks for times at which the patient is rested and alert
- Setting time limits (using alarms and timers) for working at difficult tasks to avoid fatigue and minimize mistakes

Environmental compensation for higher level traumatically brain-injured patients resembles *environmental control* for confused and agitated patients. The primary difference is one of intent. The intent of *environmental control,* as the label implies, is to bring a patient's agitated, confused, and maladaptive behaviors under control. The patient does not plan, initiate, or use environmental control procedures in a purposeful way. The patient's behavior is controlled by the environment, rather than the other way around. The intent of *environmental compensation* is to provide strategies, prompts, or cues to enhance a patient's performance in certain contexts or in certain cognitive or linguistic domains. The patient typically participates in planning the compensations, is actively trained in their use, and uses them in a purposeful and goal-directed way.

Positive Everyday Routines. Ylvisaker and Feeney (1998) described a comprehensive intervention program for persons with traumatic brain injury that incorporates aspects of restorative intervention, compensatory strategies, and environmental compensation. Ylvisaker and Feeney's program is based on the concept of *positive everyday routines*. Ylvisaker and Feeney describe positive everyday routines as "a functional and highly contextualized approach to rehabilitation" representing "collaborative alliances with everyday people" (p. 99). They advocate positive everyday routines for brain-injured persons who have chronic mild to severe disabilities in cognitive, executive system, behavioral, and communication domains—disabilities that overlap and intermingle in their negative effects on a brain-injured person's daily life. Everyday routines are routines "that occur in the course of everyday social, familial, vocational, and recreational life and involve everyday communication partners, including family members, friends, work supervisors, and teachers" (Ylvisaker, Szekeres, & Feeney, 2001, p. 757). Everyday routines are similar to *habits*—chains of behaviors that do not require effortful deliberation or planning. Positive everyday routines are highly practiced and environmentally supported chains of behaviors that facilitate the brain-injured person's successful participation in activities of everyday life despite cognitive or communicative deficits that otherwise would compromise or prevent participation.

Interventions to provide brain-injured persons with positive everyday routines are based on several premises (Ylvisaker & Feeney, 1998):

- Assessment occurs in natural contexts, is ongoing and collaborative (involves the clinician, the brain-injured person, and family members or significant others), and involves testing hypotheses about the brain-injured person's performance and what can be done to improve it.
- The most effective intervention occurs in meaningful contexts and is designed to influence routines in those contexts.
- Brain-injury rehabilitation requires an integrative, collaborative approach to intervention.

- Effective rehabilitation simultaneously addresses impairment, disability, and handicap (or in contemporary WHO terminology, impairment, activity, and participation).
- In the absence of meaningful engagement in chosen life activities, all interventions eventually will fail.

Everyday routines include the situations or settings in which routines are used, the sequences of events and activities in which routines are embedded, the materials needed to accomplish the routines, and the language or other forms of communication that accompany routines. Ylvisaker and Feeney describe everyday routines as follows:

- They are structured around the brain-injured person's own meaningful goals.
- They are infused into everyday activities.
- The brain-injured person is given enough practice that strategic behavior becomes automatic.
- Everyday people are trained in how they can facilitate improvement and support the brain-injured person's adaptive strategies and compensations.
- The brain-injured person's life experiences are adequately organized from task to task and from day to day.
- The brain-injured person is responsible for effective performance of strategies.
- Successful performance is richly and naturally rewarded.
- The brain-injured person is an active participant in determining the goals of activities, creating plans to achieve goals, monitoring her or his performance, evaluating results, and determining what works and what does not.

The positive everyday routine approach to intervention is designed to ensure that the effects of intervention transfer seamlessly to the brain-injured person's daily life and that the strategies and compensations acquired during intervention persist when formal intervention ends.

GENERAL CONCEPTS 11-5

- Most early treatment programs for adults with traumatic brain injuries relied on *drill activities* designed to stimulate and enhance mental processes. When it became obvious that stimulation programs were not effective, other approaches took center stage. Current treatment programs usually combine elements of *functionally oriented treatment, cognitive rehabilitation,* and *behavior therapy.*
- *Sensory stimulation* is a common form of treatment for comatose or semicomatose patients, although currently there is no empiric verification of its effectiveness.
- Environmental control is an important part of treatment for confused and agitated patients, whose confusion and agitation may be reduced by making their environments stable, secure, and predictable.
- Orientation training may be appropriate for patients who are confused but who can attend to orientation training procedures and remember orientation information for more than a few minutes. Orientation training may include environmental prompts (e.g., signs, calendars), overt reminders by caregivers and patient-care personnel, passive orientation drills, or active orientation training.
- *Behavior management* techniques may control problem behaviors and enhance desired behaviors by manipulating antecedent stimuli, response contingencies, and setting events.
- *Medications* may be prescribed for traumatically brain-injured patients to control agitation and restlessness, improve alertness and attention, manage depression, diminish psychotic symptoms, or control seizures. Dosages and effects must be monitored carefully to ensure that the medications do not adversely affect the patient.
- Cognitive-communicative intervention may be *restorative* (designed to repair damaged cognitive processes) or *compensatory* (designed to help the brain-injured persons,

family members, and significant others reduce the effects of cognitive-communicative impairments on daily life).
- Compensatory approaches to cognitive-communicative rehabilitation often include *component training*, in which individual cognitive processes are treated with repetitive drill activities. Component training may be appropriate for traumatically brain-injured patients with reasonably good attention and memory. Treatment of attentional impairments occupies a prominent place in component training, although the benefits of attention training for brain-injured persons have not been definitively established.
- Memory improvement programs for adults with traumatic brain injury generally have failed to generate meaningful improvements in memory beyond the treatment programs themselves. Consequently, memory drills for improving retrospective memory largely have been abandoned in favor of compensatory approaches. Restorative training of prospective memory, however, may provide meaningful benefits.
- Absent or limited appreciation of the existence, nature, severity, and effects of physical, behavioral, and cognitive impairments *(unawareness)* is a common consequence of traumatic brain injury. Crosson has described a three-level hierarchic model of awareness that often is used to structure intervention. The three levels in Crosson's model are *intellectual awareness, emergent awareness,* and *anticipatory awareness.*
- Prigitano and Klonoff differentiate between *unawareness* and *denial.* Patients who are unaware often are puzzled when told of their limitations. Patients who deny disability often become angry when told of their limitations. Unawareness is considered a direct effect of brain injury. Denial is considered to represent a patient's coping strategies.

Continued

GENERAL CONCEPTS 11-5—cont'd

- Several interventions designed to increase brain-injured persons' awareness of their limitations have been described in the literature. Their effectiveness remains to be determined.
- Several interventions designed to improve brain-injured persons' reasoning and problem-solving have been described in the literature. There is limited evidence for the effectiveness of some interventions, but definitive evidence of effectiveness awaits future research.
- Treatment of visuospatial processing impairments may be appropriate for brain-injured persons who have problems discriminating visual stimuli or analyzing spatial relationships. Treatment may include scanning drills, figure-ground discrimination tasks, and mental manipulation of visual stimuli.
- Most traumatically brain-injured persons' linguistic and communicative deficits are the result of impairments in cognitive processes that support language and communication (attention, memory, reasoning, abstract thinking, and problem-solving). Such linguistic and communicative deficits are best treated by treating the processes underlying them.
- Compensatory training is appropriate when component treatment does not rectify impairments that interfere with a traumatically brain-damaged individual's daily life competence.
- *External compensations* are changes in the environment initiated by an agent other than the patient. They are appropriate for patients who are oriented and responsive but unaware of their impairments.
- *Situational compensations* are appropriate for patients who are aware of their impairments but do not recognize problems as they occur. These patients are taught to use compensatory strategies habitually in certain situations.
- *Recognition compensations* are appropriate for patients who can recognize problems when they occur but do not anticipate

them. These patients are trained to invoke a strategy when they perceive that a problem of a given nature is occurring.
- *Anticipatory compensations* are appropriate for patients who can anticipate problems before they occur. These patients are taught to invoke a strategy at the first signs of an impending problem.
- *Time-pressure management (TPM)* may help brain-injured persons' compensate for mental slowness by attending to strategic, tactical, and operational aspects of daily life tasks.
- Compensatory techniques for memory impairment can be divided into *internal strategies* (e.g., mnemonic devices, imagery) or *external aids* (e.g., checklists, calendars, electronic organizers). Internal strategies best compensate for impaired retrospective memory. External aids are more practical for traumatically brain-injured adults than internal strategies (which require substantial cognitive resources). External aids best compensate for impaired prospective memory.
- Sohlber and Mateer assert that the choice of an external memory aid should consider *organic factors, personal factors, situational factors,* and *historical factors.*
- Training in planning and problem-solving typically entails structured practice and coaching in simulated or actual everyday situations. Positive everyday routines and time-pressure management may contribute to improved planning and problem-solving in daily life.
- Modifying a traumatically brain-injured individual's daily life environment may help to minimize the effects of the individual's impairments on daily life competence and participation.
- Ylvisaker and Feeney's *positive everyday routines approach* to intervention is designed to provide brain-injured persons with highly trained and relatively automatic strategies to enhance their performance in specific activities of everyday life.

GROUP TREATMENT

Group treatment is an integral part of intervention for most patients with traumatic brain injuries, provided they can participate in group activities without disrupting them. (This usually means patients at RLAS Level V and above.) Group treatment provides a number of benefits, not all of which are related to improvements in cognitive and behavioral adequacy. Some of these auxiliary benefits include helping patients overcome feelings of isolation and loneliness, increasing patients' self-confidence and sense of self-esteem, and helping patients express and deal with negative feelings such as anger and hostility.

Groups for traumatically brain-injured patients may serve several purposes, either separately or in combination (most frequently, *support, self-assessment, communication, cognitive rehabilitation, generalization,* and *education;* less frequently, *sensory stimulation* and *orientation*).

Group sensory stimulation activities for patients with traumatic brain injuries are controversial, owing in part to the questionable efficacy of sensory stimulation for individual patients. Sensory stimulation groups usually are made up of patients who are confused but not extremely agitated. Group sessions typically are short (30 minutes or less) and include a mix of sensory stimulation and orientation. Sensory stimulation may consist of recorded music, radio or television programs, or televised sporting events, movies, slide shows, and the like. Group stimulation activities sometimes are supplemented with tactile, taste, or movement stimulation of individual patients.

Group orientation activities are most appropriate for patients at RLAS levels V and VI. Group orientation activities are similar to those for patients in sensory stimulation groups, except that patients actively participate by acknowledging and repeating the information provided by the group leader and support staff. Some basic interactional skills, such as acknowledging and taking turns, also may receive attention.

Orientation activities may include activities in which the group leader and support staff:

- Greet each patient by name and announce to the group each patient's name and an item or two of interest about each patient
- Announce the date, day of week, and time of day (often supported by visual aids such as a large clock and calendar)
- Give the name of the treatment facility, its location, and its purpose
- Describe the current weather and give the weather forecast

Group support activities are most appropriate for patients at RLAS Level VI and above. Participation in support activities with other traumatically brain-injured patients may help individual patients dispel feelings of isolation, loneliness, and having been unfairly singled out by fate. Observing other group members who are coping with their impairments and progressing may help motivate individual patients. Support from other group members may help individual patients deal with failure and overcome disappointments. By providing a forum for expression of feelings, group activities may help individual patients express and deal with feelings of anger, rage, hostility, and frustration.

Group self-assessment activities are most appropriate for patients at RLAS Level VII and above, although some Level VI patients may profitably participate. Participation in self-assessment activities may help traumatically brain-injured patients develop a more realistic sense of their abilities and disabilities. Group experiences may serve this function both for patients who minimize or deny their impairments and who have unrealistic expectations and for patients who exaggerate their impairments and minimize or ignore their remaining strengths. (One-on-one treatment, with its highly structured format and the presence of a supportive and helpful clinician, sometimes gives patients an unduly optimistic impression of their potential success in daily life activities.) Group experiences also may provide opportunities for individual patients to observe and evaluate others' successful and unsuccessful performance as a prelude to evaluating their own performance. (Traumatically brain-injured patients, like those with right-hemisphere brain injuries, usually are better at evaluating others' behavior than they are at evaluating their own.)

Group communication activities are most appropriate for patients at RLAS Level VI and above. Group communication activities may provide traumatically brain-injured patients with a sheltered but realistic context in which to work on interpersonal interactions. Group members may practice conversational and pragmatic skills such as turn-taking, topic maintenance, requesting, asserting, and clarifying, repairing conversational breakdowns, and monitoring and responding to others' verbal and nonverbal communication. Feedback concerning appropriate and inappropriate behavior may come from group leaders or, more important, from other group members. Role-playing activities in which participants act out and discuss daily life problem situations are a common vehicle for providing participants with practice to develop communicative and interactional skills. Group review and discussion of the role-plays provides the opportunity for group members to exchange opinions and ideas regarding appropriate and inappropriate behavior in communicative interactions.

Erlich and Sipes (1985) described a communication group format for traumatically brain-injured adults in which group activities center around videotaped role-plays. Target behaviors are specified by group leaders in advance of each role-play. Group leaders make the first videotape, in which they act out a common problem situation to illustrate appropriate and inappropriate behaviors. Then the interactions are replicated by group members in a second videotaped role-play. The videotaped role-plays are reviewed and commented on by the group, with emphasis on behaviors that contribute to or interfere with communicative success.

Group members are assigned personal goals in each interaction, and members' successes and failures relative to their goals are discussed by the group. Erlich and Sipes's group format addresses *nonverbal communication* (voice inflection, facial expression, eye contact, posture, gesture), *communication in context* (topic initiation, topic maintenance, responsiveness to social context), *message repair* (awareness of communication failure, appreciation of listener needs, clarification strategies), and *cohesiveness* (organization and sequencing of information, temporal and spatial integrity).

Sohlberg and Mateer (1989) describe several group activities for working on traumatically brain-injured patients' communication skills, including a collaborative drawing task in which group members are divided into pairs. One participant in each pair draws, out of sight of the other, three simple geometric shapes in two colors. Then the participant who drew the shapes tells the other how to reproduce the drawings without seeing them. When the second participant has finished, they compare drawings and discuss communicative successes and failures. In another activity, participants wear hats labeled with phrases such as *ignore me* or *talk down to me*. (Group members cannot see what is printed on the hat they are wearing.) The group members discuss a topic and respond to each participant according to what is printed on the hat. After the discussion, each member tries to guess what is printed on her or his hat, and the group talks about what happened and how they felt.

Group cognitive rehabilitation activities may address attention, memory, reasoning, problem-solving, and visual processing, either individually or in combination. Activities may resemble those used in one-to-one treatment activities, but group members may be divided into teams that compete with one another, collaborate on solving problems posed by the group leader, or take turns in game-like activities that call on the cognitive processes that are the focus of the day. Competition among teams to finish a task first or to finish a task with the highest accuracy often has a prominent place in cognitive rehabilitation group activities, both to motivate group members to participate and to keep levels of interest and attention high.

Generalization of skills, attitudes, strategies, and behaviors acquired in one-to-one treatment to less structured and more natural contexts is an objective of most group activities. Generalization is targeted by means of group activities in which members may practice in the group what that they have learned in one-to-one treatment.

Instruction about the physical, cognitive, emotional, psychosocial, and vocational effects of brain injury often is incorporated into group activities. Some instruction may be didactic, with group leaders providing group members with instruction and handouts. Videotapes or films about the effects of traumatic brain injury may be shown to and discussed by the group. Group exercises in which group members make lists of changes in their own lives caused by their brain injury, present the lists to the group, and discuss them with the group also may serve an educational purpose. Guest speakers such as physicians, social, workers, vocational counselors, or survivors of traumatic brain injury may talk to the group and lead group discussions.

Efficacy of Group Activities

There is little objective evidence for the efficacy of group treatment of adults with traumatic brain injuries, although numerous anecdotal reports have appeared in the literature. The situation has not appreciably changed since Deaton (1991) concluded her discussion of group interventions for traumatically brain-injured adults as follows:

> At present, the most glaring gaps in the use of group interventions have to do not with the availability of various models and formats, but rather with the documentation of group effectiveness in improving cognitive skills in particular, as these skills generalize to other social environments. This remains the most significant issue needing to be addressed in future work in this area. (p. 199)

By far the most controversial purpose of group treatment is that of sensory stimulation. The appropriateness of sensory stimulation for groups of traumatically brain-injured patients is questionable because, as noted earlier, there is little evidence that sensory stimulation of individual patients hastens their return to consciousness or accelerates their recovery of orientation to person, place, and time.

Group experiences for patients at RLAS Level III and below seem unlikely to provide benefit, because these patients are at best only dimly aware of other group members and are unlikely to contribute to or benefit from a group experience. Proponents might argue that group stimulation, like individual patient stimulation, is unlikely to do harm and should be provided because it may do some good. Proponents also might argue that stimulation groups represent a cost savings over individual patient stimulation. Whether the possible good merits the time and expense of professionals to provide the stimulation remains an important question, and one might argue that providing an ineffective treatment more cheaply is no bargain.

Although there is no convincing evidence for the efficacy of purely orientation groups, the fact that participants are actively responding to the group leaders and to other group members suggests that the group experience may enhance participants' orientation and help them get started on the road toward interpersonal adequacy. However, it is unlikely that patients who qualify for purely orientation groups receive much benefit from the group experience itself. Consequently, the primary advantage of putting them into a group for orientation may be cost savings. Whether orientation groups require professionals as leaders, however, seems questionable.

The widespread use of group activities to provide support, facilitate self-assessment, improve communication, enhance cognitive processing, promote generalization, and educate traumatically brain-injured patients about the effects of brain injury, plus the presence of numerous anecdotal reports of the positive effects of such group activities, provide some support for their efficacy. At present, there is no compelling reason to reject such group activities for traumatically brain-injured adults, provided group members are appropriately selected (they must have adequate comprehension, expressive abilities, and intellectual function to participate, and they must be able to control disruptive behavior), there is at least some degree of homogeneity among group members, and activities and objectives are appropriately selected and matched to the group. However, as Deaton has noted, there is an immediate and pressing need for objective verification of the effectiveness of group treatment for traumatically brain-injured adults.

COMMUNITY INTEGRATION

The final stage of rehabilitation for many traumatic brain-injury patients is access to and participation in family, vocational, and community settings. Successful community integration may take several months, and usually takes place in residential facilities *(transitional living facilities)* where a group of traumatically brain-injured patients lives around the clock. Traumatically brain-injured persons in transitional living facilities spend their daytime hours in activities to prepare them for reentry into the community. Less often, preparation for community integration takes place in day treatment centers, where participants spend their daytime hours, returning home at the end of each workday.

Community integration programs differ across facilities and across brain-injured persons. However, most programs are directed toward a common set of objectives:

- Provide participants with a supportive context in which to practice and perfect strategies for increasing their daily life competence
- Prepare participants for carrying out routine self-care activities (e.g., personal hygiene, eating, sleeping, grooming) in daily life

- Develop participants' interest in domestic, vocational, leisure, and social activities and develop participants' ability to perform them
- Establish routines for commonly occurring daily life domestic, vocational, leisure, and social activities and train participants to perform them
- Train participants to allocate appropriate amounts of time for daily activities and to use time constructively
- Evaluate participants' competence for vocational, school, and leisure activities
- Place participants in appropriately structured work, school, and leisure activities
- Enlist family members, significant others, teachers, supervisors, employers, and others to facilitate and enhance participants' successful participation in daily life social, work, school, and leisure activities

These objectives may be realized by means of a combination of one-on-one training, group activities, and structured experiences in real-life situations. Participants typically spend part of the day working on specific behavioral strategies for increasing daily life competence and part of the day in group activities wherein they practice daily living skills, discuss problems and potential solutions, and provide communal social and emotional support. Sometimes participants spend time in real life or simulated vocational, school, or social settings in which they may practice strategies for success in work, school, or social activities. Family members, employers, and other individuals who are significant in a participant's daily life may play a part in such activities.

Community integration programs typically represent the combined efforts of teams of occupational therapists, recreational therapists, speech-language pathologists, vocational counselors, neuropsychologists, social workers, and other professionals. As the brain-injured person progresses, the team gradually withdraws structured intervention, training, and support and expects increasing independence on the part of the brain-injured person. Discharge from the facility and return to home, family, work, or school mark the end of formal rehabilitation for most participants, although counseling visits may continue for some.

Effects of Community Integration Programs on Social Participation

> *Life it is not just a series of calculations and a sum total of statistics, it's about experience, it's about participation, it is something more complex and more interesting than what is obvious. (Daniel Libeskind)*

Although participation in meaningful daily life activities is an important aspect of brain-injured persons' well-being and quality of life, few studies of cognitive-communicative interven- tion have included measures of social participa- tion as outcome measures. Most have measured the effectiveness of rehabilitation in terms of improvement in test scores or ratings of improvement in cognition and communication by brain-injured participants, clinicians, or significant others. Publication of the *Commu- nity Integration Questionnaire* (*CIQ*; Willer, Rosenthal, Kreutzer, Gordon, & Rempel, 1993) together with the World Health Organization's emphasis on participation has, however, stimu- lated clinicians and investigators to assess the effects of rehabilitation on community integra- tion for traumatically brain-injured adults.

The CIQ consists of 15 items relating to par- ticipation in home-based activities, social activi- ties, and work activities (Box 11-5). Since its publication, the CIQ has become a widely used general measure of community integration

---

Box 11-5	*The Community Integration Questionnaire*

Home Integration Section

1. Who usually does shopping for groceries or other necessities in your household?

Yourself	(2)
Yourself and someone else	(1)
Someone else	(0)

2. Who usually prepares meals in your household?

Yourself	(2)
Yourself and someone else	(1)
Someone else	(0)

3. In your home who usually does normal every-day housework?

Yourself	(2)
Yourself and someone else	(1)
Someone else	(0)

4. Who usually cares for the children in your home?

Yourself	(2)
Yourself and someone else	(1)
Someone else	(0)
No children in home	(Score is average of items 1, 2, 3, 5)

5. Who usually plans social arrangements such as get-togethers with family and friends?

Yourself	(2)
Yourself and someone else	(1)
Someone else	(0)

Social Integration Section

6. Who usually looks after your personal finances, such as banking or paying bills?

Yourself	(2)
Yourself and someone else	(1)
Someone else	(0)

Can you tell me approximately how many times a month you now usually participate in the following activities outside your home?

7. Shopping

5 or more	(2)
1-4 times	(1)
Never	(0)

Continued

From Willer, B., Rosenthal, M., Kreutzer, J.S., Gordon, W.A., Rempel, R. (1993). Assessment of community integration following rehabilitation for traumatic brain injury. *Journal of Head Trauma Rehabilitation, 8,* 75-87.

Box 11-5	*The Community Integration Questionnaire—cont'd*

8. Leisure activities such as movies, sports, restaurants, etc.

5 or more	(2)
1-4 times	(1)
Never	(0)

9. Visiting friends or relatives

5 or more	(2)
1-4 times	(1)
Never	(0)

10. When you participate in leisure activities do you usually do this alone or with others?

Mostly alone	(0)
Mostly with friends who have head injuries	(1)
Mostly with family members	(1)
Mostly with friends who do not have head injuries	(2)
With a combination of family and friends	(2)

11. Do you have a best friend with whom you confide?

Yes	(2)
No	(0)

Productivity Section

12. How often do you travel outside the home?

Almost every day	(2)
Almost every week	(1)
Seldom/never	(0)

13. Please check the answer below that best corresponds to your current (during the past month) work situation.

Full-time (more than 20 hours per week)

Part-time (less than or equal to 20 hours per week)

Not working, but actively looking for work

Not working, not looking for work

Not applicable; retired due to age.

14. Please check the answer below that best corresponds to your current (during the past month) school or training program situation.

Full-time

Part-time

Not attending school or training program

Not applicable; retired due to age

15. In the past month, how often did you engage in volunteer activities?

5 or more times

1 to 4 times

Never

Scoring: Items 13-15 are combined to form one variable, *Jobschool,* using the following scoring system. The Productivity score = Item 12 + Jobschool variable.

Not working, not looking for work, not going to school, no volunteer activities (0)

Volunteers 1 to 4 times a month AND not working, not looking for work, not in school (1)

Actively looking for work AND/OR volunteers 5 or more times per month (2)

Attends school part-time OR working part-time (less than 20 hours per week (3)

Attends school full-time OR works full-time (4)

Works full-time AND attends school part-time OR attends school full-time AND works part-time (less than 20 hours per week) (5)

If retired, score as:

In the past month, how often did you engage in volunteer activities?

5 or more	(4)
1-4 times	(2)
Never	(0)

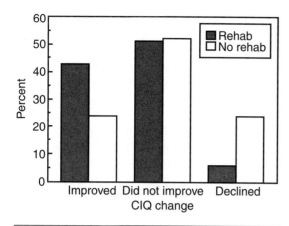

Figure 11-14 ■ Pretest-posttest changes in *Community Integration Questionnaire (CIQ)* ratings for a group of traumatically brain-injured adults who received comprehensive brain-injury rehabilitation *(Rehab)* and a group of brain-injured adults who received no rehabilitation *(No Rehab)*. (Data from Cicerone, K.D., Dahlberg, C., Malec, J.F., & associates [2005]. Evidence-based cognitive rehabilitation: Updated review of the literature from 1998 through 2002. *Archives of physical medicine and rehabilitation, 86,* 1681-1692.)

following traumatic brain injury. Studies of the validity, sensitivity, and reliability of the CIQ suggest that it is reasonably robust in all three characteristics. (However, a revised and more sensitive CIQ is currently under development in a cooperative effort among several centers in the United States.)

Cicerone (2004) compared changes in CIQ ratings reported in three studies of 148 traumatically brain-injured adults who had received some form of comprehensive brain-injury rehabilitation with changes in CIQ ratings for a group of 21 brain-injured adults in one study who had received no rehabilitation. The results of Cicerone's comparison are summarized in Figure 11-14.

Almost half the participants who participated in cognitive-communicative rehabilitation made meaningful improvement on the CIQ following intervention, but slightly more than half did not improve, and about 5% declined in CIQ ratings. The results were favorable, however, when compared with results for those who did not participate in cognitive-communicative rehabilitation. Only about one-fourth of those who did not participate in cognitive-communicative rehabilitation improved in CIQ ratings, and another one-fourth declined in CIQ ratings, leading Cicerone to conclude that cognitive-communicative rehabilitation may be as important in preventing declining social participation as it is in increasing social participation.

The limited evidence available concerning the relationship between postacute rehabilitation for traumatic brain injury and community integration (social participation) permits the following conclusions:

- Level of cognitive ability and community integration (as measured by the CIQ) are, at best, weakly related.
- Level of cognitive ability and social participation are weakly related.
- Changes in cognitive abilities are greatest in the months immediately following brain injury.
- Changes in social participation are greatest 1 year or more after brain injury.
- Subjective well-being and quality of life have been neglected as indicators of outcome.
- The relationship between cognitive and physical abilities and judgments of well-being and quality of life are stronger for persons with recent head injuries than for persons 1 year or more postinjury.
- Rehabilitation may be important not only for increasing the social participation of brain-injured adults but also for preventing declines in social participation in the years following injury.

WORKING WITH THE FAMILY

Providing support, reassurance, information, and direction to family members is an important part of the clinical management of persons with traumatic brain injuries. The family's need for support, reassurance, and information is greatest in the acute postinjury interval, and their need for direction is greatest in the middle and later stages of recovery. Polinko (1985) has divided the time following traumatic brain injury into three stages: *injury to stabilization, return to consciousness,* and *rehabilitation.*

For the family, the first stage *(injury to stabilization),* when the patient remains unconscious, is a period of apprehensive waiting. The patient is in the care of strangers and is surrounded by an intimidating array of monitors and support systems. The family may have been told that the patient may not recover. They watch for the first signs of consciousness and often misinterpret the patient's purposeless activity as purposeful behavior. According to Polinko, this is a time of shock and denial with occasional episodes of panic, and family members need extensive support and reassurance. During this time, family members also need objective information about what has happened and what the outcome is likely to be, but they may have difficulty assimilating it because of their emotional state. Consequently, information may have to be reiterated a number of times. As time goes on, denial gives way to bargaining, in which family members attempt to strike a deal with a deity or with fate by promising acceptance of the patient's condition, acts of contrition, changes in attitudes, or changes in behavior, if only the patient survives.

The second stage *(return to consciousness)* usually brings feelings of relief that the patient will live, together with apprehension about the extent to which the patient will recover. Family members continue to watch anxiously for hopeful signs and may continue to misinterpret incidental patient behaviors as signs of recovery.

Because the patient's emergence from coma often occurs rapidly, family members may be led into overly optimistic predictions about the patient's eventual recovery. Educating family members about the usual course of recovery from traumatic brain injury and helping them separate true prognostic indicators from fallacious ones is an important part of the clinician's responsibility during this stage.

By the time the third stage *(rehabilitation)* is reached, most families have accommodated to the accident and its aftermath and have moved past the stage of denial to reasonably realistic expectations about the future. The beginning of structured intervention activities usually is a time of increased hope and optimism for family members, often leading to optimistic expectations of what will be accomplished. This time of hope and optimism often gives way to anxiety, confusion, and eventually anger with the patient and with professional staff as the patient's recovery fails to meet expectations. The unpredictable nature of recovery from traumatic brain injury adds to the family's confusion and sometimes to their anger. When periods of rapid recovery alternate with periods of little change, family members may accuse the patient of slacking off, or they may accuse clinicians of not doing their job. When it becomes apparent that the patient will not recover to premorbid levels, the family will need help in planning how they will cope with a future that includes an impaired family member.

As time goes on, families usually return to a semblance of normal functioning. Family members who once stayed with the patient during major parts of the day return to work, and the patient no longer is the central focus of family life. Responsibility for the patient may be divided among family members. One family member may assume primary responsibility for visiting the patient and interacting with caregivers, and another may take responsibility for dealing with financial and logistic adjustments. During this time, the family may need the help of psychologists, neuropsychologists, social workers, rehabilitation therapists, speech-language pathologists, and community service agencies in setting up a long-term plan for incorporating the brain-injured patient into family life in a way that is maximally beneficial for the patient and the family. Throughout the course of the patient's recovery, the family will need continuing and conscientious assistance from all members of the patient-care team to survive the mental, emotional, and physical consequences of the patient's injury.

GENERAL CONCEPTS 11-6

- Group treatment may help patients overcome feelings of isolation and loneliness, increase patients' self-confidence and sense of self esteem, and help patients express and deal with negative feelings such as anger and hostility, provided the patients can attend and participate in group activities without disrupting them.

- Group treatment may provide *sensory stimulation* and promote *orientation* of more severely impaired patients with traumatic brain injuries. For higher-level patients, group activities may *provide psychological support, promote realistic self-assessment and personal goals, provide communication practice* in a controlled environment, *enhance cognitive abilities* in game-like activities, *provide for generalization* of skills to group settings, or *provide instruction* about aspects of brain injury and its effects on individuals and families.

- There is no empiric evidence for the efficacy of group treatment for adults with traumatic brain injuries. Many anecdotal reports suggest that some group treatment activities may be beneficial for some traumatically brain-injured individuals, but specification of *what, when,* and *who* remains to be accomplished.

- Reentry into family, vocational, and community settings is the final stage of rehabilitation for many traumatic-brain-injury patients.

Preparation for community reentry usually takes place in residential transitional living facilities. Treatment activities in transitional living facilities are carried out by teams of professionals.

- The *Community Integration Questionnaire (CIQ)* is a widely used general measure of community integration following traumatic brain injury.

- Limited evidence suggests that brain-injured persons' cognitive abilities and community integration are weakly related, that changes in social participation are greatest 1 year or more postinjury, and that rehabilitation may both increase social participation and prevent declines in social participation in the years following injury.

- Providing support, reassurance, information, and direction to family members is an important part of the clinical management of patients with traumatic brain injuries. The family's needs for support, reassurance, information, and direction change as the traumatically brain-injured family member recovers. Support and reassurance are important in the early stages of the brain-injured family member's recovery. The family's need for information and direction becomes greater as the patient's survival is assured, and issues of coping and management become salient.

THOUGHT QUESTIONS

Question 11-1 Mary Jones slips on the ice at her front door and hits her head on the concrete step. She does not lose consciousness but immediately gets up, goes into the house, and tells her husband what happened. Except for some swelling and a small laceration at the back of her head, she appears to be fine. Thirty minutes later she complains of a severe headache. She takes two aspirin. She complains that she feels nauseous and still has the headache 45 minutes after taking the aspirin. She vomits and complains of a stiff neck 15 minutes after that.

Speculate about the neurologic events that might explain Mary's symptoms.

Question 11-2 Jerry Smith is a 25-year-old man who was riding his motorcycle along a rural road at approximately 50 mph. As he approached a farm driveway, a pickup truck pulled out into his path. He braked and swerved to avoid the truck, but he lost control and was thrown from the motorcycle, which was at that time traveling about 30 mph. He was thrown forward, flipped upside-down, and struck the door of the pickup with his upper back and the back of his head. He was wearing a motorcycle helmet.

What would you expect the location and nature of his head injuries to be? How would your answer change if he were not wearing a helmet?

Question 11-3 You receive a referral for a 23-year-old male who is 9 days posttraumatic brain injury in a motor vehicle accident. He emerged from coma two days ago and is now at Rancho Los Amigos Level 4. The referring neurologist wishes you to evaluate the patient and make recommendations. You have a 1-hour time interval in your schedule in which you can see this patient.

Summarize what you would plan to do in your initial contact with the patient. What are your preliminary thoughts regarding prognosis? What information contributes to them?

Question 11-4 You have been asked to evaluate Ronald, a 20-year-old man who is now 6 months posttraumatic brain injury received in a motor vehicle accident. At the time of his injury, he was a sophomore at a state university where he majored in environmental studies and received mostly grades of B and some grades of A. He was injured in his college town, which is in another state, and received his postaccident medical care and 6 weeks of rehabilitation in that city. Since his discharge from the rehabilitation facility, he has been living locally at home with his parents. He wishes to return to college at the beginning of the next term, 3 months from now, to resume his studies. He feels that he is ready to return to school, but his parents insist on a professional opinion regarding his potential for success at school before they agree to pay for his college expenses. You have a report from the rehabilitation institute that contains standardized achievement test scores obtained at the time of Ron's discharge from that facility:

- Mathematics: Grade 12+
- Spelling: Grade 10
- General knowledge: Grade 12+
- Reading comprehension (sentences): Grade 12+
- Reading comprehension (paragraphs): Grade 9

The report also states that at discharge Ron was capable of living independently—he competently performed activities of daily life without supervision, organized his daily schedule, remembered and kept appointments, and interacted appropriately with those around him.

What additional information would you need to offer an opinion about Ron's potential success at school? How would you get the information you need? (Assume that Ron's parents are willing and able to pay for extensive testing, if needed, and that Ron has agreed to participate.)

Dementia

The mind I love must have wild places, a tangled orchard where dark damsons drop in the heavy grass, an overgrown little wood, the chance of a snake or two, a pool that nobody's fathomed the depth of, and paths threaded with flowers planted by the mind. (Katherine Mansfield)

DEFINING DEMENTIA

Dementia is a common consequence of several degenerative central nervous system diseases, especially central nervous system diseases that affect older adults. Dementia is marked by diffuse impairment of memory, intellect, and cognition. Alterations in behavior and personality are common, and physical impairments such as movement disorders or sensory disturbances often accompany dementia.

The most widely used definition of dementia in the United States is that of the *Diagnostic and Statistical Manual of Mental Disorders-IV* (*DSM-IV*; American Psychiatric Association, 1994). Individuals diagnosed as having dementia according to the DSM-IV definition must exhibit the following:

- Impaired short-term memory
- Impaired long-term memory
- At least one of the following characteristics:
  - Impaired abstract thinking
  - Personality change
  - Impaired judgment
  - Impaired constructional abilities
  - Impaired language
  - Impaired praxis
  - Impaired visual recognition

The *International Classification of Diseases* (*ICD-10*; World Health Organization, 1992) is more widely used internationally than DSM-IV. The ICD-10 defines dementia as follows:

Dementia is a syndrome due to disease of the brain, usually of a chronic or progressive nature, in which there is disturbance of multiple higher cortical functions, including memory, thinking, orientation, comprehension, calculation, learning capacity, language, and judgement. Consciousness is not clouded. Impairments of cognitive function are commonly

accompanied, and occasionally preceded, by deterioration in emotional control, social behaviour, or motivation. Dementia produces an appreciable decline in intellectual functioning, and usually some interference with personal activities of daily living, such as washing, dressing, eating, personal hygiene, excretory and toilet activities.

To qualify as dementia, the person's impairments must meet the following criteria:
- Insidious in onset
- Not caused by delirium, schizophrenia, or major depression
- Acquired (which distinguishes dementia from congenital conditions such as mental retardation)
- Persistent (which distinguishes dementia from transitory states such as delirium or confusion)
- Affects several areas of mental function (which distinguishes dementia from focal impairments such as aphasia or psychiatric disturbances)
- Severe enough to interfere with work, social activities, and relationships with others

Albert and associates (1974) and Cummings and Benson (1984) have commented that the DSM-IV criteria for diagnosing dementia are insensitive to the intellectual impairments of persons with dementia caused by subcortical brain damage.

Many of the early signs of dementia are exaggerated forms of the minor day-to-day lapses of normal adults.
- *Memory failure.* Normal adults occasionally forget an appointment, miss a deadline, forget a neighbor's name, or forget a birthday or anniversary. Adults with dementia may not

remember making an appointment, may forget that they have a deadline, may not recognize a neighbor as a neighbor, or may not have any idea whose birthday is July 12.

- *Disorientation.* Normal adults occasionally forget what day of the week it is and occasionally get lost in unfamiliar places. Adults with dementia routinely may not know what day it is, may not know if it is morning, afternoon, or evening, and may get lost in their own neighborhood or even in their own home.

- *Lapses in judgment.* Normal adults occasionally run a red light, dress inappropriately for the weather, or unintentionally violate social conventions. Adults with dementia may fail to notice red lights, wear a wool overcoat on a hot day, or address strangers on the street as close friends or relatives.

- *Difficulty performing activities of daily life.* Normal adults occasionally get distracted and leave the casserole in the oven too long or forget to provide towels for overnight guests. Adults with dementia may forget that they made the casserole and not only forget the towels but also forget that they have overnight guests.

- *Difficulty performing mentally challenging tasks.* Many normal adults are challenged by having to balance a checkbook, program a videocassette recorder, or double a recipe. Adults with dementia may be unable to perform simple calculations, remember what a videocassette recorder is used for, or keep the steps in a recipe in order.

- *Misplacing things.* Normal adults occasionally misplace regularly used articles such as purses, keys, and cordless telephones. Adults with dementia may put regularly used items in odd places, such as a purse in the refrigerator or the car keys in the cookie jar and later will have no idea how they got there.

- *Apathy and loss of initiative.* Normal adults sometimes get mentally worn down by work, social obligations, housecleaning, and other activities of daily life, but most recover their initiative as time passes. Adults with dementia may abandon, avoid, and withdraw from

previously enjoyed activities and never return to them.

- *Changes in mood.* Normal adults typically experience a range of emotions in response to life events. Adults with dementia may exhibit rapid changes in mood that occur for no apparent reason or for trivial reasons.

Dementia usually begins late in life, and its incidence increases rapidly with age. Approximately 2% of 65-year-olds are likely to be affected by dementia, whereas approximately 20% of 80-year-olds are likely to be so affected (Evans & associates, 1989; Katzman, 1976; Kokmen & associates, 1989). Alzheimer's disease accounts for more new cases of dementia than any other single cause (Figure 12-1).

Dementia is the most common single diagnosis for nursing home residents. Estimates of its prevalence differ greatly because of differences in where samples are obtained, variable definitions of dementia, and differences in the ages of the persons studied. In the year 2000, the United States population contained about 37 million adults older than age 65. Because of declining birth rates and longer life expectancy, the proportion of elderly persons in the world population is increasing, and with it the incidence of age-related illnesses, including dementia.

According to Jorm, Korten, and Henderson (1987), the presence of dementia in the U.S. population doubles with every 5-year increment in age after age 65. Gao and associates (1998) suggest, however, that the number of new cases of dementia is not consistent across age groups but declines in the oldest age groups. According to Gao and associates, the number of new cases of dementia triples from age 55 to age 64, doubles from age 65 to age 74, and increases by 1.5 times from age 75 to age 95 (Figure 12-2). Gao and associates suggest that the slowing incidence rates for the oldest age groups may be because individuals with dementia die earlier, leaving biologically stronger individuals (who presumably would be less likely to develop dementia) disproportionately well-represented in the oldest age groups.

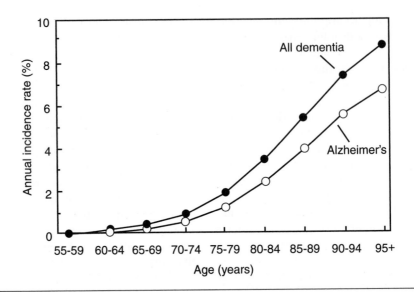

Figure 12-1 ■ Yearly percent incidence of dementia and Alzheimer's disease by 5-year age increments. (Data from Gao, S., Hendrie, M.B., Hall, K.S., & Hui, S. [1998]. The relationships between age, sex, and the incidence of dementia and Alzheimer disease. *Archives of General Psychiatry, 55,* 809-815.)

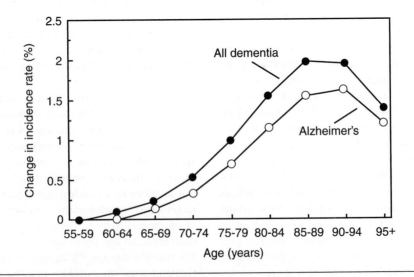

Figure 12-2 ■ Change in yearly incidence of dementia and Alzheimer's disease as a function of age. The slowing rate of incidence in the oldest age groups may represent the effects of attrition for persons who are susceptible to Alzheimer's disease, who may be less healthy and die earlier. (Data from Gao, S., Hendrie, M.B., Hall, K.S., & Hui, S. [1998]. The relationships between age, sex, and the incidence of dementia and Alzheimer disease. *Archives of General Psychiatry, 55,* 809-815.)

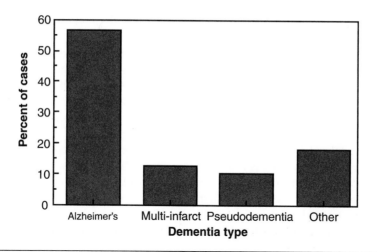

Figure 12-3 ■ Probable cause of dementia for persons referred for evaluation of dementia. Pseudodem. = pseudodementia (depression, reversible dementias); Other = Parkinson's disease, Huntington's disease, tumor, etc. (Data from Clarefield, A.M. [1988]. The reversible dementia: Do they reverse? *Annals of Internal Medicine, 109,* 472-478. Clarefield obtained these estimates by reviewing 32 published reports of diagnoses for persons referred for evaluation of dementia.)

Dementia often occurs as the primary (or only) symptom of neurologic disease, as in Alzheimer's disease and Pick's disease. Vascular disease sometimes causes dementia, and dementia often appears in the late stages of extrapyramidal diseases such as Huntington's disease or Parkinson's disease. Depression, metabolic disorders, nutritional deficiencies, drug overdoses or drug side-effects, infections (encephalitis, meningitis), and poisoning with toxic substances (mercury, lead, arsenic) also may lead to dementia. Some dementias (e.g., those caused by metabolic and nutritional disorders, drugs, infections, or toxins) are reversible, but most are irreversible and progressive.

Reversible dementia tends to occur in younger persons. Approximately 20% of dementias occurring in persons younger than 65 are reversible, but only about 5% of dementias occurring in persons older than 65 are reversible (Cummings & Benson, 1983).

Dementia syndromes can be divided into three major categories, based on the location of pathologic changes in the central nervous system. *Cortical dementias* are caused by changes in the cerebral cortex. *Subcortical dementias* are caused by changes in the basal ganglia, thalamus, and brain stem. *Mixed dementias* are caused by changes in both cortical and subcortical structures. The most common causes of cortical dementia are Alzheimer's disease and Pick's disease. The most common causes of subcortical dementia are Parkinson's disease and vascular disease. The most frequent single cause of dementia is Alzheimer's disease (Figure 12-3).

SUBCORTICAL DEMENTIA

Impairments of cortical functions (memory, intellect, language) appear early in cortical dementia but not until the late stages of most subcortical degenerative diseases. Motor impairments are prominent in the early stages of subcortical dementia. The first signs of dementia in persons with subcortical disease typically appear months to years after the appearance of the motor impairments caused by the subcortical disease, presumably when pathologic changes have progressed from subcortical structures to the brain cortex.

Parkinson's Disease (Parkinsonism)

Parkinson's disease (also known as *paralysis agitans* or *primary parkinsonism*) is a degenerative disease affecting nuclei in the midbrain and brain stem. Parkinson's disease was first described in 1817 by James Parkinson, a British paleontologist and surgeon. Parkinson's disease sometimes is called *idiopathic parkinsonism*, because the cause of the neural degeneration in Parkinson's disease is not known. Another variant, called *Parkinson-plus disease* or *multiple-system degeneration*, includes diseases in which the major symptoms of Parkinson's disease are accompanied by other symptoms of central nervous system pathology. Progressive supranuclear palsy, described later in this chapter, is an example of a Parkinson-plus disease.

The term *idiopathic* means *"of unknown cause."* Diseases that resemble Parkinson's disease, but whose causes are known, are called *secondary parkinsonism*. Parkinsonism is a generic label for several diseases in which tremor, muscle rigidity, and slowness of movement are present.

The primary symptoms of Parkinson's disease are disturbances of movement and include muscle rigidity, tremor, slowness or abolition of movement, and loss of balance. Parkinson's disease affects about 1% of the U.S. adult population and is slightly more likely to affect men than women. Parkinson's disease usually appears between the ages of 50 and 65 years.

Neuropathology. Parkinson's disease is caused by deterioration of *dopaminergic* (dopamine-producing) neurons in the basal ganglia and the brain stem (especially in a part of the basal ganglia called the *substantia nigra*). *Dopamine* is a neurotransmitter that inhibits neuronal activity and prevents unintended movements. When 60% or more of the dopamine-producing neurons in the brain are destroyed, the first symptoms of Parkinson's disease emerge. The symptoms include the following:

- Resting tremor ("pill rolling" tremor of the hands often is often the first sign of tremor to appear)
- Muscle rigidity (persons may complain of unusual stiffness and difficulty moving)
- Slowness of movement and difficulty initiating movement *(bradykinesia)*
- Postural instability (impaired balance)

Although the causes of the neuronal degeneration in Parkinson's disease are not known, the causes of some kinds of secondary parkinsonism are known. An influenza epidemic in 1918 and 1919 was followed by development of parkinsonism in some survivors. Some cases of secondary parkinsonism have been attributed to poisoning with heavy metals (manganese, lead, mercury) or poisoning with aluminum, carbon monoxide, or cyanide. Recently a form of parkinsonism has developed in individuals who have used heroin contaminated with a neurotoxin called MPTP. Repeated minor head trauma such as that incurred by boxers can cause a Parkinson's-like condition called *pugilistic parkinsonism.*

Medical Management. The primary treatment for Parkinson's disease is administration of *levodopa (L-dopa)*, a chemical precursor to dopamine, which the body converts to dopamine. Treatment with levodopa or similar medications suppresses tremor and slows mental deterioration for about two-thirds of persons with Parkinson's disease. Other medications, such as *deprenyl* (which slows the breakdown of dopamine in the body) and *bromocriptine* (which mimics the effects of dopamine) sometimes are used to control the symptoms of parkinsonism. Many patients with Parkinson's disease eventually reach the point at which their disease progresses despite medications, at which time their mental functions also deteriorate.

Two relatively new surgical procedures sometimes may help patients whose symptoms cannot be controlled with medications. In *pallidotomy,* tissue in the basal ganglia (the globus pallidus, hence the name *pallidotomy*) is surgically destroyed to relieve tremor and rigidity. *Fetal tissue transplant* is a controversial experimental technique in which dopamine-producing tissues from human fetuses are transplanted into the brains of patients with parkinsonism to replace lost dopaminergic neurons.

Evolution. Parkinson's disease is characterized by slowly progressive deterioration of motor and mental functions. The usual first symptom of Parkinson's disease is tremor, but sometimes immobility and "poverty of movement" (Adams & Victor, 1981) appear before tremor develops. As Parkinson's disease progresses, memory, problem-solving, abstract reasoning, and other mental functions requiring sustained mental effort become increasingly compromised. Affect becomes progressively flattened, and many patients become depressed. Significant dementia develops in 15% to 20% of patients with Parkinson's disease (Levin, Tomer, & Rey, 1992) and up to 30% develop some signs of dementia (Duffy, 2005).

Cognition and Communication. The usual first complaint of persons with Parkinson's disease is that their voice has become weak and that others cannot hear them in noisy environments. As the disease progresses, speech rate increases, and articulation becomes progressively more indistinct. Rapid, stuttering-like repetitions of syllables, words, and phrases may predominate. *Micrographia* (extremely small writing) is common in the early stages of Parkinson's disease. Drooling and swallowing impairments may appear in the middle stages. Vocabulary, syntax, and grammar usually are preserved until the very late stages of the disease. In the late stages of Parkinson's disease, comprehension of complex verbal materials may begin to deteriorate, and the affected individual may have difficulty in tasks requiring sustained attention and mental effort. Although some persons with Parkinson's disease become profoundly demented by the very late stages of their disease, most retain sufficient intellect to function adequately in familiar environments with caregiver supervision. Most persons with Parkinson's disease die within 15 to 20 years of the onset of their disease.

Huntington's Disease

Huntington's disease is an inherited degenerative neurologic disease first described in print (in 1872) by George Huntington, an American general practitioner. The disease soon became known as *Huntington's chorea* to highlight the movement disorder that characterizes the disease. Because there are several other signs of Huntington's disease, and because chorea is not always present, the label *Huntington's disease* has replaced *Huntington's chorea*. The genetic abnormality responsible for Huntington's disease apparently originated in Britain, and seventeenth-century British immigrants probably carried the abnormality to many parts of the world, including the United States and Canada. Diagnostic markers for Huntington's disease *(the HD triad)* include chorea, cognitive decline, and neurobehavioral symptoms (e.g., personality changes, agitation, depression, paranoia, delusions). In the United States, Huntington's disease affects about 1 person in 20,000.

> Huntington was never on a medical faculty and apparently never published another article, but his name is well known because of his accurate description of the disease that bears his name.

Neuropathology. Huntington's disease is characterized neuropathologically by loss of neurons in the caudate nucleus and the putamen, patchy loss of cortical neurons in the frontal and temporal lobes, with occasional extension of neuron loss to the cerebellum.

Medical Management. There is no cure for Huntington's disease. Medical intervention is most effective in controlling the movement disorder and the emotional and psychological effects of the disease. Antidepressants may be prescribed for depression; antipsychotics for delusions, hallucinations, or paranoia; and anxiolytics for anxiety and agitation. Antipsychotic medications may diminish the severity of chorea, at least in the early stages of Huntington's disease, but they may exacerbate depression or agitation, and at high dosages or with prolonged use may cause parkinsonian symptoms to appear.

Evolution. Huntington's disease usually appears between age 40 and age 60, but the symptoms of about 10% of patients begin before 20 years of age. Huntington's disease progresses inexorably, and most patients die by 15 to 20 years after onset. The juvenile-onset form of the disease usually progresses more rapidly, with death occurring 5 to 10 years after onset.

The first symptoms of Huntington's disease usually are involuntary movements *(chorea)*. The first choreic movements are undramatic and may be attributed to simple nervousness. The affected person appears clumsy, restless, and fidgety. As time passes, the choreic movements become more obvious and personality changes develop:

> Patients begin to find fault and complain about everything and to nag other members of the family; they may be suspicious, irritable, impulsive, eccentric, or excessively religious, or may exhibit a false sense of superiority. (Adams & Victor, 1981, p. 804)

Irritability and emotional outbursts are common. Mental deterioration follows, often becoming salient several years after the first signs of chorea. When mental deterioration begins, memory typically is affected first, followed by slowing of intellectual functions and compromised attention. Progressive motor impairments, dementia, and incontinence eventually culminate in institutionalization, followed by death from infection or poor nutrition 15 to 20 years after onset.

Cognition and Communication. Dysarthria caused by chorea is the most common commu-

nicative impairment in the early to middle stage of Huntington's disease. When chorea affects the muscles of articulation or respiration, irregular interruptions of speech and voice occur. As a patient's chorea increases, speech intelligibility declines and *dysphagia* (swallowing impairment) often develops. Language usually is preserved until the late stages of Huntington's disease, except for language tasks requiring sustained attention, memory, and judgment. In the final stages, persons with Huntington's disease become mute, incontinent, and profoundly demented.

Progressive Supranuclear Palsy

Progressive supranuclear palsy (PSP) was first described as a clinical diagnosis by Steele, Richardson, and Olszewski in 1964. Progressive supranuclear palsy is a rare disease (affecting about 1 in 20,000 adults in the United States). It usually begins between age 50 and age 80, with peak incidence in the early 60s. Progressive supranuclear palsy resembles Parkinson's disease in the presence of rigidity and slowness of movement, but it differs from Parkinson's disease in the absence of tremor and in the presence of rigidity affecting muscles of the neck and trunk, rather than the muscles of the limbs. Nevertheless, Lees (1990) claims that as many as 12% of patients with progressive supranuclear palsy are first diagnosed as having Parkinson's disease. Men develop progressive supranuclear palsy slightly more often than do women.

Neuropathology. Progressive supranuclear palsy is caused by neuronal loss, neuronal abnormalities, and proliferation of glial cells throughout the brain stem and basal ganglia. Cortical neurons are largely spared. Early symptoms of progressive supranuclear palsy include paralysis of muscles responsible for downward gaze, rigidity of neck muscles, and facial muscle weakness. As progressive supranuclear palsy advances, the patient loses vertical and lateral eye movements. The patient's limbs become stiff and rigid, dysarthria appears, and swallowing becomes difficult.

The combination of neck rigidity and paralysis of downward gaze produces early difficulties with walking for patients with progressive supranuclear palsy, because they cannot see their feet. Patients report frequent falls, usually backward. Adams and Victor (1981) report the experience of a large man with progressive supranuclear palsy who fell repeatedly, wrecking furniture as he fell, but whose stance and gait appeared normal in the neurologic examination. Some neurology texts allude to the *"dirty tie" sign,* caused by patients' inability to see food dropped as they eat.

The affected person's personality typically changes as supranuclear palsy progresses. Some become apathetic and seemingly euphoric. Others become restless and irritable. Depression is common. Dementia, characterized by slowing of mental processes and increasing forgetfulness, appears in the middle to late stages. In the final stages the affected person becomes mute, immobile, and helpless.

Medical Management. The cause of progressive supranuclear palsy is unknown, although viruses or slowly acting toxins are considered possible causes. Recent studies suggest that some forms of the disease may have a genetic origin. There is no effective medical treatment for progressive supranuclear palsy. Levodopa and similar medications sometimes provide temporary improvement, but no medical regimen provides long-term benefit. Medications to manage psychological and neurobehavioral sequelae of progressive supranuclear palsy (e.g., depression, anxiety) may be appropriate.

Evolution. The first symptoms of progressive supranuclear palsy are subtle. The patient reports frequent falls and complains of stiffness (rigidity) in neck and trunk muscles. As the disease advances, the patient may complain of double vision (the first signs of ocular muscle weakness) and changes in mood. As the disease continues, the patient loses up-and-down eye movements, muscle rigidity progresses to the patient's arms and legs, and *pseudobulbar palsy* (exaggerated palatal and laryngeal reflexes, drooling, swallowing disturbances, and heightened emotionality) appears. By this stage of the disease many patients become apathetic, and some are clinically depressed. During the late stages of the disease, the patient loses side-to-side eye movements, facial muscles become rigid, and walking becomes impossible because of frequent falls. Almost all patients with very late-stage progressive supranuclear palsy are bedridden or confined to a wheelchair and require full-time care. Most die within 4 to 7 years after diagnosis, either from aspiration pneumonia or from respiratory failure as a result of central nervous system dysfunction.

Cognition and Communication. Dysarthria appears early and can be severe even in the early stages of progressive supranuclear palsy. The affected person's speech becomes slow and littered with stuttering-like repetitions, and the person's voice intensity diminishes. Slowly progressive dementia often begins in the middle to late stages, but language usually remains well-preserved until the very late stages, at which time the person's speech becomes unintelligible. Mutism is common in the very late stages of progressive supranuclear palsy.

Human Immunodeficiency Virus Encephalopathy

Acquired immunodeficiency syndrome (AIDS) is a complex of signs and symptoms caused by infection with the *human immunodeficiency virus (HIV)* transmitted by body fluids (primarily blood and semen). The virus weakens the immune system, leading to the appearance of various opportunistic diseases, including bacterial, parasitic, and fungal infections and several forms of cancer. According to the World Health Organization, about 22 million adults are living with HIV infections worldwide, most in developing countries. Most AIDS patients are younger than age 35. More than 90% of deaths from AIDS occur in individuals younger than age 50.

Opportunistic infections are infections made possible by a patient's lowered resistance. One of the hallmarks of AIDS is the occurrence of opportunistic infections.

Neuropathology. AIDS Dementia Complex (also called *HIV encephalopathy)* is the most common neurologic consequence of AIDS. As many as 70% of persons with AIDS develop AIDS dementia complex (Aminoff, Greenberg, & Simon, 1996). Aids dementia complex is caused by infection of the brain with the human immunodeficiency virus. The infection causes pathologic changes in the subcortical white matter and basal ganglia—changes that eventually progress to the cortex (Navia, Jordan, & Price, 1986). HIV infection of the brain produces a pattern of impairment in which early symptoms (weakness, slowness, rigidity, dyskinesia) are characteristic of extrapyramidal pathology, and later developing symptoms (impaired perception, memory, intellect, and language) signify cortical involvement. The exact cause of these pathologic changes is unknown, but neurotoxins triggered by the virus are likely candidates. AIDS dementia complex usually develops late in the course of AIDS, but it sometimes appears early, and occasionally it is the first sign of AIDS.

Medical Management. There is no cure for AIDS or for AIDS dementia complex. However, a number of drugs have been shown to prolong AIDS patients' lives, and there are preliminary indications that these drugs also may lessen the severity of dementia in patients with AIDS dementia complex. Currently most practitioners believe that a combination of powerful HIV antiviral drugs provides the best treatment for AIDS. HIV often builds up resistance to a single drug, but combining two antiviral drugs greatly reduces the rate at which the virus develops resistance to them. More than a dozen HIV antiviral drugs have been approved for use in the United States. The search continues for more effective drugs that may control or even cure the disease.

Evolution. The onset of AIDS dementia complex is variable. Usually it begins insidiously and progresses slowly, but occasionally onset is abrupt and progression is rapid (Price & Perry, 1994). First the affected person becomes forgetful and apathetic and has difficulty concentrating and carrying out complex mental tasks. As AIDS progresses, motor impairments representing combinations of subcortical pathology (weakness, rigidity, ataxia) and cortical pathology (spasticity, hyperreflexia, primitive reflexes) appear, followed by seizures and incontinence. Cognitive impairments prevent the person with AIDS dementia complex from working and maintaining a household. Impairments in visuospatial abilities, abstract thinking, and reasoning appear. Persons in the final stages of AIDS dementia complex are mute, disoriented, incontinent, immobile, and require around-the-clock nursing care. Without aggressive medical treatment, death usually occurs within 6 months after the onset of central nervous system pathology, usually from aspiration pneumonia or opportunistic infection.

Cognition and Communication. In the early stages of AIDS dementia complex, speech and language generally are within normal limits, although careful testing may reveal subtle impairments in word retrieval and in comprehension of complex printed and spoken materials. As AIDS progresses and motor systems are affected, spontaneous speech becomes slow, labored, sparse, and dysarthric, the affected person gets lost in conversations, and comprehension of printed and spoken materials declines. As dementia progresses into later stages, spontaneous speech is limited to single words and short phrases, and the affected person comprehends only highly familiar spoken or printed material. In the final stages the affected person's speech is limited to a few overused words and phrases, comprehension of even simple printed materials is nonfunctional, and comprehension of speech is limited to comprehension of short and simple utterances.

Identifying Subcortical Dementia

Most subcortical dementias are delayed consequences of extrapyramidal system disease and are preceded by characteristic impairments of volitional movements (e.g., the rigidity, tremor, and slowed movements of Parkinson's disease, the choreiform movements of Huntington's disease, the eye and trunk muscle paralysis of progressive supranuclear palsy).

Identifying subcortical dementia is somewhat less ambiguous than identifying cortical dementia, because several extrapyramidal diseases often progress to dementia. When signs of mental decline appear in otherwise healthy persons who have extrapyramidal disease, the signs may signal the onset of progressive dementia. Assessment of these persons' dementia usually is preceded by assessment and treatment of speech impairments (e.g., dysarthria) and motor impairments (e.g. chorea) that appear earlier. A few persons who have extrapyramidal disease experience intellectual deterioration before detectable motor impairments appear. No pre-existing disease points to a diagnosis of dementia for these individuals, and the clinician must base the diagnosis on the pattern and progression of the individual's mental impairments. The diagnostic routine for these persons resembles the diagnostic routine for patients with cortical dementia (discussed later).

CORTICAL DEMENTIA
Alzheimer's Disease

Alzheimer's disease is the fastest growing and most expensive clinical population in the United States (Bayles, Kazniak, & Tomoeda, 1987). About 4 million adults in the United States have Alzheimer's disease. Alzheimer's disease affects 5% to 10% of the over-65 population and from 15% to 30% of the over-80 population in the United States (Clarke & Witte, 1990). Alzheimer's disease accounts for 50% to 70% of all progressive dementias (Cummings, 1990). Alzheimer's disease is more common in women than in men, especially in older age groups (Figure 12-4).

Neuropathology. Alzheimer's disease was first described by Alois Alzheimer, a German professor of neuropathology, who reported autopsy findings from a 56-year-old patient who had died following several years of severe dementia. Alzheimer examined the patient's brain at autopsy and found several pathologic changes which he described in a paper published in 1906. These pathologic changes came to define the disease.

At the time, Alzheimer was a psychiatrist and neuro-pathologist at the Frankfurt "asylum for lunatics and epileptics." Alzheimer died of heart failure at age 51.

Alzheimer described three microscopic changes in brain neurons: *neurofibrillary tangles, neuritic plaques,* and *granulovacuolar degeneration.* These changes are detectable only by direct examination of brain tissue; they are not visible on computerized tomography (CT) scans or magnetic resonance imaging (MRI) scans. It is not known whether the neuronal abnormalities are themselves the cause of dementia or are a consequence of other neurochemical processes that actually cause the dementia, but generally it is believed that the abnormalities interfere with normal neuronal functions and contribute to dementia either directly or indirectly.

In the late stages of Alzheimer's disease the brain shrinks, the ventricles become larger, and the sulci become wider (Hedera and Whitehouse, 1995). These changes are the result of neuron loss and are visible on CT or MRI scans.

Neurofibrillary Tangles. *Neurofibrils* are threadlike structures normally found in the cell bodies, dendrites, axons, and sometimes in the synaptic endings of neurons in the brain. In Alzheimer's disease, the neurofibrils become twisted, tangled, contorted, and clumped together. These changes are easily seen with a

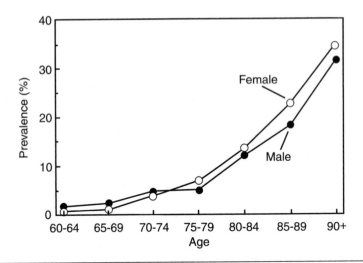

Figure 12-4 ▪ Prevalence of Alzheimer's disease by age and sex. (Based on data from Melzer, D., Pearce, K., Cooper, B., & Brayne, C. [2000]. In J. Stevens, & J. Rafferty. *Health care needs assessment: The epidemiologically based needs assessment reviews.* Oxford: Radcliffe Medical.)

standard microscope. Neurofibrillary tangles are not unique to Alzheimer's disease. Neurofibrils may be present in the brains of persons with Parkinson's disease, in the brains of persons with progressive supranuclear palsy, and occasionally in the brains of elderly persons with no obvious neurologic disease. Neurofibrillary tangles may be a neuron's nonspecific reaction to central nervous system damage (Cummings & Benson, 1983; Bayles, Kaszniak, & Tomoeda, 1987).

Neuritic Plaques. Neuritic plaques (sometimes called *senile plaques* or *dendritic plaques*) are "minute areas of tissue degeneration consisting of granular deposits and remnants of neuronal processes" (Cummings & Benson, 1992, p. 67). Neuritic plaques tend to concentrate in the cortex and subcortical regions of the brain. Regions affected by neuritic plaques have greatly reduced concentrations of functioning neurons. Neuritic plaques sometimes are found in the brains of persons with Down syndrome or Creutzfeldt-Jakob disease (a rare disease characterized by progressive degenera-

tion of corticospinal nerve fibers) and in the brains of some normal elderly adults, but they are far more common in the brains of persons with Alzheimer's disease.

Granulovacuolar Degeneration. Granulovacuolar degeneration is a pathologic process in which small fluid-filled cavities containing granular debris appear inside nerve cells. The pyramidal neurons in the *hippocampus* (a deep brain structure that seems to be important in memory) most frequently are affected, accounting, at least in part, for the insidious deterioration of memory common in Alzheimer's disease. Granulovacuolar degeneration may be present in several neurologic diseases other than those causing dementia. Granulovacuolar degeneration occasionally appears in the brains of normal elderly persons, but Tomlinson and Henderson (1976) contend that if 10% or more of hippocampal neurons are affected, dementia always is present.

Other Abnormalities. Lower than normal levels of *acetylcholine* (a neurotransmitter) have been noted in the brains of individuals with

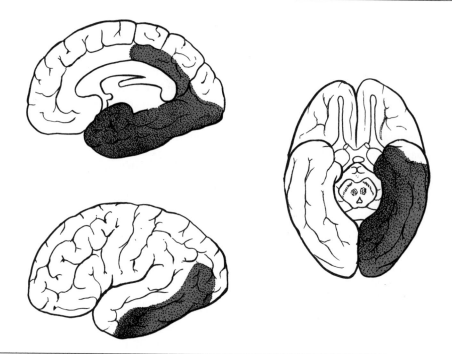

Figure 12-5 ■ Cortical brain regions most often affected by Alzheimer's disease. The darker shading represents the cortical regions most frequently affected.

Alzheimer's disease—a significant difference because acetylcholine is believed to play an important part in memory. Abnormal levels of aluminum have been found in neurofibrillary tangles and neuritic plaques, but it is not known what potential role aluminum might play in causing or perpetuating Alzheimer's disease.

The neuropathologic changes in Alzheimer's disease are not diffuse and equally distributed throughout the brain, but most frequently affect the temporoparietal-occipital junctions and the inferior temporal lobes (Figure 12-5). The frontal lobes, the motor and sensory cortex, and the occipital lobes are usually spared.

Medical Management. The cause of Alzheimer's disease is unknown, although several causes have been proposed, including aluminum poisoning, disturbed immune function, infection with a slow virus, and genetically transmitted disturbance of neuronal functions.

Some cases of early-onset Alzheimer's dementia have a familial pattern, apparently caused by a genetic defect transmitted from parents to children.

The development of symptoms in Alzheimer's disease differs somewhat among individuals, suggesting that not all cases of Alzheimer's disease are caused by the same pathologic process. Although no medical treatment prevents or cures Alzheimer's disease, some symptoms of the disease may be amenable to treatment. Persons with Alzheimer's disease may be given tranquilizers to control combativeness and aggression or antidepressants to lessen depression. Diet and fluid intake may be monitored and managed to prevent dehydration and maintain adequate nutrition. The environment of persons with Alzheimer's disease may be manipulated to stimulate them, to maintain orientation and cognition, and to prevent social isolation. Counseling and other support services may be provided to the person with Alzheimer's disease and his or her family.

During the past decade, scientists have been searching for the causes of Alzheimer's disease and have been working to develop effective medical treatments. Although a few medical treatments (neurotransmitter augmentation, nerve growth enhancement, antiinflammatory medications) have shown promise, no large-scale clinical trials have identified an effective treatment, and the search for prevention, control, and cure continues. The drug tacrine *(Cognex)* reportedly improves cognition for some persons with Alzheimer's disease, but its toxic side effects (liver damage) preclude its long-term use. The drug donepezil *(Aricept)* has fewer side effects and may improve cognition and general functioning. Two drugs, rivastigmine and galantamine, are under U.S. Food and Drug Administration review. These drugs do not cure or slow the progression of Alzheimer's disease, but they provide some improvement in cognition and behavior for persons with mild to moderate Alzheimer's disease. They may not be effective for those in the advanced stages of the disease.

Some recent reports suggest that caffeine may slow or even prevent the appearance of Alzheimer's disease. Coffee growers and distributors eagerly await the results of additional research.

Evolution. The development of Alzheimer's disease is characterized by progressive deterioration of intellect. The first symptoms are subtle and include lapses of memory (usually the first signs of the disease), faulty reasoning, poor judgment, disorientation except in familiar environments, and alterations of mood (depression, apathy, irritability, suspiciousness). Personality

and interpersonal behaviors are largely unaffected during the early stages of the disease, although the affected person may withdraw from social contact. Mental impairments become more obvious as Alzheimer's disease progresses. Intellect and cognition become increasingly impaired, and disturbances of language and communication appear. The affected individual becomes restless and agitated, gets lost even in familiar environments, and wanders off when not supervised. Episodes of incontinence appear. These symptoms gradually worsen, and the final stages leave the individual with profound motor deficits (rigidity or spasticity), complete incontinence, and loss of almost all intellectual and cognitive abilities. Motor abilities usually are spared until the very late stages of Alzheimer's disease, at which time signs of pyramidal system involvement (weakness, paralysis) may appear. Persons who have Alzheimer's disease usually die of aspiration pneumonia or infection 5 to 10 years after their disease is diagnosed.

Cognition and Communication. Language is less affected than cognition, memory, and intellect in the early stages of Alzheimer's disease. As Alzheimer's disease progresses, increasingly obvious impairments in language and communication appear. For most persons with Alzheimer's disease, the early language impairments reflect the effects of the disease on memory and intellect and do not represent specific language impairment (aphasia). There may be some similarities between the communicative abilities of persons with early-stage Alzheimer's disease and persons with anomic aphasia and between persons with late-stage Alzheimer's disease and persons with Wernicke's aphasia (Hier, Hagenlocher, & Schindler, 1985). However, persons with Alzheimer's disease always have conspicuous problems with memory and intellect that clearly separate them diagnostically from persons with aphasia.

As a general rule, the communicative performance of persons with Alzheimer's disease depends on the amount of mental effort

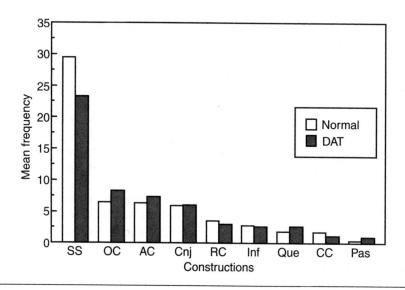

Figure 12-6 ■ Mean frequency of syntactic structures in the speech of normal adults and in the speech of adults with dementia. *SS,* Simple sentences; *OC,* other complements; *AC,* adverbial clauses; *Cnj,* conjunctions; *RC,* relative clauses; *Inf,* Infinitivals; *Que,* questions; *CC,* complex comparatives; *Pas,* passives. (Data from Kempler, D., Curtiss, S., & Jackson, C. [1987]. Syntactic preservation in Alzheimer's disease. *Journal of Speech and Hearing Research, 30,* 343-350.)

required. Communicative activities that require greater mental effort are affected first and most dramatically. Language processes that require little mental effort (grammar, syntax, social conventions) usually are preserved until the very late stages of Alzheimer's disease.

> Although persons with Alzheimer's disease usually do not have significant problems with language, their impaired memory may compromise their retention of what they read or hear and cause them to forget what they have previously said. Persons with early-stage Alzheimer's disease often annoy caregivers by failing to remember what they have been told for more than an hour or so and by their propensity to tell the same story or ask the same question over and over.

Early Stages. Phonology, syntax, articulation, and voice quality are well preserved in the speech of persons with early Alzheimer's disease, although mild word retrieval problems, occasional verbal paraphasias, and subtle comprehension impairments may appear early. When word retrieval failures occur, persons with early Alzheimer's disease usually recognize and repair them, often by talking around the missing word (e.g., ...*and she was pushing the baby in a wagon...no, that's not it...in a cart...no...in a stroller, going down the street...*). Persons with early-stage Alzheimer's disease may complain that they sometimes cannot think of the right word as they speak or write and that their spelling is not what it used to be. Persons with early-stage Alzheimer's disease make few grammatical errors in speaking or writing, and their production of syntactic structures in speech matches that of normal elderly speakers (Kempler, Curtiss, & Jackson, 1987; Figure 12-6).

Persons with early-stage Alzheimer's disease typically have functional reading comprehension for newspapers and magazines, although their reading rate is slow, and they have difficulty comprehending and retaining long or complex materials. They may miss the meaning of complex syntactic structures (e.g., passive sentences, comparatives), and they may fail to recognize low-frequency words. Highly practiced speech responses (e.g., counting, reciting the alphabet, reciting the days of the week) are preserved, but responses calling for sustained attention and mental flexibility (e.g., explaining proverbs, comprehending abstract material) are compromised early.

Persons with early-stage Alzheimer's disease are adequate conversationalists. They usually observe conversational conventions such as turn-taking and eye contact. As speakers, persons with early-stage Alzheimer's disease tend to talk too long, drift from the topic, repeat material unnecessarily, and make tangential and irrelevant comments. As listeners, they have difficulty following conversations in which topics or speakers change, and they may fail to get the point of nonliteral material such as humor, irony, or sarcasm.

Middle Stages. As persons with Alzheimer's disease progress into the middle stages of the disease, communicative impairments become more obvious. Word retrieval failures in spontaneous speech become more frequent, and the persons' success in repairing them declines. Sentence fragments and ungrammatic sentences begin to appear in the person's spontaneous speech. Reading rate continues to decline and eventually becomes nonfunctional for all but the most familiar material. Most persons in the middle stages of Alzheimer's disease abandon recreational reading.

Conversations with persons in the middle stages of Alzheimer's disease become more difficult. Some become apathetic and withdraw from conversational interactions. Most become passive conversational partners, allowing others to set the topic, tone, and content of conversations and offering trivialities, automatisms, and irrelevant comments in place of information-bearing contributions. Unnecessary repetition of ideas increases, and the individual gets lost even in simple conversations on familiar topics. Conformity with conversational conventions deteriorates. Turn-taking violations become more frequent, although most individuals retain a general sense of when to talk and when to listen. Comprehension of nonliteral material is grossly impaired.

Late Stages. Communicative performance of persons in the late stages of Alzheimer's disease is severely compromised. Reading is nonfunctional, although the affected person may recognize some highly familiar words. Writing is nonfunctional, although some individuals may be able to complete simple, overlearned sequences (numbers, the alphabet) if given the first items in the sequence. Comprehension of spoken materials is limited to simple familiar phrases and words. Speech consists primarily of single words and sentence fragments, which are often bizarre, devoid of meaning, and repeated in robotlike fashion. Syntax begins to break down, and stereotypic utterances (e.g., *great day in the morning … great day in the morning*) and neologisms (e.g., *take it down the cranbibby*) appear. Persons in the late stages of Alzheimer's disease generally are unaware of errors, and they make no attempt to revise or correct them.

Persons in the late stages of Alzheimer's disease are nonfunctional conversationalists. They fail to observe social conventions (e.g., greetings and farewells) and are insensitive to conversational rules such as those governing turn-taking, topic maintenance, eye contact, and relevance. These individuals tend to dwell on personal experiences (usually past events, and often misinterpreted) regardless of their conversational partner's intent. In the very late stages of Alzheimer's disease, some individuals become mute and others become *echolalic* (endlessly repeating what others say) or *palilalic* (endlessly repeating a self-generated word or phrase).

Those who still speak are limited to a few overused words produced indiscriminately and without regard to listeners. By the final stages of Alzheimer's disease, the individual loses all orientation to self and surroundings and does not use language in any meaningful way.

Table 12-1 summarizes the progression of communication impairment as Alzheimer's disease progresses.

Pick's Disease (Frontal Lobe Dementia)

Some individuals become demented as a consequence of pathologic changes in the frontal lobes. The most common cause of dementia-causing frontal lobe pathology is *Pick's disease,* but cases of frontal lobe dementia have been reported in which the pathologic changes symptomatic of Pick's disease are not present. However, Neary and associates (1988) suggest that these anomalous cases actually may represent a form of Pick's disease.

Pick's disease was first described in 1892 by Arnold Pick, a professor of psychiatry at the University of Prague. Pick's disease is a progressive degenerative disease beginning in the cerebral cortex of the frontal lobes. It is a rare disease, affecting less than 1% of the United States population and accounting for only about 2% of dementia cases. Pick's disease usually begins between the ages of 40 and 60, although it appears sporadically in younger or older persons.

Neuropathology. Pick's disease is characterized by two neuronal abnormalities: proliferation of enlarged neurons *(Pick cells)* and the presence of *Pick bodies* within neurons. (*Pick bodies* are dense globular formations in the neuron cytoplasm. They are about the same size as the cell nucleus and contain numerous neurofibrils.) The progression of Pick's disease is marked by shrinkage of the brain (typically confined to the posterior inferior frontal lobes and the anterior superior temporal lobes) together with loss of neurons and proliferation of glial cells throughout the cortex. The cause of Pick's disease is unknown, although a genetic component (suggested by a pattern of familial inheritance) may be present in 20% to 50% of cases.

Medical Management. At present there is no cure for Pick's disease, and its treatment, like that of Alzheimer's disease, is symptomatic, consisting of medications to control changes in mood and temperament, together with behavioral intervention to maintain the person's orientation and to manage the person's daily life behavior.

Evolution. Pick's disease is commonly first diagnosed as stress, depression, or Alzheimer's disease, with the diagnosis changing as early subtle symptoms become more dramatic. The progression of symptoms in Pick's disease differs from the progression of symptoms in Alzheimer's disease. In Alzheimer's disease, intellect is compromised early, and personality is spared until the late stages. In Pick's disease, alterations in personality and emotion usually are the first symptoms to appear. Alterations in personality and emotion are closely followed by apathy and indifference toward the affected person's usual interests and activities. The ability to independently plan, initiate, and follow through on familiar activities declines, although the person may be able to carry out the activities when prompted by others. Social behavior deteriorates, and the affected person becomes impulsive, disinhibited, and inappropriately jocular, makes inappropriate comments (often sexual in nature), talks indiscriminately with strangers, laughs inappropriately, and generally behaves with "loss of personal propriety" (Cummings & Benson, 1992). Some persons with Pick's disease become hyperoral, making overeating and weight gain a common problem.

As Pick's disease progresses, judgment and insight become progressively more impaired, and obsessional, ritualistic behaviors appear (e.g., repeated hand washing, folding and refolding articles of clothing). Some persons with Pick's disease become profoundly apathetic, sitting placidly for hours unless directed by a caregiver to perform an activity. Others become

TABLE 12-1	**Effects of Alzheimer's Disease on Communication**

Early Stages

Sounds	Used correctly
Words	May omit a meaningful word, usually a noun, when talking in sentences
	May report trouble thinking of the right word; vocabulary is shrinking
Grammar	Generally correct
Content	May drift from the topic
	Reduced ability to generate series of meaningful sentences
	Difficulty comprehending new information
	Vague
Use	Knows when to talk, although may talk too long on a subject
	May be apathetic, failing to initiate a conversation when it would be appropriate to do so
	May have difficulty understanding humor, verbal analogies, sarcasm, and indirect and nonliteral statements

Middle Stages

Sounds	Used correctly
Words	Difficulty thinking of words in a category
	Anomia in conversation
	Difficulty naming objects
	Reliance on automatisms
	Vocabulary noticeably diminished
Grammar	Sentence fragments and deviations common
	May have difficulty understanding grammatically complex sentences
Content	Frequently repeats ideas, forgets topic, talks about events of past or trivia
	Fewer ideas
Use	Knows when to talk
	Recognizes questions
	May fail to greet
	Loss of sensitivity to conversational partners
	Rarely corrects mistakes

Late Stages

Sounds	Generally used correctly, but errors are not uncommon
Words	Marked anomia, poor vocabulary, lack of word comprehension
	May make up words and produce jargon
Grammar	Some grammar is preserved but sentence fragments and deviations common
	Lack of comprehension of many grammatical forms
Content	Generally unable to produce a sequence of related ideas
	Content may be meaningless and bizarre
	Subject of most meaningful utterances is the retelling of a past event
	Marked repetition of words and phrases
Use	Generally unaware of surroundings and context
	Insensitive to others
	Little meaningful use of language
	Some patients are mute; some are echolalic

From Bayles, K.A. (1994). Management of communication disorders associated with dementia. In R. Chapey (Ed.) *Language intervention strategies in adult aphasia.* Baltimore: Williams and Wilkins (p. 542).

profoundly restless, fidgeting and pacing for hours unless a caregiver intervenes.

Cognition and Communication. Changes in cognition and communication in Pick's disease differ from those seen in Alzheimer's disease. In Alzheimer's disease, memory and orientation are compromised early, but language remains relatively intact until the late stages. In Pick's disease, memory and orientation usually are well preserved until the late stages of the disease, but language breakdown appears early and remains prominent in the middle and late stages of the disease. Word retrieval failures, impaired confrontation naming, circumlocution, and use of generic words for specific words (e.g., *I got the thing and did that other, but it wasn't there*) are common expressive abnormalities. Echolalia and verbal stereotypies (e.g., *mama-mama-mama, me-me-me*) may be present. The individual may tell the same story over and over, unaware of the repetition.

Comprehension impairments for both spoken and printed materials are prominent in the middle stages of Pick's disease and become progressively more profound as Pick's disease progresses. By the final stages, persons with Pick's disease are mute and profoundly demented, with severely impaired memory, orientation, and cognition, and many exhibit motor rigidity. Persons with Pick's disease usually die from aspiration pneumonia or infection 6 to 12 years after their disease is diagnosed.

Differentiating Pick's Disease from Alzheimer's Disease

Mendez and associates (1993) suggested that Pick's disease can be differentiated from Alzheimer's disease by the following characteristics:

- Onset of symptoms in Pick's disease begins before age 65.
- Personality change is among the first symptoms observed in Pick's disease.
- Persons with Pick's disease are hyperoral (eat excessively, indiscriminately put things in mouth).

- Persons with Pick's disease are impulsive and lack social inhibitions.
- Persons with Pick's disease roam or wander when left unsupervised. (*Author's note:* Persons with Alzheimer's disease also roam and wander, but not until later in the disease.)

Mendez and associates assert that if three of the foregoing characteristics are present, Pick's disease is the appropriate diagnosis.

Kertesz and Munoz (2000) identified the following differences between early Pick's disease and early Alzheimer's disease:

- Personality and language change are much more common in early Pick's disease.
- Memory impairments are much more prevalent in early Alzheimer's disease.
- Persons with early Pick's disease have significantly greater impairment in activities of daily living (e.g., grooming, bathing, managing personal affairs).

Primary Progressive Aphasia

Mesulam (1982b) described six right-handed patients who experienced slowly progressive language impairments without the behavioral and mental impairments of dementia. Mesulam called the collection of signs and symptoms experienced by the six patients *slowly progressive aphasia.* According to Mesulam, five of the six patients exhibited "anomic aphasia" at onset, and the sixth exhibited "pure word deafness" at onset. All six experienced gradually progressive impairments of reading, writing, and comprehension. Four experienced no signs of nonlinguistic mental deterioration within 5 to 11 years of onset. Two experienced gradual onset of dementia 7 years or more after onset. Neuropsychologic test results were consistent with involvement of the left perisylvian region. Cortical biopsy of one patient showed no pathologic conditions such as those seen in Alzheimer's dementia.

Other reports of patients with mild, slowly increasing aphasia with no apparent general mental decline followed Mesulam's report (Duffy, 1987; Heath, Kennedy, & Kapur, 1983;

Kertesz, Hudson, MacKenzie, & Munoz, 1994; Kirshner & associates, 1987), and the label *primary progressive aphasia* came to replace *slowly progressive aphasia*. Primary progressive aphasia begins gradually, with word retrieval problems in speaking and writing. As the condition progresses, word retrieval failures become prominent, comprehension of spoken and written language deteriorates, and arithmetic abilities decline. Many persons with primary progressive aphasia can perform normally in daily life activities that do not require language (e.g., home maintenance, travel, participation in sports and other recreational activities, graphic arts), provided their impairments do not extend to other aspects of cognitive function.

Many persons who are diagnosed with primary progressive aphasia begin to experience impairments in memory, attention, reasoning, and executive function 2 to 10 years after diagnosis of primary progressive aphasia (the average is about 5 years). Brain autopsy of persons with primary progressive aphasia typically shows nonspecific degeneration of brain tissues, usually in the temporoparietal region of the language-dominant hemisphere. Occasionally granulovacuolar degeneration, neurofibrillary tangles, or Pick's bodies are found.

A variant of primary progressive aphasia begins with insidious onset of impaired programming and sequencing of speech movements. Duffy (2005) has suggested the label *primary progressive apraxia of speech* for cases in which apraxia of speech is the first, the most prominent, or the major manifestation of degenerative neurologic disease. (See Chapter 13 for discussion of apraxia of speech.)

MIXED DEMENTIA
Vascular Dementia

Vascular disease is an important cause of dementia in adults. In the United States, vascular disease is second to Alzheimer's disease as a cause of dementia, accounting for 15% to 20% of all dementia cases. The prevalence of vascular dementia, like that of Alzheimer's dementia, increases with age but increases less rapidly than does the prevalence of Alzheimer's dementia (Figure 12-7).

Neuropathology. Diagnosis of vascular dementia is complicated and sometimes controversial. The basic requirement for the diagnosis is the presence of dementia and evidence of cerebrovascular disease. Pure vascular dementia is relatively uncommon. Most persons diagnosed with vascular dementia actually have a combination of vascular dementia and Alzheimer's dementia. Dickson (2001) found concomitant Alzheimer's disease in 77% of persons diagnosed with vascular dementia who later came to autopsy.

Most persons with vascular dementia have a history of hypertension, heart disease, or both, and histories of multiple strokes are common. The first symptoms of vascular dementia typically are abrupt in onset and generate focal neurologic signs (perceptual, motor, or sensory impairments) which represent the localized effects of the first incident. Subsequent incidents produce a stepwise progression of symptom development as additional focal impairments are added with each new incident. The slow accumulation of neurologic events eventually produces diffuse cerebral involvement and dementia. Personality and intellect usually are preserved until the late stages of vascular dementia, although depression, irritability, and emotional lability may appear early.

The most common vascular dementia syndrome is *multi-infarct dementia*. As the label suggests, multi-infarct dementia is caused by repeated infarcts, usually at different locations in the brain. Three etiologic subgroups of multi-infarct dementia have been described in the literature. They are *lacunar state, multiple cortical infarcts,* and *Binswanger's disease.* Lacunar state and Binswanger's disease represent primarily subcortical pathology, but multiple cortical infarcts (not surprisingly) represent primarily cortical pathology.

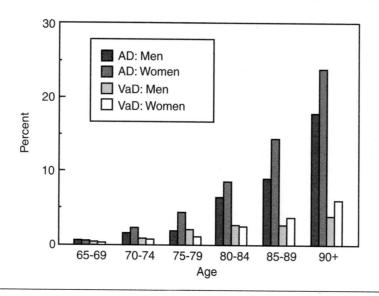

Figure 12-7 ■ Percentage of men and women with Alzheimer's dementia (AD) and vascular dementia (VaD) by age group. (Based on data from Lobo, L, Launer, L.J., Fratiglioni, L., & associates. [2000]. Prevalence of aphasia and major subgroups in Europe: A collaborative study of population-based cohorts. *Neurology, 54* [S5], 54-59.)

Lacunar state is caused by multiple small infarcts in the arteries supplying the basal ganglia, thalamus, midbrain, and brain stem. The first symptoms are subcortical in nature and include dysarthria, swallowing disturbances, pseudobulbar palsy, weakness, and sometimes tremor, because the extrapyramidal system and brain stem structures are affected. Intellect and language are preserved until late in the course of lacunar state. Dementia eventually appears in 70% to 80% of persons with lacunar state (Celesia & Wanamaker, 1972).

Multiple cortical infarcts are caused by a series of thrombotic or embolic occlusions of cortical arteries. Each occlusion causes focal neurologic symptoms, and multiple occlusions yield an increasingly diffuse pattern of impairment, eventually culminating in cortical dementia. The symptoms depend on the cortical areas involved in each incident and include those commonly associated with cortical damage (e.g., aphasia, apraxia, neglect). Hemiparesis and hemiplegia commonly are associated with cortical infarcts, but dysarthria and swallowing impairments, which typically are associated with subcortical pathology, are not.

Binswanger's disease is a rare disease caused by multiple infarcts in subcortical white matter, usually in individuals with severe hypertension. The infarcts are a consequence of thrombotic or embolic occlusion of penetrating arteries from the cortex that supply subcortical white matter tracts. The first symptoms of Binswanger's disease are focal, but repeated infarcts yield more pervasive mental and physical impairments, eventually culminating in dementia. Clinically, the symptoms of Binswanger's disease resemble lacunar state, but the onset of symptoms is slow, combinations of cortical and subcortical neurologic signs are common, and motor impairments appear somewhat later in Binswanger's disease than in lacunar state.

Vascular dementia sometimes follows heart attacks causing brain ischemia, or it may follow chronic subdural, subarachnoid, or intracerebral hematomas, and (rarely) it is associated with diseases such as autoimmune disease (lupus erythematosus) or infections such as Lyme disease. About 60% of persons with vascular dementia die within 5 years of diagnosis. Mortality of persons with vascular dementia is greater than mortality of persons with Alzheimer's dementia, probably due to the risks associated with cerebrovascular disease.

DSM-IV criteria for diagnosis of vascular dementia require the following characteristics:

1. *Memory impairment* (impaired ability to learn new information or to recall previously learned information) is present, plus one or more associated cognitive disturbances— aphasia, apraxia, agnosia, or impaired executive functioning.
2. The cognitive deficits cause significant impairment in social or occupational functioning and represent a significant decline from a previous level of functioning.
3. Focal neurologic signs are present, plus symptoms or laboratory evidence of cerebrovascular disease that is etiologically related to the disturbance.
4. The deficits do not occur during delirium.

The *Hachinski Ischemia Index* (Hachinski, Lassen, & Marshall, 1974) is a widely used set of criteria for identifying vascular dementia. It is quick and easy to complete and has been shown to differentiate reliably between vascular dementia and Alzheimer's disease (Table 12-2).

Medical Management. Medical management of patients with vascular dementia focuses on preventing additional cerebrovascular incidents by prescribing anticoagulants to lessen the chance of blood clots, controlling hypertension and cholesterol levels, managing diabetes, and recommending that smokers stop smoking. Some drugs that are helpful in lessening the severity of Alzheimer's dementia may be useful in managing vascular dementia (perhaps

TABLE 12-2	The Hachinski Ischemia Index
Feature	Score
Abrupt onset	2
Stepwise deterioration	1
Fluctuating course	2
Nocturnal confusion	1
Relative preservation of personality	1
Depression	1
Somatic complaints	1
Emotional lability	1
History of hypertension	1
History of stroke	2
Evidence of atherosclerosis	1
Focal neurologic symptoms	2
Focal neurologic signs	2
Total score	

NOTE: Total score = 4 or less: likely Alzheimer's disease. Total score = 5 to 7: Uncertain diagnosis. Total score = 8 or greater: likely vascular dementia. *Symptom*: reported by the person. *Sign*: observed by the examiner.

From Moroney, J.T., Bagiella, E., Desmond, D.W., Hachinski, V.C., & associates. (1997). Meta-analysis of the Hachinski Ischemia Score in pathologically verified dementias, *Neurology, 49,* 1096-1105.

because most vascular dementia patients have coexisting Alzheimer's dementia).

Evolution. The symptoms of vascular dementia occasionally mimic those of Alzheimer's dementia, but the acute onset of symptoms, fluctuating severity of symptoms, and a history of hypertension and stroke help to differentiate it from Alzheimer's dementia. Persons with vascular dementia often have patchy patterns of impairment and somewhat better preserved immediate memory than do persons with Alzheimer's dementia. Unlike persons with Alzheimer's dementia, persons with vascular dementia tend to remain aware of their disabilities, even in advanced stages of dementia, making them more susceptible to depression than are persons with Alzheimer's dementia.

Cognition and Communication. The cognitive and communicative impairments of persons with vascular dementia resemble those of persons with Alzheimer's dementia (problems with recent memory, abstract thinking, reasoning, and problem-solving). Depending on the sites affected by the neuropathology of vascular dementia, affected individuals may exhibit gait disturbance (if the basal ganglia and related structures are affected), loss of bowel and bladder control (if deep brain or brain stem structures are affected), speech motor control problems (if deep brain or brain stem structures are affected), and language formulation and comprehension problems (if cortical regions important for language are affected). If the frontal lobes are affected by neuropathology (which is often), the affected individual may be apathetic and lack behavioral initiative.

Lewy Body Dementia

Lewy body dementia (also known as *dementia with Lewy bodies, diffuse Lewy body disease,* and *senile dementia of the Lewy type*) was first described in 1996 as a syndrome with specific diagnostic characteristics. Lewy body dementia is now considered one of the most common progressive dementias, accounting for 10% to 15% of all cases, behind Alzheimer's dementia (50% to 65%) and vascular dementia (20% to 25%).

Neuropathology. Lewy body dementia is caused by proliferation of *Lewy bodies* (development of abnormal protein deposits in neuron cell bodies). The two major consequences of this proliferation are (1) loss of dopamine producing neurons in the substantia nigra, similar to that seen in Parkinson's disease and (2) loss of acetylcholine producing neurons throughout the brain, similar to that seen in Alzheimer's disease. Loss of dopamine producing neurons produces motor impairments (rigidity, lack of spontaneous movement) similar to the motor impairments of Parkinson's disease. Loss of acetylcholine producing neurons causes mental deterioration similar to that seen in Alzheimer's

disease. (Lewy bodies also are found in the brains of persons with Parkinson's disease and Alzheimer's disease.) Diagnosis of Lewy body dementia is complicated by the presence of granulovacuolar degeneration and neurofibrillary tangles—classic neuropathologic signs of Alzheimer's disease. Not surprisingly, early-stage Lewy body dementia is often confused with Alzheimer's dementia.

Lewy bodies were described in 1914 by Frederick Lewy, a neuropathologist and a colleague of Alois Alzheimer.

Medical Management. There is no cure for Lewy body dementia, and there is no way to slow its progression. Medical management is palliative and focuses on managing the cognitive, motor, and psychologic symptoms produced by the disease. Pharmacologic treatment often is beneficial, but the prescribing clinician must balance treatment of motor signs with treatment of cognitive impairments, because medications that are effective in treating the motor signs may cause hallucinations or psychosis, whereas medications that are effective in treating the cognitive and psychologic signs may cause worsening of motor impairments. Cholinesterase inhibitors may be prescribed to treat cognitive symptoms, and levodopa may help those who have muscle rigidity and lack of spontaneous movement.

Evolution. Lewy body dementia usually develops after age 75 but may appear in persons as young as 40 years of age. Unlike Alzheimer's dementia, Lewy body dementia affects males and females in approximately equal proportions. The first signs of the disease usually are impairments of memory, visuospatial abilities, and attention, which may fluctuate in severity. Visual hallucinations, frequent falls, and fainting may appear early, as do muscle rigidity and paucity of spontaneous movement. (Some clinicians consider cognitive decline within 1 or 2 years after diagnosis of Parkinson's disease confirmation of Lewy body dementia.) The cognitive and motor impairments of Lewy body dementia inevitably progress. The average survival after diagnosis of Lewy body dementia is about 8 years.

Cognition and Communication. Several studies of persons with Lewy body dementia have suggested that these individuals have impairments in visuospatial abilities, language, attention, working memory, and executive functions similar to the impairments of persons with Alzheimer's dementia, but with memory somewhat better preserved. Most of these studies did not verify that the persons diagnosed with Lewy body dementia did not also have Alzheimer's dementia (a differential diagnosis that can be verified only by examining brain tissue at autopsy). The primary exception is a study by Kraybill, Larson, Tsuang, and associates (2005) who studied tissue samples from the brains of 135 persons who had been diagnosed with dementia prior to death. The 135 persons had been participants in a large community-based study of dementia. Each had received comprehensive neuropsychologic assessment, a consensus diagnosis of dementia at intake, and annual physical and neuropsychologic assessments thereafter.

Neuropathologic study of the brain tissues indicated that 48 persons (36% of the study group) had pathologic changes consistent with Alzheimer's disease, 65 (48% of the study group) had pathologic changes consistent with combined Alzheimer's and Lewy body disease, and 22 (16% of the study group) had pathologic changes consistent with Lewy body disease alone. Kraybill and associates also analyzed the records of comprehensive neuropsychologic testing of participants. The results suggested that persons with both Alzheimer's and Lewy body pathologic changes had more severe memory impairments and had more rapid rates of cognitive decline than persons with only Lewy body pathologic changes. The results of neuropsychologic testing suggested that persons with only Lewy body pathologic changes

may have had somewhat greater impairments in executive function and divided attention than did those with Alzheimer's disease alone or those with Alzheimer's disease in combination with Lewy body disease.

Frontotemporal Dementia

In the mid 1990s, descriptions of dementia following pathologic changes in the frontal and temporal lobes began to appear in the medical literature. The accumulation of reports eventually led to publication of criteria for diagnosis of a syndrome called *frontotemporal dementia* (McKhann, Albert, Grossman, & associates, 2001). The criteria distinguished among five dementia subtypes characterized by abnormal neuronal inclusions, neuron loss, and structural abnormalities in brain tissues. The five categories share a common characteristic—neuropathologic changes in the frontal and temporal lobes. The five categories represent a mix of cortical, subcortical, and cortical-subcortical pathologic conditions. Despite McKhann and associates' attempt to clarify the diagnosis, frontotemporal dementia remains poorly defined and lumps persons with heterogeneous neuropathologies and heterogeneous cognitive and behavioral characteristics into a single category. An intimidating list of subtypes of frontotemporal dementia has accumulated (e.g., Pick's disease, progressive lobar degeneration, progressive aphasia, semantic dementia, dementia lacking distinctive histopathological features, progressive subcortical gliosis, atypical presenile dementia, non-Alzheimer's lobal atrophy, supranuclear palsy, corticobulbar degeneration, and others). The validity and clinical utility of *frontotemporal dementia* as a coherent diagnosis has yet to be established.

OTHER CAUSES OF DEMENTIA
Normal Pressure Hydrocephalus

Normal pressure hydrocephalus (sometimes called *nonobstructive* or *communicating hydrocephalus*) usually is caused by physiologic conditions that interfere with resorption of cerebrospinal fluid (CSF) from the brain ventricles and the spinal cord. The compromised resorption causes accumulation of excess CSF in the ventricles and spinal cord, increases intracranial pressure, and causes the ventricles to enlarge. Increased intracranial pressure eventually inhibits production of CSF by the choroid plexus and forces CSF into brain tissue, at which time intracranial pressure gradually decreases, often to normal levels. The ventricles, however, remain enlarged.

The preferred medical treatment of persons with normal pressure hydrocephalus is *shunting,* in which a hollow needle connected to a flexible tube is inserted into a ventricle, and excess CSF is siphoned off, usually into the thorax, where it is eventually resorbed. About two-thirds of those so treated improve, and about one-third show no change in symptoms or worsen, usually as a result of complications (e.g., bleeding, infection).

Persons with normal pressure hydrocephalus typically exhibit dementia, gait disturbance, and urinary incontinence. The gait disturbance exhibited by persons with normal pressure hydrocephalus is unusual. The person is unsteady while standing and has difficulty initiating walking, appearing as if "glued to the floor" (Aminoff, Greenberg, & Simon, 1996, p. 55). Once initiated, walking is slow and shuffling. The person easily performs leg movements (kicking, bicycling, walking) to command while lying down or sitting but is unable to do so when standing and bearing weight on the legs (a condition called *apraxia of gait*).

The dementia exhibited by persons with normal pressure hydrocephalus is first characterized by slowing of mental functions, impaired memory, emotional dullness, and mild attentional impairments. Focal impairments (e.g., aphasia, agnosia) are uncommon. Most individuals recover spontaneously following placement of a ventricular shunt; some stabilize at levels of mild to moderate dementia, and a few progress to global cognitive dysfunction, muteness, and

total obliviousness to surroundings, followed by death from infection or respiratory failure.

Creutzfeldt-Jakob Disease

Creutzfeldt-Jakob disease is a rare and invariably fatal disease that causes rapidly progressing dementia and neuromuscular disorders. It is caused by invasion of the central nervous system by protein particles called *prions* (for *proteinaceous infectious particle*). Prions are thought to transform normal brain proteins into an infectious and deadly form by altering the shape of molecules in healthy proteins. Most cases of Creutzfeldt-Jakob disease are sporadic—there is no known source of infection and no pattern of familial infections, although in about 10% of cases there may be a familial pattern of infection. At this time the only documented mode of transmission from person to person is by unintended consequences of medical procedures using prion-tainted human tissues (grafts, transplants) or contaminated surgical instruments. However, there is widespread belief in the scientific community that ingestion of prion-infected animal tissue (primarily from beef cattle) is responsible for many cases of Creutzfeldt-Jakob disease.

A prion-caused disease called *kuru* was common in the Fore tribe in Papua, New Guinea during the 1950s and early 1960s. Kuru was essentially eliminated when the tribe stopped the ritual handling and eating of deceased relatives' brains and internal organs.

Infection with the prion causing Creutzfeldt-Jakob disease causes widespread neuron loss and proliferation of glial cells throughout the brain, together with the appearance of numerous microscopic cavities throughout the brain. These cavities cause the brain to become soft and spongy. For this reason Creutzfeldt-Jakob disease sometimes is called *subacute spongiform encephalopathy.* Creutzfeldt-Jakob disease resembles several diseases of animals, including *scrapie* in sheep and goats, *chronic wasting disease* in deer and elk, and *bovine spongiform encephalopathy* in cattle (popularly known as *mad cow disease*). All are thought to be caused by prions. Although at this time there is no direct evidence of transmission of prion-caused diseases from animals to humans, many scientists believe that consumption of beef from infected cattle was responsible for an increase in Creutzfeldt-Jakob disease in England in the early 1990s.

Creutzfeldt-Jakob disease is rare in the United States, affecting about 1 in 1 million inhabitants. It can occur at any age, although most cases are adults in their 50s and 60s. There is no effective treatment for Creutzfeldt-Jakob disease; once contracted, the disease is rapidly progressive and invariably fatal, with death occurring within 1 year of the first symptoms.

Persons who are in the early stages of Creutzfeldt-Jakob disease exhibit a variety of signs and symptoms, but dementia is almost always present. Memory impairments, slowing of mental processes, impaired reasoning and problem-solving, insomnia, and flattened affect are prominent early in the disease. Neuromuscular abnormalities (extrapyramidal signs, cerebellar ataxia, myoclonus) quickly develop as Creutzfeldt-Jakob disease progresses. Hallucinations, confusion, and delusions often follow. The individual's condition rapidly deteriorates. Changes in intellect, behavior, and affect are rapid, often being obvious from week to week and sometimes from day to day. Persons with Creutzfeldt-Jakob disease eventually become completely unresponsive to stimulation and die, usually from an infection (most often pneumonia).

OCCASIONAL CAUSES OF DEMENTIA

Other progressive neurologic diseases sometimes lead to dementia, although often it is not clear if the disease causes dementia or if the dementia is the result of a different pathologic process. Persons in the late stages of amyotrophic lateral sclerosis or multiple sclerosis sometimes develop mild to moderate dementia. Brain tumors and chronic subdural hematomas may lead to dementia if they cause chronic elevation of intracranial pressure. Bacterial or viral infections of the brain (e.g., meningitis, encephalitis) may cause dementia. Dementia from tumors, hematomas, or infections often is reversible with appropriate medical or surgical intervention.

Prolonged (3 years or more) hemodialysis (usually for kidney failure) occasionally is associated with slowly progressive dementia (called *dialysis dementia*). The earliest neurologic signs typically are dysarthria, myoclonus of muscles, and seizures, with dementia developing later. At first the symptoms of dialysis dementia are confined to times immediately following dialysis sessions, but as time goes on the symptoms persist and eventually become continuous.

GENERAL CONCEPTS 12-1

- Dementia is characterized by diffuse impairment of *memory, intellect,* and *cognition* appearing late in life, developing gradually, and worsening over time.
- Dementia syndromes can be divided into three major categories: *cortical dementia,* *subcortical dementia,* and *mixed dementia.* Impairments of memory, intellect, and language appear early in cortical dementia. Motor impairments appear early in subcortical dementia.

- *Parkinson's disease, Huntington's disease, progressive supranuclear palsy,* and *AIDS* are the most common causes of subcortical dementia. *Alzheimer's disease* is the most common cause of cortical dementia. *Pick's disease* also causes cortical dementia. *Vascular disease* is the most common cause of mixed dementia.

- Alzheimer's disease is the single most common cause of dementia, accounting for up to 70% of all dementia. Vascular disease is the second most common cause of dementia, accounting for 15% to 20% of all dementia.

- Alzheimer's disease is characterized by three microscopic changes in the brain: *neurofibrillary tangles, neuritic plaques,* and *granulovacuolar degeneration.* There is no effective medical treatment for Alzheimer's disease.

- The speech and language of patients in the early stages of Alzheimer's disease resembles that of patients with *anomic aphasia* (impaired word retrieval, subtle comprehension problems, fluent, syntactically correct speech). The speech and language of patients in the middle stages of Alzheimer's disease resembles that of patients with moderate *Wernicke's aphasia* (semantic paraphasias, empty and excessive speech, moderate to severe comprehension problems). The speech and language of patients in the late stages of Alzheimer's disease is generally nonfunctional. Comprehension of all but the simplest and most familiar material is grossly impaired, and speech consists mostly of single words and automatisms, usually devoid of meaning.

- Several diseases characterized by frontal lobe degeneration may cause dementia. Pick's disease is the most common cause of

dementia associated with frontal lobe pathology. Pick's disease sometimes is misdiagnosed as Alzheimer's disease. However, changes in personality (impulsivity, diminished social inhibitions) and deterioration of language are more common in early Pick's disease, whereas memory impairment is more common in early Alzheimer's disease.

- *Primary progressive aphasia,* sometimes called *slowly progressive aphasia,* is characterized by gradual deterioration of language functions with no apparent decline in other cognitive functions. Many patients diagnosed with primary progressive aphasia develop impairments in memory, attention, reasoning, and executive function 2 to 10 years after the appearance of aphasia.

- Vascular disease is an important cause of dementia in adults, accounting for 15% to 20% of all dementia in the United States. The most common vascular dementia syndrome is *multi-infarct dementia.*

- *Lewy body dementia* now is one of the most common progressive dementias, ranking behind Alzheimer's dementia and vascular dementia in prevalence.

- *Frontotemporal dementia* is characterized by abnormal neuronal inclusions, neuron loss, and structural abnormalities in the frontal and temporal lobes. The validity and clinical utility of frontotemporal dementia as a coherent diagnosis has yet to be established.

- Patients with *hydrocephalus, Creutzfeldt-Jakob disease, amyotrophic lateral sclerosis, multiple sclerosis,* or who experience prolonged *kidney dialysis* sometimes develop dementia, although these conditions account for a very small proportion of all cases of dementia.

PSEUDODEMENTIA

Many nondemented elderly adults become clinically depressed because of illness, physical limitations, changes in lifestyle, or social and financial difficulties. The symptoms of depression (cognitive impairments, loss of appetite, difficulty sleeping, social withdrawal, and apathy) may mimic those of dementia (a condition called *pseudodementia*). Accurate and timely diagnosis of depression in elderly adults is crucial, because medications and psychotherapeutic intervention often lessen or eliminate the depressive symptoms. Ripich and Ziol (1998) offered the following diagnostic guidelines for discriminating pseudodementia from true dementia:

- Pseudodementia has an identifiable onset with rapid symptom development. True dementia has insidious and gradual onset with slow symptom development.
- Persons with pseudodementia make little effort to perform clinical tests. Persons with true dementia (in early stages) try hard to prove themselves adequate on tests.
- The test performance of persons with pseudodementia is highly variable from test to test and day to day, even on tests of equivalent difficulty. The test performance of persons with true dementia is consistent across tasks and test occasions.

Several rating scales and questionnaires have been developed to assess the presence and severity of depression in elderly adults. The *Geriatric Depression Scale* (Brink & associates, 1982; Sheikh & Yesavage, 1986) may be useful for estimating the severity of depression in normal elderly adults or adults with mild dementia. The long form consists of 30 questions related to feelings and mood (e.g., *Are you basically satisfied with your life? Do you often feel helpless? Do you frequently worry about the future?*). The short form consists of 15 questions taken from the long form. The long form permits users to categorize respondents as *normal, mildly depressed,* or *severely depressed,* based on the number of answers suggesting

depression. The short form permits users to categorize respondents as *normal* or *suggestive of depression.* Because the Geriatric Depression Scale requires the potentially depressed person to answer questions reliably, it is not suitable for persons with moderate or severe dementia, and it may not be suitable for persons with mild dementia who deny feelings of depression.

The *Cornell Scale for Depression in Dementia* (Alexopoulos & associates, 1988; Table 12-3) is better suited for documenting depressive signs in persons with dementia, because it relies on family member or caregiver ratings. The ratings are based on the family member's or caregiver's observations during the week prior to the rating.

The 19 signs of the Cornell Scale (see Table 12-3) provide a useful list of signs likely to be associated with depression in older adults.

DELIRIUM AND DEMENTIA

Delirium (sometimes called *confusional state*) is a (usually transient) condition in which a person experiences confusion, disordered thinking, disorientation, agitation, hyperactivity, distractibility, and sometimes delusions and hallucinations. The onset of delirium usually is rapid, taking place within hours to a few days. Delirium can arise from various causes, including those in the following list:

- Medication (especially antidepressants, antipsychotics, anxiolytics)
- Infections
- Metabolic disorders
- Surgery, anesthesia
- Substance withdrawal (e.g., alcohol, cocaine, barbiturates)
- Kidney or liver disease
- Toxins (e.g., heavy metals, food poisoning)

Delirium in elderly adults sometimes follows sudden environmental changes (changes in surroundings, location, activities, caregivers), but by far the most common cause of delirium in

TABLE 12-3 The Cornell Scale for Depression in Dementia

Mood-Related Signs		Score		
Anxiety (anxious expression, ruminations, worrying)	a	0	1	2
Sadness (sad expression, sad voice, tearfulness)	a	0	1	2
Lack of reactivity to pleasant events	a	0	1	2
Irritable, easily annoyed, short-tempered	a	0	1	2
Behavioral Disturbance				
Agitation (restlessness, hand wringing, hair pulling)	a	0	1	2
Retardation (slow movements, slow speech, slow reactions)	a	0	1	2
Loss of interest (less involved in activities in last 1 month)	a	0	1	2
Multiple physical complaints	a	0	1	2
Physical Signs				
Loss of appetite (eats less than usual)	a	0	1	2
Weight loss (score 2 if greater than 5 lbs. in 1 month)	a	0	1	2
Lack of energy (fatigues easily, does not sustain activities—acute change in less than 1 month)	a	0	1	2
Cyclic Functions				
Diurnal mood variation (symptoms worse in morning)	a	0	1	2
Difficulty falling asleep (later than usual)	a	0	1	2
Multiple awakenings from sleep	a	0	1	2
Awakens earlier than usual	a	0	1	2
Ideational Disturbance				
Suicidal thoughts (life not worth living, suicidal wishes, suicide attempts)	a	0	1	2
Self-deprecation (self-blame, poor self esteem, feelings of failure)	a	0	1	2
Pessimism (anticipates the worst)	a	0	1	2
Mood congruent delusions (delusions of poverty, illness, or loss)	a	0	1	2

Total Score (>7 = Probable depression)

Scoring System: a = unable to evaluate, 0 = absent, 1 = mild or intermittent, 2 = severe.
From Alexopoulos, G.S., Abrams, R.C., Young, R.C., & Shamoian, C.A. (1988). Cornell scale for depression in dementia. *Biological Psychiatry, 23,* 271-284.

elderly adults is medications. Delirium should be suspected whenever elderly adults who are taking medications suddenly become confused, especially if the person's medication regimen has changed recently.

Although the behavioral manifestations of delirium may resemble those of dementia, rapid onset and rapid progression of symptoms, the presence of delusions or hallucinations, and the presence of identifiable precipitants should point to a diagnosis of delirium. However, delirium sometimes appears in adults who have

dementia. Whenever an adult with confirmed dementia suddenly exhibits rapid worsening of intellect, behavior, and personality, the person's history should be examined to rule out delirium or the occurrence of another pathologic event such as stroke.

IDENTIFYING DEMENTIA

Identifying the subtle signs of early-stage cortical dementia is a challenge. Persons in the early stages of cortical dementia rarely have motor impairments, and they do not exhibit overt signs of mental decline that point unequivocally to a diagnosis of dementia. They usually arrive at the clinician's office with vague complaints of forgetfulness, mental slowing, apathy, depression, fatigue, and similar nonspecific symptoms. The reports of family members often are not helpful in diagnosing dementia, because family members tend to focus on the most disruptive alterations in behavior and overlook the subtle signs of cognitive decline that signal the beginning of dementia.

Identifying cortical dementia in its beginning stages requires comprehensive testing to detect subtle disturbances of intellect and cognition. The most sensitive tests for detecting early cortical dementia are mentally challenging tests that require abstraction, analysis, integration of information, reasoning, and problem-solving. Highly practiced and automatic activities (e.g., counting, reciting the days of the week, reciting the alphabet) or structured tasks with highly constrained responses (e.g., confrontation naming, phrase and sentence repetition, copying) are too easy to be useful for detecting early dementia. The most sensitive tests of language and communication are tests requiring mental flexibility and creativity, such as generative naming (e.g., *Tell me all the words you can think of that start with the letter _____.*), story telling or story retelling, or comprehension of abstract or implied spoken or printed material.

Identification of middle-stage and late-stage cortical dementia usually poses no great clinical challenge to experienced practitioners. Persons in the middle and late stages of cortical dementia exhibit such striking impairments of intellect, orientation, and behavior that a careful review of the person's history, an interview with the affected person, an interview with family members and caregivers, and a brief assessment of orientation, memory, and intellect usually are sufficient to confirm the presence of dementia.

One diagnostic question that occasionally confronts speech-language pathologists is whether a person has dementia or is aphasic. Persons with early-stage cortical dementia are most likely to be confused with persons who have anomic aphasia because of their word retrieval problems and their subtle comprehension impairments. Persons with middle-stage cortical dementia are most likely to be confused with persons who exhibit Wernicke's aphasia because of their vague, empty, paraphasic, and circumlocutory speech and their significant comprehension impairments.

Physicians and other healthcare personnel sometimes use the label *aphasia* in a broad sense to refer to any language impairment caused by brain damage, whether or not it is the person's primary impairment. Speech-language pathologists use the label in a narrow sense to refer to specific patterns of language impairment disproportionate to any other cognitive or behavioral impairments the person may have.

The key to differential diagnosis of dementia versus aphasia is administering nonverbal tests of intelligence and problem-solving. Persons with aphasia do better on nonverbal tests than on verbal tests, whereas persons with dementia perform poorly on both. Additional diagnostic help may come from knowledge of the onset and progression of symptoms. Dementia usually is insidious in onset and develops slowly, with gradual worsening from subtle impairments of memory, reasoning, and problem-solving to gross impairments of intellect, personality, and behavior. Aphasia usually is abrupt in onset, and symptoms develop rapidly, peaking within a few minutes to a few hours, followed by slow improvement over weeks to years.

GENERAL CONCEPTS 12-2

- The symptoms of *depression* (cognitive impairment, loss of appetite, difficulty sleeping, social withdrawal, and apathy) sometimes are mistaken for symptoms of dementia (a condition called *pseudodementia*). However, depression differs from

GENERAL CONCEPTS 12-2—cont'd

dementia in several ways. Depression usually has an identifiable onset with rapid symptom development; patients with depression make little effort to perform on clinical tests; and the performance of patients with depression is highly variable from test to test.

- The symptoms of *delirium* (a transient confusional state) sometimes resemble symptoms of dementia. However, delirium, unlike dementia, usually has an identifiable precipitant (e.g., changes in medications, infections, metabolic disorders); symptoms appear abruptly and progress rapidly; and delusions and hallucinations are common.

- Some of the symptoms of dementia may resemble some symptoms of aphasia, but patients with dementia do poorly on verbal and nonverbal tests, whereas patients with aphasia do better on verbal tests than on nonverbal tests. Dementia has insidious onset, and symptoms slowly worsen, whereas symptoms of aphasia appear abruptly and gradually improve.

ASSESSMENT OF PERSONS WITH DEMENTIA

My thoughts are whirled like a potter's wheel. I know not where I am nor what I do. (William Shakespeare, King Henry VI)

Rating scales occupy a prominent place in the assessment of persons with confirmed dementia. Rating scales provide a quick (but not very sensitive) estimate of intellectual abilities, competence in activities of daily living, or both. Most rating scales permit the user to identify the presence of moderate to severe dementia but are insensitive to subtle intellectual decline. Consequently, most rating scales are not suitable for

evaluating persons with suspected early-stage dementia. Detecting the subtle signs of early dementia requires standardized, sensitive, and reliable tests of cognitive and linguistic performance administered by a specialist trained in their administration and interpretation.

Most dementia rating scales require little or no specialized training to complete and can be completed after observing the person with dementia, interviewing family members and caregivers, or both. More than a dozen scales for rating dementia severity have been published, of which six or eight are in fairly general use. Three popular rating scales are the *Blessed Dementia Scale* (*BDS*; Blessed, Tomlinson, & Roth, 1968), the *Global Deterioration Scale* (*GDS*; Reisberg & associates, 1982), and the *Clinical Dementia Rating* (Morris, 1993).

The *Blessed Dementia Scale* uses information obtained from family members, caregivers, and the person's medical record to estimate the person's ability to get along in daily life activities. The BDS has two sections (Table 12-4). In one section the performance of eight daily life activities is rated. In the other section, 14 aspects of the person's behavior and personality are rated. For some items (eating, dressing, sphincter control) the severity of the person's impairments, as well as their presence, is rated. Increasing scores on the BDS represent increasing severity of impairment. The maximum possible score is 28. Persons scoring below 4 are considered unimpaired; scores of 4 to 9 represent mild impairment; and scores of 10 or higher represent moderate to severe impairment (Eastwood, Lautenschlaeger, & Corbin, 1983).

The *Global Deterioration Scale* describes seven levels of dementia representing increasing severity of intellectual impairment (Table 12-5). The GDS is completed by a clinician after interviewing the person with dementia, family members, and caregivers. Ratings are based on general descriptions of behavior provided in the GDS, and raters must use subjective judgment and intuition to arrive at a rating, because few persons with dementia are likely to match the

TABLE 12-4 The Blessed Dementia Scale	
Feature	Score
Changes in Performance of Everyday Activities	
1. Unable to perform household tasks	1
2. Unable to cope with small sums of money	1
3. Unable to remember short lists of items, e.g., in shopping	1
4. Unable to find way about indoors	1
5. Unable to find way about familiar streets	1
6. Unable to interpret surroundings	1
7. Unable to recall recent events	1
8. Tends to dwell in the past	1
Changes in Habits	
9. Eating	
Messily with spoon only	1
Simple solids, e.g., biscuits	2
Has to be fed	3
10. Dressing	
Occasionally misplaced buttons, etc.	1
Wrong sequence, commonly forgetting items	2
Unable to dress	3
11. Sphincter control	
Occasional wet beds	1
Frequent wet beds	2
Doubly incontinent	3
12. Increased rigidity	1
13. Increased egocentricity	1
14. Impairment of regard for feelings of others	1
15. Coarsening of affect	1
16. Impairment of emotional control	1
17. Hilarity in inappropriate situations	1
18. Diminished emotional responsiveness	1
19. Sexual misdemeanor (appearing first in old age)	1
20. Relinquishes hobbies	1
21. Diminished initiative or growing apathy	1
22. Purposeless hyperactivity	1

From Blessed, G., Tomlinson, B.E., & Roth M. (1968). The association between quantitative measures of dementia and senile change in the cerebral gray matter of elderly subjects. *British Journal of Psychiatry, 114,* 791-811. © 1968 The Royal College of Psychiatrists.

TABLE 12-5 Stages of the Global Deterioration Scale and Clinical Characteristics of Persons at Each Stage

GDS Stage	Clinical Phase	Clinical Characteristics
1. No cognitive decline	Normal	The patient has no complaints of memory impairment, and there is no evidence of memory impairments in the clinical interview.
2. Very mild cognitive decline	Forgetfulness	Subjective complaints of memory impairment, such as forgetting where one has placed familiar objects, or forgetting formerly well-known names. No objective evidence of memory impairment in the clinical interview. No objective impairment in work or social situations. Patient is appropriately concerned with regard to symptoms.
3. Mild cognitive decline	Early confusional	The patient exhibits the first obvious impairments. Exhibits more than one of the following: (1) The patient gets lost when traveling to an unfamiliar location. (2) Co-workers are aware of patient's impairments. (3) Family or caregivers note word-retrieval and naming impairments. (4) The patient does not remember information from recently-read printed material. (5) The patient has unusual difficulty in remembering names upon introduction to new people. (6) The patient loses or misplaces items of value. (7) Attentional impairments are obvious in clinical testing. Objective evidence of the patient's memory impairment is observable only with an intensive interview conducted by a trained professional. The patient exhibits impaired performance in demanding work and social situations. The patient begins to deny impairments and exhibits mild to moderate anxiety.
4. Moderate cognitive decline	Late confusional	The patient exhibits obvious impairments in a careful clinical interview. Impairments consist of: (1) Diminished knowledge of current and recent events (2) Mild impairment in giving personal history (3) Attentional impairments on difficult tasks (4) Impaired ability to travel, handle personal finances, and so on The patient usually has minimal or no impairments in: (1) Orientation to time and person (2) Recognition of familiar persons and faces (3) Ability to travel to familiar locations

Continued

Modified from Reisberg, B., Ferris, S.H., DeLeon M.J., and associates (1982). The global deterioration scale for assessment of primary degenerative dementia. *American Journal of Psychiatry, 139,* 1136-1139.

TABLE 12-5	Stages of the Global Deterioration Scale and Clinical Characteristics of Persons at Each Stage—cont'd	
GDS Stage	Clinical Phase	Clinical Characteristics
5. Moderately severe cognitive decline	Early dementia	The patient can no longer survive without assistance from others. In a clinical interview the patient cannot provide major, relevant, current information (such as address or telephone number, the names of close members of their family, the name of the high school or college from which they graduated). The patient frequently exhibits some disorientation to time (date, day, season) or place. The patient knows his or her own name and usually knows the names of their spouse and children. They eat and toilet themselves unassisted but may need assistance in choosing what to wear.
6. Severe cognitive decline	Middle dementia	The patient may occasionally forget the name of their spouse or primary caregiver. The patient is largely unaware of recent events and experiences but retains sketchy knowledge of his or her past life. The patient is generally disoriented to time and place. The patient usually requires assistance with activities of daily living and may be incontinent. The patient may retain the ability to travel to familiar locations, but cannot travel to unfamiliar locations without assistance. The patient remembers his or her own name and recognizes familiar persons. Personality and emotional changes become obvious, and may include: (1) Delusional behavior, such as accusing their spouse of being an imposter, talk to imaginary persons, or to their own image in the mirror (2) Obsessive behavior, such as continual repetition of a simple cleaning activity (3) Anxiety, agitation, and occasional violent behavior (4) Loss of willpower, because the patient cannot maintain thought long enough to determine a purposeful course of action.
7. Very severe cognitive decline	Late dementia	The patient loses all verbal ability. Speech may consist only of grunting. The patient is incontinent of urine and requires assistance with eating and toileting. The patient loses the ability to walk. Generalized neurologic signs and symptoms are obvious.

descriptions precisely. The GDS provides for relatively coarse estimates of intellectual level. However, it covers a wide range of levels of impairment, and ratings are easy to make and fairly reliable. Consequently, it occupies a place in rating dementia similar to the place occupied by the *Rancho Los Amigos Scale of Cognitive Levels* (Hagen & Malkamus, 1979; Hagen, 1997) for rating cognitive functioning following traumatic brain injury.

The *Clinical Dementia Rating* describes six domains of cognitive and functional performance: *memory, orientation, judgment and problem-solving, community affairs, home and hobbies,* and *personal care* (Table 12-6). The ratings are made by a skilled clinician, based on interviews of the person with dementia and a reliable informant (e.g., a family member). The interviews are conducted according to a standard protocol. The author of the CDR recommends that raters receive 6 to 9 hours of training in its use to ensure reliability. Online training materials are available at the Washington University School of Medicine Alzheimer's Disease Research Center website (www.alz.washington.edu).

The foregoing scales provide global estimates of dementia severity. Such scales often are used in clinical practice and research to track an individual's progression through levels representing increasing severity of impairment. A few scales focusing on an individual's functional abilities in activities of daily life have been developed. Most are completed by caregivers or other informants who have knowledge of the individual's level of daily life functioning. The *Instrumental Activities of Daily Living Scale* (*IADL*; Lawton & Brody, 1969) is widely used in clinical practice and research. A caregiver uses the IADL to rate the designated individual's performance in 8 activities of daily living (Box 12-1). Such ratings of functional performance complement global ratings of impairment by providing information about the rated person's independence in specific activities typical of everyday life.

Language and Communication

Comprehensive Test Batteries. Speech-language pathologists make perhaps their most important contribution to management of dementia by administering standardized and reliable tests to identify communicative strengths and weaknesses and to provide dependable baseline measures against which the progression of dementia and the effects of interventions can be assessed. Tests of language and communication supplement tests of verbal and nonverbal intelligence, tests of immediate and remote memory, and tests of attention and perception to provide a comprehensive description of the impairments of persons with dementia.

The *Arizona Battery for Communication Disorders of Dementia* (*ABCD*; Bayles & Tomoeda, 1991) is a clinical assessment instrument for identifying and quantifying communicative deficits of persons with dementia (specifically those caused by Alzheimer's disease). The ABCD contains four screening subtests to evaluate speech discrimination, visual perception and literacy, visual fields, and visual agnosia, plus 14 subtests to evaluate mental status, linguistic expression, verbal memory, linguistic comprehension, and visuospatial construction. The subtests in the ABCD are based on the authors' research on the language performance of 175 normal older adults and 300 adults with dementia-producing illnesses. The ABCD is standardized on 50 adults with Alzheimer's disease and 50 age-matched normal adults. The ABCD appears to be an efficient and informative instrument for assessing communicative disabilities of persons with either suspected or confirmed dementia, and the authors report that the ABCD correlates with several other measures of dementia severity.

In-depth evaluation of speech, language, and communicative abilities may include a comprehensive aphasia test such as the *Boston Diagnostic Aphasia Examination* (*BDAE*; Goodglass,

TABLE 12-6   The Clinical Dementia Rating Scale

	None 0	Questionable 0.5	Mild 1	Moderate 2	Severe 3
			Impairment Level and CDR Score (0, 0.5, 1, 2, 3)		
Memory	No memory loss or slight inconsistent forgetfulness	Consistent slight forgetfulness; partial recollection of events; benign forgetfulness	Moderate memory loss (more marked for recent events); defect interferes with everyday activities	Severe memory loss; only highly learned material retained; new material rapidly lost	Severe memory loss; only fragments remain
Orientation	Fully oriented	Fully oriented except for slight difficulty with time relationships	Moderate difficulty with time relationships; oriented for place at examination; may have geographic disorientation elsewhere	Severe difficulty with time relationships; usually disoriented to time, often to place	Oriented to person only
Judgment and Problem Solving	Solves everyday problems and handles business and financial affairs well; judgment good in relation to past performance	Slight impairment in solving problems, similarities, and differences	Moderate difficulty in handling problems, similarities, and differences; social judgment usually maintained	Severely impaired in handling problems, similarities, and differences; social judgment usually impaired	Unable to make judgments or solve problems

	Independent function at usual level in job, shopping, volunteer and social groups	Slight impairment in these activities	Unable to function independently at these activities although may still be engaged in some; appears normal to casual inspection	No pretense of independent function outside home; appears well enough to be taken to functions outside a family home	No pretense of independent function outside home; appears too ill to be taken to functions outside a family home
Community Affairs	Independent function at usual level in job, shopping, volunteer and social groups	Slight impairment in these activities	Unable to function independently at these activities although may still be engaged in some; appears normal to casual inspection	No pretense of independent function outside home; appears well enough to be taken to functions outside a family home	No pretense of independent function outside home; appears too ill to be taken to functions outside a family home
Home and Hobbies	Life at home, hobbies, and intellectual interests well maintained	Life at home, hobbies, and intellectual interests slightly impaired	Mild but definite impairment of function at home; more difficult chores abandoned; more complicated hobbies and interests abandoned	Only simple chores preserved; very restricted interests, poorly maintained	No significant function in home
Personal Care	Fully capable of self-care		Needs prompting	Requires assistance in dressing, hygiene, keeping of personal effects	Requires much help with personal care; frequent incontinence

Score only as decline from previous usual level due to cognitive loss, not impairment due to other factors.
From Morris, J.C. (1993). The Clinical Dementia Rating Scale (CDR). Current version and scoring rules. *Neurology, 43*, 2412-2414.

Box 12-1	The Instrumental Activities of Daily Living Scale (IADL)

A. Ability to use telephone
1. Operates telephone on own initiative; looks up, dials numbers, etc.
2. Dials a few well-known numbers
3. Answers telephone but does not dial
4. Does not use telephone at all

B. Shopping
1. Takes care of all shopping needs independently
2. Shops independently for small purchases
3. Needs to be accompanied on any shopping trip
4. Completely unable to shop

C. Food preparation
1. Plans, prepares, and serves adequate meals independently
2. Prepares adequate meals if supplied with ingredients
3. Heats, serves, and prepares meals or prepares meals but does not maintain adequate diet
4. Needs to have meals prepared and served

D. Housekeeping
1. Maintains house alone or with occasional assistance
2. Performs light daily tasks such as dishwashing, bed making
3. Performs light daily tasks but cannot maintain acceptable level of cleanliness
4. Needs help with all home maintenance tasks
5. Does not participate in any housekeeping tasks

E. Laundry
1. Does personal laundry completely
2. Launders small items, rinses stockings, etc.
3. All laundry must be done by others

F. Mode of transportation
1. Travels independently on public transportation or drives own car
2. Arranges own travel via taxi but does not otherwise use public transportation
3. Travels on public transportation when accompanied by another
4. Travel limited to taxi or automobile with assistance of another
5. Does not travel at all

G. Responsibility for own medication
1. Is responsible for taking medication in correct dosages at correct time
2. Takes responsibility if medication is prepared in advance in separate dosage
3. Is not capable of dispensing own medication

H. Ability to handle finances
1. Manages financial matters independently (budgets, writes checks, pays rent and bills, goes to bank), collects and keeps track of income
2. Manages day-to-day purchases but needs help with banking, major purchases, etc.
3. Incapable of handling money

From Lawton, M.P., and Brody, E.M. (1969). Assessment of older people: Self-maintaining and instrumental activities of daily living. *Gerontologist, 9,* 179-186.

Kaplan, & Barresi, 2001) or the *Western Aphasia Battery* (*WAB*; Kertesz, 1982) to measure general language abilities and to track change in language abilities over time. A test of functional communication such as *Communicative Activities in Daily Living—Second Edition* (*CADL-2;* Holland, Frattali, & Fromm, 1999) may be administered to estimate daily life communicative ability and to provide a baseline measure against which future changes in functional communication may be compared.

The WAB and *Communicative Abilities in Daily Living* (*CADL;* Holland, 1980) have been used to evaluate communicative abilities of persons with dementia, and some normative information has been published (Appell, Kertesz, & Fishman, 1982; Fromm & Holland, 1989; Murray & associates, 1984).

Comprehension and Retention of Spoken Language. Information from a comprehensive test battery may be supplemented by the results of additional tests that sample specific speech, language, and communicative abilities. A receptive vocabulary test such as the *Peabody Picture Vocabulary Test* (Dunn & Dunn, 1997) may be administered to detect subtle changes in receptive vocabulary. Bayles and associates (1989) reported that performance on the Peabody Picture Vocabulary Test dependably discriminated adults with mild Alzheimer's disease from normal elderly adults.

A *delayed story retelling task,* in which the examiner tells a short story then later asks the person with dementia to retell it, may be administered to evaluate encoding, retention, and recall of verbal material. Bayles and associates (1989) reported that delayed story recall was the single most useful test for discriminating persons with mild Alzheimer's disease from normal elderly adults. Normal elderly adults recalled, on average, 96% of the information from the stories, whereas adults with mild Alzheimer's disease recalled only about 2% of the information, and adults with moderate Alzheimer's disease recalled none of the information.

A spoken sentence comprehension test such as the *Test of Auditory Comprehension of Language* (Carrow-Woolfolk, 1999) or a sentence comprehension subtest from an aphasia test battery may help detect sentence-level comprehension impairments, although most persons with early-stage dementia are likely to have difficulty only on syntactically complex items. A test of discourse comprehension such as the *Discourse Comprehension Test* (Brookshire & Nicholas, 1993) may estimate comprehension and short-term retention of directly and indirectly stated main ideas and details from spoken stories. Persons with mild dementia are likely to have the most difficulty with implied details, are likely to have minor difficulty with stated details, and are likely to have little difficulty with main ideas, either stated or implied. As dementia progresses, deficient performance is likely to extend to main ideas, with implied main ideas affected first.

Speech Production. A generative naming test may be administered to evaluate mental flexibility and attention. The most sensitive generative naming tests for persons who are in the early stages of dementia are those in which the person is asked to provide examples of a given semantic category (e.g., animals or fruits) in a fixed time interval (usually 1 minute). Persons in the early stages of dementia usually do beter on generative naming tests in which they provide words beginning with a given letter than on category membership tests, although performance on beginning-letter tests declines as dementia progresses (Butters & associates, 1987).

The *Boston Naming Test* (*BNT*; Kaplan, Goodglass, & Weintraub, 2001) may be administered to evaluate confrontation naming. The BNT is sensitive to word retrieval impairments and disturbed visual recognition in early-stage dementia. Performance on the BNT usually is superior to performance on generative naming tests for persons at early and middle stages of dementia. (Most persons with late-stage dementia are unable to perform either test.)

A sample of connected speech elicited by a pictured scene such as the *cookie theft* picture from the BDAE provides information about the person's ability to make sense of a pictured situation and formulate and produce a cohesive and topically relevant narrative. Persons in the early stages of dementia may exhibit word retrieval failures, insert tangential comments, and have difficulty staying on topic. As dementia progresses into the middle stages, word retrieval failures become more common, neologisms appear, and gross failures to maintain a coherent topic and convey a central theme become evident. By the late stages of dementia, the person's responses contain little more than automatisms, stereotypic words and phrases, and tangential and irrelevant comments. The following transcripts trace the decline in connected speech as Alzheimer's dementia progresses:

At diagnosis:

C: Now, Mrs. ___, I'd like you to tell me what's going on in this picture.

P: Well, there's a woman...a mother...she's managing the...she's drying the dishes, but she isn't...she doesn't know that the sink is too full and it's flouting...no...it's drailing or going onto the floor. She'll notice it when her feet get wet, I guess. And behind her there there's two kids, a boy and a girl. The boy is up on a bench...a chair...that's not it but you know what I mean. And the one there is going to tip over, and the girl is laughing about it, and it looks like the top one there was stealing cookies while the mother is off lost in space. The mother. She's dishing the dishes. Is that what you mean?

C: That's it. Thank you very much.

Early stage, approximately 3 years after diagnosis:

C: Now, Mrs. ___, I'd like you to tell me what's going on in this picture.

P: I don't care for this one. Can we do a different one?

C: Let's do this one. It's one of my favorites. I hope you don't mind.

P: Well, all right. If you like it. What was it again?

C: Tell me what's going on in this picture.

P: Well, there's a woman there, and she's up to something. She's not looking at that other there, and I don't know why it's going and going and going, and she's never mind, and they must have had a meal or a dinner or something, and she's up to...dishes. Dishes and dishes. I wouldn't know... Is that it?

C: Can you tell me anything more?

P: Well there's these here little ones. A boy and a sister. Little urchins or scapegoats. He's up to it, and she's laughing and laughing and all that, and I guess they must be playing some sort of game or contest or something, but it's not clear to me why, and their mama doesn't look like she's in the game or anything, and that's about all I have to say about that.

C: Thank you. That was perfect.

Middle stage, approximately 5 years after diagnosis:

C: Now, Mrs. ___, I'd like you to tell me what's going on in this picture.

P: This looks like an indeling one. A real American art machine.

C: Can you tell me what's happening there?

P: Yes I can. They're so scabble-de-goo that I wonder what all will come of it. They don't have the sense that God gave a goose, if you ask me, and I don't know why that other one there is not in the measure of this one, but it doesn't matter because this one here is laughing and playing, and I don't know why you never know about them these days. But anyway, if they were for me, I'd have to squelge and anoint that one there, because I can't stand it when there's such chess and mirvir. Is that what you mean?

C: Thank you. That's exactly what I mean.

Late stage, approximately 9 years after diagnosis:

C: Now, Mrs. ___ here's a picture that tells a story. Look at it and tell me what's happening in this picture.

P: Never mind.

C: Can you tell me what's happening here?

P: I said never mind.

C: Mrs. ___, can you do me a big favor? Tell me what's happening here.

P: Oh, all right. It looks like somebody lost the way and was the other way. Not under and over, but imbulation.

C: Can you tell me anything more?

P: That's the usual something for under and over. And that's all.

C: Thank you very much. You did fine.

According to Bayles and associates (1989) discriminating adults with mild dementia from normal elderly adults requires at least the following tests:

- Delayed story retelling
- Mental status (orientation to time, place, person, and general knowledge)
- Pantomime expression
- The Peabody Picture Vocabulary Test

(All are included in the *Arizona Battery for Communication Disorders of Dementia*.)

HELPING PEOPLE COPE WITH DEMENTIA

Pain of mind is worse than pain of body.
(Latin proverb)

The progressive nature of irreversible dementia rules out restoration of lost abilities as a practical clinical objective for most persons with dementia. As the person's neurologic condition deteriorates, mental functions inevitably decline. Efforts at restoring declining intellectual capacities are no match for the implacable loss of neuronal function taking place. The clinical effort becomes a holding action in which the advancing effects of neurologic disease are lessened by helping the person with dementia and his or her caregivers and family members control the effects of dementia on daily life. The clinical objectives of intervention are (a) to minimize the disruptive effects of the dementia on the person with dementia and to support caregivers and family members, (b) to ensure the safety of the person with dementia and keep her or him healthy, and (c) to provide support and direction for the person with dementia, caregivers, and family members. Accomplishing these objectives requires the coordinated efforts of professionals in several disciplines, including medicine, nursing, speech-language pathology, occupational therapy, recreational therapy, physical therapy, neuropsychology, clinical psychology, social work, and dietetics, plus the person with dementia, family members, and caregivers.

The magnitude and nature of the problems, stresses, and issues faced by the family inexorably increase as the intellectual and behavioral impairments of the person with dementia progress from annoying to enervating. Clinicians who intend to provide appropriate and effective care for persons with dementia and their families must understand what the person with dementia and his or her family experience as dementia progresses. Only by matching clinical efforts with the needs of the affected person, family members, and caregivers can clinicians provide the best and most effective care for those who struggle with dementia and for those who share that struggle.

The first symptoms of dementia usually are subtle and may be overlooked by the family. The person with dementia becomes forgetful, irritable, and inattentive but remains oriented and socially appropriate. The first symptoms of dementia may be interpreted by family members as depression, stubbornness, or normal aging. As the person's gradual decline continues, family members may remain unaware that something ominous is happening, until the person's deteriorating intellect and changing behavior begin to interfere seriously with family life.

As the family's concern deepens, they seek professional help in finding out what is wrong. The diagnosis of dementia almost always begins a time of intense stress for the affected person and family members, during which counseling and support for the affected person and her or his family is crucial. The person with dementia often goes through a time of frustration and anger about what has been lost, combined with worry and anxiety about the future. As time goes on, the person with dementia may become depressed and apathetic and withdraw from family and friends, with intervals of self-imposed social isolation punctuated by angry outbursts over trivial incidents. The person with dementia needs help in dealing with feelings of grief and anger about what is happening, help with diffuse anxiety about the future, and a plan for coping with the future. The family needs information about what is happening and about the probable course of the affected person's illness. The family, like the person with dementia, needs help in dealing with the grief, anger, and anxiety that almost invariably follow the diagnosis (Box 12-2).

During the very early stages of dementia, most symptoms are inconveniences, and families often spontaneously adapt to them. They no longer permit the person with dementia to run errands unaccompanied, because they discover

Box 12-2	Family Interview 1

**Interview with the Wife of a Person
with Early Alzheimer's Dementia**
It took us a while to realize what was happening. George was always real easy-going, you know. Nothing got under his skin. Then—it must have been a year or so ago—little things started to set him off. Like—this is the first one I remember—one morning when George got up we were out of coffee. He had gone to the store the day before and forgot to get coffee, though he knew we were out. Well, anyway—when things like that happened, he usually would just shrug it off, you know—like ordinarily he would have just gone to the store to get more coffee. But this time he got really ticked off. He was slamming cupboard doors and swearing—which was really strange, because George never used profanity—and he started yelling at me and telling me I was no good. Finally I just left him there in the kitchen and walked over to the neighbors, and when I came back about an hour later, George was all settled down, and he had gone out and got the coffee. That's the first real incident I recall, but as I think back there were other times before that. Little things—nothing dramatic. Like, he'd always been a real reader—a book a week, and he stopped doing that. And he'd forget things, like the grandkids coming over for the day. And he seemed to have lost interest in socializing with our friends. But what really got me to thinking something was really wrong was when he started thinking the neighbors were spying on him. He'd close all the blinds so they couldn't see in, and I'd come by and open them up again. But next time I'd come by, the blinds would be closed again. Then he started threatening to confront the neighbors about their spying. And so I took him to see Dr. Wells, and he did some tests and suggested we make an appointment at the university. And so we went there, and that's when we found out that George probably had Alzheimer's.

that she or he tends to get lost. They take away the car keys, because they sense that impaired judgment and slow reactions place the person with dementia and other drivers in danger. They gradually assume responsibilities for shopping, paying bills, and housecleaning, and they take over the affected person's legal and financial affairs. They shape family routines around the affected person's eccentricities. If the person with dementia lives alone, the family keeps track of her or him with frequent telephone calls and visits, but gradually the family is forced to assume more responsibility, until they decide that the person with dementia must move in with a family member. This decision often is precipitated by a dramatic incident (the person with dementia starts a fire by leaving a stove or iron unattended, gets lost and is picked up by the police, or enters neighbors' houses uninvited).

As dementia progresses, lapses of memory increase in frequency and duration, until they constitute a profound impairment in storing and retrieving new information. The person with dementia begins to neglect self-care and has to be reminded, cajoled, or nagged to bathe, keep clothing clean, and maintain oral hygiene. Progressive impairments in judgment, attention, and memory put the person with dementia and others at risk when he or she uses gas stoves, ovens, power tools, ladders, or machinery. The person becomes progressively more anxious, depressed, and irritable and withdraws from interactions with family members and others. Periodic violent emotional outbursts may occur. The person takes frequent naps during the day and wakes up and wanders about during the night. For some, the wake-sleep cycle is completely reversed, and the person sleeps all day and is awake all night. Some individuals become indifferent to food and fail to maintain adequate caloric and fluid intake without supervision. Others become gluttonous, eating continuously and indiscriminately unless they are supervised.

During the middle stages of dementia, the person with dementia and family members must

---

| Box 12-3 | *Family Interview 2* |

Interview with the Wife of a Person with Middle-Stage Alzheimer's Disease

Well, it's pretty much like living with a stranger. Actually, a child who's also a stranger. But a child remembers things, and you can reason with a child. That's not true with Harry anymore. He doesn't remember, and when you remind him he blows his top. He blames me for all the problems, and that hurts. And Jim and Nancy [son and daughter] think I'm exaggerating, because when they come over, Harry gets on his best behavior, and he's very good at covering up when he wants to. Then as soon as they leave he's back to his old self again. They notice that Harry forgets things and that a lot of times what he says doesn't make sense, but they say that's just normal aging. So I'm not getting much support from them. Sometimes I just think, Oh what's the use!

---

cope with increasingly severe mental impairments and the disruptive effects of the impairments on family relationships and routines. Family members are distressed by the affected person's increasing mental impairments and unpredictable changes in mood. Family members may be angry and resentful about the burden that has been imposed on them, although they are unlikely to openly express or acknowledge their anger and resentment, and they may feel guilty about their feelings. Family relationships and routines are disrupted as caregivers become increasingly responsible for the person with dementia and are forced to neglect other activities and responsibilities (Box 12-3).

As the affected person's deterioration progresses and his or her appreciation of reality declines, depression and apathy may give way to hyperactivity, wandering, and stereotypic repetitive behaviors. The person with dementia can no longer be left alone and requires continuous supervision. Family members take responsibility for bathing the affected family member and supervising his or her oral hygiene. When incontinence develops, the burden of care esca-

lates. Additional deterioration may bring verbal abusiveness, aggressiveness, and episodes of threatened or actual physical violence, further disrupting family relationships and increasing family members' anger, resentment, and guilt.

This phase of the person's illness requires continuing education, support, and therapy for the family. Family members need education about why the person with dementia behaves disruptively and about how disruptive behaviors can be controlled or eliminated. Family members need help in setting up a safe, predictable, and stable environment for the person with dementia. They may need help in dividing caregiving responsibilities among family members, and they may need encouragement and direction in taking advantage of respite care and day care services and support groups. As the burden of care escalates, family members need help in planning for and accomplishing placement in an extended care facility (nursing home). Throughout this phase of the person's illness, family members need help in dealing with their feelings of resentment, anger, apprehension, and guilt. Guilt becomes especially prominent as the family begins to contemplate placement in an extended care facility.

Most persons with dementia are cared for at home until the burden becomes intolerable, at which time they are placed in a nursing home. The period of at-home care may range from 1 or 2 to 10 or 15 years, depending on how rapidly dementia progresses, and on the family's tolerance for the disruptions caused by the person's dementia.

Most persons with dementia spend their last years in an extended care facility. Although the physical burden of care has been alleviated by extended care placement, the emotional burden carried by family members continues, often augmented by feelings of guilt over abandoning a family member to the care of strangers and by feelings of loss that accompany the person's departure from home. As the affected person's physical condition becomes more fragile, family members are faced with decisions about whether heroic measures should be used to sustain the person's life. During this time, family members need continuing help in resolving their often conflicting feelings about their own needs and their obligations to the affected person and in making decisions about when and how to end procedures for prolonging the person's life (Box 12-4).

The death of the person with dementia does not end the family's need for advice, support, and reassurance. The period of mourning following the death of the affected family member may be brief, perhaps because the family has been mentally preparing for the person's demise for months or years. Although the mourning period may be short, the grief felt by family members may be intense, owing perhaps to the release of emotional tensions that have built up over years of the person's illness. Professional counseling and support during this period may help family members acknowledge and understand their feelings and their reactions to what they have been through and may help them reconstruct and repair family relationships that have been damaged or distorted by the pressures of caring for the person with dementia.

MANAGEMENT ISSUES

Early Stages

Memory Impairments. Memory impairments characteristically are the first and most troublesome of the affected person's early symptoms. These early memory impairments typically affect *declarative memory* (memory for the past, such as the names of children, or yesterday's visit by a family member) and *prospective memory* (remembering to do things at specific times, such as keeping an appointment or bringing in the mail). Early-stage dementia usually does not affect *procedural memory* (how to do things, such as how to make coffee), at least for procedures that are well-practiced and not too complex. Impaired declarative memory is most annoying to early-stage persons with dementia, but impaired prospective memory is most annoying to their caregivers.

> Attentional impairments may interfere with completion of well-remembered procedures by persons with dementia. Those who are interrupted or distracted while performing a remembered procedure may forget where they were in the procedure and may either start again from the beginning or abandon the procedure in confusion.

A person with early-stage dementia may forget to bring the groceries in from the car on returning from a shopping trip, but if reminded, the person has little difficulty carrying out the procedures involved in bringing the groceries in and putting them away. However, the person with early-stage dementia may exhibit signs of

---

Box 12-4	*Family Interview 3*

Interview with the Husband of a Person with Late-Stage Alzheimer's Disease

(Interviewer: What led you to place Mrs. Baxter in a nursing home?)

Well, it was probably several things. Things were just gradually getting worse, and I was getting near the end of my rope. She'd get up in the middle of the night and roam around. We had to put key locks—the ones you can lock from inside with a key—on all the doors going outside to keep her from getting out of the house in the middle of the night. And she was having accidents—wetting herself and now and then messing herself. But I could handle that. Then one day I came home, and she was asleep on the couch and the house was full of smoke. She had put a loaf of bread in a plastic bag in the oven and set the oven as high as it would go. Then she must have forgot about it and took a nap. The oven was a terrible mess—we were lucky it didn't start a fire. So the kids and I sat down and talked things over, and we decided that she should go to a home where she could be supervised 24 hours a day. She had become a danger to herself and to others. It was the hardest thing I've ever done in my life, but it had to be done. It's the best thing for her and for me and for the family. I still feel guilty about it though.

memory impairment and confusion such as the following:

- Forget the shopping list, forget to consult the shopping list when at the store, or misplace the list while shopping
- Forget the names of brands customarily purchased and return home with other brands
- Retrace a route down aisles previously taken and place items in the shopping cart that duplicate items previously placed there (but the person is unlikely to forget the shopping procedure, such as pushing the cart down the aisles, placing items in the cart, and taking the items to the checkout counter)
- At home the next day, may forget having purchased the groceries and may return to the store and purchase the same list of groceries

It is not unusual for caregivers to feel that the affected person's memory lapses can be resolved if he or she would just try harder. They may badger the person with well-intentioned but misguided admonitions to remember important items and may drill the person on the information, not understanding that neither admonitions nor drills are solutions. Caregivers can help the person with dementia cope with memory impairments by maximizing the orderliness and predictability of the person's living environment (more on this later).

> I'll tell her something and she's saying yes-yes and then 10 minutes later she's acting like I never said it. I don't think she pays enough attention. I tell her to listen and even have her say it back to me. She'll do it but then later on it's like it never happened. Sometimes I think she's just trying to get my goat.

Impaired Language and Communication.
Persons in the early stages of dementia usually have sufficient language comprehension and speech to manage routine daily life interactions. However, subtle attention and memory impairments compromise retention of spoken or printed materials. Comprehension deteriorates in noisy and distracting environments or when several people are talking, and intermittent word retrieval failures create annoying gaps in output, although they do not seriously interfere with communication. Persons in the early stages of dementia (and their families and caregivers) need help in identifying how communication is affected by the person's impairments, assistance in identifying the most important targets for management, help with devising strategies for working around the person's communication impairments, and direction in putting the strategies into practice.

> The main thing I notice is how he's gotten sort of vague. Like his thinking is fuzzy or something. He's always been a very precise speaker, but now he hesitates and fumbles and stumbles around. And he misses words. Like this morning when he was talking about getting the car serviced, and he called the car the bathtub. …I think he mostly understands what people say, but sometimes he misses things. Especially if you tell him several things in a row, like what we're having for dinner or what we need from the store. I think maybe he's not paying enough attention.

Anxiety and Depression.
Anxiety and depression are common in persons with early stage dementia. Anxiety typically begins as the person senses loss of control and independence in daily life activities. The person's anxiety is perpetuated by fear of what the future may bring, uncertainty about coping with upcoming difficult or stressful events, perception of unwanted changes in social status and interpersonal relationships, and a variety of other concerns about an uncertain future or an unsatisfactory present.

> You know, she's always been an upbeat kind of person, but now it's like she's drawing into a shell. It's like she's pulled down some sort of inner curtain between herself and the world outside. Disconnected herself. She doesn't fuss or cry or things like that. Disconnected—emotionally disconnected. That's how it seems.

Behavior Change. The onset of dementia typically brings with it alterations in the person's behavior. Some become apathetic and lose interest in activities that formerly were an important part of life. Others become hyperactive and seemingly unable to sit still, ceaselessly pacing about the house and engaging in ritualistic, obsessive activity (e.g., repeatedly asking the same questions, raising and lowering window shades, opening and closing drawers and cupboards).

Many persons in the early stages of dementia become irritable and easily frustrated. Minor annoyances and petty inconveniences precipitate angry outbursts and sometimes threatened or real physical aggression. Some persons in the early stages of dementia experience exaggerated mood swings, laugh excessively at minimally amusing or neutral material, or are propelled into tears by innocuous events.

> She's always been pretty calm and collected. I was the one who would fly off the handle, and she was the one to tell me to take it easy and calm down. But that's changed. Now it seems like she's just generally harder to get along with. Seems like she's never satisfied. She complains a lot, even about trivial things, which she never used to do. And that irritates me, and we usually end up arguing, but we never seem to get things straightened out.

Denial. Persons in the early stages of dementia often deny or minimize their impairments. Memory lapses are explained away, blamed on others, or denied. Impairments in reasoning, problem-solving, and sustained attention are dismissed. Denial usually arises from the person's need to appear normal, but it annoys caregivers and complicates the person's daily life. These persons need coaching in constructive alternatives to denial. Sometimes what seems to be denial arises from the person's genuine confusion about the specifics of an event or a situation or by the person's faulty memory. These troubled individuals need help with interpreting and remembering events and situations, not advice about denial.

> I think he's gotten more defensive lately. When he slips up, he usually finds a way to pass it off or shift the blame. Like last week he forgot to take our bill payments to the post office. When I asked him about it he said I was the one who was supposed to take them, even though I clearly remember him agreeing to do it. And just now, when we were talking to the other doctor, he said he wasn't having any problems with his urine, but we both know that he's had several accidents in the last few months. I'm having to just bite my tongue and not argue with him, because it doesn't do any good. But I think it's unhealthy for him to be so defensive.

Excess Disability. Sometimes the functional impairments exhibited by persons who have early-stage dementia exceed the limitations attributable to cognitive impairments (a phenomenon called *excess disability*). Excess disability may be caused by coexisting illness, by coexisting emotional and psychologic states (e.g., anxiety or depression), by medication, or by environmental influences, including how the person is treated by caregivers. Removing or abating the causes of excess disability (treating coexisting illness or coexisting emotional and psychologic states, modifying medications, and changing the person's environment) may have remarkable positive effects on the person's performance in activities of daily life.

Caregivers sometimes unintentionally contribute to excess disability by rewarding dependent behavior and ignoring or discouraging independent behavior. This often happens when a caregiver, frustrated by how long the person with dementia takes to perform an activity or by how imperfectly she or he performs it, takes over an activity the person is capable of performing. For example, a caregiver may dress the person, take over meal planning and preparation, or arrange vacations and outings without the person's participation, thereby increasing dependence and contributing to the person's sense of helplessness and incompetence.

Excess disability can be reduced by adapting daily life activities and responsibilities to the person's ability level. The person who can no longer independently plan meals may help caregivers plan menus. The person who can no longer arrange a vacation may help caregivers choose where to go, how long to stay, and what to do. Including the affected person in such activities helps the person feel competent, respected, and needed.

Sleep Disturbances. Most people sleep less as they get older, and disrupted sleep patterns are particularly common in dementia. Sleep medications commonly are prescribed to normalize disrupted sleep-wake cycles, probably more often than necessary. Adjusting the person's daily schedule and sleep environment may normalize the person's sleep pattern and should be tried before medications are prescribed. Even when medications are prescribed, changes in daily schedules and in the person's sleep environment can lower the dosage needed. Sleep schedules often can be normalized by cutting back on the number of naps taken during the day, going to bed at the same time every night, getting mild exercise early in the evening, and keeping doors and windows in the bedroom closed while sleeping.

> I feel tired all the time. I hardly ever get a good night's sleep, because she's constantly getting up in the middle of the night and rummaging around. That wakes me up, and I have to get up and talk her back to bed. But I'm never sure she'll stay there, so I lay there awake until I hear her snoring. Then it takes me a while to get back to sleep. This usually happens once or twice every night. If I could get some help with that it would really help me.

Health. The mental impairments associated with dementia often disrupt normal eating and drinking habits and compromise judgment about nutrition and fluid intake. Consequently, maintaining adequate nutrition and fluid intake is an important part of general healthcare for persons with dementia. Ensuring that the person has properly fitting dentures and maintaining oral hygiene are additional important, but sometimes overlooked, aspects of care.

Other illnesses often accompany dementia. Diabetes, heart disease, pulmonary disease, kidney failure, and metabolic or chemical imbalances are common in both the normal elderly and those who have dementia. Persons with dementia are particularly susceptible to bacterial and viral infections; therefore, prevention and treatment of infections is an important part of a general program of healthcare. Providing hearing aids for hard-of-hearing individuals and properly fitting eyeglasses for those with impaired vision prevent sensory deprivation and contribute to constructive interaction with the environment. Providing canes, walkers, crutches, or wheelchairs provides physically impaired persons with the mobility needed to get around.

Middle Stages

When a person enters the middle stages of dementia, impairments of memory and attention increase in severity and affect more dimensions of daily life. Ironically, the affected person's awareness of the severity and extent of the impairments diminishes as the impairments become more pronounced. Caregivers are likely to be experiencing heightened feelings of loss, anxiety, anger, and hostility as the affected person's impairments become more profound and the burden of care shifts increasingly to caregivers. Physical care problems now become more salient as the person becomes more confused, neglects self-care, sleeps less, wanders more, and perhaps experiences bowel and bladder incontinence. Incidents of hostility, verbal abuse, and actual or threatened physical violence increase in frequency. Caregivers become resigned, despondent, and tired of coping with the affected person's ever increasing impairments and with increasingly frequent troublesome behaviors.

Troublesome Behaviors. Rabins, Mace, and Lucas (1982) surveyed the families of 55 persons with irreversible dementia to find out what families considered the major problems in caring for the family member who had dementia. Their results of the survey are summarized in Figure 12-8. The five most frequently reported troublesome behaviors were *memory disturbance, catastrophic reactions, demanding and critical behavior, night waking,* and *hiding things.* The five behaviors most frequently reported as major problems were *physical*

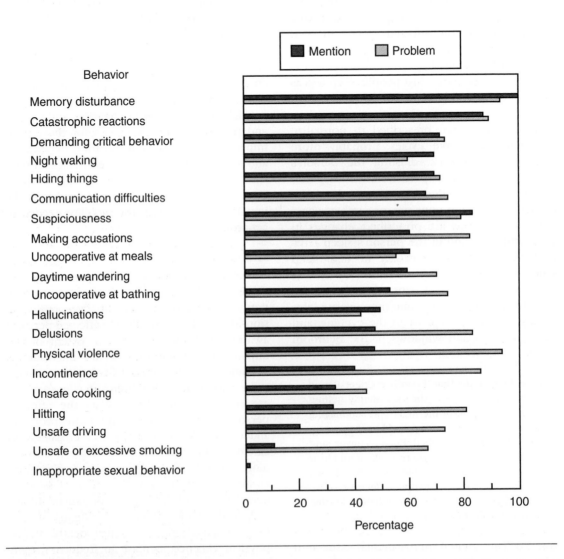

Figure 12-8 ■ Percentage of families reporting the occurrence of problem behaviors and the percentage considering a behavior to be a problem (Data from Rabins, P.V., Mace, N.L., & Lucas, M.J. [1982]. The impact of dementia on the family. *Journal of the American Medical Association, 248,* 333-336.)

violence, memory disturbance, catastrophic reactions, incontinence, and *delusions.* Every respondent reported the presence of memory failure, and almost all (88%) considered it a major problem. However, fewer than half of the respondents (47%) reported the presence of physical violence, but almost all (94%) who reported it considered it a major problem. Only 11% reported unsafe or excessive smoking, but two-thirds of those reporting it considered it a major problem. Clearly, the perceived importance of a troublesome behavior is not determined by its frequency of occurrence alone, but it reflects the amount of emotional stress or inconvenience the behavior causes for family members.

As the person progresses into the middle and late stages of dementia, behavior becomes less predictable. Emotional outbursts are triggered by trifling events. The person becomes sullen, hostile, and uncooperative for no apparent reason. He or she resists the caregiver's help with self-care, then complains of caregiver neglect. The person's volatility in mood and behavior heighten caregiver stress.

> It used to be that he gave some sign that he was about to blow his top. I could see it coming, so usually I could distract him, and he'd calm down. Now it seems like I never know what's going to set him off. We'll be going along okay, then, bam! he's hollering and shaking his fist at me and telling me I'm no good. I'm always walking on pins and needles. There's nothing I can do to keep the explosions from happening, and that's hard to take.

Insight, Judgment, and Orientation. As the person progresses into the middle stages of dementia, problems with insight, judgment, and orientation become salient. The person needs continual supervision. Independent access to appliances, tools, the telephone, and the outdoors must be increasingly restricted. The restrictions irritate and anger the person with dementia, who by now lacks insight into the reasons for the restrictions.

> He's always liked puttering around the house, but he got so that we couldn't trust him not to get hurt or do something that might flood or burn down the house. For example, one day he was building something out of copper pipe, and he was using one of those propane torches to solder with, and he went off and got the mail and was sitting in the house looking through a magazine, and the torch was sitting in the garage blazing away. Fortunately, I went out in the garage and saw it, but he could have burned the house down. So now we don't let him use the torch or any of his power tools unless there's someone there to watch him. He's not at all pleased about it, but that's the way it's got to be.

Physical Dependence. The affected person's physical dependence on caregivers steadily increases as dementia progresses. The person with dementia no longer carries out personal care activities without assistance and must be helped with bathing, dressing, toileting, and grooming. The person's medication regimen must be supervised carefully. Diet and fluid intake must be monitored and adjusted to ensure adequate nutrition and hydration. The affected person's interest in leisure activities declines, and the caregiver becomes the person's primary source of stimulation.

> It's like a 24-hour-a-day-job. There's just no letup. It's up to me to get everything done. Get her up. Get her dressed. Make her meals. It just goes on and on. Sometimes Martha [a daughter] or Fran Elliott [a neighbor] come in and takes over, to give me a break. That helps. But it really wears on a person. To have total responsibility for someone else—it's like carrying this 500-pound weight around on your back, day after day. I don't resent it, and I'm not feeling sorry for myself. But sometimes I wonder if I'm strong enough. Mentally, I mean.

Language and Communication. Communication becomes increasingly one-sided as the person progresses into the middle stages of dementia. The affected person no longer initiates conversations but becomes a passive conversational partner. The person's responses consist primarily of trivialities and automatisms (e.g., *you don't say, gracious sakes*) or tangential comments, but the he or she makes no substantive contribution to either the content or the continuity of the conversation.

We have what you might call conversations, but there's no real connection. You know what I mean? She says things, but it's like there's nothing behind what she says. Thoughtwise, I mean. She's pleasant enough, and I'm sure she's trying, but there's nothing there. No matter what we talk about, she says pretty much the same things. Empty. And like I said, no real connection.

Late Stages

Persons in the late stages of dementia are no longer capable of collaborating in programs to enhance quality of life and to maximize participation in daily life activities. Helping persons at this stage of dementia means helping their caregivers manage troublesome behaviors, ensure the person's health and security, and maintain the person's participation in daily life activities consistent with the person's intellectual and psychologic abilities.

GENERAL CONCEPTS 12-3

- *Rating scales* provide a quick but not very sensitive way to identify the presence of moderate to severe dementia. Detecting mild dementia requires sensitive and reliable tests of cognitive and linguistic performance administered by a qualified professional.
- Most dementia rating scales are designed to provide global estimates of impairment. A few rating scales for estimating the daily life functional independence of persons with dementia have been published.
- The *Arizona Battery for Communication Disorders of Dementia (ABCD)* is a standardized assessment battery for identifying and quantifying the communicative impairments of adults with dementia. Aphasia test batteries and standardized tests of speech, language, and comprehension may be administered to obtain detailed information about the language and communicative abilities of adults with dementia.

- The most sensitive tests for detecting early dementia are tests that require effortful mental processing. Bayles and associates reported that the best combination of tests for detecting mild dementia is delayed story retelling, mental status, pantomime expression, and the Peabody Picture Vocabulary Test.
- In the early stages of dementia, the person's memory lapses, personality changes, and behavioral changes are primarily inconveniences, and caregivers usually find ways to adapt to them or to work around them, often with professional guidance. As the person's dementia progresses, caregiver burden increases as troublesome behaviors become more frequent, the person begins to neglect self-care, and the person's impaired judgment place the person and others at risk. Eventually caregiver burden becomes intolerable, at which time the person is likely to be transferred to an extended care facility.

GENERAL CONCEPTS 12-3—cont'd

- Memory impairments usually are the first symptoms of Alzheimer's dementia. The impairments typically affect declarative memory and prospective memory but largely spare procedural memory. As dementia progresses, memory impairments become more profound, until all aspects of memory are grossly impaired in the very late stages of dementia.

- Persons in the early stages of Alzheimer's dementia retain sufficient language and communicative abilities to get along in daily life, although subtle problems in comprehension and word retrieval may prove annoying. As dementia progresses, comprehension impairments become more obvious, word retrieval failures in speech become more obvious, the person's contributions become less relevant and less efficient, and violations of communicative rules and conventions become more frequent. By the very late stages of dementia, the affected person has lost essentially all volitional communication.

- Many persons with dementia become anxious and depressed, first in response to the diagnosis of dementia and later in response to changes in abilities, social status, and personal relationships. Anxiety and depression often diminish as the dementia progresses and the person becomes less attuned to the environment and to personal relationships.

- Persons in the early stages of dementia often deny or minimize impairments they are aware of. As the dementia progresses, the affected person becomes less aware of impairments and consequently neither denies nor acknowledges them.

- Troublesome behaviors (e.g., wandering, hiding things, aggression) and sleep disturbances begin to appear in the early stages of dementia and increase in frequency and magnitude as the dementia progresses. Troublesome behaviors add to caregiver stress in proportion to the amount of inconvenience or disruption the behaviors create. Helping caregivers manage troublesome behaviors is an important objective of intervention.

- Sometimes persons who have dementia exhibit functional impairments that exceed the limitations imposed by the dementia (excess disability). Excess disability can be caused by coexisting illness, emotional states, medications, and the person's environment, including how they are treated by caregivers. Caregivers may contribute to excess disability by encouraging dependent behavior and discouraging independent behavior (usually unintentionally).

- Sleep disturbances and health problems, including problems with nutrition and fluid intake, often affect persons in the early stage of dementia.

- As a person moves into the middle stages of dementia, the person's awareness of his or her impairments diminishes, troublesome behaviors appear, insight, orientation, and judgment deteriorate, and the person with dementia becomes more dependent on caregivers, who must supervise and assist most activities of daily life.

- Persons in the late stages of dementia no longer are capable of active participation in daily life activities and must depend on caregivers for ensuring their health, safety, and well-being.

INTERVENTION

Early Stages

Intervention for persons in the early stages of dementia represents a three-way collaboration among the affected person, the caregiver, and the clinician. Persons in the early stage of dementia are intensely aware of their impairments and willingly participate in programs to help them compensate for or work around the impairments. Most can identify problems they would like addressed and can help the clinician select intervention strategies. Caregivers participate in planning the intervention program, practice compensatory strategies with the affected person, help to modify the person's daily life environment to facilitate the person's performance, monitor the person's performance, and help with modifications to the intervention program as the person's needs change. The clinician instructs the person with dementia and caregivers about the nature of the person's problems, helps the person with dementia and the caregivers select targets for intervention, directs the design and implementation of the intervention program, and supervises changes in the intervention program as the need arises.

Memory Impairments. The problem for persons in early-stage dementia is with recalling past experiences (*episodic memory,* sometimes called *explicit memory*) and remembering to do things in the present (*prospective memory*) but not with remembering how to do familiar procedures (*procedural memory,* sometimes called *implicit memory*). (Their problem is remembering *that,* not remembering *how.*) Activities that call on implicit memory, such dressing and bathing, typically are less affected by dementia than are activities that call on explicit memory, such as modifying behavior based on previous experience.

Spaced-retrieval training is a memory training procedure in which participants are trained to perform newly taught procedures, recognize newly taught stimuli, or remember to do something at a designated time, with gradually increasing time intervals between training and performance. If the target activity is a procedure, the participant is taught the procedure by demonstration and practice under conditions in which errors are minimized or eliminated (*errorless learning*). Then the time between practice and performance gradually is increased. If the target activity is recall of specific information, the participant is asked to repeat the information immediately after the trainer, who provides cues and prompts to limit or eliminate errors on the part of the participant. Then the time between practice and recall of the information is gradually increased. If the target activity is a prospective-memory task (e.g., remembering to attend a group session at a specified time), the participant is trained to remember to perform the designated activity over progressively longer time intervals.

Camp (1989) first described spaced-retrieval training for persons with dementia. Camp's report was followed by more than a dozen studies, all of which reported improved memory performance by participants (Bird, 2001; Brush & Camp, 1998; Cherry & Simmons-D'Gerolamo, 2004, 2005; Hawley & Cherry, 2004: McKitrick, Camp, & Black, 1992; and others). Hopper, Mahendra, Kim and associates (2005) divided spaced retrieval training approaches into two types. In *cue-behavior association,* participants are trained to perform specified actions (e.g., putting glasses in a case, handing a coupon to the trainer, reading and performing task instructions) in response to verbal or nonverbal cues. In *face/object-name associations,* participants are trained recognize faces or to select objects from an array in response to their spoken names.

Hopper and associates reviewed 15 studies of spaced-retrieval training, all of which reported positive results. Several of the studies also reported that participants retained new learning after delays ranging from several days to 3 months, and a few reported generalization of training across stimuli and contexts. Hopper and associates cautioned, however, that methodologic shortcomings in the studies compromise interpretation of the results.

> Although the results of the reviewed studies were overwhelmingly positive, methodological shortcomings warrant cautious interpretation of the findings. Lack of specification of participant characteristics decreases generalizability of the findings. Also, more attention must be paid to including inter-rater reliability judgments...These judgments are particularly important in treatment studies in which dependent measures are based solely on behavioral observations. (p. xxxii)

Hopper and associates made the following recommendations for clinical practice:

- Candidates for spaced-retrieval training are persons with mild to severe dementia who have declarative memory impairments resulting from dementia and who can engage in structured training tasks.
- Training sessions should be administered weekly or more often and should teach verbal responses and/or skills needed by the person with dementia. Caregivers should be trained in the responses and behaviors expected of the person with dementia to enhance generalization to everyday contexts.
- Spaced-retrieval training may improve the acquisition, retention, and generalization of trained information or skills and may provide for retention of learned information or skills for intervals ranging from 1 day to several months. Spaced-retrieval training is unlikely to improve global cognitive functioning or general memory function.

Errorless learning is an important component of spaced-retrieval training (and of several other approaches to training persons with impaired declarative memory). Baddeley and Wilson (1994) suggested that persons who have impaired declarative memory (which they called *explicit memory*) do not spontaneously eliminate errors during learning, because their explicit-memory impairments prevent them from remembering previous errors and their consequences. Baddeley and Wilson also speculated that repetition of error responses by persons with explicit-memory impairments actually may strengthen the error responses. Errorless learning is designed to capitalize on the preserved implicit memory of persons with dementia and to eliminate interference created by their repetition of error responses.

The basic principle governing errorless learning is that every learning trial must end with a correct response. Ensuring that every learning trial ends with a correct response is believed to exploit implicit memory while minimizing the deleterious effects of explicit-memory impairments. Although the conceptual foundations of errorless learning are consistent with what is known about learning, memory, and dementia, the evidence for its effectiveness relative to other interventions consists primarily of opinion, anecdote, and a few case studies. Well-controlled clinical trials to document the true value of errorless learning have yet to be reported.

External Memory Aids. External memory aids help persons with dementia compensate for impaired prospective memory. *Electronic organizers* (personal information managers) with built-in alarms help with prospective memory by signaling the person with dementia and displaying textual reminders of appointments and other time-based responsibilities. *Pocket-sized checklists* remind the person with dementia of scheduled obligations which the person can check off when the obligations are satisfied.

Some external memory aids help with declarative memory—usually with memory for personal information (e.g., addresses, phone numbers, names, dates). Bourgeois (1990) described the use of *memory books* and *memory wallets* (pocket-sized books) for persons who have dementia but who can read and retrieve items of information from printed materials. Memory books may contain personal information,

Today is June 27, 2006

Things to do today.

10:00   Dentist appointment
12:00   Lunch
2:00   Exercise class
4:00   Pick up mail
5:00   Watch TV news
6:00   Dinner
8:00   Watch Lawrence Welk on TV

Our address is 612 Carefree Way
Our telephone number is (944) 222-4344
Our son's name is Ben Smith
Our son's phone number is (944) 234-5677
Our daughter's name is Andrea Gannon
Our daughter's phone number is (828) 434-8777
Our doctor's name is Dr. Gambel
Doctor Gambel's phone number is (944) 222-8965

Figure 12-9 ■ A page from a typical memory book for use by a person with dementia.

photographs of family members or familiar locations, printed sentences relating to the person's daily life, or other personal material. The books provide cues and context for persons with dementia and a source of topics for conversational partners of persons with dementia. Figure 12-9 shows a page from a typical memory book.

Bourgeois (1990, 1992) reported that providing memory books to persons with dementia improved the factual content of their conversation and that the improvements were maintained across time. Bourgeois also noted that users did not require extensive training in the use of the memory books. Most began using their memory book immediately after getting the book and receiving an explanation of how it could be used. The scope and complexity of the information included in memory books can be matched to the person's needs and abilities and can be adjusted as the person's ability to use them changes. Caregivers and family members should be trained to help the memory book user use the book to facilitate conversations and promote self-care.

Bourgeois (1992) reported that providing memory books diminished the daily life frequency of memory-related problem behaviors, such as repeated questions and demands. Caregivers were trained to respond to repeated questions or demands by directing the person with dementia to the memory book or to printed messages on a memo board or card. Caregivers reported that redirection lessened the frequency of repeated questions and demands. Bourgeois also cited anecdotal reports from caregivers suggesting that some persons using a memory aid spontaneously learned to use it to avoid asking a question or repeating a demand.

Bourgeois, Camp, Rose, and associates (2003) reported that persons with mild to moderate dementia can be trained to make use of external memory aids by spaced-retrieval training and by structured cueing hierarchies. In spaced-retrieval training, participants were trained to use external memory aids (e.g., a list of daily activities) with gradually increasing time intervals between clinician prompts (e.g., *"What can you do to know what activity you should do?"*) until the participant made the correct target response (e.g., *"Look at my memory book."*) to the clinician's first prompt in three consecutive sessions spaced 24 hours apart. In cueing-hierarchy training, participants were trained with a standard hierarchy of cues of increasing power until the participant made the correct target response to the clinician's first prompt in three consecutive sessions spaced 24 hours apart. Both training methods were effective in training participants to perform the targeted behaviors, although spaced-retrieval training appeared to be slightly more effective. Bourgeois and associates concluded that external aids can be used successfully by persons with dementia if well-structured strategy training for their use is provided.

Modifying the person's daily life environment can help most persons in the early to middle stages of dementia cope with declining memory. Some environmental modifications target prospective memory:

- A schedule of activities that remains constant from day to day
- An alarm watch worn by the person or an alarm clock set to sound when it is time to perform given activities (often accompanied by a checklist to permit the person to keep track of which activities have been completed)
- Checklists posted in strategic locations to remind persons to accomplish scheduled activities and to permit them to check off completed activities (e.g., checklists next to exit doors listing things the person is to do when leaving, such as turning off lights, closing windows, and getting the car keys)

Some environmental modifications help the person with procedural memory:

- Items used in an activity are kept together (e.g., coffee pot, filters, and coffee are kept on the same shelf). Arranging the items in the order they are used helps some persons keep procedural steps in order.
- Checklists for complex procedures are posted where the procedure is to be accomplished. Steps in the procedure are listed in chronologic order (e.g., the steps in sorting the laundry, washing the clothes, and drying the clothes are posted next to the washer).

Bourgeois (1991) identified several advantages of external memory aids for persons with dementia:

- External memory aids are useful in daily life, and their use by the person elicits natural positive reinforcement.

- External memory aids enhance the person's interaction with the environment by providing many opportunities for daily use.
- External memory aids can be modified to meet the changing needs of the person with dementia or his or her caregivers or to accommodate changes in the person's ability to use them.
- External memory aids are tangible, permanent prompting mechanisms that are immediately accessible to the person with dementia.

Bourgeois also commented that the best self-prompting memory aids are likely to be those the person used before developing dementia, because using the old memory aid may be in the person's repertoire of automatic skills. Portable memory aids are useful, however, only if the person remembers to use the aid. Consequently, their usefulness typically disappears by the time the person is in the late stages of dementia.

Confusion. Intermittent episodes of confusion often occur during the early stages of dementia. The first episodes are frightening to the person with dementia and worrisome to family members, although they do not seriously compromise the person's safety or well-being. As dementia progresses and episodes of confusion increase in frequency and magnitude, the episodes may threaten the person's safety (e.g., the person gets lost and ends up in an unsafe neighborhood, drives the wrong way down a one-way street, or takes medications intended for another family member). Managing confusion is an important aspect of intervention for persons in the early stages of dementia. When confusion can no longer be managed adequately, restrictions on the person's independence and freedom of movement become necessary. Many of the procedures for managing memory impairments also make persons with dementia less vulnerable to confusion, but strategies that focus more directly on confusion may be useful:

- A large calendar may be posted in a highly visible location. The person with dementia then circles the correct day upon arising in the morning. If the person cannot remember to do this, caregivers may do it.

- The person with dementia wears a watch that shows the date and time with AM and PM indicated.
- Doors and drawers in cabinets, dressers, and bureaus are labeled with their contents.
- Personal possessions are kept in a consistent location and put back when not in use.
- Maps and printed instructions depicting familiar routes are prepared and given to the person with dementia before she or he sets out.
- The person carries a card on which are printed constructive responses to disorientation (e.g., *Stop. Stay calm. Think about where you came from and where you are going. Look around for helpful cues, such as street signs and house numbers. Try retracing your path until you see something familiar. If you are still confused, ask someone for help.*).

Every adult should carry an identification card showing the person's name, address, home telephone number, and the name of someone to notify in case of emergency. Adults with dementia should carry a card with that information, plus the names and telephone numbers of several close relatives or caregivers.

Impaired Communication. Persons who are in the early stages of dementia remain functional communicators in most everyday situations, although subtle problems with word retrieval and impaired comprehension of spoken and printed materials may prove annoying to the affected person and to caregivers. Persons in the early stages of dementia typically are acutely aware of their communicative miscues and readily cooperate with remedial programs. These individuals can learn strategies to prevent, work around, or repair communicative mishaps, provided that the strategies do not demand greater

mental flexibility, creativity, attention, and memory than the person has available.

Some communicative strategies can be characterized as *adaptive* (Clark & Witte, 1990). *Adaptive strategies* are used to regain control when communication failure occurs. The person who fails to understand a spoken message might ask the speaker to repeat the message, speak more slowly, or write it. The person who has difficulty finding words or problems organizing speech output might ask the listener for help (e.g., *Bear with me and give me a little more time. I'm having difficulty organizing my thoughts.*). The person who loses track of the topic of a conversation might ask the conversational partner to remind them of the topic (e.g., *I seem to have lost my train of thought. What was it we were talking about?*).

An appealing characteristic of adaptive behaviors such as these is that they do not strike conversational partners as abnormal, because they resemble what normal adults do when they stumble in a conversation. The major hindrance to their use by persons with early-stage dementia is the person's reluctance to engage in behaviors that might mark them as impaired. Persuasion may be needed to get the person to try the strategies, but once he or she discovers how much easier it is to use the strategies than to expend energy on concealment and to bear the consequences of communication failure, persuasion no longer is needed.

Other communication strategies are *facilitative* (Clark & Witte, 1990). *Facilitative strategies* are used to prevent or repair communication failure. Facilitative strategies allow persons with dementia to circumvent communication breakdown caused by word retrieval failure, comprehension impairments, and compromised ability to organize and communicate thoughts coherently. A person who experiences word retrieval failure might circumlocute (e.g., *I had the letter all ready to go, but I didn't have a...with flaps...you lick it and seal it...an envelope.*), use semantic self-cueing (e.g., *My wife doesn't want me to drive so she hides the lock... ring...lock...keys.*), or use phonemic self-cueing (e.g., *They played hard, but they lost the team...tame...game.*).

Clark and Witte recommend what they call *script strategies* to help persons with early-stage dementia maintain topic and cohesion in spoken discourse. The person learning a script strategy is trained to organize spoken discourse according to the parts of a story (theme, setting, characters, events, actions, consequences, and outcomes). However, many persons with mild dementia may be overwhelmed by the terminology and the memory demands of the script strategy. Giving them a set of questions makes it easier: *What is it about? Where did it happen? Who was there? What happened? What is the point?* The questions can be printed on a card if the person has difficulty remembering them or keeping them in order.

Clark and Witte recommend what they call *life-experience strategies* to help persons who have difficulty expressing abstract ideas. By illustrating abstract ideas with life experiences, persons with dementia may convey the abstract character of their ideas without explicitly conveying the abstraction. For example, a person who wishes to communicate the concept of *trust* might say:

> When I was young I knew I could always depend on Mom and Dad. Even when I didn't agree with them I knew that they wanted what was best for me and would never mean to do anything to hurt me. That's an important thing to have between people.

Group Activities. Group activities may be a useful addition to intervention programs for persons in the early stages of dementia. Rationales and procedures differ across programs, but all share similar goals:

- Stimulate self-expression
- Stimulate cognitive processes
- Promote social interaction
- Enhance feelings of self-worth

Structured group activities may provide a comfortable environment in which persons with dementia can try out newly acquired communicative strategies. Group activities may provide a supportive climate in which to talk about problems, feelings, and emotions. Group activities may provide a venue in which stories of success and failure may be shared. Group activities may enhance feelings of self-esteem and self-worth by helping participants feel that they are actively helping themselves and other group participants. Group activities may stimulate participants' remaining intellect by involving them in activities such as planning trips or outings, discussing problems, role-playing daily life situations, and playing games such as *password* or *twenty questions.*

Support groups for families and caregivers are an important part of intervention in the early stages of dementia. Participants in family and caregiver support groups may be provided with information about the nature and course of dementia, support in dealing with the emotional effects of a family member's dementia, guidance in accessing community services and resources, and information about how to maintain and enhance the functional abilities of the person with dementia. Support groups often work to reduce caregivers' sense of social isolation by increasing the quantity and quality of caregivers' social contacts, and support groups often provide advice, instruction, and training in problem-solving, behavior management, and adaptive techniques.

Brodaty, Green, and Koschera (2003) and Cooke, McNally, Mulligan, and associates (2001) reviewed published studies of support groups (which they called *psychosocial interventions*) for caregivers of persons with dementia. Cooke and associates concluded that the reviewed studies provided "little evidence that interventions consistently produce positive benefits for dementia caregivers in terms of improved psychological well-being, burden, or social outcomes" (p. 132). Brodaty and associates concluded that caregiver interventions "have modest but significant effects on caregiver knowledge, psychological morbidity, and other main outcome measures (such as coping skills and social support)" (p. 663), although they found many limitations in the scientific quality of the studies they reviewed. Both groups saw the need for improvements in the quality of studies of psychosocial support for caregivers. Cooke and associates commented, "In order to advance our understanding, a systematic approach to investigations of interventions with caregivers

is required, where components are carefully contrasted in appropriately designed studies of sufficient size" (p. 132). Neither group concluded that psychosocial intervention for caregivers has no value, but both concluded that there is little strong evidence confirming its value. As is true for many other interventions for persons with dementia and their caregivers, there is an urgent need for well-designed studies to establish the value of psychosocial interventions for caregivers of persons with dementia.

GENERAL CONCEPTS 12-4

- Activities that call on implicit (procedural) memory are less affected by dementia than are activities that call on explicit (declarative) memory.
- The effects of early-stage dementia memory impairments may be lessened by teaching compensatory memory strategies, by providing portable memory aids, and by modifying the environment to provide prompts and cues that lessen the effects of the memory impairments on the person's daily life.
- *Spaced-retrieval training* is a memory training procedure in which participants learn to perform procedures, recognize stimuli, or remember to do an assigned task with gradually increasing time intervals between training and performance.
- Errorless learning is an important aspect of many interventions for persons with impaired explicit memory. Errorless learning is designed to capitalize on the preserved implicit memory of persons with dementia and to eliminate interference created by their repetition of error responses.
- External memory aids (e.g., memory books, to-do lists, etc.) help many persons with

dementia compensate for impaired declarative and prospective memory.
- Organizing the living environments of persons with dementia by increasing predictability and regularity may help them cope with impaired memory.
- Confusion can be lessened by controlling the person's environment and providing prompts and cues to enhance orientation.
- *Adaptive* and *facilitative* communicative strategies may help persons with early-stage dementia maintain communicative abilities. *Script* strategies may help persons with early-stage dementia maintain topic and cohesion in discourse. *Life-experience* strategies may help persons with early-stage dementia express abstract ideas.
- *Group treatment* is a common component of intervention programs for early-stage dementia patients. The goals of group treatment usually include stimulating self-expression and cognitive processes, promoting social interaction, and enhancing patient feelings of self-worth.

Middle Stages

As the person with dementia progresses into the middle stages, caregiver burden increases. The affected person becomes less able to monitor behavior and to adjust it to the needs of others. Behavioral conflicts between the affected person and the caregiver increase in frequency and magnitude. The person's ability to remember and use previously acquired compensatory strategies declines. Environmental modifications that once helped the person compensate for impaired attention and memory lose their power. The person's awareness of impairments declines, and she or he no longer is capable of active participation in intervention programs. Intervention goals change from helping the person find ways to compensate for impairments to helping caregivers find ways to keep the person physically and mentally active and oriented, to promote the person's psychologic well-being, and to facilitate communication between the person with dementia and caregivers.

Intervention now requires collaboration between the clinician and caregivers. The caregivers and the clinician work together to identify targets for intervention and to rank them in order of importance. Targets for intervention include behaviors that caregivers wish to modify or control and skills caregivers wish to maintain or enhance. When targets for intervention have been selected, the clinician and caregivers work together to devise procedures to accomplish the objectives of intervention. Then caregivers practice the procedures, and the clinician monitors and gives feedback and advice. The intervention procedures are modified and adjusted based on caregivers' experiences and are organized into a comprehensive intervention program. Caregivers put the program into operation, and the clinician monitors the results and suggests alterations and adjustments as needed.

Environmental control becomes increasingly important as the person with dementia is governed less and less by internal reasoning and judgment and more and more by the external environment. Environmental prompts and cues that previously helped the person with dementia compensate for impairments lose their power as she or he becomes increasingly inattentive to the prompts and cues and becomes increasingly distracted by incidental stimuli. Maintaining environmental control requires intensification of stimuli that govern the affected person's behavior. Environmental cues are made more striking. Color and attention-getting graphics are added to checklists, posters, signs, and calendars. Caregivers increasingly direct the person's attention toward environmental prompts and cues.

As the ability to remember and use adaptive and compensatory strategies declines, intervention focuses on preserving the affected person's use of the most effective strategies. The remaining strategies may be simplified, and more powerful external cues may be incorporated to keep them within the person's repertoire.

As impairments become more pronounced, supervision increases, and the affected person's independence in risky activities is curtailed. Control of major financial decisions is assumed by caregivers, but the person with dementia may be permitted the freedom to make routine financial decisions (e.g., spending on incidental self-care items or personal clothing) in consultation with caregivers.

Managing Troublesome Behaviors. Caregivers for persons in the middle and late stages of dementia face numerous problems related to the person's declining intellect, exaggerated mood swings, and changes in behavior. Although the decline in the affected person's abilities cannot be arrested or reversed, the effects of intellectual impairments can be minimized, mood swings can be diminished, and distressing behaviors often can be controlled or eliminated by environmental manipulation and behavior management techniques similar to those used with severely impaired traumatically brain-injured adults.

Combative, aggressive, and accusatory behaviors rank high on caregivers' lists of problems as the person reaches the middle stages of dementia. Caregivers are better equipped to manage the person's problem behaviors if they understand that emotional outbursts, aggression, and physical attacks often are predictable, based on previous incidents, that they frequently are preceded by warning signs, and that they often represent the person's response to being pushed beyond his or her ability to deal with a situation or event. Many times such outbursts can be eliminated by removing their precipitating stimuli.

> A man with dementia became violently angry when he saw his wife paying the monthly bills, perhaps because he felt that she was usurping his role as head of the household. The wife realized what precipitated her husband's outbursts and began paying the bills while her husband took his usual morning nap. This change in routine eliminated the outbursts.

Warning signs can be diverse and tend to be idiosyncratic. They range from subtle signs such as increased body rigidity, aversion of gaze, or increased respiration rate to more obvious behaviors such as crying and arguing. Teaching caregivers to recognize such warning signs and to respond to them by slowing the pace of the activity, doing something else, or diverting the person's attention can reduce the frequency of such outbursts.

If caregivers understand that emotional outbursts of the person with dementia may be an involuntary response to demanding or too-difficult situations, their responses to the outbursts are likely to change in constructive ways. They are less likely to regard the person as stubborn and uncooperative and are less likely to see the person's emotional outbursts as a personal affront. They are more likely to look for what pushed the person out of control and are more likely to eliminate or control the precipitating stimuli. Understanding that accusations and suspicion may be the person's attempts to account for misplaced possessions, forgotten appointments, and unexpected changes in routine may lead caregivers to increase the predictability and orderliness of the person's environment, rather than argue with the person about the accuracy of the person's suspicions.

Finally, caregivers should know that hostile and aggressive behavior can be caused by physical pain or illness and that persons with dementia who exhibit sudden increases in aggressive behavior may need medical evaluation. Because some medications may cause increased aggressiveness, changes in mood or diminished tolerance for frustration that occur when medications are begun or dosages changed should be evaluated by a physician. Sometimes medication may be prescribed to control violent behavior, but because of their depressive effects on alertness and general mental functioning, they should be prescribed only when behavioral methods fail to provide sufficient control.

Mace and Rabins (1991) described six ways in which caregivers may manage disruptive behaviors and maintain appropriate behavior for persons who are in the middle to late stages of dementia. They call their suggestions *The Six Rs of Behavior Management:*

- **Restrict.** If the person is doing something undesirable, try to get her or him to stop, especially if the person might harm self or others. Do not be confrontational or argumentative. Be calm and reasonable.

- **Reassess.** Ask yourself: Might a physical illness or drug reaction be causing the problem? Is the person having difficulty seeing or hearing? Is something upsetting the person? Can the annoying situation or person be removed? Would a different approach upset the person less?

- **Reconsider.** Imagine how things seem from the person's point of view. It is understandable that a person becomes upset when things happen that do not make sense.

- **Rechannel.** Look for a way that the behavior can continue in a safe and nondestructive way. The behavior may be important to the person in a way that we do not understand.
- **Reassure.** Take time to reassure the person that things are all right and that you still care for her or him. Take time to reassure yourself that you are doing the best you can in a difficult and demanding situation.
- **Review.** Afterward, think about what happened and how you managed it. What can you learn from this experience that will help you next time? What led up to the behavior? How did you respond to it? What did you do right? What might you try next time?

Communication. As the person progresses into the middle stages of dementia, communication strategies previously used by the person to compensate for impaired comprehension and word finding are neglected or forgotten and the person becomes less and less capable of managing communicative interactions. Automatisms and stereotypic utterances become more frequent; the informational content of the person's speech declines; and the person has difficulty following the gist of everyday conversations. The person rattles on about trivial past events and neglects conversational behaviors such as turn-taking and eye contact. Reminding the person to use previously learned communicative strategies may have transitory effects on the person's communicative behavior, but the effects soon evaporate, leaving the person rattling on and the caregiver frustrated.

Because many persons in the middle stages of dementia cannot acquire new communicative strategies and because many cannot dependably use previously learned strategies, intervention often focuses on preserving the person's residual communicative abilities to the extent permitted by the person's declining intellect.

The focus of intervention now shifts away from training the person to use communicative strategies and toward stimulating the person, maintaining the person's remaining communica-

tive abilities, and preserving the person's interest in communicating. Intervention is now caregiver-centered. The caregiver carries out the day-to-day requirements of the intervention program. The clinician trains the caregiver, monitors progress, gives encouragement and advice, and helps the caregiver modify the intervention program as the affected person's communicative abilities change.

The clinician helps the caregiver make the transition from communicative partner to facilitator and supporter of the affected person's communicative behavior. The traditional concept of communication as a two-way exchange of information is revised to emphasize the role of communication in maintaining the relationship between the caregiver and the person with dementia, maintaining the person's ability to communicate, and preserving the person's willingness to participate in communicative interactions. The caregiver no longer arranges conversations to orient the person or to train him or her to use compensatory strategies, although if the person uses previously learned strategies, the caregiver reinforces their use. Instead of instructing, training, and correcting, the caregiver behaves in the following way:

- The caregiver accepts the person's contributions at face value. The caregiver treats the person as a conversational partner whose ideas and opinions are important, although what the person says may not make complete sense. The caregiver does not correct, argue, or test the person by asking him or her to repeat what the caregiver has said. The caregiver may restate, repeat, or paraphrase *some* of the person's contributions to verify the person's communicative intent.
- The caregiver adapts her or his contributions to the comprehension level of the person with dementia. The caregiver keeps sentences short, uses simple and concrete vocabulary, and puts only one idea in each sentence. The caregiver speaks slowly and distinctly (but not artificially) and adds redundancy to

utterances by repeating key elements and paraphrasing information. The caregiver clearly establishes the topic at the beginning of conversations and repeats or paraphrases the topic periodically thereafter, or whenever the person with dementia seems to be losing the topic. The caregiver clearly signals topic changes (e.g., *Now let's talk about something different. Let me tell you about...*).

- The caregiver encourages participation of the person with dementia by periodically asking for her or his opinion and by asking questions that can be answered in a few words and that limit the number of alternative responses from which the person must choose. Two-choice questions (yes/no, either/or) are useful, but caregivers must use them sparingly, because overuse may turn the conversation into a drill.

- The caregiver communicates respect for the person with dementia and interest in what the person contributes. Demonstrating respect and interest often proves a more powerful incentive for the person's participation in conversations than positive comments following individual utterances.

- The caregiver sets aside consistent times every day for structured conversation with the person who has dementia. The caregiver chooses topics that are relevant and interesting to the person and to which the person is likely to have something to contribute. If the person reads and gets some information from newspaper or magazine articles, the caregiver may select an article the person has read and add props such as photographs or illustrations to increase interest and enhance participation. The caregiver may use photographs or personal memorabilia relating to significant life experiences to stimulate the affected person's desire to communicate. The caregiver may guide these conversations but does not overtly attempt to control the relevance or accuracy of what the person with dementia says. However, the caregiver may guide the person in less obvious ways, such as by repeating main ideas in a conversational manner.

- The caregiver ensures that incidental communicative interchanges (e.g., comments, rhetorical questions, exclamations, and the like) are not neglected. Off-hand comments (e.g., *I'm so tired today.*), rhetorical questions (e.g., *Is it going to rain, I wonder?*), exclamations (e.g., *What a miserably hot day!*), and the like are a common part of the everyday life of adults who live together. When the person with dementia neither initiates such incidental interchanges nor overtly responds to them, caregivers are likely to forgo them, further isolating the person from the daily give-and-take that is an important part of normal adult-to-adult relationships.

Group Activities. Group activities provide structured stimulation and structured interactions for persons in the middle stages of dementia. Group activities for persons in the middle stages of dementia who live at home typically are offered at day treatment centers, rehabilitation centers, university clinics, and the outpatient departments of some medical facilities. Group activities for these individuals usually have the following goals:

- Preserve orientation
- Stimulate cognitive processes
- Preserve and stimulate communicative abilities
- Reinforce appropriate interpersonal behavior

Reminiscence Activities. Reminiscence is often used in group activities to facilitate communication for persons in the middle to late stages of dementia. Reminiscence activities are designed to capitalize on participants' remote memory, which usually is preserved until the very late stages of dementia. Reminiscence activities combine verbal stimulation with visual and auditory materials such as photographs, maps, newspaper clippings, music, personal possessions, and sound effects to facilitate and enhance communication among group members. Activities often are organized around significant historical events (e.g., the Great Depression of the 1930s) or topics (e.g., pets).

Typically the group leader (often a speech-language pathologist) asks each group member to talk about what they remember about the topic. Participants and the group leader encourage and reinforce participants' contributions, and the group leader provides prompts and cues as needed.

Kim, Cleary, Hopper, and associates (2006) reviewed 6 studies of reminiscence therapy for persons with dementia published between 1987 and 2002. Kim and associates listed several methodologic concerns related to the studies:

- Lack of control groups, small groups of study participants, nonrandom assignment of participants to groups, participant attrition, poor control of procedures, inadequate descriptions of study participants
- Subjective judgments of outcome, in which facilitation depended on the facilitator's skill and rapport with group members
- Failure to report inter-rater reliability regarding treatment implementation or data collection
- Failure to ensure that raters did not know when participants were receiving reminiscence therapy
- Failure to establish causal relationships between treatments and outcomes

Despite these shortcomings Kim and associates offered the following conclusions:

- Group reminiscence therapy may contribute to improved cognitive functioning as measured by the *Mini Mental State Examination.*
- Group reminiscence therapy may contribute to improved discourse.
- Group reminiscence therapy may contribute to increased well-being in persons with dementia and their caregivers.
- The social nature of the activities may be an important factor in promoting positive outcomes related to cognition, communication, and well-being.

Kim and associates considered reminiscence therapy appropriate for persons who have episodic memory impairments caused by mild to moderate progressive dementia, have some ability to participate in verbal communication, can attend to and tolerate social interaction without disrupting group activities, and have vision and hearing adequate for reminiscence therapy activities.

Following a comprehensive search of major healthcare databases, Woods, Spector, Jones, and associates (2005) found four published studies of reminiscence therapy that reported objective data and met basic criteria for experimental controls. They noted that the results of the four studies suggested significant improvements in participants' cognition, mood, and behavior following intervention, together with lessened caregiver strain and increased caregiver knowledge of participants' backgrounds, but they concluded with the following cautionary statement:

> Although there were a number of promising indications, in view of the limited number and quantity of studies, the variation in types of reminiscence work reported, and the variation in types of reminiscence work, the review highlights the urgent need for more and better-designed trials so that more robust conclusions may be drawn. (p. 2)

GENERAL CONCEPTS 12-5

- As a person with dementia moves into the middle stages of dementia, reliance on compensatory strategies declines, and environmental control becomes increasingly important.
- Aggressive and accusatory behaviors usually become important concerns as a person progresses into the middle stages of dementia. Helping caregivers understand why these behaviors occur and providing them with the means to control the behaviors is an important part of intervention for persons in the middle stages of dementia.

Continued

GENERAL CONCEPTS 12-5—cont'd

- In the middle and late stages of a person's dementia, the purposes of communication between the caregiver and the person with dementia become to stimulate the person, to maintain the person's remaining communicative abilities, and to preserve the person's interest in communicating. Communication no longer serves the traditional purpose of exchange of information, and the caregiver no longer uses communication to orient the person with dementia or to teach the person new strategies. The caregiver treats the person as a conversational partner whose contributions are important regardless of their accuracy or relevance.

- *Reminiscence activities* often are used to facilitate communication in group activities for persons in the middle to late stages of dementia. Reminiscence activities combine verbal stimulation with visual and auditory materials such as photographs, newspaper clippings, music, and personal possessions to facilitate and enhance communication among group members.

Late Stages

Helping Caregivers of Persons with Late-Stage Dementia Who Live at Home. The focus of intervention for caregivers of persons with late-stage dementia who live at home is on environmental control and management of behavioral contingencies. (Most persons with late-stage dementia are cared for in nursing homes or other extended-care facilities. Clinical management for these individuals is discussed in the following section.) The objective of at-home care for persons with late-stage dementia is to maintain the person's ability to carry out familiar and well-learned daily life routines and to help the person participate in life experiences to the extent permitted by the person's cognitive and physical abilities.

A structured approach to at-home care is important. The caregiver and the clinician make a list of behavioral routines that caregivers would like to see the person with dementia maintain, then rank the list in order of importance to the person and the caregiver. The list is limited to simple and highly familiar everyday routines the person with dementia has practiced repeatedly throughout adulthood (e.g., bathing, brushing teeth, hanging up clothes). A small set of target routines is selected from the highest ranked items, and an intervention program is formulated. The intervention program focuses on eliciting the routines by means of environmental stimuli and maintaining the behaviors in the routines by applying contingencies to the behaviors.

Environmental cues are used to elicit the routines. The person's daily life environment may be modified to make naturally occurring cues more prominent (e.g., placing the person's toothbrush and toothpaste on the bathroom counter where the person will see them on arising), or new and salient cues may be invoked to elicit the desired routine (e.g., taping to the bathroom mirror a colored picture of a person brushing teeth). The person's completion of behavioral routines may be reinforced by natural consequences (the toothpaste tastes good and the person's mouth feels clean) but may require additional contingencies provided by caregivers (e.g., *I see you brushed your teeth. That's great! Because you did such a good job, I have a special treat for you at breakfast.*).

Intervention and Management for Institutionalized Persons with Dementia

Numerous programs for maintaining and enhancing the cognitive, communicative, and social functioning of institutionalized persons with dementia have been described in the literature. Although the specifics differ, most fall into one of two general categories. One category *(environmental manipulation)* consists of programs that manipulate the characteristics of the living environment to maintain and enhance the person's cognitive status, communicative competence, and social participation. The other category *(behavior management)* consists of programs that manipulate specific response-eliciting stimuli and response contingencies to increase the frequency of desired behaviors and to diminish the frequency of undesired behaviors. Although designed primarily for institutionalized persons in the middle to late stages of dementia, most of the principles and procedures of these programs should be useful for persons with middle-stage to late-stage dementia who are cared for in the home.

Environmental Manipulation

Reality Orientation. Perhaps the oldest and most common approach to management of institutionalized persons with dementia is called *reality orientation. Reality orientation* seeks to preserve and enhance cognitive functioning and social adequacy by repeatedly exposing persons with dementia to information about the daily life environment (e.g., what day it is, what the weather is like, activities for the day). The information is provided orally by staff during interactions with residents and is posted in printed and/or pictorial form at strategic locations. Reality orientation is designed to help residents attend to and remember environmental information by repeatedly stimulating them with the information, usually in both spoken and printed form and enhanced by bright colors, attention-getting graphics, and so forth.

Numerous anecdotal reports suggest that reality orientation enhances orientation and promotes appropriate social interactions for persons with dementia, provided that several criteria are met:

- The orientation information is not too complex. Few persons with significant dementia attend to or understand complex printed lists, schedules, and instructions.
- Each posted informational item presents a single piece of information in an attention-getting format. Persons with dementia are more likely to attend to the information if it is enhanced with vivid color and illustrated with appealing drawings.
- Caregivers ensure that persons with dementia attend to the information. Training caregivers to routinely call attention to orientation information is crucial.
- The information is accessible to the person with dementia when the person needs it. A poster in the lounge that gives the schedule of activities for the day will not help a person who is elsewhere in the facility and needs to know what is on the schedule.
- The information is actually relevant to the person with dementia. It may be less important that the person know that the date is March 21 than to know that a party is scheduled for 2:00 that afternoon.

Milieu Therapy. Milieu therapy sometimes is combined with reality orientation. *Milieu therapy* endeavors to enhance alertness and increase appropriate social behavior by making the environment more interesting and more conducive to social interactions. Environmental changes in milieu therapy range from simple adjustments such as providing refreshments during activity periods to more complex changes such as rearranging furniture, adding plants, pictures, and other decorative items, introducing pets, and providing conversational partners.

A few controlled studies have shown that milieu therapy can increase the frequency of socially appropriate behaviors (Blackman, Hoover, & Pinkston, 1976; Quatrocchi-Tubin & Jason, 1980). However, Cartensen and Erickson (1986) report that although milieu therapy may increase the frequency of appropriate behaviors (e.g., sitting quietly, speaking, listening, touching), it also may increase the frequency of inappropriate behavior (e.g., bizarre, nonsensical utterances, verbal harassment and threats, physical violence). It may be necessary to combine milieu therapy with behavior management to ensure that desired behaviors are enhanced, and undesired behaviors are minimized.

Functional Maintenance Intervention. As the label suggests, *functional maintenance intervention* is designed to slow or prevent deterioration of function in persons with dementia. Functional maintenance programs are common in long-term care facilities, where they specify the way in which skilled rehabilitation services are provided to residents, including residents who have dementia. Functional maintenance programs are short-term interventions designed and monitored by clinicians and carried out by staff and caregivers. Functional maintenance programs are individualized interventions that require (1) assessing the individual's current abilities and needs, (2) designing an intervention program to maintain maximum functioning, and (3) training staff and caregivers to carry out the program. Clinicians monitor the effects of the program and may periodically modify the program to accommodate the changing needs of the recipient. Speech-language pathologists often design and implement programs to preserve an individual's ability to communicate basic needs and to interact with staff and others. The U.S. Healthcare Financing Administration (HCFA), which oversees Medicare and Medicaid, requires that a functional maintenance program must relate to a decline in the recipient's functional status, that intervention is required to maintain gains from rehabilitation, and that there is a reasonable expectation of improvement as a result of intervention. If these requirements are not met, HCFA will deny reimbursement.

Montessori-Based Intervention. *Montessori-based intervention* is based on the philosophy and educational methods of Maria Montessori. Montessori-based methods for persons with dementia are designed to maintain and enhance physical, cognitive, and social abilities. Activities are designed to capitalize on preserved procedural (implicit) memory abilities of persons with dementia by guiding the person through activities designed to enhance sustained attention, facilitate adaptive behavior, and encourage socially appropriate behavior. Participants may engage in activities such as constructing words and sentences from anagram tiles, sorting pictures or objects according to specified rules, constructing designs with colored tiles, and reading stories and answering story-related questions. There is limited, primarily anecdotal evidence suggesting that Montessori-based intervention is effective in facilitating participation in daily living activities for persons with dementia (Camp, Judge, Bye, & associates, 1997; Gorzell, Kaiser, & Camp, 2003; Orsulic-Jeras, Judge, & Camp, 2000), but as this is written, no controlled large-scale investigations of its effectiveness have been published.

Simulated Presence Therapy. *Simulated presence therapy* is a patented, commercially marketed program in which a family member or someone well-known to the person with dementia makes an audiotape recording of positive events in the life of the person with dementia. The person with dementia wears a hip-pack containing a continuous play audiotape player and listens to the tape through headphones. A few studies of simulated presence therapy have been published (Camberg, Woods, Ooi, & associates, 1999; Miller, Vermeersch, Bohan, & associates, 2001; Peak & Cheston, 2002; Woods & Ashley, 1995).

Woods and Ashley (1995) concluded that simulated presence therapy lessens agitated behavior and increases social interaction but does not affect aggressive behaviors. Peak and Cheston (2002) reported reduced anxiety and increased social interaction for three participants, but worsened well-being for a fourth participant. Woods, Ooi, and associates (1999) reported significantly reduced agitation in a group of 54 persons with dementia who received simulated presence therapy.

In a review of simulated presence therapy, Bales, Kim, Chapman, and associates (2006) concluded that it has "positive effects" on agitated and withdrawn behaviors of persons with moderate to severe dementia and noted that simulated presence therapy appears most effective for persons who have retained communication skills. Livingston, Johnston, Katona, and associates (2005) were less positive about the benefits of simulated presence therapy. After reviewing published studies of simulated presence therapy, they gave it a rating of *D*, which denotes *expert opinion without explicit critical appraisal, or based on physiology, bench research or general principles, rather than the results of controlled clinical trials.*

Behavior Management. Whereas environmental manipulation seeks to affect the overall level of orientation, cognitive status, communication, and social participation of persons with dementia, behavior management focuses on specific categories of behavior to diminish undesirable behaviors (e.g., shouting, hitting, wandering) and to augment desirable behaviors (e.g., bathing, grooming, participating in activities). Behavior management relies heavily on the consequences for responses. Positive consequences may be delivered contingent on instances of desirable behaviors *(positive reinforcement),* and negative consequences may be delivered contingent on instance of undesirable behaviors *(punishment).* Positive reinforcement may use intangible consequences such as caregiver praise and attention or coupons that may be exchanged for items such as sweets, cigarettes, or trinkets. Punishment may entail removal of positive consequences contingent on specified behaviors (called *negative reinforcement*), intervals of time-out in which the person with dementia is ignored or isolated, verbal reproof, or a combination of several negative consequences.

Sometimes undesirable behaviors may be controlled or eliminated by providing positive consequences for behaviors that are incompatible with the undesirable behaviors. For example, a person with dementia who wanders might receive positive consequences for participating in games, hobbies, or group activities. Positively reinforcing a desired behavior that is incompatible with an undesirable behavior and negatively reinforcing the undesirable behavior may have stronger effects on behavior than either positive reinforcement or negative reinforcement alone.

No large-scale, well-controlled studies confirm the effectiveness of behavior management for adults in the middle to late stages of dementia, although several small-group and single-case studies suggest that behavior management procedures are effective in diminishing the frequency of specific undesired behaviors and increasing the frequency of specific desired behaviors (Allen-Burge, Stevens, & Burgio, 1999; Coyne & Hoskins, 1997; Heard & Watson, 1999; Hussian, 1988; Stokes, 1990; Vaccaro, 1988; and others). However, the durability of changes in behavior achieved by means of behavior management is not well established. Few published reports address the issue of maintenance—that is, whether the behavior changes achieved by means of behavior management persist when response contingencies are discontinued. The maintenance issue is important because some published studies report that modified behaviors revert to pretreatment levels when response contingencies are no longer in force (Allen-Burge, Stevens, & Burgio, 1999; Spector & associates, 2000).

The literature suggests that environmental manipulation has somewhat more dependable and more powerful effects on the behavior of adults with dementia than does behavior management. However, those who write about environmental manipulation generally agree that it, like behavior management, generally is effective only while the manipulations are in place. If the environmental manipulations are discontinued, the behaviors affected by the manipulations usually return to pretreatment levels. At this time, a combination of environmental manipulation and behavior management appears to provide the best means of modifying and maintaining behavior change for adults in the late stages of dementia. Additional research clearly is needed to clarify the effectiveness and efficiency of existing behavior management procedures and to propose new procedures or combinations of procedures to create and maintain behavioral changes in adults who are in the late stages of dementia.

In Chapter 11, Ylvisaker and associates (2001) questioned the effectiveness of traditional, consequence-based behavior management for persons who have traumatic brain injuries. They noted that traumatically brain-injured persons do not store the internal markers needed to learn contingencies, have impulsiveness that overrides the effects of response-contingent training, have impaired working memory that prevents them from learning connections between antecedent events and consequences, and have impaired behavioral initiation that prevents them from performing actions learned by consequence-based intervention. It seems likely that Ylvisaker and associates' comments may apply to persons who are in the middle to late stages of dementia. Consequence-based behavior management may have short-term effects on the behavior of persons with middle-to-late-stage dementia, but the effects are likely to disappear when the contingencies are removed, and even the short-term effects may disappear as a person moves into the late stage of dementia.

Effectiveness of Interventions for Persons with Dementia

Clinical and scientific literature has described dozens of interventions to maintain and enhance participation in activities of daily life by persons with dementia. Most are supported by some evidence of clinical utility and effectiveness, although the evidence consists primarily of anecdotes, opinions, case reports, and studies that often suffer from flaws in design and execution. It is clear that some interventions have significant positive effects, but we do not know which interventions have positive effects, which individuals benefit from a given intervention, or under what conditions an intervention is effective. That knowledge will come only from well-designed clinical trials, which are urgently needed to establish the legitimacy of interventions to help those who suffer from dementia and to develop more efficient and more effective interventions for individuals with dementia, their family members, and their caregivers.

GENERAL CONCEPTS 12-6

- In the very late stages of dementia, intervention focuses almost exclusively on environmental control to stimulate the affected person and preserve the person's remaining cognitive and communicative abilities, using enhanced environmental prompts and cues.
- Intervention programs for institutionalized persons with dementia typically depend on environmental control, behavior management, or a combination of the two.
- *Reality orientation* seeks to preserve and enhance cognitive functioning and social adequacy by exposing persons with dementia to information about the daily life environment.
- *Milieu therapy* endeavors to enhance alertness and increase appropriate social behavior by making the environment more interesting and more conducive to social interactions.
- *Functional maintenance programs* are short-term interventions designed and monitored by clinicians and carried out by staff and caregivers. They are designed to slow or prevent deterioration of function in persons with dementia.

GENERAL CONCEPTS 12-6—cont'd

- *Montessori-based methods* are designed to maintain and enhance physical, cognitive, and social abilities by guiding the person with dementia through activities designed to enhance sustained attention, facilitate adaptive behavior, and encourage socially appropriate behavior.
- *Simulated presence therapy* is a program in which the person with dementia listens to an audiotape recording of positive life events made by a family member or someone well-known to the person with dementia.

- The evidence suggests that environmental control and behavior management can be effective in modifying and controlling the behavior of persons with dementia, but the durability of the changes achieved has not been clearly established.
- Controlled investigations are needed to evaluate the effectiveness of existing procedures and to devise new procedures for managing persons who are in the late stages of dementia.

THOUGHT QUESTIONS

Question 12-1 You are preparing for a first interview with the spouse of a man with suspected early-stage Alzheimer's dementia. You may ask 10 questions during the interview. List the questions you would choose to ask and tell why you would ask each question.

Question 12-2 The following items resemble items that might be found in a screening test of mental status. Arrange them in what you think would be increasing order of difficulty for persons with moderate Alzheimer's dementia. Briefly describe the rationale for your ordering of items.

Count backward from 20 to 1.

How old are you?

What does *a stitch in time saves nine* mean?

What is your name?

Who is the current U.S. President?

Point to the ceiling, then to the floor, and then blink three times.

What day of the week is it?

Who was the first U.S. President?

What is your phone number?

Say *please put the groceries in the refrigerator.*

Tell me the days of the week, beginning with Sunday.

How would your uncle's daughter be related to you?

Question 12-3 The following utterances were produced as patients described the BDAE *cookie theft* picture (see Figure 5-19). The patients had the following diagnoses:

Broca's aphasia

Wernicke's aphasia

Conduction aphasia

Right-hemisphere syndrome

Alzheimer's dementia

Match the utterances with the diagnoses. (Some utterances may fit more than one diagnosis.)

(1) the mother is drinking...no...the mother is drying the cups and the plates...or the dishes.

(2) If you don't know what's going on there I'm not going to be the one to tell you.

(3) The wasker...waster...walter...water is running on the floor.

(4) There's a window with some curtains and a woman looking out.

(5) I can't tell you what it is. My eyes aren't what they used to be.

(6) Cookies and...and...swipe...kids...and mother ...and...and...dishes and water...and floor...

(7) There's a major biskelorum happening there in that frenellation...

(8) ...and the...what do you call it...the dripper...or the spigot...or the hydrant...its flushing...or rushing on the floor...

Motor Speech Disorders

If all my possessions were taken from me with one exception, I would choose to keep the power of communication, for by it I would soon regain all the rest. (Daniel Webster)

The label *motor speech disorders* refers to a collection of speech disturbances that are consequences of pathologic conditions in the nervous system that affect planning, organization, control, and execution of speech movements. Motor speech disorders include *apraxia of speech,* in which planning and organization of speech movements are impaired, and the *dysarthrias,* in which the execution and control of speech movements are impaired.

APRAXIA OF SPEECH

The label *apraxia of speech* first appeared in the literature in the late 1800s and early 1900s as part of a syndrome called *oral apraxia.* During the first half of the twentieth century, writers began separating apraxic speech movements from apraxic nonspeech movements, and labels such as *apraxic dysarthria, peripheral motor aphasia, articulatory dysarthria,* and *apraxia of vocal expression* were applied to the speech syndrome, and labels such as *buccofacial apraxia, facial apraxia,* and *oral nonverbal apraxia* were applied to the nonspeech syndrome. Darley (1969) settled on the label *apraxia of speech* for the speech syndrome, and since then speech-language pathologists and many others have used this label for the collection of articulatory impairments described by Darley, Aronson, and Brown (1975):

> Apraxia of speech is a distinct motor speech disorder distinguishable from the dysarthrias (speech disorders due to impaired innervation of speech musculature) and aphasia (a language disorder due to impairment of the brain mechanism for decoding and encoding the symbol system used in spoken and written communication). Apraxia of speech is a disorder of motor speech programming manifested primarily by errors in articulation and secondarily by compensatory alterations of prosody. The speaker shows reduced efficiency in accomplishing the oral postures necessary for phoneme production and the sequences of those postures for production of words. The disorder is frequently associated with aphasia but also may occur in isolation. Oral (nonspeech) apraxia may co-occur. (p. 267)

Neuropathology

The presence of apraxia of speech almost always signifies a pathologic condition affecting the language-dominant hemisphere—usually in the posterior frontal lobe (in, around, or under Broca's area), sometimes in the parietal lobe, and occasionally in both the frontal and parietal lobes. Stroke is the leading cause of apraxia of speech in adults, but apraxia of speech also may appear as a consequence of degenerative nervous system diseases (e.g., multiple sclerosis), traumatic brain injury, or brain tumor (Figure 13-1).

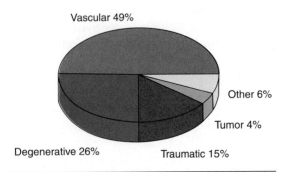

Figure 13-1 ■ Causes of dysarthria for 155 Mayo Clinic patients with a primary diagnosis of apraxia of speech. (Data from Duffy, J.R. [2005]. *Motor speech disorders: Substrates, differential diagnosis, and management* [2nd ed.]. St. Louis: Elsevier.)

Related Findings

Most patients with apraxia of speech also have hemiparesis or hemiplegia, spasticity, exaggerated reflexes, and somesthetic sensory impairments contralateral to the side of the brain injury (the right side for right-handed individuals). Many patients with apraxia of speech also have buccofacial apraxia, although either may occur in isolation. Some patients with apraxia of speech also have limb apraxia. (See Chapter 8 for descriptions of buccofacial apraxia, limb apraxia, and their neurophysiologic bases.)

Apraxia of speech usually occurs in combination with nonfluent (Broca's) aphasia. In fact, descriptions of the speech characteristics of Broca's aphasia often resemble descriptions of apraxia of speech (Benson, 1979a: Goodglass & Kaplan, 1983; Wertz, LaPointe, & Rosenbek, 1984).

> Speech production is effortful, usually limited to word groupings of one to three words produced with labored articulation. Quality of articulation varies as a function of the familiarity of the words in the message. That is, these patients often have a subset of well-practiced words that they produce with perfectly normal articulation. Articulation also may be facile in the utterance of conversational stereotypes (e.g., *"I can't say it"*) but distorted during attempts at more difficult or uncommon words. (Goodglass, 1993, pp. 202-203)

When apraxia of speech accompanies Broca's aphasia, the patient's speech may be agrammatic and telegraphic, as Benson notes. Most patients with Broca's aphasia plus apraxia of speech also exhibit word retrieval impairments and subtle to moderate comprehension impairments, which are not characteristics of apraxia of speech in isolation.

Apraxia of speech sometimes (although rarely) occurs in the absence of aphasia or other communicative impairments. Duffy (2005) reported that apraxia of speech appeared as the only apparent communication disorder in about 8% of a group of 48 patients for whom reliable diagnoses of apraxia of speech and other communicative impairments were available. Patients with apraxia of speech usually are aphasic as well. Duffy (2005) reported that 72% of a sample of 155 Mayo Clinic patients with a primary diagnosis of apraxia of speech also had evidence of aphasia. Duffy commented that these data do not mean that 28% of persons who have apraxia of speech have no aphasia, because the sample did not include patients with a primary diagnosis of aphasia and a secondary diagnosis of apraxia of speech. If patients with apraxia of speech as a secondary diagnosis were to be included in a sample, the percentage of patients exhibiting both apraxia of speech and aphasia would be greater than 78%—probably greater than 90%.

Dysarthria also is a frequent companion to apraxia of speech. Duffy (2005) reported that 29% of the 155-patient Mayo Clinic sample of patients with a primary diagnosis of apraxia of speech also exhibited dysarthria—usually appearing as unilateral upper motor neuron dysarthria or spastic dysarthria. As was true for the patients with a primary diagnosis of apraxia of speech, the patients with a primary diagnosis of dysarthria did not include those with dysarthria as a primary diagnosis and apraxia of speech as a secondary diagnosis. We know that, on average, more than 3 of 10 patients with apraxia of speech also will be dysarthric, although we do not know how many more than 3 in 10 will have both conditions.

Speech Characteristics

Apraxia of speech is characterized by highly variable articulation errors embedded in a pattern of speech made slow and effortful by trial-and-error gropings for the desired articulatory postures. The off-target productions usually are complications of articulatory performance, that is, substitutions (many of them unrelated to the target phoneme), additions, repetitions, and prolongations. Less frequently the errors are simplifications, that is, distortions and omissions. Errors are most often on consonants occurring initially in words, predominantly on those phonemes and clusters of phonemes requiring more complex muscular adjustment. Errors are exacerbated by increase in length of words and the linguistic and psychologic "weight" of a word in a sentence. They are not significantly influenced by auditory, visual, or instructional set variables. Islands of fluent, error-free speech highlight the marked discrepancy between efficient automatic-reactive productions and inefficient volitional-purposive productions. (Darley, Aronson, & Brown, 1975, p. 267)

McNeil, Robin, and Schmidt (1997) described two general phonemic characteristics of the speech of persons with apraxia of speech:

- Lengthened consonants and vowels and lengthened time intervals between sounds, syllables, and words (often perceived as sound substitutions, misplaced stress, and other prosodic abnormalities)
- Errors are relatively consistent in their locations within utterances and are consistent in type

McNeil, Robin, and Schmidt did not include substitutions, additions, repetitions, and omissions in their description of apraxia of speech characteristics as did Darley, Aronson, and Brown.

Apraxia of speech (sometimes called *verbal apraxia*) resembles other forms of ideomotor apraxia in several ways. It is not caused by weakness, paralysis, or sensory loss in the speech muscles. Unplanned, automatic speech usually is less clumsy and effortful than speech requested by the examiner. Speech elicited in natural contexts is less effortful and sounds more nearly normal than speech elicited in artificial contexts (such as a typical speech evaluation).

Several characteristics of apraxia of speech differentiate it from neurogenic communicative impairments that otherwise resemble it (particularly dysarthria and aphasia). Two important identifying characteristics are *articulatory error patterns* and *consistency of errors*.

Articulatory Error Patterns. Darley, Aronson, and Brown (1975) and Wertz, LaPointe, and Rosenbek (1984), among others, have described characteristic articulatory error patterns of

patients with apraxia of speech. These error patterns define relationships between articulatory or linguistic variables and error probabilities. Wertz, LaPointe, and Rosenbek (1984) described the following error patterns:

- Substitution errors are more frequent than distortion, omission, or addition errors. Kearns and Simmons (1988) suggest, however, that what listeners perceive as substitutions actually may be extreme phonetic distortion errors.
- Many substitution errors replace an easy-to-articulate sound with a more difficult one.
- Errors are more likely to be errors in placement of the articulators than errors of voicing, manner, or resonance.
- Most errors resemble the target sound.
- Consonant clusters are more likely to be in error than single consonants.
- Front-of-the-mouth sounds are more likely to be correct than back-of-the-mouth sounds.

Wertz, LaPointe, and Rosenbek (1984) suggested that the following characteristics are true for apraxic speakers as a group but may not always be true for an individual apraxic speaker:

- Voiceless sounds are more frequently substituted for voiced sounds than vice versa.
- *Anticipatory errors* (producing a sound before it occurs in a word or phrase, as in *thoothbrush* for *toothbrush*) are more frequent than either *perseverative errors* (inappropriately repeating a sound in a word or phrase, as in *manina* for *manila*) or *metathetic errors* (transposing adjacent sounds, as in *tevelision* for *television*).
- Consonant errors are more frequent than vowel errors.

Consistency of Errors. Darley, Aronson, and Brown (1975), Wertz, LaPointe, and Rosenbek (1984), Kearns and Simmons (1988), and others have identified *articulatory inconsistency* as an important feature of apraxia of speech. Articulatory inconsistency is manifested as correct articulation of phonemes at one time and incorrect articulation of the same phonemes at other times. Inconsistency in articulation often is related to variations in the context in which the phonemes are produced. A phoneme may be articulated correctly in one phonemic context (e.g., when the same phoneme is repeated in words or phrases, as in **Don Did the Dishes**) and misarticulated in another (e.g., when contrasting phonemes occur in words or phrases, as in **Don Bought a Car**).

Apraxic speakers' articulation usually is better in natural situations than in artificial ones. An apraxic patient's production of *see you later* is likely to be better when the patient is actually leaving than when asked by a clinician to say it in the middle of a treatment session. This phenomenon is related to what Darley, Aronson, and Brown (1975) referred to as *islands of fluent, error-free speech,* in which an apraxic speaker produces occasional fluent words, phrases, or sentences in the midst of effortful, struggling speech. Such periods of fluent speech in an overall context of nonfluent speech help to differentiate apraxia of speech from the dysarthrias, in which such intermittent periods of correct articulation rarely occur. (The primary exceptions are dysarthrias accompanying cerebellar ataxia and some dysarthrias caused by extrapyramidal disease, wherein speech may be intermittently dysarthric and nearly normal.)

Posterior Apraxia of Speech

Several writers (Buckingham, 1979; Deutsch, 1984; Square, Darley, & Sommers, 1982; and others) have described a *posterior apraxia of speech* syndrome caused by damage in the anterior parietal lobe or the anterior parietal-temporal region. Patients exhibiting this syndrome are less likely to be weak or paralyzed on one side but are more likely to exhibit contralateral somesthetic sensory impairments than patients with apraxia of speech following frontal lobe injury.

The speech characteristics of patients with posterior apraxia of speech differ in several respects from the speech of patients with apraxia of speech caused by frontal lobe damage. Square, Darley, and Sommers (1982) reported that the speech errors of patients with posterior apraxia of speech include more substitutions and fewer distortions than the speech of patients with apraxia of speech caused by frontal lobe damage. Deutsch (1984) reported that the speech errors of patients with posterior apraxia of speech include more transpositions of sounds and syllables (e.g., *tevelision* for *television*) than the speech of patients with apraxia of speech caused by frontal lobe damage. The speech of patients with posterior apraxia of speech often is described as less effortful, more fluent, and having more nearly normal prosody than the speech of patients with apraxia of speech caused by frontal lobe damage.

The concept of posterior apraxia of speech has come under fire from some writers who assert that the syndrome does not represent an apraxia but is part of the symptom-complex of *conduction aphasia* (Buckingham, 1992; Canter, 1973). According to these writers, patients who speak effortlessly and with normal prosody between instances of breakdown are more accurately described as exhibiting *conduction aphasia* than posterior apraxia of speech, and their speech errors are more accurately described as literal paraphasias than as apraxic errors. Regardless of the labels one chooses, it seems clear that there are differences in speech output between patients with damage in the posterior frontal lobe and patients with damage in the anterior parietal or temporal lobes of the language-dominant hemisphere (McNeil, Robin, & Schmidt, 1997).

- Patients with frontal lobe damage speak slowly and with great effort, distorted consonants and vowels are prominent, and runs of normal speech are rare. Patients with parietal-temporal lobe damage speak fluently and with little effort, and runs of normal speech are common.

- Patients with frontal lobe damage exhibit consistent prosodic disturbances—prolonged interword intervals, prolonged vowels, and prolonged articulatory movement durations.

The prosodic characteristics of patients with parietal-temporal lobe damage are variable but usually are within a normal range.

- Patients with frontal lobe damage tend to make the same kinds of errors in the same locations from trial to trial. Patients with parietal-temporal lobe damage tend to make different kinds of errors and make them at different locations from trial to trial.
- Patients with frontal lobe damage tend not to move toward correct productions on repeated attempts. Patients with parietal-temporal lobe damage tend to move toward correct productions on repeated attempts.

Although arguments about what constitutes apraxia of speech and what constitutes conduction aphasia are not settled, almost all of the literature on treatment for apraxia of speech is based on patients with frontal lobe or frontal-parietal damage. In what follows, the reader may assume that the label *apraxia of speech* refers to that group of patients.

TESTING FOR APRAXIA OF SPEECH

Tests to detect apraxia of speech typically include the following:

- Producing nonspeech oral movements, in isolation and in sequence; these tests are sensitive to the presence of *buccofacial apraxia*
- Producing speech movements, in isolation and in sequence
- Producing words with increasing phonologic complexity
- Producing phonologically complex phrases and sentences

Tests for limb apraxia usually complement tests for buccofacial apraxia and apraxia of speech. Tests for limb apraxia typically require sequential movements of hand and arm, such as waving good-bye or flipping a coin. As noted in Chapter 8, limb apraxia is more severe distally than proximally. Consequently, test items requiring wrist and finger movements (e.g., flipping a coin, winding a watch) are more sensitive to limb apraxia than test items requiring only

shoulder and arm movements (e.g., saluting, thumbing a ride). Because many patients with limb apraxia are paralyzed on one side, tests for limb apraxia should include movements that can be demonstrated with one arm and hand.

Box 13-1 lists tasks for identifying buccofacial apraxia, apraxia of speech, and limb apraxia.

INTERVENTION

Speak properly, and in as few words as you can, but always plainly; for the end of speech is not ostentation, but to be understood. (William Penn)

According to Rosenbek and Wertz (1972), treatment for patients with apraxia of speech should:

- Concentrate on the disordered articulation and, therefore, be different from the language stimulation and auditory and visual processing therapies appropriate to the aphasias
- Emphasize the relearning of adequate points of articulation and the sequencing of articulatory gestures
- Provide conditions such that the apraxic patient can advance from limited, automatic-reactive speech to appropriate, volitional purposive communication

Rosenbek and Wertz were addressing treatment of apraxia of speech. This does not imply that "therapies appropriate to the aphasias" are not appropriate for patients who are both apraxic and aphasic.

Most apraxic speakers can produce individual sounds and one syllable words correctly and with little effort, but problems arise when they are called on to produce multisyllabic utterances and phonologically complex words. Speech that is smooth and effortless when the apraxic patient produces short and phonologically simple utterances becomes slow, halting, and riddled with articulatory missteps when utterances are long and phonologically complex.

Apraxic speakers' problems do not arise because they cannot hear or discriminate the

Box 13-1	**Screening Tasks for Identifying Apraxia of Speech and Related Conditions**

Nonverbal Oral Movements
(Examiner may demonstrate, if necessary.)
Cough.
Stick out your tongue.
Puff out your cheeks.
Pucker your lips.
Smile.
Click your teeth.

Nonverbal Oral Movement sequences
(Examiner may demonstrate, if necessary.)
Lick your lips all the way around.
Show me how you would blow out a candle.
Pucker your lips, then smile.
  One time.
  Three times in succession.
Click your teeth, pucker your lips, then smile.
  One time.
  Three times in succession.

Repetition of Syllables
Say *puh-puh-puh-puh* as long as you can and as fast
  as you can.
Say *tuh-tuh-tuh-tuh* as long as you can and as fast as
  you can.

Say *kuh-kuh-kuh-kuh* as long as you can and as fast
  as you can.
Say *puh-tuh-kuh puh-tuh-kuh* as long as you can
  and as fast as you can.

Repetition of words
Say: *bob dad pop kick gag lap mat rap*
Say: *gingerbread snowman artillery impossibility*
Say each 3 times in succession: *gingerbread artillery*
  impossibility

Repetition of Phrases
Say: *Please put the groceries in the refrigerator.*
Say: *The shipwreck washed up on the shore.*
Say: *Nelson Rockefeller drives a Lincoln*
  Continental.

Limb Movements
Show me how you would comb your hair.
Show me how you would wave good-bye.
Show me how you would play a piano.
Show me how you would wind a watch.
Show me how you would flip a coin.

NOTE: See also Dabul, 2000; Darley, Aronson, & Brown, 1975; Disimoni, 1989; Duffy, 2005; Wertz, LaPointe, & Rosenbek, 1984.

sounds of speech—apraxic speakers do not need auditory discrimination training. Some early studies of apraxic speakers suggested that many were deficient in oral sensation and oral form identification (Guilford & Hawk, 1968; Larimore, 1970; Rosenbek, Wertz, & Darley, 1973), but subsequent studies have failed to replicate those findings (Deutsch, 1981; Square & Weidner, 1976). Sensory abnormalities sometimes coexist with apraxia of speech, but the abnormalities do not appear strongly related to its severity, making work on oral sensation a questionable treatment option for most apraxic patients.

Patients with Severe Apraxia of Speech

Characteristics at Intake. Most patients with severe apraxia of speech have no volitional

speech. Many emit stereotypic speech responses during the first month or two after onset. These stereotypic responses usually disappear by 2 months after onset, unless the patient also is severely aphasic. Most patients with severe apraxia of speech have moderate to severe buccofacial and limb apraxia. They almost always are hemiparetic or hemiplegic, and most are at least moderately aphasic.

Progression of Treatment. Treatment of severely apraxic patients begins at elemental levels. Many cannot phonate voluntarily. Most who can phonate cannot produce vowels, and few can produce consonant-vowel syllables. Early stages of treatment usually are concerned with developing volitional vocalization and a small repertoire of vowels and consonant-vowel syllables. Treatment procedures often make use of *phonetic placement* (use of drawings, models, descriptions, or mechanical positioning of the patient's articulators), *phonetic derivation* (deriving a new speech sound from a non-speech movement or position; for example, deriving a *buh* sound by having the patient close the lips, puff air, and vocalize), and *progressive approximation* (deriving a new speech sound from one the patient can make; for example, moving from *mah* to *bah*).

Phonetic contrasts (training a series of syllables or words in which elements in the series differ by a single feature; for example, *pan - tan - fan - van*) may help expand a patient's speech repertoire. Severely apraxic speakers usually are poor imitators. Consequently, imitation drills may not be appropriate, although *integral stimulation* (e.g., *watch me and do what I do*) may be useful for some patients.

Some severely apraxic speakers occasionally utter single words, but the words are likely to have little or no communicative value and are likely not to be under the speaker's volitional control. Helm and Barresi (1980) have suggested that such words can be brought under the patient's control and have described a program called *voluntary control of involuntary utterances (VCIU)* for incorporating the involuntary utterances into treatment. In *VCIU* the clinician writes on cards words that the patient spontaneously produces, then asks the patient to read the words when shown the cards. Words the patient reads correctly are retained; those the patient reads incorrectly are discarded. When a set of words the patient can read correctly has been identified, the patient is asked to produce the words when shown pictures or given prompts (e.g., *What's the opposite of night?*). When the patient consistently produces the words in response to the pictures and prompts, the words are incorporated into conversational interactions.

Alternative communication devices such as communication boards and communication books may be used to provide a means of communication for patients with severe apraxia of speech, at least on a temporary basis. Severely apraxic patients' use of gestural communication also may be emphasized and trained. Education and counseling of those who care for the patient are crucial aspects of treatment for severely apraxic patients.

Outcome. As noted earlier, apraxia of speech usually accompanies Broca's aphasia, although occasionally a patient appears with mild to moderate apraxia of speech and no detectable aphasia. Whether a patient who is both apraxic and aphasic will benefit from treatment depends both on the severity of the apraxia and the severity of the aphasia. The more severe the patient's impairments (after the first 3 or 4 weeks after onset), the poorer the prognosis for recovery. As noted earlier, patients who have no volitional speech, emit stereotypic speech responses, and are severely aphasic a month or more after onset are unlikely to recover functional speech, even with intensive treatment.

Only a small proportion of patients who remain severely apraxic at 3 or more months after onset develop more than rudimentary functional speech. Some patients with severe apraxia of speech who are also severely aphasic (and usually hemiplegic) end up in nursing homes. For these patients, it may be particularly important to develop a means of rudimentary communication between the patient and caregivers.

Patients with Moderate Apraxia of Speech

Characteristics at Intake. Patients with moderate apraxia of speech usually have some volitional speech at 1 to 2 months after onset. Stereotypic utterances may be present immediately after onset, but they disappear as the patient recovers. Many patients with moderate apraxia of speech exhibit mild to moderate buccofacial and limb apraxia. Almost all are hemiparetic or hemiplegic. Mild to moderate aphasia often accompanies the patient's apraxia of speech.

Progression of Treatment. Because patients with moderate apraxia of speech usually have some volitional speech, treatment usually begins at the syllable, word, or phrase level. Most patients with moderate apraxia of speech actively participate in treatment. They are motivated to recover. They work independently. They learn and can generalize what they learn to new situations. They may participate in setting goals and organizing treatment, and they often take responsibility for independent practice. Patients with moderate apraxia of speech usually move quickly from single-syllable to multiple-syllable speech production. Consequently, treatment activities can emphasize volitional control of sequenced articulatory movements, together with manipulations of rate, pauses, and intonation.

Wertz, LaPointe, and Rosenbek (1984) recommend *contrastive stress drill* for the early phases of treatment for patients with moderate apraxia of speech, and they suggest that oral reading may be suitable in later phases. In *contrastive stress drills,* the clinician makes a statement such as *"Bake a pie"* and then asks the patient questions such as *"DO WHAT to a pie?"* or *"Bake a WHAT?"* The patient answers each question, putting emphatic stress on words that answer the question *("BAKE a pie").*

Many patients with moderate apraxia of speech can learn a problem-solving approach to communication, in which they learn to anticipate difficult words and difficult speaking situations, recognize communication failure when it occurs, and respond to communication failure in a planned and systematic way.

Outcome. Most patients with moderate apraxia of speech regain functional speech, although speech tends to be slow and agrammatic. Many continue slow improvement in speech over many years—even after formal treatment has ended. Most return home following discharge from the primary care medical facility, and most function independently in common daily life activities. A few whose work does not depend heavily on speech may return to work, but most do not.

Patients with Mild Apraxia of Speech

Characteristics at Intake. Many patients with mild apraxia of speech at the end of the first month or so after onset spontaneously recover enough speech to be functional talkers in daily life. Most patients with mild apraxia of speech are mildly aphasic, but a few show no signs of measurable aphasia.

Progression of Treatment. Patients with mild apraxia of speech usually profit from articulation drills, instruction in strategic approaches to communication, and instruction on how to cope with the communicative disruptions created by their slow speech rate and articulatory miscues. Treatment usually consists of repetition drills coupled with exercises in which the patient formulates and produces phrases, sentences, and multiple-sentence utterances. The emphasis of treatment is on increased articulatory agility, improved articulatory accuracy, and closer-to-normal prosody and rate.

Outcome. Most patients with mild apraxia of speech return home. Some may return to work. Almost all communicate independently in most daily life situations, but they speak slowly, with exaggerated effort, and often miss articulatory targets.

General Principles of Treatment

McNeil, Robin, and Schmidt (1997) offer several principles for treating apraxia of speech:

- Intensive treatment is required. Treatment should consist of massed practice over a long interval (weeks, months, or years).
- Many repetitions are needed to stabilize newly acquired responses and make them automatic.
- The patient should revert to a neutral position between trials. A brief rest interval should occur before the patient begins a new series of trials.
- Treatment should progress systematically through a hierarchy of task difficulty (e.g., nonspeech movements to syllables, to sequences of syllables, to words, to sequences of words).

- Treatment of prosody (rhythm, stress, intonation) should accompany articulation treatment.
- Treatment should provide successful experiences for the patient. Successful communication, not perfection, is the goal.

Several of McNeil and associates' principles for treatment of apraxia of speech apply equally to treatment of other communication disorders and have been discussed elsewhere in this book.

Stimulus Manipulations and Response Accuracy

Automaticity. Overlearned sequences (counting, reciting the alphabet, reciting the days of the week) may be surprisingly easy for some patients who are severely apraxic and can produce little or no volitional speech. For these patients, drills with overlearned sequences may increase oral agility and oral motor control in preparation for work on volitional production of less automatic words and phrases.

Many apraxic patients do well as they count from 1 to 10 but are tied in knots by the multisyllabic numbers above 10. An apraxic patient who was asked to count to 20 gave the following response: *One...two...thee...four...five...six...seven...eight...nine... ten...neeleven...telve...thriteen...tritheen...thirty-teen...forty-teen...five-tithy-teen...*

Visibility, Length, and Articulatory Complexity. Visible and motorically simple articulatory movements are easiest for apraxic speakers. Visibility and complexity interact to some extent, because visible movements tend to be motorically simpler than nonvisible movements. As word length increases, the probability of apraxic speech errors increases (Johns & Darley, 1970; Shankweiler & Harris, 1966), although short words with complex articulation may be more difficult than long words without complex articulation. Apraxic errors tend to increase as the distance between successive points of articulation increases (Wertz, LaPointe, & Rosenbek, 1984).

Rate. Apraxic speakers' articulatory selection and sequencing impairments make it impossible for them to speak at their old normal rate, but many try to push their articulators beyond their capacity. An important early goal of treatment for such impatient apraxic speakers is to convince them that by talking slower they will talk better. Helping the patient understand that a few well chosen and carefully articulated words yield better communicative success than a flood of poorly articulated words helps. Showing the patient that slow, controlled speech is less effortful than fast, poorly controlled speech also helps. Providing experiences in which slow, controlled speech leads to successful communication in daily life usually puts the patient's doubts to rest. Most apraxic patients eventually adopt a slow, highly controlled and carefully monitored speaking style. Getting the patient to this stage is an important early clinical responsibility.

Delay. Many apraxic patients have difficulty keeping mental articulatory plans in place over time. This phenomenon often becomes apparent in articulation drills in which the clinician says a word, phrase, or sentence that the patient then repeats. Apraxic patients who do well when permitted to reproduce the clinician's model immediately often break down if they must delay their responses for 10 to 30 seconds. Clinicians sometimes build greater reserve capacity into apraxic patients' speech production by gradually increasing the time the patient must wait between the clinician's model and the patient's response.

Context. For most apraxic speakers, the phonologic characteristics of the word or phrase in which a particular sound is located affects the likelihood that it will be produced correctly. There is some evidence that the first sound in a word is more likely to be produced correctly than subsequent sounds (Shankweiler & Harris, 1966; Trost & Canter, 1974). However, others have failed to confirm this effect (Dunlop &

Marquardt, 1977; Johns & Darley, 1970; LaPointe & Johns, 1975).

The linguistic context in which a word is produced usually affects how difficult it is for an apraxic speaker. Placing a word in a frequently occurring phrase usually makes it easier. For example, the word *coffee* is likely to be easier if it is elicited by a phrase such as *I want a cup of…* than if it is elicited by a picture. Situational context also may affect apraxic speakers' success. Most speak better to friends and relatives (and clinicians) than they do to strangers. Most speak better face-to-face than on the telephone. Most speak better when they express their own knowledge, opinions, and wishes than they do when they must speak about topics prescribed by others.

Cues. The nature of cues provided to apraxic patients has strong effects on their success in producing speech. In general, the probability of successful responses increases as more information about target responses is provided by the cues. Love and Webb (1977) studied the effects of three cues on picture naming by patients with Broca's aphasia and apraxia of speech. The cues were a sentence with the target word missing, the first sound of the target word, and the printed target word. They found that, on the average, providing the first sound of the target word was most successful in eliciting the target word (60% success). Sentence completion was the next most effective cue (34% success), followed by the printed word (28% success). The differences were statistically significant except the difference between sentence completion and printed word cues.

Love and Webb do not report whether individual subjects all generated the same hierarchy as the group. It is unlikely that they did. Furthermore, it seems likely that many of Love and Webb's subjects' were both apraxic and aphasic, with word retrieval impairments complicating their attempts to produce spoken words (a probability to which Love and Webb allude). Love and Webb's results do, however, show that cues may have strong effects on the accuracy of apraxic speakers' retrieval and production of single words. Love and Webb's hierarchy also may provide a starting point for clinicians who wish to construct a cueing hierarchy for an individual patient.

Rosenbek and associates (1973) proposed an eight-step continuum of cues for treatment of patients with apraxia of speech. The continuum gradually reduces the salience of cues while gradually increasing response requirements:

1. The clinician and patient produce the target utterance in unison.
2. The clinician says the target utterance. The patient says the utterance while the clinician silently mouths the utterance.
3. The clinician says the utterance. The patient says the utterance.
4. The clinician says the utterance. The patient says the utterance several times in succession.
5. The patient reads the target utterance aloud from a printed card.
6. The patient studies the utterance printed on a card. The card is taken away. The patient says the utterance.
7. The clinician asks a question that is answerable with the target utterance. The patient says the target utterance.
8. The clinician and patient interact in a role-playing situation in which previously practiced utterances are appropriate. The patient says the utterances when appropriate.

Clinicians can add additional levels to Rosenbek and associates' continuum by imposing delayed-response requirements at some or all of the steps in the continuum.

Wambaugh and associates (2004) described *sound production treatment,* a systematic treatment to facilitate apraxic speakers' correct production of specific sounds targeted for intervention. Sound production treatment combines clinician modeling, imitation and repetition by the patient, minimal-pair contrasts (e.g., night/might), clinician cues for articulatory placement, and feedback. Sound production treatment employs a six-step basic hierarchy:

1. The patient produces a target phrase or word following the clinician's spoken model.
2. Step 1 is repeated with an added printed cue (a letter representing the target sound).
3. The patient produces the target word with integral stimulation (e.g., *watch me and do what I do*) for up to three attempts.
4. The patient produces the target word following articulatory placement cues and a spoken model from the clinician.
5. The patient produces the target sound in isolation following the clinician's spoken model.
6. The next item is presented.

If the patient correctly produces the target on any step, he or she is asked to produce it again before the clinician proceeds to the next step. The hierarchy may be modified depending on a particular patient's needs and to accommodate targets of different complexities.

Wambaugh (2004) and Wambaugh and associates (1998, 1999a, 1999b, 2004) have reported several single-case studies in which positive effects of sound production treatment were obtained, as well as evidence of generalization from trained to untrained sounds, generalization to untrained contexts (e.g., from single words to sentences), and limited maintenance of treatment effects following cessation of treatment. Because of its systematic nature, sound production treatment appears a promising addition to interventions for apraxia of speech. When, for whom, and to what extent it is effective awaits additional investigation.

Stimulus Modality. Most treatment programs for apraxic patients manipulate the modalities in which stimuli are delivered, although not all do so systematically. Despite the frequently encountered assertion that multimodality stimulation is better than unimodality stimulation, no experimental evidence supports the claim, and the assertion almost certainly does not apply to every apraxic patient. Some patients are confused rather than helped by the addi-

tional information provided by multimodality stimulation.

Visual stimulation in apraxia treatment consists primarily of two procedures. The most common is *integral stimulation* (e.g., *watch me and do what I do*). If integral stimulation fails to increase visual input, the clinician may add *mirror work,* in which the clinician and patient sit side side-by-side facing a mirror as the patient repeats the clinician's models. The clinician directs the patient's attention toward visual aspects of speech production, such as lip and jaw position, rounding, and so forth. Sometimes videotapes of the patient speaking may take the place of the mirror, but the clinician-patient visual monitoring procedure resembles that for mirror work. Some apraxic patients' performance improves when visual input is embellished with mirrors or videotapes. Mirror and videotape work sometimes helps patients with impaired oral tactile sensation or impaired position sense by allowing them to see the position of their articulators as they speak. Others seem confused by the additional information and do worse when they watch themselves talk than when they do not.

Emphasizing the patient's attention to tactile and kinesthetic stimuli during speech sometimes improves the accuracy of apraxic patients' speech. (This does not imply that tactile stimulation by itself, outside of speech activity, is likely to be beneficial; usually it is not.) Clinicians sometimes enhance kinesthetic stimulation by manually touching, positioning, or moving the patient's jaw, tongue, and lips. Clinicians typically use manual manipulations to help the patient position the articulators for specific sounds and gradually eliminate the manipulations as the patient becomes proficient at volitionally producing the targeted sounds. Clinicians usually resort to manual manipulation when integral stimulation and mirror work fail to produce the intended performance (although they often combine mirror work and manual manipulation).

An intervention called *prompts for restructuring oral muscular phonemic therapy (PROMPT)* emphasizes kinesthetic and tactile feedback in articulation training. (Presumably the authors were sufficiently enamored by the acronym to ignore the syntactic awkwardness of the label.) PROMPT was originally developed for use with children diagnosed with oral apraxia (Chumpelik, 1984) but has been extended to adults with apraxia of speech (Square, 1986; Square, Chumpelik, & Adams, 1986). PROMPT procedures require systematic placement of a clinician's fingers on the recipient's face and throat to cue articulatory positions and manner of articulation (e.g., stops vs. continuants). The cues are designed to regulate muscle tension, jaw position, lip placement, tongue position, and breath-stream management. The tactile cues are provided in sequences designed to guide the recipient's production of syllables and words, beginning with short, phonologically simple utterances and gradually increasing their length and phonologic complexity.

Competence in PROMPT procedures requires extensive training and practice. Consequently, it has not been widely used in interventions for adults who have apraxia of speech or dysarthria. PROMPT's focus on kinesthetic and tactile feedback and its element-by-element arrangement of tasks suggest that it may be appropriate for patients with persisting severe apraxia of speech who fail to respond to other interventions. Clinicians may use elements of the PROMPT approach to design interventions for specific patients.

Although the *auditory modality* is not usually written about in treatment of apraxia of speech (Wertz, LaPointe, & Rosenbek, 1984 is an exception), most treatment programs depend strongly on the patient's auditory self-monitoring as he or she talks. Most clinicians encourage apraxic patients to concentrate on listening to what they say and how they say it, believing that the additional information coming into the patient's ears will improve what comes out of the patient's mouth. Clinicians also typically teach patients to evaluate each utterance to tell if it is adequate (not necessarily *correct*). Few clinicians spend time training *auditory discrimination* (teaching the patient to identify phonemic differences in words spoken by the clinician), but many spend time training the patient to tell how their own productions differ from targets. Pointing out consistent mismatches (e.g., syllable transpositions, articulatory substitutions) often accelerates progress.

Meaningfulness. In general, the more meaningful a speech response is, the easier it is for an apraxic speaker. Consequently, most clinicians structure treatment around meaningful words, phrases, and sentences. Dabul and Bollier (1976), however, recommend that treatment for patients with apraxia of speech should begin by concentrating on production of nonmeaningful articulatory sequences to teach the patient volitional control of speech production prior to attempts at meaningful words. There is no conclusive evidence for either position. Majority opinion at this time seems to favor using real words as soon as possible. However, if an apraxic patient is having trouble moving from isolated sounds to sound sequences in real words, the clinician might consider using Dabul and Boller's strategy to see if it might help the patient bridge the gap.

Neurobehavioral Reorganization Approaches to Treatment

Rosenbek, Collins, and Wertz (1976) and Rosenbek (1978) have described two innovative procedures for enhancing apraxic patients' speech production—*intersystemic reorganization* and *intrasystemic reorganization.*

Intersystemic Reorganization. Intersystemic reorganization adds nonspeech behaviors (tapping, gesturing, pantomiming) to speech to facilitate speech production for apraxic individuals. (For example, a patient might pantomime the act of raising a glass and drinking from it while saying, *a drink of water.*) Intersystemic reorganization takes apraxic patients through a predetermined sequence of activities (Rosenbek & LaPointe, 1978):

- The clinician and the patient compile a set of simple, meaningful, and easily recognizable gestures.
- The patient learns to recognize each gesture and its associated word or phrase when the gesture and the word or phrase are produced by the clinician.
- The patient learns to imitate each gesture. (Rosenbek and associates stress the importance of feedback from the clinician at this stage, because they have observed that many apraxic patients have difficulty judging the adequacy of their own gestures.) The clinician may manipulate the patient's hand and arm to bring about a gesture, or the patient may be given real objects to use in the movement.
- When the patient can produce each gesture without effort, he or she learns to combine each gesture with a word or phrase.
- When the patient can reliably and appropriately produce speech and gesture combinations inside and outside the clinic, the gestures may be gradually deemphasized.

Rosenbek and associates recommend that even at the last stage of treatment patients should be encouraged to continue using gestures for self-cueing and self-correction of errors.

According to Rosenbek and associates, patients who cannot learn gestures, patients who cannot learn to pair gestural and speech responses, and patients who are severely aphasic are not candidates for intersystemic reorganization. Rosenbek and associates commented that patients who are severely aphasic usually do no better when treated using intersystemic reorganization than when they are treated using other procedures.

Wertz, LaPointe, and Rosenbek (1984) described an intersystemic reorganization treatment program for moderate apraxia of speech in which speech is combined with tapping gestures. They call this program *gestural reorganization*. In gestural reorganization, the patient is trained to emphasize the rhythm or pacing of speech by pairing tapping movements with speech. Gestural reorganization typically proceeds through an eight-step continuum:

- *Step 1: Explaining the program's purpose.* This step is necessary for patients who may be reluctant to add gestures to speech because they do not wish to appear abnormal. A patient may be told that the gestures are to help them get started and that gestures may be phased out eventually. The clinician may compare gestures to other prosthetic devices such as eyeglasses and hearing aids.
- *Step 2: Diagnostic treatment.* The clinician and the patient identify one or more simple, repetitive gestures that the patient can do reliably (e.g., tapping one finger, tapping with all the fingers on one hand, tapping one foot, tapping one hand against a thigh). The patient is trained to do the gesture in isolation. Then the patient is trained to use the gesture while producing a simple nonsense syllable or word.
- *Step 3: Stabilizing the gesture.* The clinician and the patient increase the patient's volitional control of the gesture by manipulating the rate, complexity, and length of tapping and by inserting delays between the clinician's model and the patient's response.
- *Step 4: Pairing gesture and speech.* The patient is trained to pair speech and gesture for simple speech responses. The clinician taps and says words or phrases. The patient and the clinician tap and say the words or phrases together.
- *Step 5: Fading cues.* The clinician gradually fades out cues. The clinician may tap only at the beginning of utterances, tap only for the most important words, or may tap only for difficult words. The clinician may speak more softly or may speak only for some words in each utterance.
- *Step 6: Gesture and contrastive stress.* The clinician asks questions to which the patient responds by tapping simultaneously with

speech. (Contrastive stress drill is described earlier in this chapter.)

- *Step 7: Greater volitional-purposive control.* The patient answers questions and produces phrases and sentences in response to a variety of clinician prompts, some of which may resemble conversational behaviors.

- *Step 8: Fading the gesture.* For patients who do not spontaneously stop using gestures while they speak, but could do so, the clinician may help the patient move away from gesture with drills containing successively larger proportions of utterances unaccompanied by gestures. Patients may be advised to resort to gesture when they encounter difficulty getting words out.

Helm (1979) described a simple apparatus for gestural reorganization, called a *pacing board*. The pacing board described by Helms is about 14 inches long and 2 inches wide. It is divided by ridges into eight sections (Figure 13-2). Patients are trained to tap out rhythm and stress patterns from left to right on the pacing board. Then speech and tapping are combined, and the length and complexity of tapped speech responses gradually increase. As a patient becomes proficient at speaking with the full-size pacing board, a pocket-size pacing board may be substituted, and more natural tapping or gestures gradually may replace tapping on the pacing board.

Intrasystemic Reorganization. Intrasystemic reorganization elicits speech movements by shifting the locus of control from one level of

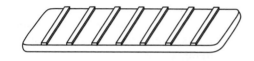

Figure 13-2 ■ A pacing board similar to the one described by Helm (1979).

the motor system to another. The shift usually is from automatic action to volitional action. The typist who slows down and types words syllable by syllable when typing unfamiliar or complicated words uses intrasystemic reorganization. (The typist who subvocally spells words while typing uses intersystemic reorganization.) Many treatment activities for apraxic patients qualify as intrasystemic reorganization, although they are not so labeled. Teaching patients to speak slowly and with consciously controlled articulatory movements is one example of intrasystemic reorganization. Teaching them to speak with exaggerated prosody and teaching them to concentrate on kinesthetic feedback during speech are other examples.

There are no reliable data to support the efficacy of reorganization in eliciting speech from apraxic patients or in reinstating speech that apraxic patients are likely to use in daily life communication, and there are no data comparing reorganization with other treatments. Anecdotal reports suggest that reorganization is effective in eliciting speech from many apraxic patients and that it makes meaningful changes in the daily life communicative ability of some of them. Intersystemic reorganization provides a way to elicit volitional speech; intrasystemic reorganization provides a way to polish it.

Melodic Intonation Therapy. Melodic intonation therapy (*MIT*; Sparks, Helm, & Albert, 1974; Sparks & Holland, 1976) was designed to elicit speech from severely aphasic (and apraxic) patients who have little or no volitional speech by increasing the participation of the nondominant hemisphere in speech activities. (The nondominant hemisphere is thought to be important for perception and production of musical and rhythmic material.) MIT places the patient in structured drills in which phrases are produced with exaggerated stress, rhythm, and pitch, and the patient taps out the rhythm of each phrase while producing the phrase (e.g., *...cup...of...CO...fee,* spoken with rising intonation and emphatic stress on *CO*).

In MIT the patient is trained to utter propositional phrases and sentences, using sung intonation patterns that are similar to the natural intonation patterns of the spoken phrases or sentences. First the clinician intones sentences and helps the patient tap the stress patterns of the sentences in unison with the clinician's utterances. Then the patient and clinician intone the sentences and tap their stress patterns together. Then the clinician gradually fades her or his participation in production and tapping until the patient is intoning and tapping phrases in response to the clinician's intoned model without assistance from the clinician. If a patient cannot tap and say the phrase, some clinicians substitute gesture for tapping.

When the patient's simultaneous intonation and tapping have stabilized, speech production moves away from melody toward natural prosody. First, there is a transition from melodic intonation to *sprechgesang* (speech song), in which words are no longer sung but are spoken with exaggerated inflection. The next transition is from *sprechgesang* to natural prosody.

Having a patient tap or gesture while speaking is a form of intersystemic reorganization; having a patient speak rhythmically and with exaggerated intonation is a form of intrasystemic reorganization.

According to Sparks, Helm, and Albert (1974), MIT is appropriate for patients with the following characteristics:

- Auditory comprehension is better than verbal expression. (Spontaneous recognition and self-correction of errors by the patient is considered a favorable sign.)
- The patient is emotionally stable and has good attention span.
- The patient has severely impaired verbal output and has little or no ability to name, repeat, or complete sentences.
- The patient makes vigorous attempts at self-correction.

- The patient emits clearly articulated, stereotyped utterances.

There are no controlled evaluations of the efficacy of MIT, either by itself or relative to other treatment approaches, although in 1994 a committee of the American Academy of Neurology described MIT as "promising." Anecdotal reports suggest that MIT is effective in eliciting speech from patients who otherwise cannot produce volitional speech. The most significant problem with MIT appears to be generalization of speech learned in the clinic to daily life. Little generalization of what patients learn in MIT to other activities usually occurs until the patient is in the final stages of MIT, and many patients do not make it to the final stages. A particularly difficult transition seems to be the transition from sung phrases to *sprechgesang*.

Nonspeech Communication Systems

Some severely apraxic patients never regain enough volitional speech to permit them to communicate even simple messages by talking. Nonspeech communication systems may help some of them communicate. However, many severely apraxic patients also have significant aphasia, which may compromise their ability to use alternative communication systems that depend on verbal skills. Some patients with severe apraxia of speech may learn gesture and pantomime as part of reorganization. The gestures and pantomime may function both as a substitute for speech and as a facilitator for the patient's production of speech. Some patients with severe apraxia of speech may learn to use sign languages, either temporarily as they are reacquiring speech or as a permanent substitute. Producing such signs also may facilitate speech through intersystemic reorganization. Other patients with severe apraxia of speech may regain basic communication by using an alternative communication device. Alternative communication devices are described later in this chapter.

GENERAL CONCEPTS 13-1

- *Apraxia of speech (verbal apraxia)* is characterized by variable articulatory errors and trial-and-error articulatory groping in a context of slow and effortful speech.
- Apraxia of speech usually is caused by damage in posterior regions of the frontal lobe in the language-dominant brain hemisphere.
- Patients with apraxia of speech often exhibit Broca's aphasia, which adds *agrammatism* and *telegraphic speech* to the signs of apraxia of speech.
- *Limb apraxia* and *buccofacial apraxia* often accompany apraxia of speech.
- Patients with apraxia of speech often have contralateral motor and sensory impairments (weakness, paralysis, spasticity, exaggerated reflexes, diminished somesthetic sensation).
- Apraxia of speech is characterized by slow, effortful speech, articulatory inconsistency, distorted articulatory substitutions, and strong effects of context on articulatory accuracy.
- *Posterior apraxia of speech* is said to be caused by parietal-temporal lobe damage. Many practitioners consider the speech errors of patients with posterior apraxia of speech to be the *literal paraphasias* of individuals with *conduction aphasia.*
- Treatment of patients with severe apraxia of speech typically begins with sound or syllable production and may require use of *phonetic placement, phonetic contrasts,* or *integral stimulation* to facilitate speech.
- Treatment of patients with moderate apraxia of speech usually begins at the word or phrase level and may involve *contrastive stress drill* in early phases. *Relaxation training* may help some speak with less effort.

- Treatment of patients with mild apraxia of speech usually consists of speech production drills with phrases, sentences, and multiple-sentence utterances, plus training in coping and compensatory strategies.
- Emphasizing attention to tactile and kinesthetic feedback helps many apraxic speakers talk better.
- Visible, short, and motorically simple speech materials are easiest for apraxic speakers.
- Slowing an apraxic speaker's rate of speech usually improves the quality of the person's speech and lessens the person's effort in producing speech.
- Delay imposed between a stimulus and an apraxic speaker's responses usually compromises response accuracy. Delay may be used in treatment to increase an apraxic speaker's reserve capacity.
- Familiar and natural linguistic and situational contexts and meaningful content usually facilitate speech for apraxic speakers.
- Many treatment programs for apraxia of speech employ cueing hierarchies in which cues of gradually decreasing power are systematically provided.
- *Intersystemic reorganization* enhances apraxic speakers' speech by incorporating nonspeech behaviors into speech production. *Intrasystemic reorganization* enhances apraxic speakers' speech by moving control from one level of the motor system to another.
- Some severely apraxic speakers may need augmentative or alternative communication systems for functional communication.

DYSARTHRIA

Dysarthria is a generic label for a group of speech disorders caused by impaired control of the muscles responsible for speech. Darley, Aronson, and Brown (1975) define dysarthria as follows:

> Dysarthria is a collective name for a group of speech disorders resulting from disturbances in muscular control over the speech mechanism due to damage of the central or peripheral nervous system. It designates problems in oral communication due to paralysis, weakness, or incoordination of the speech musculature. It differentiates such problems from disorders of higher centers related to the faulty programming of movements and sequences of movements (apraxia of speech) and to the inefficient processing of linguistic units (aphasia). (p. 246)

As Darley, Aronson, and Brown assert, dysarthria is caused by weakness, paralysis, or incoordination of the muscles required for speech. Weakness or paralysis of speech muscles most often is caused by damage in the pons and medulla (damage that affects lower motor neurons serving the speech muscles) or by damage in nerve fibers that connect motor neurons to the speech muscles. Sometimes dysarthria may be a consequence of nerve-muscle junction disease (e.g., myasthenia gravis), muscle disease *(myopathy)*, or psychosomatic conditions (wherein the physiologic mechanisms responsible for speech are unimpaired). Dysarthria often accompanies progressive neurologic diseases. When it does, the dysarthria usually worsens as the neurologic disease progresses. Dysarthria caused by destruction of motor neurons or nerve fiber tracts is irreversible, as are most dysarthrias caused by diseases affecting nerve-muscle junctions and diseases of muscles.

Darley, Aronson, and Brown (1975) divided dysarthrias among six types which reflect the nature of the underlying neuropathology and the nature of the motoric disturbances caused by the neuropathology (Table 13-1).

TABLE 13-1	Types of Dysarthria
Type	Neuropathology
Spastic	Upper motor neurons (usually bilateral)
Flaccid	Lower motor neurons
Ataxic	Cerebellar system
Hypokinetic	Extrapyramidal (usually Parkinson's disease)
Hyperkinetic	Extrapyramidal (chorea, dystonia)
Mixed	Multiple motor systems

Types were described by Darley, Aronson, and Brown (1975).

Upper Motor Neuron Damage

Unilateral damage to *upper motor neurons* (neurons in the motor cortex that connect to motor nuclei in the brain stem) or to *corticobulbar tracts* (fibers that connect cortical motor neurons to motor nuclei in the brain stem) usually does not cause persisting dysarthria, because most of the speech muscles receive input from the motor cortex in both brain hemispheres. The muscles of the pharynx, larynx, tongue, and jaw are bilaterally innervated. Consequently, pathologic conditions affecting upper motor neurons in one brain hemisphere usually cause only transitory weakness of pharyngeal, laryngeal, tongue, and jaw muscles. The external muscles of the lower face (those involved in facial expression) receive most of their input from the contralateral motor cortex. Consequently, pathologic conditions affecting the motor cortex or corticobulbar tracts serving the external muscles of the lower cause weakness or paralysis of the muscles, including those serving the lips.

Patients with unilateral upper motor neuron damage typically exhibit mild dysarthria in which sounds that depend on lip position or lip movements are imprecise because of weak lip muscles. Speech intelligibility usually is affected minimally by unilateral upper motor neuron damage.

Now and then a patient with what seems to be unilateral upper motor neuron damage experiences persisting dysarthria, a condition Duffy (2005) calls *unilateral upper motor neuron dysarthria.* According to Duffy, unilateral upper motor neuron dysarthria has received little attention in the literature because it was considered a mild and temporary problem and because it often occurs together with aphasia or apraxia of speech. Darley, Aronson, and Brown (1975), for example, asserted that unilateral pathology in upper motor neurons produces only transitory speech disturbance that resolves within the first month after onset. Duffy (2005), however, asserts that unilateral upper motor neuron pathology sometimes creates persisting mild dysarthria and that unilateral upper motor neuron dysarthria is encountered at a rate similar to the incidence of other dysarthria types seen in a large multidisciplinary practice—occurring as a primary communicative diagnosis in about 9% of all patients with a primary diagnosis of dysarthria.

> Sometimes severe dysarthria persists following an apparent unilateral stroke. Duffy (2005) suggests careful examination of such patients to rule out the possibility of bilateral brain damage. "Persistent severe dysarthria following a unilateral stroke should raise suspicion about a lesion or lesions on the other side of the brain." (p. 260)

Strokes in the brain hemispheres are the primary cause of unilateral upper motor neuron dysarthria. In a Mayo Clinic sample of 98 patients with a primary diagnosis of unilateral upper motor neuron dysarthria, 90% had experienced strokes (Duffy, 2005; Figure 13-3). The reported incidence of unilateral upper motor neuron dysarthria is somewhat greater following left-hemisphere stroke than following right-hemisphere stroke. Duffy (2005) reported that 61% of the Mayo Clinic sample of 98 patients

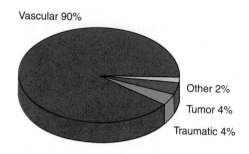

Figure 13-3 ■ Causes of dysarthria for 98 Mayo Clinic patients with a primary diagnosis of unilateral upper motor neuron dysarthria. (Data from Duffy, J.R. [2005]. *Motor speech disorders: Substrates, differential diagnosis, and management* [2nd ed.]. St. Louis: Elsevier.)

with unilateral upper motor neuron dysarthria had left-hemisphere damage, whereas 34% had damage in the right hemisphere. Duffy cautioned, however, that the difference may be an artifact of referral bias—patients with left-hemisphere damage, who are likely to be aphasic, may be more likely to come to medical attention than are patients with right-hemisphere damage. Regardless of the proportions of patients with unilateral upper motor neuron dysarthria who have left-hemisphere versus right-hemisphere damage, it is clear that damage in either hemisphere can cause unilateral upper motor neuron dysarthria.

Patients with unilateral upper motor neuron dysarthria exhibit motor and sensory deficits typical for patients with strokes in the brain hemispheres—contralateral hemiparesis or hemiplegia, contralateral sensory loss, contralateral facial weakness, and spastic muscles. The speech of patients with unilateral upper motor neuron dysarthria is characterized by imprecise articulation that usually does not seriously compromise intelligibility, occasional irregular articulatory breakdowns, slightly slower-than-normal speech rate, harsh or strained voice

Box 13-2	*Characteristics of Unilateral Upper Motor Neuron Dysarthria*

Distinguishing Speech Characteristics
Mild articulatory imprecision
Slow to normal speech rate
Harsh-strained voice quality
Occasional hypernasality
Occasional irregular articulatory breakdown
Diminished vocal loudness

Related Signs
Hemiparesis, hemiplegia
Spastic muscles
Exaggerated reflexes
Pseudobulbar state
Unilateral weakness of lower face

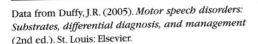

Data from Duffy, J.R. (2005). *Motor speech disorders: Substrates, differential diagnosis, and management* (2nd ed.). St. Louis: Elsevier.

quality, and (sometimes) weak voice. Hypernasality occasionally may be present. Box 13-2 lists salient characteristics of unilateral upper motor neuron dysarthria.

In contrast to the sporadic appearance of dysarthria following unilateral upper motor neuron damage, bilateral upper motor neuron damage usually creates persisting dysarthria. Bilateral upper motor neuron damage leaves the muscles responsible for articulation, voice, and resonance hypertonic and hyperreflexive, with reduced strength and range of movement. Patients who have bilateral upper motor neuron damage typically experience bilateral facial weakness or paralysis, drooling, bilateral hemiparesis, slowness of movement, and dysarthria. Dysarthria from bilateral upper motor neuron pathology often appears as part of a syndrome called *pseudobulbar state,* in which the affected patient is dysarthric, has impaired swallowing *(dysphagia),* and has poor control of laughing or crying. The most common cause of bilateral upper motor neuron dysarthria is multiple strokes. Traumatic brain injuries, tumors, and demyelinating diseases such as multiple sclerosis are less common causes.

Darley, Aronson, and Brown (1975) call dysarthria caused by bilateral upper motor neuron pathology *spastic dysarthria.* According to Darley, Aronson, and Brown, spastic dysarthria affects phonation, articulation, resonation, and prosody. Spastic laryngeal muscles create strained-strangled-harsh voice quality. Spastic articulatory muscles lose their agility, leading to imprecise consonant articulation, especially for consonants requiring rapid or complex articulatory movements. Spastic velopharyngeal muscles stiffen the velum and prevent it from occluding the velopharyngeal opening, creating hypernasality. Spastic laryngeal muscles vibrate at a slower-than-normal rate, reducing vocal pitch. Hypertonic laryngeal muscles impair vocal flexibility, diminish variability in pitch and loudness, and create strained-strangled-harsh voice quality. Reduced movement of muscles in the chest wall and abdomen compromise respiratory support for speech and contribute to weak voice and short utterances. Box 13-3 lists the salient features of spastic dysarthria.

Strokes and degenerative diseases are the most common causes of spastic dysarthria. Together they account for about 70% of cases. Traumatic brain injury and demyelinating disease are less common causes (Figure 13-4).

Cranial Nerve Damage

Pathologic conditions in the pons and medulla often cause dysarthria by damaging cranial nerves or the nuclei of cranial nerves supplying the facial, oropharyngeal, and laryngeal muscles. If cranial nerves serving the speech muscles are damaged, *flaccid dysarthria* follows. Pathologic conditions affecting cranial nerves can come from several sources. Strokes or tumors in the brain stem may cause flaccid dysarthria if cranial nerve nuclei are affected. Degenerative diseases may cause flaccid dysarthria if motor nerves or speech muscles are affected. Traumatic injuries to the head and neck, surgery on the cervical spine, or *carotid endarterectomy* (surgery to remove plaque from a carotid artery) may injure cranial nerves, creating flaccid dysarthria. Muscle diseases such as muscular dystrophy and degenerative diseases such as amyotrophic lateral sclerosis are less common causes of flaccid dysarthria (Figure 13-5).

Damage to cranial nerves or their nuclei causes flaccid paralysis and fasciculations in muscles on the same side of the body as the damaged nerve, followed by gradual muscle atrophy. The signs of cranial nerve damage depend on whether the pathology affects cranial nerve fiber tracts or the cranial nerve

Box 13-3	**Characteristics of Spastic Dysarthria**

Distinguishing Speech Characteristics
Imprecise consonants
Strained-strangled voice
Slow rate

Other Speech Characteristics
Monopitch
Reduced stress
Monoloudness
Low pitch
Hypernasality
Short phrases
Distorted vowels
Pitch breaks
Continuous breathy voice
Excess, equal stress

Related Signs
Hypertonus (spasticity)
Hemiparesis, hemiplegia
Exaggerated reflexes
Pseudobulbar state

Data from Darley, F.L., Aronson, A.E., & Brown, J.R. (1975). *Motor speech disorders.* Philadelphia: W.B. Saunders; Duffy, J.R. (2005). *Motor speech disorders: Substrates, differential diagnosis, and management* (2nd ed.). St. Louis: Elsevier; and Rosenbek, J.C., & LaPointe, L.L. (1985). The dysarthrias: Description, diagnosis, and treatment. In D.F. Johns (Ed.). *Clinical management of neurogenic communication disorders* (2nd ed.). Boston: Little, Brown and Company.

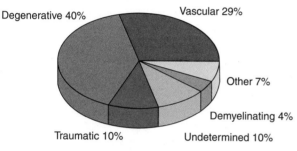

Figure 13-4 ■ Causes of dysarthria for 144 Mayo Clinic patients with a primary diagnosis of spastic dysarthria. (Data from Duffy, J.R. [2005]. *Motor speech disorders: Substrates, differential diagnosis, and management* [2nd ed.]. St. Louis: Elsevier.)

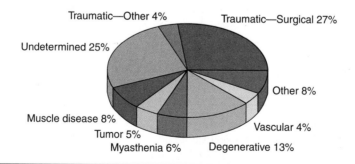

Figure 13-5 ■ Causes of dysarthria for 154 Mayo Clinic patients with a primary diagnosis of flaccid dysarthria. (Data from Duffy, J.R. [2005]. *Motor speech disorders: Substrates, differential diagnosis, and management* [2nd ed.]. St. Louis: Elsevier.)

nucleus. Pathologic conditions affecting cranial nerve fiber tracts cause paralysis of the muscles served by the nerve. Pathologic conditions affecting the cranial nerve nucleus cause paralysis of the muscles served by the nerve, often accompanied by spastic hemiparesis or hemiplegia of the contralateral arm and leg. This combination of signs happens because corticospinal fiber tracts connecting to muscles in the contralateral arm and leg pass through the brain stem next to the cranial nerve nuclei, so that pathology affecting cranial nerve nuclei often impinges on corticospinal fibers serving the contralateral arm and leg (Figure 13-6).

> Corticospinal fibers decussate below the cranial nerve nuclei. Therefore, pathologic conditions affecting cranial nerve nuclei on the left side of the brain stem create right-sided hemiplegia, and vice versa.

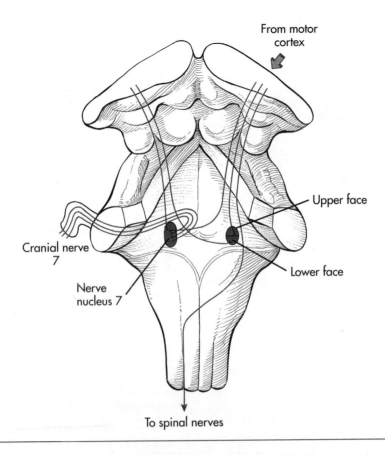

Figure 13-6 ■ Diagram of cranial nerves and their nuclei. A lesion that destroys a cranial nerve nucleus often destroys corticospinal tract fibers that descend alongside the nucleus. Muscles that depend on the destroyed cranial nerve nucleus are paralyzed on the side of the lesion. Because the corticospinal tract decussates below the level of the cranial nerve nuclei, a lesion that destroys a cranial nerve nucleus and adjacent corticospinal fibers causes contralateral paralysis of muscles that are innervated by spinal nerves (such as the muscles of the arm and leg).

Pathologic conditions affecting the motor branch of the *facial nerve (CN 7)* cause weakness or flaccid paralysis of the ipsilateral eyelid muscles and the muscles of facial expression in the lower face. Pathologic conditions affecting the sensory branch of CN 7 cause loss of taste in the anterior two-thirds of the tongue.

Pathologic conditions affecting CN 7 often create a syndrome called *Bell's palsy.* Bell's palsy is a facial nerve syndrome in which the eyelid muscles and the muscles of facial expression on the side of the affected nerve are paralyzed. Bell's palsy is caused by inflammation of CN 7, which passes through a narrow bony channel as it leaves the skull. Inflammation causes CN 7 to swell. Swelling compresses the nerve in the channel. Paralysis and sensory loss in the ipsilateral face follow. Usually Bell's palsy resolves spontaneously within a few days or weeks, but sometimes it does not resolve. When Bell's palsy persists, the patient's facial muscles atrophy and droop and the patient loses automatic eye blinks on the affected side. Loss of automatic eye blinks causes irritation of the eye because the eye no longer is moistened by tears. The patient may have to wear a bandage over the affected eye to control the irritation.

Unilateral facial nerve damage usually has relatively minor effects on speech. Weakness, slowness, and restricted movement of the muscles that purse and retract the lips may cause imprecise articulation of sounds requiring lip movements *(p, b, m, f, v, w, wh)*. Weakness of muscles that tighten the cheeks may make sounds requiring oral breath pressure *(p, b, t, k)* weak and indistinct. These articulatory flaws usually have only minor effects on intelligibility. The speech of patients with unilateral facial nerve pathology usually is intelligible, although the speaker and her or his listeners may find the speaker's articulatory imprecision a minor annoyance.

Bilateral facial nerve damage has much more serious consequences for speech than does unilateral facial nerve damage. Weakness of the muscles of mastication inhibits jaw movement. Paralysis of lip muscles causes severe distortions of sounds requiring lip closure or lip rounding. Vowels requiring lip rounding are distorted. Sounds requiring oral breath pressure are weak and indistinct, and the patient's cheeks may flutter as the patient speaks.

Some patients with bilateral facial paralysis use a finger to prop up a sagging jaw or may use a finger to push up the lower lip to make sounds that require lip closure (Duffy, 2005).

Pathologic conditions affecting the *glossopharyngeal nerve (CN 9)* reduce or abolish the gag reflex and weaken or paralyze the (ipsilateral) muscles that elevate the palate and larynx, plus the muscles that constrict the pharynx. Tactile sensation to the posterior wall of the pharynx and the back of the tongue on the side of the nerve damage may be reduced or abolished. Dysphagia is a common consequence of CN 9 damage. Pathologic conditions affecting CN 9 may cause hypernasality by limiting velopharyngeal elevation and constriction.

Because CN 9, CN 10 (the vagus nerve), and CN 11 (the spinal accessory nerve) travel side by side as they leave the medulla and exit the skull, pathologic conditions affecting CN 9 usually affect CN 10 and CN 11 also.

Pathologic conditions affecting the *vagus nerve (CN 10)* cause paralysis of the muscles of the soft palate on the side of the nerve damage, creating mild to moderate hypernasality of sounds requiring oral breath pressure. Pathologic conditions affecting the recurrent laryngeal branch of CN 10 cause unilateral vocal-fold paralysis, producing weak and breathy or hoarse voice, reduced vocal pitch, pitch breaks, and *diplophonia* (the presence of two pitches or tones in the voice). If the sensory branch of CN 10 is damaged, pharyngeal sensation is impaired, and the mechanics of swallowing may be compromised.

Pathology affecting the *spinal accessory nerve (CN 11)* usually has no direct effects on speech, because CN 11 innervates external muscles of the neck and shoulders rather than muscles directly involved in speech. Bilateral accessory nerve pathology may have indirect effects on speech if muscle weakness causes shoulder and head droop that interferes with respiration and phonation.

Pathologic conditions affecting the *hypoglossal nerve (CN 12)* cause (usually mild) ipsilateral weakness of the tongue. Patients with CN 12 damage have difficulty protruding their tongue, which deviates to the weak side because the muscles on the strong side pull the tongue out while the weak side lags behind. These patients also have difficulty moving the tongue laterally toward the side of the nerve damage because the weakened muscles on that side cannot move the tongue against the resistance created by the resting tone of the contralateral tongue muscles.

CN 12 damage typically causes imprecise articulation of sounds that depend on tongue movements. The effects of unilateral hypoglossal nerve pathology typically are mild and do not seriously compromise intelligibility. Bilateral hypoglossal nerve damage has more serious consequences. Sounds that require elevation of the tongue *(k, g, s, sh, tch, r, l)* are particularly sensitive to the effects of bilateral hypoglossal nerve damage. If tongue weakness is severe, vocal resonance may be affected because the immobile tongue changes the customary shape of the oropharyngeal cavity during speech. CN 12 damage may affect swallowing if the patient cannot control the movement of food during chewing and cannot position the food bolus before swallowing it.

Box 13-4 lists the salient characteristics of flaccid dysarthria.

Box 13-4	Characteristics of Flaccid Dysarthria

Distinguishing Speech Characteristics
Hypernasality
Imprecise consonants
Continuous breathy voice
Nasal emission
Audible inspirations

Other Speech Characteristics
Monopitch
Harsh voice
Short phrases
Monoloudness

Related Signs
Hypotonus (flaccidity)
Diminished reflexes
Muscle fasciculations
Muscle atrophy

Data from Darley, F.L., Aronson, A.E., & Brown, J.R. (1975). *Motor speech disorders*. Philadelphia: W.B. Saunders; Duffy, J.R. (2005). *Motor speech disorders: Substrates, differential diagnosis, and management* (2nd ed.). St. Louis: Elsevier; and Rosenbek, J.C., & LaPointe, L.L. (1985). The dysarthrias: Description, diagnosis, and treatment. In D.F. Johns (Ed.). *Clinical management of neurogenic communication disorders* (2nd ed.). Boston: Little, Brown and Company.

Spinal Nerve Damage

Pathologic conditions affecting cervical and thoracic spinal nerves sometimes compromise respiratory support for speech by weakening or paralyzing respiratory muscles. Spinal nerve damage affecting spinal nerves C3, C4, and C5, which innervate the muscles of the diaphragm, is especially likely to compromise respiratory support. Damage in spinal nerves T2 through T12, which innervate muscles of the thoracic and abdominal wall, usually has less striking effects on respiratory support, unless it occurs in combination with pathology of cervical spinal nerves.

If respiratory muscles are significantly weakened by spinal cord damage, the patient cannot draw enough air into the lungs to maintain adequate breath pressure at the vocal folds. The effects of respiratory insufficiency often are intensified by weakness and hypotonia in laryngeal muscles, which fail to fully adduct the vocal folds. Incomplete adduction of the vocal folds causes inefficient use of the patient's limited air supply. Patients who have insufficient respiratory support for speech speak in short utterances separated by effortful inhalations. These patients usually have weak voices and breathy voice quality, particularly at the end of utterances. The voices of patients with respiratory insufficiency usually have abnormally low pitch and have little variability in pitch and loudness, giving them a monotonous quality.

Extrapyramidal System Damage

Darley, Aronson, and Brown (1975) divided dysarthrias caused by extrapyramidal system damage into two categories—*hypokinetic dysarthria* and *hyperkinetic dysarthria*. Both kinds of dysarthria are caused by damage in and around the basal ganglia, but they differ in the nature of the abnormal movements that follow the damage.

Hypokinetic dysarthria is characterized by slow volitional speech movements and difficulty initiating volitional speech movements (a phenomenon called *bradykinesia*), rigidity of muscles supporting speech, and tremor in muscles supporting speech and respiration.

Hypokinetic dysarthria most often is associated with degenerative neurologic disease—usually Parkinson's disease. About three-fourths of all cases of hypokinetic dysarthria are related to degenerative disease (Duffy, 2005). Brain damage associated with vascular disturbances in the basal ganglia and frontal lobe white matter account for about 10% of cases (Figure 13-7).

Hypokinetic dysarthria sometimes appears as a consequence of other nervous system diseases such as progressive supranuclear palsy and Wilson's disease. Occasionally it appears following anoxia, drug overdose, or repeated blows to the head. (See Chapter 12 for more on Parkinson's disease and related conditions.)

Muscle rigidity is a prominent symptom of Parkinson's disease. The rigidity affects muscles

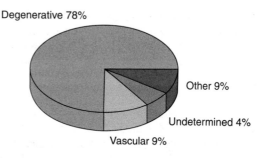

Degenerative 78%

Other 9%

Undetermined 4%

Vascular 9%

Figure 13-7 ■ Causes of dysarthria for 167 Mayo Clinic patients with a primary diagnosis of hypokinetic dysarthria. (Data from Duffy, J.R. [2005]. *Motor speech disorders: Substrates, differential diagnosis, and management* [2nd ed.]. St. Louis: Elsevier.)

of ambulation, respiration, speech, and facial expression. Rigid respiratory muscles compromise respiration. The patient's utterances are short and are separated by long pauses for breath. Rigid laryngeal muscles resist vibration and do not fully adduct the vocal folds. The patient's voice is strained and breathy. Respiratory insufficiency, rigid laryngeal muscles, and incomplete adduction of the vocal folds compromise vocal intensity. The patient's voice is weak, sometimes breathy. Rigid articulatory muscles restrict range of articulatory movement. The patient's speech is imprecise and indistinct. The initiation and timing of articulatory movements is disrupted. The patient's speech is highly variable, with periods of normal rate alternating with rushes of rapid and indistinct speech, punctuated by inappropriately placed pauses. Box 13-5 lists the salient characteristics of hypokinetic dysarthria.

Persons with Parkinson's disease often have great difficulty taking the first steps when attempting to walk, but once they get going, they walk faster and faster with smaller and smaller steps until they are shuffling rapidly along on tiny steps. When persons with Parkinson's disease talk, they often have difficulty getting speech started, but once started, speak faster and faster until their speech becomes a blur of run-together words. The speech disturbances and the gait disturbances of persons with Parkinson's disease may relate to the same problem of initiating and controlling the rate of volitional movements.

Hyperkinetic dysarthria is caused by damage in the basal ganglia. The damage causes involuntary, uncontrollable movements of muscles serving speech and respiration. Darley, Aronson, and Brown (1975) described two kinds of hyperkinesia—*quick hyperkinesia* and *slow hyperkinesia*. *Quick hyperkinesias* (myoclonus, tics, chorea, ballism) are characterized by rapid, unpatterned, unsustained, or briefly sustained involuntary movements. *Slow hyperkinesias* (athetosis, dystonia) are characterized by sustained involuntary movements that build slowly to a peak before gradually subsiding. Muscle tone waxes and wanes in slow hyperkinesias, producing distorted postures of the head, trunk, and limbs.

Duffy (2005) asserts that *hyperkinetic dysarthrias* (plural) is an appropriate label for this category of speech disturbances—a label that reflects the existence of different kinds of movement disorders that may cause hyperkinetic dysarthria.

The involuntary movements associated with hyperkinetic syndromes affect speech when the movements affect muscles of respiration, phonation, or articulation. Involuntary movements of respiratory muscles cause uncontrolled changes in breath pressure at the vocal folds, and vocal intensity fluctuates. When involuntary movements disrupt the timing, force, and amplitude of speech movements, articulation breaks down. Patients affected by hyperkinetic dysarthria speak slowly and pause often. Their speech has an uneven, jerky quality because normal variations in loudness and pitch are exaggerated by the involuntary movements of respiratory muscles. The articulation of patients with hyperkinetic dysarthria often has an intermittently

Box 13-5	***Characteristics of Hypokinetic Dysarthria***

Distinguishing Speech Characteristics
Monopitch
Reduced stress
Monoloudness
Blurring of consonant distinctions
Short rushes of speech

Other Speech Characteristics
Rapid rate, inability to modify rate
Harsh voice
Low pitch
Inappropriate silent intervals

Related Signs
Muscle rigidity
Slowness of movement
Tremor
Masked facies*
Festinating gait†
Stooped posture

*Masked facies: Rigidity of facial muscles, which causes a masklike countenance devoid of expression.
†Festinating gait: Walking begins with slow steps. Steps increase in rate and become smaller until the patient shuffles with short, rapid steps.

Data from Darley, F.L., Aronson, A.E., & Brown, J.R. (1975). *Motor speech disorders.* Philadelphia: W.B. Saunders; Duffy, J.R. (2005). *Motor speech disorders: Substrates, differential diagnosis, and management* (2nd ed.). St. Louis: Elsevier; and Rosenbek, J.C., & LaPointe, L.L. (1985). The dysarthrias: Description, diagnosis, and treatment. In D.F. Johns (Ed.). *Clinical management of neurogenic communication disorders* (2nd ed.). Boston: Little, Brown and Company.

explosive quality because involuntary movements of the speech muscles exaggerate articulatory movements.

"Of all the types of dysarthrias, it [hyperkinetic dysarthria] is probably the one in which visual observation during speech helps to define the disorder because involuntary movements of the jaw, face, and tongue so obviously explain so many of its deviant perceptual characteristics." (Duffy, 1995, p. 351)

Box 13-6	*Characteristics of Hyperkinetic Dysarthria*

Quick Hyperkinetic (Chorea)

"… a highly variable pattern of interference with articulation; episodes of hypernasality; harshness and breathiness; and unplanned variations in loudness." (Darley, Aronson, & Brown, 1975, p. 210).

Distinguishing Speech Characteristics
Prolonged intervals between phonemes
Abnormal silent intervals
Variable rate
Distorted vowels, prolonged phonemes
Excess loudness variation

Other Speech Characteristics
Imprecise consonants
Monopitch
Harsh voice
Monoloudness
Short phrases
Irregular articulatory breakdown
Excess, equal stress or reduced stress
Hypernasality
Strained-strangled-hoarse voice
Voice stoppages

Related Signs
Quick, unsustained involuntary movements
Sudden respiratory inspiration or expiration
Dysphagia (swallowing impairments)

Slow Hyperkinetic (Dystonia)

"… the hyperkinetic dysarthria of dystonia shares with ataxic dysarthria and the hyperkinetic dysarthria of chorea characteristic and marked irregularities in precision of articulation, control of loudness, maintenance of steady rate, and efficiency of phonation." (Darley, Aronson, & Brown, 1975, p. 222)

Distinguishing Speech Characteristics
Prolonged intervals between phonemes
Abnormal silent intervals
Irregular articulatory breakdown
Prolonged phonemes
Excess loudness variation

Other Speech Characteristics
Short phrases
Reduced stress
Voice stoppages
Slow rate
Imprecise consonants
Distorted vowels
Harsh voice
Strained-strangled-hoarse voice
Monopitch, monoloudness

Related Signs
Slow, sustained, unpredictable involuntary movements

NOTE: The visual characteristics of hyperkinetic movement disorders (jerks, tics, spasms, distorted postures) are diagnostically confirmatory of the disease syndrome. Speech abnormalities occur in conjunction with the movement disorders and are physiologically compatible with the movement disorders, but usually are not the primary means of diagnosing the underlying disease.

Data from Darley, F.L., Aronson, A.E., & Brown, J.R. (1975). *Motor speech disorders*. Philadelphia: W.B. Saunders; Duffy, J.R.. (2005). *Motor speech disorders: Substrates, differential diagnosis, and management* (2nd ed.). St. Louis: Elsevier; and Rosenbek, J.C., & LaPointe, L.L. (1985). The dysarthrias: Description, diagnosis, and treatment. In D.F. Johns (Ed.). *Clinical management of neurogenic communication disorders* (2nd ed.). Boston: Little, Brown and Company.

Box 13-6 lists salient characteristics of hyperkinetic dysarthria.

In terms of cause, hyperkinetic dysarthria is the most mysterious form of dysarthria. Duffy (2005) reported that the cause of dysarthria for approximately two-thirds of a sample of 141 patients with a primary diagnosis of hyperkinetic dysarthria was unknown. Toxic/metabolic conditions and degenerative disease accounted for the largest percentages of known causes (Figure 13-8).

Cerebellar Damage

Pathologic conditions affecting the cerebellum disrupt motor coordination and timing, usually accompanied by loss of muscle tone. The

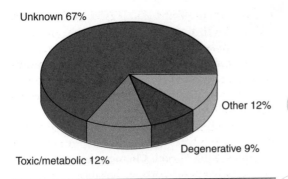

Unknown 67%

Other 12%

Degenerative 9%

Toxic/metabolic 12%

Figure 13-8 ▪ Causes of dysarthria for 141 Mayo Clinic patients with a primary diagnosis of hyperkinetic dysarthria. (Data from Duffy, J.R. [2005]. *Motor speech disorders: Substrates, differential diagnosis, and management* [2nd ed.]. St. Louis: Elsevier.)

Box 13-7	***Characteristics of Ataxic Dysarthria***

Distinguishing Speech Characteristics
Inconsistent consonant misarticulation
Excess, equal stress (scanning speech)
Irregular articulatory breakdown
Irregular, excessive loudness variability
Excessive rate variability

Other Speech Characteristics
Harsh voice
Prolonged phonemes
Prolonged interphonemic intervals
Falling intonation on vowels

Related Signs
Hypotonus
Diminished reflexes
Intention tremor
Dysmetria*

scant-like
slurred
speech &
drunken quality

*Dysmetria: Inaccurate trajectory of goal-directed movements, causing overshoot or undershoot of targets.

Data from Darley, F.L., Aronson, A.E., & Brown, J.R. (1975). *Motor speech disorders.* Philadelphia: W.B. Saunders; Duffy, J.R. (2005). *Motor speech disorders: Substrates, differential diagnosis, and management* (2nd ed.). St. Louis: Elsevier; and Rosenbek, J.C., & LaPointe, L.L. (1985). The dysarthrias: Description, diagnosis, and treatment. In D.F. Johns (Ed.). *Clinical management of neurogenic communication disorders* (2nd ed.). Boston: Little, Brown and Company.

affected person's volitional movements are slow and awkward (a condition called *ataxia*). The range and force of movements are distorted (a condition called *dysmetria*), causing movements to have a jerky and segmented quality (a condition called *decomposition of movement*). The intentional limb movements of patients with cerebellar damage are disturbed by coarse tremor at right angles to the direction of movement. The tremor disappears when the muscles are at rest. Darley, Aronson, and Brown (1975) called the dysarthria associated with cerebellar pathology *ataxic dysarthria,* an appellation that has continued to the present.

The speech of patients with ataxic dysarthria is characterized by anomalous force, timing, and amplitude of movements. Ataxic respiratory muscles create uncontrolled changes in breath pressure at the vocal folds, causing irregular and sometimes explosive changes in vocal pitch and loudness. Ataxic articulatory muscles periodically disrupt articulation. The speech of a patient with cerebellar ataxia may alternate between normal nasal resonance and hypernasality as ataxic velopharyngeal muscles fluctuate in the force and amplitude of movement.

Box 13-7 lists salient characteristics of ataxic dysarthria.

Ataxic dysarthria may be caused by several pathologic conditions affecting the cerebellum. Cerebellar degeneration and demyelinating diseases account for about half the cases of ataxic dysarthria. Vascular disease affecting the cerebellum accounts for 13% of cases (Figure 13-9).

Anterior Horn Cell Disease

Several neurologic diseases are characterized by degeneration of anterior horn cells in the spinal cord. Most also cause degeneration of motor neurons serving cranial nerves, and some

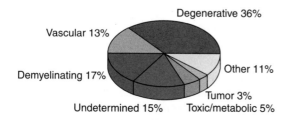

Degenerative 36%

Vascular 13%

Other 11%

Demyelinating 17%

Tumor 3%

Undetermined 15%   Toxic/metabolic 5%

Figure 13-9 ■ Causes of dysarthria for 166 Mayo Clinic patients with a primary diagnosis of ataxic dysarthria. (Data from Duffy, J.R. [2005]. *Motor speech disorders: Substrates, differential diagnosis, and management* [2nd ed.]. St. Louis: Elsevier.)

extend to the corticospinal and corticobulbar tracts. Degeneration of anterior horn cells causes symptoms typical of lower motor neuron disease—flaccid paralysis, fasciculations of muscles, and eventual muscle atrophy. Anterior horn cell disease, by itself, has only indirect effects on speech. Weakness of respiratory muscles or muscles of the shoulders and rib cage may compromise breath support for speech, reducing vocal intensity and shortening the amount that the speaker can say on a single breath. When anterior horn cell disease affects cranial nerves, corticospinal tracts, or corticobulbar tracts, movements of the speech muscles may be weak and slow, affecting articulation, speech rate, speech prosody, and vocal quality. Almost all anterior horn cell diseases are progressive (except for poliomyelitis). Consequently, many patients require augmentative or alternative communication systems during the final stage of the disease.

Spinal Nerve Disease

Spinal nerves sometimes are affected by inflammatory or destructive disease. Inflammatory spinal nerve diseases (such as Guillain-Barre syndrome) usually affect the longest nerves first. Limb muscles are affected before

muscles in the torso, and distal limb muscles are affected before proximal limb muscles. Motor fibers usually are affected before sensory fibers. Spinal nerve diseases produce symptoms typical of lower motor neuron disease—weakness, hypotonia, fasciculations, diminished reflexes, and variable sensory impairment. As is true for anterior horn cell disease, spinal nerve disease usually affects speech indirectly by compromising respiration. However, if the disease extends into the brain stem or corticobulbar tracts, speech movements may be directly affected, with changes typical of lower motor neuron pathology.

Guillain-Barre syndrome is a progressive but self-limiting autoimmune disease characterized by axonal demyelination and progressive muscle weakness. Recovery usually begins spontaneously within a few weeks of onset and may go on for months or years. Its cause is unknown, but it sometimes develops following inoculations or surgical procedures.

Diseases of the Neuromuscular Junction

Diseases of the neuromuscular junction are characterized by abnormalities in the neurotransmitters responsible for transmission of nerve impulses across synapses. The abnormalities are related to deficiency or excess of neurotransmitters or to alterations in the sensitivity of receptor cells to the neurotransmitters. *Myasthenia gravis* is the most common of the neuromuscular junction diseases. Myasthenia gravis is caused by autoimmune-mediated damage to the acetylcholine receptors on muscle cells, which interferes with neuromuscular transmission. Symptoms of myasthenia gravis include generalized but fluctuating muscle weakness (with a predilection for the extraocular, pharyngeal, oral, and proximal limb muscles), rapid muscle fatigue, and quick recovery of strength when muscles are rested. Myasthenia gravis often causes a unique flaccid dysarthria syndrome in which the patient's speech intelligibility deteriorates as the patient talks, but recovers with rest.

Injection of drugs that enhance acetylcholine uptake (Tensilon, neostigmine) causes dramatic improvement in the speech of patients with myasthenia gravis. The patient's dysarthria improves or disappears within 30 to 60 seconds after Tensilon injection, or within 10 to 15 minutes after neostigmine injection. The effects of Tensilon last 4 to 5 minutes and the effects of neostigmine last for 2 or 3 hours. (The differences in rate and duration of symptom remission exist because Tensilon is injected into a vein and neostigmine is injected into a muscle.)

Primary Diseases of Muscle

Some diseases damage muscle fibers and produce atrophy of muscles and flaccid dysarthria. *Myotonic dystrophy* is a common inherited muscle disease that affects muscles responsible for speech. *Myositis,* an acquired inflammatory muscle disease, usually does not affect speech but may affect respiratory muscles and sometimes produces swallowing problems. When myopathy affects muscles serving respiration and speech, characteristic signs of muscle weakness appear. If the patient's respiratory muscles are affected, the patient's utterances are short, long pauses occur between utterances, and vocal intensity is diminished, because the patient does not possess the respiratory drive needed for normal utterance length and vocal intensity. If the patient's laryngeal muscles are affected, the patient's voice is weak and breathy, because weakened laryngeal muscles cannot fully adduct the vocal folds and maintain the muscle tension needed for normal voice. If the patient's velopharyngeal muscles are affected the patient is hypernasal, and if the patient's articulatory muscles are affected the patient's articulation is slow and indistinct.

Sensory Loss

Damage to sensory branches of the cranial nerves or to the sensory cortex may impair sensation in the face, mouth, and neck, sometimes causing transient speech disturbances, usually lasting no more than a few weeks. Persisting dysarthria from sensory disturbance alone is rare. However, when sensory disturbances are superimposed on coexisting motor impairments, the resulting dysarthria may be more severe than if the sensory disturbance were not present. A normal motor system usually has enough resilience to compensate for sensory disturbances, but an impaired motor system often does not.

Disorders of Multiple Motor Systems *spastic & flaccid d*

What Darley, Aronson, and Brown called *mixed dysarthria* is common in clinical practice. According to Duffy (2005) about 30% of patients with a primary diagnosis of dysarthria seen at Mayo Clinic over an 11-year interval had mixed dysarthria. Mixed dysarthrias often are caused by combinations of neurologic events (e.g., multiple strokes, stroke plus demyelinating disease) and by diseases that affect more than one component of the motor system (e.g., amyotrophic lateral sclerosis).

Mixed dysarthrias represent a heterogeneous group of speech disorders and neurologic diseases. Virtually any combination of two or more of the pure dysarthria types is possible, and in any particular mix any one of the components may predominate. In spite of its heterogeneity, and the fact that sorting out the various components of mixed dysarthrias can be quite difficult, many mixed dysarthrias are perceptually distinguishable. And, like the pure forms, they may be the first, or among the first signs of neurologic disease. (Duffy, 2005, p. 276)

Combinations of spastic dysarthria and flaccid dysarthria are common in mixed dysarthria. Duffy (2005) reported the distribution of dysarthria types in a sample of 300

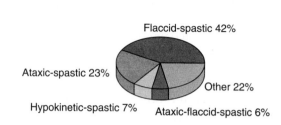

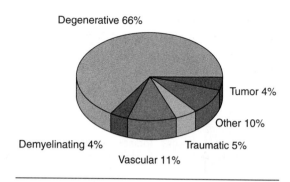

Figure 13-10 ■ Distribution of dysarthria types in a sample of 300 Mayo Clinic patients with a primary diagnosis of mixed dysarthria. (Data from Duffy, J.R. [2005]. *Motor speech disorders: Substrates, differential diagnosis, and management* [2nd ed.]. St. Louis: Elsevier.)

Figure 13-11 ■ Causes of dysarthria for 406 Mayo Clinic patients with a primary diagnosis of mixed dysarthria. (Data from Duffy, J.R. [2005]. *Motor speech disorders: Substrates, differential diagnosis, and management* [2nd ed.]. St. Louis: Elsevier.)

patients with a primary diagnosis of mixed dysarthria. Flaccid-spastic and ataxic-spastic combinations accounted for about two-thirds of the cases of mixed dysarthria in the sample (Figure 13-10). No other combination accounted for more than 7% of the sample. (*Other* in Figure 13-10 represents combinations that each accounted for less than 5% of the sample.)

Degenerative disease, especially amyotrophic lateral sclerosis (ALS), was the most common cause of mixed dysarthria in the Mayo Clinic sample, accounting for about two-thirds of cases. Vascular disease was the second most common cause, accounting for slightly more than 10% of cases. Demyelinating disease, traumatic brain injury, and tumor were occasional causes (Figure 13-11).

The distribution of dysarthria types involved in mixed dysarthria is strongly influenced by the presence of ALS. The presence of ALS patients in the Mayo Clinic group of patients with mixed dysarthria increased the proportion of patients with flaccid dysarthria and spastic dysarthria. When patients with ALS (who characteristically experience a mix of flaccid and

spastic dysarthria) were removed from the group, the proportion of these two dysarthria types decreased, and the proportions of other types of dysarthria increased. Flaccid and spastic dysarthrias were by far the most common types in the group of ALS patients (Figure 13-1?

Dysarthria Versus Apraxia of Speech

Determining if a patient's speech abnormalities represent dysarthria or apraxia of speech usually is not difficult for experienced practitioners. Information from the neurologic examination may point to an appropriate diagnosis. Damage in or near the cortex of the language-dominant hemisphere suggests *apraxia of speech*. Damage in the basal ganglia, brain stem, or peripheral nerves suggests *dysarthria*. Normal oral and velopharyngeal muscle strength and range of movement for simple nonspeech movements suggest *apraxia of speech*. Impaired muscle strength and range of movement for simple nonspeech movements suggest *dysarthria*. Hemiparesis, spasticity, and exaggerated limb reflexes are signs of damage in the cortex or in corticobulbar or corticospinal tracts. Their presence

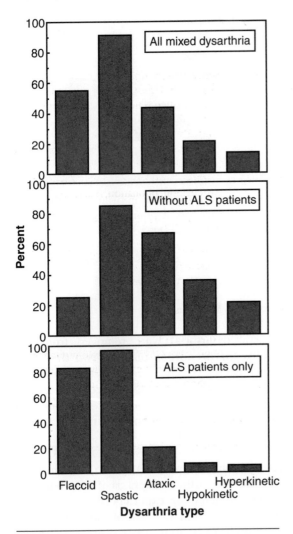

Figure 13-12 ■ Distribution of dysarthria types in a group of 300 patients with a primary diagnosis of mixed dysarthria *(top),* in a subgroup of patients without amyotrophic lateral sclerosis (ALS; *middle),* and in a subgroup of patients with ALS *(bottom).* (Extrapolated from data in Duffy, J.R. [2005]. *Motor speech disorders: Substrates, differential diagnosis, and management* [2nd ed.]. St. Louis: Elsevier.)

suggests that associated motor speech abnormalities are likely to represent *apraxia of speech.* Signs of aphasia (e.g., agrammatism, impaired comprehension, word retrieval failure) also suggest that associated motor speech abnormalities represent *apraxia of speech.*

Apraxia of speech and dysarthria affect speech processes in different ways. Because apraxia of speech is primarily a motor planning and articulatory sequencing problem and not a problem with muscle strength and range of movement, apraxic speakers' articulation and prosody sound abnormal, but their phonation and resonation sound normal or nearly normal. Because dysarthria is a product of weak or uncoordinated muscles, articulation, phonation, resonation, prosody, and sometimes respiration are abnormal.

The speech errors made by apraxic speakers differ from those made by dysarthric speakers. Most apraxic speech errors are distorted sound substitutions; dysarthric speech errors tend to be distortions and omissions. Apraxic speakers often substitute a complex sound for a simple sound (e.g., substituting *ch* for *k*). Apraxic speakers often produce simple sounds and sound sequences without error, but have trouble with complex sounds or with phonologically complex sound sequences, exhibiting effortful groping for articulatory positions. Dysarthric speakers usually have equivalent difficulty and make errors on the same sounds regardless of the length and phonologic complexity of the utterances, and effortful groping is unusual. Apraxic speakers often produce repeated articulatory false starts, often fruitless. Dysarthric speakers usually do not produce large numbers of false starts, perhaps because they have learned that their speech errors are relatively consistent across time and contexts. Imitation is unusually difficult for apraxic speakers. Imitation usually is easier than spontaneous speech for dysarthric speakers. Apraxic speakers

TABLE 13-2	Major Differences between Apraxia of Speech and the Dysarthrias	
Feature	Apraxia of Speech	Dysarthria
Neuropathology	Cortical, language-dominant hemisphere	Subcortical, peripheral
Neurologic signs	Aphasia, hemiparesis, hemiplegia, spasticity, exaggerated reflexes	Rigidity, dyskinesia, flaccid paralysis, diminished reflexes, fasciculations, atrophy[*]
Motor signs	Strength, range of movement, coordination are normal in nonverbal oral movements	Strength, range of movement, coordination are impaired in nonverbal oral movements
Related conditions	Aphasia, buccofacial apraxia, limb apraxia	Dysphagia, dyskinesia, rigidity, hypotonus[†]
Speech processes affected	Articulation, prosody	Articulation, phonation, resonation, prosody
Distinguishing speech errors	Distorted substitutions, transpositions	Distortions, omissions
Speech error pattern	Variable, unpredictable, intervals of error-free speech	Consistent, predictable. No intervals of error-free speech
	Automatic speech better than highly planned speech	No effect of automaticity[‡]
Speech sounds in error	Consonants, primarily in phonologically complex utterances	Most consonants
	Vowels may be distorted	Vowels often distorted[§]
Effects of length, complexity	Longer, phonologically complex utterances more likely to elicit errors	Short, phonologically simple utterances and long, phonologically complex utterance equally affected

[*]These differences are true for dysarthria in general. Specific dysarthria types may differ in some features.
[†]Depending on the type of dysarthria.
[‡]Some patients with hyperkinetic dysarthrias may have intervals of relatively good speech, but these intervals are not predictable based on automaticity, phonologic complexity, etc.
[§]However, more complex consonants are harder for most dysarthric speakers.

often repeat sounds and syllables. Dysarthric speakers usually do not.

Apraxic speakers typically produce what Darley, Aronson, and Brown (1975) called *islands of error-free speech,* in which automatic, unplanned utterances such as verbal asides and editorial comments (e.g., *wait a minute, well whaddya know*) are produced without error. Most dysarthric speakers do not experience such interludes of error-free speech. (The arti-

culatory accuracy of patients who have ataxic or hyperkinetic dysarthria often varies across time, but the variation is related to physiologic changes in neuromotor control, not to the automaticity or phonologic complexity of what is said.) Table 13-2 summarizes the major differences between apraxia of speech and the dysarthrias.

Apraxia of speech and dysarthria sometimes co-occur. The most frequent combination is apraxia of speech plus unilateral upper motor neuron dysarthria. The resulting speech disturbance has elements of apraxia of speech, plus elements of unilateral upper motor neuron dysarthria—mild but consistent articulatory imprecision and (sometimes) mild strained-strangled-harsh voice quality. Bilateral damage in the brain hemispheres sometimes results in apraxia of speech plus spastic dysarthria, wherein slow speech rate, moderate to severe articulatory imprecision, and strained-strangled-harsh voice quality are superimposed on the signs of apraxia of speech. Co-occurrence of apraxia of speech and other dysarthria types is less common. When such combinations do co-occur, the presence of apraxia may be indicated by intervals of improved speech that are related to the linguistic or situational context in which the speech is produced.

Apraxia of speech is less often encountered in large multidisciplinary medical facilities than is dysarthria. Duffy (2005) reviewed the records of over 6,000 Mayo Clinic patients with a pri-

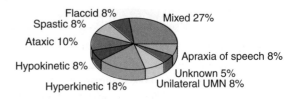

Figure 13-13 ■ Distribution of apraxia of speech and dysarthria types in a group of 6,101 Mayo Clinic patients with a primary diagnosis of neurogenic motor speech disorder. (Data from Duffy, J. R. [2005]. *Motor speech disorders: Substrates, differential diagnosis, and management* [2nd ed.]. St Louis: Elsevier.)

mary diagnosis of neurogenic motor speech disorder to determine the proportions of patients who were diagnosed as having apraxia of speech or the various types of dysarthria. Apraxia of speech was the primary diagnosis for 8% of the patients, and dysarthria was the primary diagnosis for 87% (Figure 13-13).

GENERAL CONCEPTS 13-2

- *Dysarthria* is a generic label for a group of speech impairments caused by weakness, paralysis, incoordination, or sensory loss in muscle groups responsible for speech.
- The most common cause of dysarthria is weakness or paralysis of muscles used in speech.
- Unilateral damage to upper motor neurons usually does not cause persisting dysarthria, because most of the muscles responsible for speech are bilaterally innervated.
- A few patients may develop mild but persisting *unilateral upper motor neuron dysarthria* following apparent unilateral upper motor neuron damage.
- Bilateral damage in upper motor neurons usually causes persisting *spastic dysarthria.*

- Damage in the pons and medulla almost invariably causes *flaccid dysarthria* because of damaged nuclei for cranial nerves serving speech muscles. Pathologic conditions affecting cranial nerve fibers cause *flaccid paralysis* of muscles served by the nerves.
- Flaccid dysarthria often follows damage to the *glossopharyngeal nerve (CN 9),* the *vagus nerve (CN 10),* and the *hypoglossal nerve (CN 12)* because these cranial nerves supply muscles that are important for speech. Damage to the *facial nerve (CN 7)* or the *spinal accessory nerve (CN 11)* do not usually cause significant dysarthria, because the muscles they innervate do not have major responsibilities for speech production.

GENERAL CONCEPTS 13-2—cont'd

- Pathologic conditions affecting the extra-pyramidal system often cause *hypokinetic* or *hyperkinetic dysarthria,* plus associated motor abnormalities (impaired volitional movements, muscle rigidity, uncontrollable involuntary movements).
- *Parkinson's disease* is a common disease of the extrapyramidal system which causes *hypokinetic dysarthria,* characterized by weak, strained, and breathy voice, rushes of rapid speech, and indistinct articulation.
- Pathologic conditions affecting the *basal ganglia* often cause *hyperkinetic dysarthria,* in which speech and respiration are compromised by sporadic involuntary movements of muscle groups.
- *Cerebellar damage* often causes *ataxic dysarthria,* in which relatively well-controlled speech is punctuated by intervals of dysarthria caused by aberrations in the force and amplitude of respiratory and articulatory movements.
- *Degenerative neurologic diseases* often cause *mixed dysarthria.* Mixed dysarthria usually represents a combination of spastic and flaccid signs.
- Diseases affecting *anterior horn cells* or *spinal nerves* sometimes affect speech by com-promising muscles of respiration. Patients with anterior horn cell or spinal nerve disease speak softly, in short utterances, and with abnormally long pauses between utterances, because of respiratory insufficiency.
- Diseases of the *neuromuscular junction* often cause dysarthria. The most common of these diseases is *myasthenia gravis.* The speech of patients with myasthenia gravis becomes increasingly dysarthric the longer they speak. The dysarthria diminishes or disappears with rest.
- *Sensory loss* in structures involved in speech may produce transient mild speech impairments but rarely causes significant dysarthria. However, sensory loss superimposed on coexisting motor speech impairments usually increases the severity of dysarthria.
- Dysarthria may be differentiated from apraxia of speech by the types of speech errors, consistency of speech errors, the presence of intervals of error-free speech, and the effects of context on articulatory accuracy. *Phonation* and *resonation* usually are normal in apraxia of speech but abnormal in dysarthria.

EVALUATION

Dysarthric patients arrive at the speech-language pathologist's office because their speech sounds abnormal to physicians, nurses, family members, or the patients themselves. The speech-language pathologist's assessment of a dysarthric patient usually has five purposes:

- To determine if the patient's speech is abnormal
- To evaluate the nature and severity of speech abnormalities
- To determine the cause(s) of speech abnormalities
- To determine if treatment is appropriate
- To identify potential directions for treatment

Because dysarthria is a problem with speaking, it seems logical that one should look to the mouth for its source. The mouth is an appropriate place to begin, but the search also must extend to the throat, chest, and abdomen and to the pharynx and nasal cavities. Speech requires breath, so assessment of dysarthria includes assessment of respiration. Speech requires voice, so assessment of dysarthria includes assessment of vocal-fold function. Speech requires control of nasal resonance, so assessment of dysarthria includes assessment of the muscles of the posterior pharynx and the soft palate. Speech requires shaping an air stream into consonants and vowels, so assessment of dysarthria includes assessment of how well the tongue, lips, and jaw move, and how quickly and accurately they reach their targets.

Structured assessment of dysarthria usually begins with administration of a *motor speech examination* in which respiration, phonation, resonance, prosody, and articulation are systematically evaluated. Phonation and resonance typically are estimated with a rating scale with which the examiner judges characteristics such as pitch, loudness, voice quality, and nasality. Prosody typically is estimated with a rating scale with which the examiner judges characteristics such as rate, phrase length, stress, and intonation. Respiration may be estimated indirectly with measures such as forced expiration time, sustained phonation time, or maximum utterance length, although phonation time and utterance length are affected by the efficiency of glottal closure as well as by the adequacy of breath support. Articulation is measured with a combination of rating scales and scoring of articulation in speech-production tasks (syllable repetition, word repetition, phrase repetition and spontaneous speech). Figure 13-14 shows a form for rating speech produced by dysarthric individuals.

Structured assessment of dysarthric patients often begins with assessment of respiration, phonation, resonation, and articulation, both individually and as the processes interact. Assessment of dysarthria is as much a search for interactions among processes supporting speech as it is an identification of abnormalities in speech itself.

Evaluating Respiratory Support

Characteristics of Normal Respiration. In neurologically normal adults, respiration for biologic purposes and respiration for speech differ in subtle but important ways. In normal passive breathing, the person's diaphragm provides most of the respiratory force by contracting during inhalation. Contraction of the diaphragm compresses the abdominal contents downward, increases the volume of the chest cavity, and creates negative pressure in the lungs. Muscles in the chest wall and shoulder girdle elevate the shoulders and rib cage, adding to the volume of the chest cavity and increasing negative pressure in the lungs. Outside atmospheric pressure then pushes air into the lungs. Exhalation during normal passive breathing is produced by relaxation of shoulder, chest, and abdominal muscles. The relaxed muscles permit the rib cage to return to its resting position and allow the upward pressure of the abdominal contents to push the relaxed diaphragm upward.

The forces present during passive breathing do not create enough breath pressure for speech, so normal speakers boost respiratory drive by actively contracting the abdominal muscles (Hixon, 1987). During passive breathing, normal adults inflate the lungs to about 20% of total capacity, but when they speak they inflate them to from 35% to 60% of total capacity (Hixon, 1987). The usual respiratory pattern during speech consists of quick inhalation to about 60% of lung capacity, followed by slow exhalation until the lungs reach about 30% of total capacity, at which time the speaker takes another breath. The normal ratio of inhalation to exhalation is about 1 to 6—that is, the expiratory phase lasts about six times as long as the inspiratory phase (Yorkston, Beukelman, & Bell, 1988).

Passive Respiration. A patient's posture and general appearance may suggest potential respiratory insufficiency. Patients who slouch and bend forward at the waist when standing or

Rating Scale for Motor Speech Disorders

Phonation
Overall pitch: Very low ☐ Somewhat low ☐ Normal ☐ Somewhat high ☐ Very high ☐
Pitch breaks: Often ☐ Sometimes ☐ Never ☐
Monotone, monopitch: Severe ☐ Moderate ☐ Normal ☐
Tremor: Severe ☐ Moderate ☐ Normal ☐
Loudness: Very loud ☐ Somewhat loud ☐ Normal ☐ Somewhat soft ☐ Very soft ☐
Uncontrolled changes in loudness: Often ☐ Sometimes ☐ Never ☐
Diminishing loudness with sustained phonation: Severe ☐ Moderate ☐ Normal ☐
Harsh voice (rough,raspy): Severe ☐ Moderate ☐ Normal ☐
Hoarse voice (wet,gurgly): Severe ☐ Moderate ☐ Normal ☐
Breathy voice: Severe ☐ Moderate ☐ Normal ☐

Respiration
Forced inspiration, expiration: Often ☐ Sometimes ☐ Never ☐
Audible inhalation: Often ☐ Sometimes ☐ Never ☐
Audible exhalation: Often ☐ Sometimes ☐ Never ☐
Utterance length: Very short ☐ Somewhat short ☐ Normal ☐

Resonace
Very hyponasal ☐ Somewhat hyponasal ☐ Normal ☐ Somewhat hypernasal ☐ Very hypernasal ☐
Nasal emission: Severe ☐ Moderate ☐ Mild ☐ None ☐

Prosody
Rate: Very slow ☐ Somewhat slow ☐ Normal ☐ Somewhat fast ☐ Very fast ☐
Rate: Very variable ☐ Somewhat variable ☐ Normal variability ☐ Less than normal variability ☐
Intermittent fast rate: Often ☐ Sometimes ☐ Never ☐
Stress: Reduced ☐ Excessive ☐ Uncontrolled Changes ☐ Normal ☐ Less than normal ☐
Excessive pauses: Between phrases ☐ Between words ☐ Within words ☐
Short rushes of speech: Often ☐ Sometimes ☐ Never ☐

Articulation
Imprecise consonants: Often ☐ Sometimes ☐ Never ☐
Weak plosive consonants: Severe ☐ Moderate ☐ Mild ☐ None ☐
Distorted vowels: Often ☐ Sometimes ☐ Never ☐
Prolonged phonemes: Often ☐ Sometimes ☐ Never ☐
Repeated phonemes: Often ☐ Sometimes ☐ Never ☐
Irregular articulatory imprecision: Often ☐ Sometimes ☐ Never ☐

Consistency of errors
Phoneme errors: Consistent ☐ Inconsistent ☐
Syllable/word errors: Consistent ☐ Inconsistent ☐
Intervals of fluent, error-free speech: Many ☐ Some ☐ None ☐

Error Correction
Attempts to correct errors: Often ☐ Sometimes ☐ Never ☐
Successful error correction: Often ☐ Sometimes ☐ Never ☐

Spontaneous Speech versus Repetition
Spontaneous speech better ☐ Repetition better ☐ No difference ☐

Intelligibility
10% or less ☐ 11% - 25% ☐ 26% - 50% ☐ 51% - 75% ☐ 76% or above ☐

Overall Effect on Listener
Very distracting ☐ Somewhat distracting ☐ Minimally distracting ☐ Within normal range ☐

Figure 13-14 ■ A form for rating various aspects of motor speech disorders.

sitting, or patients who sit or stand with chin lowered and head drooping may compromise respiration for speech by compressing the chest cavity and lungs. (Slouched, drooping posture often is a sign of generalized muscle weakness, which itself may compromise respiration.)

Abnormality in the rate and depth of a patient's passive respiration also may suggest respiratory insufficiency for speech. Normal passive respiration rates range from 12 to 20 cycles per minute, and movement of the shoulders or head during passive breathing is not obvious. When a patient's head and shoulders do move during passive breathing, he or she may be compensating for weak respiratory muscles. Fast, shallow breathing (in the absence of exertion or heightened emotions) also may be a sign of weakness in the muscles of respiration. Fluctuating breathing rate during passive breathing may be a manifestation of involuntary movements associated with cerebellar or extrapyramidal system pathology.

Respiration for Speech. The usual first objective in evaluating respiration for speech is to determine if comprehensive evaluation of respiratory function is necessary. The evaluation usually begins by asking the patient to produce sustained phonation and repeat long strings of syllables. Most normal adults can sustain phonation of an open vowel (e.g., *ah*) for 8 to 10 seconds and can produce at least 15 to 20 monosyllables on a single breath. If a patient can sustain effortless phonation of an open vowel with normal loudness for 4 to 5 seconds and can say 5 or 6 consonant-vowel syllables on a single breath with normal loudness, respiration is likely to be at least minimally adequate for speech, and direct work on respiration may not be needed.

Patients with 4- to 5-second maximum phonation times will be able to say only short phrases (one to three words) on a single breath. For these patients, respiration may be worked on indirectly by increasing the number of words the patient can say on a single breath.

If the patient fails to meet sustained-phonation criteria, the clinician cannot immediately conclude that the problem is with respiratory support, because sustained phonation requires not only that the patient impound an adequate air supply, but that the respiratory muscles be strong enough to generate functional subglottic air pressure, and that laryngeal muscles be strong enough and agile enough to keep the vocal folds adducted against the pressure of the breath stream. Problems with vocal-fold adduction usually are obvious during phonation. If the vocal folds are not closing, the patient's voice sounds weak and breathy. If the vocal folds are hypertonic, the patient's voice sounds harsh and strangled.

Respiratory Pressure and Flow. Sophisticated instruments are available for measuring respiratory pressure and flow. Most are not commonly available clinically. However, two inexpensive and relatively simple instruments for measuring breath pressure and flow can be constructed.

Netsell and Hixon (1978) described a *U-tube manometer* suitable for measuring breath pressure (Figure 13-15). The manometer is a U-shaped glass tube fastened to a board. The tube is half-filled with colored water and is calibrated in centimeters (see Netsell and Hixon for specifications). A flexible tube is attached to one end of the U-tube. A rigid T-shaped tube serves as a mouthpiece and bleed tube. The patient blows into the mouthpiece, and breath pressure displaces the column of water. The leak tube provides a constant escape for the air stream so that the tested person must maintain continuous air flow to sustain displacement of the water. According to Netsell and Hixon, an individual who can maintain a 5 cm displacement of the water column for 5 seconds has sufficient breath pressure for basic speech processes (*the 5 for 5 rule*).

Hixon, Hawley, and Wilson (1982) suggested a similar but simpler device. A tall drinking glass (12 cm or more) is filled with water. The glass is calibrated in centimeters (Figure 13-16). A drinking straw is affixed to the glass so that

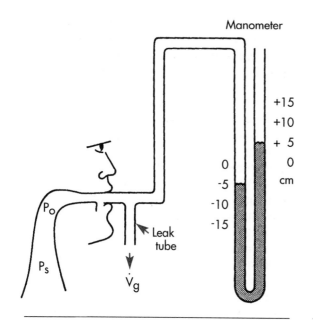

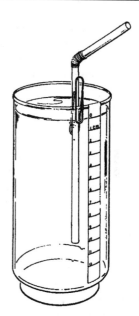

Figure 13-15 ■ A U-tube manometer. The patient blows into the mouthpiece. A leak tube permits a constant amount of air to escape. The height of the liquid in the U-tube is determined by the amount of breath pressure the patient can sustain. (From Netsell, R., & Hixon, T. J. [1978]. A noninvasive method for clinically estimating subglottal air pressure. *Journal of Speech and Hearing Disorders, 43,* 326-330.)

Figure 13-16 ■ A water-glass manometer. The deeper the straw is in the water, the more breath pressure is needed to sustain a string of bubbles at the deep end of the straw. (From Hixon, T. J., Hawley, J. T., & Wilson, K. J. [1982]. An around-the-house device for the clinical determination of respiratory driving pressure. *Journal of Speech and Hearing Disorders, 47,* 413-415.)

it reaches a prescribed depth (e.g., 5 cm). An individual blowing into the straw must maintain breath pressure equal to the depth to which the straw is inserted in the water to generate a stream of bubbles at the end of the straw. By inserting the straw to 5 cm, one can evaluate whether a patient meets the 5 for 5 rule.

Phonation

Laryngeal Mechanics. Assessment of laryngeal muscle function often precedes assessment of phonation. To determine the functional integrity of muscles that adduct the vocal cords, the examiner may ask the patient to cough, grunt, or produce *glottal stops* (voiceless grunts) individually and several times in succession. Weak, breathy, or indistinct coughs, grunts, and

glottal stops suggest weakness of vocal cord adductor muscles, impaired respiratory drive, or both. Patients with compromised respiratory support often produce sharper glottal stops and grunts than coughs, because grunts and glottal stops require less respiratory drive than coughs. Patients with compromised vocal-fold adduction produce weak and indistinct coughs, grunts, and glottal stops (Duffy, 2005). The presence of *inhalation stridor* (a rasping sound during inhalation) suggests weakness in the muscles that separate *(abduct)* the vocal cords. *Phonation Time and Voice Quality.* The typical first step in evaluating phonation is to ask the patient to sustain an open vowel (e.g., *ah*) until the patient runs out of breath, while the clinician times the duration of the patient's phonation. As the patient phonates, the clinician also evaluates the loudness, pitch, and quality of the patient's voice. Phonation times below 12 to 15 seconds are considered low and suggest problems either with glottal valving or with breath support for speech.

Damage in cranial nerves, especially the laryngeal branches of the vagus nerve, may cause weakness or paralysis of laryngeal muscles. The weakened muscles cannot fully adduct the vocal folds, leading to air wastage and to diminished phonation time, plus breathy and weak voice quality and abnormally low pitch.

Bilateral damage to upper motor neurons causes strained-strangled-harsh voice quality. Spastic laryngeal muscles constrict the glottal opening, increase glottal resistance to airflow, and reduce maximum phonation time. Most patients with bilateral upper motor neuron pathology have sufficient respiratory drive to produce 5 to 10 seconds of sustained phonation, although with strained, strangled, and harsh quality.

Most patients with cerebellar pathology can produce 5 to 10 seconds of sustained phonation, although voice quality is likely to be abnormal, and both loudness and quality may fluctuate. Abnormalities in coordination of respiration and vocal-fold adduction may cause aspiration of voiced sounds or strained, strangled voice quality at the onset of phonation.

Extrapyramidal diseases may affect vocal-fold adduction, shortening phonation time and affecting voice quality. Maximum phonation times for patients with extrapyramidal disease range from substantially reduced (3 to 4 seconds) to normal, depending on the efficiency of glottal valving and the degree to which respiratory muscles are affected.

Patients with Parkinson's disease typically have breathy, hoarse voices, with maximum phonation time reduced by laryngeal muscle rigidity. Patients with Parkinson's disease often begin phonation normally but sound progressively more strangled as they continue to phonate. These patients' phonation often ends either in a whisper or in a squeak. Patients with movement disorders caused by extrapyramidal disease (e.g., tremor, dystonia, chorea) typically experience altered vocal pitch, loudness, and quality during episodes of involuntary movements. The alterations may be either slow or rapid or continuous or intermittent, depending on the nature of the patient's movement disorder. Patients affected by tremor produce regular, cyclic perturbations of pitch and loudness. Patients with chorea produce irregular prolonged distortions of vocal pitch and loudness during episodes of choreiform movement.

Vocal Flexibility and Coordination. Assessing phonation time and voice quality provide information about the efficiency of laryngeal valving and the adequacy of respiratory support for speech. Continuous phonation requires that the vocal folds be adducted and kept in a constant state of tension, but continuous phonation does not provide much information about how well the laryngeal muscles accomplish the movements required for speech. That information is obtained by asking the patient to change vocal pitch and loudness in designated ways. A patient may be asked to do the following:

- Count aloud from 1 to 10, beginning in a whisper and ending in a shout, and from 1 to 10 beginning in a shout and ending in a whisper
- Progressively change the pitch of an open vowel up and down a musical scale
- Count aloud, beginning with the lowest pitch the patient can produce and gradually increasing pitch until the patient can go no higher
- Say short sequences of numbers aloud, alternating loud and soft voice or high and low pitch
- Repeat sentences at a whisper, normal loudness, and a shout
- Read a paragraph or story aloud with exaggerated emphatic stress

The changes in pitch and loudness achieved by the patient in these tasks may be compared with what the patient does in less-structured speech tasks such as conversational speech. Many dysarthric patients sound better in structured tasks when their attention is focused on controlling the pitch and loudness of their speech than in unstructured tasks in which they must attend to other components (e.g., formulating ideas, taking turns) in addition to controlling vocal pitch and loudness.

A patient's ability to coordinate respiration and speech may be evaluated by asking the patient to do the following:

- Produce a series of short vowels (e.g., *uh-uh-uh*, *ee-ee-ee*)
- Alternate aspirate-vowel and voiced continuant-consonant pairs (e.g., *huh-muh huh-muh*)
- Alternate voiced and voiceless consonant-vowel pairs (*puh-buh puh-buh*)

Vocal flexibility almost always is reduced if a patient has significant dysarthria. Reduced vocal flexibility may have several sources (e.g., upper motor neuron or lower motor neuron damage, cerebellar damage, extrapyramidal damage). Poor coordination between respiration and voice onset usually is a sign of pathologic conditions affecting the extrapyramidal system or cerebellum.

Velopharyngeal Function and Resonation

Velopharyngeal structures isolate the pharyngeal and oral cavities from the nasal cavity during swallowing and during production of denasalized speech sounds. Although the exact means by which velopharyngeal closure is achieved differs across individuals (Yorkston, Beukelman, Strand, & Bell, 1999), closure is accomplished primarily by movement of the *velum* (soft palate) up and back to meet the posterior pharyngeal wall and by movement of the lateral pharyngeal walls toward the midline to meet the sides of the velum. Sometimes the posterior pharyngeal wall may move forward toward the velum (Croft, Shprintzen, & Rakoff, 1981). When normal speakers produce denasal sounds, velopharyngeal muscles contract to prevent air leakage from the oral cavity into the nasal cavity. When normal speakers produce nasal sounds, the velopharyngeal muscles relax, opening the nasopharyngeal port and allowing some of the air stream to pass into the nasal cavity, adding nasal resonance.

Velopharyngeal Mechanics. The examiner begins assessment of a patient's velopharyngeal muscles by observing the palate and pharynx at rest. Bilateral palatal droop suggests bilateral weakness of the muscles that elevate the palate. Unilateral platal droop suggests weakness of palatal muscles (served by CN 9 and CN 10) on the drooping side. Spontaneous rippling or dimpling of palatal muscles suggests loss of input from CN 9 and CN 10. Sporadic or rhythmic movements or pulsations of the resting palate suggest a pathologic condition affecting the basal ganglia or cerebellum.

The examiner may indirectly assess velopharyngeal mechanics by asking the patient to puff out her or his cheeks with air. Inability to perform this action, especially when attempts are accompanied by nasal air escape, suggests poor velopharyngeal closure. However, success in puffing out the cheeks does not prove velopharyngeal closure. Some patients with weak velopharyngeal muscles compensate by pushing the velum up with the back of the tongue. A *tongue-anchor test* (Dalston, Warren, & Dalston, 1990; Fox & Johns, 1970) may identify such patients. In the tongue-anchor test, the patient must protrude her or his tongue between closed lips while puffing out the cheeks. This maneuver prevents the patient from using the tongue to occlude the velopharyngeal opening.

The examiner may listen for nasal escape of air as the patient sustains phonation or repeats syllables, phrases, or sentences containing stop consonants. Because it is not always easy to hear nasal air escape under these conditions, examiners sometimes supplement audition with vision by holding a bit of fluff or a cold mirror under the patient's nostrils while the patient phonates or speaks. If the fluff moves or the mirror clouds, nasal emission is confirmed. However, these tests yield positive results only when nasal emission is severe.

The examiner may assess velopharyngeal mechanics visually by asking the patient to produce a sustained *ah* several times with her or his mouth open wide. The examiner watches through the patient's open mouth for movement of the palate and oropharynx as phonation begins and ends. A patient's failure to elevate the palate during phonation suggests bilateral weakness in palatal muscles. Asymmetric elevation suggests unilateral weakness of palatal muscles on the drooping side.

Resonance. The examiner may assess velopharyngeal function in speech by asking the patient to produce sustained phonation and repeat syllables while the examiner listens for hypernasality, nasal escape of air, and distorted consonants. Judging hypernasality by listening is difficult. Perceptual judgment of hypernasality can be unreliable because such judgments are sensitive to other deviant speech characteristics. Patients with severe articulatory disturbance may be judged hypernasal even if their velopharyngeal function is normal (Moll, 1968). Patients who speak loudly may be judged hypernasal more often than patients who speak softly (Yorkston, Beukelman, Strand, & Bell, 1999). Consequently, perceptual judgments of hypernasality routinely should be supported by visual assessment of velopharyngeal function.

One simple test for hypernasality is for the examiner to alternately pinch and release the patient's nostrils as the patient produces a sustained vowel. If the patient is hypernasal, the sound of the vowel changes as the nostrils are occluded and opened. Although simple, the pinch test does not always predict hypernasality in connected speech. Some patients can successfully occlude the velopharyngeal port during sustained phonation but cannot do so during the more complex movement patterns of connected speech. The examiner could, of course, pinch and release the patient's nostrils as the patient produces connected speech. If hypernasality is severe, the examiner will hear changes

in vocal resonance as the patient's nostrils are pinched, but the pinch test is not sensitive to mild or moderate hypernasality. Fortunately, mild to moderate hypernasality, either alone or with mild articulatory imprecision, does not usually compromise intelligibility. Hypernasality is a concern for patients whose velopharyngeal incompetence is severe enough to significantly affect speech intelligibility.

Velopharyngeal incompetence causes distortion of consonants, especially consonants that require interruption or constriction of the air stream (stop consonants such as *p* and *b* and continuants such as *s* and *sh*). When velopharyngeal muscle function is compromised, stop consonants and continuants are indistinct and may be accompanied by nasal escape of air. Voiced consonants are indistinct and hypernasal. When articulation of consonants that require oral breath pressure (stops and continuants) is worse than articulation of other sounds, velopharyngeal incompetence is the likely reason.

Articulation

Articulatory Mechanics. Assessment of articulatory mechanics typically precedes assessment of speech-sound production, and visual examination of muscles at rest precedes evaluation of muscles in action. The examiner begins by looking for drooping, atrophy, or involuntary movements of the patient's facial muscles at rest. Then the examiner asks the patient to open her or his mouth and notes whether the patient's tongue rests on the midline and whether dimpling, rippling, or involuntary movements of the tongue are present. Off-midline resting position and dimpling or rippling may suggest weakness of CN 12; involuntary movements suggest pathologic conditions affecting the extrapyramidal system or the cerebellum.

Next the examiner tests the strength and range of movement of the patient's jaw muscles. The examiner asks the patient to open and close his or her jaw several times and watches for slowness, restricted movement, or deviation from the midline. Then the examiner grasps the patient's chin and resists the movements as the patient opens and closes his or her jaw and moves it from side to side. Then the examiner notes the speed and timing of jaw movements while the patient opens and closes the jaw several times. Weakness and restricted range of movement suggest weakness of the masseter muscles (served by CN 5). Irregular rate and timing of jaw movements may suggest problems in the extrapyramidal system or cerebellum.

The examiner evaluates the patient's lip movements and strength as the patient purses, protrudes, and retracts his or her lips, both when unopposed and when the examiner resists the movements with a tongue depressor. Asymmetrical lip retraction and protrusion and weakness on one side of the lips suggest damage affecting CN 7 on the side of the weakness.

Some patients who smile asymmetrically when they smile in response to the examiner's request produce symmetric smiles when they smile spontaneously. This phenomenon suggests that one motor system performs volitional smiles (sometimes called *pyramidal smiles*) and another motor system performs spontaneous smiles.

The examiner evaluates the patient's tongue movements and tongue strength in several ways. The examiner may ask the patient to protrude his or her tongue and move it from side to side. If the patient succeeds, the examiner may ask the patient to repeat the movements while the examiner resists the movements with a tongue depressor. The examiner also may ask the patient to push out each cheek with his or her tongue. If the patient succeeds, the examiner may resist the movement by pushing against the patient's cheek as he or she pushes. Deviation from the midline on tongue protrusion suggests weakness of tongue muscles on the side toward which the tongue deviates. Restricted range of tongue movement to one side or weakness on one side when the

examiner resists side-to-side movement suggests weakness of tongue muscles on the side of the restricted range of movement or weakness.

Speech Movements. Syllable and phrase repetition are the primary tools with which the examiner evaluates the patient's articulatory accuracy. The examiner chooses syllables and phrases to highlight the contribution of the various mechanical processes to the speech the patient produces. The examiner evaluates lip closure by asking the patient to repeat bilabial consonant-vowel combinations (e.g., *puh-puh-puh, buh-buh-buh*). The examiner evaluates tongue-tip elevation by asking the patient to repeat syllables that require contact of the tongue tip with the alveolar ridge (e.g., *tuh-tuh-tuh, duh-duh-duh*). The examiner evaluates elevation of the back of the tongue by asking the patient to repeat syllables that require contact of the back of the tongue with the posterior palate (e.g., *kuh-kuh-kuh, guh-guh-guh*). The examiner evaluates articulatory flexibility and coordination by asking the patient to repeat strings of syllables with changing articulation points (e.g., *puh-tuh-kuh, duh-buh-guh*). The examiner evaluates articulatory accuracy in connected speech by asking the patient to repeat multisyllabic words (e.g., *gingerbread-gingerbread-gingerbread,* or *artillery-artillery-artillery*), phrases (e.g., *the National Republican Convention*), and sentences (e.g., *Nelson Rockefeller drives a Lincoln Continental*).

Articulation Versus Intelligibility. Standard articulation inventories such as those used to evaluate children rarely are useful in evaluating patients who are dysarthric. Articulatory deviations in dysarthria usually are part of a constellation of respiratory, phonatory, and resonance disturbances. Consequently, clinicians are more interested in which impaired speech processes account for a patient's pattern of articulatory impairment than in which sounds are in error. The goal of treatment for most dysarthric patients is intelligibility rather than articulatory accuracy. Because articulatory accuracy has only a general relationship to intelligibility, measuring intelligibility usually provides more useful information than measuring articulatory accuracy.

Yorkston, Beukelman, Strand, and Bell (1999) offered three objections to the use of traditional articulation inventories with dysarthric speakers:

- A judge's perceptions of articulatory accuracy may not reflect the adequacy of the patient's articulatory movements.
- Articulation inventories fail to discriminate between sounds that are accurate and sounds that are distorted but still within phoneme boundaries.
- When judges know the target words, as in traditional articulation inventories, they are likely to overestimate a patient's articulatory accuracy.

Yorkston and associates (1999) advocate use of the *phoneme identification task* as a substitute for traditional articulation inventories. In the phoneme identification task, a dysarthric speaker is recorded while reading aloud a list of single words and sentences. The list is designed to elicit 57 target phonemes. A judge (not the examiner) listens to the recording and identifies the target phonemes, using the following procedure:

- A word or sentence is played.
- The judge is shown a card on which a word with the target phoneme missing is printed, and she or he is asked to identify the missing phoneme.
- The judge rates the patient's production of the target phoneme using a four-point scale, ranging from *no basis for a guess* to *correct, undistorted.*

Intelligibility

Yorkston and Beukelman (1981) published an assessment tool called *Assessment of Intelligibility of Dysarthric Speech.* The test has two sections. One measures single-word intelligibility; the other assesses sentence intelligibility and speaking rate. In the *phoneme identification task,* a patient's oral reading of 57 single words each containing a target sound is recorded. Each word is selected by the examiner before the test from a corpus of similar sounding words. One or more judges (not the examiner) then listen to the recording and either write down each word they hear or choose each word they hear from a set of seven words similar in sound to the target word.

In the *sentence intelligibility task* the patient reads aloud 22 sentences, ranging in length from 5 to 15 words. One or more judges (not the examiner) then listen to the recording and write down the sentences. Judges' transcriptions are scored by the examiner to yield several measures:

- Percent intelligibility
- Speech rate for sentences (words per minute)
- Intelligible words per minute
- Unintelligible words per minute
- Communicative efficiency ratio (intelligible words per minute divided by normal speech rate of 190 words per minute)

Assessment of Intelligibility of Dysarthric Speech may provide reliable estimates of speech intelligibility if administered and scored according to instructions. The measures obtained with Assessment of Intelligibility of Dysarthric Speech may be useful for predicting a speaker's intelligibility in daily life, for measuring changes in intelligibility over time, and for planning treatment to improve a speaker's intelligibility. Patients who are both aphasic and dysarthric may have difficulty with the sentence-production part of the test because of reading impairments, impaired auditory comprehension and retention, or paraphasic errors in oral reading. Consequently, Assessment of Intelligibility of Dysarthric Speech may not be practical for patients who are both dysarthric and more than mildly aphasic.

Computerized versions of the phoneme identification task and the sentence intelligibility task have been developed (Yorkston, Beukelman, & Tice, 1998).

GENERAL CONCEPTS 13-3

- Comprehensive assessment of dysarthria requires assessment of *respiration, phonation, resonation, articulation,* and their interactions.
- Respiration for speech requires that normal passive exhalation be assisted by active contraction of the muscles of the diaphragm to produce sufficient breath pressure for speech.
- Comprehensive assessment of respiration for speech entails measurement of respiratory pressure and flow in nonspeech activities, assessment of *sustained phonation,* and assessment of *breath support* for speech as the patient produces words, phrases, and connected speech.
- Coughs, grunts, and glottal stops provide indications of the adequacy of glottal valving in nonspeech activities.
- Abbreviated sustained phonation times suggest a problem either with respiratory support or with glottal valving for speech. Several neurologic conditions may affect glottal valving for speech, including *spastic vocal folds* (caused by bilateral upper motor neuron pathology), *flaccid vocal folds* (caused by lower motor neuron pathology), *rigid vocal folds* (caused by Parkinson's disease), and *intermittent contractions of vocal folds* (caused by extrapyramidal system or cerebellar pathology).
- Dysarthric patients' control of voice and articulation often is better in highly structured tasks such as continuous phonation and production of single syllables and short phrases than in less structured tasks such as story telling or conversation. Assessment of patients with dysarthria should assess performance both in structured tasks and in unstructured tasks.
- Visual examination of the palate at rest and during vowel production provides information about the integrity of velopharyngeal

muscle functions. Asking the patient to puff out his or her cheeks provides an indirect indication of velopharyngeal competence in nonspeech activities.
- *Hypernasality, nasal escape of air,* and *distorted consonants* during production of denasalized speech sounds are signs of impaired velopharyngeal closure. One of the easiest tests for hypernasality is to alternately pinch and release the patient's nostrils as the patient speaks, listening for changes in the quality of the patient's speech as the nostrils are alternately occluded and opened.
- Poor articulation of consonants requiring oral breath pressure and good articulation of other consonants is a sign of inadequate velopharyngeal closure.
- Drooping, atrophy, or involuntary movements of facial muscles, off-midline resting tongue position, and dimpling or rippling of the tongue suggest loss of innervation in the affected muscles.
- The examiner evaluates the strength, timing, and range of movement of the jaw, lips, and tongue by asking the patient to move them freely and against resistance applied by the examiner.
- *Standard articulation inventories* are not commonly used in assessing the speech of dysarthric patients. *Syllable and phrase repetition* is the most commonly used way to assess these patients' articulatory accuracy.
- Intelligibility, rather than articulatory accuracy, is the primary concern for most patients with significant dysarthria.
- *Assessment of Intelligibility of Dysarthric Speech* (Yorkston & Beukelman, 1981) provides a consistent procedure for assessing the intelligibility of single words and sentences produced by dysarthric speakers. It includes a *phoneme identification test* and a *sentence intelligibility test.*

INTERVENTION

Speak the speech, I pray you, as I pronounced it to you, trippingly on the tongue. (Shakespeare)

Dysarthria is a consequence of neurologic diseases that cause weakness, slowness, incoordination, diminished range of movement, or sensory loss in structures that participate in speech. Some patients do not have the muscle strength or range of movement needed for normal speech. Others may have the muscle strength but not the coordination. Still others may lack the respiratory support necessary for normal speech.

There is no single treatment for dysarthria. Treatment of dysarthria must take into account both the causes of a patient's dysarthria and the nature of the patient's speech disturbances. Some treatments may focus on causative mechanisms; others may focus on the speech disturbances themselves.

The goal of dysarthria treatment is to maximize the dysarthric patient's communicative effectiveness and efficiency. This goal can be achieved in various ways—for example, by improving the physiologic support for speech, by direct work on speech, by environmental control, by education and counseling, by providing compensatory techniques or alternatives to speech, by providing prosthetic support, or by medical or surgical intervention.

Treatment of dysarthric patients may rely on indirect approaches that improve the quality of a patient's speech by improving the patient's muscle strength and agility, the patient's respiratory efficiency, or the integrity of the patient's sensory feedback, rather than working directly on speech. *Indirect treatment* may include sensory stimulation, muscle strengthening, modifying muscle tone, or modifying respiration. *Direct treatment* may include modifying phonation, modifying resonation, modifying articulation, or modifying prosody. Treatment for most dysarthric patients combines indirect and direct

procedures. If a patient is severely dysarthric and can produce little or no volitional speech, treatment may focus on physiologic support for speech. If a patient can produce some voice, approximate a few vowel sounds, and produce a few articulatory movements, treatment may focus on production of speech. Exercises to strengthen muscles and increase muscle agility and range of movement may be appropriate for these latter patients, but usually as an adjunct to direct work on speech.

The more severe a patient's dysarthria, the more likely it is that the clinician will work to strengthen muscles and improve sensory function outside the context of speech. Patients with mild or moderate dysarthria may get stronger muscles and improved sensory function from treatment, but usually by controlled speaking practice rather than by stimulation of oral structures or by movement exercises in isolation.

Indirect Treatment Procedures

Sensory Stimulation. Sensory stimulation is designed to increase motor control for speech by increasing the amount and fidelity of sensory feedback from oral structures. Sensory stimulation may include brushing, stroking, vibrating, or applying ice to a patient's lips, tongue, pharyngeal walls, or soft palate. There is little empiric evidence that sensory stimulation improves motor performance in dysarthria, and its use remains controversial, except, perhaps, for stimulation of the soft palate.

Rosenbek and LaPointe (1985) suggested that massaging and lifting the soft palate concurrent with a patient's attempts to raise it may improve velopharyngeal competence. Johns (1985) reported that movement of the lateral pharyngeal walls toward the midline sometimes increases following installation of palatal prostheses. Johns attributed the movement to increased sensory feedback generated by contact of the pharyngeal walls with the prosthesis. However, Dworkin and Johns (1980), after reviewing various approaches to managing velopharyngeal insufficiency, assert that neither stimulation nor muscle strengthening are likely to be effective if palatal insufficiency is caused by neurologic impairment.

It may be that clinicians' willingness to use stimulation to address velopharyngeal incompetence comes as much from the absence of other methods as from belief in the effectiveness of stimulation. Stimulation of the soft palates and pharyngeal walls of dysarthric patients with velopharyngeal incompetence no doubt will continue, at least until something better comes along. *Muscle Strengthening.* Muscle strengthening exercises are designed to improve respiratory support, phonation, articulation, and resonance by enhancing the strength and range of movement of weak muscles. There is no convincing evidence that muscle strengthening by itself is an effective treatment for dysarthria, but it appears to benefit at least some dysarthric patients (Liss, Kuehn, & Hinkel, 1994; Massengill & associates, 1968; Powers & Starr, 1974; Yules & Chase, 1969).

Rosenbek and LaPointe (1978) suggest that muscle strengthening is appropriate for patients with severe flaccid dysarthria and severely compromised physiologic support for speech. They recommend muscle strengthening when adjustment of posture, muscle tone, and respiration are ineffective and when direct treatment of articulation, phonation, and prosody leave the patient unintelligible. However, they recommend muscle strengthening only if a patient remains in treatment for several weeks and can carry out assignments outside the clinic. In practice, muscle strengthening usually is reserved for patients with weak muscles and severe flaccid dysarthria who can produce little intelligible speech or can produce speech only in fragments and under ideal conditions.

It is important that clinicians not exaggerate the importance of muscle strength for adequate speech intelligibility. Intelligible speech rarely requires forceful muscle activity. In fact, forceful articulatory movements such as those seen in

ataxia, dystonia, and chorea actually may diminish intelligibility. Agility and range of movement are more important for intelligible speech than is strength. Consequently, muscle strengthening exercises that include movement *(isotonic exercises)* usually are more effective than muscle strengthening exercises that require pushing against stationary resistance *(isometric exercises)*. As a general rule, clinicians should move from isometric to isotonic movements as soon as a patient can accomplish short sequences of simple movements. Muscle strengthening exercises should move on to agility and range-of-motion exercises as soon as the muscles have enough strength to perform the exercises at low levels of speed and efficiency.

Liss, Keuhn, and Hinkel (1994) have suggested that changes in muscle strength seen in the early stages of strength training are a result of *neural adaptation* (increased rate of firing of motor neurons and participation of previously nonparticipating motor neurons) rather than increased muscle mass. These neural adaptations apparently are movement-specific—the trained movements must closely match the target movements in direction, force, range, and velocity. These findings suggest that strength-training exercises such as those in which a patient pushes against a tongue depressor with tongue or lips are unlikely to produce beneficial changes in speech precision, agility, or endurance, whereas training exercises that mimic speech movements may produce beneficial neural adaptations (Hageman, 1997; Liss, Kuehn, & Hinkel, 1994).

If a dysarthric patient with weak speech muscles can produce a vowel or two and approximate a few consonants, muscle strengthening may be supplemented by direct work on speech production. Patients whose muscles do not have the strength, agility, or range of movement to talk but who can produce a few speech sounds usually develop increased strength, agility, and range of movement in the muscle groups needed for speech as quickly (and more efficiently) if they are talking than if they are moving speech structures against resistance or in nonspeech movement drills.

Modifying Muscle Tone. Some dysarthric patients exhibit abnormalities in muscle tone that interfere with speech intelligibility. Some are hypertonic. Hypertonicity appears as *spasticity* when patients have upper motor neuron pathology and as *rigidity* in Parkinson's disease. Both kinds of hypertonicity are constant over time and are uniform across affected muscle groups. Hypertonicity also appears as a result of extrapyramidal diseases such as dystonia and chorea. In dystonia and chorea, muscle tone waxes and wanes and may move from muscle group to muscle group. Abnormally low resting muscle tone (hypotonicity) typically follows lower motor neuron or peripheral nervous system damage. Hypotonicity usually is constant over time and does not move from muscle group to muscle group.

Several procedures for relaxing hypertonic muscles have been described in the clinical literature. *Progressive relaxation* reduces a patient's overall level of muscle tension. *Shaking* and *chewing* exercises may help the patient relax speech muscles. Lying down while speaking helps some hypertonic patients by lowering overall muscle tension. *Biofeedback,* in which the electrical activity in selected muscle groups is amplified and converted to auditory or visual signals that are monitored by the patient, may help some patients relax selected muscles. Hypertonicity associated with extrapyramidal pathology (e.g., Parkinson's disease) may respond to muscle-relaxing medications. (Hypertonicity associated with extrapyramidal disease usually does not respond to behavioral intervention.)

Hypotonicity in dysarthric patients' muscles typically is treated by raising the patient's overall muscle tension. Sometimes simply asking the patient to push harder at speaking improves the intelligibility of patients with flaccid dysarthria. Sometimes intelligibility is enhanced if the patient pushes or pulls against a stationary resistance while speaking (e.g., pushing down on a table or on the arms of a chair or wheelchair, clasping the hands and pulling).

Adjusting Posture and Speaking Position. Modifying posture and speaking position may improve a dysarthric patient's speech, especially when weakness is present in major muscle groups. Straightening a slouching patient's posture and bracing or supporting a patient's drooping head may improve the mechanical base for speech. Cervical collars, body braces, slings, and restraints, singly or in combination, may move a weak patient into a more efficient position for speech. Posture and positioning adjustments are most useful for patients with weak neck and trunk muscles who have difficulty sitting up and maintaining erect head position.

When a patient has been positioned in an appropriate speaking posture, stabilization and support of selected muscle groups may add to speech intelligibility. A cervical collar or neck brace may support a patient who cannot maintain erect head position. A girdle, stomach band, or stomach board may stabilize and support weak abdominal muscles. (*Stomach boards* are boards, usually fastened across the arms of a wheelchair, against which the patient can press her or his abdomen and increase breath pressure for speech.) Patients with involuntary movements may wear cervical collars, neck braces, or body braces to limit the movements.

Postural adjustment, positioning, stabilization, and support require collaboration with the patient's physician, because these procedures may have side-effects. Abdominal banding or girdling may compromise respiration and predispose a patient to pneumonia. Cervical collars and neck braces may compress muscles and nerves in the patient's neck and shoulders.

Enhancing Respiratory Capacity and Efficiency. Respiratory capacity may be problematic for patients with generalized muscle weakness, as in demyelinating disease, spinal nerve pathology, and diseases of the neuromuscular junction. Increasing respiratory capacity for these patients may improve their speech, but only if they use the breath stream efficiently. Respiratory capacity often is less important to speech than is efficient use of the air stream. If a patient's glottal valving, velopharyngeal porting, and articulation are poor, increasing respiratory capacity will do little for the intelligibility of speech, although it may increase its loudness. (But making unintelligible speech louder is not a practical clinical goal.)

Treatment for enhancing respiratory support takes several forms. Postural adjustment, positioning, and stabilization may improve the mechanical base for respiration. Muscle strengthening may strengthen the muscles of respiration. Increasing muscle tone (e.g., pushing and bearing down) may increase respiratory drive. Enhanced glottal valving and increased articulatory precision may indirectly improve respiratory support.

Exercises focused on respiration may be beneficial. Controlled exhalation, in which the patient slowly exhales a uniform stream of air for a prescribed time, with the time interval gradually increasing, may improve a patient's respiratory capacity and enhance her or his control of exhalation. Direct treatment of respiration usually is an early phase of treatment, and the focus usually moves to speech production as soon as the patient achieves basic respiratory support for speech.

Direct Treatment Procedures

In *direct treatment procedures,* speech is produced under controlled conditions designed to systematically improve speech intelligibility. Treatment of dysarthric patients usually includes both indirect and direct procedures, and indirect procedures tend to fade into direct procedures, as when controlled exhalation leads into controlled phonation. Direct treatment procedures tend to overlap and merge one into another, as when controlled phonation progresses into articulation drills. Direct treatment procedures may address phonation, res-

onation, articulation, or prosody, either singly or in combination.

Technically, one cannot treat speech—one treats speech by changing the amplitude, speed, or accuracy of movements that generate speech or by improving the laryngeal mechanics necessary for phonation. Even "direct" treatment procedures are indirect, in this sense.

Phonation. Procedures designed to enhance phonation emphasize efficient laryngeal valving of the air stream and adjusting utterance length to the patient's respiratory capacity. Controlled phonation is the primary vehicle for increasing a dysarthric patient's laryngeal efficiency. The clinician often begins by asking the patient to produce prolonged vowels with gradually increasing prolongation. When the patient's vowel production has stabilized, she or he may be trained to produce strings of vowels or consonant-vowel syllables, with the length of the strings gradually increasing as the patient masters the shorter strings. Changes in loudness and pitch then may be superimposed to enhance respiratory control.

Patients who can say short phrases but do not have enough respiratory support for normal phrasing may benefit from training in use of *optimal breath groups* (Linebaugh, 1983). An optimal breath group is the number of syllables a patient can comfortably produce on one breath. Training a patient to speak using optimal breath groups follows a three-step sequence: (1) determine the patient's optimal breath group, (2) teach the patient to limit the number of syllables per breath to the optimal breath group, and (3) gradually increase the length of the optimal breath group by enhancing respiratory control and glottal valving.

For patients whose glottal valving is compromised by spastic laryngeal muscles, procedures for reducing laryngeal tension (e.g., relaxation training, laryngeal massage, postural support) may supplement active training in voicing. When voice intensity is problematic in dysarthria, it usually is a problem of too little rather than too much. Dysarthric patients may be helped to talk louder by improving respiratory support (e.g., teaching appropriate breath groups, positioning, bracing, banding, bearing down), by increasing the efficiency of phonation, or by speech exercises in which patients volitionally adjust the loudness of their voices. Visual feedback (e.g., feedback provided by a loudness meter or an oscilloscope tracing) may help these patients volitionally adjust the intensity of their vocalizations.

Contrastive stress drill (Rosenbeck & LaPointe, 1985) is a popular way of giving dysarthric patients training in volitional control of voice intensity. The clinician says a sentence, such as *"Bob hit Bill"* and then asks the patient questions such as *"WHO hit Bill?"* or *"WHAT did Bob do?"* The patient answers each question, putting emphatic stress on elements that answer the questions (e.g., *BOB hill hit Bill"* or *"Bob HIT BILL").*

Some dysarthric patients cannot achieve functional vocal intensity no matter how hard they try and no matter how expert their trainer and coach. A portable voice amplifier may be the answer for these patients. Portable voice amplifiers help some patients with weak voices communicate in noisy environments, at a distance from listeners, or with listeners who have impaired hearing. Portable voice amplifiers consist of a throat-mounted or headset-mounted microphone connected to a small amplifier and speaker that can be carried in a pocket, worn on a strap or belt, or attached to a wheelchair or bed. Portable voice amplifiers range in cost from less than a hundred dollars to several hundred dollars. More expensive units generally produce better sound quality.

Not every patient who needs amplification needs optimum sound quality. Patients with good articulation and good voice quality may get along well with an inexpensive unit. Patients with imprecise articulation, poor voice quality, or both may need a unit with very good sound

quality. Not all dysarthric patients with weak voices are candidates for a voice amplifier. Patients with intelligible speech but weak voices who fail to benefit from behavioral intervention to increase voice loudness are the best candidates, for as Rosenbek and LaPointe (1985) caution, amplifying unintelligible speech only produces louder unintelligible speech.

Increasing *vocal pitch range* may be appropriate for some patients, particularly those with flaccid dysarthria. Procedures for increasing pitch range include the following:

- Phonation with gradually rising and falling pitch
- Counting aloud with rising or falling pitch
- Reciting the alphabet or the days of the week with rising or falling pitch
- Producing sequences of syllables or words with gradually rising or falling pitch
- Contrastive stress drill
- Asking questions (for rising pitch) and making assertions (for falling pitch) with exaggerated intonation

Maintaining *constant pitch* may be important for patients whose pitch fluctuates because of variability in the force, timing, and amplitude of movements (as in cerebellar ataxia). Procedures for controlling unintentional pitch changes include continuous phonation while keeping pitch constant and continuous phonation with slowly rising or falling pitch.

Resonance. Speech resonance is affected by the size and configuration of the oral cavity and by the size of the opening between the oral cavity and the nasal cavities. Although aberrations in the shape of the oral cavity, by themselves, may change speech resonance, the changes are primarily cosmetic and affect speech quality rather than speech intelligibility. However, aberrations in the shape of the oral cavity often are related to abnormal positioning of the jaw, tongue, and lips, so that articulatory errors are superimposed on resonance abnormalities—a combination that may seriously compromise intelligibility. By far the most serious aberration in speech resonance is hypernasality. Hypernasality has two effects. It produces excessive nasal resonance. More importantly, however, it distorts or destroys sounds that depend on oral breath pressure because the air required to produce them escapes through the patient's nose.

Improving velopharyngeal competence usually creates dramatic improvements in hypernasal patients' speech intelligibility. Most behavioral procedures for minimizing hypernasality rely on *ear training* to teach a patient to recognize hypernasality, combined with *pushing and bearing-down exercises* to increase muscle tension and stimulate contraction of velopharyngeal muscles. Behavioral procedures such as these are practical if hypernasality is mild to moderate. If hypernasality is severe, prosthetic or surgical management may be appropriate.

Palatal lift prostheses are an appropriate option for patients whose hypernasality does not respond to behavioral intervention. Palatal lift prostheses are constructed by a prosthodontist, usually in collaboration with a speech-language pathologist. The body of the prosthesis consists of an acrylic plate that covers the hard palate and a palatal lift extension also made of acrylic. The palatal lift extension is shaped to press the patient's soft palate up and back. The prosthesis is attached to the patient's upper teeth by wires.

Prosthesis: A fabricated device that substitutes for a missing body part or physically compensates for deficient physical function. From a Greek word meaning *"an addition."*

Not every patient with velopharyngeal insufficiency is a candidate for a palatal lift. Patients with the following characteristics are the best palatal lift candidates (Netsell & Rosenbek, 1985; Rosenbek & LaPointe, 1985; Yorkston, Beukelman, Strand, & Bell, 1999):

- Patients who are extremely hypernasal, who cannot achieve velopharyngeal closure, and for whom behavioral intervention has been unsuccessful
- Patients whose soft palates and pharyngeal muscles are not spastic, because spastic muscles resist pressure and may dislodge the prosthesis
- Patients who have teeth to which the prosthesis can be anchored. Prostheses have been fitted to dentures but are not practical if the lift dislodges the dentures
- Patients who have reasonably good articulation and phonation (hypernasal patients with severe articulatory or phonatory deficits generally are as unintelligible after the prosthesis is in place as they were before the prosthesis is fitted)
- Patients who cooperate by wearing and caring for the prosthesis (some patients do not tolerate the discomfort associated with wearing the prosthesis or the inconvenience of caring for it)
- Patients who do not have swallowing impairments (palatal prostheses sometimes interfere with swallowing)
- Patients without degenerative disease (although fitting a prosthesis to these patients may provide temporarily increased intelligibility, the effects eventually are negated by the progression of the disease)

Articulation. Improving articulation was for many years the core of treatment for dysarthria because dysarthria was considered to be little more than defective articulation. However, as Rosenbek and LaPointe (1985) assert, "Articulation is being forced to share its popularity with other speech processes ... and dysarthria is coming to mean speech—not articulation—deficit" (p. 294). Most dysarthric patients receive articulation treatment. However, few receive *only* articulation treatment.

The primary goal of management is to maximize the effectiveness, efficiency, and naturalness of communication. (Duffy, 2005, p. 436)

Treatment for improving articulation may include imitation, *phonetic derivation* (deriving sounds that a patient cannot say from those that she or he can say), *phonetic placement* (physically adjusting or positioning a patient's articulators), and sequential repetition of sounds, syllables, and words. Articulation exercises usually focus on *speech movements* (production of syllables or words) rather than on *fixed positions* (individual sounds), although severely dysarthric patients may work on producing fixed articulatory positions. When a patient's articulatory movements are imprecise, he or she may be taught to exaggerate the movements, which usually adds to their precision. When a patient cannot produce an articulatory movement, a compensatory movement may be taught. Work on precision often is combined with slowing the patient's speech rate. Slower speech rate allows the patient more time to make articulatory adjustments, and it allows the patient's listeners more time to decode what the patient is saying.

Prosody. Intervention to alter the prosodic characteristics of dysarthric patients' speech may focus on rate, loudness, or pitch (intonation). A patient's speech rate may be adjusted by altering *articulation rate* (the rate at which individual speech sounds are produced), or by altering the number, placement, or duration of pauses. Dysarthric patients who have abnormally slow speech typically cannot talk faster, because their slow speech reflects their physiologic limitations, making rate manipulation impractical for them. Some dysarthric patients who have abnormally fast speech may benefit from rate-control techniques that slow them down.

Several techniques are available for modifying speech rate. Most require the patient to speak in unison with an external timing stimulus. The clinician may tap, gesture, or speak along with the patient. The patient may speak to the beat of a metronome or a flashing light. The patient may tap, use a pacing board, drop beads in a cup, gesture, or produce other non-speech movements in unison with speaking. Teaching the patient to speak with exaggerated articulation and to exaggerate emphatic stress (contrastive stress drill) also may slow the patient's speech rate.

Beukelman and Yorkston (1977) used a first-letter-pointing procedure to slow the speech rate of two severely dysarthric speakers. Each was given a board on which the alphabet, numerals from 0 to 9, and several phrases (e.g., *end of sentence, end of word*) were printed. Each speaker was trained to point to the first letter of each word as he said it. Both dysarthric speakers spoke more slowly and with greater intelligibility when using the first-letter procedure than when speaking without it. Beukelman and Yorkston attributed the effects of the procedure to (1) increased information provided to listeners by the first letter of each word and (2) the dysarthric speaker's slower speech rate.

Manipulation of pause placement and duration may improve intelligibility for patients who do not benefit from rate control. If a patient is trained to produce optimal breath groups, pauses may occur automatically, but the pauses may not be at syntactic or semantic boundaries. These patients sound more natural and are easier to understand if they are trained to pause at phrase, clause, or sentence boundaries. When a patient has learned to pause at syntactic boundaries, the duration of the pauses may be adjusted to maximize the speaker's intelligibility.

GENERAL CONCEPTS 13-4

- Treatment of dysarthria may entail modification of underlying processes (*indirect procedures*) or modification of speech (*direct procedures*). Indirect procedures include *sensory stimulation, muscle strengthening, modifying muscle tone,* and *modifying respiration.* Direct procedures include *modifying phonation, modifying resonation, modifying articulation,* and *modifying prosody.*

GENERAL CONCEPTS 13-4—cont'd

- There is no convincing evidence for the effectiveness of sensory stimulation in the treatment of dysarthria, although sensory stimulation remains a common practice of many who treat dysarthric patients.
- Muscle strengthening exercises may be appropriate for patients with severe dysarthria. Patients who can produce syllables or short phrases with reasonable intelligibility may benefit more from speech production exercises than from muscle strengthening.
- Relaxation exercises, shaking, chewing, and biofeedback may help dysarthric speakers with hypertonic speech muscles. Asking the patient to increase overall muscle effort or asking the patient to push and bear down may help dysarthric speakers with hypotonic speech muscles increase vocal loudness and enhance articulation.
- Improved respiratory capacity and efficiency for speech may be obtained by adjusting the dysarthric patient's posture and position, supporting weak muscles, or by controlled exhalation and blowing exercises.
- Dysarthric patients' phonation may be treated by improving glottal valving, teaching optimal breath groups, contrastive stress drills, or vocal pitch change drills.
- Dysarthric patients' hypernasality may be treated by combining ear training with pushing or bearing-down exercises, palatal lift prostheses, or occasionally surgical procedures.
- Dysarthric patients' impaired articulation may be treated by drills involving imitation, phonetic derivation, phonetic placement, or sequential repetition. Slowing dysarthric patients' rate of speech and teaching them to exaggerate articulatory movements also may improve their intelligibility.

Environmental Control and Education

Most dysarthric speakers eventually discover that intelligibility in the speech clinic, where rooms are quiet and well-lit and where the dysarthric speaker is face-to-face with the clinician, is no guarantee of intelligibility in daily life, where rooms may be poorly lit and noisy, and where listeners may not always be nearby or looking at the speaker. Skilled clinicians know this and teach dysarthric speakers how to compensate for less-than-ideal speaking conditions. When a dysarthric speaker reaches reasonable levels of intelligibility in the controlled environment of the clinic, the clinician may broaden the treatment program to maximize communication in less-than-ideal speaking situations. This usually requires a combination of environmental control and behavioral compensation.

A dysarthric patient and caregivers may be trained to use environmental controls to minimize the adverse effects of environmental variables on speech intelligibility. The most effective controls relate to ambient noise, lighting, and the spatial relationships between speaker and listeners. Controlling ambient noise is a simple but often overlooked way to improve a dysarthric speaker's communicative success. Turning the television set and radio down or off and closing windows and doors to shut out outside noise are simple ways to diminish ambient noise. A family may install draperies or other acoustic treatments to control ambient noise levels in a dysarthric speaker's home. Controlling lighting and the position of a dysarthric speaker relative to listeners also may enhance a dysarthric speaker's communicative effectiveness. Lighting and the speaker's position may be adjusted so that listeners can see the speaker's face.

Dysarthric speakers may be trained to monitor listeners' comprehension by maintaining eye contact and, if necessary, asking listeners whether they understand. They also may be trained when and how to repeat, simplify, paraphrase, or exaggerate articulatory movements (especially when they perceive communication breakdown). Those around the dysarthric speaker may be taught to control the situational variables described previously; to indicate either gesturally or verbally to the dysarthric speaker when they do not understand; and to ask the dysarthric speaker to slow down, exaggerate articulatory movements, repeat, paraphrase, or simplify when he or she fails to communicate.

Medical and Surgical Treatment

Medical Treatment. Some conditions that cause dysarthria are medically treatable. When medical treatment is an option, usually it precedes behavioral intervention. If medical treatment succeeds, behavioral intervention may not be needed. Medically treatable conditions causing dysarthria include extrapyramidal diseases such as Parkinson's disease, irritative and inflammatory processes causing peripheral nerve dysfunction, and some metabolic and nutritional disturbances.

Parkinson's disease is caused by deficiencies in certain neurotransmitters (dopamines) and often responds to medications such as levodopa (L-dopa) that replenish the missing neurotransmitters and diminish or eliminate the motor effects of the disease, including dysarthria. Movement disorders (e.g., chorea, dystonia) sometimes respond to tranquilizers and related medications, although complete remission of symptoms with medication is unusual. Some facial paralyses are treatable with steroids. Some neurologic conditions caused by abnormalities in central nervous system metabolism (e.g., Wilson's disease) are medically treatable. When medical treatment of a dysarthric patient's neurologic disease is effective, the patient's dysarthria often improves enough to make direct treatment of dysarthria unnecessary. However, medical treatment often lessons but does not eliminate dysarthria, making behavioral treatment necessary, either in conjunction with or following medical treatment.

Wilson's disease is an inherited disease in which copper accumulates in body tissues, especially the brain, kidneys, liver, and eyes. Wilson's disease is treated with penicillamine, which removes the copper deposits.

Teflon Injections and Surgical Treatment. When structural abnormalities produce severe hypernasality, physical modification of velopharyngeal structures may be appropriate. Teflon may be injected into the posterior pharyngeal wall to reduce velopharyngeal insufficiency. Teflon injections may lessen mild to moderate hypernasality and are an option if behavioral modification of hypernasality is not successful. Injection of Teflon into the vocal folds may improve voice quality for patients with dysphonia caused by incomplete adduction of the vocal folds.

Surgical treatment of velopharyngeal insufficiency may compensate for severe velopharyngeal incompetence, although most practitioners consider surgery a last resort, used only if less invasive approaches fail. The most common surgical procedure for lessening velopharyngeal incompetence is the *posterior pharyngeal flap* procedure. In the pharyngeal flap procedure, bands of muscle tissue are detached from the posterior pharyngeal walls and attached to the soft palate. When the pharyngeal wall muscles contract, the bands shorten, pulling the soft palate toward the pharyngeal walls.

Pharyngeal flap procedures are fairly common interventions for children with cleft palates. Their use to treat hypernasality in dysarthria is controversial. Gonzalez and Aronson (1970) assert that prosthetic management of velopharyngeal insufficiency usually produces better results than surgery. Hardy and associates (1961) make a similar assertion regarding management of velopharyngeal insufficiency in children. Miniami and associates (1975) did pharyngeal flaps on five dysarthric patients with *"palatal paresis,"* and reported disappointing results. However, after reviewing the literature and summarizing his own experience with surgical remediation of velopharyngeal insufficiency, Johns (1985) concluded that surgical management "holds great promise for a large number of dysarthric patients" (p. 175).

Augmentative and Alternative Communication

Some severely dysarthric patients do not regain enough intelligible speech to communicate even simple messages by talking. Nonspeech communication systems may enable many of these patients to communicate. Some systems (called *augmentative communication systems*) supplement speech to render it more intelligible to listeners. Voice amplifiers, described previously, are the most common augmentative system for dysarthric speakers. Other systems (called *alternative communication systems*) replace the patient's own speech as a means of communication. Alternative communication systems fall into three general categories: *gesture and pantomime, communication boards and communication books,* and *mechanical and electronic devices.*

Gesture and Pantomime. Some dysarthric patients may enhance communication by pairing gesture or pantomime with speech. Patients whose speech is at least moderately intelligible are the best candidates for augmentation with gesture or pantomime. Natural gestures that accompany speech (called *illustrators;* e.g., gestures meaning *stop, come here,* or *be quiet*) require no training for users and are understood by untrained communication partners, making them a good choice for patients whose speech is at least moderately intelligible and for whom the gestures supplement rather than replace speech. Gesture and pantomime may replace speech for severely dysarthric patients with

little intelligible speech. However, these patients usually communicate better when they are provided with a communication board, a communication book, or an electronic communication device.

Sign languages may be practical for some dysarthric patients who have the cognitive ability and the motivation to learn and use them. A major problem with most sign languages is that the signs are not comprehensible to untrained message recipients, so that patients who use them cannot communicate with untrained persons. *Amerind (American Indian Sign;* Skelly, 1979) is an exception. Amerind consists of signs that do not depend heavily on verbal skills, and most Amerind signs are comprehensible to message recipients without extensive training. Sign languages, including Amerind, require manual dexterity. Patients with weak, paralyzed, or incoordinated limbs are unlikely to be successful users.

Communication Boards and Communication Books. Communication boards and communication books are similar in content, but they differ in form. A communication board is an array of symbols on a durable surface. A communication book is a collection of symbols arranged in book form. The symbols in either can be pictures, icons, letters, words, or phrases. The user points to the symbols, either one at a time or in sequence. Figure 13-17 shows examples of two kinds of communication boards. At the top is a simple board containing pictorial symbols and printed words. At the bottom is a more complex board containing letters, numerals, and words.

Communication boards and communication books containing letters, words, and phrases are best suited for patients whose language is relatively well preserved. The board shown at the bottom of Figure 13-17 would not be appropriate for patients who have language impairments, but it could be used by many dysarthric patients if they have the motor ability to point

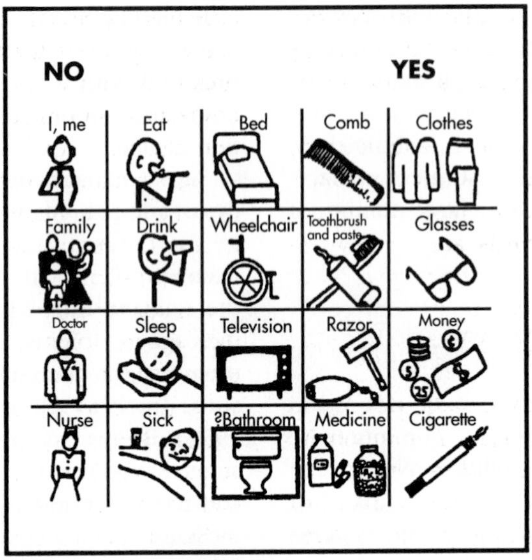

I CAN HEAR PERFECTLY	PLEASE REPEAT AS I TALK (THIS IS HOW I TALK BY SPELLING OUT THE WORDS)	WOULD YOU PLEASE CALL
A AN HE	AM ARE ASK BE BEEN BRING CAN	ABOUT ALL
HER I IT ME	COME COULD DID DO DOES DON'T	AND ALWAYS
MY HIM SHE	DRINK GET GIVE GO HAD HAS HAVE	ALMOST AS
THAT THE THESE	IS KEEP KNOW LET LIKE MAKE MAY	AT BECAUSE
THEY THIS WHOSE	PUT SAY SAID SEE SEEN SEND SHOULD	BUT FOR FROM
WHAT WHEN WHERE	TAKE TELL THINK THOUGHT WANT	HOW IF IN
WHICH WHO WHY	WAS WERE WILL WISH WON'T WOULD -ED	OF ON OR
YOU WE YOUR	-ER -EST -ING -LY -N'T -'S -TION	TO UP WITH

A B C D E F G H I J K L M N O P Qu R S T U V W X Y Z 1 2 3 4 5 6 7 8 9 10 11 12 30	AFTER AGAIN ANY EVEN EVERY HERE JUST MORE ONLY SO SOME SOON THERE VERY

SUN. MON. TUES. WED. THUR. FRI. SAT. BATHROOM	PLEASE THANK YOU MR. MRS. MISS MOTHER DAD DOCTOR	GOING OUT START OVER END OF WORD	$¢½(SHHH!!)?

Figure 13-17 ■ Communication boards. The upper one is a picture communication board suitable for a patient with moderate to severe language impairment. The lower one is a more complex board containing words and phrases that would be appropriate for a patient with good language abilities and sufficient finger and arm dexterity to point to letters and words at a reasonably fast rate.

to the symbols on the board. The board shown at the top of Figure 13-17 would be usable by many language-impaired patients, because its symbols are nonverbal.

Versions of communication boards that do not require the user to directly select symbols have been developed. The simplest is the *eye gaze board.* Eye gaze boards are used when speechless patients have good language abilities but cannot move their limbs to directly select symbols from a board (e.g., patients who are quadriplegic following cervical spinal cord injuries). Eye gaze boards allow these patients to indicate letters, words, phrases, or symbols by looking at them. Message recipients watch the patient's eye movements and say what they believe the patient is looking at. The patient signals correct choices, usually by blinking. Because it is difficult for message recipients to tell exactly where a patient is looking, eye gaze boards have to be large, with large spaces between symbols. For this reason eye gaze boards cannot contain very many items. Most eye gaze boards contain an alphabet, numbers, and perhaps a few key words or phrases. Many are printed on transparent plastic sheets, or have cutouts through which message recipients can monitor the user's eye movements.

Mechanical and Electronic Devices. Mechanical and electronic devices for augmenting or replacing speech differ in cost, complexity, portability, and output. They range in cost from less than a hundred dollars to several thousand dollars. They range in portability from small hand-held devices to large units that cannot be carried but may be attached to a wheelchair or bed. The most common units are portable electronic devices that translate key-press input into messages that are shown on display screens, printed on paper, or translated into speech output. Some generate literal representations of what is entered on the keyboard or touch-screen, and what the auditor sees is what the user has entered. Other units translate codes entered by the user into programmed output messages; (e.g., a three-digit code entered by the

user might generate a five- or six-word phrase). Some (especially the hand-held devices) require finger dexterity and coordination to operate keyboards or touch-screens, and most require that the user read, spell, or remember codes, making them unsuitable for use with most aphasic patients, patients with moderate to severe cognitive impairments, or patients with poor motor control.

An adaptive device such as a joystick (a lever that moves in all directions and controls the movement of a cursor or the elements of an onscreen display) or a scanning system (with which items to be selected are displayed sequentially and the user selects items with a switch or key-press) may permit users with reduced manual dexterity to use many alternative communication systems. Adaptive devices such as head pointers, which permit users to control cursor movements and operate touch-screens by head movements, provide access to alternative communication systems for users who cannot move their limbs to operate keyboards, touch-screens, switches, or joysticks.

The current term for communication devices that provide speech output (prerecorded, digitized speech or computer-generated, synthesized speech) is *speech generating device (SGD).* This term currently is used by Medicare in documents related to coverage and reimbursement policies. Speech generating devices sometimes are called *voice-output communication devices (VOCDs).*

Figure 13-18 shows a portable speech generating device with which the user selects desired speech outputs by touching symbols on the display screen.

Considerations in Selecting Augmentative or Alternative Communication. Selecting a communication system for a dysarthric patient requires consideration of the patient's perceptual, motor, and language abilities, because different communication systems are compatible with different user abilities and preferences and different levels of user skill.

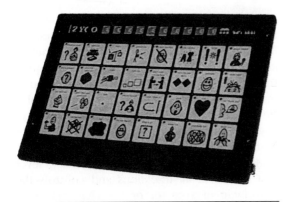

Figure 13-18 ■ A portable speech generating device. The user selects speech output by touching symbols on the display screen. (Courtesy Zygo Industries, Inc., Portland, OR.)

O'Keefe, Brown, and Schuller (1998) surveyed users of communication aids to find out what characteristics were most important to them. The four most important characteristics were the following:

- **Ease of learning.** Users preferred systems with designs that made it easy for users and caregivers to learn, use, and maintain the system.
- **Flexibility.** Users preferred systems that could easily be adapted to the unique needs of individual users, that could be modified or upgraded as a user's needs changed, and that had easy-to-access and reliable technical support.
- **Reliability.** Users preferred systems that were durable, did not fail, and were easily replaced when repairs were needed.
- **Understandability.** Users preferred systems with output that is understandable to a wide range of listeners without the need for special training or accommodation.

Silverman (1983) described several variables that should be considered when selecting an alternative or augmentative system:

- *Cost* (when resources for purchasing are limited). Funding agencies such as Medicare have strict rules governing the kinds of devices they will pay for. Patients with limited financial resources may not be able to afford an expensive system. (Medicare and many private insurers do, however, pay for speech generating devices under specified conditions.)
- *Amount of training.* If the system is to be a permanent one, extensive training may be appropriate. If the system is for temporary use or if an alternative means of communication is needed immediately, systems that require extensive training may not be appropriate.
- *Interference* (the extent to which using the system interferes with other activities). A system that requires the patient to sit at a fixed terminal and use both hands to operate it is more disruptive than a portable system that can be operated with one hand.
- *Intelligibility of the output.* This can affect both the time required to make a system functional and the situations in which it can be used by the patient. Systems that generate output that is intelligible to untrained recipients require less time to become operational and are useful in more places than systems producing symbols whose meanings recipients must be taught. Systems that print messages on tape or in displays cannot be used in the dark, over the telephone, or when patient and auditor are more than a few feet apart. Systems that generate messages on illuminated displays can be used in the dark but not over the telephone or at a distance. Systems that generate speechlike output may be unintelligible in noisy environments and may not be intelligible over the telephone, depending on the fidelity of the system's output and the fidelity of the telephone system.
- *Acceptability.* The acceptability of the system to user and recipients affects the extent to which it will be used in daily life. If the device or system is costly, cumbersome, complicated, or unnatural, it may be discarded in

favor of less costly, less cumbersome, and more effective ways to communicate. Some devices produce synthesized speech that sounds artificial. Users may prefer a device that produces digitized natural speech and permits the user to choose a voice representing a person of similar sex and age to the user.

GENERAL CONCEPTS 13-5

- Control of the dysarthric patient's everyday speaking environment is an important but sometimes overlooked component of treatment. Keeping ambient noise levels low and ensuring that the dysarthric speaker's face is visible to listeners may significantly enhance listeners' comprehension of the dysarthric patient.
- Some diseases causing dysarthria (e.g., Parkinson's disease) are treatable with medications. The medications usually have beneficial effects on dysarthria, but behavioral treatment of dysarthria may be needed when medication does not completely resolve a patient's dysarthria.
- Teflon injections, palatal lifts, and pharyngeal flaps may be appropriate for treating patients with severe hypernasality. These procedures usually are employed only when hypernasality is severe and when behavioral treatment fails to make the patient's speech sufficiently intelligible for daily life communication.
- Some patients with severe dysarthria may need *augmentative* or *alternative communication systems* to permit them to communicate in daily life. Speech amplifiers, gesture, and pantomime may *augment* a patient's limited speech. Communication boards, communication books, and electronic devices may *replace* speech for severely impaired dysarthric speakers who have the manual dexterity needed to use them.

THOUGHT QUESTIONS

Question 13-1 Speculate as to the potential motor speech disorder likely to be exhibited by:
- A patient with a history of atrial fibrillations
- A patient with ten years of participation in professional boxing
- A patient with a family history of Huntington's chorea
- A patient with a traumatic brain injury incurred in a motor vehicle accident
- A patient with a 10-year history of transient ischemic attacks

Question 13-2 A 57-year-old woman comes to a neurology clinic with the following complaints.

"I've been having increasing trouble getting up out of a chair, and now I'm having trouble turning over in bed."

"Sometimes I have trouble walking. It's like I'm glued to the floor. It takes me three or four tries to get going."

"It seems like my voice has gotten fainter, and I'm hoarse most of the time. At first I thought it was allergies or a cold or something, but it hasn't gone away. People complain that they can't hear me when there's noise in the background. And it seems like I'm beginning to stutter or something. I'll repeat things over and over—sounds and words."

The neurologist conjectured that the patient's complaints suggested neurologic disease and dysarthria—a conjecture borne out by a subsequent neurologic examination. What was the disease? What was the dysarthria type? Explain your reasoning.

Question 13-3 How might the focus of treatment differ for patients with apraxia of speech caused by damage in or near Broca's area *(frontal apraxia of speech)* versus patients with "apraxia of speech" caused by damage in temporoparietal regions *(posterior apraxia of speech)*?

Question 13-4 What do you think Darley, Aronson, and Brown (1975) meant by "islands of error-free speech" in the speech of patients with apraxia of speech? Which characteristics of speech do you think they were thinking of? Write your own definition—try to make it specific to apraxia of speech and exclude the dysarthrias.

Question 13-5 A 56-year-old man is referred to you by a neurologist who asks you for help in diagnosing the nature of the man's speech impairment. The man's neurologic examination is within normal limits, except for questionable bilateral slowness of arm and hand movements. Your examination yields the following results:

- Normal strength and range of movement of tongue, lips, and jaw
- Normal movement of palate and pharynx at beginning of phonation; visible tensing of palatal, pharyngeal muscles on sustained phonation
- Normal cough, grunt, glottal stop
- Articulation is normal for syllables, words, sentences, paragraphs
- Normal voice quality, intonation, and loudness for single syllables and words
- Unable to control voice loudness in longer speech segments; initial words in phrases, sentences, and connected speech are produced at normal loudness, but loudness quickly increases as speech continues until the patient is shouting loudly; spontaneous speech, repetition, and series speech (counting, etc.) are affected; articulation and resonance are not affected by changes in loudness
- No evidence of aphasia or cognitive impairment

The patient reports that the changes in his speech occurred gradually over several months. He says that he knows that he shouts but cannot help it and is embarrassed by it. He reports no history of head injury, significant medical problems, or diagnosed neurologic problems. He works for a railway company as a laborer. His duties include repairing and maintaining the rail line, spraying weeds and grasses along the right-of-way with herbicides, and periodically checking switches and signal systems to ensure reliable operation.

Standard Medical Abbreviations

The following list contains some frequently encountered medical abbreviations. Most medical establishments have a list of standard abbreviations for use in their facilities, but the lists differ to some extent across establishments, and individual physicians often use idiosyncratic abbreviations that may force the reader to engage in reasoning, detective work, or both to deduce what the abbreviations mean.

~	approximately
Δ	change
≃	consistent with
†	death
↘	decrease
°	degree
≤	equal to or less than
>	greater than
<	less than
♀	female
♂	male
—	negative
#	number
%	percent
%ile	percentile
+	positive
1°	primary
2°	secondary
∴	therefore
c̄	with
Ø	without
AAROM	active assisted range of motion
abn	abnormal
a.c.	before meals

ACA	anterior communicating artery, anterior cerebral artery
ADL	activities of daily living
ad lib	as desired
AIDS	acquired immunodeficiency syndrome
AK,AKA	above the knee, above-knee amputation
alc, ETOH	alcohol
ALS	amyotrophic lateral sclerosis
AMA	against medical advice, American Medical Association
amb	ambulatory
AMI	acute myocardial infarction
angio	angiogram
ant	anterior
ante	before
AODM	adult onset diabetes mellitus
AP	anteroposterior
ARD	acute respiratory disease
ARF	acute renal failure
ASA	aspirin
ASAP	as soon as possible
ASCVD	arteriosclerotic cardiovascular disease
ASHD	arteriosclerotic heart disease
AV	arteriovenous, atrioventricular
AVM	arteriovenous malformation
b.i.d.	twice a day
bil	bilateral
BK	below the knee
bm	bowel movement
BM	bone marrow
BMR	basal metabolism rate
BP	blood pressure

BRP	bathroom privileges	DT	delirium tremens
bs	bowel sounds	DTR	deep tendon reflex
BS	breath sounds	DU	diabetic urine
BUN	blood urea nitrogen	Dx	diagnosis
bx	biopsy	ECA	external carotid artery
C	Celsius, centigrade	ECG, EKG	electrocardiogram
CA	cardiac arrest	ECT	electroconvulsive therapy
CA, ca	carcinoma	EEG	electroencephalogram
Ca+	calcium	EENT	eye, ear, nose, throat
CABG	coronary artery bypass graft	EMG	electromyogram
CAD	coronary artery disease	ENT	ear, nose, throat
cal	calorie	EOM	extraocular movements
CAT	computerized axial tomography	ER	emergency room
cath	catheter	ETOH	ethanol (alcohol)
CBC	complete blood count	exam	examination
CBS	chronic brain syndrome	ext	external, exterior
cc	cubic centimeter	F	Fahrenheit
CC	chief complaint	FB	foreign body
CHF	congestive heart failure, chronic heart failure	FBS	fasting blood sugar
		FH	family history
CHI	closed head injury	fib	fibrillation
cm	centimeter	fl, fld	fluid
CMT	continuing medication and treatment	FU	follow-up
		FUO	fever of unknown origin
CN	cranial nerve	fx	fracture
CNS	central nervous system	GB	gall bladder
c/o	complains of	gen	general
COLD	chronic obstructive lung disease	GI	gastrointestinal
cont	continue(d)	gm	gram
COPD	chronic obstructive pulmonary disease	gr	grain
		GSW	gunshot wound
CPR	cardiopulmonary resuscitation	GTT	glucose tolerance test
CRF	chronic renal failure	GU	genito-urinary
CSF	cerebrospinal fluid	GYN	gynecology
CT	computerized tomography	h, hr	hour
cu	cubic	HA	headache
CV	cardiovascular	Hb	hemoglobin
CVA	cerebrovascular accident	HB	heart block
CXR	chest X-ray	HBP	high blood pressure
d	day	HCM	health care maintenance
DNR	do not resuscitate	HCVD	hypertensive cardiovascular disease
DNT	did not test		
DOA	dead on arrival	HEENT	head, eyes, ears, nose, throat
DOE	dyspnea (shortness of breath) on exertion	Hg	mercury
		Hg, Hgb	hemoglobin
d/t	due to	HH	homonymous hemianopsia

H/O	history of	NG	nasogastric
H&P	history and physical	NKA	no known allergies
HPI	history of present illness	no.	number
HR	heart rate	noc.	night
hs	bedtime	NP	neuropsychiatric
HTN	hypertension	NPO, npo	nothing by mouth
hx	history	N/S	neurosurgery
H₂O	water	NSC	not service connected
ICA	internal carotid artery	N&V	nausea and vomiting
ICP	intracranial pressure	OBS	organic brain syndrome
ICU	intensive care unit	OD	officer of the day
IM	intramuscular	OD	overdose
imp	impression	OM	otitis media
inc	increase	OOB, oob	out of bed
inf	inferior	OP	outpatient
I&O	intake and output	OPD	outpatient department
IU	international unit	OPT	outpatient treatment
IV	intravenous	OR	operating room
kg	kilogram	OT	occupational therapy
KJ	knee jerk	oz.	ounce
L, l	left	$\underline{p}$	pulse
lab	laboratory	p	after
lat	lateral	PA	posteroanterior
LCA	left coronary artery	PAR	postanesthesia recovery room
LE	lower extremity	path	pathology
liq	liquid	PC	presenting complaint
LMD	local medical doctor	p.c.	after meals
LOC	loss of consciousness	PCA	posterior cerebral artery
LOM	limitation of motion	PCN	penicillin
LOS	length of stay	PE	physical examination
LP	lumbar puncture (spinal tap)	PEG	percutaneous endoscopic
LPN	licensed practical nurse		gastrostomy
L&W	living and well	per	by
MCA	middle cerebral artery	PERLLA	pupils equal, round, reactive to
MH	marital history		light and accommodation
MI	myocardial infarction	PET	positron emission tomography
ml	milliliter	PH	past history
mm	millimeter	PI	present illness
mHg	millimeters of mercury	PMD	personal medical doctor
MRI	magnetic resonance image	PMH	past medical history
MS	multiple sclerosis	PMR	physical medicine and
MVA	motor vehicle accident		rehabilitation
NA	not applicable	p.o.	by mouth
NAD	no acute distress	POD	postoperative day
neg	negative	pos.	positive
neuro	neurologic, neurology	post.	posterior

PR	pulse rate	SI	seriously ill
preop	preoperative	SOB	shortness of breath
prep	preparation	s/p	status post
prn, p.r.n.	as needed	spec	specimen
PROM	passive range of motion	ss	one-half
Psych	psychiatry	SSN	Social Security number
Psychol	psychology	stat	immediately
pt	patient	surg	surgery
PT	physical therapy	Sx	symptoms
PTA	prior to admission	Sz	seizure
PX	physical	T	temperature
q.a.m.	every morning	TB, TBC	tuberculosis
q.d.	every day	TBI	traumatic brain injury
q.h.	every hour	temp	temperature
q.i.d.	four times per day	TIA	transient ischemic attack
q.o.d.	every other day	t.i.d.	three times per day
R, r	right	TPR	temperature, pulse, respiration
RBC	red blood cell	tx	transplant
RIND	reversible ischemic neurologic deficit	Tx	treatment
		UA	urinalysis
RMS	rehabilitation medicine service	UCHD	usual childhood disease
RN	registered nurse	VD	venereal disease
RND	radical neck dissection	VDRL	Venereal Disease Research Laboratory Test (for VD)
r/o	rule out		
ROM	range of motion	VF	visual field
RR	respiration rate	v fib	ventricular fibrillations
Rt	right	VHD	valvular heart disease
RT	radiation therapy	VS	vital signs
RT	recreational therapy	W	white
RTC	return to clinic	w. wk	week
Rx	therapy	WBC	white blood cells
s, sec	second	WD	well developed
s	without	WDWN	well developed, well nourished
SAB	subarachnoid bleed	WNL	within normal limits
SAH	subarachnoid hemorrhage	wt	weight
SC	service connected	w/u	workup
SCI	spinal cord injury	Y/O	year old
SH	social history	yrs	years

Glossary

Acceleration injury Brain injury caused when the moving head strikes a stationary surface or the stationary head is struck by a moving object in a way that causes the head to move quickly from its resting position. *Linear acceleration injury* is caused by forces that propel the head on a linear path. *Angular acceleration injury* is caused by forces that propel the head at an angle from the path of the impact and cause it to rotate. (See also *coup injury, contrecoup injury, diffuse axonal injury, translational trauma.*)

Activity limitation The effect of an impairment on a person's access to activities of daily life. (See also *impairment, disability, handicap.*)

Afferent Sensory.

Agnosia Inability to recognize stimuli in a sensory modality in spite of intact sensation in the modality. Several varieties of agnosia have been described in the literature, including *auditory agnosia, visual agnosia, tactile agnosia,* and combinations such as *auditory-verbal agnosia* and *visual-verbal agnosia.*

Agrammatism Speech in which content words (mainly nouns, verbs, adjectives) are present, but most function words (articles, prepositions, conjunctions) are missing. A common characteristic of the speech of adults with Broca's aphasia.

Agraphia (dysgraphia) Impaired writing.

Alertness, phasic Rapidly occurring changes in receptivity to stimulation.

Alertness, tonic Ongoing receptivity to stimulation.

Alexia (dyslexia) Impaired reading.

Alexia without agraphia A rare syndrome in which the patient cannot read but can write. Usually caused by isolation of the visual cortex from Wernicke's area.

Alzheimer's disease A progressive neurologic disease characterized by increasing dementia.

Amnesia Loss of memory, inability to remember.

Anesthesia Complete loss of sensation.

Aneurysm Balloonlike bulges in an artery caused by weakness in the arterial wall. Aneurysms are susceptible to hemorrhage.

Angiography (arteriography) A laboratory procedure by which blood vessels can be visualized. A contrast medium is injected into the bloodstream and a series of X-ray exposures is made to determine the condition of the patient's blood vessels.

Angular gyrus A prominent gyrus near the temporo-parietal-occipital junction, at the posterior end of the Sylvian (lateral) fissure. Damage in the region of the angular gyrus often causes problems with reading and arithmetic abilities.

Anomia Inability or impaired ability to retrieve and produce words.

Anosognosia Denial of illness. Often a symptom of right-hemisphere brain pathology.

Anterior horn cells Spinal motor neurons, located in the anterolateral part of the spinal cord.

Anton's syndrome (visual anosognosia) A condition in which a person is blind because of bilateral destruction of the visual cortex *(cortical blindness)* but denies being blind.

Aorta The main artery from the heart.

Aphasia A language impairment that crosses all input and output modalities. Can be divided into various syndromes.

Apraxia Disruption of volitional movement sequences in the absence of sensory loss, weakness, paralysis, or incoordination of the muscles involved in the movements. Usually a consequence of damage in the premotor cortex. (See also *ideational apraxia, ideomotor apraxia, buccofacial apraxia, limb apraxia, verbal apraxia, dressing apraxia,* and *constructional apraxia.*)

Aqueduct A channel or opening.

Arachnoid villi Sites at which cerebrospinal fluid is resorbed into the venous blood.

Arcuate fasciculus A major fiber tract that connects the temporal lobe with regions in the frontal lobe in each hemisphere. The arcuate fasciculus in the left hemisphere is considered the major pathway by which information from the language centers in the temporal lobe reach the frontal lobe for conversion into spoken or written output.

Arteriography See *angiography.*

Arteriosclerosis See *atherosclerosis.*

Arteriovenous malformation (AVM) Convoluted collections of weak, thin-walled veins and arteries on the brain's surface or within the brain.

Association cortex Cortical areas that are adjacent to the sensory or motor cortex. The association cortex is thought to play an important part in integrating motor or sensory information from adjacent cortical areas and input from other regions of the brain.

Association fibers Nerve fibers connecting adjacent regions of the cortex.

Astereognosis (tactile agnosia) Inability to recognize otherwise familiar objects by touch, although the sense of touch is intact.

Astrocytoma A common, relatively benign glioma.

Ataxia Clumsiness and incoordination of movements caused by cerebellar damage.

Atherosclerosis (arteriosclerosis) A disease process in which arterial walls become roughened and covered with fatty deposits. These deposits are called *atherosclerotic plaque.*

Athetosis Slow, sinuous, writhing, and uncontrollable muscle movements.

Atrophy Shrinkage and wasting away of tissues.

Attention, alternating The ability to shift attention from one stimulus to another or from one aspect of a stimulus to another.

Attention, divided The ability to attend to more than one activity simultaneously.

Attention, selective The ability to maintain attention on selected stimuli in the presence of competing or distracting stimuli. Sometimes called *focused attention.*

Attention, sustained The ability to maintain attention on selected stimuli over time.

Auditory cortex A region of cortex on the top surface of each temporal lobe (the gyrus of Heschl). It has primary responsibility for auditory perception.

Axon The conducting process of a nerve cell (neuron).

Ballism See *chorea.*

Basal ganglia Several nuclei in the diencephalon, near the thalamus. They are responsible for regulation of major muscle groups that make postural adjustments and compensate for inertial forces during movement. Depending on who is writing about them, the basal ganglia include the *caudate nucleus, putamen, globus pallidus, subthalamic nucleus,* and *substantia nigra.*

Basilar artery An artery that connects the two vertebral arteries to the posterior part of the *circle of Willis.* It progresses upward on the front surface of the pons and supplies blood to the pons.

Bell's palsy Ipsilateral paralysis of lower facial muscles caused by compression of the facial nerve (CN 7).

Binswanger's disease A rare disease, caused by multiple infarcts in subcortical white matter.

Biopsy Removal of a sample of tissue for laboratory analysis.

Brain abscess A cavity in the brain caused by infection with bacteria, fungi, or parasites.

Brain stem A stalklike structure at the base of the brain, atop the spinal cord. It contains centers that regulate some vital functions and contains most cranial nerve nuclei. Anatomists divide it into the midbrain (upper), pons (middle), and medulla (lower).

Broca's aphasia An aphasia syndrome characterized by nonfluent speech, good comprehension, and poor repetition.

Broca's area A region of the cortex just anterior to the lower end of the primary motor cortex. Damage in Broca's areas is said to cause *Broca's aphasia.*

Buccofacial apraxia Ideomotor apraxia of the oral musculature.

Bulbar Relating to the brain stem, especially the pons.

Calcarine fissure A deep groove in the occipital lobe of each hemisphere. It is important because the visual cortex is adjacent to it.

Caloric testing A diagnostic test in which cold or warm water is introduced into the external auditory canal. Patients with vestibular pathology respond with characteristic patterns of *nystagmus.*

Capgras syndrome The belief that friends, family, or acquaintances have been abducted and replaced by imposters.

Carotid arteries There are two external carotid arteries and two internal carotid arteries. The external carotid arteries supply blood to the face. The internal carotid arteries supply blood to the brain via the *circle of Willis.*

Catastrophic reaction A sudden and intense emotional outburst, usually anger, sometimes crying, or (rarely) laughing. Catastrophic reactions usually are a brain-injured patient's response to being pushed beyond his or her limits.

Central fissure A deep groove that divides each brain hemisphere into roughly equal front and back halves. Sometimes called the *fissure of Rolando.*

Central nervous system (CNS) The brain, brain stem, cerebellum, and spinal cord.

Cerebellum A structure that looks like a miniature brain and lies beneath the posterior temporal lobes. It is important in integration and coordination of volitional movements.

Cerebral aqueduct A long narrow passageway between the third and fourth ventricles. Occlusion of the cerebral aqueduct is a common cause of *hydrocephalus* (enlarged ventricles). The cerebral aqueduct sometimes is called the *aqueduct of Sylvius.*

Cerebral arteries There are three cerebral arteries in each hemisphere. They are called the *anterior, middle,* and *posterior* cerebral arteries, which serve the front, middle, and posterior parts of the hemisphere, respectively.

Cerebral dominance The belief that one hemisphere has primary responsibility for speech and language (the left hemisphere in right-handers).

Cerebral plasticity The ability of the brain to reassign functions served by one area to a different area, usually in response to brain injury. Cerebral plasticity is greatest in infants and declines steadily with age.

Cerebrospinal fluid (CSF) A clear, colorless fluid that fills the ventricles and surrounds the brain, brain stem, cerebellum, and spinal cord.

Cerebrovascular accident (CVA) Temporary or permanent disruption of brain function due to interruption of its blood supply. Sometimes called *stroke* or, more recently, *brain attack.*

Cerebrum What we usually think of as the brain. The two brain hemispheres.

Chorea A disease that causes quick and forceful involuntary movements *(choreiform movements). Ballism* is an extreme form of chorea, in which the limbs are flung wildly about by the involuntary movements. (The word *ballism* comes from the same root as *ballistic.*)

Choreoathetosis A combination of choreiform and athetoid movements. (See *chorea* and *athetosis.*)

Choroid plexus Structures in the ventricles that produce cerebrospinal fluid.

Circle of Willis A heptagonal arrangement of arteries at the base of the brain that connects the inter-nal carotid arteries and the basilar artery to the cerebral arteries. It is thought to serve as a "safety valve" for occlusions below the circle of Willis.

Circumduction A characteristic gait of patients with hemiplegia *(circumducted gait).* The patient swings the leg outward from the hip in a semicircular movement without flexing the knee.

Circumlocution Literally, *talking around* words that an individual is unable to say. Patients with conduction or Wernicke's aphasia often use circumlocution to communicate the sense of words they cannot retrieve.

Cistern A cavity or space for storage of fluids.

Clasp-knife phenomenon The tendency of spastic muscles to resist stretching when the examiner first moves the patient's limb and to gradually become less resistant as the examiner continues to move the patient's limb at a constant rate.

Coagulation time The time it takes for blood to clot. Laboratory tests of coagulation time are useful in treating patients with occlusive vascular disease.

Coherence The overall unity or point of discourse.

Cohesion The degree to which words in discourse relate to one another.

Coma Prolonged loss of consciousness.

Commissural fibers (commissures) Nerve fibers that cross between the brain hemispheres. The corpus callosum is the major commissure in the brain. The anterior and posterior commissures are minor ones.

Commissurotomy Surgically cutting the corpus callosum.

Computerized tomography (CT scanning) A radiologic test in which a computer constructs cross-sectional images of internal body structures by analyzing information from a series of X-ray exposures made at consecutive horizontal levels of a body part.

Concreteness Failure to appreciate abstract, indirect, nonliteral meanings of messages, events, or situations.

Conduction aphasia An aphasia syndrome characterized by fluent speech, fair comprehension, and poor repetition.

Confrontation naming Naming objects, pictures, color swatches, and the like.

Constructional apraxia A misnomer. Inability to copy geometric shapes. Usually a disorder of visuospatial perception and integration rather than a motor planning disorder.

Constructional impairment Inability to copy geometric shapes or three-dimensional constructions.

Contralateral On the other side. In neurology, the term usually means on the other side of the body from the nervous system disease.

Contrast Any of several fluids that may be introduced into internal spaces (usually blood vessels) or tissues to make structures easier to see in laboratory imaging studies.

Contrastive stress drill A treatment for dysarthria and apraxia of speech in which the patient is coached to produce utterances with exaggerated emphatic stress on certain words, as in Bob hit BILL.

Contrecoup injury Brain injury on the opposite side of the brain from the impact.

Corpus callosum The major commissure connecting the brain hemispheres. Almost all neural communication between the hemispheres goes via the corpus callosum.

Cortex The neuron-rich outer layer of the brain hemispheres. The cortex makes possible "higher mental processes" (thinking, reasoning, calculating, and so on).

Corticobulbar Going between the cortex and the brain stem.

Corticopontine Going between the cortex and the pons.

Corticospinal Going between the cortex and the spinal cord.

Coup injury Brain injury at the site of impact.

Cranial nerves Peripheral nerves that serve muscles and sensory receptors in the head and neck. Most connect with the central nervous system in the brain stem.

Cranial vault The inside of the skull. It contains the brain and cerebellum. It is divided into compartments by sheets of dura. The two major dural sheets are the *falx cerebri* and the *tentorium cerebelli.*

Creutzfeldt-Jakob disease A degenerative disease in which brain tissues become soft and spongy *(spongiform encephalopathy).*

Decomposition of movement Movements that have a jerky, segmented quality, often seen following cerebellar damage. A component of *ataxia.*

Decussate To cross the midline. Refers to the crossing of pyramidal tracts from one side of the central nervous system to the other at the medulla.

Delirium Altered consciousness and mentation. Sometimes called *acute confusional state.*

Dementia Diffuse impairment of intellect and cognition caused by any of several diseases and conditions.

Dementia, cortical Dementia caused by pathology affecting the cerebral cortex.

Dementia, mixed Dementia caused by a combination of cortical and subcortical pathology.

Dementia, subcortical Dementia caused by pathology affecting the basal ganglia, thalamus, and brain stem.

Dendrite Short, hairlike receptive processes of a nerve cell (neuron).

Dermatome A region of skin innervated by a cranial or spinal sensory nerve.

Diagnosis The act of assigning a label to a disease or condition.

Diaschisis Disruption of brain function in areas remote from an area of injury but connected to it by nerve pathways.

Diencephalon A deep central region within the brain hemispheres. Contains the thalamus and basal ganglia. It plays an important part in the regulation and integration of motor activity and sensory experience.

Differential diagnosis Discriminating a disease or condition from others that may resemble it.

Diffuse axonal injury Disseminated damage to nerve cell axons caused by *angular acceleration.*

Diplopia Double vision. Often caused by weakness or paralysis of muscles responsible for moving one eye, which prevents the two eyes from fixating on the same point.

Disability The effects of a structural or functional abnormality on a skill or ability (e.g., poor ambulation caused by paralysis). *Disability* was changed to the politically neutral *activity* in the most recent World Health Organization schema. (See *impairment, handicap.*)

Disconnection syndrome A unique pattern of impairments caused by interruption of fibers in the corpus callosum, which isolates the language-competent hemisphere from the non-language-competent hemisphere.

Distal Away from the trunk.

Double simultaneous stimulation Simultaneously stimulating sensory receptors at symmetrical points on both sides of the body. Patients with subtle sensory impairments report stimulation only on the unaffected side.

Dressing apraxia A misnomer. Dressing apraxia is not a true apraxia. It usually is seen in patients with nondominant-hemisphere pathology and is caused by disruptions of body schema, impaired appreciation of the relationship of the body to surrounding space, and, sometimes, neglect.

Dysarthria Any of several speech abnormalities caused by nervous system damage that affects movement or sensation within body parts involved in speech.

Dyskinesia Abnormal and involuntary muscle movements, often seen as a consequence of extrapyramidal disease. (See also *tremor, chorea, ballism, dystonia, myoclonus, fasciculations, fibrillations, tics*.)

Dyslexia, deep A reading impairment in which the individual cannot analyze words phonologically but must depend on whole-word reading to recognize words.

Dyslexia, surface A reading impairment in which the individual cannot make use of whole-word recognition in reading but must depend on phonologic analysis to recognize words.

Dysmetria Slow and awkward movements. A component of *ataxia*.

Dystonia Persisting involuntary contractions of muscles, sometimes called *torsion spasm*.

Echolalia A tendency to repeat back what is said. A common characteristic of patients with *posterior isolation syndrome*.

Edema Swelling.

Effectiveness Whether treatment causes a meaningful change in patients' daily life adequacy.

Efferent Motor.

Efficacy Whether treatment causes a significant change in patients' performance on one or more objective measures.

Egocentrism Inability to view events and situations from another's point of view.

Electroencephalography (EEG) A laboratory test in which the electrical activity of the brain cortex is measured and converted to a pen tracing on a moving strip of paper.

Electromyography (EMG) A procedure in which fine needle electrodes are inserted into muscles and the electrical activity in the muscles is recorded.

Ellipsoidal deformation Deformation of the restrained skull caused by the impact of a slow-moving object possessing a large surface area.

Embolus A fragment that travels through a blood vessel. If an embolus lodges and occludes an artery, it causes an embolic stroke.

Emotional lability Exaggerated emotional responses to stimuli. Unusually wide swings in emotional tone.

Empty speech Speech that is syntactically correct but conveys little or no overall meaning. Often a result of substituting general words such as *thing* or *stuff* for more specific words.

Encephalopathy Pathology affecting the brain and meninges.

Epidural Between the dura mater and the skull.

Evoked cortical potentials A laboratory procedure in which a computer averages the electrical activity of the brain cortex from many sites on the skull and produces a record of systematic changes in the electrical activity that occur with presentation of auditory, visual, or tactile stimuli.

Excess disability A person's functional impairments are greater than expected based on that person's physical, cognitive, and psychologic status.

Executive function A label for a collection of cognitive processes. The cognitive processes subsumed under the label usually include *response flexibility, abstract thinking, planning, reasoning,* and *problem-solving*.

Extrapyramidal system That part of the motor system not composed of corticobulbar or corticospinal tracts. Includes the basal ganglia and related structures.

Falx cerebri A rigid sheet of dura mater that goes from front to back within the longitudinal cerebral fissure. It often is called the *falx* for efficiency.

Familial Diseases that have a greater than normal occurrence in families but do not have a known genetic inheritance pattern. The exact probability that offspring of parents who have the disease will inherit the disease cannot be calculated. (See also *hereditary*.)

Fasciculations Involuntary movements that cause visible movements of muscle fibers.

Fasciculus A fiber tract that connects regions in different lobes of the brain. The three major fasciculi are the *arcuate fasciculus,* the *uncinate fasciculus,* and the *cingulum*.

Feedback Information provided contingent on responses. *Incentive feedback* depends on response consequences that have primary reinforcing (or punishing) power. *Information feedback* has no intrinsic reinforcing or punishing power but provides information to an individual about the closeness of responses to a target. (See also *reinforcement.*)

Festinating gait Short rapid steps. A common consequence of Parkinson's disease.

Fibrillations Contractions of a single muscle fiber or small group of fibers, too small to be seen but detectable with sensitive instruments.

Fissure A deep sulcus.

Fluency When used to classify adults with aphasia, *fluency* refers to the prosodic or melodic characteristics of speech. Adults with fluent aphasia speak with essentially normal rate, intonation, pauses, and emphatic stress patterns. Adults with nonfluent aphasia speak slowly, with diminished intonation, abnormally placed and excessively long pauses, and diminished variation in emphatic stress. Fluent aphasia is associated with postcentral damage, and nonfluent aphasia is associated with precentral damage.

Focal Affecting a limited region within the nervous system. The opposite of *diffuse.*

Foramen An opening. There are several foramina in the skull, through which blood vessels and nerves pass. The major foramen is the *foramen magnum,* through which the brain stem passes. There are many foramina in the spinal cord, between the vertebrae, through which nerves and blood vessels pass (the intervertebral foramina).

Frontal lobe dementia See *Pick's disease.*

Frontal lobes Make up approximately the anterior one-third of the brain. The frontal lobes provide the initial impetus for overt behavior.

Fugue state A period of disturbed consciousness, lasting from minutes to days, in which the patient goes about regular activities of daily living but has no subsequent memory for what happened during the period.

Functional communication Communication in daily life.

Gag reflex Coughing or choking when the posterior tongue or pharyngeal walls are touched.

Generalization Transfer of learned skills, behaviors, or responses from one setting to another.

Generative naming (word fluency, category naming) Providing names according to a category suggested by the examiner. For example, "*Tell me all the words you can thing of that begin with the letter* F" or "*Tell me all the vegetables you can think of.*" (Usually limited to a 1-minute interval.)

Geographic disorientation Inability to identify one's geographic location, even though one recognizes one's personal surroundings. An occasional consequence of right-hemisphere brain damage.

Glial cells Form the supporting tissue of the brain, which is called *glia.* Most of the cells in the brain are glial cells.

Glioblastoma multiforme A common, very malignant tumor of glial cells.

Glioma A tumor that arises in brain glia.

Granulovacuolar degeneration Neuronal abnormalities seen in Alzheimer's disease, other neurologic diseases, and in some normal elderly. Small fluid-filled cavities appear within nerve cells, and nerve cell function is adversely affected.

Gray matter Nervous system tissues made up primarily of cell bodies and dendrites. It is actually pinkish-gray in color.

Gyrus A "hill" on the surface of the brain. (Plural = gyri.)

Gyrus of Heschl A strip of cortex on the top surface of each temporal lobe. Also known as the *primary auditory cortex.*

Handicap The effects of a structural or functional abnormality on an individual's ability to carry out daily life roles and responsibilities. For example, diminished ability to earn a living as a consequence of hemiplegia. *Handicap* was changed to the politically neutral *participation* in the most recent World Health Organization schema. (See also *impairment, disability.*)

Hematoma Accumulation of blood from a hemorrhage.

Hemianopsia (hemianopia) Blindness in one-half of the visual field. *Homonymous hemianopsia* is blindness in the same (right or left) half of the visual field in each eye. *Heteronymous hemianopsia* is blindness in different halves of the visual field in each eye.

Hemiplegia Paralysis of an arm and a leg on one side of the body.

Hemorrhage Bleeding. Accumulation of blood from a hemorrhage is called a *hematoma.*

Hereditary Diseases that have a known genetic inheritance pattern. The probability that offspring of parents who have the disease will inherit the disease can be calculated, and "family trees" showing inheritance patterns can be constructed.

Herniation Displacement of brain tissue by swelling or space-occupying lesions such as tumors or brain abscesses.

Heuristic processes "Top-down" comprehension processes, in which listeners and readers use general knowledge, intuition, and guessing to arrive at the meaning of spoken or printed verbal materials.

Homonymous The corresponding halves of the visual fields or retinae.

Homunculus *"Little man."* A drawing of a human figure showing topographic representation of the motor cortex.

Huntington's disease A hereditary neurologic disease characterized by progressive chorea and dementia.

Hydrocephalus Enlargement of the cerebral ventricles. Hydrocephalus usually is caused by obstruction of an intraventricular passageway but also can be a result of brain atrophy. The former is called *obstructive hydrocephalus,* and the latter is called *nonobstructive hydrocephalus.*

Hyperesthesia Abnormal sensitivity to stimulation.

Hypertonia Abnormally high levels of tension in resting muscles.

Hypesthesia (hypoesthesia) Diminished sensation.

Hypoperfusion Diminished blood supply to the brain caused by insufficient blood volume or pressure.

Hypotonia Abnormally low levels of tension in resting muscles.

Ideational apraxia Inability to carry out movement sequences because of loss of the concept, knowledge, or idea of what the movements are intended to accomplish.

Ideomotor apraxia Inability to carry out movement sequences because of loss of the ability to organize the motor plans or patterns for the movements.

Impairment A structural or functional abnormality within an individual (e.g., paralysis). *Impairment* was changed to the politically neutral *body function and structure* in the most recent World Health Organization schema. (See also *disability, handicap.*)

Infarct Death of tissue caused by loss of blood supply.

Insula A patch of the cortex folded into the lateral fissure, sometimes called the *island of Reil.* The operculum surrounds the insula.

Integral stimulation A treatment procedure in which the patient imitates the clinician's model (e.g., *"Watch me and do what I do"*).

Internal capsule That section of corticobulbar and corticospinal tracts that lies within the basal ganglia.

International Classification of Functioning, Disability, and Health (ICF) A revised coding and classification system developed by the World Health Association to replace the ICIDH-2 (see the following entry). The ICF considers disability and functioning the product of interactions between *health conditions* (e.g., diseases, disorders, and injuries), *personal factors* (e.g., age, education, experience, coping styles), and *environmental factors* (e.g., social attitudes, legal and social policies, building design, climate).

International Classification of Impairments, Disabilities, and Handicaps-2 (ICIDH-2) A classification and coding system developed by the World Health Organization to quantify the effects of health conditions on individuals. The ICIDH-2 defined *body functions* as *"the physiological or psychological functions of body systems;"* it defined *body structures* as *"anatomic parts of the body such as organs, limbs, and their components;"* it defined *activity* as *"the execution of a task or involvement in a life situation in a uniform environment;"* and it defined *participation* as *"the execution of a task or involvement in a life situation in an individual's current environment."*

Intersystemic reorganization (gestural reorganization) A treatment for apraxia of speech in which patients are taught to execute nonspeech movements simultaneously with speech—for example, gesturing the act of drinking from a glass while saying, *"Drink some water."*

Intracerebral Within the brain.

Intrasystemic reorganization A treatment for apraxia of speech in which the locus of control of speech movements is shifted to another part of the system used to produce speech—for example, speaking slowly and with exaggerated articulation.

Intraventricular foramen A short passageway between each lateral ventricle and the third ventricle for movement of cerebrospinal fluid, sometimes called the *foramen of Munro.*

Ipsilateral On the same side. (See also *contralateral.*)

Ischemia Lack of oxygen in tissues.

Isolation syndrome An aphasia syndrome caused by isolation of the central region of the language-dominant hemisphere from the rest of the brain. (See also *transcortical motor aphasia* and *transcortical sensory aphasia.*)

Isometric Pushing against immovable resistance.

Isotonic Pushing against a movable resistance.

Jargon Nonsensical utterances, such as *"There's a navy dog flying in the hoghouse this morning,"* in which words are uttered in syntactically legitimate strings, but which have no overall meaning. The strings may contain *neologisms.*

Lacunar state A progressive neurologic disease caused by successive small infarcts in the midbrain and brain stem.

Lateral apertures Two openings from the fourth ventricle into the subarachnoid space, sometimes called the *foramina of Luschka.*

Lateral cerebral fissure A deep groove that separates the temporal lobe in each hemisphere from the frontal and parietal lobes, sometimes called the *fissure of Sylvius* or the *frontotemporoparietal fissure.*

Lenticular nucleus The putamen and globus pallidus (basal ganglia).

Lewy bodies Abnormal protein deposits in neuron cell bodies. Proliferation of Lewy bodies is a cause of *Lewy body dementia.*

Limb apraxia Ideomotor apraxia of the arm and hand. Limb apraxias usually are more severe *distally* (away from the trunk) than *proximally* (near the trunk).

Localization An approach to understanding the functional architecture of the nervous system by relating neurologically damaged patients' symptoms to damaged regions of the nervous system. When damage in a given part of the nervous system consistently causes certain impairments, the impaired function is attributed to the damaged part.

Logorrhea See *press of speech.*

Longitudinal cerebral fissure The deep groove at the apex of the cerebrum that separates the hemispheres. (Sometimes it is called the *superior longitudinal fissure* or *interhemispheric fissure;* perhaps it should be called the *superior longitudinal interhemispheric cerebral fissure.*)

Loose training Generalization training in which stimulus conditions, response requirements, and reinforcement contingencies are permitted to vary to increase generalization from the training environment to other environments.

Lower motor neuron Another name for the peripheral nervous system.

Lumbar puncture (spinal tap) A procedure in which a needle is inserted into the spinal column and a sample of cerebrospinal fluid is removed and analyzed for the presence of bacteria, viruses, parasites, or abnormalities in its chemical composition.

Lumen The open passageway in a blood vessel.

Macula The region in the central retina that provides the greatest visual acuity.

Macular sparing The presence of a small region of intact vision near the center of a visual field in which a person is otherwise blind. Macular sparing is common when visual field blindness is caused by destruction of the visual cortex in one brain hemisphere.

Magnetic resonance imaging (MRI scanning) A laboratory test that uses a strong magnetic field and a computer to create images of internal structures based on differences in the chemical composition of body tissues.

Manometer An instrument for measuring breath pressure.

Masked facies Rigidity of facial muscles, causing fixed, unchanging facial expression. A prominent characteristic of Parkinson's disease.

Median apertures Two openings from the fourth ventricle into the subarachnoid space, sometimes called the *foramina of Magendie.*

Mediation Elicitation of one response by another (usually internal) response—for example, saying the names of letters to oneself while writing complex words.

Medulla The bottom third of the brain stem. Contains five cranial nerve nuclei, plus some centers concerned with hearing and balance. Pyramidal tract fibers *decussate* (cross the midline) here.

Melodic intonation therapy (MIT) A treatment procedure for patients with severe speech production impairments in which melody and exaggerated intonation are used to facilitate speech.

Memory, declarative What we know about things (names, faces, places, situations, and so on).

Memory, episodic Memory for personally experienced events.

Memory, long term (Sometimes called *secondary memory.*) The third stage in some models of memory. It has large (perhaps infinite) capacity, and information in it decays slowly if at all. Considered a repository for our knowledge and sense of self.

Memory, procedural What we know about how to do things (make coffee, paint a window, and so on).

Memory, prospective The ability to remember to do things at certain points in time (remembering to remember).

Memory, retrospective Memory for past experiences and for knowledge acquired in the past.

Memory, semantic Stored general knowledge.

Memory, sensory (Sometimes called *sensory register.*) The first stage in some models of memory, in which the traces of stimuli are briefly stored. The traces decay quickly and cannot be maintained by rehearsal.

Memory, short-term (Sometimes called *primary memory.*) The second stage in some models of memory, in which information can be maintained by rehearsal. Without rehearsal, information decays within a few minutes. Short-term memory has limited capacity. Only a few items of information can be stored there at one time.

Memory, working A mental space in which the processing of information coming from short-term memory or retrieved from long-term memory takes place.

Memory loss, posttraumatic Loss of memory for a period of time following brain injury. (Sometimes called *anterograde amnesia.*)

Memory loss, pretraumatic Loss of memory for events immediately preceding brain injury. (Sometimes called *retrograde amnesia.*)

Meninges The membranes between the skull and the brain. The toughest one lines the skull and is called the *dura mater.* (Think of DURable. Also, remember that if protection is the key, it makes sense that nature would put the toughest one on the outside.) The weblike one is the *arachnoid* (think spider). The one on the surface of the brain is the *pia mater.* To keep them in order, think *PAD* (for pia, arachnoid, dura).

Meningioma A tumor in the meninges.

Mesencephalon (midbrain) A deep brain region that makes up the upper third of the brain stem. Contains several nuclei, including those for the cranial nerves that move the eyes.

Metastasis The process by which a tumor appears at a secondary site from the location of the original tumor.

Monoplegia Paralysis of one limb.

Motor cortex A strip of brain cortex just ahead of the central fissure. It is responsible for initiating most volitional motor activity.

Myasthenia gravis A neurologic disease caused by damage to the acetylcholine receptors on muscle cells. Characterized by abnormally rapid muscle fatigue with use.

Myelin Fatty material surrounding the axons of neurons.

Myelogram A laboratory procedure that permits visualization of the spinal cord. Contrast medium is injected into the subarachnoid space around the spinal cord and a series of x-ray exposures is made to visualize the structure of the spinal cord and surrounding tissues.

Myelopathy Pathology affecting the spinal cord.

Myoclonus Fine, rapid, irregular twitching movements caused by contractions of groups of muscle fibers. Usually observable as dimpling or rippling of the skin over the muscle fibers.

Myopathy Disease of muscle.

Myositis Inflammation of muscle.

Necrosis Death of tissue.

Neglect Inattention to some part of surrounding space. Most often seen as inattention to one-half of surrounding space *(hemispatial neglect)*. A common consequence of nondominant-hemisphere pathology.

Neologisms Nonword utterances (e.g., "*mandernost*") that follow the phonologic conventions of the language. Neologisms often are heard in the speech of adults with severe Wernicke's aphasia or global aphasia.

Neuralgia Pain caused by inflammation of a nerve.

Neuritic plaques Neuronal abnormalities seen in Alzheimer's disease, other neurologic diseases, and in some normal elderly. Neuritic plaques are small areas of nerve cell degeneration, primarily occurring in cortical and subcortical brain regions.

Neurofibrillary tangles Neuronal abnormalities seen in Alzheimer's disease, other neurologic diseases, and in some normal elderly. Neurofibrillary tangles are filamentous bodies seen in the nerve cell body, dendrites, axon, and sometimes in synaptic endings.

Neuron A nerve cell.

Neurotransmitter Any of several chemical compounds that are involved in the transmission of nerve impulses between nerve cells.

Nonacceleration injury Brain injury caused when the stationary head is struck by a moving object.

Norms Any of several statistics that summarize the test performance of a sample of individuals representing a population to which the norms apply. Sample means and standard deviations are the minimum normative statistics needed to relate the performance of an individual to a norm group.

Nucleus A group of neurons in the brain or spinal cord that are differentiated from surrounding tissue by cell type or by surrounding zones of nerve fibers.

Nystagmus Rhythmic oscillation of the eyes, sometimes caused by weakness in the muscles that move the eyes and sometimes caused by disturbances of balance and equilibrium.

Occipital lobes The rearmost portions of the brain hemispheres. The visual cortex is located in the occipital lobes.

Olfactory cortex A region of the cortex on the inferior surface of each frontal lobe. It has principal responsibility for the sense of smell.

Operculum The patch of brain cortex surrounding the insula.

Ophthalmoplegia Paralysis of muscles responsible for eye movements.

Optic chiasm The point at which the crossing fibers in the human visual system cross. It is located at the base of the brain near the pituitary gland.

Orientation Awareness of one's surroundings. Orientation is customarily subdivided into orientation for *person, place,* and *time.*

Outcome The long-term (final) result of treatment.

Palilalia Involuntary repetition of words and sentences.

Palmar reflex Sometimes called the *grasp reflex.* A pathologic reflex elicited by stroking the palm of the hand. The hand closes involuntarily, and the fingers grasp the object used to stroke the palm.

Palsy Another word for *paralysis.*

Papilledema Swelling of the optic disk in the back of the eye, suggesting increased intracranial pressure, inflammation of the optic disk, or ischemia of the optic disk.

Paraphasia Errors in speaking made by aphasic persons. *Literal (phonemic) paraphasias* are errors in which a speaker substitutes one sound in a word for another, such as saying *spomb* for *comb. Verbal (semantic) paraphasias* are errors in which a speaker substitutes one word for another, such as saying *cup* for *glass.*

Paraplegia Paralysis of both legs.

Paresis Muscle weakness.

Paresthesia Abnormal sensations (such as tingling, burning) in the absence of stimulation.

Parietal lobes The part of the brain hemispheres behind the central fissure and above the lateral fissure. The parietal cortex is important for somesthetic sensation (skin, muscle, joint, and tendon sensation).

Parkinson's disease A degenerative disease affecting neurons in the midbrain and brain stem.

Participation limitation The effect of an impairment on a person's participation in activities of daily life. (See also *impairment, disability, handicap.*)

Passage dependency The degree to which answering questions that test comprehension of discourse depends on having read or heard the discourse.

Patellar reflex A normal reflex elicited by tapping the patellar tendon just below the kneecap. The lower leg jerks upward when the patellar tendon is tapped. Diminished patellar reflexes may be a sign of peripheral nerve damage or muscle weakness; exaggerated patellar reflexes may be a sign of upper motor neuron damage.

Percentile A score that represents the percent of individuals in a norm group that fall above or below the score. For example, a score that places an individual at the 95th percentile means that 94% of the norm group received lower scores.

Perimetry A procedure for testing vision in all quadrants of the visual fields with a specialized instrument called a *perimeter.*

Peripheral nervous system (PNS) Consists of the cranial nerves and spinal nerves. The peripheral nervous system is sometimes called the *lower motor neuron.*

Perseveration Repetition of a response when it is no longer appropriate, as when a patient calls a comb a *comb* but continues to call subsequent objects *comb.*

Persistent vegetative state A condition in which the individual has sleep-wake cycles but makes no purposeful responses to the environment.

Pharyngeal flap A surgical procedure for alleviating hypernasality.

Phonetic contrast Drills in which a patient produces a series of sounds, syllables, or words that systematically change by a single articulatory feature.

Phonetic derivation A treatment procedure in which a new speech sound is obtained by modifying a sound the patient can produce.

Phonetic dissolution Distortion of speech sounds caused by articulatory breakdown. Sometimes resembles literal paraphasia, but literal paraphasia typically is characterized by substitution of one correctly articulated sound for another, whereas phonetic dissolution is characterized by distortions of sounds.

Phonetic placement A treatment procedure in which drawings, models, or physical positioning are used to help a patient place the articulators in position for making a sound.

Phrenology A nineteenth century pseudoscience in which personal attributes were said to be related to head shape and contours.

Pick's disease (frontal lobe dementia) A progressive degenerative disease affecting the brain cortex. It is characterized by the presence of *Pick bodies* (dense globular formations within nerve cells) and *enlarged neurons* in the brain. Pick's disease is an important cause of cortical dementia.

Plantar reflex Sometimes called the *plantar extensor* or *Babinski reflex*. A pathologic reflex elicited by forcefully stroking the sole of the foot, causing the toes to bend upward and fan out. The *plantar flexor* reflex, in which the toes bend downward and do not fan, is the normal response to this stimulation.

Plaque (arteriosclerotic plaque, atherosclerotic plaque) Fatty deposits on the inner walls of arteries.

-plegia A suffix denoting *paralysis.*

Pons The middle third of the brain stem. Contains three cranial nerve nuclei plus some nuclei concerned with balance and hearing.

Positron emission tomography (PET) A laboratory procedure in which the metabolic activity of the brain is measured by introducing a metabolically active compound (usually glucose) tagged with a mildly radioactive element and measuring the regions in which the compound concentrates.

Posterior horn cells Spinal sensory nerves, located in the posterolateral part of the spinal cord.

Posttraumatic memory loss See *memory loss, posttraumatic.*

Pragmatics Language in use.

Premotor cortex A strip of brain cortex in the posterior frontal lobes said to be important for planning volitional movements.

Press of speech (logorrhea) Excessive verbosity. Patients with mild to moderate Wernicke's or conduction aphasia are likely to exhibit press of speech.

Pretraumatic memory loss See *memory loss, pretraumatic.*

Progressive approximation A treatment procedure in which a new response is created by stepwise modification of an existing response.

Progressive supranuclear palsy (PSP) A progressive disease characterized by degeneration of brain stem neurons, causing increasingly severe motor impairments, especially in muscles served by cranial nerves.

Projection fibers Nerve fiber tracts that connect the brain, brain stem, and spinal cord. They can be either motor (efferent) or sensory (afferent).

Proprioception The ability to tell the position of the head and limbs without seeing them.

Prosody The melodic characteristics of speech—rate, intonation, and stress patterns.

Prosopagnosia Inability to recognize faces.

Prospective research Research in which the design is established prior to subject intake, and subject intake and experimental procedures are defined in advance.

Proximal Near the trunk.

Pseudobulbar affect Exaggerated emotional responses to minimally emotional stimuli. Often an early (but usually transitory) consequence of brain damage.

Pseudodementia Presence of behavioral and cognitive signs (cognitive impairment, loss of appetite, difficulty sleeping, social withdrawal, apathy) that are signs of dementia but are caused by depression, illness, or other nondementing conditions.

Pure word deafness An auditory impairment in which the individual loses the ability to comprehend spoken verbal materials despite intact hearing but retains the ability to recognize nonverbal auditory stimuli.

Pyramidal system The neural system that is responsible for initiating most volitional movement. It is made up of the motor neurons in the motor cortex together with projection fibers that connect the motor cortex to the brain stem and spinal cord. It is sometimes called the *upper motor neuron.*

Quadrantanopsia Blindness in less than half of the visual field in each eye. (See also *hemianopsia.*)

Quadriplegia Paralysis of both arms and both legs.

Quality of life A concept denoting a person's access to and successful participation in personally relevant activities of daily living, plus the person's personal well-being and satisfaction with his or her conditions of daily living.

Reduplicative paramnesia The belief that two or more identical persons, places, or things exist in different locations. An occasional consequence of right-hemisphere brain damage.

Reflex A spontaneous and uncontrollable movement in response to stimulation. The two major categories of reflexes are *superficial reflexes,* which are elicited by touching, stroking, or brushing the surface of body parts, and *deep reflexes,* which are elicited by tapping or suddenly stretching muscles or tendons. (See also *gag reflex, swallow reflex, plantar reflex, palmar reflex, sucking reflex, patellar reflex.*)

Regional cerebral blood flow (rCBF) A laboratory procedure for measuring blood flow by introducing mildly radioactive substances into the bloodstream and analyzing their concentration by means of sensitive detectors and a computer.

Reinforcement *Positive reinforcement* is delivering positive consequences following desired behaviors in order to increase their frequency. *Negative reinforcement* is removing negative consequences following desired behaviors in order to increase their frequency.

Resource allocation A model of cognitive processing in which mental operations depend on allocation of processing resources from a limited-capacity pool. Performance deteriorates if the demands for processing resources exceed the capacity of the pool.

Responsive naming Providing names in response to questions such as *"What do you drink coffee from?"* or requests such as *"Tell me what you use for digging a hole."*

Retention span The amount of information that can be held in primary memory at one time (from four to ten items for most normal adults).

Reticular formation Structures in the central core of the brain stem that regulate the individual's overall level of consciousness.

Retrospective research Research in which information about subjects is gathered from preexisting records.

Rigidity Resistance of muscles to movement in any direction. A prominent characteristic of Parkinson's disease.

Scanning speech The slow, regular, and monotonous speech of persons with cerebellar ataxia.

Scripts (Sometimes called *schemata.*) Mental representations of familiar daily life routines or situations, such as eating in a restaurant, going to a party, or shopping for groceries.

Sedimentation rate The rate at which blood cells sink in a liquid. Sedimentation rate is an indicator of clotting potential.

Seizure Episodes of disturbed consciousness caused by abnormal patterns of neuronal discharge in the brain. In *generalized seizures (convulsions, tonic-clonic seizures, grand mal seizures),* the patient loses consciousness, with spasmodic contractions of most muscle groups. In *partial seizures (focal seizures),* the patient does not lose consciousness, and only some muscle groups are affected by spasmodic contractions. In *absence seizures (petit mal seizures),* the patient does not lose consciousness and does not experience spasmodic muscle contractions but does not respond purposefully to stimulation.

Sequential modification Generalization training in which stimulus conditions, response requirements, and reinforcement contingencies are gradually changed to resemble a target environment, to increase generalization from the training environment to the target environment.

Sign An objective indicator of illness or disease observed by an examiner (See *symptom.*)

Slowly progressive aphasia Gradual development of language impairment over months to years without concomitant impairment of memory and cognition. Impaired memory and cognition often develop months to years after the first signs of language impairment.

Social validation A procedure for evaluating the clinical significance of changes created by a treatment program, in which the effects of treatment on an individual's daily life performance are evaluated.

Somatosensory cortex A strip of brain cortex just behind the central fissure. It is responsible for skin, muscle, joint, and tendon sensation.

Somesthetic sensation Sensation from the skin, muscles, joints, and tendons.

Spastic catch A sudden increase in muscle tension when spastic muscles are quickly stretched by the examiner.

Spasticity Abnormally high levels of tension in resting muscles caused by upper motor neuron damage.

Spinal nerves Peripheral nerves that supply muscles and sensory receptors in the trunk and limbs. Motor nerves have their cell bodies in the anterolateral part of the spinal cord (anterior horn cells), and sensory nerves have their cell bodies in the posterolateral part (posterior horn cells).

Stenosis Narrowing, as of an artery.

Steppage gait A characteristic gait of patients with paralysis of muscles in the front of the lower leg, causing the foot to hang down as the patient walks. The patient lifts the legs abnormally high so that the toes will clear the ground.

Stereognosis The ability to identify objects by touch.

Stereotypies, verbal Repetitive, noncommunicative utterances made by brain-injured patients (*me-me-me, wuna-wuna-wuna,* and the like). Often one indicator of severe aphasia.

Stridor Audible inhalation.

Stroke Temporary or permanent disruption of brain function due to interruption of its blood supply. Sometimes called *cerebrovascular accident (CVA)* or *brain attack.*

Subarachnoid Between the arachnoid and the pia mater.

Subclavian arteries Two large arteries branching off from the aorta. The vertebral arteries originate at the subclavian arteries.

Subcortical aphasia Aphasia that apparently is caused by damage in and around the basal ganglia. We do not know if the damaged subcortical regions directly participate in language, or if subcortical aphasia is caused by interfering with the function of other language-competent brain regions.

Subdural Between the dura mater and the arachnoid.

Sucking reflex A pathologic reflex elicited by touching or stroking on or near the lips, causing the lips to make involuntary sucking movements.

Sulcus A "valley" on the surface of the brain. (Plural = sulci.) See also *fissure.*

Swallow reflex Swallowing when the posterior tongue or pharyngeal walls are touched.

Symptom Indicators of illness or disease experienced by the patient. (See *sign.*)

Synapse The point at which an axon of one nerve cell meets the dendrite of another, where transmission of nerve impulses takes place by means of chemicals called neurotransmitters.

Syncope Fainting.

Telegraphic speech Speech in which function words are left out. (See *agrammatism.*)

Temporal lobes Make up approximately the bottom third of each hemisphere, beneath the lateral cerebral fissure. The left temporal lobe plays an important role in language and audition.

Tentorium cerebelli A rigid sheet of dura that separates the cerebellum from the base of the brain. It is often called the *tentorium* for efficiency. Neurologists sometimes use the terms *supratentorial* and *subtentorial* to describe vertical locations in the cranial vault.

Testing the limits Deviating from standard test procedures to determine the underlying reasons for a patient's deficient performance on a test.

Thalamus A pair of egg-shaped nuclei in the diencephalon. They are important for integration of sensory information, for regulating motor behavior, and they may regulate the overall activity of the cortex.

Theory of mind The ability to appreciate others' state of knowledge.

Thrombosis Accumulation of a plug of material at a specific site in a blood vessel. If it grows large enough to occlude a cerebral artery, it causes a thrombotic stroke.

Tic douloureux Shooting, lancelike pains associated with inflammation of the trigeminal nerve *(trigeminal neuralgia).*

Tics Stereotypic repetitive movements such as blinking, coughing, or sniffing. Tics usually are not related to nervous system pathology.

Tongue-anchor test Protruding the tongue through closed lips while pushing out the cheeks with impounded air.

Topographic impairment (topological disorientation) A state of confusion regarding surrounding space and how one relates to it. A frequent consequence of right-hemisphere brain damage.

Torsion spasm See *dystonia.*

Toxemia Inflammation or poisoning of brain tissue by foreign substances.

Transcortical aphasia—mixed An aphasia syndrome characterized by profound comprehension impairment, little or no functional language, but good repetition.

Transcortical motor aphasia (anterior isolation syndrome) An aphasia syndrome characterized by good comprehension, sparse speech output, and good repetition.

Transcortical sensory aphasia (posterior isolation syndrome) An aphasia syndrome characterized by poor comprehension, fluent but echolalic speech, and good repetition.

Transcranial Doppler ultrasound A laboratory test in which sound waves are transmitted into the head and a computer measures blood pressure and flow by analyzing changes in the frequency of the reflected sound waves.

Transient ischemic attack (TIA) A temporary disruption of cerebral circulation that causes a transient disturbance of motor, sensory, or mental functions.

Translational trauma Brain damage caused by acceleration of the head by outside forces.

Tremor Cyclic, small amplitude involuntary movements, usually more severe in *distal* (away from the trunk) muscles than in *proximal* (near the trunk) muscles.

Trigeminal neuralgia See *tic douloureux.*

Trismus Excessive and uncontrollable contraction of the muscles of mastication.

Upper motor neuron Another name for the pyramidal system.

Validity The degree to which a test actually measures what it purports to measure. *Content validity* is an indicator of how well the items in a test represent the domain of concern. *Construct validity* is an indicator of how well the content of a test relates to an established model, theory, or concept of the skill, process, or structure to which the test relates.

Vasospasm Constriction of arteries by contraction of muscles in the arterial wall.

Ventricles (cerebral ventricles) Fluid-filled cavities within the brain. There are four of them—two *lateral ventricles*, a *third ventricle*, and a *fourth ventricle.*

Verbal apraxia (apraxia of speech) Disruption of the motor plans for speech articulation. Verbal apraxia often accompanies Broca's aphasia. (See also *apraxia.*)

Vertebrae Bony plates surrounding the spinal cord. From top to bottom they are classified into *cervical, thoracic, lumbar,* and *sacral* divisions.

Vertebral arteries Two arteries that begin at the subclavian arteries and progress upward on the front side of the medulla. They supply blood to the medulla and, via the basilar artery, to the posterior part of the circle of Willis.

Vestibular-reticular system A diffuse neural system. It is responsible for balance and orientation of the body in space and for general states of attention and alertness.

Visual cortex A region of the cortex in each occipital lobe. It has principal responsibility for visual perception.

Wernicke's aphasia An aphasia syndrome characterized by fluent but empty speech, poor comprehension, and poor repetition.

Wernicke's area A region of the cortex in the vicinity of the temporo-parietal-occipital junction. Damage in Wernicke's areas is said to cause *Wernicke's aphasia.*

Wernicke's encephalopathy A neurologic disease caused by thiamine deficiency and usually associated with alcoholism.

White matter Nervous system tissues made up primarily of nerve axons. It is white because of the presence of *myelin.*

Word fluency See *generative naming.*

Responses to Thought Questions

## CHAPTER 1

Response to Question 1-1 Mrs. Redmond's impairments are likely to be less severe than those of Mr. Johnson.

- She is younger. Her arterial system is likely to be in better health than that of Mr. Johnson, and her nervous system is likely to be physiologically more resilient than that of Mr. Johnson.
- Her stroke was in the watershed region of the left hemisphere. Collateral supply of blood from the posterior cerebral artery may provide an alternative to the blood previously supplied by the middle cerebral artery.
- The arteries in the watershed region are small in diameter and serve small cortical areas compared with arteries in the more central regions of the hemisphere. Consequently, the volume of brain tissue affected by Mrs. Redmond's stroke is likely to be less than the volume of brain tissue affected by Mr. Johnson's stroke.

Mrs. Redmond should experience greater neurologic recovery than Mr. Johnson, and her recovery should progress at a faster rate than that of Mr. Johnson, for the reasons enumerated above, which speak to the rate of recovery from nervous system injury as well as to the initial severity of symptoms.

Response to Question 1-2 This is a classic scenario for cerebral hemorrhage. Cerebral hemorrhages tend to occur in hypertensive patients and often occur during periods of exertion, which causes blood pressure to increase, puts pressure on arterial walls, and adds to the risk of bleeding. The delayed onset of Mr. Carillo's symptoms also is consistent with cerebral hemorrhage. Symptoms of hemorrhage often develop slowly, appearing only after enough bleeding has occurred to increase intracranial pressure (unless the hemorrhage is a massive one, in which severe headache and coma occur quickly).

Response to Question 1-3 These patients complain of leg weakness and loss of sensation because the primary motor cortex for the leg (located high on the convexity of the primary motor cortex) and the primary sensory cortex for the leg (high on the primary somatosensory cortex) are pressed against the falx cerebri. The pressure causes the patient's symptoms. The patient's symptoms will affect the leg contralateral to the side on which the motor and sensory cortices are being pressed against the falx cerebri. This usually suggests a mass lesion (tumor, abscess, etc.) in the brain hemisphere contralateral to the side of the patient's symptoms. The mass lesion presses against brain tissue, squeezing it against the inner surface of the skull and displacing brain tissue from regions of high pressure to regions of low pressure—in this case across the falx cerebri into the other side of the cranial vault.

Response to Question 1-4 Harry's symptoms—excruciating pain caused by stimulation of nerves in the face—suggest trigeminal neuralgia *(tic douloureux). Tic douloureux* is characterized by momentary episodes of intense, excruciating pain following sensory stimulation of receptors in the cheek, nose, or mouth with heat, cold, touch, or movement. The intensity and sudden appearance of Harry's symptoms suggest inflammation of the maxillary branch of the trigeminal nerve. Harry saw a neurologist, who concluded that Harry's symptoms were related to trigeminal neuralgia and prescribed an antiinflammatory medication. Harry's symptoms resolved the day after he began taking the medication. Harry also transferred his dental care to Dr. Luck.

Response to Question 1-5 Those who discovered and publicized this phenomenon attribute it to differences in traffic patterns between the United States and England. In the United States, vehicle drivers sit on the left side of the vehicle. If they drive with the window open, outside air blows across the left side of the face. In England, vehicle drivers sit on the right side of the vehicle, and air from an open window blows across the right side of the face. It is known that exposure to cold sometimes leads to inflammation of the facial nerve, causing it to swell. Combining this information leads to the conclusion that the difference in laterality between the two countries is related to driving habits. (If this hypothesis is true, then one would expect that northern regions of the two countries should show a greater disparity in laterality than warmer regions if the culprit is indeed cold air, but as far as I can determine, no one has addressed this possibility.)

CHAPTER 2

Response to Question 2-1 The events described here represent a typical scenario in which a patient seen in the first few hours after a stroke presents a somewhat confusing picture in terms of the probable location, extent, and (sometimes) etiology of the patient's neurologic signs and reported symptoms. The probability is high that this patient has had a stroke in the left hemisphere, probably embolic (because of his history of heart disease). The finding of mild hemiparesis and Wernicke's aphasia are somewhat inconsistent, because one ordinarily wouldn't expect a patient with Wernicke's aphasia (and temporal lobe injury) to be hemi-

paretic. It is important to remember that stroke patients seen in the first few hours (and sometimes days) after stroke may exhibit signs that do not point to the location of the stroke, and sometimes may not accurately indicate its nature (occlusion vs. hemorrhage, thrombus vs. embolus). Also remember that one often sees signs that are caused by the generalized immediate consequences of brain injury—swelling, neurotransmitter release, diaschisis—that may confuse one's attempts at localization in the first few days after onset. The co-occurrence of hemiparesis (usually mild) and Wernicke's aphasia is fairly common in the first few hours or days after injury.

One might be tempted to hypothesize that this man's neurologic signs either (a) require two lesions (one in the temporal lobe and one near the motor cortex) or (b) require a large lesion that extends to the motor cortex. There is a problem with each of these hypotheses. It would be unusual for two strokes to occur close enough in time to create the two lesions suggested by (a), and a preexisting "silent" stroke is unlikely because a stroke either in Wernicke's area or the motor cortex would cause symptoms that would send the patient to his physician. The problem with (b) is that the massive lesion envisioned would generate severe impairments (global aphasia) rather than the relatively mild symptoms exhibited by this patient.

There is a more troublesome inconsistency in this report. One would not expect left hemianopia to occur along with the other signs, all of which point to damage in the left hemisphere. I can think of two possible explanations. (1) The neurologist made a mistake, and it was really a right hemianopia (these things do happen!). (2) The hemianopia was the result of an old "silent" lesion in the right hemisphere.

Note that the patient's arm was weaker than his leg. This points to damage low in the hemisphere. If the leg were weaker than the arm, one would suspect damage high in the hemisphere. Can you see why?

Response to Question 2-2 This patient apparently understands the task—he repeats three "words" according to instructions, but the "words" are not real words. That means that a test of memory for words cannot depend on the patient's saying the words. I would see if I could circumvent the patient's output problem by giving him an alternative way of responding. I'd try the test again, but instead of asking the patient to say the words back to me, I would ask him to choose the words I said from an array of printed words. If that worked, I would give him three new words to remember and would subsequently test his memory for the words by asking him to choose them from an array of printed words.

If the patient could not choose the words I said from an array of printed words, I would ask him to choose them from an array of pictures containing pictures of the test words plus several additional pictures. If that worked, I would give him three new words to remember and would subsequently test his memory for the words by asking him to choose pictures representing the words from an array of pictures.

If the patient could neither choose words I said from an array of printed words or from an array of pictures (a word recognition/comprehension impairment), I might try to circumvent the patient's comprehension impairment by showing him drawings of the three stimulus items, asking him to remember them, and subsequently test him with an array of pictures.

Response to Question 2-3 That the patient's symptoms are localized to one side of the body (*hemianesthesia*) suggests central nervous system pathology. The sudden onset of symptoms and their presence on awakening suggest an acute event such as stroke as the cause of the symptoms. However, the absence of other signs of central nervous system pathology (e.g., motor impairments, speech, language, or cognitive impairments, visuospatial impairments) makes a central nervous system etiology implausible. If a central nervous system source for the

patient's symptoms is eliminated, then pathology affecting the peripheral nervous system becomes a candidate. However, peripheral neuropathy rarely, if ever, creates symptoms that affect all of one side of the body, leaving the other side asymptomatic. A typical pattern for peripheral neuropathy is for symptoms to appear distally (in hands and feet) and progress proximally (toward the trunk), because the longest fibers tend to be the first ones affected by peripheral neuropathy. Most peripheral neuropathies develop slowly, over days and weeks, rather than abruptly, as in this case. Finally, the patient's failure to report vibration when bony structures near the midline, but on the left, seems unusual, because if sensitivity to vibration on the right side were intact, the patient should sense vibratory stimulation on the left side of the midline via bone conduction to sensory receptors on the right side. This patient's symptoms do not match patterns that would be expected based on the structure of the nervous system. The probability that their source is functional rather than organic seems high.

Response to Question 2-4 Patients with loss of sensation and position sense and patients with vestibular abnormalities typically are more stable when standing with eyes open than when standing with eyes closed because they use visual information to compensate for the lack of positional information from the legs or the vestibular system. When these patients close their eyes they lose this compensatory information, and their unsteadiness increases, usually dramatically (a phenomenon called *Romberg's sign*). Patients with cerebellar ataxia are as unsteady with eyes open as with eyes closed, because their unsteadiness arises from inability to maintain constant levels of muscle tension and inability to quickly adjust muscle tension to subtle changes in posture—impairments that are not alleviated by the presence of visual feedback.

Response to Question 2-5 The symptoms reported by the patient and his wife suggest a pathologic condition affecting the patient's frontal lobes. The patient's complaint of a frontal headache suggests irritation or inflammation of the frontal meninges or the frontal lobe. The patient's report of a change in visual acuity suggests involvement of optic fibers passing beneath the frontal lobe. The wife's description of impulsivity, distractibility, and social inappropriateness are consistent with dysfunction of the frontal lobes. The neurologic examination also points to frontal lobe dysfunction. The patient's loss of visual acuity in his left eye together with abnormal pallor of the left optic disc suggest a pathologic condition in or beneath the left frontal lobe that compromises the left optic nerve. The patient's loss of olfaction on the left also suggests an inferior left frontal lobe location. Weakness in muscles of the right-side lower face and exaggerated tendon reflexes on the right suggest involvement of the left motor cortex or descending motor pathways.

The neurologist concluded that the findings were consistent with a space-occupying lesion at the base of the left frontal lobe—probably a tumor pressing on the left optic nerve and the left olfactory nerve, with swelling causing pressure on the left motor cortex or on descending pyramidal tract fibers. Laboratory tests confirmed the presence of a meningioma at the base of the patient's left frontal lobe. Surgical removal of the meningioma resulted in gradual resolution of the patient's neurologic signs and reported symptoms, except for the patient's diminished visual acuity in his left eye, which improved but did not return to its premorbid level.

CHAPTER 3

Response to Question 3-1 *What I would do next*. I would say, *"I'm pleased to meet you, Mrs. Olson. I'll come back another time and we can talk again"* or something to that effect, and leave. I would see little to be gained by more attempts to get her to respond. I would talk with the patient's nurse to find out if this is a typical behavior pattern and to find out if there are times of the day in which Mrs. Olson is more alert and responsive. When her medical record becomes available I would review it. I would look in progress notes for evidence of her alertness, responsiveness, and orientation; I would read the physician's report of her medical history, signs, and symptoms, and I would look through the doctor's orders to see if Mrs. Olson is on any medications that might explain her lethargy and somnolence.

I would put a note such as the following in the Progress Notes: *I saw Mrs. Olson at bedside this day. She opened her eyes and attended when touched but did not respond to my verbal requests. Assessment of speech, language, and cognition awaits her improved alertness and responsiveness. I will see her at bedside daily to monitor her progress and will schedule more extensive testing when her alertness and responsiveness permit.* I would cross-reference it with an entry in the Doctors Orders, such as: *See speech pathology preliminary report in Progress Notes.*

Potential reasons for Mrs. Olson's unresponsiveness: (1) Mrs. Olson is only one day into recovery from a probable right-hemisphere stroke. She may be experiencing general effects of brain injury (brain swelling, reduction in cerebral blood flow, diaschisis, etc.) that diminish her responsiveness and alertness. Such general effects often are present in the first few days following moderate to severe brain injury from strokes. (2) Mrs. Olson may be depressed. Sometimes patients are so traumatized by their personal catastrophe that they withdraw behaviorally and emotionally. (3) Mrs. Olson may be receiving medications that depress her level of responsiveness and alertness (not likely, because physicians do not routinely prescribe sedative or tranquilizing drugs for patients who are in the early postonset phase of stroke recovery).

Response to Question 3-2 The only situation in which a brain-injured adults' performance (or anyone else's) on a small number of test items is likely to be as accurate as their performance on a large number is when a patient's responses are extremely homogeneous, such as when all responses are correct or when all responses are errors. When responses are extremely homogeneous the results of testing will be equivalent, regardless of the number of items in the test. As performance becomes less homogeneous, the accuracy with which a small number of test items represents the brain-injured adult's true performance level usually declines.

An exception might be when a patient's performance is very symmetric across time. What symmetry means in this context is that a patient who misses 20% of test items always misses every fifth item, and a patient who misses 50% of test items always misses every second item. Under these conditions, one would need five items in a test to specify the true performance of a patient who misses 20% of test items, and would need only two items to specify the true performance of a patient who misses 50% of test items. (But one would have to know, somehow, that the patient's performance is symmetric, which ordinarily would require sampling performance across a fairly large number of items.)

Brain-injured adults' performance is never this orderly. For most, performance fluctuates unpredictably across test items. A patient who misses 25% of test items may miss the first two, get the next eight right, miss one, get seven right, miss two, and so on. For this reason, brain-injured adults' performance rarely matches their overall error percentage in any small block of items (five or fewer) and may only approximate their true performance level across large blocks of items (20 or 30).

Some brain-injured adults have difficulty "tuning in" to new tasks in a test situation. Their responses to initial test items are inaccurate, delayed, and/or distorted but improve as the test continues, provided that the characteristics of test stimuli and the response requirements do not change. If brain-injured adults with "tuning in" problems are tested with only a few items, their performance is worse than it would be if more items were administered. Someone who

did not get tuned in until the sixth item would produce only error scores if tested with a 5-item test, but would get 50% correct if tested with a 10-item test. (Presumably the last five items would all be correct. In practice, there usually is more gradual improvement in performance from initial test items to later ones.)

Other brain-injured adults seem to develop "noise buildup" or "fatigue" across test items. Their responses to initial test items are prompt and accurate, but as the test progresses their performance deteriorates. These persons' performance looks better on a short test than on a long one, because the test ends before the noise buildup or fatigue sets in.

It is important to understand that when a brain-injured adult's test performance is affected by processing abnormalities such as tuning in problems or noise buildup, the test may not be a valid measure of what the test is designed to measure. Suppose a clinician were to administer a 20-item written spelling test to a brain-injured patient with a tuning-in problem. (The words in the test are approximately equal in frequency of occurrence and spelling difficulty.) The patient misses the first 4 items, gets the next item correct, misses the next 2, and gets the remaining 13 correct. The patient's overall score is 70% correct. Has the clinician tested the patient's knowledge of how to spell the tested words? Probably not, because the patient's performance looks suspiciously like a tuning-in problem. The clinician could test this hypothesis by retesting with the same words in inverted order, putting the first words last and the last words first. If a tuning-in problem were responsible for the patient's performance, the patient will miss items that he previously spelled correctly and will spell correctly items that he previously missed.

The point is that brain-injured adults' test performance often represents some combination of impaired component skills and information-processing abnormalities, behavioral tendencies, or both. It is important to separate these influences to ensure that a brain-injured adult's test performance represents the person's competence in the skill targeted by the test (e.g., spelling, arithmetic, sentence comprehension) and not the character of the brain-injured adult's information processing or behavioral tendencies. (Lezak's comments on *testing the limits* in this chapter relate to this issue.)

Response to Question 3-3 The test contains 10 items, which ordinarily would be sufficient for a screening test, provided the items were homogeneous. Unfortunately for potential users of this test, these items are not homogeneous. Frequency of occurrence differs widely across test items, from *the* (frequency approximately 1 per 15 words) to *perambulator* (frequency less than 1 per million words). Parts of speech also differs across test items. There are three nouns, two pronouns, one verb, two adjectives, one adverb, and one article in the test. Phonologic complexity also differs across test items, from multisyllabic phonologically complex words (*perambulator, umbrella, seventy-two*) to single-syllable words. The level of abstractness also differs across test items, from concrete, visualizable words (*cat, umbrella*) to abstract nonvisualizable words (*its, slowly*). Each of these variables has been shown to affect brain-injured adults' performance in various language tests. Consequently, heterogeneity among test items on these variables is likely to lead to differences in performance among patients who are sensitive to different variables. Patients with phonologic encoding problems or speech motor programming problems will miss phonologically complex items. Patients who are sensitive to word frequency effects will miss low-frequency items. Patients who have problems with "little words" in English will miss articles and perhaps pronouns and adverbs. Patients who have difficulty with abstract material will miss abstract words.

Response to Question 3-4 Mr. Chambers appears an impulsive responder. He interrupts the clinician and unnecessarily repeats what the clinician says. His inappropriate verbalizations disrupt the flow of the session and may compro-

mise Mr. Chambers's performance in the task—he talks when he should be listening, and so is likely to misunderstand, misinterpret or flatout miss what the clinician says.

Some potential reasons for Mr. Chambers's behavior: (1) He is anxious and threatened by the test situation. He reacts by verbalizing excessively. (2) He is trying to compensate for impaired comprehension and retention by "jumping the gun" when he feels that he's losing the sense of what the clinician is saying. (3) His impulsive responding is caused by his brain injury. (4) He was an impulsive responder before his injury, and what we see here is simply a continuation (or exaggeration) of his pre-injury personality. (5) Some combination of (1) through (4).

What to do next? I'd try telling Mr. Chambers, *"Wait until I'm finished before you say anything,"* reminding him if necessary as the session progressed. If that didn't work, I'd interject a nonverbal cue to indicate when he should respond—hold up my hand, palm out as I give an instruction or command, and point to him when it's time for him to respond. If that didn't work, I'd end the task, engage Mr. Chambers in a short interval of social conversation to get him relaxed and settled, then try the task again, incorporating gestural cues to signal him when to respond. If that didn't work, I'd switch to a task that I knew would be very easy for him and use that task to train him to respond at appropriate times and without excessive verbalization. When I had an appropriate response pattern firmly established, I'd go back to the original task, expecting that the new response pattern would generalize to that task.

CHAPTER 4

Response to Question 4-1 The pattern of responses does not match the typical pattern of responses in retention span tests. In the typical pattern of responses, items early in the list and items late in the list are remembered better than items in the middle (phenomena called the *primacy effect* and the *recency effect,* respectively). This patient's responses show a recency effect but not a primacy effect. Studies of the serial position effect in list-learning suggest that the primacy effect is a result of the test taker's rehearsal of early items in the list. Rehearsal encodes the items in a long-term (secondary) memory store from which the items are later retrieved. The studies suggest that the recency effect occurs because the last items in the list are still in short-term (immediate) memory. Items in the middle of the list are not recalled because they have not been rehearsed sufficiently to encode them in long-term memory and are replaced in short-term memory by later test items.

How might one explain this patient's pattern of responses? Absence of a primacy effect suggests that the patient is not able to transfer early list items into long-term memory. What might cause such a failure? Perhaps the patient does not rehearse the early list items, leaving them in short-term memory where they are replaced by later items in the list. Perhaps the patient has a "tuning in" problem in which he is slow to allocate attention to items early in the list.

How could one tell which of these reasons explains the patient's performance? No doubt there are many ways, but I would begin by testing the rehearsal hypothesis. First I would show the patient how to rehearse the early items in the list by silently repeating them, and I would do a few trials in which the patient rehearses early list items. If coaching rehearsal had no effect, I would do a few training trials with three-item or four-item lists with 2 or 3 seconds between items to give the patient a bit more time to rehearse. Then I would try eight-item lists read at 1 item per second. If I still saw no primacy effect, I might try an eight-item list with 2 or 3 seconds between items. If that failed to yield a primacy effect, I would test the tuning-in hypotheses. I would use an eight-word list read at a one-word per second rate, but I would provide a countdown to prime the patient's system prior to the list—e.g., "*Here comes the list you*

are to remember. Listen for the words after I have finished counting: Five...four...three...two... one..."(word list). I'd probably provide a few training trials to get the patient into the task. (However, this procedure might pose difficulties for some patients who may be unable to clear the immediate memory buffer of the priming numbers and make the space available for the words in the test list. I would know this if the patient gave me numbers instead of, or mixed with, test words. This pattern of responses might suggest a problems with alternating attention, which would suggest yet another divergence in testing procedures.)

If neither method yielded a primacy effect, I'd probably move on to something else, unless there were an important reason for finding the source of the unusual pattern of retention span test responses.

Response to Question 4-2 The pattern of this patient's spelling responses fits the traditional definition of *perseveration.* Letters from previous words intrude into the patient's spelling of test words, with occasional correctly spelled words breaking the pattern of intrusions. Perseverative responses of this kind are fairly common in confrontation-naming tests in which a patient is asked to name a set of common objects or their pictorial representations — the patient gives the name of a previously named item for the current test item (e.g., after correctly naming *cup,* the patient calls the next several items *cups*). Most patients are aware of their perseverative errors and often try to correct them, usually with minimal success. One aphasic patient described his perseverative responses as, "*Words get stuck in my mind and I can't get rid of them. I know what I say is not going to be right, but I can't help it.*"

I have had reasonable success in helping patients compensate for this problem by inserting a 5-second to 10-second delay between the patient's response to one item and my presentation of the next item. It seems to me that the delay allows the memory traces for one item to decay before the patient's system has to cope with the next item. When an unfilled delay doesn't work, I've filled the delay with a nonsensical task, such as saying, "*one, one, one*" between stimulus items. Some patients were helped, and some found the nonsensical task intruding into their responses to test items. I have also had some success with a visualization strategy in which I tell the patient to think of how the word looks, visualize the first few letters, subvocally say the word, then say or write the word. Patients who find this strategy successful sometimes generalize its use to daily life.

Comment: The label *perseveration* denotes a pattern of responses but says nothing about the nature of the process or processes that may be responsible for the pattern. Perseveration may represent a variety of cognitive processing abnormalities, such as impaired attention, impaired self-monitoring, memory impairment, or impaired linguistic processes. Helping a patient cope with perseverative responding requires that the clinician understand the reasons for the perseveration and devise strategies to help the patient circumvent it.

Response to Question 4-3 This pattern of spelling errors is unusual. The frequency of misspellings and their magnitude are similar for common, regularly spelled words such as *everyone, cowboy, birthday,* and *today* and less common, irregularly spelled words such as *architect, thought,* and *believe.* I would expect less frequent and less dramatic errors on common regularly spelled words. It is unusual to see a pattern of spelling errors in which irregularly spelled portions of words (e.g., *ch* in *architect* and *heartache, gh* in *thought* and *eight, ie* in *believe*) are correctly spelled, whereas regularly spelled parts of words are misspelled (e.g., *tekt* in *architect, birt* in *birthday, kamp* in *campground*). This man misspells every word in the test—high-frequency words such as *today, farmer, eight,* and *cowboy* and low-frequency words such as *architect, heartache,* and *license.* I would expect that someone who comes close to the correct spelling of low-frequency, irregularly spelled words would correctly spell at least

some high-frequency, regularly spelled words. This man's pattern of spelling errors suggests that he may be intentionally misspelling the words in the test, perhaps because of pending litigation.

CHAPTER 5

Response to Question 5-1 The disparate sign is Mr. Portofino's poor reading comprehension. Ordinarily we would expect a patient with Broca's aphasia to have reasonably good auditory comprehension and that reading comprehension should also be relatively well preserved. (Poor oral reading would be expected, reflecting the patient's problems with motor aspects of speech production.) I can think of two reasons for Mr. Portofino's poor reading comprehension. The most likely reason is that the patient's comprehension of printed material was poor before Mr. Portofino's stroke occurred. A less likely reason is the presence of two lesions, one in the posterior inferior frontal lobe which created the Broca's aphasia and the hemiplegia, and another in the posterior temporal lobe which disrupted (but did not completely destroy) communication between the visual cortices and Wernicke's area (perhaps from a previous small temporal lobe stroke which Mr. Portofino did not notice because he didn't do much reading or which he chose to ignore). However, I would expect at least some partial right-side visual field blindness from a temporal lobe stroke in such a location. The most likely explanation—poor reading skills before the stroke. (A clinician probably would know of a patient's poor reading skills in advance. Clinicians routinely gather information about a patient's previous reading, writing, spelling, and arithmetic skills before formal assessment begins—*How far did you go in school? How did you do in school? Were you a good speller? Were you good at arithmetic? Did you do much reading before your stroke?*

Response to Question 5-2 Ms. Aldeberan's pattern of performance suggests a visuoperceptual problem—errors tend to be visual. Ms. Aldeberan appears to do better on longer words, perhaps because longer words provide more context. Also, the words *tomorrow, mother,* and *newspaper,* which she reads correctly, are not words with visually similar alternatives which might lead the patient with visuo-perceptual problems astray. I would expect an aphasic patient to make more semantic errors than visual errors in an oral reading task such as the one in this example—*home* for *house, today* for *tomorrow, father* for *mother,* and so on. So Ms. Aldeberan's performance is somewhat unusual for an aphasic person. Be that as it may, visual errors such as those committed by Ms. Aldeberan implicate the posterior regions of the brain (visual cortex, visual associations areas, connecting pathways), so I would expect her to exhibit a fluent aphasia. It is probably not Wernicke's aphasia, because of the absence of semantic reading errors—more likely mild (anomic) aphasia.

Response to Question 5-3 Ms. Smith's performance on Part F is better than her performance on Part E. Most aphasic persons do better on Part E than on Part F. How to explain Ms. Smith's "unusual" performance? A fatigue or tuning-out problem can't explain it, because we would expect fatigue and tuning out to affect Part F more than Part E. An attentional problem also doesn't fit with Ms. Smith's performance, because we wouldn't expect fluctuations in attention to coincide so neatly with changes in test items. Let's look at the commands in Parts E and F to see what characteristics change between Part E and Part F. The commands in Part E are syntactically simpler than those in Part F, but that should lead to poorer performance in Part F on Ms. Smith's part. The commands in Part E are longer than most of the commands in Part F. Hmm! Perhaps we're seeing the results of a retention span problem for Ms. Smith. That possibility seems strengthened by Ms. Smith's performance in Part F—her errors occur on the longer commands, and she tends to miss the final elements in the commands. She also misses preponderantly final items in Parts D and E, which fits our

hypothesis. But why doesn't she miss only the final elements in the commands in Part E? Perhaps overloading Ms. Smith's retention span generated interference that affected earlier parts of the commands. I'd go with a retention span explanation for Ms. Smith's performance. I might do some follow-up testing to test the hypothesis in more detail. (It's not all that unusual to see patients who do better on Part F of the Token Test than on Part E. And it's usually a retention span problem.)

Response to Question 5-4 **Mrs. Bloom.** Mrs. Bloom probably is aphasic. The evidence is several verbal paraphasias—*cat* for *dog; sitter* for *sofa; cleaned* for *messed; rug* for *floor.*

Some other fairly typical aphasic speech responses: *the mother is gonna...trying to get him out of there; those ones there....children...boys and girls* (false starts perhaps indicating word retrieval failure), indefinite words without referents (*got into it, he's hiding, those ones there*), and incomplete sentences (*the rest of the birthday cake*).

The presence of verbal paraphasias and fluent speech suggest Wernicke's aphasia. Mrs. Bloom's major speech deviations are inaccurate and slightly off-the-mark words, suggestive of word retrieval failure. The other deviations probably are close enough to normal not to be a problem for Mrs. Bloom in daily life interactions. However, her speech deviations are likely to prove annoying to Mrs. Bloom and to her listeners.

Mr. Jones. Mr. Jones's slow speech rate and telegraphic speech are definite indicators of Broca's aphasia. Mr. Jones's major speech deviations are extremely low speech rate, long pauses, the presence of nonword filler, use of the word *and* as a filler and continuant, and telegraphic speech, with utterances averaging about three words in length. He probably can communicate reasonably well in daily life, although with greatly reduced efficiency. His slow speech rate may cause listeners to become impatient and may compromise Mr. Jones's daily life communicative competence.

CHAPTER 6

Response to Question 6-1 I can think of several variables that might influence these mens' quality-of-life ratings:

- **Familial, social, and community support.** A person with a supportive family and supportive friends, associates, and professional personnel seems likely to have greater satisfaction with quality of life than a person without those resources. Access to community support services (e.g., stroke groups, adult community centers, transportation services for disabled persons, etc.) also seems likely to enhance judgments of quality of life.
- **History of language and communication activities.** A person who has a history of extensive reading, writing, and communicative interactions with others seems likely to experience greater dissatisfaction with quality of life after becoming aphasic than a person for whom such activities were not an important part of daily life.
- **Vocational and financial concerns.** A person who depends on income from current work, who is not financially comfortable, or both seems likely to experience the negative effects of aphasia on quality of life more intensely than a person for whom aphasia does not bring with it worries about financial matters.
- **Coping styles.** Some people have more effective coping styles than others. Some respond to problems with effective coping mechanisms. They think realistically about problems and take action to solve them. They make the problem situation better by changing how they think about it, or they develop new habits, adjust living conditions, develop compensatory strategies, or learn new skills. Others seem unable to respond effectively to problems—they avoid thinking about the problem, avoid situations in which the problem is apparent, and give up and allow the problem to dominate them. Persons with aphasia, like the rest of us, differ in how they cope with problems. Those with effec-

tive coping strategies seem likely to experience greater satisfaction with quality of life than those without effective strategies.
- **Time after onset of aphasia.** It seems to me that time after onset of aphasia may affect an aphasic person's feelings about quality of life in two ways. In the time immediately after onset, when patients and families may be in a state of emotional crisis, apprehension about the future may negatively affect the aphasic person's judgments concerning quality of life. For these reasons, some aphasic persons' judgments of quality of life may be lower in the first weeks after onset of aphasia than later, when the aphasic person and his or her family have adjusted to their changed life circumstances. Some aphasic persons' judgments of quality of life may later decline as the aphasic person and the family come to grips with the fact that the aphasic person will be left with residual disabilities for the rest of his or her life. It would not be unusual to see both effects in the same aphasic person's quality of life ratings—low ratings early after onset, with ratings increasing for weeks or months, then a dip in ratings, perhaps followed by a slow increase in ratings as the aphasic person and the family adjust to the long-term consequences of aphasia.
- **Comorbidity.** The presence of health-related conditions other than aphasia seems likely to depress aphasic persons' estimates of quality of life. Perhaps the aphasic person who gave a lower rating of quality of life in this question also was experiencing health-related conditions other than aphasia—hypertension, diabetes, pulmonary disease, heart disease, arthritis, paralysis—than the person who gave a more positive quality of life rating.

These to me are the most obvious variables. No doubt there are other equally important variables that you may think of.

Response to Question 6-2 Here is my order of complexity for the CETI items, from simpler to more complex, with discontinuities *(gaps)* noted.

1	Getting someone's attention
2	Responding to or communicating anything (including yes or no) without words
3	Communicating physical needs such as aches and pains
4	Communicating his/her emotions
5	Indicating that he/she understands what is being said to him/her
6	Saying the name of someone whose face is in front of him/her
7	Giving yes and no answers appropriately
	Gap #1
8	Understanding writing
	Gap #2
9	Having a one-to-one conversation with you
10	Having coffee-time visits and conversations with friends and neighbors
	Gap #3
11	Getting involved in group conversations about him/her
	Gap #4
12	Having a spontaneous conversation
	Gap #5
13	Participating in a conversation with strangers
14	Starting a conversation with people who are not close family
15	Being a part of a conversation when it is fast and there are a number of people involved
16	Describing or discussing something at length

I see several obvious discontinuities. Gaps #1 and #2 are created by the vagueness of the phrase *"understanding writing,"* which conceivably could mean anything from recognizing one's printed name to reading and comprehending advanced technical texts. Phrases such as, *"Reads and understands shopping lists, signs, and telephone book entries," "Reads and understands the newspaper,"* or *"Reads and understands letters from friends and relatives"* could expand this item and increase its specificity.

Gap #3 seems to me a discontinuity caused by a change in specificity from preceding to succeeding items. Items 10 and 12 describe generic conversational interactions. Item 11 describes conversations about a specific topic—the person being rated. Item 11 also seems to me largely redundant with Item 10 in terms of complexity. Gaps #4 and #5 are created by what I see as vagueness in Item 12. *"Having a spontaneous conversation"* can mean anything from a conversation with a spouse about the menu for dinner to conversation with strangers about an editorial in *The Economist.* It seems to me that Item 12 could be deleted, because it pretty much overlaps with adjacent items. I see a large discontinuity between Item #7 and Item #9. The gap might be filled by inserting items representing gradations of complexity and eliminating some overlapping items from Item #10 through Item #16.

CHAPTER 7

Response to Question 7-1 Strict *peaks* or *valleys* approaches to selecting treatment tasks risk violating three principles that I believe to be important to effective treatment of adults with cognitive-communicative impairments:

- Treatment tasks should be difficult enough to challenge the patient but not so difficult that they overwhelm the patient.
- Treatment should be directed toward mental processes that account for a patient's performance in a task or in a collection of tasks.
- Treatment should target skills that will enhance the patient's daily life communicative competence.

Task Difficulty: When a patient's peak performances represent minimal impairments, treating the peaks may produce treatment tasks in which the patient is not challenged and lead the clinician to treat where treatment is not needed—focusing on impairments so slight as to have minimal effects on the patient's daily life communicative competence. If I were to use a *treat the peaks* approach, I would establish upper performance limits for each task beyond which I would not select a task for treatment. These limits might be related either to normal performance (for example, the 75th percentile for normal adults) or to the performance of a group of brain-injured patients (for example, the 90th percentile for aphasic adults).

When the *valleys* in a patient's test performance represent tasks in which a patient's performance is severely impaired, selecting treatment tasks to represent the valleys produces treatment tasks in which error responses predominate. The patient's high error rate creates deteriorating performance. Errors cause more errors and patient frustration. A treat the valleys approach may be appropriate, however, for patients with mild impairments except for a few valleys that represent moderate impairments. Treating the valleys may challenge these patients but should not overwhelm them.

Treating Underlying Processes: Both peaks and valleys approaches run the risk of enticing clinicians to *train to the test*—to select treatment tasks that resemble the tests that led to selection of the tasks. Suppose, for example, that a patient's peak on a test battery was a confrontation naming subtest. A clinician who followed a strict treat the peaks approach might focus treatment on confrontation naming drills, without considering the relevance of naming to the patient's communicative needs and without considering whether training naming addresses any underlying cognitive processes. Both peaks and valleys approaches may lead a clinician into a fragmented approach to treatment, because a clinician may select treatment tasks based only on their relative level of difficulty for the patient, with no consideration of how the patient's test-to-test pattern of performance may point to impairments in mental processes that underlie performance on several tests.

Enhancing Patients' Daily Life Competence: Strict use of a treat the peaks or treat the valleys approach fails to take into account the daily life importance of skills or abilities sampled by the tests that are used to select treatment activities.

Both approaches also fail to consider the needs and wishes of patients and families.

Response to Question 7-2 I would reply as follows:

- Surface similarity between treatment tasks and daily life communicative interactions is no guarantee of generalization from clinic treatment to a patient's daily life environment.
- Forcing treatment activities to simulate daily life communicative interactions may lead to inefficiency and limit the effectiveness of treatment by directing treatment away from mental processes that may support a wide range of daily life communicative skills.
- The effectiveness of treatment is not indicated by how closely treatment activities resemble daily life communicative interactions but by outcome measures that document the degree to which a patient's daily life communication changes concurrent with treatment.

I would suggest to the administrator that the focus of the directive be on measuring outcome using measures that predict daily life communicative success, rather than on the form of treatment activities.

Response to Question 7-3 Clearly the clinician's repeated attempts to instruct the patient in the task are not succeeding. Perhaps the patient doesn't comprehend the clinician's instructions. Perhaps the patient is perseverating. Perhaps the patient doesn't understand the concept of opposite. The signs of trouble are there early in the interaction, and the clinician should have heeded them and taken a different tack. After the second failure (when the patient responds *white as snow*) I would simplify the task. I might make up some cards on which I print a stimulus word on one line and print an antonym and two or three foils on another line. I might underline the antonym on some of the cards and use those cards to demonstrate the task—I'd say the stimulus word, then point to the underlined antonym, saying something like, *"And this word means the opposite of..."* Then I'd try a few trials in which I said a stimulus word and had the patient point to the underlined antonym. Then I'd try a few trials in which I used cards on which the antonym was not underlined. If the patient could do this task, I would eliminate the printed stimulus word and have the patient choose antonyms for my spoken word by pointing to the appropriate word on the card. And so on. The point is, when instructions fail, I'd try simplifying the task and use demonstration plus instruction to train the task.

It seems to me that there is a larger issue here. I would question the appropriateness of this task to this patient. If the patient's comprehension impairment is so severe that he or she cannot understand the instructions for the task (which seems likely), I don't think that drilling the patient to produce antonyms is relevant to the patient's needs. With this patient I'd probably be working on comprehension, not on producing antonyms.

I'm also puzzled regarding the clinician's purpose in working on antonym production. Working on an arcane skill such as producing antonyms suggests that the clinician's intent is to reorganize the patient's semantic representations or to stimulate or revitalize the patient's semantic processing skills. However, the patient's responses suggest that the patient's semantic representations and semantic processes are in reasonably good condition—the phrases the patient produces are normal semantic associations. I would focus treatment on other issues. If the patient's problem is with understanding the concept of opposite, and I felt it important to teach that concept—which I think unlikely—I'd teach it nonverbally, rather than with antonyms.

Response to Question 7-4

Several aspects of this interaction deserve comment. The clinician persists with confrontation naming drill in the face of four consecutive unacceptable responses by the patient. (That the responses are *unacceptable* is clear from the clinician's feedback. The patient's responses are not necessarily *wrong*.) There seem to me two potential reasons

for the patient's failures at confrontation naming in this series. (1) The patient may not understand the task, although this seems unlikely, because the patient gives semantically related words on each trial. (2) The patient cannot retrieve and say the target words but gets semantically related words instead. This seems likely to me.

I would question why the clinician insists on an exact match between stimuli and the patient's responses, because producing semantically related words when retrieval goes awry might permit the patient to communicate reasonably well in daily life, where such substitutions might work quite well to get the patient's meaning across to listeners. I also would wish to evaluate the patient's word retrieval in connected speech—sometimes patients who have word retrieval problems in confrontation naming drills do considerably better in connected speech.

I personally don't put much faith in confrontation naming drills as an effective treatment procedure. I'd probably choose to treat word retrieval with more naturalistic materials. I might have the patient provide missing words in sentences or in short samples of narrative discourse in which semantic and syntactic constraints limit the number of reasonable choices for missing words. I might use story retelling as a treatment procedure, because I would expect that having heard the words in the story might enhance the patient's word retrieval in the retellings.

I also see several procedural faults in this clinician's treatment of the patient's unacceptable responses. The clinician does not acknowledge that the patient's responses are semantically related to the target responses. He or she should. The clinician deviates from the purpose of the drill (word retrieval) and strays into word repetition when the patient does not respond appropriately. (The clinician's task is not to *correct* but to *stimulate*.) I would not ask the patient to repeat my production of word names after the patient fails to produce them on confrontation. That's not the point of the drill, and repetition is unlikely to have any effect on the patient's word retrieval. I might try providing some cues—the first sound or a rhyming word—to see what kinds of cues facilitated the patient's performance. I certainly would not permit a string of five consecutive unacceptable responses without intervening—explaining, cueing, or changing the stimulus or response requirements. The clinician and the patient are getting nowhere in this sample. It's the clinician's fault, and it's the clinician's responsibility to do something to get the treatment session on track.

CHAPTER 8

Response to Question 8-1 The absence of paralysis suggests that the primary motor cortex in the left and right hemispheres is not affected by neuropathology, nor are descending corticospinal tract fibers. (An unusual phenomenon—hemiparesis or hemiplegia almost always accompanies limb apraxia.) Neuropathology causing unilateral limb apraxia almost always is a sign of damage in the anterior corpus callosum that interrupts fiber tracts connecting the premotor cortex in the language-competent hemisphere with the motor cortex in the non-language-competent hemisphere. For right-handers this means that fibers crossing from the left hemisphere premotor cortex to the right hemisphere motor cortex have been affected. As a result, the left hand (controlled by the motor cortex in the right hemisphere) does not have access either to the motor plans set up by the left hemisphere or to the sense of the spoken commands used to test for limb apraxia. Consequently, if a right-hander exhibits unilateral limb apraxia, the left hand will be the apraxic hand. The most reasonable explanation for unilateral apraxia of the right hand and arm is that the patient is right-hemisphere dominant for language (and left-handed).

Response to Question 8-2 The examiner should test the patient's left arm and hand first because if the patient is unilaterally apraxic, the left limb will be the apraxic one. If the examiner tests the (potentially nonapraxic) right arm and hand, then requests the same movement from the (potentially apraxic) left arm and hand, the patient can watch the nonapraxic limb perform the movement and mimic the movement with the apraxic limb. If this happens, apraxia in the patient's left arm and hand will not be detected. When I test a right-handed patient with suspected limb apraxia and no hemiplegia, I routinely test the left side first, then test the right side, using the same commands but in a different order.

Response to Question 8-3 It is possible, but highly unlikely. Right-handed patients who exhibit alexia without agraphia almost always have right homonymous hemianopia because of destruction of the left-hemisphere visual cortex. (Destruction of visual pathways from the right-hemisphere visual cortex isolates the language areas in the left hemisphere from the remaining visual cortex, creating the alexia.) Alexia without agraphia in the absence of hemianopia would, I believe, require two lesions—one that cuts the crossing fibers in the posterior corpus callosum, and another that undercuts the language region (Wernicke's area) in the left temporal lobe so as to cut its connections to the left-hemisphere visual cortex without either destroying the visual cortex or extending deep enough into the temporal lobe to affect the optic radiations going back to the visual cortex. Pathology in the posterior corpus callosum implicates the posterior cerebral artery. Pathology near Wernicke's area in the left temporal lobe implicates the posterior branch of the middle cerebral artery. It would be unusual to see simultaneous strokes in both locations. It would also be unusual to see a patient with a lesion undercutting Wernicke's area who is not aphasic, because undercutting Wernicke's area should have the same effect as destroying Wernicke's area. The scenario described is possible, but highly unlikely.

Response to Question 8-4 I would expect no hemiplegia because of the likely high-parietal location of the brain damage. However, if the lesion extends into the middle regions of the motor cortex, I would not be surprised by right-sided weakness with the right arm and hand affected more than the right leg and face. (Patients with conduction aphasia rarely are paralyzed, but many have arm and hand weakness because of patchy damage in the motor cortex adjacent to the midparietal lobe.) I would test for limb and buccofacial apraxia and would expect to find bilateral limb apraxia and buccofacial apraxia resulting from disconnection of posterior language regions from anterior motor-planning regions. I would test for tactile perception and recognition *(stereognosis)* and would be watching for right-side impairments because of potential damage to the left-hemisphere somatosensory cortex and somatosensory association areas. I would expect sensory impairments to affect the patient's arm and hand and perhaps the face more than the patient's leg, because of the probable midparietal location of the patient's brain damage. I would test the patient's visual fields. If a visual field defect were present, I would expect it to affect inferior regions of right-side visual space (right inferior quadrantanopsia).

Response to Question 8-5 *Transcortical motor aphasia:* I would expect some hemiparesis—leg greater than arm, because of involvement of upper regions of the motor cortex. I also would expect elements of anterior disconnection syndrome—the patient may have difficulty verbalizing about unseen objects palpated with the hand contralateral to the language-dominant hemisphere. Limb apraxia (perhaps unilateral) may be present because of damage in the anterior corpus callosum. The patient may exhibit behavioral *inertia* (lack of responsiveness) because of frontal lobe damage. *Transcortical sensory aphasia:* I would expect contralateral somatosensory impairment, because of involvement of the parietal sensory cortex, and perhaps astereognosis, because of involvement of parietal sensory association cortex. The patient is likely to have contralateral inferior visual field

blindness because of involvement of the upper optic radiations. If the lesion extends into the visual cortex, the patient may have a right-side homonymous hemianopia. I also would expect diminished awareness of impairments, common in patients with posterior brain injury.

CHAPTER 9

Response to Question 9-1 I would guess that Mr. Murphy's poor performance on yes-no questions relates to problems in producing understandable yes-no responses. Perhaps he is severely apraxic and does not have the motor skills to produce *yes* and *no*. I would know if this were likely by his performance on other tests of speech production. However, even if Mr. Murphy were severely apraxic, I would expect him to be able to indicate *yes* and *no* by gestures (head nods, head shakes, hand gestures such as thumbs-up or thumbs-down). In my experience, few apraxic patients are so severely apraxic that they cannot indicate *yes* and *no* by some gestural means. Perhaps Mr. Murphy confuses *yes* and *no*. I would know if this were likely by his test performance— whether he indicated dissatisfaction with his responses to yes-no questions by gestures, body language, or facial expressions. It's not uncommon for aphasic patients to confuse *yes* and *no,* but when they do, they usually signal their confusion by indicating "*I know the answer, but I can't tell whether to say* yes *or* no."

If Mr. Murphy does not have reliable yes-no responses, I would see two possibilities in treatment. (1) Work around the problem. Use materials that do not require yes-no responses. (2) Find a way to give Mr. Murphy reliable yes-no responses. The first alternative, I think, would not be practical from Mr. Murphy's point of view, because he will need dependable yes-no responses in daily life. Therefore, I would be inclined to find a way for Mr. Murphy to answer yes-no questions reliably. I'd try training him with a simple task in which the *yes* and *no* responses were very obvious,' for example showing him cards on which pairs of simple geometric symbols were printed. If the symbols in a pair were the same, the appropriate response would be *yes,* and if they were not the same the appropriate response would be *no.* I'd start with natural responses—the words *yes* and *no* if Mr. Murphy could produce them, head nods and head shakes if he could not. If those responses didn't work out, I'd try a less natural response (e.g., thumbs-up and thumbs-down). If that failed, I'd put two cards on the table, on one of which was printed a smiling face and on the other of which was printed a frowning face and train Mr. Murphy to point to the smiling face to indicate *yes* and to point to the frowning face to indicate *no.*

I'd train Mr. Murphy to use whatever response we chose to begin with in the following way. I'd begin with strings of consecutive *yes* and *no* trials—say five trials in which *yes* is appropriate, followed by five trials in which *no* was appropriate, and so on, for several iterations until Mr. Murphy was consistently responding appropriately and changing from *yes* to *no* and vice versa when the sequence changed. Then I'd gradually decrease the length of strings of consecutive *yes* and *no* responses and gradually introduce randomness into the sequences. If I got Mr. Murphy to 100% accuracy with unpredictable sequences of *yes* and *no* trials using a less natural response, such as pointing to symbols or thumbs-up thumbs-down, I might try to substitute a more natural response (e.g., head nod and head shake or perhaps spoken *yes* and *no*). I would even accept *uh-huh* and *huh-uh,* or *yeah* and *nah*—something that Mr. Murphy can produce that listeners would consider equivalents to *yes* and *no.* (The goal is functionality, not elegance.)

Response to Question 9-2 The positive side of Ms. Snyder's response to the *cookie theft* picture is that she gets the overall theme of the situation and chooses words that relate to that theme. The negatives are (a) severe agrammatism, (b) mispronunciation of content words, and (c) many false starts, filler words, and interjections. Fortunately her mispronunciations are close

enough to their targets to make most words intelligible in context. For the time being, I would not work on articulatory accuracy because listeners should be able to decode her off-target productions if given some contextual support, such as knowing the topic. I'd begin by targeting her false starts and filler words and interjections. I'd put her in a structured task such as picture description, instruct her regarding what the objective is (elimination of false starts and filler), have her talk, and signal her when she inserts a false start or a filler. If signaling alone were not effective, I might slow her speaking rate and have her be certain to have a word clearly in mind before she begins an utterance. When she can speak in the structured task with little or no filler, I would gradually loosen the structure—perhaps move on to story retelling or telling about personal experiences—under conditions like those used in the first task. When Ms. Snyder could talk in a variety of contexts without false starts and fillers, I might then focus on producing more information, providing more content words, and perhaps working on communicating relationships among them, either by a few well-chosen function words or by intonation and gesture. I wouldn't directly attack Ms. Snyder's agrammatism until I felt that she had achieved maximum benefit from treatment that targeted other aspects of her speech. Then I might try training her in the use of a selected list of function words, especially prepositions. (I would not be surprised if her use of function words spontaneously increased as we eliminated filler and false starts and began working on generating more content words and establishing relationships among them.)

Response to Question 9-3 Mrs. Bloom's major speech deviations are slightly off-the-mark words, suggestive of word retrieval failure. If I were to treat Mrs. Bloom's connected speech, it seems to me that word retrieval drills may be the most appropriate avenue. I might work on decreasing Mrs. Bloom's production of completely inaccurate words and try to get her to produce words that are "in the ballpark." That way, she will communicate well, even though all her words aren't precisely what a "normal" speaker would produce. I might try training Mrs. Bloom to recognize when her words are inaccurate, rather than approximations, and teach her to repair an inaccurate word by replacing it with a word that approximates what Mrs. Bloom intends. I might train her to "talk around" words that she can't come up with and for which she can't find a word that approximates the word she needs. I'd focus on maximizing Mrs. Bloom's communicative adequacy. I wouldn't worry about whether the words she produces are precisely the ones needed, as long as they are close enough that listeners can follow what she is attempting to communicate.

Mr. Jones's major speech deviations are extremely low speech rate, the presence of many filler words, telegraphic speech, and short utterances. The first question I'd ask is whether Mr. Jones is likely to communicate adequately in daily life interactions with his present speech patterns. The answer, I think, is "*yes,*" in terms of communicating essential information. However, his slow speech rate and telegraphic speech in combination are likely to prove burdensome to listeners and are likely to be a source of ongoing frustration to Mr. Jones. Consequently, I might try (first) to increase his speech rate, and then see if I can do anything to make his speech less telegraphic. (I'd tackle speech rate first because probably it would be easier to modify than his telegraphic speech, and increasing his speech rate would likely strongly affect listeners' sense of effort as they listened to him.) Because his slow rate is likely due to motor programming problems, I'd start him off with articulation drills, in which he produced sequences of controlled articulatory complexity, first at slow rate, and then with gradually increasing speech rate. As he got better, I'd increase the articulatory complexity of the materials, dropping speech rate back each time I increased articulatory complexity. I'd try to get him up to about 100 words per minute, mini-

mum, which I think would make his speech rate pretty tolerable for most listeners. I might also try some work on improving the syntax of what Mr. Jones says by training him to produce more connecting words. However, I've not had much luck with doing this in the past, and I wouldn't expect much success here. However, I'd still try some trial treatment with this focus. Who knows? I might get lucky!

I might also experiment with decreasing Mr. Jones's use of filler words, but if eliminating fillers simply led to long pauses where the filler words had been, I'd probably back off, because Mr. Jones's speech probably would seem more natural with filler words than with an equivalent number of long silent pauses.

Response to Question 9-4 I'd (obviously!) target Mr. Osborne's comprehension of function words. I would stay away from drills with lists of function words—I wouldn't expect such drills to improve his reading comprehension or to do much beyond making Mr. Osborne frustrated. Instead I'd use printed cloze exercises to accomplish my objectives. I'd use printed texts in which function words are replaced with blanks. Mr. Osborne's assignment would be to fill in the missing words. I'd begin with simple texts with a small number of function words deleted, and I'd provide Mr. Osborne with a list of the words needed to complete each exercise, plus a few foils as in the following:

> Harry Davis was ____ a hurry. His business meeting in San Diego had lasted ____ hour longer ____ planned and Harry was worried ____ he would miss his flight back ____ Omaha. He stood on the curb ____ front of the hotel. His suitcase was ____ the sidewalk beside him. ____ was raining lightly. He waved frantically ____ the taxicabs as ____ rushed by.

Word list plus foils:

> than when that because it by he on out
> his to over of an in they beside at

I would gradually add to the list of function words, increase the length and complexity of the cloze texts, and make the choices of which words went into the blanks less obvious. To measure generalization (which I would expect) I would periodically test Mr. Osborne's reading comprehension, using passages which Mr. Osborne had not previously seen and in which passage comprehension depended on function words.

CHAPTER 10

Response to Question 10-1 Fred's experience strongly indicates cerebral hemorrhage affecting his right hemisphere as the cause of his signs and symptoms. Intense physical exertion is a common precursor to hemorrhagic strokes, because physical exertion increases blood pressure, thereby increasing the risk of rupturing a weakened arterial wall. Severe headache is a common early sign of cerebral hemorrhage but is much less common following occlusive stroke. It's hard to predict location, beyond right versus left side, although I'd lean toward surface rather than deep, based on the presence of exaggerated reflexes, neglect, and hemianopia, which point toward cortical or immediately subcortical involvement. I'd also expect greater effects from an intracerebral hemorrhage (loss of consciousness, vomiting) because of compromised midbrain functions. Fred's hemorrhage clearly is not in the brain stem. If it were, Fred would be hemiplegic rather than hemiparetic; he probably would be unconscious; and respiration, heart rate, and other vital functions would likely be affected. I'd expect the physician to order an emergency CT scan to verify what has happened and to pinpoint the location of the trouble.

That Fred remained conscious, made it to the emergency room, and apparently made it through the physician's examination without a worsening of symptoms suggests that the bleeding in Fred's brain has stopped, so the immediate threat of death or progression into coma seems relatively low. However, the next few days will be critical, and careful management will be required to stabilize Fred's physiological condition and get him on the way to recovery.

Assuming that Fred had a cerebral hemorrhage and assuming that the bleeding has stopped and also assuming that surgical intervention (e.g., clipping of an aneurysm) is not needed, I'd guess that Fred might not show a great deal of improvement in the first few weeks, but that eventually (anywhere from 2 to 6 weeks) the rate of his recovery may accelerate—a common pattern for hemorrhagic strokes. Fred is a young man. He probably doesn't have generalized vascular disease. Consequently, his brain should be relatively resilient. If he survives the next week or so without another incident, I'd expect very good recovery as the hematoma is resorbed, brain swelling diminishes, and undamaged nerve fiber tracts resume functioning. I'd guess that he might be left with some residual left-sided weakness, but I wouldn't expect his hemianopia or neglect (or other right-hemisphere signs) to persist. I'd expect Fred's recovery to be significantly better than the recovery of a patient with a right-hemisphere occlusive stroke, who is likely to be older, have a compromised vascular system, and perhaps have other medical problems. A patient with an occlusive stroke may begin the recovery process sooner than Fred, but Fred's eventual level of recovery will almost certainly be better.

Response to Question 10-2 I would expect Ms. Snyder to tend to miss the leftmost stimuli in an array, regardless of the position of an array relative to the midline of the visual space. I would expect the effects of position relative to the midline and position in an array to interact, so that the leftmost items in an array in left hemispace would be most often missed and that the rightmost items in right hemispace would be missed least frequently. In the diagram below, I have indicated the probability that Ms. Snyder would identify a square by the density of its shading—the darkest squares are those that I would expect her to report most consistently.

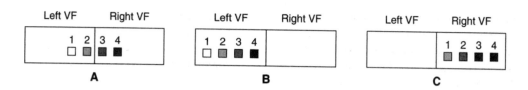

A   B   C

Ms. Snyder is likely to miss squares 1 and 2 in A, because squares 3 and 4 capture her attention. She is likely to see squares 3 and 4 in B, even though they are to the left of the midline, because there is nothing in right hemispace to capture her attention. However, squares 3 and 4 in B might capture her attention, leading her to miss squares 1 and 2, with 1 more likely to be missed than 2. I would expect Ms. Snyder to inconsistently miss squares 1 and 2 in C (*ipsilesional neglect*) for the same reasons, but, because the entire array is in right hemispace, identification of leftward squares should be better than for the array in B, above.

I would guess that many neglect patients might change their performance if given a large number of trials with these three arrays, because they would eventually learn that four squares are present on every trial. Knowing that, they might verbally cue themselves to find all four, and perhaps even count each square as they identified it. If they ended up with less than four squares on a trial, they would know that additional search is necessary, which might lead them to scan visual space (including the left side) more carefully. They might also learn that if they saw nothing, then all the squares must be to the left, which might also lead them to look leftward. If a patient failed to learn such strategies over a large block of trials, I'd worry about the patient's overall cognitive flexibility and adaptability.

Response to Question 10-3 Ms. Glindon seems alert and cooperative but also seems to deny and minimize her impairments. She comprehends and remembers what she has been told about the reasons for her hospitalization, but what she says suggests that she does not believe what she has been told and that she is unaware of or refuses to admit the physical (and perhaps cognitive) effects of her apparent stroke.

I would expect Ms. Glindon to cooperate during testing but perhaps not to try very hard, causing her test performance to underestimate her true potential. Still, I'd do an hour or so of testing to establish baseline performance, track potential recovery, and make preliminary decisions about treatment. I wouldn't expect treatment to be very effective until she gains greater awareness of her impairments and becomes motivated to work on them. I'd probably not put her in a treatment program right away but do some screening testing every 3 or 4 days to track her performance.

Ms. Glindon is only 3 days after onset of her stroke. It is possible that her awareness of her impairments may increase as she recovers. If she remains in the hospital, I'd do a daily bedside screening to see if her awareness of her impairments improves. If it did, I might schedule a few 30-minute trial treatment sessions to evaluate her response to treatment. If she's discharged from the hospital soon, I would recommend that she return in a few weeks for reevaluation. If her denial resolved, it would simplify treatment. If her denial were not to resolve, I'd probably spend a few sessions working on it. If I made progress, I'd move into a full-fledged treatment program. If not, I'd probably discharge her but might recommend reevaluation in another 4 weeks, if she's willing.

Response to Question 10-4 First, I would examine Mr. Blanding's medical records and talk with his physician and other patient care personnel to get a general sense of his impairments, his apparent cognitive and emotional state, and his on-the-ward behavior and how they have changed since onset. Then I'd interview the patient and whatever family members are available. My objectives would be to get a sense of how the patient and family members feel about Mr. Blanding's situation, their concerns, their understanding of Mr. Blanding's impairments, and to get an impression of how Mr. Blanding and family members interact. I'd also answer questions and provide some general information about what happened to Mr. Blanding and what potential outcomes might be. *(Estimated time: 30 minutes.)*

I'd try to select tests that had the most potential for indicating (a) whether Mr. Blanding needs treatment, and (b) whether he would be likely to profit from it. For (a) I'd try to test general processes that are likely to indicate the level of Mr. Blanding's communicative handicaps in daily life and which are likely to be important in a variety of cognitive-communicative activities. For (b) I'd observe Mr. Blanding in testing to evaluate his attention, retention of instructions, ability to stay on task, interpersonal behaviors, and whether he carries over learning from one task to another. I'd also be looking for signs of perceptual impairments, such as neglect and visuospatial impairment. I wouldn't administer a general test battery such as CADL, an aphasia test, or a right-hemisphere test battery (which, according to the instructions is not available anyway), but I would opt for short tests that specifically target abilities that I would be interested in. To get started, I'd plan to administer tests of the following abilities:

- **Attention:** I'd test sustained, selective, and alternating attention. I wouldn't test divided attention at this time. Divided-attention tasks demand high levels of attention and mental flexibility, and I wouldn't be concerned about it so soon after Mr. Blanding's injury. *(Estimated time: 30 minutes.)*
- **Memory:** I'd evaluate immediate memory with digit-span and word-list tests of immediate recall. I'd also administer the Rivermead Behavioral Memory Test to get a sense of

Mr. Blanding's ability to handle quasi–real life situations requiring memory for different kinds of material. *(Estimated time: 30 minutes.)*

- **Abstraction, inferences:** I'd administer several short tests to assess Mr. Blanding's ability to get beyond literal meanings and to make inferences.
  - Two stories and questions from the Discourse Comprehension Test: I'd want to know if Mr. Blanding remembers main ideas better than details (which would mean that he is sensitive to relationships among story elements), and whether his performance on implied information is dramatically worse than his performance on stated information. (If I had time, I might retest him with the DCT questions after giving several unrelated tests to assess his long-term retention of such material.)
  - Five multiple-choice items testing appreciation of idioms and metaphor
  - Two or three common proverbs which Mr. Blanding is asked to interpret

  (Estimated time: 30 minutes.)
- **Judgment, reasoning, and problem-solving**
  - To assess judgment, I'd administer five items similar to *"Suppose you are sitting in a movie theater and you smell smoke. What would you do?"*
  - To assess reasoning, I'd administer five items similar to *"What would happen if all speed limits on roads and highways were removed?"*
  - To assess problem-solving, I'd administer five items similar to *"You get up in the morning and discover that your bedroom light does not come on when you flip the switch. What would you do to find out why?"*

  (Estimated time: 20 minutes.)
- **Neglect and visuospatial abilities:** I'd administer the following tests:
  - Line bisection, clock drawing, and scene drawing to assess neglect in drawing tasks

- Reading aloud compound words, sentences and short texts (full page and two column)
- Copying 3-dimensional figures and a few multiple-choice spatial-relations test items

(Estimated time: 20 minutes.)

- **Follow-up and exploration:** In-depth exploration of significant impairments indicated by previous testing to specify their nature and severity.

(Estimated time: 30 minutes.)

- **Patient and family feedback and instruction:** An interview with the patient and family members to summarize what I found in my evaluation, make recommendations, and answer questions

(Estimated time: 30 minutes.)

I would not test for some "typical" right-hemisphere-syndrome impairments—prosopagnosia, geographic disorientation, reduplicative paramnesia, anosognosia—because I don't believe they would address the question of whether or not to treat. I also wouldn't do a formal pragmatics assessment. I'd get a sense of the patient's pragmatics from observing him in testing and interviews and watching him interact with family members. I'd get a sense of whether he denies or minimizes impairments in my interactions with him during testing and the interview.

Response to Question 10-5 Although neither individual should be permitted to drive, a driver with left neglect might be slightly safer driving in England.

Many accidents in both countries are associated with turns across oncoming traffic (left turns in the United States and right turns in England). In England oncoming traffic is on the right, and in the United States oncoming traffic is on the left. Consequently, a driver with left neglect might be better at making turns across traffic in England than in the U.S., because in England oncoming traffic would be in the driver's nonneglected visual space.

Many accidents in both countries also are associated with failure to obey traffic control signs (especially stop signs). In England traffic control signs usually are on the left-hand side of the roadway, and in the United States traffic control signs usually are on the right-hand side. Consequently, a driver with neglect would be in greater danger of failing to obey traffic control signs in England than in the United States, because in England the signs are likely to be in left hemispace.

Passing another vehicle on a 2-lane roadway would seem less risky for a driver with left neglect in England than in the United States, because in England drivers pass on the right and oncoming traffic is on the right, whereas the situation is reversed in the United States. Consequently, drivers with left neglect in England would be more likely than drivers with left neglect in the United States to see oncoming traffic before passing. However, in England the passed vehicle is on the left, while in the United States the passed vehicle is on the right. Therefore drivers with left neglect in England might be more likely to sideswipe or cut off the passed vehicle than would drivers in the United States.

Cross-traffic would present risks for drivers with left neglect in either country—vehicles coming from the left would be problematic both in England and the United States.

How about risks to pedestrians? In England a pedestrian stepping off the curb into oncoming traffic is to the left of an approaching driver. In the United States a pedestrian stepping off the curb into oncoming traffic is to the right of an approaching driver. Therefore, pedestrians stepping off a curb in England would be in greater danger from a driver with left neglect than pedestrians in the United States. (However, pedestrians who make it to the middle of the roadway and are crossing more traffic would be in greater danger in the United States.).

Drivers with left neglect in England might be more likely to run off the roadway and strike signs, lamp posts, and so forth because they would not see them, while drivers with left neglect in the U.S. might be more likely to cross into opposing traffic, with more serious consequences. However, if drivers with neglect were attracted by nonneglected hemispace, as sometimes happens, the situation would be reversed, because they would tend to drift into non-neglected hemispace.

Finally, drivers with neglect in England would be more likely to use seat belts than drivers in the United States, because in England the seat belt is on the right prior to use, but in the United States it is on the left.

Most vehicle-pedestrian accidents happen when pedestrians step off the curb. Therefore, *pedestrians* with left neglect might be safer in England than in the United States. Do you see why?

CHAPTER 11

Response to Question 11-1 Mary's case is a classic scenario for subdural hemorrhage. Subdural hemorrhages sometimes occur after relatively minor blows to the head, caused by tearing of the fragile blood vessels that traverse the space between the arachnoid and the dura mater. Mary's symptoms did not develop immediately but began to appear only when the bleeding into the subdural space began to create increased intracranial pressure. Initial headache, followed by nausea and vomiting are classic indicators of increasing intracranial pressure. Neck stiffness is also a common complaint of patients with elevated intracranial pressure, and it usually is an ominous sign. That Mary took aspirin for her headache may have contributed to her worsening condition, because aspirin, having anticoagulant properties, may exacerbate bleeding. Mary's husband should get her to a medical facility right away!

Subdural hemorrhage, and not epidural hemorrhage or subarachnoid hemorrhage, is the most likely explanation for Mary's symptoms. Epidural hemorrhages are caused by tearing or rupture of blood vessels on the surface of the dura mater. They usually require severe blows to the head, because the dura mater is not easily torn. Epidural hemorrhages are most common when the skull is fractured, causing tearing of the dura mater and its blood vessels. Subarachnoid hemorrhages usually are caused by ruptured aneurysms and not by blows to the head. However, the exact cause of Mary's symptoms can be determined only by a careful neurologic examination together with comprehensive laboratory tests (especially spinal tap) and brain imaging tests (especially CT or MRI scans). **Question:** Why might the neurologist order a spinal tap in Mary's case?

Response to Question 11-2 Jerry's head injury clearly would be translational trauma—linear acceleration because he was moving in a straight line when he hit the side of the truck. Because he was wearing a helmet, his head injury will be much less severe than if he were not wearing one. However, no helmet can protect its user against acceleration injuries when the head is moving rapidly through space and strikes an unyielding surface. The major benefit of a helmet in such a scenario is to protect against skull fracture and penetrating injuries—something for which the hard shell of a helmet is well designed. Helmets are less adept a protecting against acceleration injuries. The polyfoam liner compresses to cushion the impact of a blow (either from an object hitting the helmet or the helmet hitting an object), but the compression is not sufficient to protect the brain against acceleration injury when the head is moving rapidly through space when it strikes an object. In Jerry's case, we could expect coup (occipital) and perhaps contrecoup (frontal) damage. The amount of contrecoup damage would depend in part on what Jerry's helmeted head hit. If it hit the center of the door, which is primarily sheet metal with no reinforcing frame behind it, the sheet metal might collapse inward, slowing the rate at which Jerry's head decelerated and (perhaps) lessening the amount by which Jerry's head rebounds off the door. If Jerry's head hit the door at a reinforcing and unyielding frame member, Jerry's head would precipitously stop, and the amount of rebound would be increased, increasing the severity of both coup and contrecoup injuries. (Contrecoup injuries are most likely when the head rebounds from the impact and subsequently snaps back in the direction of the original path.) If Jerry were fortunate enough to hit the truck side window with his helmeted head, he might have even less severe head injuries. However, he might then fracture his neck or spine, depending on where his back hit the frame around the window. In addition to his head injuries, Jerry is likely to incur fractures of limbs, ribs, and (as noted) perhaps neck or spine. Neck or spine fractures are, of course, very dangerous because of the probability of subsequent paralysis, or in the case of neck fractures, the possibility of damaging vital brainstem structures that regulate respiration and other autonomic processes.

Without a helmet, Jerry would incur severe and probably fatal head injuries.

Response to Question 11-3 If I have 1 hour available, I would plan 1/2 hour for medical record review and for talking with ward personnel about the patient. In the medical record I would, of course, review the patient's history to get a sense of what happened to him the in accident and also to get a sense of his previous life. For example, had he incurred previous head injuries? Does he have a history of substance abuse? Is there evidence of aggressiveness, antisocial behavior, or other signs of problems with personality in his social history? (This information would be important both for anticipating how to approach the patient and for speculating about his eventual recovery.) I would also pay close attention to progress notes, to get a sense of the depth of the patient's "coma," how his condition changed as he emerged from coma, and what his behavior, communication, and cognition have been in the last day or so. The progress notes would also point to potential management issues such as hyperactivity, aggressiveness, assaultiveness, or the like. I would also check the physician's orders to see what medications have been prescribed—especially antiseizure medications, sedatives, or tranquilizers, which might affect the patient's responsiveness and attention span.

For the remaining 1/2 hour, I would see the patient at bedside. A patient at Rancho Los Amigos Scale level 4 who is 2 days out of coma would be unlikely to be ambulatory. He likely would be connected to monitors, feeding tubes, catheters, and such. If he were agitated and assaultive he might be restrained. I wouldn't plan to do any formal testing but would focus on getting a sense of the patient's responsiveness, attention to his environment, and general pattern of behavior (agitated, lethargic, aggressive, etc.). I would also do some probing to find out what kinds of stimuli are most effective in eliciting responses and what kinds of stimuli elicit the most purposeful responses (e.g., orientation to source of stimulation, cessation of agitated behavior, vocalization). I'd spend some time simply talking to the patient without attempting to elicit any specific responses, just to get the patient accustomed to me and the sound of my voice. I'd be making notes of my findings to help me plan what to do on my next visit.

As for prognosis, it seems to me, based on the information given, that the patient's prognosis for recovery is fair to good. He was in a coma for 7 days. The literature suggests that patients who are in a coma no longer than a week or so are likely to be left with mild to moderate residual impairments when recovery is complete. My prediction for this patient would be made somewhat rosier by the fact that he seems to be progressing rapidly—in 2 days he has moved from comatose to Rancho Los Amigos Scale level 4. I'd say the prospects for substantial recovery are good. Predicting outcome is a real guessing game at this point, but I'd expect this patient to end up with mild to moderate residual impairments. (Of course, if the patient had a history of substance abuse, previous head injuries, or other negative indicators, I'd no doubt be somewhat more pessimistic.)

Response to Question 11-4 The achievement test results suggest that Ron is functioning at reasonably high levels in most basic skills (arithmetic, general knowledge, reading comprehension for sentences). His spelling and paragraph comprehension scores are well below the level of his other test scores, suggesting that he is having problems in those areas. I'd want to gather some additional information that might reflect Ron's potential for accomplishing the kinds of tasks that would be required at school, were he to return. Important skills include the following:

- Listening comprehension for discourse (lectures, etc.)
- Note-taking skills
- Reading comprehension for college-level texts
- Ability to organize and remember information from spoken discourse and printed texts
- Spelling, grammar, and writing skills
- Test-taking ability

I would begin by administering several standardized achievement tests as follows:

- Spelling (to find out if that has improved since the previous test)
- Reading comprehension—narratives (the Nelson-Denny Reading Test or another standardized reading test that includes college-level texts)
- Discourse comprehension (the Discourse Comprehension Test to get a sense of Ron's comprehension of stated and implied main ideas and details in a controlled environment)

I would need information about Ron's performance in less structured environments in which he would be expected to obtain and retain information from spoken discourse (lectures), in which listening and note-taking are required. I might have Ron watch videotapes of speeches or lectures and take notes on their content (public television programs might provide a source for such videotapes). To see how Ron performs in less-controlled environments, in which he is surrounded by others who may be moving about, whispering, or engaging in other potentially distracting activities, I might arrange for Ron to sit in on a lecture at a local college or community organization, take notes, and bring them to me for review.

I would need information about Ron's ability to comprehend long and sometimes complex college-level printed texts, organize the information, and take organized notes that reflect the important information from the texts. I might have Ron bring in two or three textbooks from his previous college courses, assign reading passages from them, have Ron take notes and bring the notes to me for review. I might find books related to classes Ron has taken but which Ron has not previously read, and have Ron read assigned material, take notes, and bring them to me. I would time Ron in at least some of these activities to get a sense of how quickly he gets them done and whether slow reading and note-taking might prove problematic for Ron when he returns to school.

I would need to know something about Ron's study and test-taking skills. I might prepare examinations on the content of videotapes Ron has watched and made notes from, or on the content of printed materials Ron has read and made notes on. I would include multiple-choice, fill-in-the-blanks, and short essay items in the examinations to see how Ron handles each kind of test item.

I would wish to get a sense of Ron's ability to produce written discourse. I might have him write a two to three page report on a topic of interest, to get a sense of his spelling and grammar and to evaluate the coherence and relevance of what he writes. I would time at least some of Ron's written discourse production, to estimate whether slow rate might be problematic at school.

That's where I would begin. Depending on Ron's performance, I might do some follow-up evaluation in given areas, but I'd guess that the foregoing information would permit me to make recommendations regarding the appropriateness of Ron's return to school and to suggest strategies for enhancing Ron's performance (for example, that Ron tape-record lectures and listen to them a second time, during which Ron reviews and edits his original lecture notes). Depending on the results of my evaluation, I might suggest training or retraining activities to deal with weaknesses that I felt would compromise Ron's success at school. (My! This could go on forever. But I will stop here.)

CHAPTER 12

Response to Question 12-1

1. *How old is your spouse?* This would be my first question. It is a good opening question because it asks for readily recallable information and provides a good lead-in for more probing questions to follow. It also provides information that may contribute to a diagnosis, because advancing age increases the probability that a person will have Alzheimer's disease.

2. *What physical impairments or health problems does your spouse have at this time?* This question addresses the probability that the signs of the man's suspected dementia are caused by illness or other health problems.

3. *What medications is your spouse taking?* This question addresses the possibility that the signs of the man's suspected dementia are caused by medications.

4. *What significant events have occurred in your spouse's life recently?* This question addresses the probability that the signs of the man's suspected dementia represent his emotional response to a stressful life event (death, divorce, etc.).

5. *What was the first thing you noticed that made you suspect the presence of dementia?* The spouse's response to this question may provide information helpful to differential diagnosis. If the first signs were related to memory and orientation, then a diagnosis of Alzheimer's dementia becomes more probable. Altered personality and emotion (apathy, impulsivity, declining interest in social activities, etc.) may suggest Pick's disease or depression. Motor impairments may suggest subcortical pathology (Parkinson's disease, Huntington's disease, etc.).

6. *What other things have you noticed that made you suspect the presence of dementia?* The spouse's response to this question may help establish a pattern of behavior or a collection of signs that may point toward a diagnosis.

7. *Did the changes that led you to suspect dementia occur gradually (over weeks or months) or within a few days?* The spouse's response to this question may point to an identifiable precipitant (stroke, stressful life event, pain, illness, etc.) which would be inconsistent with a slowly developing dementia such as Alzheimer's dementia.

8. *Have you noticed changes in your spouse's memory (misplacing things, forgetting conversations, repeating the same story several times, etc.)?* This question addresses memory impairment—the typical first sign of Alzheimer's disease. An affirmative response would increase the likelihood of Alzheimer's disease.

9. *Have you noticed changes in your spouse's personality (worry, irritability, changes in mood, loss of interest, etc.)?* This question addresses changes in personality and mood —typical first signs of Pick's disease (and of some subcortical diseases, but motor impairments would ordinarily be obvious and not the first signs of possible dementing illness).

10. *What else have you noticed that you think may be significant?* I would end my questions with a catch-all question which invites the person being interviewed to tell me about things that may have been missed in earlier questions or to add more detail to information provided in response to other questions.

I might ask additional questions to follow up on leads provided by the spouse in responding to the other questions.

Response to Question 12-2

1. What is your name?
2. Say *please put the groceries in the refrigerator.*

3. Tell me the days of the week, beginning with Sunday.
4. Point to the ceiling, then to the floor, and blink three times.
5. Who was the first U.S. President?
6. How old are you?
7. What day of the week is it?
8. What is your phone number?
9. Who is the current U.S. President?
10. Count backward from 20 to 1.
11. How would your uncle's daughter be related to you?
12. What does *a stitch in time saves nine* mean?

Comments: Saying one's name (1) should be highly practiced and automatic—therefore very easy. Repetition and producing automatized sequences (2, 3) should also be among the easiest tasks, because they do not make demands on memory, sustained attention, or mental flexibility. Comprehension and short-term retention (4) should be relatively well preserved. (However, delayed recall would be impaired.) Memory for well learned factual information (5) often is well preserved. Many patients with moderate Alzheimer's dementia have lost track of their age (6), and most are unaware of current date and sometimes time of day (7). Few patients with moderate Alzheimer's disease remember their phone number (8) or know the name of the current President (9). (Someone who had the same phone number for many years and used it many times a day for those years might retain it because of previous "overlearning.") Tasks requiring mental flexibility and sustained attention (10, 11, 12) would likely be impossible for a person with moderate Alzheimer's dementia. My ranking of these three items is based on my sense of increasing need for sustained attention and mental flexibility across these three items. I would guess that my ranking of this list would approximate the performance of many persons with moderate Alzheimer's dementia, but I wouldn't be surprised if items moved up or down a few levels for individuals. However, I would be very surprised if items moved from the beginning of my list to the end or from the middle of the list to the beginning or end.

Response to Question 12-3

1. Mild Wernicke's aphasia or anomic aphasia; early-stage Alzheimer's dementia (verbal paraphasias)
2. Mid-stage Alzheimer's dementia; possibly right-hemisphere syndrome, but unlikely (not doing the task; inappropriate responses socially)
3. Conduction aphasia (literal paraphasias)
4. Right-hemisphere syndrome (focuses on discrete and incidental elements on right side of drawing—does not respond to central theme)
5. ??? Could be Alzheimer's; could be right-hemisphere syndrome (denial); could be anyone with visual perceptual problems
6. Broca's aphasia (agrammatism, slow speech rate, many pauses)
7. Moderate to severe Wernicke's aphasia; middle- to late-stage Alzheimer's dementia; can't differentiate with this small sample (neologisms)
8. Mild Wernicke's aphasia, moderate anomic aphasia, early-stage Alzheimer's dementia; any of the three might say this (Many verbal paraphasias, no attempted repairs)

CHAPTER 13

Response to Question 13-1 *History of atrial fibrillations:* Atrial fibrillations increase the probability of embolic stroke, so I would expect this patient's motor speech disorder to be consistent with occlusion of an artery in the brain. Emboli are most common in the cerebral arteries, so I would expect either apraxia of speech or unilateral upper motor neuron dysarthria (which might resolve over time) or perhaps spastic dysarthria, if emboli had affected cerebral arteries in both hemispheres. Cardiac emboli usually do not travel into the small diameter penetrating arteries that serve the basal ganglia, so I would not expect hypokinetic or hyperkinetic dysarthria. Although cardiac emboli in the vertebral-basilar arterial system are less common than emboli in the cerebral arteries, they do occasionally occur but do not usually travel into the small diameter arteries supplying the pons and medulla. They do, however, occasionally affect cerebellar arteries, so an ataxic dysarthria is possible.

Participation in boxing: I would definitely expect hypokinetic dysarthria. Repeated minor closed-head injury to the brain commonly causes a parkinsonian syndrome—pugilistic parkinsonism, such as that exhibited by Mohammed Ali.

Family history of chorea: Too obvious! Definitely hyperkinetic dysarthria (unless another medical condition were also present, in which case one might see a mixed dysarthria; e.g., a stroke might create spastic-hyperkinetic dysarthria).

Traumatic brain injury: This is a difficult one, because traumatic brain injury can damage many different parts of the brain and nervous system. Translational trauma may cause bleeding and swelling in the brain hemispheres and lead to spastic dysarthria (not unilateral upper motor neuron dysarthria, because the bleeding and swelling should affect both hemispheres). Diffuse axonal injury could cause damage in axial regions (basal ganglia, brain stem, and cerebellum) which would cause mixed dysarthria—perhaps ataxic-flaccid or even spastic-flaccid-ataxic! If the accident physically damaged structures at the base of the skull, I would expect flaccid dysarthria, ataxic dysarthria, or a mixed flaccid-ataxic dysarthria as a result of damage to the brain stem and cerebellum. If the patient incurred a neck fracture, respiratory support might be compromised because of damage to corticospinal tracts.

History of transient ischemic attacks: Dysarthria associated with a history of transient ischemic attacks suggests that stroke is responsible for the patient's dysarthria. If the patient's transient ischemic attacks had created symptoms of cerebral artery involvement (slurred speech, confusion, comprehension impairment), then I would expect apraxia of speech, unilateral upper motor neuron dysarthria, or spastic dysarthria. If the patient's transient ischemic

attacks suggested involvement of the vertebral-basilar arteries (hemianopia, clumsiness, gait disturbances), I would expect flaccid or ataxic dysarthria or a mixed flaccid-ataxic dysarthria because of involvement of the brain stem, cerebellum, or both.

Response to Question 13-2 The patient's complaints strongly suggest the presence of Parkinson's disease. Difficulty getting out of chairs, turning over in bed, and "freezing" during walking, in combination, suggest the presence of muscle rigidity. (Difficulty getting out of chairs and turning over in bed, by themselves, do not necessarily suggest extrapyramidal disease. "Freezing" during walking is a classic parkinsonian sign.) Weak voice and hoarseness are common complaints of patients with parkinsonian syndromes. Stuttering-like repetitions also are common complaints. My diagnosis: *Parkinson's disease* and *hypokinetic dysarthria.*

Response to Question 13-3 Differences in speech errors and speaking behavior between persons with the anterior syndrome and persons with the posterior syndrome suggest problems at different stages of speech formulation and production, which would mandate different approaches to treatment.

The speech errors of persons with the anterior syndrome appear to be more *motoric* than *mental.* Persons with the anterior syndrome exhibit high levels of muscular effort as they struggle to force the articulators into the appropriate movement patterns. Their articulatory movements are slow, clumsy, and effortful, and their attempts at self-correction are slow and labored. Persons with the anterior syndrome behave as if they are aware of misarticulations while they are in the act of producing them. They sometimes stop in the middle of a syllable or word and attempt to correct an error. Their self-correction efforts tend to focus on a single sound or syllable, suggesting that they know exactly which sounds are in error. They often insert a neutral vowel between syllables and words. These behaviors suggest immediate, online awareness of errors.

The speech errors of persons with the posterior syndrome appear to be more *mental* than *motoric*. Persons with the posterior syndrome speak fluently, with little evidence of muscular effort. Their attempts at self-correction are fluent and effortless, though not always successful. Persons with the posterior syndrome behave as if they must hear what they have said before they can attempt repairs. Their self-correction behaviors tend not to target specific sounds but typically consist of repeated attempts at a multisyllabic word or phrase with no particular focus on specific sounds. Their shotgun approach to self-correction suggests that they may not appreciate exactly which sounds are in error. Articulatory errors in successive repair attempts often occur at different locations and represent different kinds of errors (substitutions, transpositions, etc.).

The problem for persons with the *anterior syndrome* seems to be that the speech muscles are not following orders—the orders are correct, but execution is flawed. The problem for persons with the *posterior syndrome* seems to be that the speech muscles are following orders. The orders, however, are incorrect.

It seems to me that the speech impairments of persons with the anterior syndrome may represent problems organizing and executing speech movements, whereas the speech impairments of persons with the posterior syndrome may represent problems retrieving and/or retaining the phonological images of words and, perhaps, in getting the neural representations of those images to the premotor cortex for execution. Persons with the anterior syndrome work very hard at getting their articulators to do what they want them to do and are irritated rather than surprised by their speech errors. Individuals with the posterior syndrome have no problem getting the words out, but they are repeatedly surprised by what they say. (Although most have a general sense that phonologically complex material is difficult for them. They often precede an attempt at phonologically complex material with comments such as "*Oh*

boy! This will be a tough one!" Interestingly, the comments almost always are fluent, effortless, and phonologically correct.)

It seems to me that treatment procedures such as phonetic placement, phonetic derivation, articulation drills, and reorganization are appropriate when a patient's problems relate to the motoric aspects of speech (the anterior syndrome) but are not appropriate for persons with the posterior syndrome, whose problems relate to phonologic retrieval, retention, or encoding. I agree in general with those who assert that the speech characteristics of "posterior apraxia of speech" may be appropriately called *literal paraphasia* and that they represent problems in phonologic retention, retrieval, and transmission, rather than a motoric impairment. It seems to me that "posterior apraxia of speech" is a part of the syndrome of *conduction aphasia*. For such patients I would work on their aphasia as well as on their speech production. I would work on auditory comprehension (which almost always is impaired in conduction aphasia) and perhaps on word retrieval. I might include repetition drills in which patients had to delay their responses to words and phrases, to build up their short-term retention of phonologic information. I might include oral reading drills in which I had a patient underline words they thought might be difficult and then help them devise strategies to produce them. If a patient showed indications of limited retention span (and many patients with conduction aphasia do), I might do some work on short-term retention of digits or word lists—especially word lists containing phonologically complex words.

Response to Question 13-4 I doubt that Darley, Aronson, and Brown ever published a formal definition for *islands of error-free speech*. In their writings they use descriptors such as *fluent* and *well-articulated*. Although they have not, as far as I know, defined what they meant by *fluent*, contemporary usage at the time used *fluency* to refer to the prosodic characteristics of speech—rate, timing, intonation, and emphatic stress. My guess is that Darley,

Aronson, and Brown had these characteristics in mind when they used the word *fluent.*

Substituting *normal rate, timing, intonation, and emphatic stress* for *fluent* yields a more specific label—*islands of well-articulated speech with normal rate, timing, intonation, and emphatic stress.* The new label does a fairly good job of differentiating apraxia of speech from the dysarthrias, except for hyperkinetic dysarthria, because some individuals with hyperkinetic dysarthria may speak fluently and without articulatory errors between incidents of involuntary movement. Some individuals with ataxic dysarthria may have intervals of relatively well articulated speech but with abnormal intonation and emphatic stress patterns, making the *islands* label inappropriate for their speech patterns. Individuals representing other dysarthria types (spastic, flaccid, hypokinetic) typically do not experience intervals of well articulated speech or intervals of speech with normal intonation and stress patterns, making the islands label clearly not appropriate for their speech patterns.

My definition of *islands of error-free speech:* intervals during which speech is correctly articulated, spoken with normal rate, and in which timing, intonation, and stress patterns are normal. This definition doesn't separate the phenomenon seen in apraxia of speech from the intervals of error-free speech experienced by some individuals with hyperkinetic dysarthria, but that's not much of an issue, because the movement disorders experienced by individuals with hyperkinetic dysarthria clearly identify them as not having apraxia of speech.

Response to Question 13-5 The patient's normal neurologic examination and the absence of weakness in oral, pharyngeal, and laryngeal muscles and normal range of movement in those muscles rule out pathology in upper or lower motor neurons. The patient's normal articulation and resonance also suggest that upper and lower motor neurons are functioning adequately. The absence of gait disturbance, dysmetria, and scanning speech and the patient's normal articulation argue against cerebellar pathology. This leaves the extrapyramidal system as a potential location for neuropathology. The patient's speech abnormality does not represent either classic hypokinetic dysarthria or classic hyperkinetic dysarthria. The patient's runaway voice loudness resembles, in some respects, Parkinson's disease patients' runaway speech rate. Patients with Parkinson's disease often speak at a normal rate as they begin to talk, but their rate increases as they continue speaking until they are speaking extremely rapidly—so rapidly that their articulators can no longer keep up, and their articulation becomes blurred and indistinct. This patient, it seems to me, exhibits a similar phenomenon, except that vocal loudness (rather than speech rate) gets out of control. I would guess that this patient had damage or neurochemical abnormalities in his basal ganglia, perhaps related to his exposure to toxic chemicals in the pesticides he handled during his work.

Another alternative might be that this patient's speech abnormality is psychogenic, but this explanation appears less likely. This patient's speech abnormality doesn't fit what one typically sees in psychogenic voice disorders, which tend to show up as aphonia and hoarseness. This patient's speech abnormality developed gradually. Psychogenic disorders tend to develop rapidly, over hours to a few days, and often in response to a present or an anticipated life stress.

I might suggest that the neurologist try a trial regimen of treatment with an antiparkinsonian medication to see if medication eliminated the patient's abnormal voice. If the patient's symptoms were controlled by the medication, it would support a diagnosis of extrapyramidal system pathology. (However, it would still be possible that the effects of the medications represented placebo effects. That possibility could be eliminated only by a placebo phase before treatment with antiparkinsonian medications.)

Bibliography

Adamovich, B. (1990, June). *A comparison of FIM evaluations by nurses and speech pathologists.* Paper presented at the Clinical Aphasiology Conference, Santa Fe, NM.

Adamovich, B. B., & Brooks, R. A. (1981). A diagnostic protocol to assess the communication deficits of patients with right hemisphere damage. In R. H. Brookshire (Ed.), *Clinical Aphasiology Conference proceedings* (pp. 244-253). Minneapolis, MN: BRK Publishers.

Adamovich, B. B., & Henderson, J. (1992). *Scales of cognitive ability for traumatic brain injury.* Chicago: Riverside.

Adams, C. (2002). Practitioner review: The assessment of language pragmatics. *Journal of Child Psychology and Psychiatry, 43,* 973-987.

Adams, J. H., Graham, D. I., Scott, G., & associates. (1980). Brain damage in fatal non-missile head injury. *Journal of Clinical Pathology, 33,* 1132-1145.

Adams, M. J., & Collins, A. (1979). A schema-theoretic view of reading. In R. O. Freedle (Ed.), *New directions in discourse processing.* Norwood, NJ: Ablex.

Adams, R. D., & Victor, M. (1981). *Principles of neurology* (2nd ed.). New York: McGraw-Hill.

Agranowitz, A., Boone, D., Ruff, M., & associates. (1954). Group therapy as a method of retraining aphasics. *Quarterly Journal of Speech, 40,* 170-182.

Albert, M. L. (1973). A simple test of visual neglect. *Neurology, 23,* 658-664.

Albert, M. L., Feldman, R., & Willis, A. (1974). The subcortical dementia of progressive supranuclear palsy. *Journal of Neurology, Neurosurgery, and Psychiatry, 37,* 121-130.

Albert, M. L., Goodglass, H., Helm, N. A., & associates. (1981). *Clinical aspects of dysphasia.* New York: Springer-Verlag.

Alexander, M. P., & Lo Verme, S. R. (1980). Aphasia after left hemisphere intracerebral hemorrhage. *Neurology, 30,* 193-202.

Alexander, M. P., Naeser, M. A., & Palumbo, C. (1987). Correlations of subcortical CT lesion sites and aphasia profiles. *Brain, 110,* 961-991.

Alexopoulos, G. S., Abrams, R. C., Young, R. C., & Shamoian, C. A. (1988). Cornell scale for depression in dementia. *Biological Psychiatry, 23,* 271-284.

Alfano, D. P. (1994). Recovery of function following brain injury. In M. A. J. Finlayson & S. H. Garner (Eds.), *Brain injury rehabilitation: Clinical considerations* (pp. 34-56). Baltimore: Williams & Wilkins.

Allen-Burge, R., Stevens, A. B., & Burgio, L. D. (1999). Effective behavioral intervention for decreasing dementia-related challenging behavior in nursing homes. *International Journal of Geriatric Psychology, 14,* 213-228.

American Academy of Neurology. (2001). Practice parameter: The management of concussion in sports. *Neurology 1997, 48,* 581-585.

American Psychiatric Association. (1994). *Diagnostic and statistical manual of mental disorders* (Rev. 4th ed.). Washington DC: American Psychiatric Association.

Aminoff, M. J., Greenberg, D. A., & Simon, R. P. (1996). *Clinical neurology* (3rd ed.). Stamford, CT: Appleton & Lange.

Andrews, P. J. D., Piper, I. R., Dearden, N. M., & associates. (1990). Secondary insults during intrahospital transport of head injured patients. *Lancet, 1,* 327-330.

Annegers, J. F., Grabow, J. D., Kurland, L. T., & associates. (1980). The incidence, causes, and secular trends of head trauma in Olmsted County, Minnesota. *Neurology, 30,* 912-919.

Ansell, B. J., & Keenan, J. E. (1989). The Western neurosensory stimulation profile: A tool for assessing slow-to-recover head-injured patients. *Archives of Physical Medicine and Rehabilitation, 70,* 104-108.

Appell, J., Kertesz, A., & Fishman, M. (1982). A study of language functioning in Alzheimer patients. *Brain and Language, 17,* 73-81.

Appelros, P. Karlsson, G. M., Thorwalls, A., Tham, K., & Nydevik, I. (2002). Unilateral neglect: Further validation of the baking tray task. *Journal of Rehabilitation Medicine, 36,* 256-261.

Arciniegas, D. B., & Silver, M. M. (2006). Pharmacotherapy of posttraumatic cognitive impairments. *Behavioral Neurology, 17,* 25-42.

Arguin, M., & Bub, D. (1993). Modulation of the directional attention deficit in visual neglect by hemispatial factors. *Brain and Cognition, 22,* 148-160.

Armus, S. R., Brookshire, R. H., & Nicholas, L. E. (1989). Aphasic and non-brain-damaged adults knowledge of scripts for common situations. *Brain and Language, 36,* 518-528.

Aronson, M., Shatin, L., & Cook, J. C. (1956). Sociopsychotherapeutic approach to the treatment of aphasic patients. *Journal of Speech and Hearing Disorders, 21,* 352-364.

Arthur, G. (1947). *A point scale of intelligence tests.* New York: The Psychological Corporation.

Aten, J., Caliguiri, M., & Holland, A. (1982). The efficacy of functional communication therapy for chronic aphasic patients. *Journal of Speech and Hearing Disorders, 47,* 93-96.

Aten, J. L., & Lyon, J. (1978). Measures of PICA subtest variance: A preliminary assessment of their value as predictors of language recovery in aphasia. In R. H. Brookshire (Ed.), *Clinical Aphasiology Conference proceedings* (pp. 106-116). Minneapolis, MN: BRK Publishers.

Backus, O., & Dunn, H. (1952). The use of a group structure in speech therapy. *Journal of Speech and Hearing Disorders, 17,* 116-122.

Baddeley, A. D. (1986). *Working memory.* London: Oxford University Press.

Baddeley, A. D. (1996). The fractionization of working memory. *Proceedings of the National Academy of Science, 93,* 13468-13472.

Baddeley, A., Harris, J., Sunderland, A., & associates. (1987). Closed head injury and memory. In H. S. Levin, J. Grafman, & H. M. Eisenberg (Eds.), *Neurobehavioral recovery from head injury* (pp. 295-317). New York: Oxford University Press.

Baddeley, A. D., & Hitch, G. J. (1974). Working memory. In G. A. Bower (Ed.), *Recent advances in learning and motivation.* New York: Academic Press, 47-90.

Barber, J. B., & Webster, J. C. (1974). Head injuries: A review of 150 cases. *Journal of the National Medical Association, 66,* 201-204.

Barco, D. P., Crosson, B., Bolesta, M. M., & associates. (1991). Training awareness and compensation in postacute head injury rehabilitation. In J. S. Kreutzer & P. H. Wehman (Eds.), *Cognitive rehabilitation for persons with traumatic brain injury: A functional approach* (pp. 129-146). Baltimore: Paul H. Brookes.

Barlow, D. H., & Herson, M. (1984). *Single-case experimental designs: Strategies for studying behavior change* (2nd ed.). New York: Pergamon Press.

Barton, M., Maruszewski, M., & Urrea, D. (1969). Variation of stimulus context and its effect on word finding ability in aphasics. *Cortex, 5,* 351-365.

Basso, A., Capitani, E., & Vignolo, L. A. (1979). Influence of rehabilitation on language skills in aphasic patients: A controlled study. *Archives of Neurology, 36,* 190-196.

Basso, A., Lecours, A. R., Morashini, S., & associates. (1985). Anatomo-clinical correlations of the aphasias as defined through computerized tomography: Exceptions. *Brain and Language, 26,* 201-229.

Bate, A. J., Mathias, J. L., & Crawford, J.R. (2001). Performance on the test of everyday attention and standard tests of attention following severe traumatic brain injury. *The Clinical Neuropsychologist, 15,* 405-422.

Bayles, K. A., Boone, D. R., Tomoeda, C. K., & associates. (1989). Differentiating Alzheimer patients from the normal elderly and stroke patients with aphasia. *Journal of Speech and Hearing Disorders, 54,* 74-87.

Bayles, K. A., Kaszniak, A. W., & Tomoeda, C. (1987). *Communication and cognition in normal aging and dementia.* Boston: College-Hill.

Bayles, K.A., Kim, E., Chapman, S.B., & associates. (2006). Evidence-based practice recommendations for working with individuals with dementia: Simulated presence therapy. *Journal of Medical Speech-Language Pathology, 14,* xiii-xvi.

Bayles, K. A., & Tomoeda, C. (1991). *Arizona battery for communication disorders of dementia* (Research ed.). Tucson, AZ: Canyonlands Publishing.

Benson, D. F. (1979a). *Aphasia, alexia, and agraphia.* New York: Churchill-Livingstone.

Benson, D. F. (1979b). Aphasia. In K. M. Heilman & E. Valenstein (Eds.) *Clinical neuropsychology* (pp. 22-58). New York: Oxford University Press.

Benton, A.L. (2003). *Benton Visual Retention Test-Fifth Edition,* San Antonio, TX: Psychological Corporation.

Benton, A. L., Smith, K. C., & Lang, M. (1972). Stimulus characteristics and object naming in aphasic patients. *Journal of Communication Disorders, 5,* 19-24.

Bergner, M. Bobbitt, R. A., Carter, W. B., & associates. (1981). The Sickness Impact Profile: Development and final revision of a health status measure. *Medical Care, 19,* 787-805.

Bernstein-Ellis, E., & Elman, R.J. (2007). *Group treatment of neurogenic communication disorders: The expert clinician's approach.* San Diego, CA: Plural.

Beukelman, D. R., & Yorkston, K. (1977). A communication system for the severely dysarthric speaker with an intact language system. *Journal of Speech and Hearing Disorders, 62,* 265-270.

Bird, M. (2001). Behavioural difficulties and cued recall of adaptive behavior in dementia. *Neuropsychological Rehabilitation, 11,* 357-375

Bisiach, E. (1966). Perceptual factors in the pathogenesis of anomia. *Cortex, 2,* 90-95.

Bisiach, E., Capitani, E., Luzzati, C., & associates. (1981). The brain and conscious representation of reality. *Neuropsychologia, 19,* 545-551.

Bisiach, E. and Luzzatti, C. 1987: Unilateral Neglect of Representational Space. *Cortex, 14,* 129-133.

Bisiach, E., Luzzati, C., & Perani, D. (1979). Unilateral neglect: Representational schema and consciousness. *Brain,* 102, 609-618.

Bisiach, E., Pizzamiglio, L., Nicco, D., & Atonnucci, G. (1996). Beyond unilateral neglect. *Brain, 119,* 851-857.

Blackman, D. K., Hoover, M., & Pinkston. E. M. (1976). Increasing participation in social interactions of the institutionalized elderly. *The Gerontologist, 16,* 69-76.

Blessed, G., Tomlinson, B. E., & Roth, M. (1968). The association between quantitative measures of dementia and senile change in the cerebral gray matter of elderly subjects. *British Journal of Psychiatry, 114,* 791-811.

Blonder, L. X., Bowers, D., & Heilman, K. M. (1991). The role of the right hemisphere in emotional communication. *Brain, 114,* 1115-1127.

Bloom, L. M. (1962). A rationale for group treatment of aphasic patients. *Journal of Speech and Hearing Disorders, 27,* 11-16.

Bloom, R. L., Borod, J. C., Obler, L. K., & associates. (1992). Impact of emotional content on discourse production in patients with unilateral brain damage. *Brain and Language, 42,* 153-164.

Bogner, J. A., Corrigan, J. D., Stange, M., & Rabold, D. (1999). Reliability of the Agitated Behavior Scale. *Journal of Head Trauma Rehabilitation, 14,* 91-96.

Boll, T. J. (1994). Neurologically impaired adults. In F. E. Miltersen & S. M. Turner (Eds.), *Diagnostic interviewing* (2nd ed., pp. 345-372). New York: Plenum.

Bond, M. R. (1976). Assessment of the psychosocial outcome of severe head injury. *Acta Neurochirurgica, 34,* 57-70.

Bonin, G. von. (1962). Anatomical asymmetries of the cerebral hemisphere. In V. B. Mountcastle (Ed.), *Interhemispheric relationships and cerebral dominance* (pp. 122-135). Baltimore, MD: Johns Hopkins Press.

Boning, R. A. (1990). *Specific skill series* (4th ed.). New York: Macmillan/McGraw-Hill.

Borkowski, J. G., Benton, A. L., & Spreen, O. (1967). Word fluency and brain damage. *Neuropsychologia, 5,* 135-140.

Boser, K. I., Weinrich, M., & McCall, D. (2000). Maintenance of oral production in agrammatic aphasia: Verb tense morphology training. *Neurorehabilitation and Neural Repair, 14,* 105-118.

Bowen, A., McKenna, K., & Tallis, R.C. (1999). Reasons for variability in the rate of occurrence of unilateral spatial neglect after stroke. *Stroke, 30,* 1196-1203.

Bourgeois, M. S. (1990). Enhancing conversational skills in patients with Alzheimer disease using a prosthetic memory aid. *Journal of Applied Behavior Analysis, 23,* 31-64.

Bourgeois, M. S. (1991). Communication treatment for adults with dementia. *Journal of Speech Language and Hearing Research, 34,* 831-844.

Bourgeois, M. S. (1992). Evaluating memory wallets in conversations with persons with dementia. *Journal of Speech Language and Hearing Research, 35,* 1344-1357.

Bourgeois, M.S., Camp, C., Rose, M., & associates (2003). A comparison of training strategies to enhance use of external aids by persons with dementia. *Journal of Communication Disorders, 36,* 361-378.

Bower, G. H., Black, J. B., & Turner, T. J. (1979). Scripts in memory for texts. *Cognitive Psychology, 11,* 177-220.

Bowers, S. A., & Marshall L. F. (1980). Outcome in 200 consecutive cases of severe head injury treated in San Diego County: A prospective analysis. *Neurosurgery, 6,* 237-242.

Boyd, T. M., & Sauter, S. W. (1994). Route finding: A measure of everyday executive functioning in the head-injured adult. *Applied Cognitive Psychology, 72,* 171-181.

Bryden, M. P., & Ley, R. G. (1983). Right hemispheric involvement in imagery. In E. Perecman (Ed.), *Cognitive processing in the right hemisphere* (pp. 111-123). New York: Academic Press.

Brink, T. L., Yesavage, J. A., Lum, O., & associates. (1982). Screening tests for geriatric depression. *Clinical Gerontologist, 1,* 37-44.

Brismar, B., Engstrom, A., & Rydberg, U. (1983). Head injury and intoxication: A diagnostic and therapeutic dilemma. *Acta Chirugica Scandinavia, 149,* 11-14.

Brodaty, H. Green, A., & Koschera, A. (2003). Meta-analysis of psychosocial interventions for caregivers of people with dementia. *Journal of the American Geriatric Society, 51,* 657-664.

Brooks, D. N. (1984). Cognitive deficits after head injury. In D. N. Brooks (Ed.), *Closed head injury: Psychological,* *social, and family consequences* (pp. 44-73). New York: Oxford University Press.

Brooks, N. (1989). Closed head trauma: Assessing the common cognitive processes. In M. Lezak (Ed.), *Assessment of the behavioral consequences of head trauma* (pp. 61-86). New York: A.R. Liss.

Brookshire, R. H. (1972). Effects of task difficulty on naming performance of aphasic subjects. *Journal of Speech and Hearing Research, 15,* 551-558.

Brookshire, R. H. (1975). Effects of prompting on spontaneous naming of pictures by aphasic subjects. *Journal of the Canadian Speech and Hearing Association, Autumn,* 63-71.

Brookshire, R. H. (1976). Effects of task difficulty on sentence comprehension performance of aphasic subjects. *Journal of Communication Disorders, 9,* 167-173.

Brookshire, R. H., Krueger, K., Nicholas, L., & associates. (1977). Analysis of clinician-patient interactions in aphasia treatment. In R. H. Brookshire (Ed.), *Clinical Aphasiology Conference proceedings* (pp. 181-187). Minneapolis, MN: BRK Publishers.

Brookshire, R. H., & Nicholas, L. E. (1984). Comprehension of directly and indirectly stated main ideas and details in discourse by brain-damaged and non-brain-damaged listeners. *Brain and Language, 21,* 21-36.

Brookshire, R. H., & Nicholas, L. E. (1985). Consistency of the effects of rate of speech on brain-damaged subjects' comprehension of information in narrative discourse. In R. H. Brookshire (Ed.), *Clinical aphasiology: Vol. 15* (pp. 262-271). Minneapolis, MN: BRK Publishers.

Brookshire, R. H., & Nicholas, L. E. (1993). *The discourse comprehension test.* Minneapolis, MN: BRK Publishers.

Brookshire, R. H., & Nicholas, L. E. (1995). Performance deviations in the connected speech of adults with no brain damage and adults with aphasia. *American Journal of Speech-Language Pathology, 4,* 118-123.

Brookshire, R. H., Nicholas, L. E., & Krueger, K. M. (1978). Sampling of speech pathology treatment activities: An evaluation of momentary and interval sampling procedures. *Journal of Speech and Hearing Research, 21,* 652-667.

Brookshire, R., Nicholas, L., Redmond, K., & associates. (1979). Effects of clinician behaviors on acceptability of patients' responses in aphasia treatment sessions. *Journal of Communication Disorders, 12,* 369-384.

Brown, J. I., Fischco, V. V., & Hanna, G. (1993). *The Nelson-Denny reading test.* Chicago: Riverside.

Brown, J. W. (1972). *Aphasia, apraxia, and agnosia: Clinical and theoretical aspects.* Springfield, IL: Charles C. Thomas.

Brownell, H., & Friedman, O. (2001). Discourse ability in patients with unilateral left and right hemisphere brain damage. In R. S. Berndt (Ed.), *Handbook of neuropsychology* (2nd ed., pp. 189-203). New York: Elsevier.

Brownell, H., Griffin, R., Winner, E., & associates. (2000). Cerebral lateralization and theory of mind. In S. Baron-Cohen, G. Tager-Flusberg, & D. J. Cohen (Eds.), *Understanding other minds* (2nd ed., pp. 306-333). New York: Oxford University Press.

Brownell, H., Pincus, D., Blum, D., & associates. (1997). The effects of right-hemisphere brain damage on patients' use of terms of personal reference. *Brain and Language, 57,* 60-79.

Brownell, H., Potter, H. H., Bihrle, A. M., & associates. (1986). Influence of deficits in right-brain-damaged patients. *Brain and Language, 27,* 310-321.

Brownell, H. H. (1988). The neuropsychology of narrative comprehension. *Aphasiology, 2,* 247-250.

Brush, J., & Camp, C. J. (1998). Using spaced-retrieval training as an intervention during speech-language therapy. *Clinical Gerontologist, 19,* 51-64.

Brust, J. C., Shafer, S. Q., Richter, R. W., & associates. (1976). Aphasia in acute stroke. *Stroke, 7,* 167-174.

Bryan, K. L. (1989). *The right hemisphere language battery.* Leicester, GB: Far Communications.

Bryan, K. L. (1995). *The right hemisphere language battery* (2nd ed.). London: Whurr Publishers.

Buckingham, H. W. (1979). Explanation in apraxia with consequences for the concept of apraxia of speech. *Brain and Language, 8,* 202-226.

Buckingham, H. W. (1992). Phonological production deficits in conduction aphasia. In S. E. Kohn (Ed.), *Conduction aphasia* (pp. 76-116). Hillsdale, NJ: Earlbaum.

Burgess, P. W., & Shallice, T. (1997). *Hayling Sentence Completion Test.* Suffolk, England: Thames Valley Test Company.

Burns, M. (1997). *Burns brief inventory of communication and cognition.* San Antonio: The Psychological Corporation.

Busch, C., & Brookshire, R. H. (1982). *Aphasic adults auditory comprehension of yes-no questions.* Unpublished manuscript.

Bushnik, T., Hanks. R. A., Kreutzer, J., Rosenthal, M. (2003). Etiology of traumatic brain injury: Characterization of differential outcomes up to one year postinjury. *Archives of Physical Medicine and Rehabilitation, 84,* 255-262.

Butfield, E., & Zangwill, O. L. (1946). Re-education in aphasia: A review of 70 cases. *Journal of Neurology, Neurosurgery and Psychiatry, 9,* 75-79.

Butters, N., Granholm, E., Salmon, D. P., & associates. (1987). Episodic and semantic memory: A comparison of amnesic and disoriented patients. *Journal of Clinical and Experimental Neuropsychology, 9,* 479-497.

Butterworth, B. Howard, D., & Mcloughlin, P. (1984). The semantic deficit in aphasia: The relationship between semantic errors in auditory comprehension and picture naming. *Neuropsychologia, 22,* 409-426.

Buxbaum, L. J., Ferraro, M. K., Veramonte, B. A., & associates (2004). Hemispatial neglect: subtypes, neuroanatomy, and disability. *Neurology, 62,* 749-756.

Camberg, L., Woods, P., Ooi, W. L., & associates (1999). Evaluation of simulated presence: A personalized approach to enhancing well-being in persons with Alzheimer's disease. *Journal of the American Geriatrics Society, 47,* 446-452.

Camp, C. J. (1989). Facilitation of new learning in AD. In G. Gilmore, P. Whitehouse, M. Wykle (Eds.). Memory and aging: Theory, research, and practice. New York: Springer Verlag (pp. 212-225).

Camp, C. J., Judge, K. S., Bye, C. A., & associates (1997). An intergenerational program for persons with dementia using Montessori methods. *Gerontologist, 37,* 688-692.

Cancelliere, A. E. B., & Kertesz, A. (1990). Lesion localization in acquired deficits of emotional expression and comprehension. *Brain and Cognition, 13,* 133-147.

Candelise, L., Landi., G., Orazio, E. N., & associates. (1985). Prognostic significance of hyperglycemia in acute stroke. *Archives of Neurology, 42,* 409-426.

Canter, G. J. (1973). *Dysarthria, apraxia of speech, and literal paraphasia: Three distinct varieties of articulatory behaviors in the adult with brain damage.* Paper presented at the annual convention of the American Speech and Hearing Association, Detroit.

Caplan, D. (1987). *Neurolinguistics and linguistic aphasiology.* New York: Cambridge University Press.

Caplan, D., Baker, C., & DeHaut, F. (1985). Syntactic determinants of sentence comprehension in aphasia. *Cognition, 21,* 117-125.

Caplan, L. R. (1993). *Stroke: A clinical approach.* Boston: Butterworth-Heinemann.

Cappa, S. F., Cavalotti, G., Guidotti, M., & associates. (1983). Subcortical aphasia: Two clinical CT-scan correlation studies. *Cortex, 19,* 227-242.

Cappa, S. F., Cavalotti, G., & Vignolo, L. (1981). Phonemic and lexical errors in fluent aphasia: Correlation with lesion site. *Neuropsychologia, 19,* 171-177.

Cappa, S. F., & Vignolo, L. A. (1979). Transcortical features of aphasia following left thalamic hemorrhage. *Cortex, 15,* 121-130.

Caramazza, A., & Zurif, E. B. (1976). Dissociation of algorithmic and heuristic processes in language comprehension: Evidence from aphasia. *Brain and Language, 3,* 572-582.

Carlsson, G. S., Svardsudd, K., & Welin, L. (1987). Long term effects of head injuries sustained during life in three male populations. *Journal of Neuropsychology, 67,* 197-205.

Carney, N., Chesnut, R.M., Maynard, H., & associates. (1999). Effect of cognitive rehabilitation on outcomes for persons with traumatic brain injury: A review. *Journal of Head Trauma Rehabilitation, 14,* 277-307.

Caronna, J., & Levy, D. (1983). Clinical predictors of outcome in ischemic stroke. In H. J. M. Barnett (Ed.), *Neurologic clinics: Cerebrovascular disease* (pp. 103-117). Philadelphia: W.B. Saunders.

Carrow-Woodfolk, E. (1999). *Test for auditory comprehension of language* (3rd ed.). Austin, TX: Pro-Ed.

Cartensen, L. L., & Erickson, R. J. (1986). Enhancing the social environments of elderly nursing home residents: Are high rates of interaction enough? *Journal of Applied Behavior Analysis, 19,* 349-355.

Carver, R. P. (1973). Reading as reasoning: Implications for measurement. In W. H. MacGinitie (Ed.), *Assessment problems in reading* (pp. 173-195). Newark, DE: International Reading Association.

Cassidy, T. P., Burce, D. W., Lewis, S., & Gray, C. S. (1999). The association of visual field deficits and visuo-spatial neglect in acute right-hemisphere stroke patients. *Age and Ageing, 28,* 257-260.

Cassidy, T. P., Lewis, S., & Gray, C. S. (1998). Recovery from visuospatial neglect in stroke patients. *Journal of Neurology, Neurosurgery and Psychiatry, 64,* 555-557.

Celesia, G. G., & Wanamaker, W. M. (1972). Psychiatric disturbances in Parkinson disease. *Diseases of the Nervous System, 33,* 577-583.

Centers for Disease Control and Prevention. (1995). CDC quality of life as a new public health measure: Behavioral risk factor surveillance system. Atlanta, GA: U.S. Department of Health and Human Services.

Centers for Disease Control and Prevention. (1997). *Traumatic brain injury: Colorado, Missouri, Oklahoma, and Utah, 1990-1993* (MMWR Report #46, pp. 8-11). Atlanta, GA: Centers for Disease Control and Prevention, U.S. Department of Health and Human Services.

Centers for Disease Control and Prevention. (2001). *Traumatic brain injury: Mortality and morbidity.* Atlanta, GA: National Center for Health Statistics, U.S. Department of Health and Human Services.

Centers for Disease Control and Prevention. (2005). *Stroke: Facts and statistics.* Atlanta, GA: National Center for Heart Disease and Stroke Prevention, U.S. Department of Health and Human Services.

Cermak, L. S. (1975). Imagery as an aid to retrieval in alcoholic Korsakoff patients. *Cortex, 11,* 163-169.

Chall, J. S. (1983). *Stages of reading development.* New York: McGraw-Hill.

Chamberlain, E. (2003). Test review: The behavioural assessment of the dysexecutive syndrome (BADS). *Journal of Occupational Psychology, Employment, and Disability, 5,* 33-37.

Cherney, L. and Halper, A. (2001). Visual neglect in right-hemisphere stroke: A longitudinal study. *Brain Injury, 15,* 585-592.

Cherney, L. R., Halper, A. S., & Miller, T. K. (1991). Treatment of communication problems. In A. S. Halper, L. R. Cherney, & T. K. Miller (Eds.), *Clinical management of communication problems in adults with traumatic brain injury* (pp. 57-131). Gaithersburg, MD: Aspen.

Cherry, K. E., & Simmons-D'Gerolamo. (2004). Spaced-retrieval with probable Alzheimer's. *Clinical Gerontologist, 27,* 139-157.

Cherry, K. E., & Simmons-D'Gerolamo. (2005). Long-term effectiveness of spaced-retrieval memory training for older adults with probable Alzheimer's disease. *Experimental Aging Research, 31,* 261-289.

Chumpelik, D. (1984). The PROMPT system of therapy: Theoretical framework and applications for developmental apraxia of speech. *Seminars in Speech and Language, 5,* 139-156.

Cicerone, K. D. (2004). Participation as an outcome of traumatic brain injury rehabilitation. *Journal of Head Trauma Rehabilitation, 19,* 494-501.

Cicerone, K. D., Dahlberg, C., Malec, J. F., & associates. (2005). Evidence-based cognitive rehabilitation: Updated review of the literature from 1998 through 2002. *Archives of Physical Medicine and Rehabilitation, 86,* 1681-1692.

Cicone, M., Wapner, W., & Gardner, H. (1980). Sensitivity to emotional expressions and situations in organic patients. *Brain and Language, 16,* 145-158.

Clark, H. H., & Haviland, S. E. (1977). Comprehension and the given-new contract. In R. O. Freedle (Ed.), *Discourse comprehension and production* (pp. 1-40). Norwood, NJ: Ablex.

Clark, H. M., & Robin, D. A. (1995). Sense of effort during a lexical decision task: Resource allocation deficits following brain injury. *American Journal of Speech Language Pathology, 4,* 143-147.

Clarke, L., & Witte, K. (1990). Nature and efficacy of communication management in Alzheimer disease. In R. Lubinski (Ed.), *Dementia and communication* (pp. 238-256). Philadelphia: B.C. Decker.

Cohn, R., Neumann, M. S., & Wood, N. H. (1977). Prosopagnosia: A clinicopathological study. *Annals of Neurology, 1,* 177-182.

Collins, M. (1991). *Global aphasia.* San Diego: College-Hill Press.

Colsher, P. L., Cooper, W. E., & Graff-Radford, N. (1987). Intonational variability in the speech of right-hemisphere damaged patients. *Brain and Language, 32,* 379-383.

Cooke, D. D., McNally, K. T., Mulligan, M. J. G., & associates. (2001). Psychosocial interventions for caregivers of people with dementia: A systematic review. *Aging and Mental Health, 5,* 120-135.

Corbin, M. L. (1951). Group speech therapy for motor aphasia and dysarthria. *Journal of Speech and Hearing Disorders, 16,* 21-34.

Corkin, S. H., Hurt, R. W., Twitchell, T. E., & associates. (1987). Consequences of penetrating and nonpenetrating head injury: Posttraumatic amnesia, and lasting effects on cognition. In H. S. Levin, J. Grafman, & H. M. Eisenberg (Eds.), *Neurobehavioral recovery from head injury* (pp. 318-329). New York: Oxford University Press.

Corlew, M. M., & Nation, J. E. (1975). Characteristics of visual stimuli and naming performance in aphasic adults. *Cortex, 11,* 186-191.

Correia, L., Brookshire, R. H., & Nicholas, L. E. (1990). Aphasic and non-brain-damaged adults' descriptions of aphasia test pictures and gender-biased pictures. *Journal of Speech and Hearing Disorders, 55,* 713-720.

Courville, C. B. (1937). *Pathology of the central nervous system.* Mountain View, CA: Pacific.

Cowan, N. (1984). On short and long auditory stores. *Psychological Bulletin, 96,* 341-370.

Coyne, M. L., & Hoskins, L. (1997). Improving eating behaviors in dementia using behavioral strategies. *Clinical Nursing Research, 6,* 275-290.

Craik, F. I., & Lockhart, R. S. (1972). Levels of processing: A framework for memory research. *Journal of Verbal Learning and Verbal Behavior, 11,* 671-684.

Crary, M. A., Haak, M. J., & Malinsky, A. E. (1989). Preliminary psychometric evaluation of an acute aphasia screening protocol. *Aphasiology, 2,* 67-78.

Crary, M. A., & Rothi, L. J. G. (1989). Predicting the Western aphasia battery aphasia quotient. *Journal of Speech and Hearing Disorders, 54,* 163-166.

Crosson, B., Barco, P. P., Velozo, C. A., & associates. (1989). Awareness and compensation in postacute head injury rehabilitation. *Journal of Head Trauma Rehabilitation, 4,* 46-54.

Croft, C. B., Shprintzen, R. J., & Rakoff, S. J. (1981). Patterns of velopharyngeal valving in normal and cleft palate subjects: A multi-view videofluoroscopic and naso-endoscopic study. *Laryngoscope, 91,* 265-271.

Culton, G. L. (1969). Spontaneous recovery from aphasia. *Journal of Speech and Hearing Research, 12,* 825-832.

Cummings, J. L. (1990). Clinical diagnosis of Alzheimer disease. In J. L. Cummings & B. L. Miller (Eds.), *Alzheimer disease: Treatment and long-term management* (pp. 3-20). New York: Dekker.

Cummings, J. L., & Benson, D. F. (1983). *Dementia: A clinical approach.* Boston: Butterworth.

Cummings, J. L., & Benson, D. F. (1984). Subcortical dementia: Review of an emerging concept. *Archives of Neurology, 41,* 874-879.

Cummings, J. L., & Benson, D. F. (1992). *Dementia: A clinical approach* (2nd ed.). Boston: Butterworth-Heinemann.

Dabul, B. (2000). *The apraxia battery for adults* (2nd ed.). Austin, TX: Pro-Ed.

Dabul, B., & Bollier, B. (1976). Therapeutic approaches to apraxia. *Journal of Speech and Hearing Disorders, 41,* 268-276.

Dale, E., & Chall, J. S. (1948). A formula for predicting readability. *Educational Research Bulletin, 27,* 11-20.

Dalston, R., Warren, D. W., & Dalston, E. T. (1990). The modified tongue-anchor technique as a screening test for velopharyngeal inadequacy: A reassessment. *Journal of Speech and Hearing Disorders, 55,* 510.

Damasio, A. R. (1985). Disorders of complex visual processing: Agnosias, achromatopsia, Baliut syndrome, and related difficulties of orientation and construction. In M. M. Mesulum (Ed.), *Principles of behavioral neurology* (pp. 259-288). Philadelphia: F.A. Davis.

Damasio, A. R., & Damasio, H. (1983). Localization of lesions in achromatopsia and prosopagnosia. In A. Kertesz (Ed.), *Localization in neuropsychology* (pp. 417-428). New York: Academic Press.

Damasio A. R., Damasio H., Rizzo M., Varney N., & Gersh F. (1982). Aphasia with non-hemorrhagic lesions in the basal ganglia and internal capsule. *Archives of Neurology, 39,* 15-24.

Damico, J. (1992). *Whole language for special-needs children.* Buffalo, NY: Educom Associates.

Darley, F. L. (1969). *The classification of output disturbance in neurologic communication disorders.* Paper presented at the American Speech and Hearing Association Convention, Chicago.

Darley, F. L. (1982). *Aphasia.* Philadelphia: W.B. Saunders.

Darley, F. L., Aronson, A. E., & Brown, J. R. (1975). *Motor speech disorders.* Philadelphia, W.B. Saunders.

Davis, G. A. (1993). *A survey of adult aphasia and related language disorders* (2nd ed.). Englewood Cliffs, NJ: Prentice-Hall.

Davis, G.A. (2000). *Aphasiology: Disorders and clinical practice.* Boston: Allyn & Bacon.

Davis, G. A., & Wilcox, M. J. (1985). *Adult aphasia rehabilitation: Language pragmatics.* San Diego, CA: College-Hill.

Deaton, A. V. (1991). Group interventions for cognitive rehabilitation: Increasing the challenges. In J. S. Kreutzer & P. H. Wehman (Eds.), *Cognitive rehabilitation for persons with traumatic brain injury: A functional approach* (pp. 178-190). Baltimore: Paul H. Brookes.

De Bruin, A. F., Kiederiks, J. P. M., De Witte, L. P. and associates. (1994). The development of a short generic version of the sickness impact profile. *Journal of Clinical Epidemiology, 47,* 407-418.

DeKosky, S. T., Heilman, K. M., Bowers, D., & associates. (1980). Recognition and discrimination of emotional faces and pictures. *Brain and Language, 9,* 206-214.

Delis, D. C., Kramer, J. H., Kaplan, E., & associates. (2000). *The California verbal learning test: Second Edition.* San Antonio, TX: The Psychological Corporation.

DeRenzi, E. (1989). Apraxia. In F. Boller, J. Grafman (Eds.), *Handbook of neuropsychology,* Vol 2. Amsterdam: Elsevier, 245-263.

DeRenzi, E., & Ferrari, C. (1978). The reporter test: A sensitive test to detect expressive disturbances in aphasics. *Cortex, 14,* 279-283.

DeRenzi, E., Pieszuro, A., & Vignolo, L. A. (1966). Oral apraxia and aphasia. *Cortex, 2,* 50-73.

DeRenzi, E., & Vignolo, L. A. (1962). The token test: A sensitive test to detect receptive disturbances in aphasics. *Brain, 85,* 665-678.

Deutsch, S. E. (1981). Oral form identification as a measure of cortical sensory dysfunction in apraxia of speech and aphasia. *Journal of Communication Disorders, 14,* 65-71.

Deutsch, S. E. (1984). Prediction of site of lesion from speech apraxic error patterns. In J. C. Rosenbek, M. R. McNeil, & A. E. Aronson (Eds.), *Apraxia of speech, physiology, acoustics, linguistics, management* (pp. 113-134). San Diego: College-Hill.

Dewitt, L. D., Grek, A. J., Buonanno, F. S., & associates. (1985). MRI and the study of aphasia. *Neurology, 35,* 861-865.

Dickson, D. W. (2001). Neuropathology of Alzheimer's disease and other dementias. *Clinical Geriatric Medicine, 17,* 209-228.

Diener, E., Emmons, R.A., Larsen, R. J., & Griffin, S. (1985). The satisfaction with life scale. *Journal of Personality Assessment, 49,* 71-75.

Dikman, S. S., Machamer, J. E., Winn, H. B, & Tempkin, N. R. (1995). Neuropsychological outcome 1-year post head injury. *Neuropsychology, 9,* 80-90.

Diggs, C. C., & Basili, A. G. (1987). Verbal expression of right CVA patients. *Brain and Language, 30,* 130-147.

Diller, L., & Weinberg, J. (1977). Differential aspects of attention in brain-damaged persons. *Perceptual and Motor Skills, 35,* 71-81.

Disimoni, F. (1989). *The comprehensive apraxia test.* Dalton, PA: Praxis House Publishers.

Disimoni, F., Keith, R., & Darley, F. (1980). Prediction of PICA overall scores by short versions of the test. *Journal of Speech and Hearing Research, 25,* 511-576.

Disimoni, F., Keith, R., Holt, D., & associates. (1975). Practicality of shortening the PICA. *Journal of Speech and Hearing Research, 18,* 491-497.

Dobkin, J. A., Levine, R. L., Lagreze, H. L., & associates (1989). Evidence for transhemispheric diaschisis in unilateral stroke. *Archives of Neurology, 46,* 1333-1336.

Doricchi, F., & Angelelli, P. (1999). Misrepresentation of horizontal space in unilateral neglect. Role of hemianopia. *Neurology, 52,* 1845-1857.

Doyle, P., Goldstein, H., & Bourgeois, M. (1987). Experimental analysis of syntax training in Broca aphasia: A generalization and social validation study. *Journal of Speech and Hearing Disorders, 52,* 143-155.

Duffy, J. R. (1987). Slowly progressive aphasia. In R. H. Brookshire (Ed.), *Clinical aphasiology* (pp. 349-356). Minneapolis, MN: BRK Publishers.

Duffy, J. R. (1995). *Motor speech disorders: Substrates, differential diagnosis, and management.* St. Louis, MO: Mosby.

Duffy, J. R. (2005). *Motor speech disorders* (2nd ed.). St. Louis, MO: Elsevier/Mosby.

Duffy, J. R., Keith, R. L., Shane, H., & associates. (1976). Performance of normal (non-brain-injured) adults on the Porch index of communicative ability. In R. H. Brookshire (Ed.), *Clinical Aphasiology Conference proceedings* (pp. 32-42). Minneapolis, MN: BRK Publishers.

Dunlop, J. M., & Marquardt, T. P. (1977). Linguistic and articulatory aspects of single word production in apraxia of speech. *Cortex, 13,* 17-29.

Dunn, L. M., & Dunn, L. M. (1997). *Peabody picture vocabulary test* (Rev. ed.). Circle Pines, MN: American Guidence Service.

Dworkin, J. P., & Johns, D. F. (1980). Management of velopharyngeal incompetence in dysarthria: A review. *Clinical Otolaryngology, 5,* 61-74.

Eastwood, M. R., Lautenschlaeger, E., & Corbin, S. (1983). A comparison of clinical methods for assessing dementia. *Journal of the American Geriatrics Society, 31,* 342-347.

Eisenberg, H. M., & Weiner, R. L. (1987). Input variables: How information from the acute injury can be used to characterize groups of patients for studies of outcome. In H. S. Levin, J. Grafman, & H. M. Eisenberg (Eds.), *Neurobehavioral recovery from head injury* (pp. 13-29). New York: Oxford University Press.

Eisenson, J. (1964). Aphasia: A point of view as to the nature of the disorder and factors that determine prognosis for recovery. *Neurology, 4,* 287-295.

Eisenson, J. (1974). *Examining for aphasia.* New York: The Psychological Corporation.

Elman, R. J. (1999). Introduction to group treatment of neurogenic communication disorders. In R. J. Elman (Ed.), *Group treatment of neurogenic communication disorders: The expert clinician approach* (pp. 3-7). Boston: Butterworth-Heinemann.

Elman, R. J., & Bernstein-Ellis, E. (1995). What is functional? *American Journal of Speech-Language Pathology, 4,* 115-117.

Ellwood, P. (1988). Shattuck lecture—Outcomes management: A technology of patient experience. *New England Journal of Medicine, 318,* 1549-1556.

Erlich, J. S., & Sipes, A. L. (1985). Group treatment of communication skills for head trauma patients. *Cognitive Rehabilitation, 3,* 32-37.

Evans, D. A., Funkenstein, H. H., Albert, M. A., & associates. (1989). Prevalence of Alzheimer disease in a community population of older persons: Higher than previously reported. *Journal of the American Medical Association, 262,* 2552-2556.

Evans, R. W., Palsane, M. N., & Carrere, S. (1987). Type A behavior and occupational stress: A cross-cultural study of blue-collar workers. *Journal of Personality and Social Psychology, 36,* 1213-1220.

Ewert, J., Levin, H. S., Watson, M. C., & associates. (1989). Procedural memory during posttraumatic amnesia in survivors of severe closed head injury. *Archives of Neurology, 46,* 911-916.

Faber, M. M., & Aten, F. L. (1979). Verbal performance in aphasic patients in response to intact and altered pictorial stimuli. In R. H. Brookshire (Ed.), *Clinical Aphasiology Conference proceedings* (pp. 177-186). Minneapolis, MN: BRK Publishers.

Fasotti L., Kovacs F., Eling P. A. T. M., Brouwer W. H. (2000). Time pressure management as a compensatory strategy training after closed head injury. *Neuropsychological Rehabilitation, 10,* 47-65.

Ferber, S., & Karnath, H. (2001). How to assess spatial neglect —line bisection or cancellation tasks? *Journal of Clinical and Experimental Neuropsychology, 23,* 599-607.

Ferber, S., & Karnath, H.O. (1999). Parietal and occipital lobe contributions to perception of straight ahead orientation. *Journal of Neurology, Neurosurgery, Psychiatry, 67,* 572-578.

Ferro, J. M., Kertesz, A., & Black, S. E. (1987). Subcortical neglect: Quantification, anatomy, and recovery. *Neurology, 37,* 1487-1492.

Filley, C. M., Cranberg, L. D., Alexander, M. P., & associates. (1987). Neurobehavioral outcome after closed head injury in childhood and adolescence. *Archives of Neurology, 44,* 194-198.

Finlayson, M. A. J., & Garner, S. H. (1994). Challenges in rehabilitation of individuals with acquired brain injury. In M. Allen, M. A. J. Finlayson, & S. H. Garner (Eds.), *Brain injury rehabilitation: Clinical considerations* (pp. 3-10). Baltimore: Williams & Wilkins.

Fischer, S. Gauggel, S., & Trexler, L. (2004). Awareness of activity limitations, goal setting, and rehabilitation outcome in patients with brain injury. *Brain Injury, 18,* 547-562.

Fitch-West, J., & Sands, E. S. (1987). *Bedside evaluation screening test.* Rockville, MD: Aspen.

Fleming, J., & Strong, J. (1995). Self-awareness of deficits following brain injury: Considerations for rehabilitation. *British Journal of Occupational Therapy, 58,* 55-60.

Fleming, J., & Strong, J. (1999). A longitudinal study of self-awareness: Functional deficits overestimated by persons with brain injury. *Occupational Therapy Journal of Research, 19,* 3-17.

Flesch, R. F. (1948). A new readability yardstick. *Journal of Applied Psychology, 32,* 221-223.

Folstein, M. F., Folstein, S. E., & McHugh, P. R. (1975). Mini mental state. *Journal of Psychiatric Research, 12,* 189-198.

Fox, D. R., & Johns, D. F. (1970). Predicting velopharyngeal closure with a modified tongue-anchor technique. *Journal of Speech and Hearing Disorders, 35,* 248.

Frattali, C. M. (1992). Functional assessment of communication: Merging public policy with clinical views. *Aphasiology, 6,* 63-83.

Frattali, C. M. (1998). Assessing functional outcomes: An overview. *Seminars in Speech and Language, 19,* 198-221.

Frattali, C. M., Thompson, C. K., Holland, A. L., & associates. (1995). Functional assessment of communication skills for adults: ASHA FACS. Rockville, MD: American Speech-Language Hearing Association.

Friedman, A., & Polson, M. C. (1981). The hemispheres as independent processing systems: Limited capacity processing and cerebral specialization. *Journal of Experimental Psychology: Human Perception and Performance, 7,* 1031-1058.

Friedman, W. A. (1983). *Head injuries.* CIBA Clinical Symposia, Summit, NJ: CIBA Pharmaceutical Company.

Fromm, D., & Holland, A. L. (1989). Functional communication in Alzheimer disease. *Journal of Speech and Hearing Disorders, 54,* 535-540.

Frymark, T. (2003). FIM or foe? Functional independence measures fall short, data show. *ASHA Leader, 8,* 6-9.

Gaddes, W. H., & Crockett, D. J. (1973). *The Spreen-Benton aphasia test: Normative data as a measure of normal language development* (Research monograph #25). Victoria, British Columbia, Canada: Neuropsychology Laboratory, University of Victoria.

Gainotti, G. (1991). Frontal lobe damage and disorders of affect and personality. In M. Swash & J. Oxbury (Eds.), *Clinical neurology* (pp. 71-81). Edinburgh: Churchill-Livingstone.

Gainotti, G., & Tiacci, C. (1970). Patterns of drawing disability in left and right hemisphere patients. *Neuropsychologia, 8,* 379-384.

Gao, S., Hendrie, M. B., Hall, K. S., & associates. (1998). The relationships between age, sex, and the incidence of dementia and Alzheimer disease. *Archives of General Psychiatry, 55,* 809-815.

Gardiner, B. J., & Brookshire, R. H. (1972). Effects of unisensory and multisensory presentation of stimuli upon naming by aphasic subjects. *Language and Speech, 15,* 342-357.

Gardner, H., Albert, M. L., & Weintraub, S. (1975). Comprehending a word: The influence of speed and redundancy on auditory comprehension in aphasia. *Cortex, 11,* 155-162.

Gardner, H., Brownell, H. H., Wapner, W., & associates. (1983). Missing the point: The role of right hemisphere in the processing of complex linguistic materials. In E. Perecman (Ed.), *Cognitive processing in the right hemisphere* (pp. 169-192). New York: Academic Press.

Garner, S. H., & Valadka, A. B. (1994). Medical management and principles of head injury rehabilitation. In M. A. J. Finlayson & S. H. Garner (Eds.), *Brain injury rehabilitation: Clinical considerations* (pp. 83-101). Baltimore: Williams & Wilkins.

Gates, W. H., MacGinitie, R. K., Maria, K., & associates. (2000). *Gates-MacGinitie reading tests.* Chicago: Riverside.

Gauthier, L., Dehaut, F., & Joanette, Y. (1989). The Bells Test: A quantitative and qualitative test for visual neglect. *International Journal of Clinical Neuropsychology, 11,* 49-54.

German, D. J. (1990). *Test of adolescent/adult word finding.* Austin, TX: Pro-Ed.

Geschwind, N. (1975). The apraxias: Neural mechanisms of disorders of learned movement. *American Scientist, 63,* 188-195.

Geschwind, N., Quadfasel, F.A., & Segarra, J. (1968). Isolation of the speech area. *Neuropsychologia, 6,* 327-340.

Gilchrist, E., & Wilkinson, M. (1979). Some factors determining prognosis in young people with severe head injuries. *Archives of Neurology, 36,* 355-359.

Giles, G. M., & Clark-Wilson, J. (1993). *Brain injury rehabilitation: A neurofunctional approach.* London: Chapman & Hall.

Gillen R, Tennen H, & McKee T. (2005). Unilateral spatial neglect: relation to rehabilitation outcomes in patients with right hemisphere stroke. *Archives of Physical Medicine & Rehabilitation, 86,* 763-767.

Gilson, J. S., Gilson, R. M., Bertner, R. A., & associates. (1975). The Sickness Impact Profile: Development of an outcome measure of health care. *American Journal of Public Health, 65,* 1304-1310.

Glisky, E. L., & Schacter, D. L. (1986). Remediation of organic memory disorders: Current status and future prospects. *Journal of Head Trauma Rehabilitation, 1,* 54-63.

Gloag, D. (1985). Rehabilitation after head injury: Cognitive problems. *British Medical Journal, 290,* 834-837.

Glonig, I., Glonig, K., Haub, C., & associates. (1969). Comparison of verbal behavior in right-handed and non-right-handed patients with anatomically verified lesion of one hemisphere. *Cortex, 5,* 43-52.

Glonig, K., Trappl, R., Heiss, W. D., & associates. (1976). Prognosis and speech therapy in aphasia. In Y. Lebrun & R. Hoops (Eds.), *Recovery in aphasics* (pp. 57-64). Atlantic Highlands, NJ: Humanities Press.

Glosser, G., & Deser, T. (1990). Patterns of discourse production among neurological patients with fluent language disorders. *Brain and Language, 40,* 67-88.

Glosser, G., & Goodglass, H. (1990). Disorders in executive control functions among aphasic and other brain-damaged patients. *Journal of Clinical and Experimental Neuropsychology, 12,* 485-501.

Glosser, G., Wiener, M., & Kaplan, E. (1988). Variations in aphasic language behaviors. *Journal of Speech and Hearing Research, 53,* 115-124.

Godfrey, H., & Knight, R. (1985). Cognitive rehabilitation of memory functioning in amnesic alcoholics. *Journal of Consulting and Clinical Psychology, 43,* 555-557.

Golden, C. J. (1978). *The Stroop color and word test.* Chicago: Stoelting.

Goldman-Eisler, F. (1968). *Psycholinguistics: Experiments in spontaneous speech.* New York: Academic Press.

Goldstein, K. (1948). *Language and language disturbances.* New York: Grune & Stratton.

Golper, L. A. C., & Cherney, L. (1999). Back to basics: Assessment practices with neurogenic communication disorders. *Neurophysiology and Neurogenic Speech and Language Disorders, 9,* 3-8.

Golper, L. A. C., Thorpe, P., Tompkins, C., & associates. (1980). Connected language sampling: An expanded index of aphasic language behavior. In R. H. Brookshire (Ed.), *Clinical Aphasiology Conference proceedings,* (pp. 174-186). Minneapolis, MN: BRK Publishers.

Gonzalez, J., & Aronson, A. (1970). Palatal lift prosthesis for treatment of anatomic and neurologic palatopharyngeal insufficiency. *Cleft Palate Journal, 7,* 91-104.

Goodglass, H. (1993). *Understanding aphasia.* San Diego, CA: Academic Press.

Goodglass, H., Blumstein, S. E., Gleason, J. B., & associates. (1979). The effect of syntactic encoding on sentence comprehension in aphasia. *Brain and Language, 7,* 201-209.

Goodglass, H., & Kaplan, E. (1972, 1983). *The Boston diagnostic aphasia examination.* Philadelphia: Lea & Febiger.

Goodglass, H., & Kaplan, E. (1983). *The assessment of aphasia and related disorders* (2nd ed.). Philadelphia: Lea & Febiger.

Goodglass, H., Kaplan, E., & Barresi, B. (2001). *The assessment of aphasia and related disorders* (3rd ed.). Philadelphia: Lippincott Williams & Wilkins.

Goodglass, H., Kaplan, E., & Barresi, B. (2001a). *The Boston diagnostic aphasia examination* (3rd ed.). Philadelphia: Lippincott Williams & Wilkins.

Goodglass, H., Kaplan, E., Weintraub, S., & associates. (1976). The tip of the tongue phenomenon in aphasia. *Cortex, 12,* 145-153.

Goodglass, H., Klein, B., Carey, P., & associates. (1966). Specific semantic word categories in aphasia. *Cortex, 2,* 74-89.

Goodglass, H., & Quadfasel, F. (1954). Language laterality in left-handed aphasics. *Brain, 77,* 523-528.

Goodglass, H., & Stuss, D. T. (1979). Naming to picture versus description in three aphasia subgroups. *Cortex, 15,* 199-211.

Gordon, W. A., Ruckdeschel-Hibbard, M., Egelko, S., & associates. (1984). *Evaluation of the deficits associated with right brain damage: Normative data on the Institute of Rehabilitation Medicine test battery.* New York: Department of Behavioral Sciences, N.Y.U. Medical Center.

Gorzell, G. J., Kaiser, K., & Camp, C. J. (2003). Montessori-based training makes a difference for home health workers and their clients. *Caring, 22,* 40-42.

Gouvier, W. D., Blandon, P. D., LaPorte, K. K., & associates. (1987). Reliability and validity of the Disability Rating Scale and the Levels of Cognitive Functioning Scale in monitoring recovery from severe head injury. *Archives of Physical Medicine and Rehabilitation, 68,* 94-97.

Grafman, J., & Salazar, A. (1987). Methodological considerations relevant to the comparison of recovery from penetrating and closed head injuries. In H. S. Levin, J. Grafman, & H. M. Eisenberg (Eds.), *Neurobehavioral recovery from head injury* (pp. 43-54). New York: Oxford.

Graham, D. I., Adams, J. H., & Doyle, D. (1978). Ischemic brain damage in fatal non-missile head injuries. *Journal of Neurological Science, 39,* 213.

Graham, R. K., & Kendall, B. S. (1960). The memory for designs test: Revised general manual. *Perceptual and Motor Skills, 11*(Monograph Suppl. 2-VIII), 147-188.

Grant, D. A., & Berg, E. A. (1948). A behavioral analysis of degree of reinforcement and ease of shifting to new responses in a Weigl-type card sorting problem. *Journal of Experimental Psychology, 38,* 404-411.

Gray, L., Hoyt, P., Mogil, S., & associates. (1977). A comparison of clinical tests of yes/no questions in aphasia. In R. H. Brookshire (Ed.), *Clinical Aphasiology Conference proceedings* (pp. 265-268). Minneapolis, MN: BRK Publishers.

Greenberg, D. A., Aminoff, M. J., & Simon, R. P. (1996). *Clinical neurology* (2nd ed.). Norwalk, CT: Appleton & Lange.

Gronwall, D. M. A. (1997). Paced auditory serial addition task: A measure of recovery from concussion. *Perceptual and Motor Skills, 44,* 367-373.

Guilford, A. M., & Hawk, A. M. (1968). A comparative study of form identification in neurologically impaired and normal subjects. In A. Smith (Ed.), *Speech and hearing science research reports* (pp. 34-37). Ann Arbor, MI: University of Michigan.

Gunning, R. (1952). *The technique of clear writing.* New York: McGraw-Hill.

Haas, J., Cope, D. N., & Hall, K. (1987). Premorbid prevalence of poor academic performance in severe head injury. *Journal of Neurology, Neurosurgery, and Psychiatry, 50,* 52-56.

Hachinski, V. C., Lassen, N. A., & Marshall, J. (1974). Multi-infarct dementia: A cause of mental deterioration in the elderly. *Lancet, 2,* 207-210.

Hageman, C. (1997). Flaccid dysarthria. In M. R. McNeil (Ed.), *Clinical management of sensorimotor speech disorders* (pp. 193-215). New York: Thieme.

Hagen, C. (1997). The *Rancho Los Amigos Scale of Cognitive Levels-Revised.* Unpublished document. (Personal communication from author, 2005.)

Hagen, C., & Malkamus, D. (1979). *Interaction strategies for language disorders secondary to head trauma.* Paper presented at the annual convention of the American Speech-Language-Hearing Association, Atlanta, GA.

Hall, K., Cope, N., & Rappoport, M. (1985). The Glasgow Outcome Scale and the Disability Rating Scale: Comparative usefulness in following recovery in traumatic head injury. *Archives of Physical Medicine and Rehabilitation, 66,* 35-37.

Halliday, M. A. K., & Hasan, R. (1976). *Cohesion in English.* New York: Longman.

Halligan, P. W., Manning, L., & Marshall, J. C. (1991). Hemispheric activation via spatiomotor cueing in visual neglect: A case study. *Neuropsychologia, 29,* 165-176.

Halligan, P. W., Marshall, J. C., & Wade, D. T. (1989). Visuospatial neglect: Underlying factors and test sensitivity. *Lancet, 14,* 908-911.

Halligan, P., Wilson, B., & Cockburn, J. (1990). A short screening test for visual neglect in stroke patients. *International Disability Studies, 12,* 95-99.

Halper, A. S., Cherney, L. R., Burns, M. S., & associates. (1996). *Clinical management of right hemisphere dysfunction* (2nd ed.). Rockville, MD: Aspen.

Halpern, H. (1965). Effect of stimulus variables on dysphasic verbal errors. *Perceptual and Motor Skills, 21,* 291-298.

Hammill, D. D. (1985). *Detroit Test of Learning Aptitudes.* Austin, TX: Pro-Ed.

Hannay, H. J., Levin, H. S., & Grossman, R. G. (1979). Impaired recognition memory after head injury. *Cortex, 15,* 269-283.

Happe, F., Brownell, H., & Winner, E. (1999). Acquired theory of mind impairments following stroke. *Cognition, 70,* 211-240.

Hardy, J. C., Rembolt, R. R., Spreisterbach, D. C., & associates. (1961). Surgical management of palatal paresis and speech problems in cerebral palsy. *Journal of Speech and Hearing Disorders, 26,* 320-327.

Hart, T., & Hayden, M. E. (1986). The ecological validity of neuropsychological assessment and remediation. In B. P. Uzzell, & Y. Gross (Eds.), *Clinical neuropsychology of intervention* (pp. 21-50). Boston: Martinus Nijhoff.

Harvey, A. M., Johns, R. J., McKusick, V. A., & associates. (1988). *The principles and practice of medicine* (19th ed.). Norwalk, CT: Appleton & Lange.

Hawley, K.S., & Cherry, K.E. (2004). Spaced-retrieval effects on name-face recognition in older adults with probable Alzheimer's disease. *Behavior Modification, 28,* 276-296.

Hayes, D. P. (1989). *Guide to the lexical analysis of texts.* (Tech. Rep. Series 89-96). Ithaca, NY: Cornell University Department of Sociology.

Heard, K., & Watson, T. (1999). Reducing wandering by persons with dementia using differential reinforcement. *Journal of Applied Behavior Analysis, 32,* 381-384.

Heath, P. D., Kennedy, P., & Kapur, N. (1983). Slowly progressive aphasia without generalized dementia. *Annals of Neurology, 13,* 687-688.

Hecaen, H., & Angelergues, D. (1962). Agnosia for faces. *Archives of Neurology, 7,* 92-100.

Hecaen, H., & Assal, G. (1970). A comparison of constructive deficits following left and right hemisphere lesions. *Neuropsychologia, 8,* 289-303.

Hedera, P., & Whitehouse, P. (1995). Neurotransmitters in neurodegeneration. In D. Calne (Ed.), *Neurodegenerative diseases* (pp. 97-117). Philadelphia: W.B. Saunders.

Heilman, K. M., Schwartz, H. D., & Watson, R.T. (1978). Hypo-arousal in patients with the neglect syndrome and emotional indifference. *Neurology, 28,* 229-232.

Helm, N. (1979). Management of palilalia with a pacing board. *Journal of Speech and Hearing Disorders, 44,* 350-353.

Helm, N. A., & Barresi, B. (1980). Voluntary control of involuntary utterances: A treatment approach for severe aphasia. In R. H. Brookshire (Ed.), *Clinical Aphasiology Conference proceedings* (pp. 308-315). Minneapolis, MN: BRK Publishers.

Helm-Estabrooks, N. A. (1981). Show me the ... whatever Some variables affecting auditory comprehension scores of aphasic patients. In R. H. Brookshire (Ed.), *Clinical Aphasiology Conference proceedings* (pp. 105-107). Minneapolis, MN: BRK Publishers.

Helm-Estabrooks, N. A. (1982). *Helm elicited language program for syntax stimulation (HELPSS).* Chicago: Riverside.

Helm-Estabrooks, N., & Hotz, G. (1991). *Brief test of head injury.* Chicago: Riverside.

Helm-Estabrooks, N., Ramsberger, G., Morgan, A., & Nicholas, M. (1989). *Boston Assessment for Severe Aphasia (BASA).* Chicago: Riverside.

Hier, D., Hagenlocker, K., & Shindler, A. G. (1985). Language disintegration in dementia: Effects of etiology and severity. *Brain and Language, 25,* 117-133.

Hilari, K., Byng, S., Lamping, D. L., & Smith, S. C. (2003). Stroke and aphasia quality of life scale-39 (SAQOL-39): Evaluation of acceptability, reliability, and validity. *Stroke, 34,* 1944-1950.

Hillbom, M., & Holm, L. (1986). Contribution of traumatic head injury to neuropsychological deficits in alcoholics. *Journal of Neurology, Neurosurgery, and Psychiatry, 49,* 1348-1353.

Hixon, T. J. (1987). *Respiratory function in speech and song.* San Diego, CA: College-Hill.

Hixon, T. J., Hawley, J. L., & Wilson, J. L. (1982). An around-the-house device for the clinical determination of respiratory driving pressure. *Journal of Speech and Hearing Disorders, 47,* 413-415.

Holland, A. L. (1977). Some practical considerations in aphasia rehabilitation. In M. Sullivan & M. S. Kommers (Eds.), *Rationale for adult aphasia therapy* (pp. 167-180). Omaha: University of Nebraska Medical Center.

Holland, A. L. (1980). *Communicative abilities in daily living.* Baltimore: University Park Press.

Holland, A.L. (1991). Pragmatic aspects of intervention in aphasia. *Journal of Neurolinguistics, 6,* 197-211.

Holland, A. L. (1996). Treatment efficacy: Aphasia. *Journal of Speech and Hearing Research, 30,* S27-S36.

Holland, A. L., & Beeson, P. M. (1999). Aphasia groups: The Arizona experience. In R. Elman (Ed.). *Group treatment of neurogenic communication disorders: The expert clinician approach* (pp. 77-84). Boston: Butterworth-Heinemann.

Holland, A. L., Frattali, C. M., & Fromm, D. (1998). *Communication activities in daily living* (2nd ed.). Austin, TX: Pro-Ed.

Holland, A. L., & Ross, R. (1999). The power of aphasia groups. In R. J. Elman (Ed.). *Group treatment of neurogenic communication disorders: The expert clinician approach* (pp. 115-120). Boston: Butterworth-Heinemann.

Holtzapple, P., Pohlman, K., LaPointe, L. L., & associates. (1989). Does SPICA mean PICA? *Clinical Aphasiology, 18,* 131-144.

Hooper, H. E. (1983). *The Hooper Visual Organization Test.* Los Angeles: Western Psychological Services.

Hopper, T., & Holland. A. (1998). Situation-specific training for an adult with aphasia: An example. *Aphasiology, 12,* 933-944.

Hopper, T., Holland, A., & Rewega, M. (2002). Conversational coaching: Treatment outcomes and future directions. *Aphasiology, 16,* 745-761.

Hopper, T. Mahendra, N. Kim, E., & associates (2005). Evidence-based practice recommendations for individuals working with dementia: Spaced-retrieval training. *Journal of Medical Speech-Language Pathology, 13,* xxvii - xxxiv.

Hornak J. (1992). Ocular exploration in the dark by patients with visual neglect. *Neuropsychologia, 30,* 547-552.

Horner, J., Massey, E. W., Woodruff, W. W., & associates. (1989). Task-dependent neglect: Computed tomography size and locus correlations. *Journal of Neurological Rehabilitation, 3,* 7-13.

Howard, D., & Hatfield, F. M. (1987). *Aphasia therapy: Historical and contemporary issues.* Hillsdale, NJ: Lawrence Erlbaum.

Humphrey, M., & Oddy, M. (1981). Return to work after head injury. A review of postwar studies. *Injury, 12,* 107-114.

Hussian, R. A. (1988). Modification of behaviors in dementia via stimulus manipulation. *Clinical Gerontologist, 8,* 37-43.

Jehkonen, M., Ahonen, J. P., Dastider, P., Doivisto, A. M., Laippala, P., Vilkki, J., & Molnar, G. (2000). Visual neglect as a predictor of functional outcome one year after stroke. *Acta Neurologica Scandinavia, 101,* 195-201.

Jennett, B. (1976). Assessment of the severity of head injury. *Journal of Neurology, Neurosurgery, and Psychiatry, 39,* 647-655.

Jennett, B., & Bond, M. (1975). Assessment of outcome after severe brain damage: A practical scale. *Lancet, 1,* 480-484.

Jennett, B., & Teasdale, G. (1981). *Management of head injuries.* Philadelphia: F.A. Davis Company.

Jennett, B., Teasdale, G., Braakman, R., & associates. (1979). Prognosis of patients with severe head injury. *Neurosurgery, 4,* 283-289.

Jennett, B., Teasdale, G., Galbraith, S., & associates. (1977). Severe head injuries in three countries. *Journal of Neurology, Neurosurgery, and Psychiatry, 40,* 291-298.

Jerger, J., Weikers, N., Sharbrough, F., & associates. (1969). Bilateral lesions of the temporal lobe: A case study. *Acta Otolaryngologica, 258,* 1-51.

Joanette, Y., Brouchon, M., Gauthier, I., & associates. (1986). Pointing with the left versus right hand in left visual field neglect. *Neuropsychologia, 24,* 391-396.

Joanette, Y., & Goulet, P. (1994). Right hemisphere and verbal communication: Conceptual, methodological, and clinical issues. *Clinical Aphasiology, 22,* 1-23.

Joanette, Y. Goulet, P, & Hannequin, D. (1990). *The right hemisphere and verbal communication.* New York: Springer.

Joanette, Y., Lecours, A. R., Lepage, Y., & associates. (1983). Language in right-handers with right-hemisphere lesions: A preliminary study including anatomical, genetic, and social factors. *Brain and Language, 20,* 217-248.

Johns, D. (Ed.). (1985). *Clinical management of neurogenic communication disorders.* Boston: Little, Brown and Company.

Johns, D. F., & Darley, F. L. (1970). Phonemic variability in apraxia of speech. *Journal of Speech and Hearing Research, 13,* 556-583.

Jorm, A. F., Korten, A. E., & Henderson, A. S. (1987). The prevalence of dementia: A quantitative integration of the literature. *Acta Psychologica Scandinavia, 76,* 465-479.

Kagan, A. (1998). Supported conversation for adults with aphasia: Methods and resources for training conversational partners. *Aphasiology, 9,* 816-830.

Kagan, A., Black, S. E., Duchan, J. F., & associates. (2001). Training volunteers as conversation partners using supported conversation for adults with aphasia: A controlled trial. *Journal of Speech, Language, and Hearing Research, 44,* 624-638.

Kagan, A., & Cohen-Schneider, R. (1999). Groups in the introductory program at the Pat Arato Aphasia Center. In R. Elman (Ed.), *Group treatment of neurogenic communication disorders: The expert clinician approach.* Boston: Butterworth-Heinemann.

Kagan, A., & Dailey, G. F. (1993). Functional is not enough: Training conversation partners for aphasic adults. In A. L. Holland & M. M. Forbes (Eds.), *Aphasia treatment: World perspectives* (pp. 199-225). San Diego: Singular.

Kahneman, D. (1973). *Attention and effort.* Englewood Cliffs, NJ: Prentice-Hall.

Kalmar, K, & Giacino, J.T. (2005). The JFK coma recovery scale-revised. *Neuropsychological Rehabilitation, 15,* 454-460.

Kaplan, E., Goodglass, H., & Weintraub, S. (2001). *The Boston naming test.* Philadelphia: Lippincott Williams & Wilkins.

Kapur, N., Glisky, E. L., & Wilson, B. A. (2004). Technological memory aids for people with memory deficits. *Neuropsychological Rehabilitation, 14,* 41-60.

Karnath H. O., Fetter M. (1995). Ocular space exploration in the dark and its relation to subjective and objective body orientation in neglect patients with parietal lesions. *Neuropsychologia, 33,* 371-377.

Katsuki-Nakamura, J., Brookshire, R. H., & Nicholas, L. E. (1988). Comprehension of monologues and dialogues by aphasic listeners. *Journal of Speech and Hearing Research, 53,* 408-415.

Katz, D. I. (1992). Recovery following severe head injuries. *Journal of Head Trauma Rehabilitation, 7,* 1-15.

Katz, D. I., & Alexander, M. P. (1994). Traumatic brain injury. In D. C. Good & J. R. Couch (Eds.), *Handbook of neurorehabilitation* (pp. 493-549). New York: Dekker.

Katz, N. Hartman-Maeir, A., Ring, H., & Soroker, N. (1999). Functional disability and rehabilitation outcome in right hemisphere damaged patients with and without unilateral spatial neglect. *Archives of Physical Medicine and Rehabilitation, 80,* 379-384.

Katz, R. C., & Nagy, V. T. (1983). A computerized approach for improving word recognition in chronic aphasic adults. In R. H. Brookshire (Ed.), *Clinical Aphasiology 1983 Conference proceedings* (pp. 65-72). Minneapolis, MN: BRK Publishers.

Katz, R. C., & Nagy, V. T. (1984). An intelligent computer-based task for chronic aphasic patients. In R. H. Brookshire (Ed.), *Clinical Aphasiology 1984 Conference proceedings* (pp. 159-165). Minneapolis, MN: BRK Publishers.

Katz, R. C., Wertz, R. T., Davidoff, M., & associates. (1989). A computer program to improve written confrontation naming in aphasia. In T. E. Prescott (Ed.), *Clinical Aphasiology 1988 Conference proceedings* (pp. 321-338). Austin, TX: Pro-Ed.

Katzman, R. (1976). The presence and malignancy of Alzheimer's disease. *Archives of Neurology, 33,* 217-218.

Kay, J., Lesser, R., & Coltheart, M. (1992). *The Psycholinguistic Assessment of Language Processing in Aphasia (PALPA).* Hove, U.K.: Erlbaum.

Kay, T., & Silver, S. M. (1989). Closed head trauma: Assessment for rehabilitation. In M. Lezak (Ed.), *Assessment of the behavioral consequences of head trauma* (pp. 145-170). New York: A.R. Liss.

Kazdin, A. E. (1982). *Single-case research designs: Methods for clinical and applied settings.* New York: Oxford University Press.

Kearns, K. (1994). Group therapy for aphasia: Theoretical and practical considerations. In R. Chapey (Ed.), *Language intervention strategies in adult aphasia* (3rd ed., pp. 304-321). Baltimore: Williams & Wilkins.

Kearns, K., & Hubbard, D. J. (1977). A comparison of auditory comprehension tasks in aphasia. In R.H. Brookshire (Ed.), *Clinical Aphasiology Conference proceedings* (pp. 32-45). Minneapolis, MN: BRK Publishers.

Kearns, K. P., & Simmons, N. N. (1985). Group therapy for aphasia: A survey of V.A. Medical Centers. In R.H. Brookshire (Ed.), *Clinical Aphasiology Conference proceedings* (pp. 176-183). Minneapolis, MN: BRK Publishers.

Kearns, K. P., & Simmons, N. N. (1988). Motor speech disorders: The dysarthrias and apraxia of speech. In N. J. Lass, L. V. McReynolds, J. L. Northern, & associates (Eds.), *Handbook of speech-language pathology and audiology* (pp. 434-448). Philadelphia: B.C. Decker.

Keefe, K. A. (1995). Applying basic neuroscience to aphasia therapy: What the animals are telling us. *American Journal of Speech-Language Pathology, 4,* 88-93.

Keenan, J. S., & Brassell, E. G. (1975). *Aphasia language performance scales.* Murfreesboro, TN: Pinnacle Press.

Kempler, D., Curtiss, S., & Jackson, C. (1987). Syntactic preservation in Alzheimer disease. *Journal of Speech and Hearing Research, 30,* 343-350.

Kennedy, M. R. T. (2004). Self-monitoring recall in two tasks after traumatic brain injury: A preliminary study. *American Journal of Speech-Language Pathology, 13,* 142-154.

Kennedy, M., Strand, E., Burton, W., & associates. (1994). Analysis of first-encounter conversations of right-hemisphere-damaged adults. *Clinical Aphasiology, 22,* 67-80.

Kerns, K. A., & Mateer, C. A. (1998). Walking and chewing gum: The impact of attentional capacity in everyday activities. In R. J. Sbordone & C. J. Long (Eds.) *Ecological validity: Some critical issues for the neuropsychologist* (pp. 147-169). Boston: St Lucie Press.

Kerr, T. A., Kay, D. W. K., & Lassman, L. P. (1971). Characteristics of patients, type of accident, and mortality in a consecutive series of head injuries admitted to a neurosurgical unit. *Journal of Preventative and Social Medicine, 25,* 179-185.

Kertesz, A. (1979). *Aphasia and associated disorders: Taxonomy, localization, and recovery.* New York: Grune & Stratton.

Kertesz, A. (1982). *Western aphasia battery.* New York: Grune and Stratton.

Kertesz, A. Ferro, J. M., & Shewan, C. M. (1984). Apraxia and aphasia: the functional-anatomical basis for their dissociation. *Neurology, 34,* 40-47.

Kertesz, A., Hudson, L., McKenzie, I., & Munoz, D. (1994). The pathology and nosology of primary progressive aphasia. *Neurology, 44,* 2065-2072.

Kertesz, A., & McCabe, P. (1977). Recovery patterns and prognosis in aphasia. *Brain, 100,* 1-18.

Kertesz, A., & Munoz, D. (2000). Differences between Pick disease and Alzheimer disease in clinical appearance and rate of cognitive decline. *Archives of Neurology, 57,* 225-232.

Kim, E. S., Cleary, S. J., Hopper, T., & associates. (2006). Evidence-based practice recommendations for working with individuals with dementia: Group reminiscence therapy. *Journal of Medical Speech-Language Pathology, 14,* xxiii-xxxii.

Kimelman, M. D. Z., & McNeil, M. R. (1987). An investigation of emphatic stress comprehension in aphasia: A replication. *Journal of Speech and Hearing Research, 30,* 295-300.

Kimura, D. (1963). Right temporal lobe damage. *Archives of Neurology, 8,* 264-271.

Kinsella, G., Ford, B. (1985). Hemi-inattention and the recovery patterns of stroke patients. *International Rehabilitation Medicine, 7,* 102-106.

Kintsch, W. (1974). *The representation of meaning in memory.* Hillsdale, NJ: Lawrence Erlbaum.

Kiresuk, T. J., & Sherman, R. E. (1968). Goal-attainment scaling: A general method for evaluating comprehensive mental health programs. *Community Mental Health Journal, 4,* 443-453.

Kirshner, H. S., Tanridag, O., Thurman, L., & associates. (1987). Progressive aphasia without dementia: Two cases with focal spongiform degeneration. *Annals of Neurology, 22,* 527-533.

Klare, G. R. (1984). Readability. In P. D. Pearson (Ed.), *Handbook of reading research* (pp. 681-744). New York: Longman.

Knopman, D., Selnes, O. A., Niccum, N., & associates. (1983). A longitudinal study of speech fluency in aphasia: CT correlates of recovery and persistent nonfluency. *Neurology (Cleveland), 33,* 1170-1178.

Knopman, D. S., Selnes, O. A., Niccum, N., & associates. (1984). Recovery of naming in aphasia: Relationship to fluency, comprehension, and CT findings. *Neurology, 34,* 1461-1470.

Kokmen, E., Beard, M., Offord, K., & associates. (1989). Prevalence of medically diagnosed dementia in a defined Unites States population: Rochester, Minnesota, January 1, 1975. *Neurology, 39,* 773-776.

Kratchowill, T. R. (1978). *Single-subject research: Strategies for evaluating change.* New York: Academic Press.

Kraus, J. F. (1993). Epidemiology of head injury. In P. R. Cooper (Ed.), *Head injury* (3rd ed., pp. 1-25). Baltimore: Williams & Wilkins.

Kraybill M. L., Larson E. B., Tsuang D. W., & associates. (2005). Cognitive differences in dementia patients with autopsy-verified AD, Lewy body pathology, or both. *Neurology, 64,* 2069-2073.

Kreindler, A., Gheorghita, N., & Voinescu, I. (1971). Analysis of verbal reception of a complex order with three elements in aphasics. *Brain, 94,* 375-386.

Kremin, H. (1993). Therapeutic approaches to naming disorders. In M. Paradis (Ed.), *Foundations of aphasia rehabilitation* (pp. 261-292). New York: Pergamon.

Kreutzer, J. S., & Wehman, P. H. (Eds.) (1991). *Cognitive rehabilitation for persons with traumatic brain injury: A functional approach.* Baltimore: Brookes.

Kwakkel, G., Kollen, B., & Lindeman, E. (2004). Understanding the pattern of functional recovery after stroke: Facts and theories. *Restorative Neurology and Neuroscience, 22,* 281-299.

Lackner, J. R., & Garrett, M. F. (1972). Resolving ambiguity: Effects of biasing context in the unattended ear. *Cognition, 1,* 359-372.

Lambrecht, K., & Marshall, R. (1983). Comprehension in severe aphasia: A second look. In R. H. Brookshire (Ed.), *Clinical Aphasiology Conference proceedings* (pp. 186-192). Minneapolis, MN: BRK Publishers.

Langfitt, T. W. (1978). Measuring outcome from head injuries. *Journal of Neurosurgery, 48,* 673-678.

Langlois, J. A., Rutland-Brown, W., & Thomas, K.E. (2004). *Traumatic brain injury in the United States: Emergency department visits, hospitalizations, and deaths,* Atlanta, GA: Centers for Disease Control and Prevention, National Center for Injury Prevention and Control.

LaPointe, L. L. (1991). Base-10 response form (revised manual). San Diego: Singular. (Previously published as LaPointe, L. L. [1977]. Base-10 programmed stimulation: Task specification, scoring, and plotting performance in aphasia therapy.) *Journal of Speech and Hearing Disorders, 42,* 90-105.

LaPointe, L. L., Holtzapple, P., & Graham, L. F. (1985). The relationship among two measures of auditory comprehension and daily living communication skills. In R. H. Brookshire (Ed.), *Clinical Aphasiology Conference proceedings* (pp. 38-46). Minneapolis, MN: BRK Publishers.

LaPointe, L. L., & Horner, J. (1998). *Reading comprehension battery for aphasia* (2nd ed.). Austin, TX: Pro-Ed.

LaPointe, L. L., & Johns, D. F. (1975). Some phonemic characteristics in apraxia of speech. *Journal of Communication Disorders, 8,* 259-269.

Larimore, H. W. (1970). *Some verbal and nonverbal factors associated with apraxia of speech.* Unpublished doctoral dissertation, University of Denver.

Lawton, M.P., & Brody, E.M. (1969). Assessment of older people: Self-maintaining and instrumental activities of daily living. *Gerontologist, 9,* 179-186.

Lee, L. (1971). *Northwestern syntax screening test.* Evanston, IL: The Northwestern University Press.

Lees, A. (1990). Progressive supranuclear palsy. In J. Cummings (Ed.), *Subcortical dementia* (pp. 123-131). New York: Oxford.

Lenneberg, E. (1967). *Biological foundations of language.* New York: Wiley.

Leon, S. A., Rosenbek, J. C., Crucian, G. P. (2005). Active treatments for aprosodia secondary to right hemisphere stroke. *Journal of Rehabilitation Research and Development, 42,* 93-102.

Lesser, R. (1976). Verbal and non-verbal memory components in the token test. *Neuropsychologia, 14,* 79-85.

Levin, B. E., Tomer, R., & Rey, G. J. (1992). Cognitive impairments in Parkinson disease. *Neurologic Clinics, 10,* 471-481.

Levin, H. S., Benton, A. L., & Grossman, R. G. (1982). *Neurobehavioral consequences of closed head injury.* New York: Oxford University Press.

Levin, H. S., O'Connell, V. M., & Grossman, R. G. (1979). The Galveston orientation and amnesia test: A practical scale to assess cognition after head injury. *Journal of Nervous and Mental Disorders, 167,* 675-684.

Lewinsohn, P. M., Danaher, B. G., & Kikel, S. (1977). Visual imagery as a mnemonic aid for brain-injured persons. *Journal of Consulting and Clinical Psychology, 45,* 717-723.

Ley, R. G., & Bryden, M. P. (1979). Hemispheric differences in processing emotions and faces. *Brain and Language, 7,* 127-138.

Lezak, M. D. (1983). *Neuropyschological assessment* (2nd ed.). New York: Oxford University Press.

Lezak, M. D. (1995). *Neuropsychological assessment* (3rd ed.). New York: Oxford University Press.

Lezak, M. D., Howieson, D. B., & Loring, D. W. (2004). *Neuropsychological assessment* (4th ed.) New York: Oxford University Press.

Liepmann, H. (1908). Das krankheitsbild der apraxia. *Monatschrift f. Psychiatrie u Neurologie, 7,* 11-18.

Liles, B. Z., & Brookshire, R. H. (1975). The effects of pause time on auditory comprehension of aphasic subjects. *Journal of Communication Disorders, 8,* 221-236.

Lincoln, N., & Ellis, P. (1980). A shortened version of the PICA. *British Journal of Communication Disorders, 15,* 183-187.

Lincoln, N. B., Mulley, G. P., Jones, A. C., & associates. (1984). Effectiveness of speech therapy for aphasic stroke patients: A randomized controlled trial. *Lancet, 2,* 1197-1200.

Linebaugh, C., & Lehner, L. (1977). Cueing hierarchies and word retrieval: A therapy program. In R. H. Brookshire (Ed.), *Clinical Aphasiology Conference proceedings* (pp. 19-31). Minneapolis, MN: BRK Publishers.

Linebaugh, C. W. (1983). Treatment of anomic aphasia. In W. H. Perkins (Ed.), *Language handicaps in adults* (pp. 35-43). New York: Thieme-Stratton.

Lippert, M., Gruner, T., & Terhaag, D. (2000). Multimodal early onset stimulation (MEOS) in rehabilitation after brain injury. *Brain Injury, 14,* 585-594.

Liss, J., Kuehn, D., & Hinkel, K. (1994). Direct training of velopharyngeal musculature. *National Center for Voice and Speech: Progress Report, 6,* 43-52.

Livingstone, G., Johnston, K., Katona, C., & associates. (2005). Systematic review of psychological approaches to the management of neuropsychiatric symptoms of dementia. *American Journal of Psychiatry, 162,* 1996-2021.

Livingstone, M. G., & Livingstone, H. M. (1985). The Glasgow assessment schedule: Clinical and research assessment of head injury outcome. *International Rehabilitation Medicine, 7,* 145-149.

Lomas, J., Pickard, L., Bester, S., & associates. (1989). The communicative effectiveness index: Development and psychometric evaluation of a functional communication measure for adult aphasia. *Journal of Speech and Hearing Disorders, 54,* 113-124.

Longstreth, W. T., Koepsell, T. D., Nelson, L. M., & associates. (1992). Prognosis: Keystone of clinical neurology. In R. W. Evans, D. S. Baskin, & F. M. Yatsu (Eds.), *Prognosis of neurological disorders* (pp. 19-44). New York: Oxford University Press.

Love, R. J., & Webb, W. J. (1977). The efficacy of cueing techniques in Broca aphasia. *Journal of Speech and Hearing Disorders, 42,* 170-178.

Lucas, S. E., & Fleming, J. M. (2005). Interventions for improving self-awareness following acquired brain injury. *Australian Occupational Therapy Journal, 52,* 160-170.

Luria, A. R. (1965). Neuropsychological analysis of focal brain lesions. In B. B. Wolman (Ed.), *Handbook of clinical psychology* (pp. 42-58). New York: McGraw-Hill.

Luria, A. R. (1966). *Human brain and psychological processes.* New York: Harper & Row.

Luria, A. R. (1970). *Traumatic aphasia.* The Hague, Netherlands: Mouton.

Lyon, J. G. (1989). Communicative partners: Their value in reestablishing communication with aphasic adults. In T. Prescott (Ed.), *Clinical Aphasiology, 18,* 11-18.

Lyon, J. G. (1992). Communication use and participation in life for adults with aphasia in natural settings: The scope of the problem. *American Journal of Speech-Language Pathology, 1,* 7-14.

Lyon, J.G. (2000). Finding, defining, and refining functionality in real life for people confronting aphasia (pp. 137-161). In L.E. Worrall & C.M. Frattali (Eds.), *Neurogenic communication disorders: A functional approach.* New York: Thieme.

Lyon, J., Cariski, D. Keisler, L., & associates (1997). Communication partners: Enhancing participation in life and communication for adults with aphasia in natural settings. *Aphasiology, 11,* 693-708.

Lyon, J.G., & Shadden, B.B. (2001). Treating life consequences of aphasia chronicity. In R. Chapey (Ed.) *Language intervention strategies in aphasia and related neurogenic communication disorders* (4th ed.). Philadelphia: Lippincott, Williams & Wilkins (pp. 297-315).

Mace, N., & Rabins, P. (1991). *The 36-hour day.* Baltimore: Johns Hopkins University Press.

Macniven, E. (1994). Factors affecting head injury rehabilitation outcome: Premorbid and clinical parameters. In M. A. J. Finlayson & S. H. Garner (Eds.), *Brain injury rehabilitation: Clinical considerations* (pp. 57-82). Baltimore: Williams & Wilkins.

Major, B. J., & Wilson, K. J. (1985). *Computerized reading for aphasics.* San Diego, CA: College-Hill.

Markwardt, F. C. Jr. (1989). *The Peabody individual achievement test revised.* Circle Pines, MN: American Guidance Service.

Maroon, J. C., Lovell, M. R., Norwig, J., & associates. (2000). Cerebral concussion in athletes: evaluation by neuropsychological testing. *Neurosurgery, 47,* 659-672.

Marotta, J. J., McKeeff, T. J., Behrmann, M. (2003). Hemispatial neglect: Its effects on visual perception and visually guided grasping. *Neuropsychologia, 41,* 1262-1271.

Marshall, J. C., & Newcombe, F. (1973). Patterns of paralexia: A psycholinguistic approach. *Journal of Psycholinguistic Research, 2,* 175-199.

Marshall, R. C. (1976). Word retrieval behavior of aphasic adults. *Journal of Speech and Hearing Disorders, 41,* 444-451.

Marshall, R. C. (1998). An introduction to supported conversation for adults with aphasia: Perspectives, problems, and possibilities. *Aphasiology, 12,* 811-816.

Marshall, R. C., & Phillips, D. S. (1983). Prognosis for improved verbal communication in aphasic stroke patients. *Archives of Physical Medicine and Rehabilitation, 64,* 597-600.

Martin, R., & Feher, E. (1990). The consequences of reduced memory span for the comprehension of semantic versus syntactic information. *Brain and Language, 38,* 1-20.

Martino, A. A., Pizzamiglio, L., & Razzano, C. (1976). A new version of the Token Test for aphasics: A concrete objects form. *Journal of Communication Disorders, 9,* 1-5.

Massengill, R., Quinn, G. W., Pickrell, K. L., & associates. (1968). Therapeutic exercise and pharyngeal flap. *Cleft Palate Journal, 5,* 44-52.

Mateer, C. A., & Ojemann, G. A. (1983). Thalamic mechanisms in language and memory. In S.J. Segalowitz (Ed.), *Language functions and brain organization.* New York: Academic Press 171-191.

Mattingley, J. B., Berberovic, N., Corben, L., Lavin, M. J., Nicholls, M. E. R., & Bradshaw, J. L. (2004). The greyscales task: A perceptual measure of attentional bias following unilateral hemispheric damage. *Neuropsychologia, 42,* 387-394.

Mattingley, J. B., Bradshaw, J. L., Nettleton, N. C., & Bradshaw, J. A. (1994). Can task specific attentional bias be differentiated from unilateral neglect? *Neuropsychologia, 32,* 805-817.

McDonald, S. (1993). Viewing the brain sideways? Frontal versus right hemisphere explanations of nonaphasic language disorders. *Aphasiology, 7,* 535-549.

McKeever, W. F., & Dixon, M. F. (1981). Right-hemisphere superiority for discriminating memorized from un-memorized faces: Affective imagery, sex, and perceived emotionality effects. *Brain and Language, 12,* 246-260.

McKhann, G. M., Albert, M. S., Grossman M., & associates (2001). Clinical and pathological diagnosis of frontotemporal dementia: Report of the work group on frontotemporal dementia and Pick's disease. *Neurology, 58,* 1803-1809.

McKitrick, L. A., Camp, C. J., & Black, F. W. (1992). Prospective memory intervention in Alzheimer's disease. *Journal of Gerontology, 47,* 337-343.

McNeil, M., Odell, K., & Tseng, C. H. (1990). Toward the integration of resource allocation into a general model of aphasia. In T. Prescott (Ed.), *Clinical aphasiology* (pp. 21-39). Austin, TX: Pro-Ed.

McNeil, M. R., & Kimelman, M. D. Z. (1986). Toward an integrative information-processing structure of auditory comprehension and processing in adult aphasia. *Seminars in Speech and Language, 7,* 123-146.

McNeil, M. R., & Prescott, T. E. (1978). *Revised Token Test.* Baltimore: University Park Press.

McNeil, M. R., Robin, D. A., & Schmidt, R. A. (1997). Apraxia of speech: Definition, differentiation, and treatment. In M. R. McNeil (Ed.), *Clinical management of sensorimotor speech disorders* (pp. 311-344). New York: Thieme.

Meadows, J. C. (1974). The anatomical basis of prosopagnosia. *Journal of Neurology, Neurosurgery, and Psychiatry, 37,* 489-501.

Mendez, M. F., Selwood, A., Mastri, A.R., & associates. (1993). Pick disease versus Alzheimer disease: A comparison of clinical characteristics. *Neurology, 43,* 289-292.

Mesulam, M. M. (1982). A cortical network for directed attention and unilateral neglect. *Annals of Neurology, 10,* 309-325.

Mesulam, M. M. (1982). Slowly progressive aphasia without dementia. *Annals of Neurology, 11,* 592-598.

Metter, E. J., Riege, W. H., Hanson, W. R., & associates. (1983). Comparisons of metabolic rates, language and memory in subcortical aphasias. *Brain and Language, 19,* 33-47.

Metter, E. J., Riege, W. H., Hanson, W. R., & associates. (1984). Correlations of glucose metabolism and structural damage to language function in aphasia. *Brain and Language, 21,* 187-207.

Meyer, B. J. F. (1975). *The organization of prose and its effects on memory.* Amsterdam: North-Holland.

Meyer, B. J. F., & McConkie, G. W. (1973). What is recalled after hearing a passage? *Journal of Educational Psychology, 65,* 109-117.

Miceli, G., Silveri, M. C., Nocentini, U., & associates. (1988). Patterns of dissociation in comprehension and production of nouns and verbs. *Aphasiology, 2,* 351-358.

Miller, J. D., Sweet, R. G., Narayan, R., & associates. (1978). Early insults in the injured brain. *Journal of the American Medical Association, 240,* 439-442.

Miller, S. Vermeersch, P.W., Bohan, K., & associates (2001). Audio presence intervention for decreasing agitation in persons with dementia. *Geriatric Nursing, 22,* 66-70.

Mills, R. H., Knox, A. W., Juola, J. F., & associates. (1979). Cognitive loci of impairments of picture naming by aphasic subjects. *Journal of Speech and Hearing Research, 22,* 73-87.

Milner, B. (1971). Interhemispheric differences in the localization of psychological processes in man. *British Medical Bulletin, 27,* 272-277. (Reported in Lezak, 1995.)

Milner, B. (1975). Psychological aspects of focal epilepsy and its neurosurgical management. *Advances in Neurology, 8,* 299-321.

Miniami, R. T., Kaplan, E. N., Wu, G., & associates. (1975). Velopharyngeal incompetency without overt cleft palate. *Plastic and Reconstructive Surgery, 55,* 573-587.

Mohr, J. P., Pessin, M. S., Finkelstein, S., & associates. (1978). Broca aphasia: Pathologic and clinical aspects. *Neurology, 28,* 311-324.

Mohr, J. P., Walters, W. C., & Duncan, G. W. (1975). Thalamic hemorrhage and aphasia. *Brain and Language, 2,* 3-17.

Moll, K. L. (1968). Speech characteristics of individuals with cleft lip and palate. In D. C. Spriesterbach & D. Sherman (Eds.), *Cleft palate and communication.* New York: Academic Press.

Molloy, R., Brownell, H.H., & Gardner, H. (1990). Discourse comprehension by right-hemisphere stroke patients: Deficits of prediction and revision. In Y. Joanette & H. Brownell (Eds.), *Discourse ability and brain damage: Theoretical and empirical perspectives* (pp. 113-130). New York: Springer-Verlag.

Morris, J. C. (1993). The Clinical Dementia Rating Scale (CDR). Current version and scoring rules. *Neurology, 43,* 2412-2414.

Murdoch, B. E. (1990). *Acquired Speech and Language Disorders.* New York: Chapman & Hall.

Murray, L. L., & Clark, H. A. (2001). A comparison of relaxation training and syntax stimulation for chronic nonfluent aphasia. *Journal of Communication Disorders, 34,* 87-113.

Murray, L. L., Holland, A. L., & Beeson, P. M. (1997). Auditory processing in individuals with mild aphasia: A study of resource allocation. *Journal of Speech, Language, and Hearing Research, 40,* 792-808.

Murray, J., Marquardt, T. P., Richardson, A., & associates. (1984). Differential diagnosis of aphasia and dementia from aphasia test battery scores. *Journal of Neurological Communication Disorders, 1,* 33-39.

Myers, P. S. (1979). Profiles of communication deficits in patients with right cerebral hemisphere damage: Implications for diagnosis and treatment. In R. H. Brookshire (Ed.), *Clinical Aphasiology Conference proceedings* (pp. 38-46). Minneapolis, MN: BRK Publishers.

Myers, P. S. (1991). Inference failure: The underlying impairment in right hemisphere communication disorders. In T. E. Prescott (Ed.), *Clinical aphasiology: Volume 20* (pp. 167-180). Austin, TX: Pro-Ed.

Myers, P. S. (1994). Communication disorders associated with right-hemisphere brain damage. In R. Chapey (Ed.), *Language intervention strategies in adult aphasia* (3rd ed., pp. 513-534). Baltimore: Williams & Wilkins.

Myers, P. S. (1999). *Right hemisphere damage: Disorders of communication and cognition.* San Diego, CA: Singular.

Myers, P. S., & Mackisack, E. L. (1990). Right hemisphere syndrome. In L. L. LaPointe (Ed.), *Aphasia and related neurogenic language disorders* (pp. 177-195). New York: Thieme.

Naeser, M. A., Alexander, M. P., Helm-Estabrooks, N., & associates. (1982). Aphasia with predominantly subcortical lesion sites: Description of three capsular putamenal aphasia syndromes. *Archives of Neurology, 39,* 2-14.

Naeser, M. A., & Borod, J. C. (1986). Aphasia in left-handers. *Neurology, 36,* 471-488.

Navia, B. A., Jordan, B. D., & Price, R. W. (1986). The AIDS dementia complex: Clinical features. *Annals of Neurology, 19,* 517-524.

Neary, D., Snoden, J. S., Northern, B., & associates. (1988). Dementia of frontal lobe type. *Journal of Neurology, Neurosurgery, and Psychiatry, 44,* 409-411.

Netsell, R., & Hixon, T. J. (1978). A noninvasive method for clinically estimating subglottal air pressure. *Journal of Speech and Hearing Disorders, 43,* 326-330.

Netsell, R., & Rosenbek, J. C. (1985). Treating the dysarthrias. In J. K. Darby (Ed.), *Speech and language evaluation in neurology: Adult disorders* (pp. 87-101). New York: Grune & Stratton.

Nicholas, L. E., & Brookshire, R. H. (1983). Syntactic simplification and context: Effects on sentence comprehension by aphasic adults. In R. H. Brookshire (Ed.), *Clinical Aphasiology Conference proceedings* (pp. 166-172). Minneapolis, MN: BRK Publishers.

Nicholas, L. E., & Brookshire, R. H. (1986). Consistency of the effects of rate of speech on brain-damaged adults' comprehension of narrative discourse. *Journal of Speech and Hearing Research, 29,* 462-470.

Nicholas, L. E., & Brookshire, R. H. (1993). A system for quantifying the informativeness and efficiency of the connected speech of adults with aphasia. *Journal of Speech and Hearing Research, 36,* 338-350.

Nicholas, L. E., & Brookshire, R. H. (1995a). Presence, completeness, and accuracy of main concepts in the connected speech of non-brain-damaged adults and adults with aphasia. *Journal of Speech and Hearing Research, 38,* 145-156.

Nicholas, L. E., & Brookshire, R. H. (1995b). Comprehension of spoken narrative discourse by adults with aphasia, right-hemisphere brain damage, or traumatic brain injury. *American Journal of Speech-Language Pathology, 4,* 69-81.

Nicholas, L. E., Brookshire, R. H., MacLennan, D. L., & associates. (1989). Revised administration and scoring procedures for the Boston Naming Test and norms for non-brain-damaged adults. *Aphasiology, 3,* 569-580.

Nicholas, L. E., MacLennan, D. L., & Brookshire, R. H. (1986). Validity of multiple-sentence reading comprehension tests for aphasic adults. *Journal of Speech and Hearing Disorders, 51,* 82-87.

Nicholas, M., Obler, L. K., Albert, M. L., & associates. (1985). Empty speech in Alzheimer's disease and fluent aphasia. *Journal of Speech and Hearing Research, 28,* 405-410.

Noll, D. J., & Lass, N. D. (1972). *Use of the Token Test with children: Two contrasting socioeconomic groups.* Paper presented at the American Speech and Hearing Association Convention, San Francisco (November).

Nolte, J. (1993). *The human brain* (3rd ed.). St. Louis: Mosby.

Norman, D. A., & Bobrow, D. G. (1975). On data-limited and resource-limited processes. *Cognitive Psychology, 7,* 44-64.

Norman, D. A., & Shallice, T. (1986). Attention to action: Willed and automatic control of behavior. In R. G. Davidson, G. E. Schwartz, & D. Shapiro (Eds.), *Consciousness and self-regulation: Advances in research.* Vol. IV. New York: Plenum.

Norris, G., & Tate, R. L. (2000). The behavioural assessment of the dysexecutive syndrome (BADS): Ecological, concurrent, and construct validity. *Neuropsychological Rehabilitation, 10,* 33-45.

Ojemann, G. A. (1975). Language and the thalamus: Object naming and recall during and after thalamic stimulation. *Brain and Language, 2,* 101-120.

O'Keefe, B. M., Brown, L., & Schuller, R. (1998). Identification and rankings of communication aid features by five groups. *Augmentative and Alternative Communication, 14,* 37-50.

Ommaya, A. K., Grubb, R. L., & Naumann, R. A. (1971). Coup and contrecoup injury: Observations on the mechanics of visible brain injuries in the rhesus monkey. *Journal of Neurosurgery, 35,* 503-507.

Orsulic-Jeras, S., Judge, K. S., & Camp, C. J. (2000). Montessori-based activities for long-term care residents with advanced dementia: Effects on engagement and affect. *Gerontologist, 40,* 107-111.

Osgood, C., & Miron, M. (1963). *Approaches to the study of aphasia.* Chicago: University Park Press.

Osterrieth, P.A. (1944). Le teste de copie d'une figure complexe. *Archives de Psychologie, 30,* 206-356.

Palmese, C. A., & Raskin, S. A. (2000). The rehabilitation of attention in individuals with mild traumatic brain injury using the APT-II programme. *Brain Injury, 14,* 535-548

Pang, D. (1989). Physics and pathophysiology of closed head injury. In M. Lezak (Ed.), *Assessment of the behavioral consequences of head trauma* (pp. 1-19). New York: A.R. Liss.

Parente, R., & DiCesare, A. (1991). Retraining memory: Theory, evaluation, and applications. In J. S. Kreutzer & P. H. Wehman (Eds.), *Cognitive rehabilitation for persons with traumatic brain injury: A functional approach* (pp. 147-162). Baltimore: Brookes.

Park, N. W., & Ingles, J. L. (2001). Effectiveness of attention rehabilitation after an acquired brain injury: A meta-analysis. *Neuropsychology, 15,* 199-210.

Parkhurst, B. G. (1970). *The effects of time altered speech stimuli on the performance of right hemiplegic adult aphasics.* Paper presented at the annual convention of the American Speech and Hearing Association, New York.

Parkin, H. J. (1982). Residual learning capability in organic amnesia. *Cortex, 18,* 417-440.

Parr, S. (1992). Everyday reading and writing practices of normal adults: Implications for aphasia assessment. *Aphasiology, 6,* 273-283.

Parr, S. (1996). Everyday literacy in aphasia: Radical approaches to functional assessment and therapy. *Aphasiology, 10,* 469-479.

Pashek, G. V., & Brookshire, R. H. (1982). Effects of rate of speech and linguistic stress on auditory paragraph comprehension by aphasic individuals. *Journal of Speech and Hearing Research, 25,* 377-382.

Paul, D. R., Frattalli, C. M, Holland, A. L., & associates. (2004). *Quality of communication life scale.* Bethesda, MD: American Speech-Language-Hearing Association.

Peak, J. S., & Cheston, R. L. (2002). Using simulated presence therapy with people with dementia. *Aging and Mental Health, 6,* 77-81.

Pease, D. M., & Goodglass, H. (1978). The effects of cueing on picture naming in aphasia. *Cortex, 14,* 178-189.

Pederson, P. M., Jorgenson, H. S., Nakayama, H., & associates (1997). Hemineglect in acute stroke: Incidence and prognostic implications. *American Journal of Physical Medicine and Rehabilitation, 76,* 122-127.

Penfield, W., & Roberts, L. (1959). *Speech and brain mechanisms.* Princeton, NJ: Princeton University Press.

Phelps-Terasaki, D., & Phelps-Gunn, T. (1992). Test of pragmatic language. Austin TX: Pro-Ed.

Phillips, J. P., Devier, D. J., & Feeney, D. M. (2003). Rehabilitation pharmacology: Bridging laboratory work to clinical application. *Journal of Head Trauma Rehabilitation, 18,* 342-356.

Pierce, R. (1989). Linguistic context and aphasia treatment. In R. Pierce & M. J. Wilcox (Eds.), *Seminars in speech and language: Pragmatics of aphasia.* New York: Thieme.

Pimental, P. A., & Knight, J. A. (2000). *The mini inventory of right brain injury: Second edition.* Austin, TX: Pro-Ed.

Pizzamiglio, L., Antonucci, G., Judica, A., Montenero, P., Razzano, C., & Zoccolotti, P. (1992). Cognitive rehabilitation of the hemineglect disorder in chronic patients with unilateral right brain damage. *Journal of Clinical and Experimental Neuropsychology, 14,* 901-923.

Podraza, B. L., & Darley, F. L. (1977). Effect of auditory prestimulation on naming in aphasia. *Journal of Speech and Hearing Research, 20,* 669-683.

Poeck, K. (1983). What do we mean by phasic syndromes? A neurologist view. *Brain and Language, 20,* 79-89.

Poeck, K., Huber, W., & Willmes, K. (1989). Outcome of intensive language rehabilitation in aphasia. *Journal of Speech and Hearing Disorders, 54,* 471-479.

Polinko, P. R. (1985). Working with the family: The acute phase. In M. Ylvisaker (Ed.), *Head injury rehabilitation: Children and adolescents* (pp. 87-101). San Diego: College-Hill.

Ponsford, J., & Kinsella, G. (1992). Attentional deficits following closed head injury. *Journal of Clinical and Experimental Neuropsychology, 32,* 3-25.

Poppelreuter, W. (1917). *Die psychischen schodigringen-durch kopfschuss im kriege. 1914/1916.* Leipzig: Verlag von Leopold Voss.

Porch, B. E. (1967, 1981a). *Porch Index of Communicative Ability.* Palo Alto, CA: Consulting Psychologists Press.

Porch, B. E. (1981b). Therapy subsequent to the PICA. In R. Chapey (Ed.), *Language intervention strategies in adult aphasia* (2nd ed., pp. 283-296). Baltimore: Williams & Wilkins.

Porch, B. E. (2001). *Porch Index of Communicative Ability* (4th ed.). Albuquerque, NM: Pica Programs.

Porch, B. E., & Callaghan, S. (1981). Making predictions about recovery: Is there HOAP? In R. H. Brookshire (Ed.), *Clinical Aphasiology Conference proceedings* (pp. 187-200). Minneapolis, MN: BRK Publishers.

Porch, B. E., Collins, M., Wertz, R. T., & associates. (1980). Statistical prediction of change in aphasia. *Journal of Speech and Hearing Research, 12,* 312-321.

Povlishock, J. T., Becker, D. P., Sullivan, H. G., & associates. (1978). Vascular permeability alterations to horseradish peroxidase in experimental brain injury. *Brain Research, 153,* 233-239.

Powers, G. L., & Starr, C. D. (1974). The effects of muscle exercise on velopharyngeal gap and nasality. *Cleft Palate Journal, 11,* 28-40.

Price, R. W., & Perry, S. (1994). *HIV, AIDS, and the brain.* New York: Raven Press.

Prigitano, G., Fordyce, D., Zeiner, H., & associates. (1984). Neuropsychological rehabilitation after closed head injury in young adults. *Journal of Neurology, Neurosurgery, and Psychiatry, 47,* 505-513.

Prigitano, G. P., Klonoff, P. S. (1998). A clinician's rating scale for evaluating impaired self-awareness and denial of disability after brain injury. *Clinical Neuropsychologist, 12*, 56-67.

Prins, R. S., Snow, C. E., & Wagenaar, E. (1978). Recovery from aphasia: Spontaneous speech versus language comprehension. *Brain and Language, 6*, 192-211.

Prutting, C. A., & Kirchner, D. M. (1987). A clinical appraisal of the pragmatic aspects of language. *Journal of Speech and Hearing Disorders, 52*, 105-119.

Quatrocchi-Tubin, S., & Jason, L. A. (1980). Enhancing social interactions and activity among the elderly through stimulus control. *Journal of Applied Behavior Analysis, 13*, 159-163.

Rabins, P. V., Mace, N. L., & Lucas, M. J. (1982). The impact of dementia on the family. *Journal of the American Medical Association, 248*, 333-336.

Rader, M. A., & Ellis, D. W. (1994). The sensory stimulation assessment measure (SSAM): A tool for early evaluation of brain-injured patients. *Brain Injury, 4*, 309-321.

Rafal, R. D., & Posner, M. I. (1987). Deficits in human spatial attention following thalamic lesions. *Proceedings of the National Academy of Science, 84*, 7349-7353.

Rappaport, M., Dougherty, A.M., & Kelting, D.L. (1992). Evaluation of coma and vegetative states. *Archives of Physical Medicine and Rehabilitation, 73*, 628-634.

Rappoport, M., Hall, K. M., Hopkins, K., & associates. (1982). Disability rating scale for severe head trauma: Coma to community. *Archives of Physical Medicine and Rehabilitation, 63*, 118-123.

Raskin, S.A., & Sohlberg, M.M. (1996). The efficacy of prospective memory training in two adults with brain injury. *Journal of Head Trauma Rehabilitation, 11*, 32-51.

Raven, J. C. (1960). *The standard progressive matrices*. New York: The Psychological Corporation.

Raven, J. C. (1965). *The coloured progressive matrices*. New York: The Psychological Corporation.

Reisberg, B., Ferris, S. H., DeLeon, M. J., & associates. (1982). The global deterioration scale for assessment of primary degenerative dementia. *American Journal of Psychiatry, 139*, 1136-1139.

Regard, M. Strauss, E., & Knapp, P. (1982). Children's production on verbal and non-verbal fluency tasks. *Perceptual and Motor Skills, 55*, 839-844.

Rey, A. (1941). Psychological examination of traumatic encephalopathy. *Archives de Psychologie, 28*, 286-340; sections translated by J. Corwin & F. W. Bylsma. (1993). *The clinical neuropsychologist* (pp. 4-9).

Rey, A. (1941). Psychological examination of traumatic encephalopathy. *Archives de Psychologie, 28*, 286-340.

Rey, A. (1964). *L xamen clinque en psychologie*. Paris: Presses Universitaires de France. (Reported in Lezak, 1995.)

Ripich, D. N., & Ziol, E. (1998). Dementia: A review for the speech-language pathologists. In A. F. Johnson & B. H. Jacobson (Eds.), *Medical speech-language pathology: A practitioner guide* (pp. 467-494). New York: Thieme.

Rivers, D. L., & Love, R. J. (1980). Language performance on visual processing tasks in right hemisphere lesion cases. *Brain and Language, 10*, 348-366.

Rizzo, M., & Robin, D. A. (1990). Simultanagnosia: A defect of sustained attention yields insights on visual information processing, *Neurology, 40*, 447-455.

Robertson, I. (1990). Does computerized cognitive rehabilitation work? A review. *Aphasiology, 4*, 381-405.

Robertson, I., & North, N. (1993). Active and passive activation of left limbs: Influence on visual and sensory neglect. *Neuropsychologia, 31*, 293-300.

Robertson, J. H., Ward, T., Ridgeway, V, & Nimmo-Smith, I. (1996). The structure of normal human attention: The test of everyday attention. *Journal of the International Neuropsychological Society, 2*, 525-534.

Robey, R. R. (1994). The efficacy of treatment for aphasic persons: a meta-analysis. *Brain and Language, 47*, 582-608.

Robey, R. R. (1998). A meta-analysis of clinical outcomes in the treatment of aphasia. *Journal of Speech, Language, and Hearing Research, 41*, 172-187.

Robey, R. R., Schultz, M. C., Crawford, A. B., & associates. (1999). Single-subject clinical outcome research: Designs, data, effect sizes, and analyses. *Aphasiology, 13*, 445-473.

Robin, D., & Scheinberg, S. (1990). Subcortical lesions and aphasia. *Journal of Speech and Hearing Disorders, 55*, 90-100.

Robin, D. A., Tranel, D., & Damasio, H. (1990). Auditory perception of temporal and spectral events in patients with focal left and right cerebral lesions. *Brain and Language, 39*, 539-555.

Robertson, I., & North, N. (1993). Active and passive activation of left limbs: Influence on visual and sensory neglect. *Neuropsychologia, 31*, 293-300.

Robertson, J. H., Ward, T., Ridgeway, V, & Nimmo-Smith, I. (1994). *The Test of Everyday Attention*. Bury St. Edmunds, UK: Thames Valley Test Co.

Robertson, J. H., Ward, T., Ridgeway, V, & Nimmo-Smith, I. (1996). The structure of normal human attention: The test of everyday attention. *Journal of the International Neuropsychological Society, 2*, 525-534.

Rochford, G., & Williams, M. (1965). Studies in the development and breakdown in the use of names, IV: The effects of word frequency. *Journal of Neurology, Neurosurgery, and Psychiatry, 28*, 407-413.

Rosenbek, J. C. (1978). Treating apraxia of speech. In D. F. Johns (Ed.), *Clinical management of neurogenic communication disorders* (pp. 191-241). Boston: Little, Brown and Company.

Rosenbek, J. C., Collins, M. J., & Wertz, R. T. (1976). Intersystemic reorganization for apraxia of speech. In R. H. Brookshire (Ed.), *Clinical Aphasiology Conference proceedings* (pp. 255-260). Minneapolis, MN: BRK Publishers.

Rosenbek, J. C., & LaPointe, L. L. (1978). The dysarthrias: Description, diagnosis, and treatment. In D. F. Johns (Ed.), *Clinical management of neurogenic communication disorders* (pp. 251-310). Boston: Little, Brown and Company.

Rosenbek, J. C., & LaPointe, L. L. (1985). The dysarthrias: Description, diagnosis, and treatment. In D. F. Johns (Ed.), *Clinical management of neurogenic communication disorders* (2nd ed., pp. 97-152). Boston: Little, Brown and Company.

Rosenbek, J. C., LaPointe, L. L., & Wertz, R. T. (1989). *Aphasia: A clinical approach.* Boston: Little, Brown and Company.

Rosenbek, J. C., Lemma, M. L., Ahern, M. B., & associates. (1973). A treatment for apraxia of speech in adults. *Journal of Speech and Hearing Disorders, 38,* 462-472.

Rosenbek, J. C., & Wertz, R. T. (1972). Treatment of apraxia of speech in adults. In R. T. Wertz & M. Collins (Eds.), *Clinical Aphasiology Conference proceedings* (pp. 191-198). Madison, WI: Veterans Administration Medical Center.

Rosenbek, J. C., Wertz, R. T., & Darley, F. L. (1973). Oral sensation and perception in apraxia of speech and aphasia. *Journal of Speech and Hearing Research, 16,* 22-36.

Rosenshine, B. V. (1980). Skill hierarchies in reading comprehension. In R. J. Spino, B. C. Bruce, & W. F. Brewer (Eds.), *Theoretical issues in reading comprehension* (pp. 535-554). Hillsdale, NJ: Lawrence Erlbaum.

Rosenthal, M., Griffith, E., Bond, M., & associates. (1990). *Rehabilitation of the adult and child with traumatic brain injury.* Philadelphia: F.A. Davis.

Ross, D. G. (1996). *Ross information processing assessment* (2nd ed.). Austin, TX: Pro-Ed.

Rowley, G., & Fielding, K. (1991). Reliability and accuracy of the Glasgow Coma Scale with experienced and inexperienced users. *Lancet, 2,* 535-538.

Rubens, A. B. (1977). The role of changes within the central nervous system during recovery from aphasia. In M. Sullivan & M. S. Kommers (Eds.), *Rationale for adult aphasia therapy* (pp. 28-43). Lincoln, NE: University of Nebraska Medical Center.

Ruddier, J., Seitz, M.D., Nina, P., & associates. (2000). The role of diaschisis in stroke recovery. *Review of Neurology, 30,* 941-945.

Rusch, J. (1944). Intellectual impairment in head injuries. *American Journal of Psychiatry, 100,* 480-496.

Russell, W. R. (1971). *The traumatic amnesias.* New York: Oxford University Press.

Russell, W. R., & Spir, M. L. E. (1961). *Traumatic aphasia.* London: Oxford University Press.

Russell, W. R., & Nathan, P. W. (1946). Traumatic amnesia. *Brain, 69,* 183-187.

Rutherford, W. H. (1977). Diagnosis of alcohol ingestion in mild head injuries. *Lancet, 1,* 1021-1023.

Rotter, M. (1981). Psychological sequelae of brain damage in children. *American Journal of Psychiatry, 183,* 1533-1549.

Saint-Cyr, J. A., & Taylor, A. E., (1992). The mobilization of procedural learning: The key signature of the basal ganglia. In L. R. Squire & N. Butters (Eds.), *Neuropsychology of memory* (2nd ed.) (pp. 126-134). New York: Guilford Press.

Salvatore, A. P., Strait, M., & Brookshire, R. H. (1978). Effects of patient characteristics on delivery of Token Test commands by experienced and inexperienced examiners. *Journal of Communication Disorders, 11,* 325-334.

Sands, E., Sarna, M. T., & Shankweiler, D. (1969). Long term assessment of language function in aphasia due to stroke. *Archives of Physical Medicine and Rehabilitation, 50,* 202-207.

Sarno, M. T. (1969). *The functional communication profile.* New York: NYU Medical Center Monograph Department.

Sarno, M. T., & Levita, E. (1971). Natural course of recovery in severe aphasia. *Archives of Physical Medicine and Rehabilitation, 52,* 175-178.

Sarno, M. T., Silverman, M., & Sands, E. (1970). Speech therapy and language recovery in severe aphasia. *Journal of Speech and Hearing Research, 13,* 607-623.

Sbordone, R. J. (1998). Ecological validity of neuropsychological testing. In R.J. Sbordone & C.J. Long (Eds.) *Ecological validity: Some critical issues for the neuropsychologist* (pp. 15-41). Boston: St Lucie Press.

Schacter, D., Rich, S., & Stampp, A. (1985). Remediation of memory disorders: Experimental evaluation of the spaced-retrieval technique. *Journal of Clinical and Experimental Neuropsychology, 7,* 79-96.

Schacter, D. L., & Glisky, E. L. (1986). Memory remediation: Restorations, alleviation, and the acquisition of domain-specific knowledge. In Y. Gross & B. P. Uzzell (Eds.), *Clinical neuropsychology of intervention* (pp. 257-282). Boston: Martinus Nijhoff.

Schneider, A., Buth, C., Eisenber, N., & associates (1999). Evanston-Northwestern Healthcare: Right hemisphere screen. *Seminars in Speech and Language, 20,* 311-316.

Schretlin, D., Bobholtz, J., & Brandt, J. (1996). Development and psychometric properties of the Brief Test of Attention. *The Clinical Neuropsychologist, 10,* 80-89.

Schuell, H. M. (1957). A short examination for aphasia. *Neurology, 7,* 625-634.

Schuell, H. M. (1965, 1972). *The Minnesota test for differential diagnosis of aphasia.* Minneapolis, MN: University of Minnesota Press.

Schuell, H. M., & Jenkins, J. J. (1961). Reduction of vocabulary in aphasia. *Brain, 84,* 243-261.

Schuell, H. M., Jenkins, J. J., & Jimenez-Pabon, E. (1964). *Aphasia in adults.* New York: Harper and Row.

Segatore, M., & Way, C. (1992). The Glasgow Coma Scale: Time for a change. *Heart and Lung, 21,* 548-557.

Selnes, O. A., Knopman, D. S., Niccum, N., & associates. (1983). Computed tomographic scan correlates of auditory comprehension deficits in aphasia: A prospective recovery study. *Annals of Neurology, 13,* 558-566.

Selnes, O. A., Knopman, D. S., Niccum, N., & associates. (1985). The critical role of Wernicke area in sentence repetition. *Annals of Neurology, 17,* 549-557.

Seron, X., Deloche, G., Moulard, G., & Rousselle, M. (1980). A computer-based therapy for the treatment of aphasic subjects with writing disorders. *Journal of Speech and Hearing Disorders, 45,* 45-58.

Shallice, T. (1982). Specific impairments of planning. *Philosophical Transactions of the Royal Society of London, 298,* 199-209.

Shallice, T. (1988). *From Neuropsychology to Mental Structure.* Cambridge: Cambridge University Press

Shallice, T., & Burgess, P.W. (1991). Deficits in strategy application following frontal-lobe damage in man. *Brain, 114,* 727-747.

Shallice, T., & Warrington, E. K. (1970). Independent functioning of the verbal memory stores: A neuropsychological study. *Quarterly Journal of Experimental Psychology, 22,* 261-273.

Shankweiler, D., & Harris, K. S. (1966). An experimental approach to the problem of articulation in aphasia. *Cortex, 2,* 277-292.

Shapiro, B. E., & Danly, M. (1985). The role of the right hemisphere in the control of speech prosody in propositional and affective contexts. *Brain and Language, 25,* 19-36.

Shatz, P., & Chute, D. L. (1995). Predicting level of independence following moderate and severe traumatic brain injury. *Archives of Clinical Neuropsychology, 11,* 444-445.

Sheehan, V. (1945). Rehabilitation of aphasia in an army hospital. *Journal of Speech Disorders, 11,* 148-154.

Sheikh, J. I., & Yesavage, J. A. (1986). The Geriatric Depression Scale (GDS): Recent evidence and development of a shorter version. *Clinical Gerontologist, 5,* 165-173.

Shewan, C. M. (1988). The Shewan spontaneous language analysis system (SSLA) for aphasic adults: Description, reliability, and validity. *Journal of Communication Disorders, 21,* 103-138.

Shewan, C. M., & Canter, G. J. (1971). Effects of vocabulary, syntax, and sentence length on auditory comprehension in aphasic patients. *Cortex, 7,* 209-226.

Shewan, C. M., & Kertesz, A. (1980). Reliability and validity characteristics of the Western Aphasia Battery (WAB). *Journal of Speech and Hearing Disorders, 45,* 308-324.

Shewan, C. M., & Kertesz, A. (1984). Effects of speech and language treatment on recovery from aphasia. *Brain and Language, 23,* 272-299.

Silverman, F. H. (1983). Dysarthria: Communication augmentation systems for adults without speech. In W. H. Perkins (Ed.), *Dysarthria and apraxia* (pp. 115-121). New York: Thieme-Stratton.

Simmons-Mackie, N.N. (2000). Social approaches to the management of aphasia. In L.E. Worrall & C.M. Frattalli (Eds.). *Neurogenic communication disorders: A functional approach.* New York: Thieme, pp. 162-187.

Simmons-Mackie, N. (2001). Social approaches to aphasia intervention. In R. Chapey (Ed.) *Language intervention strategies in aphasia and related neurogenic communication disorders* (4th ed.). Philadelphia: Lippincott, Williams & Wilkins (pp. 246-268).

Simmons-Mackie, N., & Damico, J. (1996). Accounting for handicaps in aphasia: Communicative assessment from an authentic social perspective. *Disability and Rehabilitation, 18,* 540-549.

Skelly, M. (1979). *Amer-Ind gestural code based on universal American Indian hand talk.* New York: Elsevier.

Sklar, M. (1973). *The Sklar aphasia scale.* Los Angeles: Western Psychological Services.

Smith, A. (1972). *Diagnosis, intelligence, and rehabilitation of chronic aphasics. Final report.* Ann Arbor, MI: University of Michigan Press.

Smith, A. (1968). The Symbol-Digit-Modalities Test: A neuropsychologic test for economic screening of learning and other cerebral disorders. *Learning Disorders, 3,* 83-91.

Snow, P., Douglas, J., & Ponsford, J. (1995). Discourse assessment following traumatic brain injury: A pilot study examining some demographic and methodological issues. *Aphasiology, 9,* 365-380.

Sohlberg, M. M., Johnson, L., Paule, L., & associates (1994). Attention process training II: A program to assess attentional deficits for persons with mild cognitive dysfunction. Puyallup, WA: Association for Neuropsychological Research and Development.

Sohlberg, M. M., & Mateer, C. A. (1989). *Introduction to cognitive rehabilitation: Theory and practice.* New York: Guilford.

Sohlberg, M. M., & Mateer, C. A. (2001). *Cognitive rehabilitation: An integrative neuropsychological approach.* New York: Guilford.

Sohlberg, M.M., McLaughlin, K. Parese, A., & associates (2000). Evaluation of attention process training and brain education in persons with acquired brain injury. *Journal of Clinical and Experimental Neuropsychology, 22,* 656-676.

Sparks, R., Helm, N. A., & Albert, M. L. (1974). Aphasia rehabilitation resulting from melodic intonation therapy. *Cortex, 10,* 303-316.

Sparks, R., & Holland, A. L. (1976). Method: Melodic intonation therapy for aphasia. *Journal of Speech and Hearing Disorders, 41,* 287-297.

Spector, A., Orrell, M., Davies, S., & associates. (2000). Reality orientation for dementia. *Cochrane Database of Systematic Reviews, 2,* CD0001119.

Spreen, O., & Benton, A. L. (1977). *Neurosensory center comprehensive examination for aphasia.* Victoria, BC: Neuropsychology Laboratory, University of Victoria.

Square, P., Chumpelik, D, & Adams, S. (1985). Efficacy of the PROMPT system of therapy for the treatment of acquired apraxia of speech. In R. H. Brookshire (Ed.), *Clinical aphasiology: Conference proceedings,* Minneapolis, MN: BRK Publishers, 319-320.

Square, P. (1986). Efficacy of the PROMPT system of therapy for apraxia of speech: A follow-up investigation. In R. H. Brookshire (Ed.), *Clinical aphasiology: Conference proceedings,* Minneapolis, MN: BRK Publishers 221-226.

Square, P. A., Darley, F. L., & Sommers, R. K. (1982). An analysis of the production errors made by pure apractic speakers with differing loci of lesions. In R. H. Brookshire (Ed.), *Clinical Aphasiology Conference proceedings* (pp. 245-249). Minneapolis, MN: BRK Publishers.

Square, P. A., & Weidner, W. E. (1976). *Oral sensory perception in adults demonstrating apraxia of speech.* Paper presented to the American Speech and Hearing Association, Houston, Texas.

Stachowiak, F. J., Huber, W., Poeck, K., & associates. (1977). Text comprehension in aphasia. *Brain and Language, 4,* 177-195.

Stanczak, D. E., White, J. G., Gouview, W. D., & associates. (1984). Assessment of level of consciousness following severe neurological insult. *Journal of Neurosurgery, 60,* 955-60.

Stanton, K., Yorkston, K. M., Talley-Kenyon, V., & associates. (1981). Language utilization in teaching reading to left neglect patients. In R. H. Brookshire (Ed.), *Clinical Aphasiology Conference proceedings* (pp. 262-271). Minneapolis, MN: BRK Publishers.

Stedman's Medical Dictionary. (1990). Baltimore, MD: Williams & Wilkins.

Steele, J. C., Richardson, J. D., & Olszewski, J. (1964). Progressive supranuclear palsy. *Archives of Neurology, 10,* 333-359.

Stoicheff, M. L. (1960). Motivating instructions and language performance of dysphasic subjects. *Journal of Speech and Hearing Research, 3,* 75-85.

Stokes, G. (1990). Controlling disruptive and demanding behaviors. In G. Stokes, & F. Goudie (Eds.), *Working with dementia* (pp. 158-173). London: Winslow Press.

Stokes, T. F., & Baer, D. M. (1977). An implied technology of generalization. *Journal of Applied Behavior Analysis, 10,* 349-367.

Sunderland, A., Harris, J. E., & Baddeley, A. D. (1983). Do laboratory tests predict everyday memory? *Journal of Verbal Learning and Verbal Behavior, 22,* 341-357.

Sunderland, A., Wade, D. T., Langton, B, & Hewer, R. (1987) The natural history of visual neglect after stroke: Indications from two methods of assessment. *International Disability Studies, 9,* 55-59.

Swindell, C. S., Holland, A. L., & Fromm, D. (1984). Classification of aphasia: WAB type versus clinical impression. In R. H. Brookshire (Ed.), *Clinical Aphasiology Conference proceedings* (pp. 48-54). Minneapolis, MN: BRK Publishers.

Taylor, D. (2003). Measuring mild visual neglect: Do complex visual tasks activate rightward bias? *New Zealand Journal of Physiotherapy, 31,* 67-72.

Teasdale, G., & Jennett, B. (1974). Assessment of coma and impaired consciousness. *Lancet, 2,* 81-84.

Teasdale, G., & Mendelow, D. (1984). Pathophysiology of head injuries. In D. N. Brooks (Ed.), *Closed head injury: Psychological, social, and family consequences* (pp. 4-36). Oxford: Oxford University Press.

Teng, E. L., & Chui, H. (1987). The modified Mini-Mental State (3MS) Examination. *Journal of Clinical Psychiatry, 48,* 314-318.

Thompson, C., & Byrne, M. (1984). Across setting generalization of social conventions in aphasia. In R. H. Brookshire (Ed.), *Clinical Aphasiology Conference proceedings* (pp. 132-144). Minneapolis, MN: BRK Publishers.

Thompson, R. S., Rivara, F. P., & Thompson, D. C. (1989). A case control study of the effectiveness of bicycle safety helmets. *New England Journal of Medicine, 320,* 1362-1367.

Thurstone, L. L. (1944). *A factorial study of perception.* Chicago: University of Chicago Press.

Tombaugh, T. N., & Hurley, A. M. (1997). The 60-item Boston Naming Test: Norms for cognitively intact adults aged 25 to 88 years. *Journal of Clinical and Experimental Neuropsychology, 19,* 922-932.

Tomlinson, B. E., & Henderson, G. (1976). Some quantitative cerebral findings in normal and demented old people. In R. Terry & S. Gerskor (Eds.), *Neurobiology of aging.* New York: Raven.

Tompkins, C. A. (1990). Knowledge and strategies for processing lexical metaphor after right or left hemisphere brain damage. *Journal of Speech, Language, and Hearing Research, 33,* 307-316.

Tompkins, C. A. (1995). *Right hemisphere communication disorders: Theory and management.* San Diego, CA: Singular.

Tompkins, C. A., Baumgaertner, A., Lehman, M. T., & associates. (1997). Suppression and discourse comprehension in right brain-damaged adults: A preliminary report. *Aphasiology, 11,* 505-519.

Tompkins, C. A., Bloise, G. R., & Timko, M. L. (1994). Working memory and inference revision in brain damaged and normally aging adults. *Journal of Speech, Language, and Hearing Research, 37,* 896-912.

Tompkins, C. A., & Flowers, C. R. (1985). Perception of emotional intonation by brain-damaged adults: The influence of task processing levels. *Journal of Speech and Hearing Research, 28,* 527-538.

Tompkins, C. A., & Lehman, M. T. (1998). Interpreting intended meanings after right hemisphere brain damage: An analysis of evidence, potential accounts, and clinical implications. *Topics in Stroke Rehabilitation, 51,* 29-47.

Tompkins, C. A., Lehman, M. T., Baumgaertner, A., & associates. (1996). Suppression and discourse comprehension in right brain-damaged adults: Inferential ambiguity processing. *Brain and Language, 55,* 172-175.

Tompkins, C. A., Lehman-Blake, M. T., Baumgaertner, A., & associates. (2001). Mechanisms of discourse comprehension impairment after right hemisphere brain damage: Suppression in referential ambiguity resolution. *Journal of Speech, Language, and Hearing Research, 44,* 400-415.

Toth, C., & Kirk, A. (2002). Representational bias does not affect bisection of lines with a pictorially or semantically defined top by patients with left hemispatial neglect. *Brain & Cognition, 50,* 167-177.

Trost, J. E., & Canter, G. J. (1974). Apraxia of speech in patients with Broca aphasia: A study of phoneme production accuracy and error patterns. *Brain and Language, 1,* 63-79.

Trupe, E. H. (1984). Reliability of rating spontaneous speech in the Western Aphasia Battery: Implications for classification. In R. H. Brookshire (Ed.), *Clinical Aphasiology Conference proceedings* (pp. 55-69). Minneapolis, MN: BRK Publishers.

Tucker, D. M., & Frederick, S. L. (1989). Emotion and brain lateralization. In H. Wagner & A. Manstead (Eds.), *Handbook of social psychophysiology* (pp. 27-70). New York: Wiley.

Tuiman, J. J. (1974). Determining the passage dependency of comprehension test questions on five major tests. *Reading Research Quarterly, 2,* 206-233.

Tulving, E. (1972). Episodic and semantic memory. In E. Tulving & W. Donaldson (Eds.), *Organization of memory.* New York: Academic Press.

Tulving, E. (1983). *Elements of episodic memory.* Oxford: Clarendon Press.

Tweedy, J. R., & Shulman, P. D. (1982). Toward a functional classification of naming impairments. *Brain and Language, 15,* 193-206.

Ulatowska, H. K., Doyel, A. W., Freedman-Stern, R. F., & associates. (1983). Production of procedural discourse in aphasia. *Brain and Language, 18,* 315-341.

Uniform Data System for Medical Rehabilitation (1996). Buffalo, NY: University at Buffalo Foundation.

Uzzell, B. P., Dolinskas, C. A., Wiser, R. F., & associates. (1987). Influence of lesions detected by computed tomography on outcome and neuropsychological recovery after severe head injury. *Neurosurgery, 20,* 396-402.

Vaccaro, F. J. (1988). Application of operant procedures in a group of institutionalized aggressive geriatric patients. *Psychology and Aging, 3,* 22-28.

Vallar, G., & Baddeley, A. D. (1984). Phonological short-term store, phonological processing, and sentence processing: A neuropsychological case study. *Cognitive Neuropsychology, 1,* 121-142.

Vallar, G., & Perani, D. (1986). The anatomy of unilateral neglect after right-hemisphere stroke: A clinical/CT scan correlation study in man. *Neuropsychologia, 24,* 609-622.

Van Buskirk, C. (1955). Prognostic value of sensory deficit in rehabilitation of hemiplegics. *Neurology, 6,* 407-411.

Van Houten, R., Rolider, A., Malenfant, L., & associates. (1994). Prevention of brain injuries by improving safety-related behaviors. In M. A. J. Finlayson & S. H. Garner (Eds.), *Brain injury rehabilitation: Clinical considerations* (pp. 313-331). Baltimore: Williams & Wilkins.

van Straten, A., de Haan, R. J., Limburg, M., & van den Bos, G. A., (1997). A stroke-adapted 30-item version of the Sickness Impact Profile to assess quality of life (SA-SIP30). *Stroke, 28,* 2155-2161.

Van Zomeren, A. H., Brouwer, W. H., & Deelman, B. G. (1984). Attentional deficits: The riddles of selectivity, speed, and alertness. In N. Brooks (Ed.), *Closed head injury: Psychological, social, and family consequences* (pp. 74-107). Oxford: Oxford University Press.

Verfaelli, M., Bauer, R. H., & Bowers, D. (1991). Autonomic and behavioral evidence of implicit memory in amnesia. *Brain and Cognition, 15,* 10-25.

Veterans Administration. (1972). Veterans Administration cooperative study group on antihypertensive agents: Effects of treatment on morbidity in hypertension III: Influence of age, diastolic pressure, and prior cardiovascular disease; further analysis of side effects. *Circulation, 45,* 991-1004.

Vignolo, L. A. (1964). Evolution of aphasia and language rehabilitation: A retrospective study. *Cortex, 1,* 344-367.

Vignolo, L. A., Frediani, F., Boccardi, F. E., & associates. (1986). Unexpected CT scan findings in global aphasia. *Cortex, 22,* 55-70.

Wagenaar, E., Snow, C. E., & Prins, R. S. (1975). Spontaneous speech of aphasic patients: A psycholinguistic analysis. *Brain and Language, 2,* 281-303.

Waller, M. R., & Darley, F. L. (1978). The influence of context on the auditory comprehension of paragraphs in aphasic subjects. *Journal of Speech and Hearing Research, 21,* 732-745.

Walker-Baston, D., Curtis, S., Smith, P., & associates. (1999). An alternative model for treatment of aphasia: The Lifelink approach. In R. Elman (Ed.), *Group treatment of neurogenic communication disorders: The expert clinician approach* (pp. 67-75). Boston: Butterworth-Heinemann.

Wambaugh, J. L. (2004). Stimulus generalization effects of sound production treatment for apraxia of speech. *Journal of Medical Speech-Language Pathology, 12,* 77-98.

Wambaugh, J. L., Kalinyak-Fliszar, M. M., West, J. E., & associates. (1998). Effects of treatment for sound errors in apraxia of speech and aphasia. *Journal of Speech, Language, and Hearing Research, 41,* 725-743.

Wambaugh, J. L., Martinez, A. L., McNeil, M. R., & Rogers, M. A. (1999a). Sound production treatment for apraxia of speech: Overgeneralization and maintenance effects. *Aphasiology, 13,* 821-837.

Wambaugh, J., & Nessler, C. (2004). Modification of sound production treatment for apraxia of speech: Acquisition and generalization effects. *Aphasiology, 18,* 407-427.

Wambaugh, J. L., West, J. E., & Doyle, P. J. (1999b). Treatment for apraxia of speech: Effects of targeting sound groups. *Aphasiology, 12,* 731-742.

Warlow, C. P., Dennis, M. S., van Gijn, J., Hankey, G. J., Sandercock, P.A.G., Bamford, J.M., & Wardlaw, J. (1996). *Stroke: A practical guide to management.* Oxford: Blackwell Science.

Warren, R. L. (1992). Functional outcome: An introduction. *Clinical Aphasiology, 21,* 59-65.

Warrington, E. K., & James, M. (1967). Disorders of visual perception in patients with localized cerebral lesions. *Neuropsychologica, 5,* 253-266.

Watson, B. D., Miller, R. D., & Heilman, K. M. (1978). Nonsensory neglect. *Annals of Neurology, 3,* 500-508.

Watson, R. T., & Heilman, K. M. (1979). Thalamic neglect. *Neurology, 29,* 690-694.

Waxman, S. (2000). *Correlative neuroanatomy* (24th ed.). New York: McGraw-Hill.

Webb, W. G. (1990). Acquired dyslexias. In L. L. LaPointe (Ed.), *Aphasia and related language disorders* (pp. 130-146). New York: Thieme.

Wechsler, D. (1981). *Wechsler Adult Intelligence Scale Revised.* New York: The Psychological Corporation.

Wegner, M. L., Brookshire, R. H., & Nicholas, L. E. (1984). Comprehension of main ideas and details in coherent and noncoherent discourse by aphasic and nonaphasic listeners. *Brain and Language, 21,* 37-51.

Weidner, W. E., & Jinks, A. F. (1983). The effects of single versus combined cue presentations on picture naming by aphasic adults. *Journal of Speech and Hearing Disorders, 16,* 111-121.

Weigl, E. (1968). On the problem of cortical syndromes: Experimental studies. In M. L. Simmell (Ed.), *The reach of mind* (pp. 143-159). New York: Springer.

Weigel-Crump, C., & Koenigsknecht, R. A. (1973). Tapping the lexical store of the adult aphasic: Analysis of improvement made in word retrieval skills. *Cortex, 9,* 411-418.

Weiner, F. (1983). *Aphasia I: Noun association.* Baltimore: University Park Press.

Weisenburg, T. H., & McBride, K. E. (1935). *Aphasia.* New York: Commonwealth Fund.

Wener, D. L., & Duffy, J. R. (1983). An investigation of the sensitivity of the Reporter Test to expressive language disturbances (abstract). In R. H. Brookshire (Ed.), *Clinical Aphasiology Conference proceedings* (pp. 15-17). Minneapolis, MN: BRK Publishers.

Wepman, J. M. (1951). *Recovery from aphasia.* New York: Ronald Press.

Wertz, R. T., Collins, M., Weiss, D., & associates. (1981). Veterans Administration cooperative study on aphasia: A comparison of individual and group treatment. *Journal of Speech and Hearing Research, 24,* 580-594.

Wertz, R. T., Deal, J. L., Holland, A. L., & associates. (1986). Comments on an uncontrolled aphasia no treatment trial. *ASHA J, 28,* 31.

Wertz, R. T., Deal, J. L., & Robinson, A. J. (1984). Classifying the aphasias: A comparison of the Boston Diagnostic Aphasia Examination and the Western Aphasia Battery. In R. H. Brookshire (Ed.), *Clinical Aphasiology Conference proceedings* (pp. 40-47). Minneapolis, MN: BRK Publishers.

Wertz, R. T., Dronkers, N. F., & Hume, J. L. (1993). PICA intra-subtests variability and prognosis for improvement in aphasia. In M. L. Lemme (Ed.), *Clinical aphasiology, vol. 21,* (pp. 207-211). Austin, TX: Pro-Ed.

Wertz, R. T., Keith, R. L., & Custer, D. D. (1971). *Normal and aphasic behavior on a measure of auditory input and a measure of verbal output.* Paper presented at the annual convention of the American Speech and Hearing Association, Chicago.

Wertz, R. T., LaPointe, L. L., & Rosenbek, J. C. (1984). *Apraxia of speech in adults: The disorder and its management.* Orlando, FL: Grune & Stratton.

Wertz, R. T., Weiss, D., Aten, J., & associates. (1986). A comparison of clinic, home, and deferred language treatment for aphasia: A VA cooperative study. *Archives of Neurology, 43,* 653-658.

West, J. F. (1981). Group treatment for aphasia: Panel discussion. In R. H. Brookshire (Ed.), *Clinical Aphasiology: Conference proceedings 1981* (pp. 151-152). Minneapolis, MN: BRK Publishers.

West, J. F., & Kaufman, G. A. (1972). *Some effects of redundancy on the auditory comprehension of adult aphasics.* Paper presented at the annual convention of the American Speech and Hearing Association, San Francisco.

Whitely, A. M., & Warrington, E. K. (1977). Prosopagnosia: A clinical, psychological, and anatomical study of three patients. *Journal of Neurology, Neurosurgery, and Psychiatry, 40,* 395-403.

WHOQOL Group (1995). The World Health Association quality of life assessment (WHOQOL): Position paper from the World Health Organization. *Social Science and Medicine, 41,* 1403-1409.

Wilkinson, G. (1993). *The wide range achievement test* (3rd ed.). Wilmington, DE: Wide Range.

Willer, B., Rosenthal, M., Kreutzer, J. S., & associates. (1993). Assessment of community integration following rehabilitation for traumatic brain injury. *Journal of Head Trauma Rehabilitation, 8,* 75-87.

Williams L.S., Weinberger M., Harris L.E., Clark D.O., & Biller, J. (1999). Development of a stroke-specific quality of life scale. *Stroke, 30,* 1362-1369.

Williams, S. E., & Canter, G. J. (1982). The influence of situational context on naming performance in aphasic syndromes. *Brain and Language, 17,* 92-106.

Wilson, B. (1981). Teaching a patient to remember people names after removal of a left temporal tumor. *Behavioral Psychotherapy, 9,* 338-344.

Wilson, B.A. (1981). Theory, assessment, and treatment in neuropsychological rehabilitation. *Neuropsychology, 5,* 281-291.

Wilson, B.A. Alderman, N., & Burgess, P.W. (1996). Behavioral assessment of the disexecutive syndrome. Bury St. Edmunds U.K., Thames Valley Test Company.

Wilson, B. A., Cockburn, J., & Baddeley, A. (1985). *The Rivermead behavioural memory test.* Suffolk, England: Thames Valley Test Company.

Wilson, B. A., Cockburn, J., & Baddeley, A. (1999). *The Rivermead behavioural memory test extended.* Suffolk, England: Thames Valley Test Company.

Wilson, B. A., Cockburn, J., & Halligan, P. (1987). *Behavioral inattention test.* Suffolk, England: Thames Valley Test Company.

Wilson, J. A., Pentland, B., Currie, C. T., & associates. (1987). The functional effects of head injury in the elderly. *Brain Injury, 1,* 183-188.

Winner, E., Brownell, H., Happe, F., & associates. (1998). Distinguishing lies from jokes: Theory of mind deficits and discourse interpretation in right hemisphere brain-damaged patients. *Brain and Language, 62,* 89-106.

Woodcock, R. W., & Johnson, M. B. (1989). *Woodcock-Johnson psycho-educational battery revised.* Allen, TX: DLM Teaching Resources.

Woods, P., & Ashley, J. (1995). Simulated presence therapy: Using selected memories to manage problem behaviors. *Geriatric Nursing, 16,* 9-14.

Woods, B., Spector, A., Jones, C., & associates. (2005). Reminiscence therapy for dementia (Cochrane review). *The Cochrane database of systematic reviews, 2,* Article No. CD001120, DOI 10.1002/14651858.CD001120.

World Health Organization (1992). *The ICD-10 Classification of Mental and Behavioural Disorders.* Geneva.

World Health Organization. (1998). *WHOQOL-BREF:* Geneva: Programme on mental health, World Health Organization.

World Health Organization. (2000). *International classification of impairments, disabilities, and handicaps 2: prefinal draft.* Geneva: World Health Organization.

World Health Organization (2001). *ICIDH-2: International classification of impairments, disabilities, and handicaps.* Geneva: World Health Organization.

Worrall, L. (1995). The functional communication perspective. In D. Muller and C. Code (Eds.) *Treatment of aphasia.* London: Whurr Publishers.

Worrall, L. (2000). A conceptual framework for a functional approach to acquired neurogenic disorders of communication and swallowing. In L. Worrall and C. Frattali (Eds.) *Neurogenic Communication Disorders: A Functional Approach.* New York Thieme.

Worrall, L., McCooey, R., Davidson, B., & associates. (2002). The validity of functional assessments of communication and the activity/participation components of the ICIDH-2: Do they reflect what really happens in real life? *Journal of Communication Disorders, 35,* 107-137.

Worrall, L. E., & Holland, A. L. (2003). Editorial: Quality of life in aphasia. *Aphasiology, 17,* 329-332.

Wyke, M., & Holgate, D. (1973). Colour naming defects in dysphasic patients: A qualitative analysis. *Neuropsychologia, 11,* 451-461.

Ylvisaker, M. (1998). *Peer review of evidence report.* Unpublished manuscript. (Cited in Carney and associates, 1999.)

Ylvisaker, M., & Feeney, T. (1998). *Collaborative brain injury intervention: Positive everyday routines.* San Diego, CA: Singular.

Ylvisaker, M., Szekeres, S. F., & Feeney, T. (2001). Communication disorders associated with traumatic brain injury.

In R. Chapey (Ed.), *Language intervention strategies in aphasia and related communication disorders* (4th ed). Philadelphia: Lippincott Williams & Wilkins.

Ylvisaker, M., & Urbanczyk, B. (1994). Assessment and treatment of speech, swallowing, and communication disorders following traumatic brain injury. In M. A. J. Finlayson & S. H. Garner (Eds.), *Brain injury rehabilitation: Clinical considerations* (pp. 157-186). Baltimore: Williams & Wilkins.

Ylvisaker, M. S., & Holland, A. L. (1985). Coaching, self-coaching, and rehabilitation of head injury. In D. F. Johns (Ed.), *Clinical management of neurogenic communication disorders* (pp. 243-357). Boston: Little, Brown and Company.

Yorkston, K. M. (1981). Treatment of right hemisphere damaged patients: A panel presentation. In R. H. Brookshire (Ed.), *Clinical Aphasiology Conference proceedings* (pp. 281-283). Minneapolis, MN: BRK Publishers.

Yorkston, K. M., & Beukelman, D. R. (1981). *Assessment of intelligibility of dysarthric speech.* Tigard, OR: C.C. Publications.

Yorkston, K. M., Beulkelman, D. R., & Bell, K. R. (1988). *Clinical management of dysarthric speakers.* San Diego: College-Hill.

Yorkston, K. M. Beukelman, D. R., Strand, E. A., & Bell, K. R. (1999). *Management of motor speech disorders in children and adults.* Austin, TX: Pro-Ed.

Yorkston, K. M., Beukelman, D. R., & Tice, R. (1998). *Phoneme identification task: A computer program. Sentence intelligibility task: A computer program.* Lincoln, NE: Tice Technology Services. (Currently available from Madonna Rehabilitation Hospital, Lincoln, Nebraska.)

Yorkston, K. M., Dowden, P. A., Beukelman, D. R., & associates. (1986). *A phoneme identification task as a measure of perceived articulatory adequacy.* Paper presented at the third biennial Clinical Dysarthria Conference, Tucson, AZ.

Yudofsky, S. C., Silver, S. M., Jackson, W., & associates (1986). The Overt Aggression Scale for the objective rating of verbal and physical aggression. *American Journal of Psychiatry, 143,* 35-39.

Yules, R. B., & Chase, R. A. (1969). A training method for reduction of hypernasality in speech. *Plastic and Reconstructive Surgery, 43,* 180-185.

Zaidel, E. (1978). Unilateral auditory language comprehension on the Token Test following cerebral commissurotomy and hemispherectomy. *Neuropsychologia, 15,* 1-18.

Index

A

ABCD. *See* Arizona Battery for Communication Disorders of
    Dementia (ABCD)
Abilities
    cognitive and communicative, 480-481
    tests of pragmatic, 417-418
Abnormal movements, causes of, 69t
Abnormalities, cognitive and behavior, 426-430
    alternating attention, 428-429
    attentional impairments and distractibility, 427-428
    denial of impairments, 426-427
    divided attention, 429
    impaired reasoning, 430
    impulsivity, 429
    problem-solving, 430
    selective attention, 428
    sustained attention, 428
Abstract thinking, 158-159, 485
Abuse, substance, 473
Acceleration injuries, 451-454
Acoustic-vestibular mirror (CN 8), 57
Acquired immunodeficiency syndrome (AIDS), 539
Active orientation training, 494
Activities
    group, 523-524, 587-588, 592
    reading, 353t
    reminiscence, 592-593
    Strooplike, 501
    task-switching, 345-346
Activities of daily living. *See also* Instrumental Activities of
    Daily Living Scale (IADL)
Activity-participation approaches, 256
    impairment-level and, 275t
Activity-participation level, 257
    intervention, 273-275
Acute global aphasia, 334
Add-subtract alternation, 501
Adult cognitive-communicative disorders, neurological
    causes of, 35-43
    cerebral hemorrhage, 39-42
    general effects of the ischemic stroke, 38-39
    hemorrhagic stroke, 39-42
    hypoperfusion, 38
    ischemic stroke, 37-38

Page numbers followed by *b, f,* or *t,* indicate boxes, figures,
or tables, respectively

Adult cognitive-communicative disorders—*cont'd*
    recovery from ischemic and hemorrhagic strokes, 42-43
    stroke, 36-43
    transient interruptions of cerebral blood supply, 38
Adult skull, normal, 80f
Adults
    assessing with traumatic brain injuries with, 478-490
        abstract thinking, 485
        agitation, 480
        attention, 481
        cognitive and community code abilities, 480-481
        evaluation of traumatically brain injured adults,
            487-489
        executive function, 485
        language and communication, 485-487
        level of consciousness, 478-479
        memory impairments, 481-484
        orientation, 479-480
        problem solving, 485
        reasoning, 485
        responsiveness to stimulation, 478-479
        visual processing, 484
    effects on performance of brain-injured, 153b
    non-brain-injured, 88f
    test batteries for evaluation of traumatically brain
        injured, 488b
    testing with brain injuries, 115-122, 117b
    who sustain traumatic brain injuries in United States,
        446f
Adults and children, reading test for non-brain injured,
    190-192
Affect, pseudobulbar, 161
Afferent projection fibers, 19
Afferent spinal nerves, 18
Age and sex, Alzheimer's disease by, 542f
Agitation, 480
Agnosia, 319-321
AIDS. *See* Acquired immunodeficiency syndrome (AIDS)
Aids
    external, 499, 513-516
    external memory, 514, 583-585
Alertness, 137
Alexia, how brain damage produces, 313f
Allocation, resource, 260-261
Altered mental state, 76-77
Alternating attention, 138-139, 428-429
Alternating cancellation tasks, 500
Alternation, add-subtract, 501